Color Atlas and Textbook of

Hematology

Color Atlas and Textbook of
HEMATOLOGY

William R. Platt, M.D., F.C.A.P., F.A.C.P.

Chief of Pathology, U. S. Public Health Service Hospital;
Lecturer in Pathology, The Johns Hopkins University School of Medicine
Baltimore, Maryland;
Associate Professor of Pathology (Visiting Staff)
Washington University School of Medicine
St. Louis, Missouri

SECOND EDITION

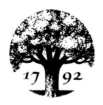

J. B. Lippincott Company
Philadelphia·Toronto

Second Edition

Copyright © 1979, by J. B. Lippincott Company

Copyright © 1969, by J. B. Lippincott Company

This book is fully protected by copyright and, with the exception of brief excerpts for review, no part of it may be reproduced in any form by print, photoprint, microfilm, or any other means, without written permission from the publisher.

ISBN-0-397-50407-1

Library of Congress Catalog Card No. 78-21851

Printed in the United States of America

2   4   6   5   3   1

Library of Congress Cataloging in Publication Data

Platt, William R.
   Color atlas and textbook of hematology.

   Includes bibliographies and index.
   1. Hematology.   2. Hematology — Atlases.   I.   Title.
[DNLM: 1.   Hematologic diseases.   2.   Hematology —
Atlases.   WH100.3 P719c]
RB145.P56 1978   616.1′5   78-21851
ISBN 0-397-50407-1

To the Family of a Man

To those who have passed on and are sorely missed—my dear wife, Shirley Ades Platt; my most beloved parents, Ida S. Platt and Louis A. Platt; my most respected and loved mother-in-law and father-in-law, Sara Fox Ades and David Ades; and my very special and precious sister-in-law, Frances Lederman Ades.

And to those whose love and devotion are very, very important to me, my children, Karen, Lois, and James; my sisters and brothers, Mildred, Morton, Irvin, George, David, and Ann and their families; and my dear wife's family, Louis Ades, Grace and Henry Levy, and Helen and Jack Benjamin and their families.

And to my dear Jeanette.

Preface

This edition is concerned, to a great extent, with the rapidly developing branch of hematology that applies improved techniques and instrumentation to the more efficient diagnosis of hematopoietic disorders. Beginning with methods of marrow culture *in vitro*, the text offers new insights into the factors involved in the regulation of hematopoiesis, for example, the ways that they have helped to delineate the group of committed progenitor cells that originate from pluripotential stem cells. The text concludes with the proposition that the progenitor cells appear to respond to long-range humoral-stimulating factors and ultimately give rise to the differentiated end cells of the hematopoietic cell lines.

This edition also mentions the minor innovation in instrumentation, the Jamshidi needle technique, that has led to an improvement in morphologic preparations of the bone marrow by providing better and more easily obtained marrow biopsy and aspirated material. This technique has resulted in less uncertainty in obtaining serial marrow studies that demonstrate the effects of combinations of chemotherapeutic agents on the hematopoietic system during and following sophisticated oncologic therapeutic approaches to the leukemias and lymphomas. New concepts that explain the relation of various intraerythrocytic enzymes, such as 2,3-DPG, to RBC metabolism are described. In addition, there are analyses of the molecular biology and bio-

physics of the erythrocyte, as they relate to several of the hemoglobinopathies, for instance, thalassemias and sickle cell disease.

This edition presents an analysis of new automatic electronic blood cell counters with a detailed description of the basic fundamentals associated with them and the part they play in the expanding role of quality control in the diagnosis of disease. A natural sequel to this is the automation of the differential cell count, from machine-stained blood films to computer-controlled, printed read-out. The relatively good reproducibility and consistency of most of the instruments on the market is an excellent reflection of the accuracy of most differential counts now being performed. It is hoped that these phases of automation will decrease the amount of repetitive, nonproductive work performed by the experienced medical technologist and will allow time for selective, more intricate work in the nonautomated aspects of hematology. This is not to imply that the skills of the morphologically oriented hematology technologist will no longer be needed. Rather there will always be a need for atypical cell interpretation, for analysis of machine-related misdiagnoses that might result from unusual hematopoietic disease manifestation, and for examination of the effect of chemotherapeutic agents on the cytologic components of the peripheral blood and bone marrow.

The introduction of a serum ferritin test by radioimmunoassay techniques is described along with its possible role in the quantitative assay of marrow iron stores, which could lead to a reduction in the necessity for bone marrow aspirations. A reevaluation of the estimation of the iron needs during infancy is also mentioned.

With the advent of increased accuracy in automated platelet counts and the new knowledge of thrombocyte metabolism and platelet kinetics, recent concepts of hemostasis and blood coagulation have been modified. New instruments measuring platelet aggregation plus semiautomated and automated coagulation instrumentation have made the diagnosis of clotting disorders (e.g., the Factor VIII disorders, hemophilia A, and Von Willebrand's disease) more accurate and developed increased understanding across the entire field of hemostasis. The use of HL-A-compatible platelets in thrombocytopenic states, platelet antibodies and immunosuppressive therapy, post-transfusion purpura, and reevaluation of idiopathic thrombocytopenic purpura of childhood are also covered.

Discussed in detail are changing concepts of lymphocyte origin, especially the localization, distribution, laboratory diagnosis, and clinical applications of T- and B-lymphocytes; the nomenclature, histopathologic classification, and staging of lymphomas and their relationship to modes of therapy; and the relationship of all of these to the use of radiotherapy or combination chemotherapy with new concepts of induction, consolidation, and maintenance. It is pointed out that these have all led to significant prolongation of survival in acute lymphocytic leukemia in childhood, certain stages and types of non-Hodgkin's lymphoma, and the staged overall Hodgkin's disease in adults. Also described are new approaches in cytogenetics, scanning electron microscopy, differential histochemical staining of leukemic states, and the use of bone marrow transplant therapy in the treatment of pancytopenia and leukemic processes.

The hematology division of the laboratory, in the final analysis, appears to be heading toward a state of complete automation, in which the entire software system is being modified to allow performance of research, parallel processing, and systems progression over extremely short time periods. In this text, the use of the computer to achieve this end is discussed in light of ways to determine for a particular laboratory functions useful to computerize, all of which are summarized and concluded from the 1977 American Society of Hematology seminar on this subject.

The audiovisual portions at the end of each chapter have been revised and updated to reflect the unlimited, excellent photographic material on hematology available from the ASCP, AFIP, and the facilities of the University of Washington—American Society of Hematology.

The addition of many new colored plates that depict aspects of leukemia and lymphoma and marrow morphologic changes associated with the chemotherapeutic approach to the leukemia and lymphoma moieties, the hematologic patterns of other hematopoietic aberrations and entities, the configurations of special stains, and other new plates have contributed to an extensive updating of an already comprehensive color atlas of hematology.

WILLIAM R. PLATT, M.D.

Acknowledgments

I am especially grateful to the people who helped to make the preparation of this book a less burdensome task. My most sincere gratitude goes to the various chiefs of the pathology departments in those schools of medicine with whom I have had the honor, privilege, and pleasure of being associated: Dr. Paul E. Lacy, Dr. Vernie Stembridge, and Dr. Robert H. Heptinstall; to Dr. Frank Vellios, Dr. William W. Sheehan, Dr. Eugene Frenkel, and Dr. Saba Demean, whose many kindnesses and encouragement were so deeply appreciated. To two excellent medical librarians whose cooperation in the bibliographical aspects of this endeavor were so greatly appreciated, Dr. Estelle Brodman, and Mrs. Mildred Langner. To Mr. Gale Spring, Ms. Nola Nelson, and Dr. Virginia Minnich, who assisted and supported the development of some of the illustrative hematologic material herein.

I sincerely appreciate the efforts expended by the following people who lent me illustrations, Kodachromes, Ektachromes, and color prints to use as needed: Dr. Raymond Alexanian, Dr. James O. Armitage, Dr. C. Robert Baisden, Dr. Asa Barnes, Dr. W. Bell, Dr. Richard D. Brunning, Dr. Samuel C. Bukantz, Dr. Brian S. Bull, Dr. J. A. Clarke, Dr. Robert D. Collins, Dr. Lockard Conley, Dr. Paul Didisheim, and Dr. Thomas F. Dutcher who has been especially kind, considerate, and most helpful in permitting the use of color prints made from his special Kodachrome slide set; Rebecca F. Dunn, Dr. Dana Boggs, Dr. Bertal E. Glader, Dr. Harvey R. Gralnick, Dr. Thomas Hale Ham, Dr. Etienne deHarven, and Dr. N. Lampen, for scanning electron micrography material, Dr. Arthur I. Hollub, Dr. Elaine S. Jaffe, Dr. John H. Kersey, Dr. George G. Klee, Dr. Patrick M. Lai, Dr. Dennis F. Leavelle, for the automation in coagulation Kodachrome slides and associated material; Dr. Raul I. Lede, Dr. Peck-Sun Lin, Dr. Aaron Polliack, Dr. Stanley S. Raphael, Dr. Irene E. Roeckel, Dr. Warner Rosenau, Dr. Gordon D. Ross, Dr. Maria Ruehsen, Dr. Ruth Saducks, Dr. Frances Sanel, Dr. Lyle L. Sensenbrenner, and Dr. Adel A. Yunis. I am particularly grateful to Dr. Sloan J. Wilson and to his associates, Mr. Irvin T. Youngberg and Dr. William E. Larsen. I am also thankful to the entire group of physicians mentioned in the first edition who contributed to and gave permission for illustrations and other hematologic material.

I sincerely appreciate the cooperation and contributions of the following people associated with various publishing companies and diagnostic and instrumentation supply organizations who were so gracious in providing permission or black and white prints, illustrations, graphs, and so forth illustrating various aspects of their products: John Aschemeier, Velma Beaman, V. Borsodi, John A. Chaya, Linde T. Clark,

Lee Cooper, Margaret Cozzolino, Nancy M. Day, Mary S. Degnan, Henry G. DiRusio, Diane Hunter, Tommye Ann Jordan, Paul R. Lundell, A. A. Marchesi, Susan E. Miller, Eleanore Mosheir, Helen M. Moore, Thomas Muich, Carolyn Nash, Gerard T. Paul, Linda Ray, Sanford L. Simons, Bonnie Van Cleven, Milton C. Paige, Jr., and Gloria M. Freeman.

I would like to express my sincere appreciation to Stuart Freeman, Editor-in-Chief, for his interest and skill in the development of this text, and to Ellen Sklar, production assistant, Niels Malmquist, production supervisor, and Laura Dabundo, copy editor, all of J. B. Lippincott Company, and to Martha Dewey, secretary, V.A. Hospital, Dallas, Texas.

Finally, I would like to extend my deepest gratitude to the following members of the secretarial and technical staff of the U.S. Public Health Service Hospital (Baltimore) whose aid, cooperation, and patience were beyond the call of duty, Anna Wassell, Jeannette Franzl, and especially to Mrs. Dorothy Blackburn, without whom the final material organization and preparation would have been most difficult.

Contents

Color Plates

Plate 1

MATURATION OF HUMAN BLOOD CELLS

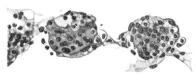

EMBRYO - MESENCHYME - BLOOD ISLANDS OF YOLK SAC

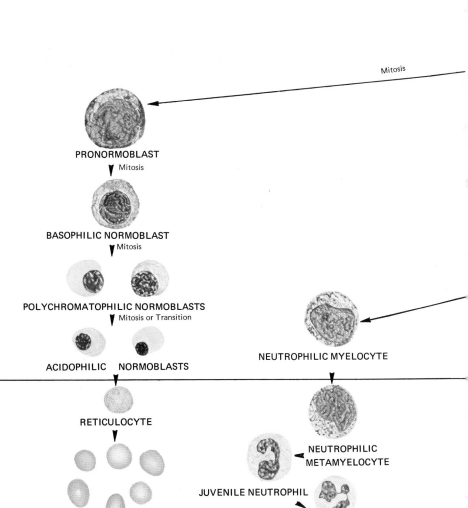

Mitosis

PRONORMOBLAST

Mitosis

BASOPHILIC NORMOBLAST

Mitosis

POLYCHROMATOPHILIC NORMOBLASTS

Mitosis or Transition

ACIDOPHILIC   NORMOBLASTS

NEUTROPHILIC MYELOCYTE

RETICULOCYTE

NEUTROPHILIC
METAMYELOCYTE

JUVENILE NEUTROPHIL

ERYTHROCYTES

PM NEUTROPHIL

Bone Marrow

Peripheral Blood Stream

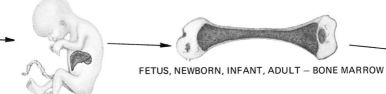

FETUS, NEWBORN, INFANT, ADULT — BONE MARROW

EMBRYO-EXTRAMEDULLARY HEMATOPOESIS—
LIVER AND SPLEEN

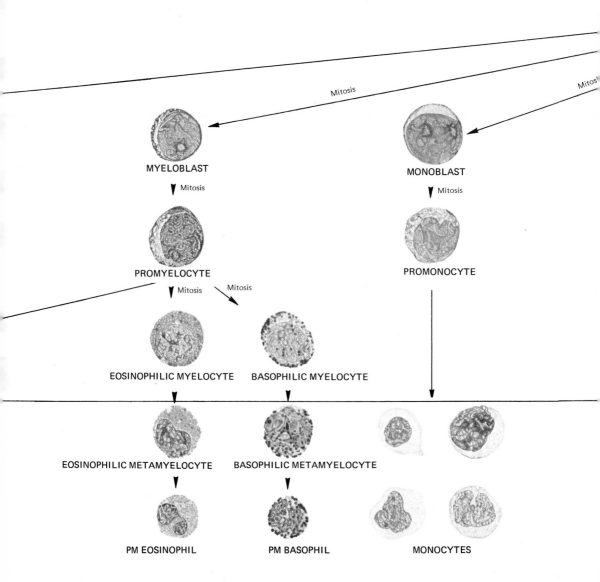

Mitosis

Mitosis

MYELOBLAST

MONOBLAST

Mitosis

Mitosis

PROMYELOCYTE

PROMONOCYTE

Mitosis   Mitosis

EOSINOPHILIC MYELOCYTE   BASOPHILIC MYELOCYTE

EOSINOPHILIC METAMYELOCYTE   BASOPHILIC METAMYELOCYTE

PM EOSINOPHIL   PM BASOPHIL   MONOCYTES

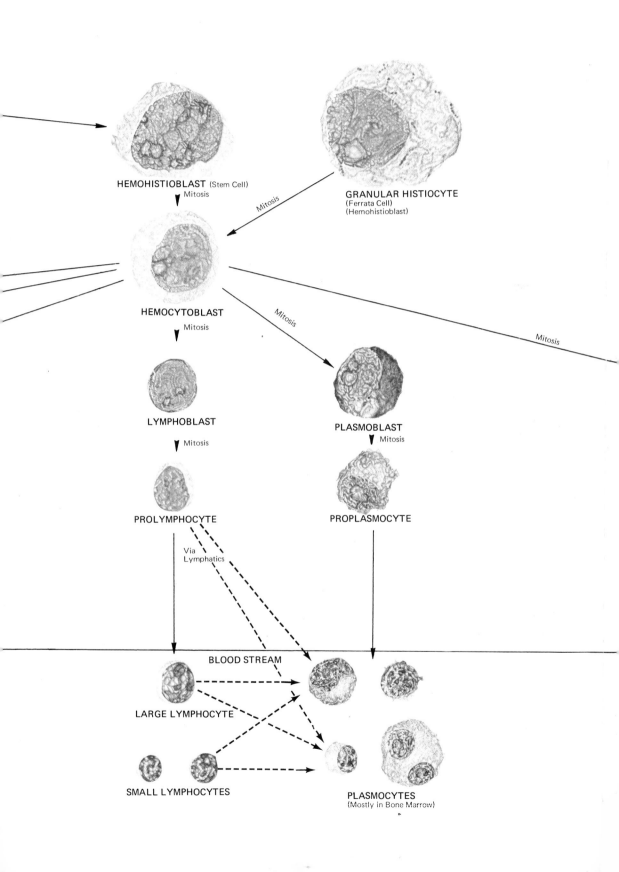

HEMOHISTIOBLAST (Stem Cell)

Mitosis

Mitosis

GRANULAR HISTIOCYTE
(Ferrata Cell)
(Hemohistioblast)

HEMOCYTOBLAST

Mitosis

Mitosis

Mitosis

LYMPHOBLAST

Mitosis

PLASMOBLAST

Mitosis

PROLYMPHOCYTE

PROPLASMOCYTE

Via
Lymphatics

BLOOD STREAM

LARGE LYMPHOCYTE

SMALL LYMPHOCYTES

PLASMOCYTES
(Mostly in Bone Marrow)

MEGAKARYOBLAST

BASOPHILIC
MEGAKARYOCYTE

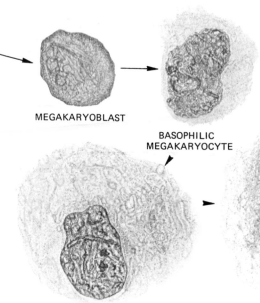

GRANULAR MEGAKARYOCYTE

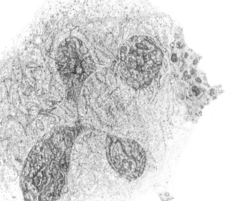

PLATELET-PRODUCING MEGAKARYOCYTE

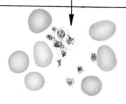

PLATELETS, WITH ERYTHROCYTES

D. L. MAGIDSON

1 *Introduction to Hematology*

DEFINITIONS

There are certain embryologic-morphologic criteria, pathophysiologic data, and diagnostic laboratory procedures involving blood that provide hematologic knowledge that is essential to the complete clinical study of any patient.

Simply stated, blood is a unique bright (arterial) to dark (venous) red fluid of variable composition circulating through the transport vessels of the body with a total volume of approximately 30 ml./kg. body weight. It participates in the physiologic and pathologic activities of all organs and is composed of a liquid called plasma in which are suspended erythrocytes (red blood cells), leukocytes (white blood cells), and thrombocytes (platelets), collectively called hemocytes. These elements of the blood have differing functions. The red blood cells are intimately associated with cardiac output, pulmonary and kidney activity, and blood vessel response in order to oxygenate body tissues. The white blood cell components participate in phagocytosis, utilizing the granulocytes and monocytes together with coexistent factors in the plasma. The lymphocytes and successor plasma cells function in the elaboration of gamma globulin fractions, which are intimately associated with antibody formation and tissue alterations. The eosinophils and basophils participate in hypersensitivity phenomena.

The platelets are initiators and co-sponsors of the coagulation process.

Clinical hematology is the division of medicine associated with diagnostic laboratory procedures and morphologic interpretations related to blood, and with the correlation of this hematologic data with the entire clinical condition of the patient. Hematology is concerned with the sum total of the interaction of the hematopoietic and the vascular systems. The hematopoietic system is that organ complex associated with the morphologic components of the blood and the manner and loci of their pathophysiologic formation and function. The vascular system can be defined as the entire arrangement of vessels operative in the circulation of all body fluids, including the heart, arteries, capillaries, veins, and lymphatics. If blood coagulation (clotting) is prevented after blood is withdrawn from the vascular system, the formed cellular elements of the blood (hemocytes) can be separated from the noncellular liquid portion (pale straw-colored plasma). Serum, on the other hand, is the amber-colored fluid that remains after separation of the clot associated with blood coagulation. It differs from plasma only by the loss of the protein fibrinogen, which is removed together with the blood cells as insoluble fibrin threads in the coagulation process.

The individual cytologic components of the blood may be defined as follows:

1

The *erythrocyte* (red blood cell) is an elastic non-nucleated biconcave discoid cell usually found in the lumina of peripheral blood vessels. It has an average life span of 80 to 120 days, an average diameter of approximately 7.2 μ, and is a pale greenish yellow when unstained (it stains eosin red with the Romanowsky or Wright stain). The main function of the erythrocyte is the carrying of hemoglobin with its associated O_2 and CO_2.

The *leukocyte* (white blood cell) is a nucleated living cell 8 to 12 μ in diameter and is found in the bone marrow and peripheral blood. It has an indefinite, variable life span. In the peripheral blood, leukocytes are mainly composed of polymorphonuclear cells (with a life span of 3 to 4 days), lymphocytes (with a life span of approximately 4.4 years or longer), monocytes (life span of approximately 2 days to 2 weeks), and occasionally plasma cells (long life span of unknown duration). Leukocytes also have certain nuclear and cytoplasmic staining and morphologic qualities when the Romanowsky stains are used. Each type of leukocyte plays some part in the protection of the body from disease—by phagocytosis and immune body formation.

The *thrombocyte* (platelet) is a morphologically irregular fragment (with an average life span of 8 to 11 days) derived from the cytoplasmic portion of megakaryocytes (parent cell usually situated in the bone marrow). It has a purple-red color with Romanowsky stains (for example, Wright's stain) and is essential for the proper coagulation of shed blood, clot retraction, and adhesion to the wall of a damaged blood vessel for the purpose of repair. Thrombocytes have recently been reported to be able to attract submicroscopic particles, and they therefore may enhance the removal of solid particles from the blood.

Any moderate to marked variation in the number, morphologic alteration, and function of one or more of the cytologic components of the blood will produce a hematologic symptom called a blood dyscrasia.

REVIEW OF VASCULAR SYSTEM AND BLOOD CONSTITUENTS

Physiology of the Vascular System

In order to understand the significance of qualitative and quantitative variations in bone marrow and peripheral blood, a brief review of the physiology of the blood and blood-forming organs seems appropriate at this point.

The main organs of hematopoiesis are the bone marrow, liver, spleen, thymus, and lymph nodes. Hematopoiesis begins during fetal life; however, under specific situations of stress the liver, spleen, thymus, and lymph nodes may revert to their fetal function and demonstrate extramedullary hematopoiesis. Fatty material occupies most of the bone marrow spaces in adult life except in the flat bones, where blood cell formation remains physiologically active; the fatty areas serve as foci of reserve hematopoiesis as the need may arise in various diseases. The main functions of the cells of the hematopoietic system are those of oxygen transport, resistance to infection, antibody production, hemorrhage cessation, and reaction to foreign material.

Reductions in cell proportions are occasionally related to physiologic aberrations —for example, reduction in oxygen supply to tissues due to reduction in hemoglobin or in red blood cells, overwhelming infection with poor host response due to a reduction in leukocytes, and petechial and hemorrhagic manifestations due to platelet deficiency. In addition, these cytopenias may affect the inter-involvement of coagulation factors I to XIII, the integrity of capillary endothelium, and the action of thrombocytes in hemorrhagic diseases. The knowledge of the relationships of the basophil to heparin and histamine production, fat metabolism, and allergic states; of the neutrophil to bacterial phagocytosis; of the lymphocyte and plasma cell to antibody production; of the eosinophil to stress (adrenocortical activity); and of the eosinophil and basophil to hypersensitivity phenomena is still complex but is rapidly developing through the impetus of immunobiologic phenomena. Hyperplasia of hematologic cellular elements may result in disturbed physiologic functions—for example, thrombotic tendencies associated with thrombocythemic and polycythemic states, organ enlargement, and pain in leukemic and lymphomatous states. Finally, atypical cytologic function may be associated with hemolysis in intrinsic red blood cell disease and with hyperglobulinemia in lymphocyte and plasma cell diseases.

Composition of Blood

Cellular elements of blood may be defined as follows (Plate 1):

In the erythrocyte, *hemoglobin* is the main functioning constituent and has a molecular weight of approximately 66,000. The function of hemoglobin is the transportation of oxygen to the tissues, the removal of carbon dioxide from the tissues, and the buffering of blood, which aids the maintenance of the constant reaction of blood. The last is accomplished by the intraerythrocytic enzyme, carbonic anhydrase, which catalyzes the carbon dioxide and transforms it into carbonic acid. The hydrogen ions of carbonic acid are then buffered by the moderately alkaline deoxyhemoglobin, and the bicarbonate ion diffused back into the plasma. In the pulmonary capillary the same process, in reverse, liberates carbon dioxide for pulmonary elimination. In addition, the amino groups of the globin fraction of hemoglobin form reversible carbamino groups with carbon dioxide and are responsible for approximately 10 per cent of carbon dioxide transport and excretion. Reticulocytes are young, slightly enlarged red cells in which the reticular or granular network is revealed by supravital

stains counterstained with Romanowsky's stain.

Thrombocytes and leukocytes have been briefly discussed above. The following are various types of leukocytes.

Granulocytes are motile polymorphonuclear cells having ameboid activity, variegated nuclear shape, and cytoplasmic granules. A juvenile or band form is a transitional cell type that developmentally is between the marrow metamyelocyte and the mature granulocyte of the peripheral blood. This form is characterized by an elongated C-shaped nuclear pattern without distinct lobe formation; the number of nuclear lobes denotes the age of the cell, with older cells having more lobes. A *neutrophilic* (polymorphonuclear) granulocyte has an average diameter of about 10 to 12 μ with two to four lobes and slightly acidophilic granules in the cytoplasm. An *eosinophilic* (polymorphonuclear) granulocyte is approximately the same size as the neutrophil, usually with two lobes. It contains large, coarse, round or oval eosinophilic granules that stain a deep pink and usually fill the cell proper. The *basophilic* (polymorphonuclear) granulocyte, which is functionally and chemically related to the mast cell, has an average diameter of 8 to 10 μ. It has a kidney-shaped or slightly lobulated nucleus and large, deep purple granules in the cytoplasm that often obscure nuclear detail.

Lymphocytes are mononuclear leukocytes originating and differentiating first in the primary lymphoid structures of the bone marrow and the thymus. They are then distributed to the secondary lymphoid organs (spleen, lymph nodes, tonsils, pharynx, and subepithelial lymphoid tissue in the gastrointestinal tract), where they are characterized by arrangement into follicles with germinal centers and where they function in specific immune responses. They have an average diameter of 12 to 15 μ in the large motile type and 7 to 8 μ in the small nonmotile type. The circular, deeply

Table 1-1. Development of Hematologic Values

Age	Hb (gm.)	Hemato- crit (%)	RBC (million per cu.mm.)	Platelets (thousand per cu.mm.)	Reticulo- cytes (%)	W.B.C. (per cu.mm.)	P.M.N. adult	Band (%)	Eosinophils (%)	Basophils (%)	Lymphocytes (%)	Monocytes (%)
Birth	17.6	55	5.5	350.0	5.0	9000–30,000 (av., 18,000)	9400 (52%)	9.1	2.2	0.6	31	5.8
24 hrs.	18.0	56	5.3	400.0	5.2	9400–34,000 (av., 19,045)	9800 (52%)	9.2	2.4	0.5	31	5.8
1 wk.	17.0	54	5.0	300.0	1.0	5000–21,000 (av., 12,279)	4700 (39%)	6.8	4.1	0.4	41	9.1
2 mos.	12.4	30	4.3	260.0	0.5	5500–18,000 (av., 11,000)	3300 (30%)	4.4	2.7	0.5	57	5.9
6 mos.	11.5	34	4.6	250.0	0.8	6000–17,500 (av., 11,900)	3300 (28%)	3.8	2.5	0.4	61	4.8
2 yrs.	12.9	40	4.8	250.0	1.0	6000–17,000 (av., 10,680)	3200 (30%)	3.0	2.6	0.5	59	5.0
6 yrs.	14.1	42	4.8	250.0	1.0	5000–14,500 (av., 8500)	4000 (48%)	3.0	2.7	0.6	42	4.7
14 yrs.	15.0	45–♂ 42–♀	5.1	250.0	1.0	4500–13,000 (av., 7900)	4200 (53%)	3.0	2.5	0.5	37	4.7
21 yrs.	15.0	45–♂ 42–♀	5.1	250.0	1.0	4500–11,000 (av., 7400)	4200 (56%)	3.0	2.7	0.5	34	4.0

basophilic chunky chromatin-containing nucleus occupies practically all available space in the cell and possesses a clear pale blue rim of cytoplasm (Wright's stain) with occasional distinct reddish-purple azurophil granules.

Monocytes are occasionally motile, large mononuclear leukocytes originating in the marrow, measuring approximately 14 to 19 μ. These cells are the major source of macrophages in sites of inflammation. They have a lobulated kidney-bean- or horseshoe-shaped pale violet nucleus with vesicular chromatin crisscrossing the nuclear strands. The nucleus is often located to one side of the cell. The cytoplasm is pale grayish blue, sometimes with an irregular outer border, sometimes vacuolated, and occasionally containing red-staining Auer bodies.

Percentage of Cellular Elements in Blood. Quality control studies of the peripheral blood show some variation in the oft-quoted "norm" values given in various texts of hematology. However, a range of values presents a more accurate approach to blood composition. For reference purposes, see Table 1-1.

Percentage of Liquid Constituents. Included among the liquid constituents are diffusible anabolic substances, diffusible catabolic substances, and nondiffusible constituents.

Because blood is the specialized fluid tissue of the transport system of the body, it contains liquid constituents in which its solid elements are suspended (Fig. 1-1). The specific gravity of whole blood averages between 1.048 and 1.066 to 1.057 in males and 1.053 in females. The specific gravity of serum is 1.026 to 1.031 and that of red blood cells is 1.092 to 1.095. The pH of normal blood is 7.35 to 7.45 (the range compatible with life is 6.8–7.8). Total blood volume in terms of body weight is greater in males than in females, chiefly owing to the higher red cell volume in the male. Average values are 75.5 ml./kg. in males and 66.5 ml./kg. in females, or a total of 5 to 6 liters or about 7 to 8 per cent of body weight. Blood cells make up 45 per cent by volume of the whole blood, and because they are

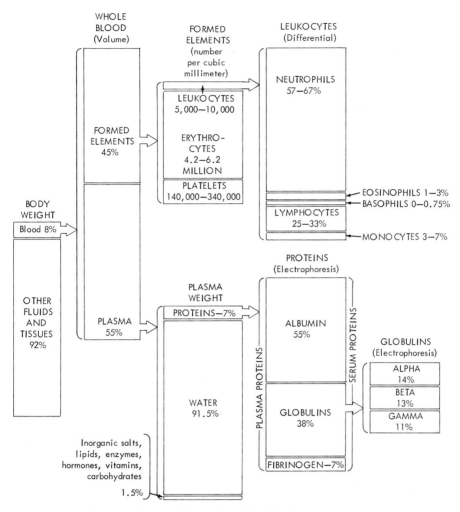

Fig. 1-1. Composition of the blood in the normal adult.

heavier than plasma, they sink to the bottom of an anticoagulated blood sample. Blood plasma, which is composed of serum plus fibrinogen, makes up 55 per cent of blood volume; water makes 91 to 92 per cent by weight of the plasma, and plasma protein, 6 to 7 per cent by weight of plasma. The plasma proteins, which are formed mainly in the liver, exert an osmotic pressure of 25 to 30 ml. of mercury, are nondiffusible, and are important in regulating blood volume and the body's fluid balance. Plasma proteins are also responsible for blood viscosity, which is important in main-

taining blood pressure. The plasma proteins are composed of: (1) Serum albumin (4%), which exerts the osmotic pressure previously described. (2) Serum globulin (2.7%). The alpha fraction is associated with the transport of bilirubin, lipids, and steroids; the beta fraction is associated with the transport of iron and copper in plasma; and the gamma fraction is associated with the production of antibodies. (3) Fibrinogen (0.3%) is the precursor of fibrin, which forms the framework of the blood clot. Also present in the plasma are regulatory and protective proteins, such as hormones, enzymes, and antibodies. *Diffusible anabolic substances* include inorganic material (0.9%), such as sodium chloride, calcium, potassium, acid carbonate (HCO_3) iodine, and iron. Also included in this category are nutritive organic materials (such as amino acids, glucose, fats, cholesterol, all of which are foodstuffs in solution absorbed from the gastrointestinal tract, from which they go to other body tissues for utilization and storage), plus respiratory gases (O_2 and CO_2). *Diffusible catabolic constituents* (such as urea, uric acid, xanthine, creatine, creatinine, and ammonia) in plasma are products of tissue activity that are transported from tissues to kidney and skin for excretion. From the preceding discussion, one can summarize the functions of blood as respiration, nutrition, excretion, maintenance of water content in tissues, and regulation of body temperature.

METHODS OF OBTAINING BLOOD FROM THE PATIENT

When a technician approaches the patient for blood withdrawal, he should radiate an attitude of confidence, self-assurance, and poise. He should explain briefly what he is going to do so that the patient will give his full cooperation. It is essential that the request slip with the name of the patient, room number, and physician's name is checked verbally with the patient, that all tubes and equipment are in readiness and properly numbered, that the patient and operator are both comfortable, and that there is good light. The technician should be sure that he has blood lancets, sharp needles of proper size, and a dry syringe or proper Vacutainer in good working condition. Material for cleansing the arm, tourniquet, containers for blood, and other equipment should be conveniently placed. If the patient is in bed, a disposable towel placed under the arm prevents the soiling of linen. It is desirable that the patient be reclining when the skin puncture is performed because he is more easily con-

trolled if he feels sick or faint. If the patient is seated, the arm should extend over the corner of a table, and be placed on a disposable towel.

SELECTION OF SITES

In selecting the site for blood withdrawal, consideration must be given to the type of laboratory test requested, the volume of blood required, and the age of the patient. For example, if both blood chemistry procedures and hematologic procedures are ordered, it is more efficient to obtain a suitable quantity of venous blood with only one venipuncture (especially in using the Vacutainer tubes with or without various types of anticoagulants). If the patient is an infant or is severely burned, adequate samples may be obtained from a skin puncture utilizing microtechniques. In the adult and child, the median basilic veins in the antecubital fossae are most suitable. The best right or left vein is selected after observation and palpation of both antecubital fossae.

Small Specimens

For small specimens from adults, the usual puncture sites are the lobe of the ear or the end or side of the distal phalanx of the third or fourth finger. The heel, great toe, or skin of the forearm below the elbow are the sites of choice in very young infants. For continued cooperation, older children should be told what type of "pinprick" to expect when a puncture is made.

The materials needed are blood lancets (heat-sterilized, disposable lancets in sealed envelopes), cotton pledgets, and alcohol (70%).

Technique. A free flow of blood should be assured by warming or rubbing the skin of the site chosen with a piece of dry cotton. The puncture site should be cleansed with 70 per cent alcohol applied with a cotton pledget, and allowed to dry. The skin is then made tense, and the needle placed on its surface. A clean, quick jab 2 to 3 mm. in depth is made with the disposable blood lancet. The first drop of blood is wiped away with a dry cotton pledget; the next drop will well up naturally. Blood is then drawn up into the dilution pipettes by capillarity. After the proper amount of blood has been obtained, a cotton pledget moderately soaked in antiseptic (70% alcohol) is lightly pressed over the puncture site until bleeding has ceased. Sterile 2 × 2 inch gauze may be used instead of the cotton pledget.

Advantages. This technique has several advantages. It is a relatively easy and painless method of obtaining volumes of blood adequate for the information desired, especially from infants. Blood may be taken more than once, even if the patient has poor veins, is uncooperative, or if patient is in shock or badly burned over a large part of his body. It is easy to control the flow of blood using this technique in patients who have a hemorrhagic disease, especially from a finger-puncture site. The disposable equipment used reduces and possibly eliminates the potential danger of transmitting infection—for example, the virus of homologous serum hepatitis.

Disadvantages. The blood count may be incorrect if:

The finger is squeezed after puncture, and the blood is diluted with tissue fluids or is concentrated by stasis. Also, squeezing enhances clotting. However, moderate pressure some distance above the puncture is allowed.

The blood flow is not free—that is, if a small amount of blood is obtained and further pressure needed. The red blood cell count and hemoglobin may be higher or lower, and hematocrit and platelet count lower (platelets lost by adherence to puncture tissue area).

Collection of the blood will be made difficult if the skin at the puncture site is not dry; that is, the blood will spread along the surface. Also, if alcohol is mixed with the blood collected, the cells will be distorted and a dilution error will be introduced.

Large Specimens

For large specimens, in which venous blood is collected, the veins in the bend of the elbow, the back of the wrist, or the ankle region are used. If the technician is confident and experienced and if repeated venipunctures are to be made for repeated tests and infusions, it is wise to use the wrist and ankle areas. However, if the vessels in these sites are not prominent, if the patient is exceedingly apprehensive (with a low threshold for pain), or if the technician is not highly proficient, the median basilic or cephalic elbow vein is best to use. In obese patients, veins that appear as faint blue lines are usually too superficial and too small and should not be used. It is best to have the patient look away as venipuncture is being performed. The patient should be comfortable and lying down, and good light should be present.

The materials needed are cotton pledgets; alcohol (70%); a tourniquet such as one made by using laboratory rubber tubing (18 in. long by ¼ in. wide) or one of the commercially available flat or tubular tourniquets; and multicolored, rubber-stoppered Vacutainers containing anticoagulants such as Sequestrene (dipotassium or tripotassium ethylenediaminetetraacetate [EDTA]), balanced oxalate (ammonium and potassium oxalate) with or without fluoride, or nonanticoagulant tubes. Sequestrene (the dipotassium or disodium salt of ethylenediaminetetraacetic acid, EDTA) is preferred for erythrocyte counts, leukocyte counts, hematocrits, and platelet counts because it maintains good morphology for 3 to 4 hours after blood is drawn. However, if it is refrigerated, blood counts may be performed for as long as 24 hours after collection in EDTA. EDTA also acts as an anticoagulant by binding calcium in the blood in a nonionized form, therefore making the calcium unavailable to the blood clotting mechanism. EDTA is used in a concentration of 1 to 2 mg./ml. of blood. The most widely used anticoagulant is a

mixture of ammonium and potassium oxalate (6 and 4 parts respectively), a total
of 2 mg./ml. of blood. It may be used for
hemoglobin and other tests for which
EDTA is used; double oxalate, not EDTA,
must be used for the "sucrose-hemolysis"
test for paroxysmal nocturnal hemoglobinuria.[4] However, the ammonium-potassium
oxalate mixture cannot be used for the
stydy of blood film preparations after remaining in the blood film for more than 2
or 3 minutes because there is rapid artifact formation and other malformations
in lymphocyte and monocyte nuclei, vacuolation in granulocyte cytoplasm, oxalate
crystal phagocytosis, and red cell crenation.
This balanced oxalate anticoagulant also
cannot be used for nitrogen (BUN) or
potassium determinations in blood chemistry. Disodium citrate (1 part of 3.8%
solution and 4 parts of blood) is only
useful in determining sedimentation rates
and in the investigation of clotting mechanisms. The oxalate and citrate anticoagulants act as EDTA does in preventing
the coagulation of blood. Heparin (0.1
mg./ml. of blood) acts as an anticoagulant
by neutralizing thrombin. It is best for preventing hemolysis in osmotic fragility tests
and does not affect the corpuscular size and
hematocrit. It is not good for blood films in
which Wright's stain is used, because it
produces a bluish background. The Vacutainer tubes are desirable because they are
disposable and only one needle stick is
needed for as much blood as is desired.
Vacutainers and similar preparations are
test tubes vacuum-sealed by a flexible
rubber stopper, which is punctured by the
rear end of a special needle held in its own
adapter when the front end of the needle
has entered the vein (see following section).
The collection tube, which utilizes this
technique, also serves as a syringe. However, if this equipment is not available,
sterile dry Luer syringes with standard
center tips are suitable (5–10 cc. volume).
Sharp needles should be 19- to 22-gauge
and 1 to 1.5 inches in length. Disposable

needles are preferred for patient's comfort,
ease of venipuncture, and avoidance of risk
of transmitting homologous serum hepatitis. Time is also saved because sharpening
and beveling needles are eliminated.

*Technique and Selection of Vein. Adults
and Children.* The puncture area is cleaned
with an alcohol sponge. A tourniquet is
placed about 2 inches above the site of
puncture so that it may be released easily.
The tourniquet should not be tightened
enough to cut off arterial circulation; that is,
the radial pulse at the wrist should be palpable. The patient should open and close his
fist a few times and then close it tightly.
Vacutainer tubes are used. If these are not
available, the plunger of a regular syringe is
pulled back to make sure that the needle is
open. The needle is checked to make certain that it is attached tightly, and the
plunger is depressed to its closed position.
The patient's arm is grasped with the technician's free hand (usually the left), and the
technician places his left thumb directly
over the vein approximately 1.5 inches
away from the intended puncture site. Gentle traction is then applied.

The syringe is held between the right
thumb and the last three right fingers. With
the needle bevel up, above, and directly in
line with the course of the vein, the needle
is inserted quickly and steadily under the
skin and then into the vein. Some prefer to
insert into the skin and vein in one complete motion. When the needle has entered
the lumen of the vein, penetration is felt to
be easier, and blood will flow freely into the
syringe. The amount of needed blood is
withdrawn by exerting gentle traction on
the plunger. Frothing and hemolysis are
avoided by withdrawing blood slowly.

The tourniquet is released and the needle
is then slowly withdrawn. A sterile gauze or
alcohol cotton pledget is applied to the
entry site and held tightly. The patient is
told to maintain pressure with his free hand
for 3 to 5 minutes to prevent bleeding and
hematoma formation. According to some
sources, it is better to elevate the patient's

arm slightly and, with a piece of dry sterile gauze or cotton over the entry site, to apply thumb pressure at the site. The needle is removed from the syringe, and the blood is carefully transferred to the proper containers. Each container is tilted so that the blood runs down the side, thus minimizing trauma and frothing. The containers are gently inverted several times to mix the blood and anticoagulant. This is especially important in cases of hyperglobulinemia, anemia, and hyperfibrinogenemia, in which leukocytes and platelets will tend to settle upon standing. Prior to manual or automated counting, the specimen should be inspected for macroscopically visible autoagglutination of erythrocytes, platelet aggregation, and the presence of clots. The plunger is pulled back, and the syringe and needle are immediately rinsed with cold water.

Infants. When the infant is crying, the external jugular vein in the neck is easily visible. The infant is wrapped in a blanket up to and including his shoulders, thus completely immobilizing his chest, trunk, and extremities. The infant is placed flat on a table with his shoulders on the edge of the table and his head turned to the side and stretched slightly downward. The external jugular or internal jugular vein becomes more prominent in this position.

A syringe with a 21-gauge needle is then placed just lateral to the outer border of the sternocleidomastoid muscle pointed toward the chest area and midway between the tip of the mastoid process and the clavicle. The needle, with bevel up, is then inserted in a direction aimed at the sternoclavicular junction just beneath the sternomastoid muscle. The needle is then withdrawn slowly, and traction is maintained on the plunger until blood begins to enter the syringe barrel.

If the foregoing procedure is not feasible, puncture of the femoral vein may be performed. The femoral artery is palpated with the index finger as it passes through the femoral canal area. With the index finger over the pulsating femoral artery, the needle, bevel up, is inserted just medial to the finger down toward the superior ramus of the ischium (bone). The needle is then pulled back slowly, and continuous traction is maintained on the plunger until blood begins to come into the syringe barrel.

Advantages. This is the easiest and most convenient method of obtaining a volume of blood adequate for a variety of tests; more than one type of test can be done with the large volume of blood obtained using this procedure—for example, hematologic, chemical, and serologic.

The sample may be divided and treated as the prescribed investigations demand. Thus, some of the sample may be mixed with anticoagulant to provide plasma or whole blood; some may be allowed to clot to provide serum and to determine accurately clotting time; some may be used to make blood films and blood cultures.

In addition, this is the fastest method of collecting samples from a large number of patients, for it allows accurate dilutions to be carried out with more leisure once the morning collection rush is over. This method also reduces the amount and variety of apparatus needed in the hospital wards.

By providing sufficient blood, this method allows various tests to be repeated in case of accident or error, or for the all-important checking of a doubtful result. It frequently allows the performance of additional tests that may be suggested by the results of those already ordered or that may occur to the clinician or clinical pathologist as afterthoughts. It reduces the possibility of error associated with the finger-puncture technique, which results from dilution with tissue juices or constriction of skin vessels by cold or emotion.

Disadvantages. This method may cause hemoconcentration with subsequent erroneous hematologic and biochemical results, all due to prolonged application of the tourniquet. Blood may fail to enter the syringe owing to collapse of a small vein. Piercing the outer coat of the vein without entering the lumen may lead to hematoma formation and subsequent pain around the puncture site. When this technique is used, blood may not be obtainable from the veins of a patient with circulatory failure. Syncope may occur in some patients after venipuncture, and continued venous oozing may occur in patients with a bleeding tendency.

Thrombosis of a vein may occur as a result of trauma or infection with the possible subsequent development of thrombophlebitis. Homologous serum jaundice may be transmitted to patients by improper handling and contamination of needle or of syringe.

Arterial puncture may occasionally occur, especially in children.

METHODS OF OBTAINING BONE MARROW[2]

Definition

Bone marrow is the heterogeneous organ located within the interstices in cancellous bone and between the trabeculae of the marrow cavities in long bones. On aspiration, bone marrow has a rusty-red color and normally has a thick fluid-like consistency with varying amounts of fatty material and pale gray-white marrow fragments.

Site of Puncture

The morphologic study of bone marrow cells is of corroborative and diagnostic value in diagnosing some blood dyscrasias, and it is even more helpful in elucidating hematopoiesis. Marrow material is best and most easily obtained from the flat bones of the body (for example, the sternum and iliac crest in adults) and from the iliac crest, spinous processes of the vertebrae, and tibia in children. The sternal area is usually not used in children because this cavity is too shallow, the chest is difficult to mobilize, the danger of mediastinal and cardiac perforation is too great, and observation of the procedure is associated with apprehen-

sion and lack of cooperation. Many hematologists now use the posterior superior iliac crest solely, especially if repeated marrow examinations are to be made.*

Bone Marrow Needles

Different types of needles are available for puncture of the marrow cavity. Most hematologists believe the safest one is a simple, short, rigid needle (to prevent bending or breaking) with a 1 to 2 mm. diameter lumen, tight-fitting stylet, short bevel, and sharp point with a permanent removable guard to prevent excessive penetration.† Infusions of blood and other fluids by way of the bone marrow may be performed using the same needle or another type in which the outer needle is fitted with an adjustable guard.[9]

A Vim-Silverman needle, or a modification of it, can be used for surgical biopsy of the bone marrow when aspiration has been unsatisfactory (for example, in "dry taps" and in myelofibrosis). This needle has a cutting edge and obtains sufficient material both for marrow imprints and for histologic study of the marrow pattern (for example, in metastatic carcinoma cells and myelophthisic disorders). The disadvantages of this needle are those of time, danger, and the frequent necessity for professional assistance from the internist, surgeon, pathologist, medical technologist, or anesthesiologist.

During the last 5 years, two marrow biopsy needles and techniques have become popular and appear to yield excellent results in both marrow aspiration and biopsy approaches. The Westerman-Jensen needle, which is supplied with finger grips, an assembly stylet, and an obturator that locks in position has had acceptance in many medical centers. The main disadvan-

---

* Rebuck, J. W.: Washington University School of Medicine Lecture Series (personal communication), 1966.
† For example, the University of Illinois sternal needle manufactured by V. Mueller & Co., 408 S. Honore Street, Chicago, Illinois 60612.

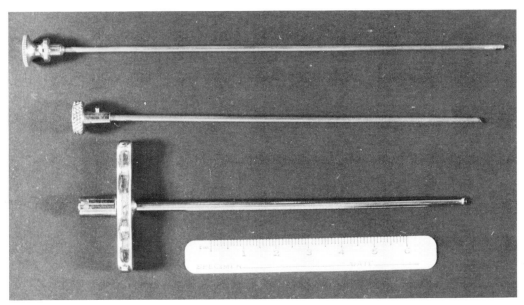

Fig. 1-2. Jamshidi Needle. From top to bottom, this photograph displays the stylette, the obturator, and the needle, which are used in performing the Jamshidi technique for bone marrow biopsy and aspiration. (Roeckel, I. E.: Diagnosis of metastatic carcinoma by bone marrow biopsy versus bone marrow aspiration. Annals of Clinical and Laboratory Science, *4:*194, 1974)

tages of this instrument have been the easy bending of the needle and its blunting from frequent use. Most recently, the Jamshidi biopsy (Fig. 1-2) aspiration needle has been demonstrated to be a particularly satisfying instrument.*[5, 11]

The posterior superior iliac spine is the site of choice since there is little danger of penetrating the bone at this site, the patient cannot see the procedure, the site is usually easy to locate, good marrow specimens can be obtained, there is minimal architecture damage to the sample, and an aspirate and biopsy specimen can be obtained at the same time. The Jamshidi needle has a uniform, external cylindrical configuration with a core of substantially constant internal diameter except for the tapered distal portion. The distal tip is beveled and has a sharp cutting edge. The interior diameter of the distal portion is tapered radially toward the cutting tip. This provides space within the interior of the instrument that has a larger diameter than the cutting tip, avoids compression of the tissues, and produces specimens without plugging the lumen of the needle. The proximal end is calibrated for syringe attachment and has finger grips. The stylet is designed to interlock, to fit the tapered internal core, and to project 1 to 2 mm. beyond the tip in order to protect the cutting edge and to provide a means of entering the marrow (Fig. 1-3*A*). These needles are available in the following sizes: Regular/Adult—4 inch, 11-gauge; Adult—4 inch, 8-gauge; Pediatric—3½ inch, 13-gauge; and Infant—2 inch, 13-gauge. Although the posterior superior iliac spine is the preferred site, some physicians prefer the proximal tibia in young children because it is easy to immobilize. In general, one should select the iliac spine, but the needle can be used in any area of bone tenderness or radiologic lesions. If aspiration is to be performed, it should be done before the biopsy since residual tissue thromboplastin may enhance clotting and make it difficult to obtain adequate smears. The marrow biopsy should be taken after the

* Kormed, Inc., 2510 Northland Drive, St. Paul, Minnesota 55120.

aspiration using the same skin incision but choosing a different location to obtain the biopsy sample.

Biopsy Procedure

Take the biopsy after the aspiration. Before using, check the cutting end of the needle. Resharpening may be necessary after approximately ten biopsies.

1. Place the patient in a right or left lateral decubitus position, with the back comfortably flexed and the top knee drawn toward the chest.

2. Locate the posterior superior iliac spine and mark with ink or thumbnail pressure (Fig. 1-3*B*).

3. Using sterile technique, prepare the skin with antiseptic and drape (Fig. 1-3*C*).

4. Infiltrate the marked area with local anesthetic, especially the periosteum which is the region of greatest sensitivity. This can be done by fixing the needle in the bone and injecting the anesthetic under pressure. Occasionally, in a very anxious patient, a tranquilizer, sedative, or analgesic may be helpful.

5. Make a 3-mm. skin incision with a scalpel blade over the marked area (1 cm. caudal and medial to the posterior superior iliac spine) to facilitate the insertion of the biopsy needle.

6. Hold the needle with the proximal end in the palm and the index finger against the shaft near the tip. This position stabilizes the needle and allows better control (Fig. 1-3*D*).

7. With the stylet locked in place, introduce the needle through the incision pointing toward the anterior superior iliac spine (laterally and cephalad) and bring it into contact with the posterior iliac spine, with the axis of projection through the posterior superior iliac spine.

8. Using gentle, but firm and steady pressure, advance the needle. Rotate the needle in an alternating clockwise-counterclockwise motion. Entrance into the marrow cavity is generally detected by decreased resistance (Fig. 1-3*E*).

9. Remove the stylet (Fig. 1-3*F*).

10. Slowly and gently advance the needle millimeter by millimeter, with clockwise-counterclockwise motion (for better cutting) until adequate marrow is obtained (Fig. 1-3*G*).

11. Pull the needle back 2 to 3 mm. and, with less pressure, direct its tip at a slightly different angle. (*Caution:* applying too much pressure may bend the needle.) Then advance the needle 2 to 3 mm. farther. This procedure insures that the specimen is severed before withdrawing the needle (Fig. 1-3*H*).

12. Rotate the needle along its axis with quick, full twists several times to the right and to the left. Slowly remove the needle with alternating rotary motions (Fig. 1-3*I*).

13. Remove the specimen with the probe. Introduce the probe only through the distal cutting end. This procedure prevents crushing the specimen, which would result were the specimen forced through the narrow distal tip (Fig. 1-3*J*).

Aspiration Procedure

Take the aspiration before taking the biopsy. The technique is the same through Step 8. After lodging the needle firmly in the bone marrow cavity, remove the stylet. With a syringe locked into the proximal portion, apply a negative pressure (Fig. 1-3*K*). The marrow specimen (.5–1 ml.) collected in the syringe is then handed to a lab technologist who will make smears or sections, as described in the next section (p. 17).

Preparing the Specimen

Aspirated Material. The medical technologist quickly makes smears as described in the next section (pp. 17-19). For histologic sections of aspirated marrow, the unused marrow material in the syringe is immediately put into Zenker's formol (1 part formaldehyde to 1 part of Zenker's solution) or into neutral buffered 10 per cent formalin solution before it clots. As a variation from (*Text continues on p. 16*)

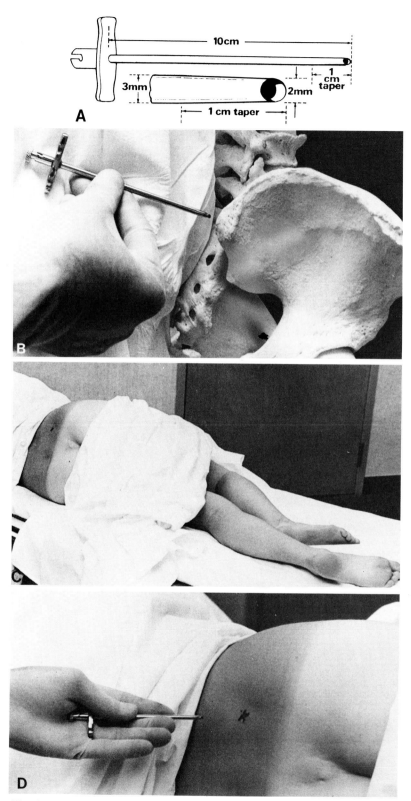

Fig. 1-3. Jamshidi technique (courtesy of Kormed, Inc.). (*Figure continues on p. 14* and *15*.)

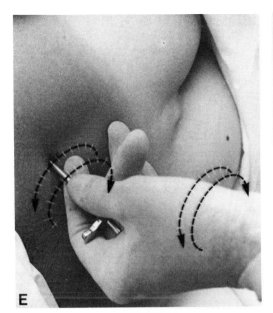

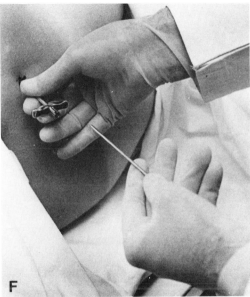

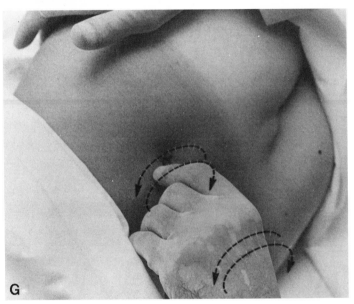

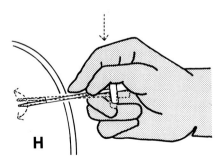

Fig. 1-3. Continued.
(See also facing page)

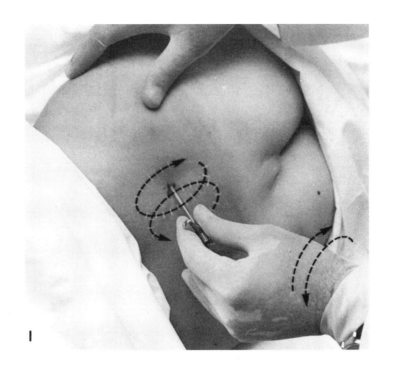

I

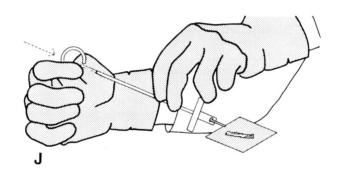

J

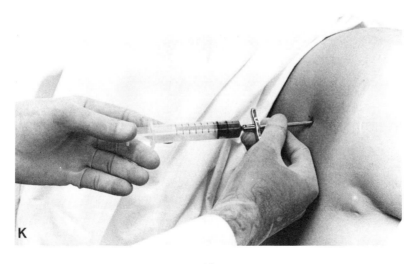

K

the EDTA or heparin technique, some technologists filter the marrow fixative mixture through filter paper, thus concentrating the particles. These are then processed in the routine manner for embedding. Sections of aspirated marrow are sometimes better than needle biopsy specimens since the latter may require decalcification and may sometimes show crushing artefacts, both of which decrease cellular detail.

Biopsied Material. Place the specimen immediately into Zenker's formol (see above) or neutral buffered 10 per cent formalin solution for fixation and decalcification and then routine histologic section processing. Autopsy marrow material is best scraped out of the sternum, ribs, vertebral bodies, and ileum and placed in 5 per cent albumin to form a uniform suspension. This is then centrifuged, and most of the supernate is removed. The remaining supernate is mixed with the marrow deposit, and smears and sections are made. Marrow cellularity, presence or absence of granulomas or metastatic tumor, iron storage, and the quantity of megakaryocytes are assessed under low- and high-power magnification.

Different staining procedures are used in various institutions (see p. 20). Routine stains include hematoxylin-eosin (H & E), Wright's, Prussian blue stain for iron, and the reticulin stain. When they are indicated, special stains for bacteria, fungi, and parasites may be used. Differential stains have come into constant use in present-day hematologic diagnosis (e.g., chloroacetate esterase and nonspecific esterase may be used to differentiate granulocytes from monocytes and granulocytic foci from lymphomatous areas). Histiocytes, megakaryocytes, and monocytes have very strong nonspecific esterase activity, whereas granulocytes and lymphocytes show minimal responses. The myeloid series of cells (granulocytes, promyelocytes, and many myeloblasts) stain strongly with chloroacetate esterase stain, while basophils and monocytes stain weakly or not at all. The cytoplasm of plasma cells stain pink with methyl green-pyronin as do megaloblasts, monoblasts, immunoblasts, Burkitt's lymphoma cells, megakaryocytes, and the plasmacytoid lymphocytes of Waldenström's macroglobulinemia. Finally, collagen stains green with most trichrome stains.

Marrow Aspiration Techniques and the Role of the Medical Technologist in Assisting the Pathologist

The simplest technique for marrow aspiration involves aspiration of the sternum at a level between the second and third ribs in the midline or of the iliac crest just beneath the anterior superior spine as the patient lies flat on his back. A marrow puncture tray is usually prepared and sterilized by the hematology laboratory department or by the central supply department of the hospital, from which it may be obtained at any time. The nurse on the floor notifies the hematology laboratory of the request for marrow examination, makes an appointment for the most suitable time, and simultaneously orders the tray from central supply. The pathologist or hematologist then requests the technologist and students to accompany him to the room of the patient, who has been sedated if he is at all apprehensive.

A marrow tray usually contains the following sterile equipment: 5 or 10 cc. hypodermic syringe, 1 or 2 cc. syringe, bone marrow needle in sterile test tube, small intradermal needle, cotton pledgets, hemostat, 2 × 2 gauze pads, a tonsil drape with suitable opening, rubber gloves, and powder (Fig. 1-4*A*).

The operator's hands are washed with soap and water and dried, and the entire procedure is explained to the patient, who lies flat in bed while preliminary pressure is applied over the point of sternal entry, marked with an X by the operator's finger nail. This pressure is explained to the patient as similar to that made by downward pressure of the needle during the actual sternal or iliac crest entry. The skin is shaved, if necessary, and then washed with 3½ per cent tincture of iodine (or other antiseptic) and then alcohol. The operator puts on gloves, and the tonsil drape is placed over the prepared area.

One-half to 1 cm. of 1 to 2 per cent procaine solution, supplied by the nurse or medical technologist, is then used to make a small intradermal bleb by the hematologist or pathologist at the X-marked point of sternal or iliac crest entry, followed by further injection into the subcutaneous area and into or above the sternal or iliac crest periosteum (Fig. 1-4*B*).

While the local anesthetic is taking effect, the operator explains that he will insert the needle, with the proper 1 to 1.5 cm. guard, and that the patient will have some pain as the needle enters the bone and also when the marrow is aspirated back into the syringe. A marrow puncture needle with stylet is then held at a 45° angle from the chest wall with the butt of the needle toward the patient's feet (Fig. 1-4*C*). The needle is then inserted into the skin directly through the anesthetized area. With a rotating or boring motion, the marrow puncture needle is then pushed into the marrow cavity; a sudden "give" in resistance usually occurs at the time of entry (Fig. 1-4*D*). The stylet is removed from the needle and a dry, sterile, tight-fitting 5 or 10 cc. syringe is attached (Fig. 1-4*E*).

Firm but gentle continuous backward pull of the plunger will usually yield thick, dark, reddish marrow fluid (Fig. 1-4*F*).

If no marrow appears, it is necessary to remove the syringe, replace the stylet and move the needle slightly further in or to another sternal or iliac crest locus 2 to 3 mm. from the first point of entry. As soon as ½ cc. of marrow appears in the syringe, the syringe is removed and given to the medical technologist, who then prepares several blood films on coverslips or slides. A drop of the marrow is quickly placed near the end of a coverslip or glass slide (Fig. 1-4*G; H*). The slide is quickly tilted, or with another syringe and needle, the excess blood is removed from the drop of marrow material, leaving pale gray-white marrow fragments and a small amount of blood (Fig. 1-4*I*).

After removal of the marrow needle, a small sterile adhesive bandage or dressing is applied with pressure over the puncture site. Thin films are made from the marrow material by coverslip technique or by pushing the fragments ahead with the edge of another slide. The excess marrow plus blood may be placed in a tube containing EDTA or heparin (1 drop of a 1:1000 solution), equal parts of each, and the clot may be placed in another tube containing fixative for histologic sectioning and possible tumor cell identification (Fig. 1-4*J*).

If desired, a second portion of marrow (1 cc.) may be obtained before removing the needle from the marrow cavity, by using a second syringe after handing the first syringe to the medical technologist. The material from the second syringe is mixed in a small test tube containing EDTA. The aspirated material is then centrifuged for 8 minutes at 2500 r.p.m., and films are made from the nucleated buffy coat layer diluted with an equal volume of plasma. This technique is of diagnostic aid in studying hypocellular marrow material.

The hematology department of the University of Rochester School of Medicine uses the following technique: one cubic centimeter of bone marrow is placed into a paraffin-lined vial that contains a small amount of powdered heparin or sodium EDTA (about the amount that clings to the tip of a glass rod); this is mixed gently but well. A couple of drops of marrow are placed in the middle of each of two glass slides (1 in. × 3 in.); a gauze sponge is used to absorb the liquid, leaving a few particles. A clean slide is placed on top of each of the glass slides so treated, squashing the marrow particles. The slides are then pulled apart by sliding the top one along the length of the bottom one. These preparations are used for the unstained and stained hemosiderin studies.

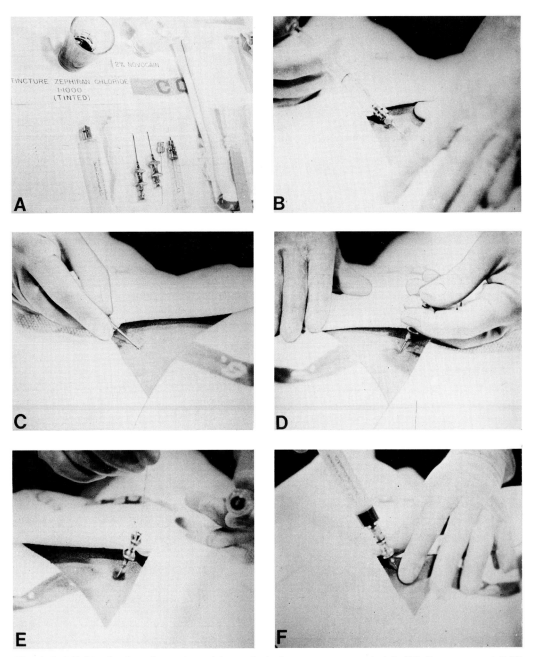

Fig. 1-4. (*A*) Standard equipment used to aspirate bone marrow material. (*B*) One per cent (1%) aqueous procaine may be used to infiltrate skin and outer periosteum. (*C*) The marrow needle is inserted in a steady boring and rotating motion into the skin and periosteum. (*D*) The marrow needle is then carefully pushed into the marrow cavity (sudden "give" sensation). (*E*) The stylet is removed from the marrow needle. (*F*) Bone marrow material is aspirated, utilizing a moderately firm backward pull on the plunger of a sterile dry syringe. (*Continued on facing page*)

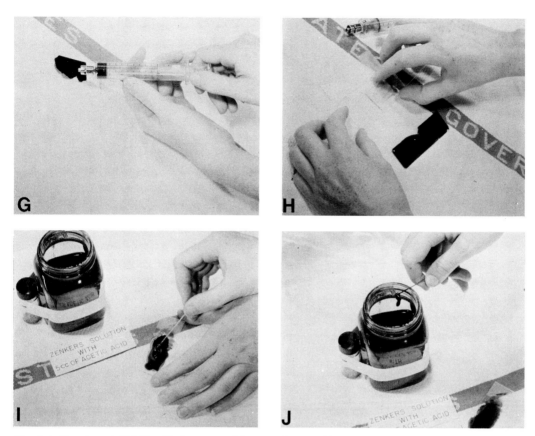

Fig. 1-4. Continued. (*G*) Needle is removed from syringe and bone marrow material is expelled onto a clean glass slide, forming a marrow aspirate pool. (*H*) Bone marrow films are made by slide spread technique (cover slips may also be used). Wright's, Giemsa and iron stains are used routinely. (*I*) The needle stylet is stirred around in the clotted marrow material; a clot is then collected. (*J*) The marrow clot is transferred to a fixation solution for histologic preparation and study. (Agress, H.: Comparative study of spreads and sections of bone marrow. Am. J. Clin. Path. *27:*282-299, 1957.)

A recently described innovation in bone marrow smearing technique involves the placing of a few drops of the aspirated spicule-laden marrow on glass slides tilted at 45° angles.[6] The bone marrow runs down the slide leaving behind the spicule. Wipe away the excess bloody material. Place a clean slide parallel to the specimen slide and gently lower it until it touches the spicule. The slides are then gently pulled away in opposite directions as the spicule spreads under the gentle pressure of the upper slide. The resulting smear will appear oval with tapered ends and will give a glistening appearance surrounded by a thin layer of blood.

As soon as possible, 1 cc. of the anticoagulated marrow is pipetted into a Wintrobe hematocrit tube and centrifuged for 8 minutes at 2500 r.p.m. The percentage of the various layers is noted (reading downward); fat layer, mixed layer, plasma layer, Myeloid:Erythroid (M:E) layer, and mature red cell layer. The fat and mixed layers are removed with a capillary pipette, and two slides are made for the unstained and stained hemosiderin studies, as previously described. The M:E layer plus an equal

Table 1-2. Quantitative Marrow Report[3, 7, 8]*

Formed Cell Elements	Normal (mean %)	Range (%)
Undifferentiated cells	0.0	0.0 – 1.0
Reticulum cells	0.4	0.0 – 1.3
Myeloblasts	2.0	0.3 – 5.0
Promyelocytes	5.0	1.0 – 8.0
Myelocytes		
Neutrophilic	12.0	5.0 –19.0
Eosinophilic	1.5	0.5 – 3.0
Basophilic	0.3	0.0 – 0.5
Metamyelocytes		
Neutrophilic	25.6	17.5 –33.7
Eosinophilic	0.4	0.0 – 1.1
Basophilic	0.0	0.0 – 0.2
Segmented granulocytes		
Neutrophilic	20.0	11.6 –30.0
Eosinophilic	2.0	0.5 – 4.0
Basophilic	0.2	0.0 – 3.7
Monocytes	2.0	1.6 – 4.3
Lymphocytes	10.0	3.0 –20.7
Megakaryocytes	0.4	0.0 – 3.0
Plasma cells	0.9	0.1 – 1.7
Erythroid series		
Pronormoblasts	0.5	0.2 – 4.2
Basophilic normoblasts	1.6	0.25– 4.8
Polychromatic normoblasts	10.4	3.5 –20.5
Orthochromatic normoblasts	6.4	3.0 –25
Promegaloblasts	0	0
Basophilic megaloblasts	0	0
Polychromatic megaloblasts	0	0
Orthochromatic megaloblasts	0	0
Myeloid: Erythroid ratio (M : E)	3–4 : 1	

*(See Plate 1)

amount of plasma is decanted with a capillary pipette, and this is placed on a paraffin-coated watch glass. This material is mixed with a glass rod. A drop of the resulting mixture is placed onto each of eight slides, and push smears are made. Six of the direct bone marrow smears (BMD) and six of the concentrated bone marrow smears (BMC) are stained. The staining time is 3 minutes with Wright's stain and 6 minutes for the buffering with distilled water. The staining times needed are occasionally shorter or longer than the times given here. The smears are washed with distilled water just long enough to float the stain off, and they are then allowed to dry in the air. The two unstained direct smears and two concentrated smears are labeled and kept for other types of staining, if needed.

Special differential diagnostic stains may be used, for example, Prussian blue (for hemosiderin concentration), peroxidase (supravital cytoplasmic granule "blast" differentiater in some instances), alkaline phosphatase stain (high concentration in normal leukocytes and low to negative in leukemic leukocytes), and PAS stains for granules in erythroleukemia. The clot left in the syringe is then placed in neutral formalin solution, after which it is sectioned in the usual manner as tissue sections and stained with hematoxylin and eosin.

Bone marrow aspiration is contraindicated in hemophilia and hemophilia-like dyscrasias. Pressure over the puncture site controls excessive bleeding, which sometimes occurs in thrombocytopenic patients.

Examination of Bone Marrow Preparations

Good bone marrow smears are characterized by thinness, their nucleated cells almost touching one another, and their elements present in high proportion with visible fatty areas and concentrated marrow foci in many areas. It is most important to examine proper loci in a marrow film for selective qualitative and quantitative study; that is, cells chosen for examination must be identifiable but not present in an area that is too thick.

Normal bone marrow in patients 1 to 21 years of age has the quantitative proportions shown in Table 1–2, and this table may serve as a guide in making the report sheet for a quantitative study (Plate 7).

REFERENCES

1. Buskard, N. A., and Gray, G. R.: Bone marrow biopsy. Experience with a new bone marrow biopsy needle (Jamshidi). Abst. No. 183, Program Booklet Am. Soc. Hematol., 1973.
2. Dacie, J. V., and White, J. D.: Erythropoiesis with particular reference to its study by biopsy of human bone marrow; a review. J. Clin. Pathol., 2:1, 1949.
3. Glaser, K., Limarzi, L. R., and Poncher, H. G.: Cellular composition of bone marrow in normal infants and children. Pediatrics, 6:789, 1950.
4. Hartmann, R. C., et al.: Diagnostic specificity of sucrose hemolysis test for paroxysmal nocturnal hemoglobinuria. Blood, 35:462, 1970.
5. Jamshidi, K., and Swaim, W. R.: Bone marrow biopsy with unaltered architecture: A new biopsy device. J. Lab. Clin. Med., 77:335, 1971.
6. Martone, J.: Bone marrow smearing technique. Laboratory Medicine, 8:24, 1977.
7. Merritt, K. K., and Davidson, L. T.: The blood during the first year of life. Am. J. Dis. Child., 46:990, 1933.
8. Shapiro, L. M., and Bassen, F. A.: Sternal marrow changes during the first week of life; correlation with peripheral blood findings. Am. J. Med. Sci., 202:341, 1941.
9. Tocantins, L. M., O'Neill, J. F., and Jones, H. W.: Infusions of blood and other fluids via the bone marrow; application in pediatrics. J.A.M.A., 117:1229, 1941.

AUDIOVISUAL AIDS*

Aspiration and Processing of Bone Marrow. Film Library Service, U.S. Naval Medical School, National Naval Medical Center, Bethesda, Maryland 20014.

Blood Collection for Pediatric Tests. (1966). M-1299. National Medical Audio-visual Center (Annex), Station K, Atlanta, Georgia, 30324.

Bone Marrow. [*four-part series*]. AFIP 24, 25, 26, and 27. Armed Forces Institute of Pathology, Audiovisual Comunications Center, Washington, D.C. 20305.

Bone Marrow Aspiration. M-1526. National Medical Audiovisual Center (Annex) Station K, Atlanta, Georgia 30324.

Bone Marrow Biopsy. (Principles of Interpretation) [100 (35 mm.) color transparencies plus descriptive booklet]. Medcom, Inc., 2 Hammerskjold Plaza, New York, New York 10017.

Bone Marrow Biopsy—Aspiration Technique. [Jamshidi needle]. BF-2116 [16 mm. standard reel]; BF-2108 [8 mm. cassette for use on Fairchild 70-07 portable projector (video tape also available upon request)]. Kormed, Inc., 2510 Northland Drive, St. Paul, Minnesota 55120.

Bone Marrow Evaluation—Pros and Cons and Cells. 247503. [51 (35 mm.) transparencies plus lecture on standard audio cassette]. Communications in Learning, Inc., 2929 Main Street, Buffalo, New York 14214.

Collection and Preparation of Bone Marrow. [35 mm. transparencies, audiocassette]. American Society of Clinical Pathologists, P.O. Box 12073, Chicago, Illinois 60612.

Formed Elements in the Microcirculation. Frederick W. Maynard, Biological Research Laboratories, Boston University, 765 Commonwealth Avenue, Boston, Massachusetts 02159.

Hematological Technique: Collecting Blood Samples. (1954). National Audiovisual Center (GSA), Washington, D.C. 20409.

Hemo the Magnificent. ASMT Education and Research Fund, Inc., 5555 West Loop South, Bellaire, Texas 77401.

Introduction to the Interpretation of Bone Marrow Sections. [videocassette program]. American Society of Clinical Pathologists, P.O. Box 12073, Chicago, Illinois 60612.

Marrow Puncture. (1953). Imperial Chemical Industries, Box 1274, 151 South Street, Stamford, Connecticut 06904.

The Story of the Blood Stream. [I, II]. ASMT Education and Research Fund, Inc., 5555 West Loop South, Bellaire, Texas 77401.

The Vacutainer System. Becton, Dickinson and Company, Inc., Film Service Dept., Rutherford, New Jersey 07070.

Venipuncture. (1952). Imperial Chemical Industries, Box 1274, 151 South Street, Stamford, Connecticut 06904 or The University of Oklahoma, Health Ser-

---

* Films unless otherwise stated.

vices Center, Audiovisual Information, Oklahoma City, Oklahoma 73190.

William Harvey and the Circulation of Blood. (1957). Burroughs Wellcome Company, 114 West 26th Street, New York, New York 10001, or M-2607-X.

National Medical Audiovisual Center (Annex), Station K, Atlanta, Georgia 30324.

Work of the Blood. University of Minnesota, Audiovisual Library Service, 3300 University Avenue, S. E., Minneapolis, Minnesota 55455.

2 Origin and Development of Blood Cells; Maturation and Enumeration of Erythrocytes

BLOOD FORMATION

Intrauterine Blood Formation

The mesenchyme or primordial connnective tissue in the embryo is the primary source of blood development, with three dynamic phases merging into one another. In the human embryo, the *megaloblastic* or *mesoblastic phase* starts sometime during the first 2 months (possibly as early as the third day) in the yolk sac, specifically in the blood islets in the area vasculosa. The mesodermal portion of the area vasculosa forms a tubular structure composed of two layers, an outer layer forming primitive vascular structures and an inner layer forming the primitive endothelial cells. The primitive endothelial cells separate from the lining of the inner layer and develop into primitive blood cells (hemocytoblasts or hemohistioblasts), possessing large nuclei having a vesicular chromatin meshwork and a thin rim of cytoplasm.

The megaloblast of Ehrlich, formed from the hemocytoblast, then protrudes into the blood vessel lumen and gradually becomes hemoglobinized (embryonic hemoglobin $\alpha_2\delta_2$) from porphyrin type precursor substances in its cytoplasm; it subsequently develops into an early nucleated red blood cell. Early nucleated red blood cells undergo mitosis in the fetal vascular system and form smaller nucleated red cells containing more hemoglobin (pronormoblast, basophilic normoblast, and others). The mature erythrocyte is finally produced by a process of normoblastic erythropoiesis and is characterized by the loss of nuclei. The foregoing process continues up to about 9 weeks of embryonic life; the hepatic phase of blood formation meanwhile begins.

The *hepatic phase* apparently begins intravascularly in the liver on or about the sixth to ninth week of embryonic life with loci of basophilic normoblasts developing from mesenchymal undifferentiated cells, which separate the hepatic cells proper. Until about the fifth month the spleen and thymus also participate in this intraluminal blood vessel process. The granular leukocytic cells begin to arise extravascularly from the mesoderm, beginning at the fourth month, and they then migrate through the capillary walls to become intravascular. Only a comparatively few white blood cells are produced up to the fifth embryonic month. Cells of lymphocyte series are produced throughout life mainly in the spleen, lymph nodes, and thymus. The spleen especially serves as the reserve organ for the bone marrow, mainly because its microcirculation appears to be well suited for blood cell formation. Erythrocytic (containing fetal hemoglobin $\alpha_2\gamma_2$ polypeptide chains) and granular leukocytic cells continue to be formed intrahepatically in diminishing numbers until the time of fetal birth.

The *myeloid phase* begins at about the fifth intrauterine month, simultaneously with the development of bone cavities;

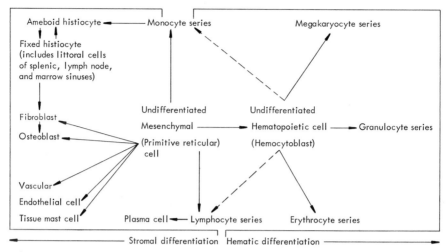

Fig. 2-1. Modified schema of the derivation of the cells of the reticular tissue. (Rappaport, H.: Tumors of the hematopoietic system. Sec. III. Fasc. 8. Washington, D.C., Armed Forces Institute of Pathology, 1966)

granular leukocytes are formed first, followed by erythrocytic-type cell formation. In the interim, there is practically no hematopoiesis from hepatic mesenchymal cells. These cells plus other somatic cells are converted into the reticuloendothelial system of cells. The lining cells (macrophage, clasmatocyte, hemohistioblast) take over new functions and, resembling large monocytes, are occasionally found in the bloodstream.

Extrauterine Blood Formation

Myeloid Tissue. Although some hepatic and splenic hematopoiesis is still present up to the fifteenth day of extrauterine life, by about the time of birth the marrow has completely taken over production of erythrocytic and leukocytic granular cells. At birth all fetal skeletal structures contain red marrow throughout; the   continue to do so until the age of 2 to 3 years.

Reticuloendothelial System. Because of the lack of relatively nonfunctioning fatty marrow reserve, any need (sudden crises such as hemorrhage and other diseases) for blood formation up to 2 or 3 years of age results in extramedullary hematopoiesis by

the reticuloendothelial cells of the liver, spleen, and occasionally kidney and retroperitoneal adipose tissues. Furthermore, most investigators believe that reticuloendothelial cells are the parent cells for all formed elements of the blood, that is, by division and maturation, the first recognizable blood cells with primitive nuclei and basophilic cytoplasm arise. These blood cells divide and mature further to produce the well differentiated erythroid and myeloid cells of the blood circulation. Controversy, however, has arisen concerning the specific site of origin (intravascular or extravascular) and the stage at which differentiation of the first cells becomes permanent enough to allow only one specific type cell to form.

Rappaport has proposed a schema of derivation of the cells of the reticular tissue (Fig. 2-1).[29] Even though it cannot demonstrate all theoretic and experimental evidence concerning the origin and interrelationships of the various cell types that develop from the primitive reticular cells, it may help to clarify the potentialities for abnormal proliferation that different cell types possess. This schema may also help elucidate the finding of mixed cellular growths and the alterations in cellular makeup seen during the development of some of the hematopoietic neoplastic diseases. As seen from this schema, embryonic mesenchyme retains a potential for hematopoietic or stromal differentiation in the adult by means of the fixed cells associated with it. These undifferentiated mesenchymal or primitive reticular cells are not confined to the hematopoietic tissues but are diffusely distributed throughout the body with the adventitia of vessels as a predilection site. According to Bloom and Fawcett, these cells are intimately associated with the argyrophilic, fibrillar framework of the hematopoietic organs.[5] These primitive cells are thought to be the precursors of all types of blood cells and connective tissue cells.

Recently, some investigators have proposed that each cellular system must be continuously replenished from a stem cell source. This is suggested especially since all blood cells are consistently and irretrievably lost to the tissues or meet their demise in the peripheral circulation, yet their numbers remain apparently constant in normal people. Therefore, it is all the more evident that a functioning stem cell in a normal person must have the capability of self-replication and the capability of differentiation. Indirect evidence points toward the presence in man of a stem cell pluripotent for granulocytes (including monocytes), megakaryocytes, and erythrocytes, but not for lymphocytes. The last-named cell may be most unusual among normal mature blood cells in the adult in that it is its own stem cell, that is, lymphocytes in the peripheral circulation can divide and apparently reproduce themselves. Modern concepts suggest a series of hematopoietic stem cell compartments — the potentiality of each succeeding compartment is more restricted than the preceding one. In other words, each of the most immature subdivisions is not in an active generative cycle, and the more differentiated cells develop from late stem cell compartments that are capable of being assayed directly. By utilizing plated peripheral blood or bone marrow cells in semi-solid media, with appropriate growth stimuli, one can obtain clonal growth of colonies containing neutrophils, eosinophils, and monocytes (macrophages). The main cell observed with this technique is the medium-sized or transitional lymphocyte. However, it is thought to be nonlymphoid in character since it is almost completely absent in lymph nodes, thymus, or thoracic duct effluence. Blood dyscrasias such as polycythemia vera, paroxysmal nocturnal hemoglobinuria, aplastic anemia, and granulocytic leukemias reflect either previous qualitative or quantitative defects (or both) of pluripotential stem cells.

Slightly fatty and relatively inactive marrow begins to appear at 5 to 7 years of age and is evident until adolescence (11–14), when the long bones begin to develop fatty marrow in their diaphyseal portions. This process gradually increases from the distal to the proximal ends of the bones until all the red marrow (except upper ends of the femur and humerus) has been replaced at approximately age 20 to 22. Full-functioning red marrow areas, producing red blood cells, granular and nongranular leukocytes, remain in the flat bones of the body — for example, sternum, vertebrae, ribs, and the ilium. That is, recent literature points toward the likelihood that lymphocytes and monocytes are also formed from a common stem cell in the bone marrow. They are also formed elsewhere, particularly in the lymph nodes, thymus, spleen, and reticuloendothelial cells.

Anatomy and Histology of Bone Marrow

The bone marrow is the largest, most widely dispersed, and least homogeneous organ in the body. Its volume is 1600 to 3000 cc. in the adult, and its location within the interstices of cancellous bone and between the trabeculae of the marrow cavities in long bones makes complete study of all the marrow an almost impossible feat.[27] It is thought that the marrow sinusoids probably substitute for the capillary bed of most organs and that these sinusoids are probably a closed system, with most of them collapsed at any one time. In cross section, the marrow structures have been likened to a wheel with a rim, spokes, and hub. The marrow sinusoids (spokes) are composed of a single layer of flattened littoral reticular cells and contain blood.

For the most part, pronormoblasts and other hematopoietic and connective tissue elements are outside the sinusoids; no lymphatics are demonstrable. The reticular lining cells themselves are unstable, and if they become phagocytic or differentiate into other cell types, they leave their position in the sinusoid, making a gap in the wall (i.e., finished cells have to pass through narrow openings in the endothelial vascular lining in order to enter the circulation). Furthermore, their instability enables them to respond to changing requirements for marrow functions of erythropoiesis, myelopoiesis, antibody and plasma protein formation, phagocytosis, lymphatic drainage, blood flow, delivery of cells to the circulation, and sequestration of cells from the circulation. The more adult erythrocytes and leukocytes, probably formed outside the marrow sinusoids, gain access to the intravascular compartment by diapedesis (red blood cells) and pseudopodesis (white blood cells).

Human adult bone marrow varies from an almost exclusively fatty tissue to the most cellular red marrow, with all gradations in between represented. As mentioned previously, in the adult, fat predominates in the shafts of the long bones, and red marrow in the cancellous heads of these bones and the flat bones. However, all gradations are often seen in a single histologic section of grossly red marrow from a health person. Not only is cellular marrow interspersed with fat but, in the cellular area, adjacent foci consist of many cell types and lie next to vascular channels filled with blood. In disease, this patchy structure is still more pronounced—for example, the lesions of multiple myeloma, metastatic neoplasms, and the lipoid histiocytoses. Usually, however, the fatty portion remains as a reservoir for hyperplasia of active red marrow and subsequent infiltration by this additional red marrow.

Interrelationship of Cells

The bone marrow is one of the chief reticuloendothelial-lymphoid structures of the body and is involved in antigen processing, cellular and humoral immunity, the production of differentiated blood cells derived from pools of self-perpetuating stem cells, and the recognition and removal of aging cells. Although there is, to some extent, general agreement that all blood cells come from the reticuloendothelial or stem cells of the bone marrow and also from the liver, spleen, thymus, blood vessels, and lymph nodes, there is considerable controversy whether all blood cells do indeed come from a single polyvalent cell known as the hemocytoblast (*monophyletic theory*). The *neounitarian theory* maintains that the lymphocyte of normal blood does not usually transform to some other cell type, but that it has such marked developmental potentialities that this change may occur in an atypical, abnormal environment, for example, tissue cultures, and experimental and pathologic conditions. Normally, however, the myeloblast acts as a granulopoietic cell, without any of its offspring ever present in the normal adult lymph node.

The *polyphyletic theory* proposes mainly that there are two or perhaps three cells of origin. That is, *dualistically,* lymphoblasts give origin to lymphocytes; myeloblasts give rise to the granulocyte, monocyte, and megakaryocyte cell series; and the pronormoblast develops into the red cell series. Schilling, a proponent of *trialistism,* agreed with the dualist group, except he believed that monocytes develop from reticuloendothelial cells lining the sinusoids of the liver and spleen.

Finally, Sabin and co-workers believed that there is a stem cell for each of several cell series; that is, primitive reticulum cells give origin to different cells depending on the environment and stimulus. Thus, myeloblasts would give rise to the granulocytic cells, lymphoblasts to lymphocytic cells, and monoblasts to monocytic cells. Sabin also proposed that cells of the red blood series were derived from the endothelial cells lining the intersinusoidal capillaries of the bone marrow. This was called the *complete theory*. In any event, there is general agreement that except in disease or embryonic life all cell formation of the erythrocyte, granulocyte, and thrombocyte series apparently occurs in the marrrow, although platelets are also derived on occasion from lung tissue. That is, according to Boggs and Chervenick there are two pools of self-perpetuating stem cells, a multipotential pool capable of differentiation in several directions and unipotential pools committed to erythropoiesis, granulopoiesis or thrombopoiesis (Fig. 2-2).[6] The formation of cells of the lymphocyte, monocyte, and plasmocyte series is shared with the lymph nodes, thymus, spleen, and other lymphoid or reticuloendothelial tissue.

Factors Governing Hematopoiesis

Hematopoietic Principle. The factors that govern the development and production of the red blood cell, white blood cell, and platelets are diverse and at the present stage of our knowledge incompletely understood. In general, it may be proposed that hematopoiesis is maintained in a steady state in which mature cell production equals mature cell loss (i.e., increased cell demands as a result of disease or physiologic change are associated with increased cell production [suggestive of a feedback control]). In terms of erythropoiesis, the marrow responds according to its own inherent capacity for proliferation and susceptibility to hypoxia and antibodies of various types. Ineffective erythropoiesis is also affected by cyanocobalamin (vitamin B$_{12}$). Leukopoiesis has direct and indirect marrow and peripheral blood relationships to infections, foreign substances, antibodies, and blood loss into body spaces, that is, through the basic stimulus of chemotaxis (nucleoproteins and nucleic acid derivatives from dead or dying granulocytes and bacteria). Newer work reveals that colony-stimulating factor (CSF) appears to be a humoral regulator of leukopoiesis.[16] This factor is produced by hematopoietic cells in liquid cultures of human bone marrow; that is, bone marrow mononuclear cells provide CSF, which supports the proliferation and differentiation of marrow elements in liquid culture.

Of all types of hematopoiesis, the least is known about thrombocytopoiesis. No specific stimulus is known. However, tissue destruction and splenic activity are somewhat related, especially in reference to the possibility that circulating antibodies directly and indirectly affect platelet production, liberation, and breakdown.

Endocrines. Red blood cell formation is probably directly related to a hormone called erythropoietin. This plasma-circulating factor has the chemical properties of a glycoprotein and is produced mainly in the kidney.[19] It is not known whether the kidney is the major site of production or is only a coproducer. The site of action is in the bone marrow, where erythropoietin is specifically required for initiation of differentiation of the stem cells into the red cell series. No red cell formation appears to be possible without erythropoietin. However, in man, kidney removal does not eliminate erythropoiesis nor does it bring about the complete disappearance of erythropoietin activity from the plasma. In fact, nonrenal erythropoietin-producing tissues (e.g., liver) may be involved,[14] or, as has been suggested, the kidney may not produce erythropoietin directly but may rather produce an enzyme that is capable of transforming a circulating erythropoietin precursor into the active hormone. In addition, the partial pressure of oxygen in some renal

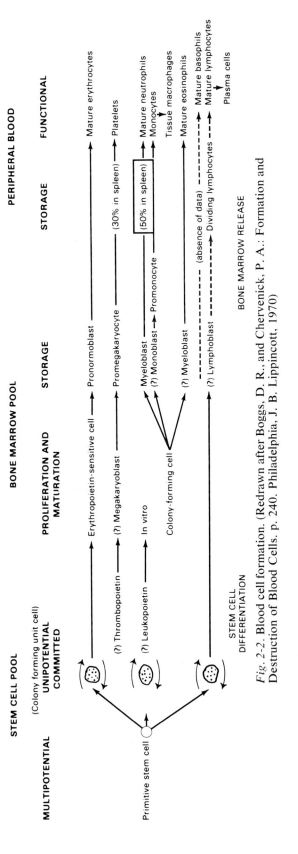

Fig. 2-2. Blood cell formation. (Redrawn after Boggs, D. R., and Chervenick, P. A.: Formation and Destruction of Blood Cells. p. 240. Philadelphia, J. B. Lippincott, 1970)

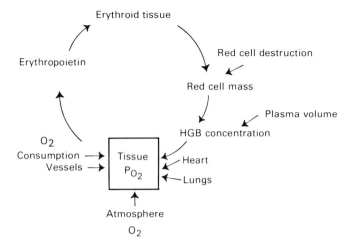

Fig. 2-3. This feedback circuit links red cell production to the tissue tension of oxygen. (Erslev, A. J.: The role of erythropoietin in the control of RBC production. Medicine, *43*:661, 1964)

and certain other cells (site unknown) appears to regulate hormone production and thus the rate of red blood cell production in the steady state of the red blood cell mass (Fig. 2-3).

In a number of clinical conditions in which severe anemia exists, the erythropoietin titer in plasma and urine may be greatly increased. This is true in several disease states in which the process of differentiation and orderly maturation of the red blood cell series is altered or interfered with in such a way that the hormone produced in response to the anemic anoxic stimulus cannot be utilized. In other clinical anemic conditions, in advanced renal disease with uremia, for example, it appears that underproduction of erythropoietin is related etiologically to the anemia. It is only in this group of anemic states that therapeutic administration of the hormone may be useful.

Other endocrine substances from the pituitary, adrenal, thymus, thyroid, and testis do not directly and specifically control red blood cell formation. At least, there is no absolute evidence showing such control, although cortisone and ACTH obviously exert some influence. The hypothalamus, diencephalon, and sympathetic nervous system also affect red blood cells through their marrow effect, but not directly.

Leukopoiesis is reportedly affected by androgenic hormones, but their role is not clear. Shen and Hoshino have observed a neutrophilia-producing factor in rats after the administration of triamcinolone.[31] Bierman and others have also recently described a stimulant to myelopoiesis in plasma, which has been designated *leukopoietin*.[4]

Release of Blood Cells into Peripheral Blood

The spleen has been shown to affect the release of red blood cells into the bloodstream, for example, in clinical hypersplenism. Other factors that affect the release of red blood cells are the level of maturation reached by the erythrocyte series and the pressure exerted by the intramarrow growth of cells of the erythrocyte series, which is affected by variations in respiration and body position. Some workers in the field believe that cell deformability may be an important factor in cell release; reticulocytes and erythrocytes are much more deformable than their precursor cells

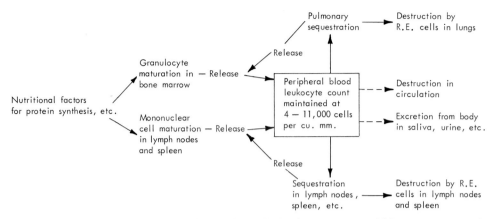

Fig. 2-4. Maintenance of a normal level of circulating leukocytes. (Whitby, L. E. H., and Britton, C. J. C.: Disorders of the Blood, ed. 9. London, J. & A. Churchill, 1963)

and their release into the peripheral blood may depend upon their ability to deform enough to traverse the fenestrations of the sinusoidal wall.[34]

Recent studies in vitro have permitted identification and biochemical characterization of the glycoprotein-colony-stimulating activity (CSA) as a humoral stimulatory substance necessary for the proliferation and differentiation in vitro of granulocytic-monocytic progenitor cells, or colony-forming cells (CFU-C). Erythroid culture techniques have characterized the clonogenic erythropoietic precursor cells, burst forming units (BFU-E), and the more differentiated erythroid colony forming units (CFU-E), and their responsiveness to erythropoietin.[17, 25]

In addition to CSA and erythropoietin, other humoral substances are known to have important effects on hematopoiesis. Although much information on endocrine moderation of blood cell production has been acquired from in vivo experiments, the above-described in vitro clonal culture methods have elicited a more detailed exposition of the direct effect of various hormones on hemopoietic cell proliferation. Steroids (androgens and glucocorticosteroids), polypeptides (thyroid hormone, and growth hormone), adrenergic agonists,

prostaglandins and other hormone types influence hematopoiesis in vitro. These endocrine interactions may be of a potentiating or inhibitory nature, but none of the hormones can substitute for the primary humoral regulators, that is, CSA or erythropoietin. Most of the endocrines involved appear to operate through receptor mechanisms as defined in other cell systems with cyclic nucleotides important in the regulation of some proliferative responses.[12, 15, 30]

The number of circulating white cells exercises some control in regulating the release of leukocytes into the bloodstream. Stimulation of the diencephalon, various endocrine glands, neutropoietin, and the splenic inhibitory influence associated with hypersplenism also play some part in the liberation and distribution of white blood cells into the peripheral blood. Cortisone especially causes an increase in circulating neutrophils and a decrease in lymphocytes, eosinophils, and basophils. The maintenance of a normal level of circulatory leukocytes is portrayed in Figure 2-4.

Finally, the regulation of the white blood cell count depends on many factors controlling production, maturation, and release from the bone marrow; distribution in peripheral blood pools; and egress to extravascular sites. Evaluation of leukopenia or leukocytosis must take all these factors into account.

According to observations made by Wintrobe and his colleagues with white cells labeled with diisopropyl fluorophosphate (DF³²P), the total blood granulocytes are distributed between two compartments in equilibrium with one another, the circulating granulocyte pool and the slightly larger pool of marginal granulocytes.[2] The term "marginal granulocytes" refers to the probable distribution of these cells along the vascular endothelium in lungs, spleen, and elsewhere in the body. The abrupt leukocytosis that follows epinephrine or exercise has been shown by these workers to be due to a shift of the white cells from the marginal compartment to the circulating compartment, and it has been postulated that steroids may have a similar effect. The mechanism perhaps justifies the term *pseudoleukocytosis*, which was applied to this response by earlier workers.[32]

A larger source of readily available granulocytes from intramedullary storage sites has been demonstrated by Craddock and his colleagues using leukophoresis techniques.[7] The total life span from the stage of myeloblast to polymorphonuclear leukocyte has been estimated using several techniques to be 8 to 12 days, during the last period of which the granulocyte exists in the bone marrow in the adult form. It is the consensus that the direction of flow is from the marrow pool to the blood to the extravascular areas without free access from the latter sites back to the bloodstream.

As previously stated (p. 29), there are endogenous stimulants to granulopoietic activity in the marrow as well as stimulants to rapid release from the readily available marrow pool—for example, androgenic hormones, the neutropoietin of Shen and Hoshino, and the leukopoietin of Bierman and colleagues. Other workers have suggested that bacterial or leukocyte products have a significant role in regulating white cell production and distribution into the peripheral blood. It is not clear which factor or factors are responsible for the leukocytosis observed in response to bacterial infection.

Although the total life-span of the granulocyte is more than a week, the half-life of disappearance of the adult granulocyte from the bloodstream has been calculated to average only 6.6 hours,[2] and it is probable that the rate of egress in sepsis is much faster. In spite of this increased disappearance rate this demand on the marrow cannot be met in the most overwhelming infections. Because the life-span of the granulocyte in the bloodstream is so short, such a demand on bone marrow lacking normal ability to mobilize reserves and to increase its rate of white blood cell production quickly results in granulocytopenia and, in a patient with sepsis, leads to serious complications.

Myeloid (marrow) tissue is also sensitive to both physical and chemical trauma—that is, many drugs and industrial products are known to be myelotoxic, but their mechanism of action and the reason for individual susceptibility are not apparent. Because the chemical nature of these agents is diverse, it is unlikely that they have one common action. Their effects may be partial or complete, transient or irreversible, and the response of patients to a given drug may vary. However, Eastwood and associates[9] have described the depressant action of nitrous oxide on myelopoiesis in animals and also in human patients with leukemia, and this depressant action apparently is predictable and does not depend on any individual sensitivity.

The megakaryocyte normally throws out pseudopodia that pass through the wall of the marrow sinusoids and become nipped off to form platelets in the circulation. Very little is known concerning the physical, chemical, or endocrine factors that govern the quantitative release of platelets into the peripheral blood. Utilizing electron microscopy, one can see that the release reaction of platelets appears to be dependent on the contractile system of the platelet, for release does not occur without contraction. The involvement of the contractile system signifies the possibility that the platelets are, in fact, muscle cells. No specific stimulus for platelet production is known. Tissue destruction, possibly splenic hormones or splenic sequestration,* adrenal cortical and medullary substances, and possibly circulating antibodies are directly and indirectly related to platelet production and liberation into the peripheral blood.

PRINCIPLES OF NORMAL CELL MATURATION

General Features[23]

Eight general statements should be made concerning normal blood cell maturation: (1) Blast cells contain no granules. (2) Blast cells contain a large nucleus and a small amount of cytoplasm. Usually the nucleus makes up ¾ to ⅞ of the cell area. (3) As cells become older, the cytoplasm becomes less basophilic; the deeper blue the cytoplasm, the younger the cell. The plasma cell is the exception to this rule. (4) As cells become older, the chromatin of the nucleus becomes heavier, and the darker the nucleus stains the heavier the chromatin is. (5) Usually as cells become older, they become smaller. The megakaryocyte is the exception. (6) Nucleoli are present in young cells and tend to disappear in mature cells. (7) There are four different types of granules seen with Wright's stain—neutrophilic, basophilic, eosinophilic, and azurophilic granules. (8) As cells become older, specific granules become less prominent and smaller (Plates 1–7).

Transformation

As blood cells develop and are distributed into the peripheral blood, cytoplasmic and nuclear variations can occur. These are seen as synchronous and asynchronous, cy-

toplasmic differentiation, nuclear maturation, and reduction in cell size.

The normal *synchronous* process of blood cell development is a dynamic transition process in which there is no assurance of conformity of cell type at any one time as observed in films made from the peripheral blood and bone marrow of any one patient. The synchronism of coordinated and concomitant parallel development of cytoplasm and nucleus may be associated with the *asynchronism* or different ratio of maturation for cytoplasm and nucleus. In this manner, typical cells associated with synchronistic cellular development may also be seen in the same blood smear together with atypical or bizarre cells formed as a result of synchronistic cytologic maturation. However, there are some basic principles of cell identification that are helpful for students just beginning the study of hematology. One principle is the need to compare all cell types with a standard such as the mature normal erythrocyte, which is approximately 7 μ in size. The other principle is that the transformation from a young to a more adult cell always involves alterations in the cytoplasm and nucleus and is usually associated with a reduction in cell size.

In the process of cytoplasmic differentiation, the youngest cells, called blast forms, are characterized by a large nucleus, prominent nucleoli, and a thin rim of cytoplasm that stains deep blue (basophilic) when subjected to the methylene blue in Wright's stain and other polychromatic stains. This basophilia of the cytoplasm is proportional to the cytoplasmic ribonucleic acid (RNA) content. As the RNA decreases in concentration, the cytoplasm becomes a paler blue and usually larger in volume with the nucleus proportionately smaller.

The granulocyte series differentiates into three types of granular cytoplasm characterized by selective individual staining properties and associated with diverse lipid and enzyme content (for example, peroxidase and alkaline phosphatase) which may

---

* Hypersplenism may act as a regulating influence on the maturation and release of platelets from the marrow.

possibly differentiate the myelocyte from the lymphocyte or monocyte cell types. At first the granules are few in number and pinkish red; as the cell matures from myelocyte to neutrophil, the granules become specific for the type of cell to be formed and have an affinity for the acid or basic portion of the dyes present in polychrome stains (most commonly Wright's stain)—for example, basophilic (dark blue, chunky) granules in the basophil, acidophilic (bright orange, chunky) granules in the eosinophil, and acidophilic-basophilic (fine, pinkish purple) granules in the neutrophil. At this stage, the nuclei change their shape and consist of two or more lobules of nuclear chromatin connected by nuclear membrane filaments. Senile polymorphonuclear leukocytes may have as many as four or five lobules (Plate 3).

The lymphocyte series shows a reduction in the nucleus-cytoplasm ratio but does not develop cytoplasmic granulation. The cells of the monocyte-plasma cell series mimic lymphocytic cell development, but occasionally they show nonspecific azurophilic granules in the cytoplasm of their more mature cells. Cells of the megakaryocyte series are also devoid of differential cytoplasmic granules during maturation; however, from the cytoplasm are formed many mature platelet structures that stain a pinkish-blue (Plates 1, 4).

Finally, a special type of maturation occurs in the erythrocyte. At first there is very little cytoplasm (hemoglobin), but at maturity the adult red blood cell has developed from the large pronormoblast having dark basophilic cytoplasm through the normoblastic phases having light basophilic to acidophilic cytoplasm, and finally the nucleus is extruded with the development of a maximum amount of salmon-colored respiratory pigment (hemoglobin), thus forming a mature erythrocyte 7 μ in diameter.

The maturation of the nuclei of blood cells is also accompanied by physiologic development in size and shape. The most immature blast nucleus is round or oval and has a high nucleus-cytoplasm ratio. At first the supporting stroma of the nucleus, called the chromatin, is lacelike, vesicular, and deep purple (rich in DNA). As the cell becomes older and matures, the chromatin network becomes coarse, clumped, and blue. The nucleoli (RNA) are reduced in number and finally disappear. In the fully mature cell, the nucleoli (Fuelgen-negative stain) are replaced by DNA heterochromatin (Fuelgen-positive stain), and the nucleus-cytoplasm ratio is low. When studying young cells, one can distinguish the more mature cell because it will be less rounded or oval than the "pro" and blast forms.

To summarize, when a young blast cell becomes a normal mature cell, there is first a loss of cytoplasmic basophilia; second, a modification and differentiation of cytoplasmic granules (azurophilic, basophilic, acidophilic, and neutrophilic), and formation of a specific cytoplasmic constituent (hemoglobin); third, reduction in nuclear size, condensation of chromatin, and reduction in the number of nucleoli; fourth, an alteration of nuclear shape; and fifth, a reduction in total cell size (Plates 1–7).

Concerning total cell size, the maturity usually varies inversely to the cell size. Thus, the more immature cell type is larger than the mature one—for example, the myeloblast is larger than the myelocyte, which in turn is larger than the polymorphonuclear leukocyte, and so on. An exception is the megakaryocyte series, in which the immature megakaryoblast is smaller than the mature megakaryocyte. Finally, as the cell becomes more mature, the nucleus becomes smaller and the chromatin material condenses so that the ratio of the amount of nucleus to the amount of cytoplasm is low in mature cells and high in immature cells.

Abnormal Cell Maturation

When hematopoiesis becomes pathologic (abnormal), one may observe mature nuclei with immature cytoplasm and vice versa, in the same cell—for example, a polymorphic nucleus with agranular cytoplasm, or ovoid nucleus with granular cytoplasm. This is called *asynchronous* development, as opposed to normal, physiologic, or synchronous maturation. When this is seen, the age of the cell is best classified according to the nuclear stage of maturation. This of course excludes nuclear abnormalities of hereditary origin—for example, *Pelger-Huet* anomaly. This anomaly is seen in granulocytes and is characterized by decreased nuclear segmentation in all formed elements associated with marked condensation of nuclear chromatin, but with normal cytoplasmic development. Occasionally, pseudo-Pelger-Huet cells are observed in the blood of patients with myeloid metaplasia and leukemia, at times after chemotherapy and usually late in the disease.

An example of bizarre granulation of hereditary origin is that seen in the cytoplasm of leukocytes associated with *Alder's anomaly*. In this anomaly there are fairly coarse, dark azurophilic granules, occasionally obscuring the nuclei. These granules replace the specific granulation in members of the granulocyte series and occupy loci in the cytoplasm of lymphocytes and monocytes. The *Reilly bodies* are considered similar to Alder's anomaly. They are observed in patients with gargoylism and consist of lymphocytic inclusions and bone marrow granules of acid mucopolysaccharide, that is, different enzymatic deficiencies lead to incomplete degradation of these protein-carbohydrate complexes, with special impairment of the carbohydrate portions. Nuclear abnormalities may consist of multiple nuclei, macronuclei, and an atypical irregular nuclear outline (instead of the normal indented ovoid pattern).

Cytoplasmic asynchronistic maturation is characterized in the myeloid series by the absence of granules or atypical granularity (minimal, azurophilic, etc.)—for example, toxic granules, Döhle's inclusion bodies in infections, and Auer bodies in leukemia. Persistent cytoplasmic basophilia and late

hemoglobin formation are also other characteristics of atypical cytoplasmic maturation cells of the erythrocyte series. Variations in size of total cellular development is also often significant—for example, giant myeloid forms in all types of leukemia, in hematopoietic factor deficiencies, and also associated with multiple nuclei. Large immature blast cells of the erythroid series are also seen in hemopoietic factor deficiencies. Small blast forms are seen in some cases of acute myeloid leukemia.

ERYTHROCYTES

Definition

An erythrocyte is the mature unit of the erythron (circulating red blood cells and their precursors in the bone marrow). The human erythrocyte is a circular, elastic, non-nucleated, eosinophilic, biconcave disk that stains red with Romanowsky stain and whose primary function is the transport of hemoglobin (34% of erythrocyte by weight). By chemical union, the erythrocyte carries oxygen and carbon dioxide from the lungs, distributing them to tissues through the capillaries. The hemoglobin is contained as an adherent component of the spongelike meshes of the interior of the red blood cell. The outer membrane of the erythrocyte is an active semipermeable structure composed mainly of stromatin (a protein) in combination with lecithin and cholesterol. This membrane retains potassium ions within the red blood cell and allows bicarbonate, chloride, and hydrogen ions to pass in and out of the cell in proportion to the ionic concentration. The membrane contains the blood group constituents and other material involved in hemolysis and agglutination. Present evidence supports the fluid "mosaic" model for normal RBC membrane architecture. This theory proposes that erythrocyte membrane proteins are embedded, but mobile, within the membrane matrix, while loosely bound by hydrophobic interaction between membrane lipid and nonpolar segments of the protein. The Rh antigen mobility aptly conforms to this model.

The erythrocyte averages 7.2 μ in diameter and 2.1 μ in thickness. The mean corpuscular volume (or average volume) is 87 cu.μ with a range of 76 to 96 cu.μ. There are 4.8 million per cu.mm. in the adult female and 5.4 million per cu.mm. in the adult male, with an average life-span of 120 days, as determined by the Ashby technique (transfusion of compatible cells of different groups) or by ^{51}Cr radioisotope tagging of red blood cells. Approximately 0.83 per cent of circulating red blood cells are destroyed daily (a reticulocyte count of 0.83% indicates a normal equilibrium of red blood cell production and destruction).

MATURATION

The maturation of the erythrocyte starts with its derivation from a multipotential cell —the *primitive stem cell* or *hemohistioblast* (Plate 2). The hemohistioblast is a large (25 to 35 μ) oval cell having a relatively large oval nucleus with regular fine vesicular reticulated chromatin. One-third of its volume is occupied by a lilac-gray cytoplasm containing minute nonspecific polychromatic granules. This cell matures into a *hemocytoblast* (20–30 μ) characterized by the same type of finely reticulated nucleus and nucleoli found in the hemohistioblast (see Plate 1). However, the irregularly outlined cytoplasm becomes smaller, bluish, and nongranular and has a varying, mottled pattern less deeply stained near the nucleus than at the periphery. Division of this hemocytoblast, under the stimulus of erythropoietin, produces one differentiated daughter cell and one undifferentiated multipotential cell. The differentiated daughter cell is found in marrow, lymph nodes, spleen, and liver; it is 25 to 35 μ in diameter with an oval to round nucleus that almost fills the cell diameter. The undifferentiated multipotential cell remains so, thereby preventing depletion of stem cells. It is not known what mechanism or factors determines which daughter cell remains undifferentiated and which starts along a maturation sequence.

The youngest specific blast cell of adult normal erythrocyte series is the *pronormoblast* (*proerythroblast* or *rubriblast*). It is an ovoid cell about twice the size of a red blood cell, and it averages 14 to 19 μ in diameter. The nucleus is light purple, vesicular, and granular with slight clumping of the chromatin. The chromatin becomes more strandlike as the cell ages. Nucleoli are one to three in number, and prominent. The cytoplasm is a granular light blue in the earlier forms, but in the more common later forms it is a thin rim of dark purplish blue. These cells average approximately 4 per cent of the nucleated red blood cells in the bone marrow. Approximately three mitotic divisions occur during the evolution of a pronormoblast into an orthochromic normoblast (Plate 2).

The *basophilic normoblast* (early *erythroblast* or *prorubicyte*) develops by mitosis and maturation in a definite quantitative sequence.[1] Most of the iron destined for hemoglobin biosynthesis is taken into the cells at the pronormoblast or basophilic normoblast stage. The basophilic normoblast is 12 to 17 μ in diameter (slightly smaller than the pronormoblast). The nucleus is a darker purple, and the chromatin clumps more markedly and is occasionally cartwheeled. Nucleoli are absent. The cytoplasm is a navy blue color. These cells constitute 1 to 4 per cent of the nucleated red blood cells of the marrow.[11, 22]

The *polychromatophilic normoblast* (late *erythroblast* or *rubricyte*) represents another stage in karyokinesis of the normoblast. It is 12 to 15 μ in diameter with a shrunken, condensed, more mature nucleus whose chromatin is blue-black, coarse, and clumped. The cytoplasm is bluish red or polychromatic, with a light area resembling hemoglobin often seen at one region near the nucleus. These cells constitute approximately 75 per cent of the nucleated red blood cells of the marrow.

The *orthochromic* or *acidophilic* *normoblast* (*normoblast* or *metarubricyte*) forms by maturation from the pronormoblast form over a period of 2 days. At this time the nucleus has become dark and homogeneous with condensed chromatin and a structureless mass described as pyknotic. This cell is unable to carry out DNA synthesis and is consequently incapable of further division. The cell is 8 to 12 μ in diameter. Successive states show a progressive diminution in cell size, an increasing tendency to eosinophilic staining of its cytoplasm owing to the acquisition of hemoglobin. The mature prototype of this cell usually has a faint polychromatic tinge with the nucleus often eccentrically placed. These cells make up about 18 per cent of nucleated red blood cells in the marrow.

The *reticulocyte* (*polychromatophilic* or *diffusely basophilic erythrocyte*) is a young erythrocyte formed by either extrusion of the nucleus from the cell by the process of active contraction,[3] or the nucleus is destroyed by fragmentation and solution apparently resulting from action by alkaline phosphatase. After loss of the nucleus, the cell usually retains some RNA, accounting for its polychromatophilic properties in Wright's stain and its reticulated bluish characteristics in cresyl blue stain. The cell is 7 to 10 μ in diameter. The marrow reticulocytes are larger and less mature, and they contain more reticulum when stained supravitally than do the peripheral blood reticulocytes. The marrow reticulocytes are found outside the sinusoids in the marrow fixed tissue. This pool of extravascular marrow reticulocytes approximately equals in number the nucleated red blood cells. With specific stimulus (for example, hypoxia), these reticulocytes shift to the peripheral blood, which, when complete, may double the total number of circulating reticulocytes. In approximately 2 days, reticulocytes mature in the circulation and number 0.0 to 1.5 per cent of the erythrocytes in the circulation. Their presence reflects the regenerative or reactive response of the bone marrow, an increase indicating accelerated hematopoiesis—for example, after 5 to 7 days of therapy for pernicious anemia or related megaloblastic anemias and after 5 to 10 days of therapy for iron deficiency anemias.

The *erythrocyte* (normocyte or red blood cell) measures 6 to 8 μ in diameter, is a buff or reddish color, and forms in 4 days from the pronormoblast. Having been formed outside the marrow sinusoids, the more adult red cells gain access to the intravascular compartment by diapedesis.[1] No adult red blood cells are present extravascularly in the normal marrow. Their biconcave discoid shape causes them to appear lighter in the center than at the periphery. Normal variants in shape occur—for example, cup-shaped, spherical, and crenated cells.

Although, logically speaking, discussion of the maturation of abnormal erythrocytes, derived from patients with liver disease, folic acid deficiency or vitamin B_{12} deficiency, does not belong in a discussion of normal maturation of cells in the erythrocyte series, their abnormal patterns are briefly described at this time because of the past confusion associated with their nomenclature. First of all, it must be remembered that cells of this type are larger than normal in all stages of development, possibly because the cells grow for longer periods without undergoing mitosis, and thus diapedesis into the circulating blood is possibly delayed. Abnormal mitoses, multiple nuclei, more cytoplasm in relation to nucleus in early forms (asynchronism), less homogeneous cytoplasm, and premature hemoglobin development with associated immature nuclei and eosinophilic cytoplasm are observed in cells in this maturation sequence.

The earliest progenitor of this series is the *promegaloblast*, which measures 19 to 27 μ in diameter. The nucleus is a light purple with an open stippled reticular chromatin pattern without the clumping found in the pronormoblast. Three to five nucleoli are present. Cytoplasm is more abundant in proportion to the amount of nuclear material, and there may be lighter staining areas around the nucleus. The *megaloblast (basophilic megaloblast)* measures 15 to 22 μ. Although it corresponds to the basophilic normoblast in development, it is larger, and the nucleus has a more finely divided chromatin with abundant sharply demarcated parachromatin and is usually eccentrically placed in the cell. There are no nucleoli; the cytoplasm is a darker intense royal blue. There is less cytoplasm than in the promegaloblast, but more than in its normal counterpart, the basophilic normo blast.

The *megaloblastic polychromatophilic normoblast (polychromatophilc megaloblast)* measures 10 to 18 μ and is therefore larger than its normal counterpart, the polychromatophilic normoblast. However, the nuclei are round and eccentric, and they still have the fine reticular chromatin, showing little tendency to clump as seen in the polychromatophilic normoblast. The cytoplasm is abundant and multicolored owing to the presence of hemoglobin (that is, pink-orange basophilia).

The *megaloblastic orthochromic normoblast (orthochromic megaloblast)* measures 8 to 15 μ and is occasionally three to four times larger than its normal counterpart, the orthochromic normoblastic. The nucleus is purplish blue, reduced in size from its predecessor, shows clumping of coarse to dense chromatin material with a slight reticular pattern still left. The cell occasionally contains two to three abnormal nuclei without nucleoli. The cytoplasm is darkly eosinophilic (pink to orange), completely hemoglobinated, and more abundant than its normal counterpart.

The *megaloblastic reticulocyte* and *megalocyte* (macrocyte, erythrocyte) measure 9 μ or more in diameter. They are a dark to light bluish orange to orange and are devoid of nuclei. Occasionally some variation in size (anisocytosis) and shape (poikilocytosis) occurs.

Materials Required to Form Erythrocytes

The preceding discussion is a fairly well defined morphologic summary of the typical and atypical maturation sequence of the erythron leading to the development of the erythrocyte. Biochemically speaking, iron, copper, protein, cobalt, and vitamins are required to form normal erythrocytes.

Iron. The total amount of iron found in the body of adults is 3.0 to 5.0 gm.[24] After absorption from the intestinal mucosa, iron is transported in the plasma in the ferric state in combination with a β-1-globulin fraction to the reticuloendothelial cells of the marrow. Approximately 55 per cent of iron is mobilized from its storage sites for hemoglobin production in the red blood cells in the bone marrow. Iron is preferentially transferred from the aforementioned iron-binding protein to immature heme-synthesizing cells.[28] It is then accepted by the reticulocyte membrane from the plasma and is first associated with the particulate fractions of the cell stroma, mitochondria, and microsomes.[20] From here it is gradually released to a transient nonhemoglobin protein phase before it is incorporated into hemoglobin.

Iron is distributed to the maturing red blood cells from the available plasma iron pool (ferric iron combined with β-1-globulin), which in turn is derived from available dietary iron, from hemoglobin iron conserved from red blood cell breakdown, and from iron stored in the reticuloendothelial tissues. The relationship of iron to hematologic disorders is described in greater detail in Chapters 3 and 8. Administration of iron results in a rise in hemoglobin, and an increase in the number of reticulocytes and red blood cells.

Copper. This element is found in minute amounts in the body (100 to 150 mg.) in two major forms: circulating serum ceruloplasmin (34 mg./100 ml.), and erythrocyte-bound copper known as erythrocuprein. Its role in normal erythropoiesis in man is related to defective biosynthesis of hemoglobin, which appears to follow impaired iron absorption, defective transfer of iron from reticuloendothelial cells and hepatocytes to plasma, and failure of the normoblast to utilize intracellular iron for hemoglobin synthesis.[21] Ceruloplasmin values are low in Wilson's disease, and serum copper levels are low in certain iron-deficiency anemias in infants, in hypoproteinemic states, and in nephrotic syndrome. Erythrocuprein levels are increased in iron-deficiency anemias, and they return to normal when iron is given.

Protein. This factor is important in erythropoiesis, especially in hemoglobin production.[35] Most of the ten essential amino acids are involved, as has been demonstrated in protein dietary restriction research.

Cobalt. This element is normally incorporated into vitamin B_{12} (cyanocobalamin) and as such is associated with erythropoiesis. However, cobalt deficiencies per se do not produce blood dyscrasias. The administration of cobalt however does stimulate erythropoiesis.[26] The effects are similar to those produced by *erythropoietin* (a substance found in the plasma of anemic patients and thought to be localized mainly in kidney substance). It is possible, therefore, that cobalt salts may stimulate an increased production of erythropoietin.

Vitamins. Portions of the vitamin B complex (citrovorum factor, folic acid, vitamin B_{12}, and pyridoxine) and possibly vitamin C are associated with proper erythrocyte formation. Deficiencies of folic acid (and its active form, citrovorum factor or folinic acid) and vitamin B_{12} (cyanocobalamin) both produce abnormal hematopoiesis— basically a macrocytic anemia in which bone marrow megaloblastic hyperplasia occurs associated with atypical leukocyte and thrombocyte formation. Vitamin B_{12} (Castle's extrinsic factor) requires an intrinsic factor found in gastric juice for facilitation of absorption of the complete combined hematopoietic principle from the gastrointestinal tract.

Pyridoxine (vitamin B_6) deficiency has been described as being associated with certain hypochromic microcytic anemias. Many investigators have believed that patients having this type of anemia cannot metabolize iron normally because of the accompanying disturbed tryptophan metabolism and xanthurenic acid excretion. However, the trytophan tolerance test has not corroborated all pyridoxine-deficiency anemia cases.

Vitamin C (ascorbic acid) possibly effects red blood cell formation owing to its participation in the conversion of folic acid to folinic acid. Nicotinic acid and riboflavin deficiencies are not clearly associated with erythropoiesis.

ENUMERATION OF ERYTHROCYTES

The general procedures involved in a red blood cell count include the pipetting of a specific, accurately measured, small amount of blood into a scrupulously cleaned pipette. The blood is then diluted up to a certain mark (101) on the same pipette with a liquid that is anticoagulatory and isotonic with the erythrocytes. After proper admixture, the resultant solution is placed in a thoroughly cleansed counting chamber (hemocytometer) and covered with a standardized, optically plane, clean coverglass. The quantity of red blood cells, in a given volume, is then counted on the stage of a light microscope. Because the accuracy obtained under optimal situations using the hemocytometer is at best ± 11 per cent, presently either the erythrocyte count is being replaced by the hematocrit (unless blood indices are required), or electronic instruments are being used that can count red blood cells with an accuracy of ± 2 per cent. Description of the use of electronic instruments begins on page 61.

The Hemocytometer

This glass instrument is composed of two counting chambers separated by a horizontal grooved canal and bordered on each side by a similar vertical moat. The improved Neubauer ruling is preferred; this consists of a double (instead of triple as in the original) line surrounding each group of 16 small squares, producing the optical phenomenon of a single translucent boundary line. The distance between the bottom of the coverglass and the surface of the chamber is 0.1 mm. This surface is ruled so that two specific areas are formed, one on each side of the horizontal trench. Each of these two largest ruled areas is square and measures 3 mm. on each side. Therefore each completely ruled chamber on each side of the transverse moat measures $3 \times 3 \times 0.1$ mm. (depth of chamber) and therefore has a volume of 0.9 cu.mm. Each ruled chamber is then divided into nine large squares; the side of every one of these is bordered by a double line and measures 1 mm. Therefore each of these chambers is 0.1 mm. $\times$ 0.1 mm. $\times$ 0.1 mm. (depth of chamber) and has a volume of 0.1 cu.mm. Each of the four corner large squares used for counting leukocytes is subdivided into 16 smaller squares, each of which measures 0.25 mm. $\times$ 0.25 mm. $\times$ 0.1 mm. (depth of chamber) and therefore has a volume of 0.00625 cu.mm. (Figs. 2-5; 2-6).

The center large square is subdivided into 25 smaller center squares separated from each other on all four sides by a double line, the outer line of which is the boundary. Each smaller center square measures 0.2 mm. $\times$ 0.2 mm. $\times$ 0.1 mm. (depth of chamber) with a volume of 0.004 cu.mm. Each smaller center square is further subdivided into 16 smallest center squares for convenience in counting red blood cells.

Hemocytometer chambers and coverglasses should meet the specifications of the National Bureau of Standards and are so marked by the manufacturer. These specifications state that the depth of the standard chamber must not vary more than ± 2 per cent (± 0.002 mm.); the length of any side of the 1 mm. squares must not exceed ± 0.01

mm. and coverglasses must be free of visible defects and optically plane on both sides within ± 0.002 mm. These are best kept clean with water, dried with soft cloth, kept in absolute ethyl alcohol, and when used again dried carefully with a soft rag.

The Red Cell Diluting Pipette

These tubular glass pipettes, used in erythrocyte counting, are carefully calibrated instruments. If desired, they may be calibrated by the gravimetric or colorimetric methods.[10, 13] A simpler approach is to purchase only pipettes certified by the National Bureau of Standards and to use these as a basis of comparison in calibrating and using other micropipettes. The allowable error of the red cell pipette is ± 5 per cent. Better still, red blood cell pipettes may be purchased and then sent to the National Bureau of Standards for calibration (for a modest charge) so that the correction factor for both a 1:100 and 1:200 dilution is obtained.* The properly calibrated pipette marks indicate a certain dilution of the sample when the pipette is filled. The volume is made up of one part in the capillary portion and 100 parts in the bulb. Blood drawn up to the 0.5 mark and diluted to the 101 mark makes a dilution of 0.5 parts in 100 (or 1:200) in the bulb section of the pipette because the cell-free contents in the capillary portion do not participate in the dilution process.

Diluting Fluids. There are several types of diluting fluids used in the laboratory. The most common ones are Gower's solution and Hayem's solution. Others used commonly include Toison's solution and Dacie's solution. Hayem's solution is composed of Na_2SO_4 (2.5 gm.), NaCl (0.5 gm.), $HgCl_2$ (0.25 gm.), and distilled water (100 ml.). Gower's solution contains anhydrous Na_2SO_4 (C.P., 12.5 gm.), glacial acetic acid (33.3 ml.), and distilled water (to 200 ml.).

---

* Capacity, Density, and Fluid Meters Section, National Bureau of Standards, Washington 25, D.C.

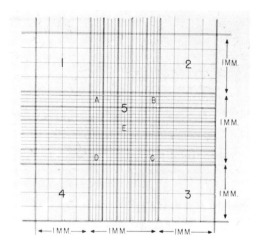

Fig. 2-5. All cells in squares 1, 2, 3, and 4 are counted for the white cell count.

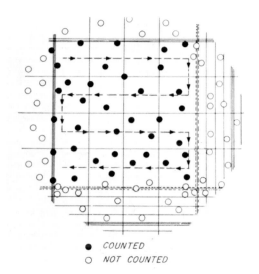

● COUNTED
○ NOT COUNTED

Fig. 2-6. This is square 1 as it would be seen using the low-power objective. Cells are counted systematically in the manner indicated. All cells (WBCs) within the large square are counted. In addition, all cells touching the upper and left outside borders are also counted. Cells touching the right and lower borders are not counted.

Toison's solution contains Na_2SO_4 (8 gm.), NaCl (1 gm.), methyl violet (0.025 gm.), glycerin (30 ml.), and distilled water (180 ml.). Dacie's solution is composed of 40 per cent solution of formaldehyde (10 ml.) and 3 per cent W/V trisodium citrate (990 ml.).

Occasionally agglutination of erythrocytes occurs in Hayem's solution and Toison's solution occasionally is contaminated by fungi, resulting in slow settling of the red blood cells. In using these solutions, clumping and rouleaux formation of red blood cells are prevented. The white blood cells are not destroyed, and therefore, if counted with the red blood cells, their addition will not cause too much variation in the total red blood cell count.

Technique of the Erythrocyte Count

1. The pipette is held horizontally, and the blood sample is introduced into the red cell counting pipette *exactly* to the 0.5 mark. Any excess blood may be pulled down to the 0.5 mark by touching the end of the pipette gently with the finger. Any blood on the outside of the pipette is wiped off.

2. The slanted (45°) pipette held between finger and bulb is gently rotated as it is filled almost to 101 mark. The pipette is raised to the vertical position, and diluting fluid is drawn slowly and exactly to the 101 mark.

3. The rubber suction tube is carefully removed, and with thumb on top of pipette and middle finger on the other end, the pipette is shaken horizontally and slantingly for 2 to 3 minutes. Frequently ends of the pipette are sealed with rubber or plastic sealing cups and placed on a pipette rotor, which utilizes the bead in the bulb to mix the solution more evenly and readily.

4. After completion of shaking, the first 4 to 8 drops from each pipette are immediately expelled and discarded to eliminate the non-blood-containing capillary fluid. The hemocytometer is then immediately loaded.

5. The clean and dry coverglass is placed accurately on the counting chamber. The partly emptied pipette is then held as if it were a pencil at an angle, and with the index finger controlling the flow at the bulb end, the tip of the pipette is brought to the edge of the placed coverglass-chamber

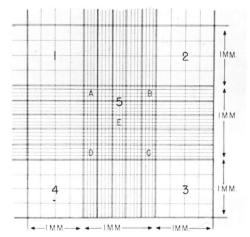

Fig. 2-7. The number of erythrocytes is obtained by counting the total number of cells in squares 5A, 5B, 5C, 5D, and 5E. Because the counting chamber is 0.1 mm. deep, each small division has a volume of 0.004 cu. mm. ($0.2 \times 0.2 \times 0.1$).

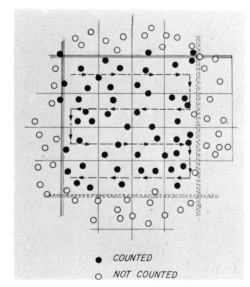

- COUNTED
o NOT COUNTED

Fig. 2-8. In this high-power view of square 5A, only the cells in black are counted. Cells are systematically counted if they lie within the confines of the area or touch the lines at the top or left side. The light cells outside the square or touching the lines at the bottom and right are not counted.

combination. The pressure of the index finger is decreased slightly, and fluid is drawn between the coverglass and the hemocytometer by capillary attraction until the chamber is filled. There should be no bubbles, and the adjacent trenches should be free of blood.

6. The hemocytometer is then placed on the microscope stage, and the cells are allowed to settle for 3 minutes. Using a $10 \times$ objective the central large square is located and surveyed to make sure the cells are evenly distributed. Then using a $40 \times$ objective and with the light reduced, cells are counted in five of the 25 smaller squares situated in the large center square—that is, the four outer smaller squares and the one centrally located smaller square located in the large center square are usually used. Because each of these smaller squares is bordered by double lines (in the improved Neubauer ruling) and each contains 16 *smallest* squares, a total of 80 of these smallest squares is counted; cells lying on and touching the top and left side boundary lines of each smallest square are included in the count, and those cells on the bottom and right side boundary are excluded (Fig.

2-7). Counting is started first in the upper left outer smaller squares followed by the upper right outer, lower right outer, lower left outer, and finally the center smaller square (Fig. 2-8). In each of the 16 smallest squares of each small square, counting is begun by starting first from left to right beginning with the first four smallest squares on the top row, then proceeding from right to left on the second row of the four smallest squares, then left to right on the third row of the four smallest squares, and finally right to left on the fourth row of the four smallest squares. The number of red blood cells for each group of the five groups of 16 squares is then recorded separately, and the results are added.

Computation and Reporting of Results

The total erythrocyte count is computed accurately only when the previously described hemocytometer-coverglass dimensions and pipette dilutions are understood.

That is, the number of red blood cells per cubic millimeter of undiluted blood is best calculated by taking into account the area counted, the depth of the chamber, and the dilution according to the formula for the red blood cell count:

Cells/cu.mm. = cells/sq.mm. × 10 × dilution.

This same formula applies to any situation in which the cells are counted in a certain number of squares and the cell count for an area of 1 sq.mm. is calculated by a simple proportion:

$$\frac{\text{Cells counted}}{\text{Area counted (sq.mm.)}} = \frac{\text{Cells/sq.mm.}}{1}$$

The number of cells counted in each square millimeter is then multiplied by ten (because the depth of the chamber is 0.1 mm., the cells in 1 sq.mm. must be multiplied by 10 to give the number of cells in 1 cu.mm. of the diluted specimen). This result is then multiplied by the pipette dilution in order to give the number of cells in each cubic millimeter of undiluted specimen.

There is another way of calculating the results. Because the central large square measures 1 sq.mm. and contains 25 small squares, and because the total number of cells counted are those in five of the 25 small squares, then cells in $5/25$ or $1/5$ of a square millimeter are counted. The dilution in the pipette is 1:200. The *depth* of the counting chamber—the distance between undersurface of the coverglass and the surface of the hemacytometer—is 0.1 mm. Therefore the number of red blood cells per cubic millimeter may be computed as follows:

Number of erythrocytes counted

$(1/5$ sq.mm.$)$ × 200 (dilution factor) × 10 (depth of counting chamber) *or*
the total count × 10,000 *or*
the total count + 0000 = Total red blood cell count in cu.mm.

Normal red blood cell counts are 4.2 to 6.0 million/cu.mm. in men, 4.5 to 5.0 million per cu.mm. in women, 4.0 to 5.8 mil-lion per cu.mm. in infants up to 3 years of age, and 4.0 to 5.2 million per cu.mm. in children.

If the patient is very anemic or if less than 400 cells have been counted, the dilution of the blood should be decreased to 1:100 by filling the pipette with blood to the 1.0 line instead of to the 0.5 line. If the patient is very polycythemic or if more than 600 cells have been counted, the dilution of the blood should be increased to 1:500 or 1:333 by filling the pipette with blood to the 0.2 or 0.3 line, respectively.

Sources of Error. The sources of error in doing erythrocyte counts include those due to equipment used, performance, and field errors.

Errors Due to Equipment. (1) Broken pipettes with chipped tips should be discarded. (2) Pipette markings should not be obscure. (3) Poorly calibrated pipettes and nonoptically planed (not flat) coverglasses can cause errors. (4) A poorly calibrated, scratched, etched, or dirty (marred by dust or oil) hemacytometer or coverglass can cause errors. After each count, they should be washed with water, dried with soft cloth, placed in absolute ethyl alcohol, and then dried with soft cloth before use. (5) An unclean or wet pipette can result in hemolysis of red blood cells and admixture with particulate debris or other red blood cells. The pipette should be washed three or four times by suction pump, with water, alcohol, and ether in that order, with air being drawn through after the ether until the inside is clean and dry. Any blood clot in a pipette not cleaned by vacuum suction should be soaked for 12 hours in water or H_2SO_4 and then loosened with a fine flexible wire.

Errors in Performance. (1) Too much pressure on finger or ear in order to obtain free-flowing blood can cause error. (2) Too much cyanosis and chilling or edema of capillary or venous puncture site can cause error. (3) Application of the tourniquet for too long a time can result in stasis of venous blood. (4) Agglutination or coagulation of erythrocytes can result from delay in diluting blood or mixing with anticoagulant. (5) Improper or irregular filling of pipette or counting chamber can result in error in dilution and final calculation. Many technicians feel that this cause for error can also be obviated by discarding the first four drops from the pipette before filling the counting chamber. (6) Failure to wipe off pipette tip can result in error, as can (7) inadequate mixing in the pipette. (8) Error can result from counting cells twice or not counting enough cells, that is, wrong borders or skipping cells. (9) Evaporation of fluid or trapped air bubbles in the counting chamber can result in error. There may be an error in calculation, in other words, a failure to consider (nonstandard) dilution or area counted.

Field Errors. These errors result from the distribution of cells in the counting chamber due to random settling of cells in different parts of the chamber. It is part of the procedure and cannot be completely eliminated. It can be reduced by counting large numbers of cells. Because the error is due to cell distribution, it varies with the square root of the number of cells counted, because error increases at a slower rate than the total number of cells counted, the percentage of error in red blood cell counts *decreases* with an increase in the number of cells counted. The combination of field error and performance error averages ±7 to 11 per cent; therefore a better normal range would be plus or minus 7 to 11 per cent of 5 million red blood cells per cu.mm.

REFERENCES

1. Alpen, E. L., and Cranmore, D.: Cellular kinetics and iron utilization in bone marrow as observed by Fe[59] radioautography. Ann. N. Y. Acad. Sci., 77:753, 1959.
2. Athena, J. W., et al.: Leukokinetic studies. III. Distribution of granulocytes in blood of normal subjects. J. Clin. Invest., 40:159, 1961.
3. Bessis, M.: Phase contrast microscopy and electron microscopy applied to the blood cells: general review. Blood, 10:272, 1955.
4. Bierman, H. R., Marshall, G. J., Maekawa, T., and Kelly, K. H.: Granulocytic activity of human plasma. Acta Haematology., 27:217, 1962.
5. Bloom, W., and Fawcett, D. W.: Blood cell formation and destruction. *In* A Textbook of Histology. ed. 8. pp. 112–143. Philadelphia, W. B. Saunders, 1962.
6. Boggs, D. R., and Chervenick, P. A.: Hemopoietic stem cells. *In* Greenwalt, T. J., and Jamieson, G. A. (eds.): Formation and Destruction of Blood Cells. p. 240. Philadelphia, J. B. Lippincott, 1970.
7. Craddock, C. G., Jr., Perry, S., and Lawrence, J. S.: Control of steady state proliferation of leukocytes. *In* Stohlman, F., Jr. (ed.): The Kinetics of Cellular Proliferation. pp. 242–259. New York, Grune & Stratton, 1959.
8. Cronkite, E. P., Flieder, T. M., Bond, V. P., Rusini, J. R., Brecher, G., and Questler, H.: Dynamics of hemopoietic proliferation in man and mice studied by H[3]-thymidine incorporation into DNA. Ann. N. Y. Acad. Sci., 77:803, 1959.
9. Eastwood, D. W., Green, C. D., Lambdin, M. A., and Gardner, R.: Effect of nitrous oxide on the white cell count in leukemia. N. Eng. J. Med., 286:297, 1963.
10. Ellerbrook, L. D.: A simple colorimetric method for calibration of pipets. Am. J. Clin. Pathol., 24:868, 1954.
11. Erslev, A. J.: The effect of anemic anoxia on the cellular development of nucleated red cells. Blood, 14:386, 1959.
12. ———: The role of erythropoietin in the control of RBC production. Medicine, 43:661, 1964.
13. Francis, D.: Calibration of micropipettes and tubes simplified. J. Lab. Clin. Med., 22:718, 1937.
14. Fried, W.: The liver as a source of extrarenal erythropoietin production. Blood, 40:671, 1972.
15. Golde, D. W., Bersch, N., and Li, C. H.: Growth hormone: species-specific stimulation of erythropoiesis in vitro. Science, 196:1112, 1977.
16. Golde, D. W., and Cline, M. J.: Regulation of bone marrow leukopoiesis. Br. J. Haematol., 26:235, 1974.
17. Gregory, C. J.: Erythropoietin sensitivity as a differentiation marker in the hemopoietic system: Studies of three erythropoietic colony responses in culture. J. Cell. Physiol., 89:289, 1976.
18. Harris, J. W.: The Red Cell. p. 124. Cambridge, Harvard University Press, 1963.
19. Jacobson, L. O.: Erythropoietin and the regulation of the red blood cell formation. Physiol. Physicians, 1:1, 1963.
20. Lajtha, L. G.: Bone marrow cell metabolism. Physiol. Rev., 37:50, 1957.
21. Lee, G. R., et al.: Iron metabolism in copper-deficient swine. J. Clin. Invest., 47:2058, 1968.
22. London, I. M.: The metabolism of the erythrocyte. Harvey Lectures Series, 56:151, 1961.
23. Minnich, V.: Identification and differentiation of blood and bone marrow cells stained with Wright's stain. Division of Hematology, Washington University School of Medicine, St. Louis, Missouri.
24. Moore, C. V., and Dubach, R.: Metabolism and requirements of iron in the human. J.A.M.A., 162:197, 1956.

25. Moore, M. A. S., Williams, N., and Metcalf, D.: In vitro colony formation by normal and leukemic human hemopoietic cells: Interaction between colony forming and colony-stimulating cells. J. Natl. Cancer Inst., *50:*591, 1973.

26. Orten, J. M., Underhill, F. H., Mugrage, E. R., and Lewis, R. C.: Blood volume studies in cobalt polycythemia. J. Biol. Chem., *99:*457, 1932–33.

27. Osgood, E. E., and Seaman, A. J.: The cellular composition of normal bone marrow as obtained by sternal puncture. Physiol. Rev., *24:*46, 1944.

28. Paoletti, C.: Rôle des β-globulins plasmatiques dans le transport du fer utilisé par les cellules erythroformatrices. C. R. Acad. Sci. [D] (Paris), *245:*377, 1957.

29. Rappaport, H.: Tumors of the hematopoietic system. Sec. III, Fasc. 8, Armed Forces Institute of Pathology, Washington, D.C., pp. 10–11, 1966.

30. Singer, J. W., and Adamson, J. W.: Steroids and hematopoiesis: III. The response of granulocytic and erythroid colony-forming cells to steroids of different classes. Blood, *48:*855, 1976.

31. Shen, S. C., and Hoshino, T.: Study of humoral factors regulating production of leukocytes. I. Demonstration of "neutropoietin" in plasma after administration of triamcinolone to rats. Blood, *17:*434, 1961.

32. Statland, B., Haegan, B., and White, J. G.: The uptake of calcium by platelet relaxing factor. Nature (Lond.), *223:*521, 1969.

33. Verglens, G.: Distribution of leukocytes in vascular system. Acta Pathol. Microbiol. Scand. [Supp.], *33:*1, 1938.

34. Weed, R. I., et al.: Metabolic dependence of red cell membrane deformability. J. Clin. Invest., *48:*795, 1969.

35. Whipple, G. H., and Robscheit-Robbins, F. S.: Dietary effects on anemia plus hypoproteinemia. J. Exp. Med., *89:*359, 1949.

36. Whitby, L. E. H., and Britton, C. J. C.: Disorders of the Blood. ed. 9. p. 16. New York, Grune & Stratton, 1963.

AUDIOVISUAL AIDS*

Basic Red Cell Morphology and Function. 247608. [24 (35 mm.) transparencies plus descriptive booklet. Lecture also recorded on a standard audiocassette] Betty Murphy, M. T. (ASCP), Communications in Learning, Inc., 2929 Main Street, Buffalo, New York 14214.

Cell Division and Growth. Abbott Laboratories, Professional Services Department, Abbott Park, North Chicago, Illinois 60064.

Hematological Technique for Charging the Hemocytometer. (1954). Medical Film Library, National Naval Medical Center, Bethesda, Maryland 20014.

Introduction to Blood Cell Morphology. (1972). [35 mm. transparencies, teaching exercise, examination, answer sheet]. American Society of Clinical Pathologists, P.O. Box 12073, Chicago, Illinois 60612.

Normal and Abnormal Peripheral Blood. Set B1. [35 mm. transparencies, manual]. A.S.H. National Slide Bank, HSLRC T252 (SB-56), University of Washington, Seattle, Washington 98195.

Normal and Pathological Erythrocytes. [I]. International Society for Hematology, James L. Tullis, M.D., 110 Francis Street, Boston, Massachusetts 02215.

Phase Microscopy of Normal Living Blood Cells. (1954). AMA Film Library, 535 Dearborn Street, Chicago, Illinois 60610.

Quality Control in Hematology. [35 mm. transparencies, audiotape]. ASCP Seminar 215-10, ASMT Education and Research Fund, Inc., 5555 West Loop South, Bellaire, Texas 77401.

---

* Films unless otherwise stated.

3 Hemoglobin

Hemoglobin is a protein moiety of 200 million to 300 million nearly spherical molecules in each red blood cell, each molecule having a molecular weight of 64,458 based on the chemical structures of its alpha and beta chains and of heme.[10] Hemoglobin is synthesized normally in the lipoprotein framework of cells of the erythrocyte series. The main function of hemoglobin is the transport of large amounts of oxygen in the circulating blood. The uptake and delivery of oxygen by the hemoglobin molecules are associated with marked rearrangement of the hemoglobin molecule, which, in turn, explains the oxygen dissociation curve.[33] Chemically, hemoglobin is composed of four coiled polypeptide porphyrin chains oriented about two axes of symmetry and bonded to a protein matrix by means of ferrous iron atoms. The four chains are of two types with two members of each type present. The ferrous atoms have six coordinate bonds, four of which are attached to the pyrrole nitrogens of the prophyrin radical. The fifth coordinate bond is attached to the imidazole nitrogen of a histidine radical in a polypeptide chain of globin. The sixth is attached by an oxygen molecule in a reversible state (Fig. 3-1).[31]

The two types of polypeptide chains are designated α and β. In the major normal adult hemoglobin (Hb A), the two α polypeptide chains are identical; the other two chains (β) are identical but different from the α chains. There are a total of 574 amino acid residues in the four polypeptide chains—141 amino acids in one α chain for a total of 282 in both, and 146 amino acids in one β chain for a total of 292 in both of these. (The sequential mapping of the amino acids has been of great importance for the identification of abnormal hemoglobins with specific amino acid substitutions.) When the four major polypeptide chains are digested with trypsin, the chains are broken at the arginine and lysine carboxyl binding sites. Roman numerals are given to the smaller peptide chains formed according to the peptide sequence in the chain, beginning with the NH_2 terminal end.

The three important *normal hemoglobin* components are: (1) *Hb A* is found in normal adult blood and is written as $\alpha_2{}^A\beta_2{}^A$. This indicates that this molecule is made up of two α chains each with a certain amino acid sequence and two β chains each with a certain amino acid sequence.[6] (2) Hb A_2, also found in normal adult red blood cells in much smaller quantities than Hb A, is composed of two α chains and two Δ chains and is written $\alpha_2{}^A\Delta_2{}^A$. (3) Fetal hemoglobin (Hb F), also a normal hemoglobin present during the first 4 to 6 months of life, consists of two α chains and two γ chains and is written as $\alpha_2{}^A\gamma_2{}^F$. In addition, other poorly understood hemoglobin components are also found in normal red blood cells in minute quantities.

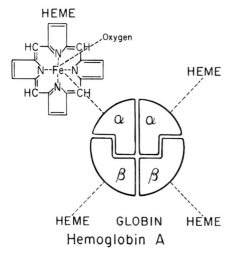

HEME

HEME

HEME   GLOBIN   HEME

Hemoglobin A

Fig. 3-1. Structure of the hemoglobin molecule (in this case, hemoglobin A). The hemoglobin molecule is composed of globin (two alpha plus two beta polypeptide chains) plus four heme (iron porphyrin complexes). (Linman, J. W.: Principles of Hematology. New York, Macmillan, 1966.)

METABOLISM

ERYTHROPOIESIS

Metabolically, hemoglobin is produced as part of the erythron in a very complex manner. Some of the complexity results because there is more than one stimulus to erythropoiesis. The fundamental stimulus to erythropoiesis and change in erythron size is hypoxia.[15] The sequence is as follows:[17] The rate of red cell production determines the size of the hemoglobin mass, which determines the circulating hemoglobin concentration. The hemoglobin concentration determines the degree of tissue oxygenation, which determines the rate of cell production. In addition, an erythrocytic enzyme (2,3-diphosphoglycerate or 2,3-DPG) affects tissue oxygen delivery by reversibly combining with deoxygenated hemoglobin and decreasing hemoglobin oxygen affinity.[52]

Examples of anoxemia controlling the volume and rate of production of red cells are the increase in red blood cells and hemoglobin associated with high altitude ascent, deficient pulmonary ventilation (pulmonary arteriovenous fistulas, pulmonary hemangiomas, and congenital heart disease with right-to-left shunts), fetus near term, and preeclampsia. Because erythropoiesis is stimulated under conditions in which oxygen delivery is not sufficient to meet oxygen demand and because oxygen delivery is restrained when the supply exceeds the demand, it was at one time assumed that a decrease in oxygen supply to the developing erythrocytes themselves hastened proliferative activity, whereas an excess of oxygen inhibited or retarded such activity. Many experiments performed to disprove this concept do not form conclusive evidence against the theory that hypoxia stimulates marrow cells directly.[40] In fact, changes in 2,3-DPG levels play an important role in adaptation to hypoxia, that is, in a number of situations characterized by hypoxemia, RBC 2,3-DPG levels increase, oxygen affinity is reduced, and delivery of oxygen to tissues is facilitated.[50] For example, in blood stored over 1 week in acid-citrate-dextrose solution (ACD) or over 2 weeks in citrate-phosphate-dextrose solution (CPD), markedly reduced 2,3-DPG levels are found. The ability of hemoglobin to release oxygen is therefore decreased. However, other investigators have found that these reduced 2,3-DPG levels are restored in the RBCs within a few hours after transfusion. Moreover, the use of CPD as a preservation fluid reduces the 2,3-DPG loss during storage. The fear, therefore, that the transfusion of stored blood might not be fully effective in tissue oxygenation is not justified, unless the clinical situation calls for massive and rapid blood replacement.[18]

Other regulatory mechanisms in addition to hypoxia exist. Some are consistent with considerable experimental evidence, and others are promulgated without direct evidence. For example, there is an erythropoiesis-stimulating factor in circulating blood called erythropoietin.[3] One worker found that this hormonal substance may be brought into play by lowered oxygen tension rather than as a simple direct effect of hypoxia.[41] This evidence was observed in parabiotically united rats. One animal was kept in lowered oxygen concentration and the other at normal oxygen concentration for several weeks. The hypoxia effects in one animal thus were transferred to the other through the parabiotic circulatory setup.[16]

Clinical proof of the results of this animal experiment was supplied by a case report. A patient had pulmonary hypertension with reversal of the shunt through a patent ductus arteriosus, producing anoxia of the lower part of the body only.[47] The patient developed polycythemia with normal white blood cell count and platelet count. At autopsy, the marrow of the well oxygenated region of the body showed erythroid hyperplasia comparable in degree to that from the anoxic region.

Other experiments on this subject have revealed that when plasma obtained from anemic (bled) rabbits was injected (in large quantities on successive days to minimize hemodilution), erythropoiesis was stimulated in the form of reticulocytosis, elevated hemoglobin level, and increases in the hematocrit and red blood cell count. Also observed were an increase in the number of nucleated red blood cells in the marrow, an increase in the plasma clearance rate of radioactive iron, and an increase in the utilization of radioactive iron by the erythrocytes.[16]

Clinically, the plasma or urine of anemic patients with hypochromic, refractory, hemolytic, megaloblastic, leukemic, or infectious patterns has been found to contain high levels of erythropoietin. However, practically no erythropoietin is found in the serum or urine of patients with chronic renal disease, leading one to suspect that the kidneys have something to do with the erythropoietin production. This was further corroborated when it was discovered that

none of the hormone is found in the blood 48 hours after bilateral nephrectomy, but is found in the plasma after ligation of both ureters.[35] By means of the fluorescent-antibody staining technique, erythropoietin was found to be localized in the glomerular epithelial cells; the juxtaglomerular apparatus cells were not stained.[11]

Another confirmatory fact pointing to an important renal source is the finding that there is an increased erythropoietin blood concentration in some renal tumor cases.[20] Some workers have suggested that there may be a minor extrarenal source of erythropoiesis-stimulating factor, possibly in the liver.[13] One disturbing factor in the whole picture is that although in starvation anemias, infections, chronic renal diseases, and neoplasms no increase in plasma erythropoietin has been demonstrated, these anemias do not respond to administration of erythropoietin-rich plasmas. This leads one to presume that there is a relative inadequacy of bone marrow responsiveness. Chemically, this erythropoietic factor is relatively heat-resistant, nondialyzable, subject to proteolytic destruction, and insoluble in ether or lipid solvents, and therefore is most likely an α-2-glycoprotein.

Injection of erythropoietin in suitable test subjects results initially in an increase in the stem cells and the most immature red cells of the marrow, and later in generalized hyperplasia, reticulocytosis, and increases in red blood cell count, hemoglobin concentration, and hematocrit value. Finally, one observes an increase in the clearance of iron through the plasma and an incorporation of iron into the hemoglobin of functionally competent erythrocytes. Therefore, it may well be that more than one factor is necessary to stimulate normal erythropoiesis and that an excess (or relative deficiency) of one or the other factor(s) can result in skipped mitoses and short-lived macrocytes, or, on the other hand, too many mitoses and short-lived microcytes.

Although there is no absolute evidence of

direct and specific control of erythropoiesis by endocrines, they do play a very important role. For example, marked hematologic alterations are consistently observed in endocrine disorders involving pituitary, adrenals, thymus, thyroid (myxedema and associated anemia), and gonads. Erythropoiesis per se appears to be regulated indirectly through effects of metabolism and oxygen requirements and not by direct effect on the marrow or direct modification of the fundamental stimulus to hypoxia. Although it appears that androgenic hormones are involved in erythropoiesis—for example, hemoglobin and hematocrit values in relation to age and sex—the mechanism whereby androgens bring about the changes is obscure. Possibly, it may be related to the increased erythropoietin secretion demonstrated in isolated kidneys perfused with androgens.[33] Indirectly, this is demonstrated by the observation that castration in adult males is followed by a diminution in hemoglobin and hematocrit values to levels normally associated with females. There is no physiologic or metabolic information, but the increased proliferation of red blood cell precursors suggests that a primary effect is through the stem cell.[14] Even if this is so, other workers believe that the endocrine effect is subject to the higher control of the central nervous system; stimulation of the hypothalamus of the rabbit often causes an increase in erythropoietin, reticulocytosis, and an increase in the red cell mass.[45]

Clinically, this may be corroborated by the observation that an increased volume of packed red cells follows the administration of androgens in patients with panhypopituitarism and hypogonadism.[22] The same elevations in hematocrit and hemoglobin concentration are also induced by androgenic therapy in patients with certain, otherwise refractory anemias (e.g., aplastic anemia, myelofibrosis, or sideroblastic anemia). In addition, a number of vasoactive hormones (vasopressin, angiotensin, 5(OH) tryptamine, norepinephrine, and prostaglandin E) have been found to stimulate erythropoiesis, possibly by decreasing blood flow to the renal hypoxic-sensing mechanism, which, thereby, induces erythropoietin secretion.[12]

Finally, cobaltous chloride and its effect on erythropoiesis should be mentioned. Brown has demonstrated an increased amount of plasma erythropoietin following the use of cobaltous chloride.[4] Because cobalt interferes with certain enzymes concerned with the transport and utilization of oxygen,[28] its use may result in a histotoxic hypoxia and possibly even cardiomyopathy. Tissue hypoxia may then stimulate the production of erythropoietin, resulting in polycythemia. However, the specific identity of the erythropoietic factor stimulated by cobalt—and that produced by bleeding or by phenylhydrazine-induced hemolytic anemia—has not been definitely established. Although some difference in effects has been noted, the final answer has not yet been established.

Heller states that in hypoxia the decrease in oxygen saturation causes the intraerythrocytic levels of 2,3-DPG to increase and to shift the oxygen dissociation curve toward the right.[19] This effect, however, is initially (in the first six hours) counteracted by respiratory alkalosis, which has the opposite effect on the hemoglobin-oxygen equilibrium and increases oxygen affinity, which leads to tissue hypoxia and a prompt increase in erythropoietin. In the presence of hypoxia for longer than 12 hours, 2,3-DPG levels continue to rise, counterbalancing the effect of alkalosis on oxygen affinity and leading to a prompt return to normal of the erythropoietin. Thus, the decline of erythropoietin level in the presence of continued hypoxia which appeared to be quite puzzling seems to be explained, and we do not have to invoke other reasons, such as consumption of erythropoietin by the hyperplastic marrow. In anemia, increased erythropoietin production should only start after the shift to the right of the oxygen dissociation curve becomes insufficient for adequate tissue oxygenation.

HEMOGLOBIN SYNTHESIS AND BREAKDOWN

The synthesis of hemoglobin is a complex process starting in the erythrocyte series in the bone marrow. Hemoglobin, a chromoprotein, is composed of globin, protoporphyrin, and ferrous iron. Globin is synthesized from natural amino acids in the diet and formed in the body, if necessary, by the breakdown of autogenous proteins. Protoporphyrin (porphyrin I and porphyrin II) is formed from succinate and glycine in the presence of certain enzymes with the subsequent synthesis of δ-aminolevulinic acid (ALA). Two molecules of this acid in the presence of ALA dehydrase unite to form porphobilinogen. By enzymatic action the porphobilinogen is converted to uroporphyrinogen III, then to coproporphyrinogen III and finally to protoporphyrin.

Iron is absorbed as ferrous iron from food and is changed to ferric iron, after which it is linked with apoferritin, a protein found in the cells of the intestinal mucosa, and forms ferritin. This ferric form combines with globulin, is carried by the bloodstream, and is stored as ferritin in the liver, spleen, and bone marrow. Iron assimilation is controlled by the saturation state of these iron stores. Simultaneously, iron from senescent red blood cells is carefully conserved by the body — only 1 mg. per day is excreted.

Protoporphyrin, assisted by ascorbic acid and reduced glutathione, unites with ferrous iron in the presence of certain enzymes and hematopoietic factors and forms heme. Heme combines with globin to form activated hemoglobin, which combines reversibly with oxygen to form oxyhemoglobin without change in iron valency. When reduced hemoglobin is exposed to oxygen at increasing pressures, oxygen is taken up until each molecule of hemoglobin has bound four oxygen molecules, also leading to the formation of a fully saturated oxyhemoglobin containing 1.34 ml. of oxygen per gram of hemoglobin.[43]

Hemoglobin breakdown is associated with two mechanisms of destruction — phagocytosis and fragmentation. With a normal life-span of 100 to 120 days, approximately 1 per cent of erythrocytes leave the circulation each day. These effete red blood cells are removed from the bloodstream by the process of phagocytosis in the reticuloendothelial cells of the bone marrow, liver, spleen, and occasionally other organs. However, the major mechanism by which erythrocytes are destroyed is fragmentation, caused by the traumatic buffeting effects of the circulation.

Other factors that contribute to erythrocyte fragmentation are splenic erythrophagocytosis and plasma-tissue hemolytic factors. Also, fragmentation occasionally occurs when the protective red blood cell enzymes are decreased or lost, or when the spherical shape and osmotic fragility of erythrocytes are altered owing to erythrocyte stagnation in the spleen. It might be mentioned that one rarely sees erythrocytic phagocytosis in the peripheral blood and bone marrow of patients having erythroblastosis fetalis and acute leukemia.

Destruction and disposal of the senescent red blood cell are accompanied by a breakdown of hemoglobin, especially in the reticuloendothelial cells of the body. At first the α methene bridge of the protoporphyrin ring is opened by oxidation leading to the formation of a green bile pigment (biliverdin-globin) called verdohemoglobin. Iron is then split off and removed by its attachment to a β-1-globulin of the plasma (siderophilin, or transferrin).

In the bone marrow, the iron-transferrin complex is used in the regeneration of hemoglobin. In the liver, spleen, and other organs it is deposited as ferritin and, when it is excessive, as hemosiderin. The protein portion of the hemoglobin molecule — *globin* — is degraded to its constituent amino acids, which enter the body metabolic pool, to be used again in protein synthesis or serve as a source of energy. Verdohemoglobin is reduced at the γ methene bridge to yield free bilirubin (orange-red, insoluble, and nonfilterable by the kidneys), which passes out of the reticuloendothelial cells into the plasma, where it is loosely bound to albumin. This bilirubin-albumin complex is carried to the liver, where it is conjugated with glucuronic acid within the liver cells. Normally most of this soluble bilirubin-diglucuronide passes into the biliary canaliculi. A small amount of this soluble, conjugated bilirubin is regurgitated back into the plasma, where it is again loosely attached to albumin. Because it is insoluble, it cannot be filtered readily by the kidneys.

From the biliary canaliculi, most of the soluble bilirubin-diglucuronide passes into the common bile duct and thence into the intestinal tract, where the bacterial flora removes the glucuronic acid, leaving the free bilirubin to be reduced in accordance with the type of bacterial flora present. One of the reduction products is urobilinogen, a colorless complex consisting mostly of stercobilinogen. When broad-spectrum antibiotics are given to patients, the bacterial flora is markedly diminished. This decreases the amount of bilirubin reduced to urobilinogen, and therefore urobilinogen excretion is reduced. Bilirubin thereby becomes the main bile pigment found in the feces. After the patient is taken off these antibiotics, the bacterial flora gradually returns, first reducing bilirubin to d-urobilinogen and then to stercobilinogen predominantly. A small amount of intestinal tract urobilinogen complex is reabsorbed and excreted again through the liver, or it appears in the urine. When feces and urine are exposed to air, they are oxidized to the urobilin group of compounds.

HEMOGLOBIN COMPOUNDS

The main function of hemoglobin in body metabolism is as a respiratory pigment in the form of oxyhemoglobin (scarlet red). As erythrocytes flow along in single file in the delicate alveolar capillaries of the lung, the partial pressure (100 torr.) of oxygen in the alveolar air converts almost all the hemoglobin in these red blood cells to oxyhemoglobin, by a process of diffusion through the erythrocytic membrane. Because the association of oxygen and hemoglobin is loose and unstable, the oxygen readily diffuses back to the tissues for oxidative purposes, and the oxyhemoglobin then becomes reduced hemoglobin (dark red). There is, then, a concomitant release of base, which binds part of the incoming carbon dioxide. Carbon dioxide is also bound as a carbamate at the free amino groups of the hemoglobin molecule. A most important portion of the carbon dioxide diffuses from the plasma into the red blood cells, where catalysis by carbonic anhydrase joins it with water to form carbonic acid, which in turn dissociates into $(H)^+$ and $(HCO_3)^-$.

Carboxyhemoglobin is one of the abnormal hemoglobin pigments incapable of carrying oxygen. It is formed when hemoglobin in the red blood cells is exposed to carbon monoxide, which has an affinity 200 times greater for hemoglobin than oxygen does. When toxic amounts of carbon monoxide are present (from automobile exhaust fumes, for example), the blood is cherry red, and anoxia may result with subsequent death caused by irreversible tissue changes. Endogenous carbon monoxide production and subsequent respiratory excretion are related to heme degradation on a one-mole-to-one-mole basis. Since there is no other source of endogenous CO, measurement of its production rate accurately quantitates the catabolism of heme compounds, and thus also the rate of hemolysis.[25] Like oxyhemoglobin, carboxyhemoglobin is seen spectroscopically at 576 μ (Plate 8).

Methemoglobin is formed when hemoglobin in its deoxygenated state (reduced hemoglobin) is oxidized to the ferric form (iron normally exists in the ferrous state in the iron porphyrin complex of the heme portion of the hemoglobin molecule. See p.

45-46). In the ferric form oxygen and iron cannot combine, and therefore when a high concentration of methemoglobin is produced in the red blood cells, it reduces the capacity of the red blood cells to combine with and transport oxygen. When approximately 15 per cent of the total hemoglobin is methemoglobin, cyanosis is produced. Methemoglobin normally makes up about 2 per cent of the hemoglobin pigments.

There are several mechanisms for maintaining hemoglobin in the normal reduced hemoglobin state. All depend on enzyme systems utilized in glucose metabolism: production of reduced diphosphopyridine nucleotide (DPNH) acting in the presence of methemoglobin reductase (a diaphorase), production of reduced triphosphopyridine nucleotide (TPNH) in the presence of glucose-6-phosphate dehydrogenase, and glutathione and its associated enzyme systems. Methemoglobinemia therefore results chemically from any one of the following mechanisms:

Acquired methemoglobinemia results from the effects of chemical or therapeutic agents that oxidize hemoglobin from ferrous to ferric state at a rate beyond the capacity for its reduction back to the ferrous state. Among these agents are the *direct oxidants* (active in vitro)—for example, nitrites, chlorates, and quinones.* *Indirect oxidants* (active in vivo) include aniline and its derivatives—for example, absorption from diapers freshly stamped with aniline marking ink and from freshly dyed shoes and blankets and from ingestion of colored wax crayons, the early sulfonamide derivatives, and acetanilid and phenacetin.

Primary or congenital methemoglobinemia is an inborn error of metabolism caused by failure of the intracellular reducing enzyme system. There are two types of hereditary methemoglobinemia. The *enzymatic type* is transmitted usually as a recessive trait, reflecting a deficiency in one or more

enzymes (for example, diaphorase or glutathione) required to reduce methemoglobin ferric iron (Fe^{+++}) to the ferrous iron (Fe^{++}) of hemoglobin. The *M type* of hereditary methemoglobinemia is characterized by a defect in the globin component of hemoglobin; there are ten types of globin with different spectral properties.

Acquired methemoglobinemia may be suspected when cyanosis is observed in patients without concomitant evidence of cardiovascular or pulmonary dysfunction, that is, if venous blood from the patient remains a chocolate brown when it is shaken vigorously in open air for 15 minutes. In other words, greater than one per cent of a patient's hemoglobin contains iron that is oxidized to ferric form, so that each molecule is thus rendered incapable of transporting oxygen. Further confirmation is obtained when a 1:100 aqueous dilution of blood examined with a hand spectroscope shows a well defined absorption band at 630 mμ that disappears almost immediately after addition of a few drops of 5 per cent KCN solution. Congenital methemoglobinemia is associated with compensatory polycythemia, a positive family history, and a spectroscopic absorption band at 630 mμ, with the M type observed at 602 or 622 mμ. Therapy, in emergencies, includes the administration of methylene blue intravenously (1 mg./kg.). Methylene blue is thought to be effective since it brings about reversion of methemoglobin by activating the pentose phosphate cycle and thereby increasing the amount of glucose metabolized in the erythrocyte. In less severe cases, oral methylene blue, 60 mg. three times daily, or ascorbic acid, 300 to 600 mg. orally daily in 3 to 4 divided doses, may be administered. Methylene blue may induce hemolysis in G-6-PD-deficient patients.

Cyanmethemoglobin is a stable abnormal hemoglobin pigment produced when ferricyanide is added to the ferrous iron of normal red blood cell hemoglobin; the ferricyanide converts the ferrous iron to the ferric iron of methemoglobin, which then

---

* Nitrates in well water and bismuth subnitrate given to infants for diarrhea may be reduced to nitrites by bowel action.

combines with KCN to produce cyan-methemoglobin. Because nitrites have a strong affinity for the cyanide in cyanhemoglobin, administration of nitrites will cause methemoglobin to form. The methemoglobin then unites with the free cyanide radical in cyanhemoglobin to form cyanmethemoglobin, which is less toxic. A cyanmethemoglobin solution of certain concentration known as Drabkin's solution is used in hemoglobinometry.

Sulfhemoglobin is an abnormal hemoglobin pigment produced by the combination of inorganic sulfides with hemoglobin in vivo. It is not normally present in red blood cells, and it does not transport oxygen. Sulfhemoglobinemia often accompanies methemoglobinemia, but unlike methemoglobin it cannot be converted to reduced hemoglobin by red blood cells. Once sulfhemoglobin is formed, it is stable and irreversible, disappearing with the red blood cells after the completion of the 120 day life span. Methylene blue and ascorbic acid cannot convert sulfhemoglobin to hemoglobin. Also, the absorption band of sulfhemoglobin is at 618 mμ and is unaltered by the addition of KCN solution. Clinically, sulhemoglobinemia is observed in patients who take oxidant drugs such as phenacetin and acetanilid. Shaking blood in the air for 15 minutes produces a mauve-lavender color.

HEMOGLOBINOMETRY

The oxygen-combining capacity of blood is directly proportional to the hemoglobin concentration rather than to the red blood cell count. Therefore hemoglobinometry—one of the most frequently performed laboratory procedures—is important as a screening test for diseases associated with anemia and for following the response of these diseases to treatment. The normal hemoglobin concentration, expressed in g./100 ml. of blood, varies widely according to the hemoglobin standard used, to the age and sex of the patient, and to the altitude of

the environment. Percentage equivalents therefore cannot be used at any time.

At sea level the normal range for males is 16 ± 2 g./100 ml. and for females it is 14 ± 2 g./100 ml. of blood. It is difficult to state at what level anemia is present because of the wide range of normal values and the variable adaptability and efficiency of the body in response to blood hemoglobin concentration. An arbitrary level of 12 g. per 100 ml. of blood, however, is acceptable.

There are many methods for determining hemoglobin concentration, among which are many unreliable techniques that are still used. All methods are indirect because it is quite difficult to crystallize and accurately weigh hemoglobin. The most commonly used methods measure hemoglobin in one of four basic ways: measurement of the oxygen-combining capacity of blood in the Van Slyke blood-gas apparatus (gasometric method); measurement of the iron content of the blood (chemical method); colorimetric measurement of the specific gravity of whole blood in copper sulfate solutions of known specific gravity and the subsequent determination of hemoglobin from previously prepared line charts (gravimetric or physical method); and colorimetric measurement of a colored derivative of hemoglobin (for example, oxyhemoglobin, acid hematin, alkaline hematin, and cyanmethemoglobin) and comparison of the unknown sample with a standard, by utilizing visual, photoelectric, or automated electronic methods.

GASOMETRIC METHOD

The gasometric method utilizes the same Van Slyke apparatus used in the estimation of carbon dioxide in blood. It is based on the principle that a given sample of blood can be equilibrated with oxygen under standard conditions of temperature and pressure. One millimole of hemoglobin weighs 68 g. because the molecular weight of hemoglobin is approximately 68,000, and 1 mM of hemoglobin contains 4 mM of iron^{++} and combines with 4 mM of oxygen.

Volumetrically, 1 mM of oxygen equals 22.4 ml. of oxygen under conditions of standard temperature and pressure; therefore, 1.34 ml. of oxygen is bound by and is equivalent to 1 g. of hemoglobin. A measured volume of blood so equilibrated is then analyzed for its content of oxygen, and from this its equivalent content of hemoglobin in grams is estimated.

Advantages. The following are advantages of the gasometric method: It is an accurate method for determining hemoglobin because a result with an error of only ±0.5 per cent can be obtained by skilled, careful technologists. This is an accurate method for the standardization of other methods and various hemoglobinometers. It measures only "active" hemoglobin (that hemoglobin which is functional and can carry oxygen).

Disadvantages. The gasometric method involves the following disadvantages: Rigid control of the technique is required.[9, 38] The gasometric method is technically demanding if an accuracy of ±0.5 per cent is to be obtained. The method is too time-consuming for practical clinical use, and in addition the apparatus is expensive. The method does not measure total hemoglobin because it does not measure the normal 2 to 10 per cent of methemoglobin, sulfhemoglobin, and carboxyhemoglobin which do not combine with oxygen.

Modification of Technique. Carbon monoxide may be substituted for oxygen in this technique. Total hemoglobin may then be determined by this method if the blood is first reduced completely by an active reducing agent. Normal values in this method are 16 ± 2 g. per 100 ml. in males, 14 ± 2 g. per 100 ml. in females.

CHEMICAL METHOD

For all practical purposes, the total iron content of blood may be regarded as being bound to hemoglobin. In the *Wong* test, iron is liberated from hemoglobin by the action of sulfuric acid and potassium persulfate. The proteins are precipitated by tungstic acid, and the iron in the protein-free filtrates is made to form ferric thiocyanate. The density of the resultant color is measured photometrically and compared with the color of a standard solution of known iron content. The density of the color is directly proportional to the amount of iron present and therefore to the amount of hemoglobin. This method typifies the basic principle of all colorimetric methods—that the optical density of monochromatic light of a colored solution is proportional to the concentration of the colored material therein (Beer's law).

The iron content of hemoglobin is 0.338 g. per 100 g. of hemoglobin (U.S.A. standard). The amounts 0.347 g. per 100 g. of hemogllbin (w/w) are now used, according to the International Committee for Standardization in Hematology (ICSH), which is also the European standard, and is computed from the molecular weight of 64,458 for hemoglobin and the atomic weight of iron with four atoms of iron per molecule of hemoglobin).[10] The European standard contains 2.5 per cent of hemoglobin iron; thus there is only a final difference of 2 per cent between both standards. Drabkin's molecular weight of hemoglobin is that of hemoglobin as it exists within the red blood cell, including the cations associated with this polyvalent amphoteric protein. On the other hand, the European standard (Braunitzer, cited in Eilers[10]) is based on the chemical structure of the globin and heme alone. Neither is correct.

The technique of the chemical method is as follows:[32] In a 50 ml. volumetric flask place 2 ml. of concentrated sulfuric acid and 0.5 ml. of oxalated blood (well mixed). It should be mixed for 2 minutes; then add 20 ml. distilled water and 2 ml. of a saturated solution of potassium persulfate (7g. + 100 ml. of water) and 2 ml. of a 10 per cent sodium tungstate solution (w/v). Mix well and add distilled water to 50 ml. mark on the volumetric flask. Filter through Whatman No. 1 filter paper.

In three small (6 × 1 ml.) test tubes place the following solutions:

	Unknown	Standard	Blank
Filtrate	20 ml.	–	–
Standard iron solution (0.1 mg./ml.)	–	1.0 ml.	–
Distilled water (deionized water may be used)	–	18.2 ml.	19.0 ml.
Concentrated sulfuric acid	–	0.8 ml.	1.0 ml.
Potassium persulfate solution	1.0 ml.	1.0 ml.	1.0 ml.
Potassium thiocyanate (146 g. q.s. to 500 ml. with distilled water)	4.0 ml.	4.0 ml.	4.0 ml.

Mix the solution in the tubes. Then read the unknown and standard against the reagent blank in a photometer, using a green light filter, or in a spectrophotometer at 540 mμ.

Preparation of Standard Iron Solution

Dissolve 0.7 g. of crystalline ferrous ammonium sulfate in approximately 50 ml. of distilled water in a liter volumetric flask. Add 20 ml. of 10 per cent H_2SO_4 (w/v); warm slightly and add $\frac{1}{10}$ N $KMnO_4$ drop by drop until a pink color that persists for at least 30 seconds is obtained. Cool to room temperature, and dilute up to 1 liter with distilled water or deionized water. The finished solution contains 0.1 mg. of iron per ml. All the reagents and distilled water or deionized water must be free of iron.

Calculations:

$$\frac{\text{Unknown reading}}{\text{standard reading}} \times \left(0.1 \times \frac{100}{0.2}\right) \text{ or } \times 50 =$$

mg. of iron/100 ml. of blood or

expressed another way:

$$\frac{\text{mg. of iron/100 ml. of blood}}{3.47 \text{ g. of hemoglobin/100 ml. of blood}}$$

Advantages. The chemical method offers the following advantages: Practically the total hemoglobin of blood is measured. It is an accurate method for determining total hemoglobin when performed by skilled hands. It is useful in providing primary standards for the colorimetric method.

Disadvantages. The chemical method involves the following disadvantages: Rigid control of the method is required, which is technically difficult and time-consuming. This method is not completely accurate; the iron content of the hemoglobin molecule is not accurately established because crystalline hemoglobin has not been prepared in an absolutely pure and dry state. Iron in the plasma, which is 1.4 per cent, is also measured, causing an error of 0.1 to 0.2 per cent in a nonanemic patient.

SPECIFIC GRAVITY OR GRAVIMETRIC METHOD

The specific gravity of blood is the ratio of the weight of a volume of blood to the weight of the same volume of water at 4° C. Drops of blood are made to fall into a series of 40 copper sulfate solutions having specific gravities from 1.035 to 1.075 at intervals of 0.001. In less accurate determinations, 16 copper sulfate solutions having specific gravities from 1.015 to 1.075 at intervals of 0.004 are used. It is then noted whether the drops of blood sink or rise in the solutions. Upon immersion, the drops of blood become coated with a layer of copper proteinate.

In this method, venous blood is released into the copper sulfate solution from a height of about 1 cm. (the blood has been drawn and previously mixed with a dry oxalate mixture, 200 mg./100 ml. of blood). From the medicine dropper or syringe and needle, the drop falls and penetrates 2 to 3 cm. below the surface. In a few seconds the drop begins to rise or continues to fall. The specific gravity of the drop does not change for another 10 to 15 seconds. If the drop is of the same specific gravity as the test solution, it will become stationary for 10 to 15 seconds and will then resume its downward course. If it is lighter, it will rise for a few seconds and then begin to sink; if it is heavier, it will continue to fall. One can also take 2 ml. of the whole blood sample, centrifuge it, remove the plasma, and determine its specific gravity by the technique just described. Both specific gravity results are corrected for the anticoagulant effect by subtracting 0.0008. A straight line connecting the values of specific gravity for plasma and whole blood on the line chart intersects the scale for hemoglobin at a point that indicates the number of grams per 100 ml. of blood.[36] The $CuSO_4 \cdot 5H_2O$ solution can be prepared from information given in the original article by Phillips and associates,[39] or it may be purchased from several commercial sources.

Advantages. The specific gravity method of determining hemoglobin concentration offers the following advantages: This method is valuable in hemoglobin screening in mass surveys and before blood is drawn from donors. It is a practical and rapid procedure in determining both plasma protein and hemoglobin concentration with considerable accuracy. Results are within plus or minus 2 per cent of the mean hemoglobin value determined by the highly accurate Van Slyke method.

Disadvantages. This method involves the following disadvantages: The copper sulfate solution is difficult to prepare accurately. Solutions must be replaced from time to time. The method assumes erroneously that the corpuscular hemoglobin concentration is constant.

Normal Values. The normal specific gravity ranges from 1.048 to 1.066. The average for men is 1.057 and for women is 1.053.

COLORIMETRIC METHODS

Derivates of hemoglobin are measured by conversion into one of several compounds (acid hematin, alkaline hematin, or cyanmethemoglobin) or by measurement of oxyhemoglobin. An unknown is compared with a standard, by utilizing visual or photoelectric instrumentation.

Direct Matching Method

Direct matching is based on the use of color standards with which the red color of whole fresh blood is matched. An example of this is the Tallqvist hemoglobin scale, which utilizes a printed color scale graded from 10 to 100 per cent. This is matched with the color of a drop of patient's blood on absorbent paper. The error is large (20 to 50 per cent) owing to the variability of the personal equation in matching red colors, especially because the percentages on the scale are not accurate. Another direct matching technique for hemoglobin measurement is that of Dare, in which blood is drawn by capillary attraction between two glass plates, one transparent and the other white and translucent. The undiluted blood color is then matched with a rotating disk of tinted glass varying in thickness and red color intensity. This also gives a large error (20 to 30 per cent), is expensive, and depends too much on the personal ability of the investigator to match visually the various intensities of red color.

Another direct matching instrument is the Spencer hemoglobinometer (Hb-meter, American Optical Co.), in which the transmission of light through a thin layer of hemolyzed blood (oxyhemoglobin) of constant depth is compared with that of a standardized glass wedge with a transmission of 540 mμ wavelength (green color). In this technique, the intensity of light is measured rather than the color itself. The advantage is that a green color has maximal sensitivity to the human eye in an instrument with a fairly constant light source. This method is quick and fairly efficient, but the instruments are expensive compared to the Sahli instruments and there is an upper limit of measurement of 20 grams of hemoglobin.

Advantages. The direct matching method offers the following advantages: The simplicity and reproducibility of this approach and the minimal equipment needed make it a good method when the photoelectric colorimeter is broken or not available recommend this technique. It is useful in screening prospective blood donors. This method can be used by a doctor in the office or on home calls.

Disadvantages. This method involves the following disadvantages: The cost is high. The physiologic variation from one eye to another causes inaccurate results. All optical and glass parts must be kept clean and free from dust and finger marks. Adequate light is needed for the color match; therefore, batteries must be constantly replaced, or a transformer must be used.

Acid Hematin Method

Another colorimetric technique is the acid hematin method, in which the red blood cells are laked in dilute hydrochloric acid, converting hemoglobin into acid hematin (a brownish yellow solution). This is then matched with brown standards in a colorimeter or comparator. Sahli instruments or tubes that are used are of various types—for example, Sahli-Hellige and Sahli-Haden (Haden-Hausser) instruments are not equally standardized. In this technique, the concentrated acid hematin is diluted with water until the color matches that of the glass standard. The concentration of hemoglobin in grams per 100 ml. of blood is read directly from the gram scale etched on the tube; the meniscus of the hematin suspension is used as the level for reading the concentration in grams per cent. The scale showing the percentage of normal hemoglobin should be disregarded because the amount of hemoglobin varies in normal patients depending on age, sex, climate, and other factors, and therefore no value can be arbitrarily fixed as the equivalent of 100 per cent hemoglobin.

Advantages. The advantage of this method is that it is inexpensive and simple once the instruments are standardized and the proper technique is used.

Disadvantages and Source of Error. The acid hematin method includes the following disadvantages and sources of error: The equipment must be standardized by time-consuming techniques, and expensive National Bureau of Standards 0.02 ml. pipettes must be purchased. A correction factor must be used for each particular make of Sahli tube and color standards (brown glass). If the end point is passed, the procedure must be started again from the beginning. The result may be affected by technical errors, which include the following: the collection of dirt, grease, or blood inside or outside the pipette; wet or improperly filled pipette; improper mixing of blood with acid; variability of light source in type and intensity; error in visual colorimetry with variation in rate and degree of color development of the acid hematin. Because of the last, the result must be read each time after the same interval for which the instrument was standardized. Also, nonhemoglobin substances (protein and lipids) in plasma and erythrocyte stroma influence the color of the acid hematin, which is a colloidal suspension and not a true solution.

Alkali Hematin Method

The alkali hematin technique is based on the fact that fairly strong alkali solutions produce a more homogeneous lipid and protein moiety than does the acid hematin method, and they therefore produce a more accurate solution. Also the inactive hemoglobin derivatives (carboxyhemoglobin, methemoglobin, and sulfhemoglobin) are converted to hematin solution, which reduces the error associated with their insolubility in acid solution. However, the fetal hemoglobin of newborn and young infants is alkali-resistant, producing an error when used in this group of patients. In the method proper, 5 ml. of 0.1 N NaOH is added to 0.05 ml. of blood, heated in a boiling water bath for 4 to 5 minutes, cooled, and read against a proper standard.

Oxyhemoglobin Method

In the oxyhemoglobin method, oxyhemoglobin is prepared by washing 0.02 ml. of blood into 5 ml. of copper-free glass-distilled aqueous NH_4OH solution (0.007 N) in a stoppered cuvette, and it is then shaken well to ensure proper oxygenation of hemo-globin. The solution is read in a photoelec-tric colorimeter using a green filter (540 mμ; 0.007 N NH$_4$OH is used as a blank). A standard curve is also set up.

Advantages. The oxyhemoglobin method offers the following advantages: It is accu-rate, and the test can be read within a few seconds, or if the solution is stoppered, it can be read up to 3 days later.

Disadvantages. This method includes the following disadvantages: The pipette must be rinsed three times with copper-free dis-tilled water or deionized water. If copper is present in distilled water, oxyhemoglobin may be converted to methemoglobin, and lower values may be obtained.

Cyanmethemoglobin Method

In cyanmethemoglobin method, a blood sample is diluted in a solution containing potassium ferricyanide and potassium cya-nide (Drabkin's solution). Hemoglobin, methemoglobin, and carboxyhemoglobin are converted to cyanmethemoglobin, which is measured colorimetrically. Ex-actly 0.02 ml. (use calibrated Sahli pipette) of whole blood is diluted with exactly 5 ml. (volumetric pipette) of Drabkin's solution.* Hemoglobin is oxidized to methemoglobin and then forms cyanmethemoglobin (the millimolar extinction coefficient of cyan-methemoglobin – hemoglobincyanide, cy-anferrihemoglobin – is taken to be 44.0 at 540 mμ).[10] The optical density (O.D.) of the resulting solution is then measured by using light in a spectrophotometer at a wave length of 540 mμ. The optical density is converted into the concentration of he-moglobin by using a constant determined from the optical densities of a series of stan-dards of known concentration.†

Stable standard cyanmethemoglobin so-lutions in concentrations representing

1:251 dilutions of whole blood containing 5, 10, and 15 g. per 100 ml. of hemoglobin are available commercially and can be kept in the laboratory for original calibration of the colorimeter and also for periodic checks (1–2 times monthly) of the accuracy of the instrument being used. In addition to the cyanmethemoglobin standards, one should check instrument performance and cyan-methemoglobin solutions by having an in-dependent photometric standard. In this way, if the photometric reading of the cyan-methemoglobin standard should change no-ticeably from one reading to another and if the copper ammonium sulfate independent standard has also been used, one can tell if the change in value is caused by a change in the instrument or hemoglobin.‡

In preparing Drabkin's solution, pipettes should be filled by using a suction bulb, and the blood should be mixed with the solu-tions by swirling. Proper precautions should be taken in the use of cyanide solu-tions and in cleaning any spillage that might occur.

Preparation of a Standard Curve. An auto-matic diluter or the rubber bulb tip of 5 ml. volumetric pipette is used to transfer 5 ml. of the concentrated standard to each of three large clean test tubes. The same pi-pette is used to transfer an additional 5 ml. of the concentrated standard into tube two. The pipette is carefully rinsed with the diluent. Five milliliters of the diluent solu-tion is pipetted into tube two and 10 ml. into tube three. The concentration of cyan-methemoglobin in tube one is the same as that stated on the standard solution. The concentration in tube two is $2/3$ that of the concentrated standard. The concentration of cyanmethemoglobin in tube three is $1/3$ that of the standard solution. The spec-trophotometer, previously set at 540 mμ, is turned on and allowed to warm up. The diluent is used as a blank, and the pho-tometer is set at zero on the optical density

---

* This may be purchased as Aculute (Ortho) tablets.
† This may be purchased commercially as Acuglobin (Ortho), or Hycel Cyanmethemoglobin Standard (Sci-entific Products). College of American Pathology Standards are accurate to within ±2 per cent of the stated concentration.

‡ Copper ammonium sulfate solution remains constant for 1 year when stored in tightly stoppered dark pyrex flasks.

scale. The optical density of each of the three dilutions of the standard is measured. The values are plotted on linear graph paper with the optical density readings on the ordinate and the hemoglobin in grams per 100 ml. on the abscissa. A table of optical densities and the corresponding hemoglobin concentrations may be prepared from this graph.

Technique. The automatic diluter is used to pipette 5 ml. of Drabkin's solution, which keeps well in a refrigerator for at least a week,[1] into a test tube. Blood is drawn into a Sahli pipette, the tip is wiped, and the blood is made to come exactly to the 0.02 ml. mark. The blood is blown into the Drabkin solution and the pipette is rinsed in the solution. The blood and solution are mixed thoroughly by rotation. The tube is allowed to stand 10 minutes. The spectrophotometer is set at 0 with a reagent blank of 5 ml. of Drabkin's solution.

The unknown solution is poured into the cuvette, and the optical density is read in the green region of the spectrum. The hemoglobin concentration is read from the standard curve or table. Standardization is done to develop a working curve, using prediluted standards of cyanmethemoglobin. This predilution is necessary because cyanmethemoglobin is not stable in high — that is, normal blood — concentrations, and it precipitates out if prepared at high concentration levels. The only way one can check one's measurement technique is to purchase a blood sample of known hemoglobin concentration, and to go through the entire procedure, comparing the results with the known value. One may check the instrument once a month by preparing a new standard curve.

Advantages. The cyanmethemoglobin method offers the following advantages: All forms of hemoglobin except sulfhemoglobin are quantitatively converted to cyanmethemoglobin on the addition of a single reagent. Solutions of cyanmethemoglobin are the most stable of the various hemoglobin pigments (9 months to 6 years without

deterioration). Cyanmethemoglobin solutions can be standardized accurately because the absorption band of cyanmethemoglobin in the region of 540 mμ (nm.) is broad rather than narrow, and its solutions therefore can be used in all types of photometers. The technique is rapid and reproducible in good hands; use of clean glassware, calibrated pipettes, and a standardized spectrophotometer can produce an accuracy of ± 2 to 3 per cent.

Disadvantages. This method involves the following disadvantages: Drabkin's solution prepared from commercial pellets deteriorates rapidly so that diluting fluid should be prepared fresh each day it is used. When it is prepared from reagent grade chemicals, Drabkin's solution is stable for at least 1 week, especially when kept refrigerated in a dark bottle. Cyanide is dangerous and must be used with precaution, although it would take ingestion of 4 to 6 L. of Drabkin's solution to produce a lethal dose. The spectrophotometer and pipette must be standardized accurately for the test to be accurate. Results may be erroneous in the determination of hemoglobin values in heavy smokers. In smokers, as much as 10 per cent of their hemoglobin is in the form of carboxyhemoglobin (HbCO). Hemoglobin bound with carbon monoxide takes fully an hour to convert completely to the cyanmethemoglobin form. Therefore, if blood with 10 per cent HbCO is tested by the cyanmethemoglobin method, the result would be about 15.4 instead of a correct 15, if measurements are taken 3 minutes after mixing. In 15 minutes the results would be 15.2; in 40 minutes, 15.1.

Cuvettes must be matched, clean, and dry without scratches. Cuvettes should give an identical reading each time they are used, and they must be placed in the well-housing the same way and direction each time they are used. Lipemic blood is a source of error because of turbidity produced when in solution. False high hemoglobin values may be seen in patients with easily precipitable globulins — for example, in multiple myeloma and Waldenström's macroglobulinemia. This error may be corrected by adding 0.1 g. of K_2CO_3 to 1 L. of Drabkin's solution; this increases the alkalinity of the reagent and allows the globulin to remain in solution.

Normal Values. The normal range of values of hemoglobin concentration are 14 to 18 g. per dl. in the male and 12 to 16 g. per dl. in the female.

AUTOMATIC METHODS OF HEMOGLOBIN DETERMINATION

IL Hemoglobinometer

The IL Hemoglobinometer (Model 231)* is an apparatus that utilizes a direct digital readout method for rapid measurement of hemoglobin concentration in the blood.† It is a spectrophotometric instrument containing a high precision interference filter with a narrow band width set precisely at 548.5 mμ (in the green region). This wavelength is used because here oxyhemoglobin and hemoglobin have equal absorptivity, and the absorptivity of carboxyhemoglobin is only slightly less (absorbance is linearly dependent on the hemoglobin concentration).

Examination of the front panel of the instrument reveals three important switch positions (Fig. 3-2). When the switch is in the "ON" position, all circuitry is turned on, but the pump will not run except on the automatic cleanout cycle. In the "PUMP" position the pump is always on. In the "AUTO" position, the pump is on only when the aspirating tube, which normally points slightly outward, is pushed to the vertical position. Hemoglobin determinations are made only when the switch is in the "PUMP" and "AUTO" positions. A measurement is made, when the instrument is calibrated, by mixing the blood sample well and thoroughly aspirating it into the in-

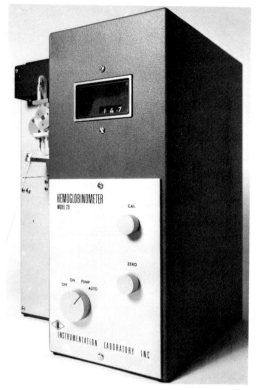

Fig. 3-2. Hemoglobinometer Model 231. (Courtesy of Instrumentation Laboratory, Inc.)

strument, when the switch is in either the "AUTO" or in the "PUMP" position.

In this method, the well mixed, unhemolyzed, whole blood sample in the collection tube is presented directly to the aspirating column of the instrument, where 100 μl. is drawn up automatically. The aspiration is continued until the digital readout gives a steady indication; this typically takes 10 to 12 seconds. During this process, an extremely accurate proportioning pump in the unit automatically dilutes—1 part blood to 10 parts diluent—and hemolyzes the sample using 1 ml. of a pH 10 buffered hemolyzing agent with a pH of 10 called Triton $\times$ 100.‡ The diluted hemolyzed blood solution then automatically flows through a cuvette, where its absorbance is measured (monitored) at 548.5 mμ(nm).

---

* Produced by Instrumentation Laboratory, Inc.
† Rosse, T. A.: Personal communication, 1967.

---

‡ Obtainable from Instrumentation Laboratory, Inc.

The current from the monitoring photo-tube is fed into a logarithmic response amplifier. This amplifier then has an output proportional to the absorbancy, which, in turn, is directly proportional to the hemoglobin concentration in the sample. The signal is then directed to an analog-digital computer for final readout on the digital counter. The sample is then removed (in the "AUTO" position the pump will stop), and the data will appear as the numerical readout on the digital counter. The next sample is aspirated, and the procedure is repeated. It is not necessary to flush the instrument between determinations.

Four separate determinations can be performed in 1 minute. Samples smaller than 100 μl. can be diluted manually, and, by bypassing the automatic system, the hemoglobin concentration can be read out on the digital counter. If one does not aspirate a sample within 30 seconds of the previous one, the pump (in the "AUTO" position) will turn on for 30 seconds to clean out the sample-handling assembly. If a sample is presented during the cleanout cycle, the cycle is automatically terminated, and begins again only after 30 seconds has passed since a sample was aspirated. The cleanout cycle is also activated 30 seconds after the switch is turned to "ON," just to ensure that no one has left a blood sample to clot in the instrument. It is considered good practice to flush the instrument with diluent after the last sample is measured. The automatic cleanout cycle prevents clots from forming because most of the blood is removed, but the best cleaning is achieved using the diluent in the sample line.

Standardization of the instrument is achieved by first aspirating a blank into the unit with the readout set to "00.0" with the "ZERO" control. A calibration dye* is then aspirated into the instrument, and the readout indication is set to the value on the label of the dye bottle, by using the "CALI-

BRATE" control. The value of the dye is set at the factory by comparing its absorbancy with that of a known hemoglobin concentration, which is determined by iron assay of washed erythrocytes with atomic absorption spectroscopy (AAS). Iron assay is used instead of the cyanmethemoglobin method because $\frac{1}{2}$ per cent accuracy is obtained with atomic absorption spectroscopy, whereas the limit of accuracy with the cyanmethemoglobin method is probably 1 per cent. For best accuracy, calibration is usually performed every 30 minutes — that is, once in every 120 determinations if one does four measurements every 1 minute. However, calibration and zero usually need only be checked every several hours. This method of standardization of the instrument has the advantage that the calibrating solution and the sample are handled in exactly the same manner.

Advantages. Use of the IL hemoglobinometer offers the following advantages: This instrument differs from conventional hemoglobin measuring systems in that it is faster—a determination is obtained in 15 seconds after sample presentation by direct digital readout. Whole blood samples are used, and therefore there is no need to convert into another type of hemoglobin by chemical means. No time-consuming aspiration and manual dilution are needed because these procedures are done automatically within the instrument. This method is therefore more economical in that it is not necessary to purchase cyanmethemoglobin or other solutions. Precision is much better than in other methods. Typical duplicates repeat within 0.1 g. per dl. of blood from hemoglobin levels of 25 g. per dl. down to zero. Full scale is 30 g. per dl. The cyanmethemoglobin method has uncertainties of about ±0.5 g. per dl. in a hemoglobin sample of 15 g. per dl. If a heavy smoker's blood is presented with 10 per cent HbCO, one would get a 14.9 g. per dl. reading using the cyanmethemoglobin method instead of the exact 15 g. per dl. This is because the absorptivity of HbCO is about 5 per cent

---

* Produced by Instrumentation Laboratory, Inc.

less than that of Hb and HbO_2. Duplicate runs do not vary more than 0.1 g. per dl. Therefore, there is much greater precision than in the cyanmethemoglobin method. The system is self-cleaning, simple, and foolproof.

Disadvantages. The only disadvantages in the use of the IL Hemoglobinometer are that the initial equipment cost is high, but not exorbitant, and occasionally the aspiration tubing becomes clogged.

AUTOMATIC ELECTRONIC BLOOD ANALYSIS

Hemalog-8 and Hemalog 8-90 (Technicon)

The Hemalog-8 is a hematology profile system that is totally automatic (Fig. 3-3). Once whole blood samples are loaded, the instrument turns out the printed results sequentially and automatically in pertinent concentration terms on a three-part pre-printed report form (Fig. 3-4). In other words, once the "OPERATE" button is pressed, the entire CBC profile, consisting of platelet count, white and red cell counts, and hemoglobin and packed cell volume (PCV or hematocrit), is printed out with virtually "hands off" operation. The three red cell indices (MCHC, MCH, and MCV) are calculated electronically from the measured parameters. Visual monitors are also provided, and the system incorporates cell-monitoring functions with appropriate visual and audio-warning signals (12 electronic alarms).

The flow system on the Hemalog-8 is depicted in diagrammatic form in Figure 3-5. On the left hand side of this diagram one sees the sampling unit which accommodates 40 EDTA anticoagulated samples in the tray. Each sample consists of 11.7 parts of whole blood added to 0.1 part of a 15 per cent K_3.EDTA solution in a 75 × 16 mm. collection tube. (A B.D. Vacutainer-Pn 4733 containing the K_3.EDTA solution can also be used). Once the sample tray is loaded, the technologist places it on the Sampler. Then by pressing the "POWER ON" push-button switch, the technologist starts the flow of pressurized reagents through the system. After approximately five minutes, the "READY" indicator lamp lights, the "OPERATE" push-button switch is pressed, and the sample probe aspirates 1.5 ml. of blood (previously mixed with a Teflon paddle) at the rate of one sample per minute. After sample aspiration, the 1.5 ml. anticoagulated whole blood sample is pumped through the stream splitter (Fig. 3-5), which provides samples for the five measurements: PBC (platelet count), WBC, RBC, HgB (hemoglobin), and the PCV. That is, the sample streams for PBC, WBCs, RBCs, and Hb are combined with their appropriate pressurized reagents and diluents before entering their respective detection devices.

For platelets, sufficient quantity of the sample is provided for a final dilution of 1:1500 in urea, which lyses the red cells; for WBCs, a final dilution of 1:100 in glacial acetic acid, which lyses the red cells takes place; and the third split is introduced into buffered saline (R-DF[1]), which dilutes the sample. This diluted mixture is then combined with Hb diluent, producing cyanmethemoglobin, which is measurable by standard colorimetric techniques. For the red cells, a further dilution in saline to 1:14,000 occurs. The PCV stream receives whole blood. The diluted streams for the PBC, WBC, and RBC tests enter through separate optical legs where cell counting is performed. The sample for the PCV passes through the manifold without dilution and enters a constantly spinning centrifuge where the cells are packed by centrifugal force (Fig. 3-6). During the cell packing process, an optical system (to be described later) constantly monitors the height of the packed red cells at the red cell buffy cost interface.

Two innovations are incorporated in the Hemalog-8 flow system. First, reagents are stored under 10 psi pressure, which determines the constant flow rate necessary for precision. A peristaltic pump is used only

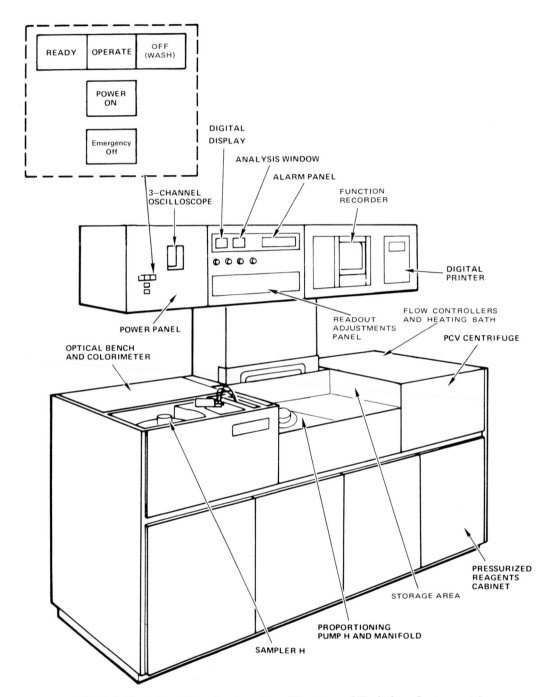

READY | OPERATE | OFF (WASH)

POWER ON

Emergency Off

DIGITAL DISPLAY

ANALYSIS WINDOW

ALARM PANEL

3-CHANNEL OSCILLOSCOPE

FUNCTION RECORDER

DIGITAL PRINTER

POWER PANEL

READOUT ADJUSTMENTS PANEL

FLOW CONTROLLERS AND HEATING BATH

PCV CENTRIFUGE

OPTICAL BENCH AND COLORIMETER

PRESSURIZED REAGENTS CABINET

STORAGE AREA

PROPORTIONING PUMP H AND MANIFOLD

SAMPLER H

Fig. 3-3. Technicon Hemalog-8 system. (Courtesy of Technicon Instruments)

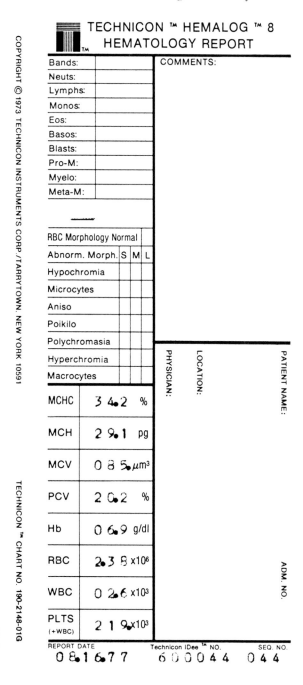

TECHNICON ™ HEMALOG ™ 8
HEMATOLOGY REPORT

Bands:	
Neuts:	
Lymphs:	
Monos:	
Eos:	
Basos:	
Blasts:	
Pro-M:	
Myelo:	
Meta-M:	

COMMENTS:

RBC Morphology Normal			
Abnorm. Morph.	S	M	L
Hypochromia			
Microcytes			
Aniso			
Poikilo			
Polychromasia			
Hyperchromia			
Macrocytes			

MCHC	3 4.2	%
MCH	2 9.1	pg
MCV	0 8 5.	µm³
PCV	2 0.2	%
Hb	0 6.9	g/dl
RBC	2.3 8	x10⁶
WBC	0 2.6	x10³
PLTS (+WBC)	2 1 9.	x10³

PHYSICIAN: LOCATION: PATIENT NAME: ADM. NO.

REPORT DATE   0 8.1 6.7 7

Technicon IDee ™ NO.   6 0 0 0 4 4

SEQ. NO.   0 4 4

Fig. 3-4. Hemalog-8 hematology report form. (Courtesy of Technicon Instruments Tarrytown, N.Y. 15091)

to aspirate the sample and pull out the waste. Second, the manifold incoporates glass tubing with periodic constrictions for improved mixing.

The counting of RBCs, WBCs, and platelets is performed in three separate chambers with filtering diaphragms for each of the counting functions. The counting principle employed is a small angle, inverse dark-field illumination of a sharply defined flow-cell view volume (Fig. 3-7). A dark-field disc prevents light from reaching the

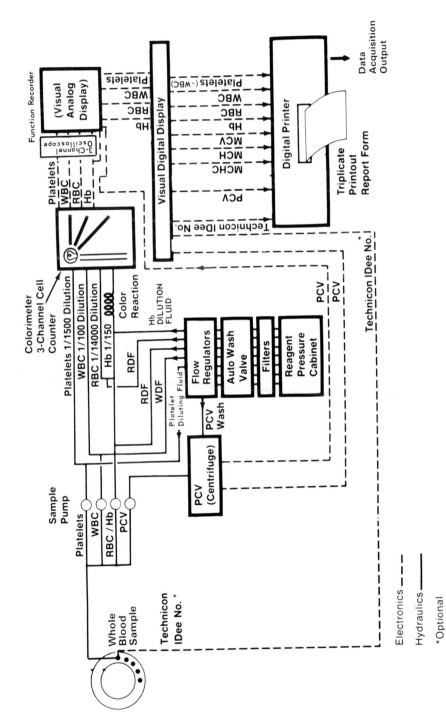

Fig. 3-5. Flowchart of structure of Hemalog-8. (Courtesy of Technicon Instruments)

Electronics — — —

Hydraulics ————

*Optional

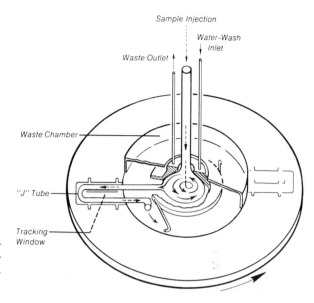

Fig. 3-6. PCV centrifuge head of Hemalog-8 centrifuge. (Courtesy of Technicon Instruments Tarrytown, N.Y. 15091)

detector except when a red blood cell, white blood cell, or platelet scatters some of the beam so that it passes around the disc. The manufacturer claims that this design reduces coincidence errors to insignificance. The sensitivity of the system enables platelet counting without separate preparation of a platelet-rich sample. However, the platelet count does include the white cell count, which is negligible when the WBC count is within normal range but which may produce errors in very high WBC levels. To prevent sample carryover and avoid clogging, the analytic channel — after efflux of each sample from the flow cell — is automatically flushed with a reverse flow-wash.

One of the most notable new features of the Hemalog-8 is the automated centrifuge hematocrit system. This involves a permanently mounted J-shaped tube which rotates continuously at about 20,000 rpm. about an axis through the top of the "J" (Fig. 3-8). When the sample valve opens, a large enough volume is injected at the top of the "J" and centrifugally forced to the base of the "J" to wash out the previously packed sample. After the sample valve

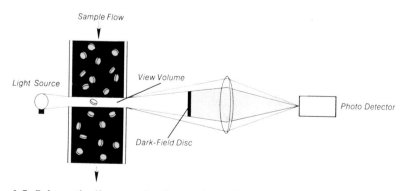

Fig. 3-7. Schematic diagram of cell counting. (Courtesy of Technicon Instruments)

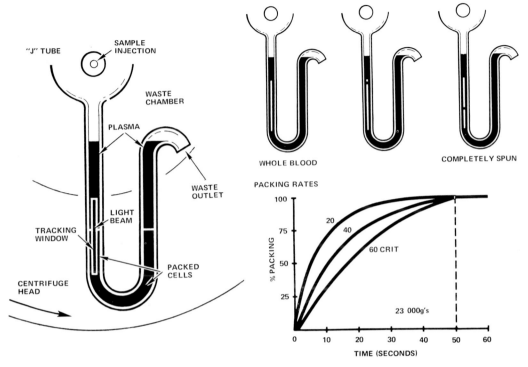

Fig. 3-8. Automated centrifuge hematocrit system of Hemalog-8. (Courtesy of Technicon Instruments)

closes and the new sample packs, an optical system detects the distance of the buffy coat-red cell interface from the base of the "J." From this, the system electronically calculates the hematocrit.

The hemoglobin determination is made by the cyanmethemoglobin method in a double-flow filter colorimeter built into one of the channels (Fig. 3-9). In order to conform to the 60-second sampling time of the Hemalog-8 system, color development of the reacting sample is catalyzed by exposure to ultraviolet light. An oscilloscope monitors the electronic counting channels; a recorder traces the functioning of all channels continuously; and a digital display of results from each test, as it is completed, is available.

As the tests are performed, the results are presented sequentially on the digital display panel. A multichannel chart recorder serves as a function monitor for the PBC, WBC, RBC, Hgb, and the PCV tests. The graphs produced allow the operator to observe and evaluate the tests in progress as the sample enters, achieves steady state, and leaves the applicable detection device. The portion of the steady-state plateau

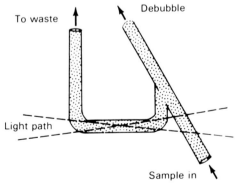

Fig. 3-9. Hemoglobin flow cell. (Courtesy of Technicon Instruments)

from which the test results are taken is identified by a notch on the curve.

The MCHC, MCH, and MCV indices are calculated by electronic counting, which utilizes the results of tests actually performed by the system as its basis. All indices are calculated using the respective Wintrobe formula:

$$MCV = \frac{Hct}{RBC}; \ MCHC = \frac{Hgb}{Hct};$$

$$MCH = \frac{Hgb}{RBC}$$

The entire profile is printed out on Z-fold report forms. The manufacturer recommends calibration of the CBC profile parameters by means of Multiple Hematology Reference II, which it can supply.

Advantages. There are a number of advantages in using the Hemalog-8. As an example of automatic electronic blood analysis, this instrument offers the advantage of automatic, rapid, simultaneous performance with particular usefulness in the inclusion of the platelet count and the lack of carryover. It is said to be free of errors of dilution and counting, and therefore its results are manifestly reproducible. Only one medical technologist is needed to operate the system. As a result, the analytical time formerly spent in separate determinations is saved, as is the clerical time that would otherwise be needed to collect data from multiple sources. The average daily opening-up procedure, which involves daily maintenance checks, preparation of references, wash cycles, and calibration takes only 30 minutes. At any time during the day from power on to accepting of samples, only 5 minutes is required, and dwell time is only $3\frac{1}{2}$ minutes. Furthermore, manual operation is very simple.

The Hemalog-8 is considered to be a reliable instrument as long as the tight maintenance of the manufacturer's service department is matched by the hospital laboratory where it will be used, and as long as meticu-

lous attention to cleanliness, which is essential for any instrument in hematology, is respected.

Built into the Hemalog-8 are mechanisms to safeguard its proper functioning. The function alarm system and the Pump Tube Leak are especially useful. In addition, an improved voltage regulator protects against low-line situations, in place of the low voltage warning system originally used. Interfacing with a laboratory computer system is now accomplished with a replaceable electronics board. As a method of hematologic quantitation of the RBC, Hgb, WBC, and platelet count, and the red-call parameters (MCV, MCHC, and MCH), the Hemalog-8 avoids the purchase of costly, breakable glassware and the cleaning that that requires, the tedium and eyestrain of microscopic quantitation, and the subjective interpretations that compromise accuracy.

Disadvantages. There are, however, several disadvantages to using the Hemalog-8. Like other automated electronic hematology cell counters and analyzers, this instrument will not be accurate with white blood cell counts over 100,000 per cu. ml. High counts must be diluted 1:2 or 1:10 with saline solution; the count is therefore multiplied by a dilution factor. Nucleated erythrocytes or platelets in very high platelet counts may be counted along with leukocytes; thus, correction must be made if they are observed in the blood film. The Hemalog-8 is unable to track hematocrit levels less than 13.5; this proves inconvenient in most general hospitals. In fact, 15 per cent of all hematocrits on electronic instruments may not be completely accurate (they should be checked with MCHC). As a result, all automated hematocrit values of 30 to 36 or below should be checked by manual centrifuge microhematocrit methods, to determine whether the indicated abnormality is due to a pathologic condition or to an abnormal plasma conductivity, when significant elevation of serum proteins is present.

Samples must initially be mixed well and

checked carefully for clots. Correlation of samples with printout and transcription of information is always open to error. This is indicative of the need for specific hematologic training in careful perusal of recording and checking of the printout. In addition, there is no easy way of obtaining results on capillary blood samples.

The working rate is only 60 samples an hour and, in view of the likelihood of downtime, this may be a problem in large laboratories. Downtime varies from short halts, due to difficulties such as occasional pump tube leaks, removal of small clots, or replacement of badly fitting reagent tops, to major halts, such as rewarming the reagent bath following accidental removal of the power supply connection or renewing the pump tube. In regard to the latter, a "PUMP TUBE LEAK" warning may be falsely activated. Experience has indicated that it is desirable to continue to pump reagents for about 5 minutes before shutdown following testing of the last sample. Occasionally, a reverse wash cycle may have to be done. Earlier manufacturer-prepared reference material for platelets tended to clump on refrigeration. A separate platelet reference stored unrefrigerated is now offered along with the reference material for the other parameters. After installation, significant replacement and service may be required during the first few months of the evaluation period. Therefore, for long-term smooth running, detailed training in the operation of the machine is necessary, and great care in maintenance is essential. For example, costly major replacement would be necessary in the event that blood was allowed to remain in the "J" tube for more than a short period. Because of the high initial cost for this equipment, many users expressed uneasiness with the use of expensive electronic printed circuit boards. There is the occasional need to change an expensive board because of the failure of a small component.

In addition, the leukocyte count should not be relied on when the differential smear shows marked lymphocytosis (from leukocytosis, chronic lymphocytic leukemia, or other causes) due to easy dissolution and breakdown of lymphocytes. Counter orifices may become plugged; therefore, cell tubes, caps, and vials should be dry, clean, and fungus- and dust-free. The machine should be checked with a background saline count daily. Since automation cell counts are slightly higher than on the hemacytometer method, both should be compared daily.

A Hemalog reference is used for hemoglobin calibration. Some workers[2] recommend using six to ten samples for standards with about 1 g. increments and starting at about 6 g. The values are determined with a spectrophotometer, by using an absorption coefficient and also by using commercially available certified cyanmethemoglobin standards. These standards are stored frozen and are prepared in amounts that last approximately 1 month. A larger volume of blood is obtained for a K, or constant; this is run with every ten specimens. A change in the percentage of transmission (T) of this sample shows instrument drift, which indicates the necessity of running a new standard curve. Some laboratories feel that Hemachrome-Fe (Uni-Tech Corp.) may take care of the objections and tediousness associated with the hemoglobin standard check just described. This preparation has been preanalyzed for total iron for use in cyanmethemoglobinometry. It is said to monitor effectively Drabkin's solution, pipettes, cuvettes, technique, and instrumentation. It is manufactured in standardized lots to provide a value specifically within the range of 48.0 to 54.8 mg. of iron or 14.2 to 18.2 g. of hemoglobin per dl. of blood.

A recent modification of the Hemalog-8 is the Hemalog 8-90, in which the speed of operation is accelerated so that 90 units per hour are counted instead of the usual 60 units per hour (Fig. 3-10). A combination instrument Technicon HS/90 system is also

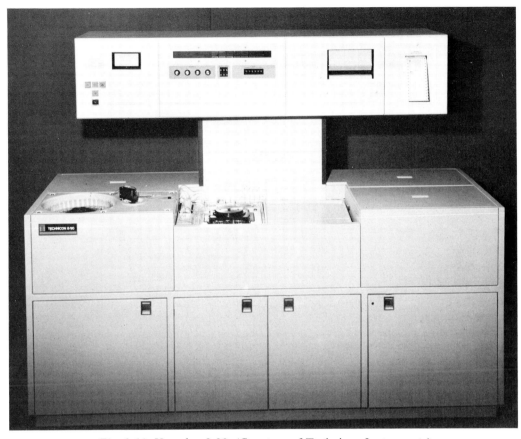

Fig. 3-10. Hemalog 8-90. (Courtesy of Technicon Instruments)

available which collates two systems, the Hemalog 8-90 (electronic counter) and the Hemalog D-90 (automated leukocyte differential counting machine). The advantages include the use of fewer reagents (25% fewer due to an increased rate) and less sample (2–5 ml.). Also, there is a dual probe, in which one probe aspirates blood for automatic electronic blood cell counting and the other probe handles the automated differential counting procedure, including fixation, staining, labeling, and dating of each slide.

Other automatic electronic cell counters include: Coulter Counter Models S and S^{SR} (Coulter), Hemac Laser Hematology Counter (Ortho Diagnostics), MK-40 and MK-3 (General Science Corp.), Hycel Counter 500 and 300 (Hycel Inc.), and Ultra Logic 800 (Clay-Adams). The first three are described on pps. 115-140.

ACCURACY OF MANUAL HEMOGLOBIN MEASUREMENTS

Some discussion has been raised concerning the accuracy and precision of manual techniques of hemoglobin measurements. Skendzel and Copeland summarized the situation by stating that most laboratories prefer to purchase a cyanmethemoglobin standard that is prepackaged and preweighed and that there has been an overall increase in the precision of hemoglobin measurements.[46] Also the value of daily control systems was demonstrated by the increased accuracy of laboratories (95% were within ±1 g,) using such control systems, and there has been a slow but steady improvement of precision in manual hemoglobin measurement. In fact, the International Committee for Standardization in Hematology in 1964 decided to increase by 2 per cent the conversion factor now used to define the U.S. standard.[7, 10] Inasmuch as the average error in optical clinical hemoglobinometry is more than 2 per cent and commercial U.S. standards need only agree within 2 per cent with the values of the reference laboratory, the contemplated 2 per cent change should occasion no concern in clinical practice.

On the other hand, Sunderman believed that iron, the metallic component of hemoglobin, should be used as a standard and not cyanmethemoglobin.[48] He further stated that iron, of certified composition, may be procured from the National Bureau of Standards, and it may then serve as a basic standard for clinical hemoglobinometry. Rice and Gambino disagreed with Sunderman.[42] Direct assay of iron by x-ray emission spectrography has presented an alternative for the determination of iron in hemoglobin.[34]

ACCURACY OF AUTOMATED HEMOGLOBIN MEASUREMENTS

Recently there has been an almost explosive development as well as widespread acceptance of automated instruments in hematology laboratories. Today less than half of the 4,600 laboratories participating in the College of American Pathologists Basic Survey use a manual cyanmethemoglobin procedure, and only 7 per cent of the 2,700 laboratories in the CAP Comprehensive Hematology Survey use this manual procedure.[24]

With the advent of automation, hemoglobinometry has continued to show improvement, particularly in the precision of the automated procedures. For example, coefficients of variation on the Coulter S instrument are of the order of 1.5 per cent nationwide, as documented in the CAP Comprehensive Hematology Survey.[23]

However, with this improved provision the question of the accuracy of the Coulter S methodologies has been raised. When comparing the performance of the Coulter S instrument with the cyanmethemoglobin procedure, an invariably consistent bias of the order of 0.3 grams per dl. in the normal range is noted. That is, when comparing the mean values for survey hemoglobin specimens measured on the Coulter S to that obtained on the manual procedure, the Coulter S measurement is invariably lower. The problem, then, is to determine which measurement is more accurate.

One logical explanation for the discrepancy is that the manual procedure calibration is straightforward; it is tentatively presumed (on the basis of the availability of a stable certified hemoglobin standard) that the mean hemoglobin level obtained by proponents of the manual procedures is correct. However, examination of the data from Coulter S users and their calibration methods reveals that less than 5 per cent of all Coulter S users calibrated their instrument using a cyanmethemoglobin procedure; the vast majority (90%) used Coulter 4C as the primary calibrator, even though this reagent is in fact a control rather than a calibrator. The relationship of Coulter 4C to a certified cyanmethemoglobin standard is a tenuous one in most cases, and it is believed by some that too much reliance has been placed on the value of this material given by the manufacturer. This becomes of extreme importance when one accepts the fact that the hemoglobin level, in particular, should be directly related to a primary standard. Therefore, one might question the accuracy of the automated Hbg instrumentation calibration procedure in those laboratories that use Coulter 4C as a calibrator rather than as a control. On the other hand, the Hbg level differences noted between manual and automated procedure could be due to a consistent bias in the laboratories using manual cyanmethemoglobin procedures. This bias would be a positive one and would require another explanation for the differences.

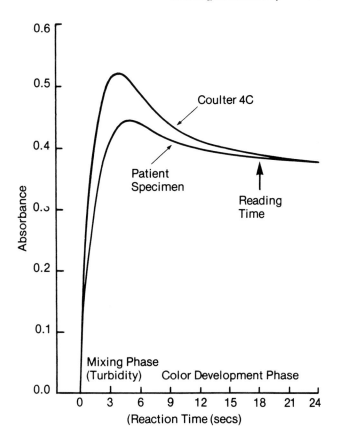

Fig. 3-11. Optical density changes in simulated Coulter S. (Courtesy of Coulter Electronics, Inc.)

An attempt at resolving the dilemma was carried out by using WHO reference methods for true hemoglobin levels on a number of the CAP Survey hemoglobin samples.[50] The results obtained indicated that the true hemoglobin level lies someplace between the mean of the methods in question. Koepke sought to explain the above by utilizing a Beckman ACTA MVI in which a flow cell was constructed that had characteristics similar to those found in the Coulter S apparatus.[23] Using the recording spectrophotometer, the experimenter determined the time (for RBCs in patient specimens and in Coulter 4C) to lyse and to come to equilibrium. This procedure of evaluation was chosen since it was thought that erythrocytes in the commercial preparations (Coulter 4C) may lyse at a somewhat slower rate due to the stabilization process of the red cell membranes. That is, if lysis of RBCs in these commercial materials occurred at a slower rate than do patient sample RBCs, the apparent hemoglobin level in all specimens subsequently measured would be somewhat higher than the true value. Therefore, there would be a tendency for specimens done on an automated machine – calibrated in this manner – to read somewhat lower. This would explain the bias noted in the CAP surveys. Since the critical measurement in the Coulter 4C is the measurement of the hemoglobin optical density by using a green filter at the 18-second time interval, when Koepke's laboratory instrumentation was used, a 3-second delay occurred in the complete RBC lysis and color development. This delay confirmed the experimenter's suspicions. In other words, if Coulter 4C is used as a calibrator, small but significant errors occur due to the delayed lysis of the stabilized RBCs (Fig. 3-11).

A possible explanation for the bias observed between the manual method and the true level of hemoglobin may be due to minor variations in the manual technique. For example, even though a calibration curve may be prepared using a spectrophotometer blanked with Drabkin's cyanmethemoglobin solution, some laboratories may use distilled water rather the Drabkin's solution for blanking the instrument. Therefore, there is an unproven possibility for a minimal positive bias in the manual measurement of hemoglobin. The Coulter S company manufacturer is now in the process of correcting such a discrepancy in order to permit the Coulter 4C to be used as an ideal calibrator rather than as a control.

In the meantime it is suggested that automated hematology instrumentation be calibrated by the procedure devised by Bull and colleagues.[6] The system, as outlined, and also as endorsed by the American Public Health Association is basically sound, and it avoids reliance on commercial materials for calibration.[5, 25, 26] The basic design of the Bull program is to use carefully measured patient specimens as secondary calibrators for the Coulter S or any other automated hematology instrument. Patient specimens are initially measured using appropriate manual techniques and, in particular, by measuring hemoglobin by the reference method. These specimens are then used tentatively to calibrate the automated hematology instrument. With this interim calibration, red cell indices are recorded on 1,000 consecutive patient specimens. The presumption is that the mean cell indices from these 1,000 patients — when they are measured in a correctly functioning and controlled, automated instrument — will agree with the generally accepted red cell indices for all people. These values should fairly closely match published data. Any significant deviations from these benchmarks indicate that the automated instrument is not accurately calibrated, and appropriate correction should be made.

This system of quality assurance takes advantage of the fact that human RBCs are inherently an internal standard. They have,

on the average, fairly precise size and hemoglobin content. These facts can then be used as the basis for an ongoing internal standard for quantitative hematology. When the final calibration of the instrument is made, the ongoing quality assurance procedure takes advantage of this internal standard by continually measuring and plotting the mean red cell indices for the quality control program. Deviations in these plots may be used as indicators of machine drift or other malfunctions. These patterns are readily identified; for example, one laboratory may analyze every group of 20 patients and when any of the mean indices of this 20-patient sample shows a significant deviation, an investigation of machine performance should be undertaken. It may be that a valve, a circuit board, a pump, or some other part of the equipment is malfunctioning. Any problem requires identification and correction before proceeding with patient samples.

Advantages. The advantages of this proposed system over the use of commercial quality control materials are: the invariability of the red cell indices when they are examined from a group (basically it is a sounder method for standardization), and this is significantly less expensive since commercial controls may cost up to several thousand dollars annually.

Disadvantages. In employing this program of quality assurance, one must purchase a desk-top programmable calculator with a capacity of about 500 programming steps and 10 storage registers, for instance, the Monroe 1860 Programmable Calculator. An interface with the Coulter S, which allows for the direct input of the Coulter data to the desk-top calculator, is commercially available.* The unit eventually generates appropriate quality assurance data without any significant amount of time required from the technologist.

An alternative to this calibration proce-

---

* S. A. Clark & Associates, P.O. Box 563, Marion, Iowa, 52302.

dure is the use of commercial materials for control but not for calibrators. Also, it is imperative that each laboratory confirm the label values on the commercial material by using its own calibrated instruments. Due to the problems with the lysis time of RBCs, as described for the Coulter instruments, even this attempt at confirmation may not be valid. However, after laboratory confirmation, these results may become secondary standards and may be used to calibrate the machine in use, but may never be used for controls on the same instrument. Other quality control materials, for example, those available in the regional multistate quality control programs, or the patient red cell indices data, may serve as appropriate quality control methodology for automated instruments. Until there are satisfactory standards for platelets or white cells, the approaches outlined by Dr. Bull appear to be the most reliable and accurate techniques for hematologic parameters.

REFERENCES

1. Barnett, R. N.: Summary report. Commission on Continuing Education (American Society of Clinical Pathology), 2:3, 1964.
2. Bell, H.: Automation in hematology—recent advances in medical technology lecture. Lawrence, University of Kansas, 1966, pp. 1-11.
3. Bonsdorff, E., and Jalavisto, E.: Humoral mechanism in anoxic erythrocytosis. Acta Physiol. Scand. 16:150, 1948.
4. Brown, T. E., and Meineke, H. A.: Presence of an active erythropoietic factor (erythropoietin) in plasma of rats after prolonged cobalt therapy. Proc. Soc. Exp. Biol. Med., 99:435, 1958.
5. Bull, B. S.: A statistical approach to quality control. *In* Lewis, S. M., and Caster, J. F., (eds.): Quality Control in Haematology. pp. 111-122. London, Academic Press, 1975.
6. Bull, B. S., Flashoff, R. M., Heilbren, D. C., and Couperus, J.: A study of various estimators for the derivation of quality control procedures from patient erythrocyte indices. Am. J. Clin. Pathol., 61:473, 1974.
7. Cannan, R. K.: Proposal for adoption of an international method and standard solution for hemoglobinometry, specifications for preparation of the standard solution and notification of availability of a reference standard solution. Am. J. Clin. Pathol., 44:207, 1965.
8. Cartwright, G. E.: Diagnostic Laboratory Hematology, ed. 3. p. 179. New York, Grune & Stratton, 1963.
9. Consolazio, C. F., Johnson, R. E., and March, E.: Metabolic Methods. p. 261. St. Louis, C. V. Mosby, 1951.
10. Eilers, R. J.: Notification of final adoption of an international method and standard solution for hemoglobinometry specifications for preparation of standard solution. Am. J. Clin. Pathol., 47:212, 1967.
11. Fisher, J. W., et al.: Localization of erythropoietin in glomeruli of sheep kidney by fluorescent antibody technique. Proc. Soc. Exp. Biol. Med., 137:327, 1971.
12. Fisher, J. W.: Erythropoietin: pharmacology, biogenesis, and control of production. Pharmacol. Rev., 24:459, 1972.
13. Gallagher, N. I., McCarthy, J. M., and Lange, R. D.: Erythropoietin production in uremic rabbits. J. Lab. Clin. Med., 57:281, 1961.
14. Gardner, F. H., and Pringle, J. C.: Androgens and erythropoiesis. Arch. Interne Med., 107:846, 1961.
15. Grant, W. C., and Root, W. S.: Fundamental stimulus for erythropoiesis. Physiol. Rev., 32:449, 1952.
16. Gray, D. F., and Erslev, A. J.: Reticulocytosis induced by serum from hypoxic animals. Proc. Soc. Exp. Biol. Med., 94:283, 1957.
17. Harris, J. W.: The Red Cell-Production, Metabolism, Destruction: Normal and Abnormal. p. 129. Cambridge, Harvard University Press, 1963.
18. Heller, P.: In vivo aging of transfused erythrocytes and 2,3-diphosphoglycerate levels [editorial comment]. Yearbook of Medicine. p. 212. Chicago, Yearbook Medical Publishers, 1974.
19. Heller, P.: pH effect on erythropoietin response to hypoxia [editorial comment]. Yearbook of Medicine. p. 216. Chicago, Yearbook Medical Publishers, 1974.
20. Jones, N. F., Payne, R. W., Hyde, R. D., and Price, T. M. L.: Renal polycythemia. Lancet, 1:299, 1960.
21. Kennedy, B. J., and Gilbertsen, A. S.: Increased erythropoiesis induced by androgenic hormone therapy. N. Engl. J. Med., 256:719, 1957.
22. Kennedy, B. J., and Gilbertsen, A. S.: Increased erythropoiesis induced by androgenic-hormone therapy. J.A.M.A., 190:104, 1964.
23. Koepke, J. A.: 1975—Intra-laboratory trials: The quarterly control survey program of the College of American Pathologists. pp. 53–68. *In* Lewis, S. M., and Caster, J. F. (eds.): Quality Control in Hematology. London, Academic Press, 1975.
24. Koepke, J. A.: The calibration of automated instruments for accuracy in hemoglobinometry. Lab World. July, 1976.
25. Koepke, J. A., Bull, B. S., Gilmer, P. R., Jr., and Goldblatt, S. A.: Quality assurance in hematology. *In* S. L. Inhorn, (ed.): Quality Assurance Practices for Health Laboratories. American Public Health Assoc. (*In press*)
26. Korpman, R. A., and Bull, B. S.: The implementation of a robust estimator of the mean for quality

control on a programmable calculator or a laboratory computer. Am. J. Clin. Pathol., 65:252, 1976.

27. Landaw, S. A., et al.: J. Clin Invest., 49:914, 1970.

28. Levy, H., Levison, V., and Schrade, A. L.: Effect of cobalt on the activity of certain enzymes in homogenates of rat tissue. Arch. Biochem. Biophys., 27:34, 1950.

29. Linman, J. W., Bethell, F. H., and Long, M. J.: Studies on the nature of the plasma erythropoietic factor(s). J. Lab. Clin. Med., 51:8, 1958.

30. Linman, J. W.: Factors controlling hemopoiesis: Erythropoietic effects of "anemic" plasma. J. Lab. Clin. Med., 59:249, 1962.

31. Linman, J. W.: Principles of Hematology. p. 18. New York, Macmillan, 1966.

32. Lynch, M. J., et al.: Medical Laboratory Technology. p. 271. Philadelphia, W. B. Saunders, 1963.

33. Malgor, L. A., and Fisher, J. W.: Effects of testosterone on erythropoietin production in isolated perfused kidneys. Am. J. Physiol., 218:1732, 1970.

34. Morningstar, D. A., Williams, G. Z., and Suutarinen, P.: The millimolar extinction coefficient of cyanmethemoglobin from direct measurements of hemoglobin iron by x-ray emission spectrography. Am. J. Clin. Pathol., 46:603, 1966.

35. Naets, J. P.: The role of the kidney in the production of the erythropoietic factor. Blood, 16:1770, 1960.

36. Page, L. B., and Culver, P. J.: Syllabus of Laboratory Examinations in Clinical Diagnosis. p. 48. Cambridge, Harvard University Press, 1960.

37. Perutz, M. F.: Stereochemistry of cooperative effects in hemoglobin. Nature, 228:726, 1970.

38. Peters, J. P., and Van Slyke, D. D.: Quantitative Clinical Chemistry II. Methods. Baltimore, Williams & Wilkins, 1932.

39. Phillips, R. A., et al.: Copper sulfate method for measuring specific gravities of whole blood and plasma. Glendale, Calif., Baxter Laboratories, 1945.

40. Powsner, E. R., and Berman, L.: Correlation of radioactive hemin formation with morphologic alterations in cultures of human bone marrow. Blood, 14:1213, 1959.

41. Reissmann, K. R.: Studies on the mechanisms of erythropoietic stimulation in parabiotic rats during hypoxia. Blood, 5:372, 1950.

42. Rice, E. W., and Gambino, S. R.: Reply to reference 30. Am. J. Clin. Pathol., 44:211, 1965.

43. Riley, R. L., Lilienthal, J. L., Jr., Proemmel, D. D., and Franke, R. E.: The relationships of oxygen, carbon dioxide and hemoglobin in the blood of man: Oxyhemoglobin dissociation under various physiological conditions. J. Clin. Invest., 25:139, 1946.

44. Rosenfield, R. E., Debrot, J., Negersmith, K. M.: Evaluation of a sequential multiple analyzer for red count, white count, hemoglobin and hematocrit. Technicon seminar paper. pp. 1-7. Sept., 1966.

45. Seip, M., Halvorsen, S., Andersen, P., and Kaada, B. R.: Effects of hypothalamic stimulation on erythropoiesis in rabbits. Scand. J. Clin. Lab. Invest., 13:553, 1961.

46. Skendzel, L. P., and Copeland, B. E.: Hemoglobin measurements in hospital laboratories. Am. J. Clin. Pathol., 44:245, 1965.

47. Stohlman, F., Jr., Rath, C. E., and Rose, J. C.: Evidence for a humoral regulation of erythropoiesis. Studies on a patient with polycythemia secondary to regional hypoxia. Blood, 9:721, 1954.

48. Sunderman, F. W.: Reply to reference 28. Am. J. Clin. Pathol., 44:212, 1965.

49. Torrance, J., et al.: Intraerythrocytic adaptation of anemia. N. Engl. J. Med., 283:65, 1970.

50. van Assendelft, O. W.: Spectrophotometry of Hemoglobin Derivatives. Assen, The Netherlands, Van Garcum & Co., 1970.

51. Wintrobe, Clinical Hematology. ed. 7. p. 102. Philadelphia, Lea & Febiger, 1974.

AUDIOVISUAL AIDS*

Hemoglobin Determination Using Cyanmethemoglobin Standards. (1965). M-769. National Medical Audiovisual Center (Annex), Station K, Atlanta, Georgia 30324.

The Iron Cycle. Marcel Bessis, M.D., Ortho Diagnostics, Raritan, New Jersey 18869.

---

* Films unless otherwise stated.

4 Hematocrit and Sedimentation Rate

HEMATOCRIT

The packed cell volume (hematocrit) is the percentage of the total volume of whole blood that is occupied by packed red blood cells when a known volume of whole blood is centrifuged at a constant speed for a constant period of time. The value thus obtained is used in the estimation of the mean corpuscular hemoglobin concentration (MCHC) and the mean corpuscular volume (MCV).

The macroscopic technique of determining the hematocrit makes use of Wintrobe hematocrit tubes calibrated from botton to top in 100 divisions (Fig. 4-1). The sample of oxalated or heparinized venous blood is thoroughly mixed by 20 to 35 slow inversions of the container. The tube is then filled to the 100 mark with blood expelled slowly from a filling pipette. The blood is introduced at the bottom of the Wintrobe tube, and the tip of the pipette is kept just below the surface of the blood as the tube is filled. The Wintrobe tube is next covered with a rubber cap and centrifuged for 30 minutes at 2260 to 2500 G or 3000 r.p.m. The bottom of the tube then contains the packed red blood cells, and on top is the buffy layer, consisting of the white blood cells and the platelets. Without shaking the specimen, one reads the number of millimeters from the bottom up, from just beneath the junction of the red blood cells and the buffy layer at the uppermost portion of the narrow black band of reduced hemoglobin. Thus,

$$\frac{\text{packed red blood cells in mm.}}{\text{whole blood specimen in mm.}(100)} \times 100 = \\ \% \text{ packed cell volume}$$

The microscopic technique (microhematocrit) utilizes so-called melting-point capillary tubes (7 cm. long × 1 mm. wide core). Commercially available dried heparin-lined tubes can be used, or tubes can be filled by capillary action with a 1:1000 dilution of commercial heparin, then placed in a 56°C drying oven or 37°C incubator until dried. They are then stored in tightly stoppered containers ready for use. Special centrifuges capable of producing 5000 to 10,000 G enable centrifugation times of 10 minutes and 5 minutes to be used (Fig. 4-2). Strumia recommends 11,000 G for 2 minutes and 28,000 G for 1 minute.

After a good, deep puncture of skin, the first two drops of blood are wiped away, and the tube is filled by capillary action to approximately 1 cm. from the end (Fig 4-3). Modeling clay (Plasticine) or the small flame of a microburner is used to seal the empty end of the tube, and a rubber gasket is attached. The filled tubes are then placed in the radial grooves of the centrifuge head with the sealed end away from the center, and the centrifuge is turned on. Because the tube is ungraduated, reasonably accurate measurement of the lengths of the columns of packed red blood cells and plasma may

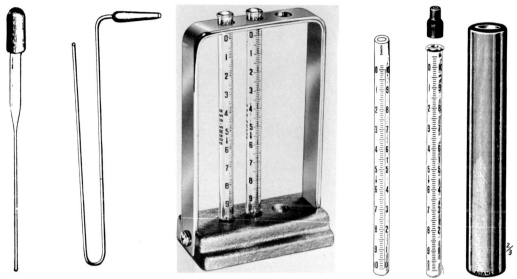

Fig. 4-1. Wintrobe hematocrit tube and accessories. (*Left to right*) Pipette, all glass; tube cleaner; Wintrobe rack; disposable Wintrobe tube; Wintrobe hematocrit and sedimentation tube with rubber cap; adapter for centrifuge shield to hold Wintrobe tube. (Courtesy of Clay-Adams, Inc.)

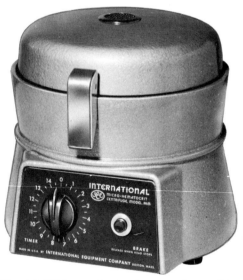

Fig. 4-2. High-speed microhematocrit centrifuge for capillary blood tubes. (Courtesy of International Equipment Co.)

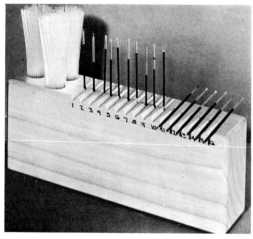

Fig. 4-3. Capillary tube holder. (Courtesy of Aloe Scientific)

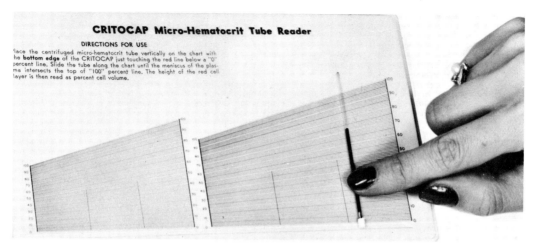

CRITOCAP Micro-Hematocrit Tube Reader

DIRECTIONS FOR USE

Place the centrifuged micro-hematocrit tube vertically on the chart with the **bottom edge** of the CRITOCAP just touching the red line below a "0" percent line. Slide the tube along the chart until the meniscus of the plasma intersects the top of "100" percent line. The height of the red cell layer is then read as percent cell volume.

Fig. 4-4. A graphic reader for the microhematocrit method. It is graduated from 0 to 100 per cent, to indicate volume of red blood cells. (Courtesy of Aloe Scientific)

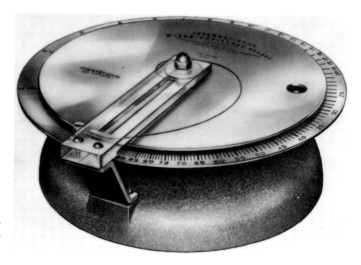

Fig. 4-5. Circular microcapillary reader. (Courtesy of International Equipment Co.)

be made by using a well-graduated millimeter rule and a low-power magnifying lens. A commercial reading device, however, is more efficient. This expresses the percentage of packed red blood cells directly from a scale without the necessity of computation (Figs. 4-4, 4-5).

The hematocrit values may also be determined by use of the automatic sequential multiple analyzer (p. 61) or the Coulter Model S. Counter (pp. 96–98). This equipment can be used automatically, rap-

idly utilizes microamounts of blood, is practically free of technician error, saves time in performance of large numbers of hematocrits, and avoids the purchase of costly, breakable glassware and the cleaning that that would require. Occasionally, the values may differ from the manual microhematocrit results; this is usually because the leukocyte count is off-scale. However, calculation of erythrocyte indices discloses the source of error.

A comparison of these macro- and micro-

Table 4-1. Normal Hematocrit Values

	Range (%)	Average (%)
Newborn	44–64	54
1 year	40–30	35
10 years	42.5–32.5	37.5
Men	40–54	47.0 (after 50 yr. = 40)
Women	37–47	42 (after 50 yr. = 37)
Pregnant women	30–40	37–39

techniques reveals that the macrotechnique can be used first to determine the erythrocyte sedimentation rate without resorting to additional techniques. This also produces more efficient separation of corpuscles into layers when the sample is ultimately centrifuged. The microhematocrit method produces a maximal packing of red blood cells, which is 2.8 per cent greater than that obtained by the macrotechnique, with a negligible value for trapped plasma. Less time is used in the microtechnique, and microcentrifuges have constant and standard performance characteristics. Also a smaller amount of blood is used, thus avoiding the need for venipuncture in shock, severe burn, and infant cases. The MCHC is higher and the MCV lower in the microtechnique.

There are several sources of error in both the macro- and microtechniques of hematocrit determination: There are sampling errors related to capillary blood (microtechnique), owing to failure to obtain free flowing blood without local pressure, excessive massage, or pressure at puncture site; edema; cyanosis; or chilling of area. Sampling errors related to venous blood (macrotechnique) may be caused by prolonged stasis due to the tourniquet, edema, cyanosis, or chilling of area; agglutination of cells or blood coagulation due to a delay in mixing with anticoagulant; inadequate amount of blood in sample; or hemolysis due to dirty or wet equipment or excessive trauma. Errors due to centrifugation result

because red blood cells must be packed optimally so that additional centrifugation does not reduce further the packed cell volume, and because trapped plasma with white blood cells and platelets may elevate the hematocrit up to 2 per cent. An increased amount of plasma trapping may be found in some anemias, especially hypochromic anemias and sickle-cell anemia.[3]

In addition, the hematocrit is unreliable immediately after even moderate loss of blood, and immediately following transfusions. The anticoagulant used must be balanced oxalate or 5 mg. of Versene per 5 ml. of whole blood. Misreading of the level of packed cells by 5 ml. may occur. Error may result from tube differences.

Normal values for hematocrit are given in Table 4–1.

The hematocrit is lowered in most anemias and in physiologic hydremia of pregnancy; it is elevated in polycythemias and hemoconcentration due to shock. The hematocrit is used mostly in determining red blood cell indices, in calculating blood volume and total red blood cell mass, and in roughly measuring the concentration of red blood cells. Additional information, such as the volume of packed white cells and platelets, may also be obtained utilizing the Wintrobe method. For example, the thickness of the layer above the packed RBCs, depends on the number of WBCs, type of WBCs, and the quantity of platelets. Smaller-sized lymphocytes and associated lymphocytosis produce a narrower layer than myeloid leukocytosis. Thrombocytopenia is associated with a narrow buffy coat, especially with associated leukopenia. The hematocrit does not measure the total red blood cell mass per se or the oxygen-carrying capacity of red blood cells.

For normal blood, the hemoglobin and erythrocyte counts may be estimated from the microhematocrit reading according to the following formulas: 1 hematocrit point = 0.34 gm. hemoglobin/100 ml. of blood. *Or* 1 hematocrit point = 107,000 red blood cells/cu.ml. of blood.

SEDIMENTATION RATE

The basic principle of the erythrocyte sedimentation rate or E.S.R. is that blood is essentially a suspension of formed elements (corpuscles) in plasma; therefore, when whole blood is mixed with an anticoagulant and placed in a perpendicular tube, the red blood cells sink because they are heavier than the plasma in which they are suspended. The speed at which the well-separated red blood cells in normal blood settle is relatively slow. However, in many diseases—for example, inflammatory, degenerative, and necrobiotic cell states—changes occur in the physicochemical properties of the plasma. These changes include alterations in the positive charge of the plasma and plasma colloids, increase in plasma fibrinogen, and variation in the concentration of plasma protein fractions and in the ratio of the differing plasma protein fractions to one another.

Changes may also occur in the erythrocyte surface; for example, a change in the surface negative electric charge of the red blood cells causes the erythrocytes to aggregate, clump, or to form rouleaux. The surface area of clumps of red blood cells is less than the total surface area of the individual erythrocytes in the tube. As a consequence of this decreased surface area, large clumps of cells fall at a faster rate. In addition, the clumping of erythrocytes produces wide spaces between the cells and cell groups, allowing the displaced plasma to rise with less retardation as the red blood cells sink. For example, there is increased clumping of erythrocytes and, therefore, an increased rate of erythrocyte fall in diseases having increased fibrinogen or globulin. Also, there is decreased erythrocyte clumping in diseases with increased albumin and, therefore, there is less of a retarding effect on the erythrocyte sinking, with subsequent slowing of the sedimentation rate.

Sequentially, then, there are three stages in erythrocyte sedimentation: the initial period of a few minutes, during which rouleau formation occurs; following this, a period of approximately 30 to 120 minutes, depending on the tube length, during which sedimentation or settling occurs at a fairly constant rate; and a period of slower rate of fall, during which packing of the sedimented red-cell column occurs. Because the sedimentation rate preparations must be set up preferably within 2 hours and not later than 6 hours after blood collection, the settling phase is the most important period. The rate becomes correspondingly reduced the longer sedimentation is delayed.

Macrotechniques

The macrotechniques are all somewhat similar. In the *Wintrobe-Landsberg method,* 5 ml. of venous blood is immediately mixed in a Wintrobe hematocrit tube containing 6 mg. of dried ammonium oxalate and 4 mg. of dried potassium oxalate. After mixing, the Wintrobe tube is filled to the 0 mark from the bottom, and the filling pipette is withdrawn as the Wintrobe tube is filled, to avoid forming air bubbles. The Wintrobe tube is placed in an exactly vertical position in a rack at room temperature. Readings are made at 15-minute intervals for 1 hour, in order to get an indication of sedimentation rate. No attempt at correction should be made, because all methods of correction for anemia are inaccurate and misleading. The *Westergren method* utilizes a pipette graduated from 0 to 200 mm. Venous blood (4.5 ml.) is mixed with 0.5 ml. of 3.8 per cent aqueous sodium citrate. The pipette is filled to the 200-mm. mark and placed in a special rack with spring clips that hold the lower end of the pipette tightly against a rubber mat in a vertical position (Fig. 4-6). In the *Rourke-Ernstene method,* heparin is used as the ideal anticoagulant, and a tube of wider lumen than the Wintrobe tube is used.

Microtechniques

In the microtechniques (Crista or Hellige-Vollmer), short, graduated tubes are used that have marks indicating proper ci-

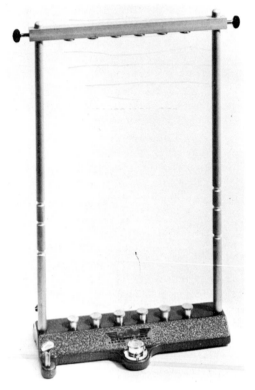

Fig. 4-6. Blood sedimentation apparatus for the Westergren method. (Courtesy of Aloe Scientific)

trate dilution. The citrate-charged pipette is allowed to fill from a skin puncture by capillary flow. The blood-citrate combination is then mixed on a celluloid plate, and the mixture is drawn up to the 0 mark. The pipette is placed in a special stand, and a reading is made after the pipette has stood for 60 minutes at room temperature.

Bull and Brailsford have described a more sophisticated and improved technique, similar to the E.S.R., which uses a new instrument, the Zetafuge.* This device augments gravitational sedimentation of erythrocytes in capillary tubes by the application of controlled centrifugation, which produces alternating compaction and dispersion of the RBCs. The tubes are placed into a plastic head, which holds them in a nearly vertical position with a slight inward

* Coulter Electronics, Inc., Hialeah, Florida 33010.

inclination. Four spin cycles at 400 r.p.m., each lasting 45 seconds, are employed. The tubes are automatically turned 180 degrees after each cycle. Figure 4-7 illustrates the zigzag path that the erythrocytes follow as the result of the procedure. The final level of RBC compaction is called the zetacrit (ZHct). A simultaneous hematocrit (Hct) value is obtained and divided by the ZHct. This ratio, expressed as a percentage, is the zeta sedimentation ratio (ZSR), that is, a ratio not of ml./hr. but of ml./dl. (vol. %). The normal range is 40 to 51 ml./dl. in both men and women. This value is related linearly to increases in fibrinogen or gamma globulin; can be done on micro quantities; is not affected by anemia; is faster than either the Westergren or Wintrobe method; can be performed on blood anticoagulated with EDTA; and need not be corrected for age, sex, or packed cell volume.[1] A brief survey comparing and contrasting the other methods is given in Table 4–2.

Sources of Error

In determining the erythrocyte sedimentation rate, errors may be introduced from several sources: The tube must be clean, dry, and free of all alcohol and ether, or else hemolysis that modifies the sedimentation may occur. An exact concentration of anticoagulant must be used (especially double oxalate). If the concentration is high, sedimentation may be slowed down or delayed. Defibrination or partial clotting with defibrination retards the sedimentation rate. The adequate mixing of specimen with anticoagulant must be ensured, and the tube must be filled accurately without bubbles. For optimal accuracy of determination, the tube diameter (2.75 to 3.25 mm.) and length (at least 100 mm.) must not vary.

In addition, the test should not be delayed more than 2 hours after the blood sample is obtained, because red blood cells tend to become spherical on standing, which makes them less inclined to form rouleau and subsequently delays sedimentation rate. The tube must not be tilted during sedimentation because an angle of as lit-

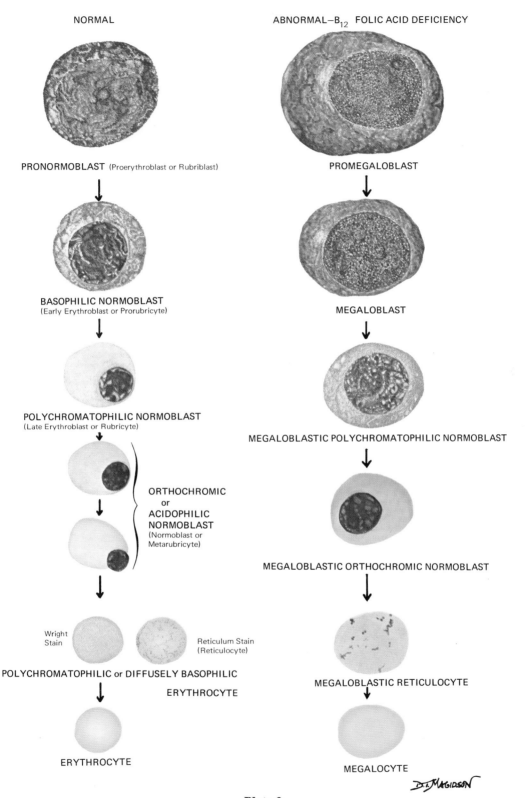

NORMAL

ABNORMAL—B$_{12}$ FOLIC ACID DEFICIENCY

PRONORMOBLAST (Proerythroblast or Rubriblast)

PROMEGALOBLAST

BASOPHILIC NORMOBLAST
(Early Erythroblast or Prorubricyte)

MEGALOBLAST

POLYCHROMATOPHILIC NORMOBLAST
(Late Erythroblast or Rubricyte)

ORTHOCHROMIC
or
ACIDOPHILIC
NORMOBLAST
(Normoblast or
Metarubricyte)

MEGALOBLASTIC POLYCHROMATOPHILIC NORMOBLAST

MEGALOBLASTIC ORTHOCHROMIC NORMOBLAST

Wright
Stain

Reticulum Stain
(Reticulocyte)

POLYCHROMATOPHILIC or DIFFUSELY BASOPHILIC

ERYTHROCYTE

MEGALOBLASTIC RETICULOCYTE

ERYTHROCYTE

MEGALOCYTE

D.L. MAGIDSON

Plate 2

SEQUENCES OF ERYTHROCYTE MATURATION

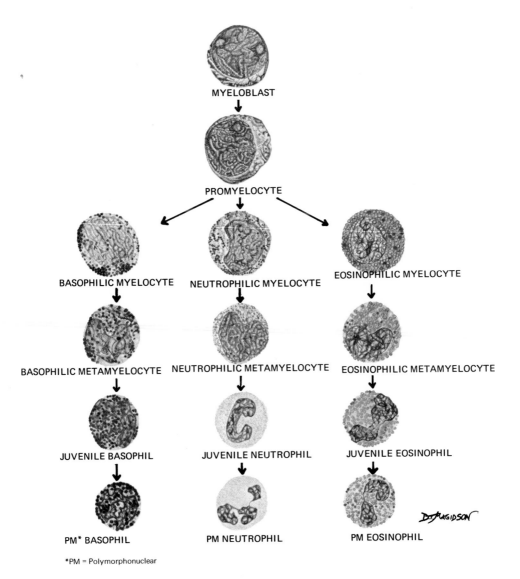

MYELOBLAST

PROMYELOCYTE

BASOPHILIC MYELOCYTE   NEUTROPHILIC MYELOCYTE   EOSINOPHILIC MYELOCYTE

BASOPHILIC METAMYELOCYTE   NEUTROPHILIC METAMYELOCYTE   EOSINOPHILIC METAMYELOCYTE

JUVENILE BASOPHIL   JUVENILE NEUTROPHIL   JUVENILE EOSINOPHIL

PM* BASOPHIL   PM NEUTROPHIL   PM EOSINOPHIL

*PM = Polymorphonuclear

Plate 3

MATURATION OF GRANULOCYTE SERIES

MATURATION OF LYMPHOCYTIC SERIES

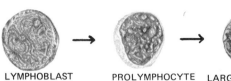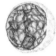

LYMPHOBLAST   PROLYMPHOCYTE   LARGE LYMPHOCYTE   INTERMEDIATE   SMALL
                (with Azure Granules)   LYMPHOCYTE   LYMPHOCYTE

MATURATION OF MONOCYTIC SERIES

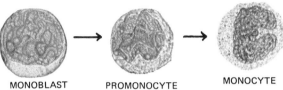

MONOBLAST   PROMONOCYTE   MONOCYTE   MONOCYTE   MONOCYTE
               (with Azure Granules)

Plate 4

MATURATION OF LYMPHOCYTE SERIES AND
MATURATION OF MONOCYTE SERIES

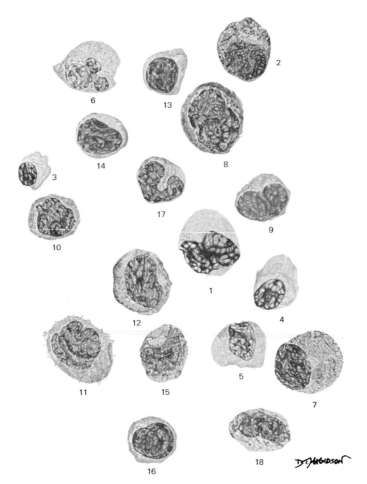

Plate 5

TYPES OF (MONONUCLEAR) LEUKOCYTES

1, Monocyte. 2, Neutrophilic myelocyte. 3, Lymphocyte. 4, Lymphocyte. 5, Monocyte. 6, Monocyte. 7, Neutrophilic myelocyte. 8, Promonocyte. 9, Lymphocyte. 10, Monocyte. 11, Monocyte. 12, Neutrophilic myelocyte. 13, Lymphocyte. 14, Lymphocyte. 15, Neutrophilic myelocyte. 16, Lymphocyte. 17, Neutrophilic metamyelocyte. 18, Neutrophilic metamyelocyte.

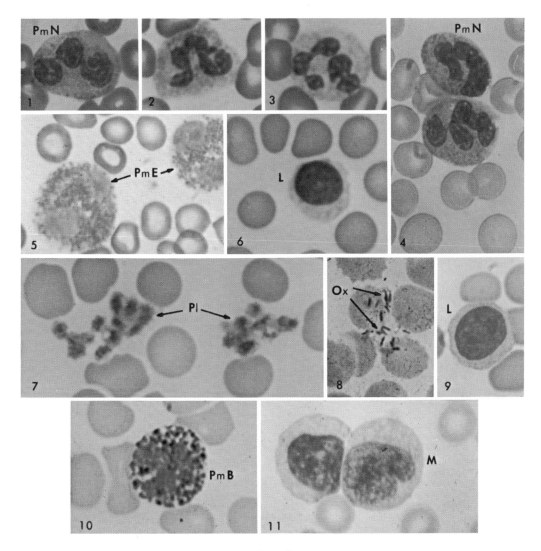

Plate 6

NORMAL BLOOD
Peripheral Blood

Lymphocytes (L), monocytes (M), oxalate crystals (anticoagulant) (Ox), polymorphonuclear basophil (PmB), polymorphonuclear eosinophil (PmE), polymorphonuclear neutrophil (PmN).

Diagnostic Features: Normally there are 50 to 70 per cent polymorphonuclear neutrophilic leukocytes (PmN), 25 to 30 per cent lymphocytes (L), 3 to 8 per cent monocytes (M), 1 to 4 per cent eosinophils (PmE), and 0 to 1 per cent basophils (PmB). Only well made blood films (Wright's stain) should be used. If the film is too thick, differentiation of cell type, especially monocytes from lymphocytes, will be very difficult; if the blood film is too thin, most of the PmNs and monocytes will be situated at the edges and tail of the blood film.

The first examination of the blood film should be made with low (× 100) or high dry magnification (× 430) to ascertain the quality of the blood film and the distribution of the WBCs. Having done this, the observer can pick out abnormal cells (e.g., normoblasts, other blast cells, plasma cells, parasites, etc.). Using the oil immersion lens one can then assess: (1) RBC size, shape and degree of hemoglobinization, presence or absence of anisocytosis, poikilocytosis, hypochromia, microcytosis, macrocytosis, polychromasia, basophilic stippling and presence of nucleated RBCs; (2) WBC maturity, atypicality, lobe quantitations in PmNs; presence or absence of toxic granulation, vacuolation, smudge and basket cells; an approximate quantitative comparative estimate of differential and total leukocyte counts; (3) Platelets—estimation of number and ratio to RBCs i.e., normal proportion of 3 to 8 platelets per 100 RBCs, also qualitative appearance and presence or absence of normal, giant or bizarre forms.

Plate 7

NORMAL BLOOD
Bone Marrow

Basophilic Myelocyte (BMc), basophilic normoblast (BNb), hemocytoblast (HcB), juvenile (Juv), lymphocyte (L), metamyelocyte (mMc), megakaryocyte (Mgk), myeloblast (Myb), neutrophilic myelocyte (NMc), orthochromic normoblast (ONb), polychromatophilic normoblast (PcNb), polymorphonuclear neutrophil (PmN), prolymphocyte (prL), promonocyte (prM), promyelocyte (prMc), pronormoblast (prNb).

Diagnostic Features: The normal film is characterized by a variegated pattern of all types of myeloid and erythroid cells which are usually present in a ratio of 4 myeloid to 1 erythroid or (4:1)

M:E. The maturation of bone marrow cells is progressive with some cells showing forms between the younger and next more mature stage. For diagnostic purposes it is not important whether the "in between" cells are placed in a younger or more mature category. The absence of a preponderance of immature cells and the presence of a variegated myeloid and erythroid pattern with a fairly normal ratio of M:E usually signifies the absence of a primary blood dyscrasia. Sufficient functioning megakaryocytes should be present without atypical nuclear and cytoplasmic patterns. Morphologically the erythrocytes should have the normal size, shape and staining qualities.

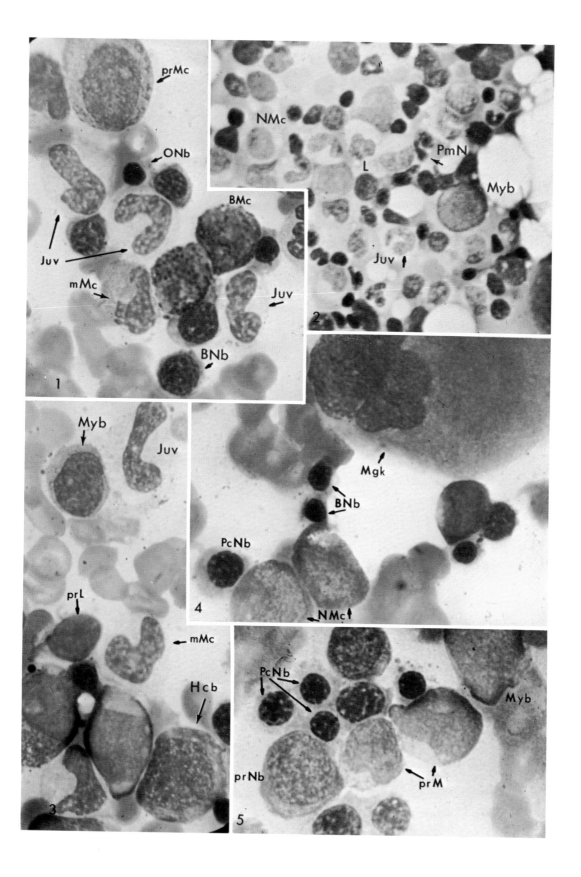

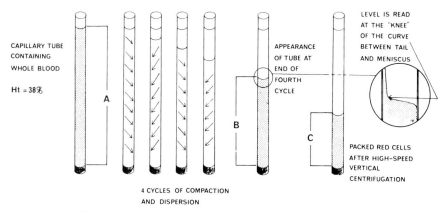

C/A % is the initial Ht (38% in this case)

C/B % is the Z.S.R. (approx. 60% in this case)
It is the Ht of the compacted blood in the portion B of the tube.

Fig. 4-7. This drawing illustrates the typical path of erythrocyte sedimentation that the Zetafuge produces. The four cycles of centrifugation alternate compaction and dispersion. The data that this process yields can be used to calculate the zeta sedimentation ratio (ZSR), which is the ratio of the hematocrit value (Hct) to the zetacrit (ZHct), or final compaction level, as a percentage. (Courtesy of Coulter Electronics, Inc.)

Table 4-2. Comparison of Methods Used to Determine Erythrocyte Sedimentation Rate

Methods	Advantages	Disadvantages
Macrotechniques		
Wintrobe-Landsberg	A simple method requiring a small amount of blood without dilution. Using the same preparation, estimation of the hematocrit, determination of microbilirubin and icterus index, and examination of smears of buffy coat can be made.	Owing to short column and use of oxalate anticoagulant, this method is not as sensitive an index of systemic disease as the Westergren method. Excess oxalate may cause sedimentation rate to appear low because oxalate retards sedimentation.
Westergren	The higher blood column of 200 mm. gives more reliable results in blood with rapid sedimentation. This method may be truly abnormal when Wintrobe is erroneously normal and is probably the most sensitive method for serial study of chronic diseases.	This method requires a large amount of blood and involves dilution with its associated sources of error. It is somewhat cumbersome and gives no more information than the Wintrobe method.
Rourke-Ernstene	This method has the most nearly linear correlation with plasma fibrinogen. Its correlation with other indicators of activity clinically has also been judged to be the most accurate.	This method is a time-consuming performance, and requires the preparation of heparin solution every few weeks.
Microtechnique Cresta or Hellige-Vollmer	Microtechniques are of value when venipuncture is impossible and blood difficult to obtain in adequate amounts, e.g., in infants, young children, and fat patients.	These are the same as those *sampling* errors associated with use of capillary blood.

Table 4-3. Normal Ranges (Average) of Erythrocyte Sedimentation Rate for 1 Hour

	Children	Men	Women
Wintrobe	5–10 mm. (1–15)	4 mm. (0–9)	10 mm. (0–20)
Westergren	—	3–5 mm. (0–9)	4–7 mm. (0–20)
Rourke-Ernstene	—	.05–0.35 mm./min.	—
Hellige-Volmer	8–10 mm. (infants)	6–8 mm.	—

tle as 3° from vertical may accelerate the sedimentation rate by as much as 30 per cent. On standing, the red blood cells aggregate along the lower side of the tube, while the plasma rises along the upper side. Consequently, the retarding influence of the rising plasma is diminished. An optimal temperature of 20° C is desirable (range 22–27° C), because sedimentation rate increases with increasing temperature. If it is necessary, the tube should be placed in a constant temperature bath of 20° C. If the blood has been kept in a refrigerator, it should be permitted to reach room temperature before the test is set up. The quantity of red blood cells in suspension affects the stability of the suspension—a decrease (anemia) in the number of red blood cells accelerates the sedimentation rate, and an increase (polycythemia) retards it. However, corrections for these may produce misleading results. In addition, anisocytosis may interfere with rouleau formation, and marked poikilocytosis, as found in sickling and pernicious anemia, may retard sedimentation.

Significance of Abnormal Values

Acceleration of the sedimentation rate (see normal ranges in Table 4–3) is a nonspecific response to tissue damage. Thus, it is only an indication of disease, and not specifically of severity. The greatest value of the E.S.R. lies in serial determinations as evidence of exacerbations or subsidence of an inflammatory process, for example, tuberculosis; subacute bacterial endocarditis; spondylitis; disseminated lupus erythematosus; rheumatic carditis; and, occasionally, neoplasia, especially when there are metastases, tumor tissue breakdown, and inflammatory tumor processes. In ectopic pregnancy, the E.S.R. remains normal until rupture of tube or detachment of embryo occurs; then it becomes rapid. The E.S.R. may be of help in differentiating myocardial infarction from angina pectoris, rheumatoid arthritis from osteoarthritis, and advanced stomach cancer from peptic ulcer. The E.S.R. is rapid in dysproteinemic states, for example, multiple myeloma.

REFERENCES

1. Bucher, W. C., Gall, E. P., and Woodworth, R.: Zeta sedimentation ratio in rheumatic disease. Am. J. Clin. Path., *64*:613, 1975.
2. Bull, B. S., and Brailsford, J. D.: The zeta sedimentation ratio. Blood, *40*:550, 1972.
3. England, J. M., et al.: Re-assessment of the reliability of the hematocrit. Br. J. Haematol., *23*:247, 1972.

AUDIOVISUAL AIDS*

Why Blood Volume. (1964). Ames Company, Division of Miles Laboratories, Inc. Elkhart, Indiana 46514.

---

* Films unless otherwise stated.

5 Maturation of Leukocytes and the Leukocyte Count

INTRODUCTION

The term leukocyte should be considered synonymous to white blood corpuscle and includes all white cells of the blood and their precursors in the blood-forming organs—myelocytic (granulocytic), lymphocytic and monocytic cells. Chemically, leukocytes are composed of water (82%), phospholipids, nucleoproteins, glycogen, lactic acid, alkaline phosphatase and other enzymes, and histamine, and traces of sodium, potassium, zinc, magnesium, calcium, chloride, inorganic phosphorus, and bicarbonate. Glycolytic metabolism in leukocytes is predominantly aerobic. Metamyelocytes and neutrophilic leukocytes, especially in infection, contain large amounts of glycogen, which is reduced in chronic myeloid leukemia and increased in polycythemia vera with leukemoid pattern. Monocytes have no glycogen. Alkaline phosphatase is elevated in neutrophils in infection, leukemoid reaction, polycythemia vera, myelofibrosis, and thrombocythemia.

Both the cell nuclei and the cytoplasm of young actively growing leukocytes contain a high concentration of nucleic acids. When these nucleic acids are attached to proteins, nucleoproteins are formed. The two most important polynucleotides are deoxyribonucleic acid (DNA) and ribonucleic acid (RNA). DNA is found in chromosomes and chromatin, is synthesized in the second half of the interphase between mitoses, and are Feulgen-positive in these structures. The nucleoli and cytoplasm (mitochondria and microsomes) contain RNA and are Feulgen-negative. Phospholipids are found mostly in neutrophilic granules, to some extent around eosinophilic granules and in monocytes. Peroxidase is found in neutrophilic granules; acid phosphatase is ten times more prevalent in neutrophils than in lymphocytes. Beta-glucuronidase is found in large amounts in neutrophils and eosinophils, but lymphocytes and leukemic cells contain little. The sulfhydryl content of leukocytes is greater than that of red blood cells and is increased in chronic myelocytic leukemia. Histamine and heparin are mostly contained in basophils with some histamine in eosinophils and neutrophils.

Leukocytes, at the time of birth, originate from a primitive stem cell or cells in the bone marrow with some production from fixed reticuloendothelial cells; in lymphoid-splenic tissue, the thymus, bone marrow (lymphocyte series); and lymphoid tissue, bone marrow, and connective tissue (monocyte series). Under abnormal conditions the reticuloendothelial cells at any tissue site may give rise to any variety of cell with occasional reversion to embryonic extramedullary blood formation in the liver and spleen.

Biologically, neutrophilic leukocytes are released from the bone marrow in response to various stimuli, and they circulate in the peripheral blood for 1 to 4 days with occasional sequestration in the liver, lungs, spleen, gastrointestinal tract, bone marrow, and striated muscle for variable periods before being destroyed. An apparent cyclic behavior of the normal blood neutrophil count (distinct from the disease, cyclic neutropenia) appears to be related to a shift of cells within the blood pools in these various loci and not to any specific physiologic periodicity.[27] Functionally, leukocytes are concerned with many different defensive and reparative activities in the body, especially in destroying invading antigens and probably in the production, or at least transportation and distribution, of antibodies. For example, because of their active ameboid locomotive properties, neutrophils are attracted by chemotaxis to areas of inflammation and bacterial proliferation (chemotaxis is the property of directional affinity in response to a liberated chemical substance), where they actively phagocytose bacteria and other foreign particles. After bacteria are ingested by neutrophils, they are destroyed by proteolytic enzymes found in their granules, after which the leukocyte itself dies and fragments into particles that are removed by phagocytes.

Among the substances chemotactic for neutrophils, activated complement components (C_{5-6}) play a major role; therefore, a defective complement system or an intrinsic neutrophil abnormality may lead to defective chemotaxis. Serum opsonins (e.g. immunoglobulins) and the cell itself are associated with bacterial recognition and, perhaps, phagocytosis; defects in the cell and in immunoglobulin can therefore be mirrored by deficient attempts at bacterial recognition and phagocytosis. In addition, specific lysosomal enzyme deficiency (e.g., peroxidase) may result in defective killing of phagocytosed organisms; the same is true of other acquired or inherited defects of cell metabolism.

Another major route of elimination of granulocytes, at least experimentally in the rat, is by removal via gastrointestinal mucosal diapedesis and by decomposition of the granulocyte in the lamina propria.[39] Eosinophils are found in increased numbers in the peripheral blood and at antigenic inflammatory loci in response to a hyperimmune or allergic reaction—for example, certain parasitic and infectious diseases and certain degenerative lesions such as polyarteritis nodosa. Basophils contain heparin, which is important in lipoprotein metabolism and in hemostasis. However, basophils have no known relationship to anticoagulation. Because basophils contain histamine, Shelley and Parnes, utilizing a new technique for absolute basophil counts, have demonstrated that a basophil count above 50/cu.mm. is a sign of allergic sensitization whereas a count below 20/cu.mm. regularly accompanies allergic reactions.[36]

Lymphocytes, according to Yoffey[42] and Rebuck,[34] migrate early and late to areas of inflammation and gradually transform to phagocytic cells with associated phagocytosis of dead bacteria and particulate debris. Lymphocytes also contribute to the formation of low concentrations of antibodies, and they possibly, by transformation to plasma cells, quickly produce large amounts.

Monocytes, like histiocytes, are derived from a primitive reticulum cell, and they circulate in certain conditions in which their macrophagic properties act specifically—for example, tuberculosis, leprosy, lipoid storage diseases, and subacute bacterial endocarditis. Some workers believe that monocytes respond to tuberculophosphatides and that their large content of lipase helps them phagocytose organisms with a lipoid capsule—for example, *Mycobacterium tuberculosis.*

However, it has been shown that monocytes have a unique sensitivity in vitro to corticosteroids, which causes them to display impaired random movement, chemotaxis, and bactericidal activity after brief exposure to low concentrations of hydrocortisone succinate.[35] Other workers showed that corticosteroid treatment of tuberculin immunized guinea pigs did not affect the transferability by lymphocytes of tuberculin sensitivity to normal recipients, but treatment of the recipients clearly affected their reactivity.[40]

Plasma cells, supposedly variants of lymphocytes, contain large amounts of gamma globulin and therefore are associated with hyperproteinemic states and in certain exanthems.

In addition, one may observe mild marrow plasmacytosis and hypergammaglobulinemia accompanying hepatic disease. This may be associated with marked proliferation of B-lymphocytes-plasmacytes which probably occurs in response to the antigenic stimulation provided by transfusion of HL-A incompatible leukocytes and platelets.[28] If the presence of plasma cells or immunoblasts (transformed lymphocytes) in the peripheral blood is suspected on clinical grounds, a smear of the buffy layer should be done. Their presence is suggestive of serum sickness, other hypersensitivity reactions, and even myeloma.

Histiocytes or reticulum cells, frequently classified as monocytes in a differential white cell count, are active phagocytes seen in certain hemolytic anemias, lymphomas, subacute bacterial endocarditis, and in certain parasitic diseases.

MATURATION OF LEUKOCYTES

Granulocyte Series (Plates 1, 3, 6, 7)

There are certain criteria for identifying cells within granulocyte series — size of cell, ratio of nucleus to cytoplasm, nuclear pattern, shape and location of nucleus, nuclear membrane, presence of nucleoli, staining reaction and structure of cytoplasm, presence of cytoplasmic granules, and type, size, and distribution of granules. Therefore, a description of blood and bone marrow cells stained with Wright's stain can best be summarized as follows (Plates 1 and 3):

1. *Stem cells (reticuloendothelial or reticulum cells)*

Size: Usually 25 to 40 μ; occasionally 10 to 15 μ, depending on the frequency of mitoses and the period of growth between cell divisions. Because they are fixed tissue cells torn away in the collection of material, their margins are irregular with blunt protoplasmic projections.

Nucleus: Round, large with finely reticulated purple-red stained nuclear chromatin.

Nucleoli: One to four, pale blue, well defined and irregular in shape; nucleus-cytoplasm ratio of 1:1.

Cytoplasm: Bluish, nongranular, with mottled or foamy structure and less deeply stained near the nucleus. Occasionally contains a few large azurophilic granules or red strands in cytoplasm.

2. *Myeloblast*

Size: 10 to 18 μ in diameter, ovoid.

Nucleus: Occupies most of cell, round or slightly ovoid with nucleus-cytoplasm ratio of approximately 6:1. It has a smooth, thin nuclear membrane with fine, reticular, evenly distributed, purplish nuclear chromatin.

Nucleoli: Two or more, distinct, ovoid, pale blue.

Cytoplasm: Very thin, deeply basophilic rim. Occasionally contains one or more red-staining rods called Auer bodies. These are also found in the monoblast but not in the lymphoblast.

3. *Progranulocyte (promyelocyte)*

Size: 12 to 20 μ, round or oval (slightly larger than myeloblast).

Nucleus: Ovoid, large, with slightly coarse clumping, light purple chromatin, especially near the nucleoli. The nucleus-cytoplasm ratio is 4:1.

Nucleoli: Two or more, less distinct, than in blast nuclei, ovoid, pale blue.

Cytoplasm: Light purple, basophilic, with few relatively large dark blue granules occasionally overlying the nucleus.

4. *Myelocyte:* No nucleoli; has granules (the myeloblast has nucleoli and no granules; the promyelocyte has nucleoli and granules).

Size: 12 to 18 μ, round or oval.

Nucleus: Round or oval, indistinct with more medium clumping of light purple chromatin than in the myeloblast or promyelocyte. The nucleus-cytoplasm ratio is approximately 2:1. The parachromatin is either blue or pink, and irregularly located.

Nucleoli: Usually absent.

Cytoplasm: Bluish pink, with early undifferentiated azurophilic granules more numerous and smaller than in the promyelocyte, or they may be differentiating into chunky orange-red (eosinophilic), blue-black (basophilic), or lilac (neutrophilic) granules, which may obscure the nuclear outline.

5. *Metamyelocyte (juvenile cell)*

Size: 10 to 18 μ, round or oval, and slightly smaller than the myelocyte. Differentiated from the myelocyte by the shape of the nucleus.

Nucleus: Indented, kidney-shaped. The nucleus-cytoplasm ratio is approximately 1.5:1.0. The nuclear chromatin is dark, purplish, and coarse or in strands.

Nucleoli: Absent.

Cytoplasm: Abundant, pinkish blue, and filled with numerous small granules (neutrophilic, eosinophilic, or basophilic).

6. *Staff cell (stab cell, band cell)*

Size: 10 to 16 μ, round or oval.

Nucleus: Maturation or condensation of its chromatin material to equal diameter bands of sausage- or horseshoe-shape with occasional areas of constriction. The nucleus-cytoplasm ratio is approximately 1:2. Nuclear chromatin is coarse and deep purple-blue.

Nucleoli: Absent.

Cytoplasm: A large amount is present, and it is pale blue or pink, with large chunky orange (eosinophilic), fine lilac (neutrophilic) or coarse large blue-black (basophilic) granules.

7. *Polymorphonuclear (segmented) granulocytes: Neutrophil, Eosinophil, and Basophil*

Size: 10 to 15 μ.

Nucleus: Those in younger cells consist of two purplish lobes separated by a thinner strand of solid, coarse nuclear chromatin; those in older cells consist of three or more lobes separated by a very thin filamentous chromatin strand. The nucleus-cytoplasm ratio is approximately 3:1. The eosinophilic and the basophilic nucleus usually have only two lobes.

Cytoplasm: Light pink to blue. The neutrophil has many small violet-pink granules; the eosinophil has large, bright yellowish-red granules; the basophil has large, coarse blue-black granules that almost completely fill the cytoplasm and frequently obscure the nucleus.

Lymphocyte Series (Plates 1, 4, 5, 6, 7)

1. *Lymphoblast:* Present normally in bone marrow on occasions but not in peripheral blood.[42]

Size: 10 to 18 μ.

Nucleus: Occupies most of the cell, round or oval. The chromatin is dark purple and aggregates along the nuclear membrane; it is coarser than in the myeloblast. The nucleus-cytoplasm ratio is 6:1.

Nucleoli: One or two indistinct light blue structures.

Cytoplasm: Deep blue with granules,

but with frequent paler perinuclear area.

2. *Prolymphocyte*

   Size: 9 to 17 μ.

   Nucleus: Ovoid, occasionally indented border. The chromatin is coarser and a darker purple and more aggregated than in the lymphoblast. The nucleus:cytoplasm ratio 4.5:1.0.

   Nucleoli: One structure, bluish.

   Cytoplasm: More than in the lymphoblast, with light to dark blue color, occasionally with azurophilic granules.

3. *Lymphocytes:* Size varies from small to large in different blood films; smaller lymphocytes seen in thick smears.

   Size: Larger lymphocytes are 8 to 16 μ; smaller ones 7 to 9 μ.

   Nucleus: Indentation is variable with otherwise rounded shape and frequently eccentrically located. Chromatin is dark purple-blue and very coarse and clumped. Parachromatin is difficult to see. The nucleus-cytoplasm ratio is 1.5 to 1.25:1.0. The nuclear membrane is sharply defined.

   Nucleoli: Absent (occasionally present).

   Cytoplasm: Light blue and varies from only a rim around the nucleus to relatively abundant amount. A perinuclear clear zone is frequent with occasional azurophilic granules in larger lymphocytes.

Monocyte Series (Plates 1, 5, 6)

1. *Monoblast:* Thought by some to be derived from myeloblasts (compare with Naegeli type of cell in monocytic leukemia). Normally not present in peripheral blood.

   Size: 12 to 20 μ.

   Nucleus: Large, round or ovoid. Light purple-pink chromatin, very fine and delicate with even and dis-

tinct nuclear membrane. The nucleus:cytoplasm ratio 1.5 to 2:1.0.

   Nucleoli: One to two.

   Cytoplasm: Deep blue without granules.

2. *Promonocyte*

   Size: 12 to 18 μ.

   Nucleus: Large lobulated to kidney-shaped. Fine, light purple, thread-like chromatin. The nucleus:cytoplasm ratio is approximately 2 to 2.5:1.0.

   Nucleoli: Zero to one.

   Cytoplasm: Gray-blue with large and small lilac-azurophilic dustlike granules.

3. *Monocyte:* Largest of normally occurring peripheral blood cells. Must be properly stained and studied in the thin part of blood films.

   Size: 12 to 16 μ

   Nucleus: Oval, notched, folded-over or horseshoe-shape. Fine lacy delicate chromatin, stains light purple-pink. The nucleus:cytoplasm ratio is approximately 2.5:1.0.

   Nucleoli: None present.

   Cytoplasm: Abundant, slate gray, with many fine lilac-colored granules.

The monocyte nucleus stains lighter than that of the metamyelocyte and prolymphocyte. Very fine lilac granules, when the cell is properly stained, also differentiate the monocyte from the metamyelocyte with its pink neutrophilic granules and the prolymphocyte and lymphocyte with their darker and occasionally chunkier azurophilic granules. The lobular, irregular, folded-over shape of the nucleus helps to differentiate the monocyte from the myelocyte with its regular, ovoid nucleus and the metamyelocyte with its slightly indented nucleus.

Plasmocyte Series (Plate 1)

1. *Plasmoblast:* Normally not present in blood and only rarely seen in normal bone marrow.

   Size: 14 to 24 μ.

Nucleus: Eccentrically placed; somewhat egg-shaped, usually in the narrower pole of the cell. The chromatin is reticulated, purplish, and relatively coarse. The nucleus:cytoplasm ratio is approximately 1:1 or 2:1.

Nucleoli: One to three large nucleoli with a blue base.

Cytoplasm: Relatively abundant; moderate to deeply basophilic with occasional areas of mottling.

2. *Proplasmocyte*

Size: 14 to 22 μ.

Nucleus: Eccentric egg to ovoid shape; purplish somewhat coarser chromatin. The nucleus:cytoplasm ratio is approximately 2:1.

Nucleoli: One to two and large.

Cytoplasm: Abundant, bright to light blue with lighter perinuclear halo frequently present.

3. *Plasmocyte (plasma cell):* Egg-shaped; narrower on one end than the other.

Size: 8 to 18 μ.

Nucleus: Ovoid, eccentrically located, usually in the small end of the cell. Chromatin is purplish, extremely coarse, and clumped with distinct sparse parachromatin. The nucleus:cytoplasm ratio is approximately 1:2.

Nucleoli: None.

Cytoplasm: Deep blue with pale perinuclear halo near one side of nucleus. Vacuoles are present near the cell border.

ENUMERATION OF LEUKOCYTES

The general principle of the hemocytometer method involves the use of an acid solution that hemolyzes the erythrocytes but does not alter leukocytes or nucleated red blood cells (with or without a nuclear staining dye). The acid solution is used to dilute blood in a special white blood cell pipette. The diluted fluid-blood mixture is placed in the hemocytometer (counting chamber), covered with a special coverglass, and allowed to settle (see pp. 38-39 for additional description). The leukocytes are then counted under the microscope. The pipette, hemocytometer, and coverglass must meet the accuracy specifications of the National Bureau of Standards, and of course must be clean before used. The cell count must be corrected to the exact leukocyte count if the blood smear shows nucleated red blood cells.

The Hemocytometer

The hemocytometer consists of a rectangular piece of thick glass that has two ruled areas in the center of the upper surface. The two ruled areas are separated from each other by moats and two raised transverse bars (see Figs. 2-5, 5-2). One transverse bar is located on each side of the ruled area. An optically corrected and standardized plane coverglass is placed on the raised bars making a depth of exactly 0.1 mm. between the lower surface of the coverglass and the surface of the ruled area. The improved hemocytometers with Neubauer ruling are preferred.

The ruled area is a square 3 mm. on a side. This square is divided first into nine squares, each 1 × 1 mm., called "large squares." Each corner of the ruled area contains a square that is 1 × 1 mm. and that is divided into 16 squares, each of which is $\frac{1}{4} \times \frac{1}{4}$ mm., and is called an "intermediate square." In the center of the ruled area is a square that is 1 × 1 mm. and is divided into 25 groups of 16 small squares each—that is, into 400 "small squares," each $\frac{1}{20} \times \frac{1}{20}$ mm. Therefore the volume above each square is:

large square = 1 × 1 × 0.1 mm. = 0.1 cu.mm. (Fig. 2-4)

intermediate square = $\frac{1}{4} \times \frac{1}{4} \times 0.1$ = 0.00625 cu.mm.

small square = $\frac{1}{20} \times \frac{1}{20} \times 0.1$ = 0.00025 cu.mm.

The volume above the entire ruled area is 3 × 3 × 0.1 mm. = 0.9 cu.mm.

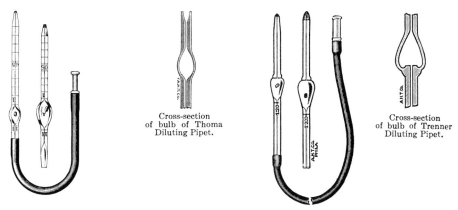

Fig. 5-1. Diluting pipettes for counting blood cells. (*Left*) Thoma pipettes and cross-section; (*right*) Trenner automatic pipettes and cross-section. (Courtesy of Arthur H. Thomas Co.)

White blood cells are counted in the four corner large squares using the lowpower objective. The count in each large square should not vary more than ten cells. The rule for including or excluding cells is to count the cells that touch the left and upper outer line and disregard the cells that touch the right and lower inner line. After use, both the counting chamber and coverglass are washed in distilled or deionized water and detergent, then water. They are then dried with a soft cloth and placed in absolute ethyl alcohol. They are dried before use again. The pipette after use, is attached to a suction cleaner through water, alcohol, and commercial ether, and it is allowed to dry.

Types of Leukocyte Diluting Pipettes

The Trenner automatic pipette has a white bead and a "21" mark above the bulb. It is made by fusing a separately made bulb on the end of a piece of straight capillary tubing, the upper end of which ends suddenly in a polished and ground surface at right angles to the longitudinal axis. The volume of the capillary tubing is exactly $1/20$ of the total volume of the bulb. It has the advantage of allowing the capillary tube to be filled by capillary attraction, with the blood automatically stopping at the end of the tube, thus providing accurate control of the blood column. However, these pipettes are more expensive and more fragile than other white blood cell pipettes (Fig. 5-1).

The Thoma pipette consists of a graduated capillary tube having a volume of one unit with calibrated markings at 0.1 unit. There is a mixing bulb containing a white glass bead located just above the capillary tube. On top of the bulb is another capillary tube with an engraved mark of "1" (Fig. 5-1).

The Unopette System* is stated to eliminate the major sources of error—those of drawing blood to a mark accurately and making an accurate dilution. The basis of this system is a self-filling, disposable glass micropipette, combined with a plastic container, and prefilled with a suitable diluent. From a single blood sample (0.013 ml.), determinations of the hemoglobin, erythrocytes, white blood cells, and platelets can be quickly and easily made (Fig. 5-2). Comparison with standard pipette counts proved to have a high index of correlation except platelet counts, which gave consistently lower results.[17]

---

* Manufactured by Becton-Dickinson & Co. of Rutherford, New Jersey.

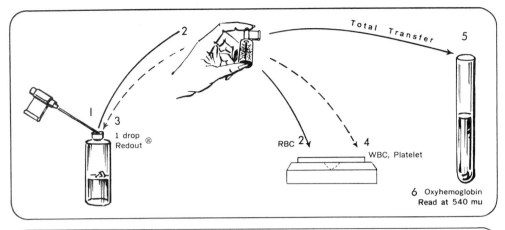

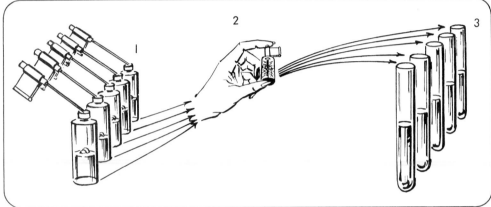

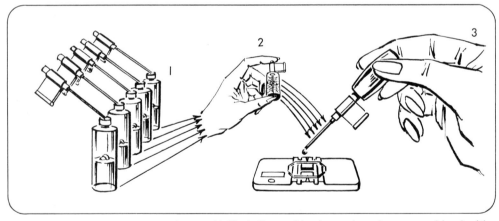

Fig. 5-2. Unopette system showing a self-filled, disposable glass micropipette, combined with a glass container, prefilled with a suitable diluent. From a single blood sample (0.013 ml.), a hemoglobin, RBC, WBC, and platelet count can be quickly and easily performed. (Manufactured by Becton-Dickinson & Co., of Rutherford, N.J.)

General Considerations

White blood cell pipettes are calibrated just like those for erythrocytes — by gravimetric or colorimetric methods (see p. 38). If there is not enough time available for calibration, it would be advantageous to purchase one set each of red blood cell pipettes and white blood cell pipettes, counting chambers, and coverglass certified by the National Bureau of Standards, using the noncalibrated pipettes for comparison with the calibrated ones.

In order to understand the final dilution in the white blood cell pipette, one must refer to a pipette while reading this description. The bottom part or stem is divided into ten parts that measure the volume or level of the blood sample column; the fifth division is marked 0.5, and the tenth is marked 1.0. The volume of the mixing bulb extends up to an 11.0 mark on the stem located above the intermediate mixing bulb. This volume is 20 times the volume of the stem at the 0.5 mark and ten times the volume at the 1.0 mark. Therefore when blood is drawn to the 0.5 mark and the diluting fluid to the 11.0 mark, the blood dilution is 1:20 and the dilution factor is 20. When blood is drawn to the 1.0 mark and the diluting fluid to the 11.0 mark, the blood dilution is 1:10 and the dilution factor is 10.

One may use a simple 2 per cent acetic acid diluting solution to lake all the red blood cells. In order to distinguish the white blood cell diluting fluid bottle from the erythrocyte diluting fluid bottle, and also in order to stain the nuclei and therefore identify better the leukocytes, Turk's solution (1 ml. of 1% aqueous gentian violet, 2 ml. glacial acetic acid, and distilled water to 100 ml.) is preferred.

The sources of error are the same as in the erythrocyte count except that the dilution factor in leukocyte counts is smaller than in the red blood cell count. This influences the error factor in that if only four large squares are counted using normal blood, there is an allowable error of ±20 per cent; if eight large squares are counted using normal blood, there is an allowable error of ±15 per cent. Thus the error decreases as the total leukocyte count and the number of cells included in the count increases. Diluting fluid contaminated with debris and impurities may also be a source of error; this can be avoided by frequent filtering of diluting fluid. If oxalated or heparinized blood is left standing too long before a count is made, the white blood cells may clump causing error. Finally, nucleated red blood cells will be counted if present, and a correction should therefore be made for this.

Computation and Reporting of Results

The technique of the leukocyte count is as follows: Blood is drawn exactly to the 0.5 mark in the white blood cell pipette. Blood adhering to the external surface of the pipette is wiped off. The 2 per cent acetic acid solution or Turk's solution is drawn up exactly to the 11 mark. The pipette is shaken in a rotor machine, preferably for 3 minutes. The first 3 to 4 drops of the mixed solution are expelled from the pipette and discarded. Both sides of the counting chamber are loaded from the one pipette. The number of white blood cells in each of the four large corner squares in each chamber is counted under low power. All the considerations of pipetting, shaking, filling the chambers, and counting described in the enumeration of red blood cells should be remembered (see p. 39).

As previously mentioned, the volume of diluted blood contained in one large square (1 × 1 × 0.1 mm.) is 0.1 cu.mm. The following formula may therefore be used for calculating the white blood cell count: Number of cells/cu.mm. = number of leukocytes counted × 1/vol. in which the cells are counted × the dilution. Eight large squares are counted (four large squares on each side of the hemacytometer), each of which has a volume of 0.1 cu.mm. Thus the volume in which the cells are counted is equal to 8 × 0.1 or 0.8 cu.mm. The dilution is 1 to 20; therefore, cell count = number of cells counted in eight large squares × 1.25 × 20, or the number of cells counted × 25% cell count/cu.mm.

If four large squares are counted, then the number of cells counted in four large squares × 2.5 × 20 or the number of cells counted × 50 = the white blood cell count/cu.mm. If the total white blood cell count is below 2500/cu.mm., the blood is drawn to the 1.0 mark (instead of the 0.5 mark) and diluted to the 11 mark. This makes a dilution of $1/10$ (instead of $1/20$). Therefore, the number of cells counted in eight large squares is then multiplied by 12.5 (instead of 25). If four large squares are counted at the dilution of $1/10$, this amount is multiplied by 25 (instead of 50). If there is marked leukocytosis (for example, in leukemia and leukemoid reactions in infections), a dilution of $1/200$ or $1/100$ is made in the red cell pipette. The number of cells counted in eight large squares is then multiplied by 250 ($1/200$ dilution) or 125 ($1/100$ dilution). The number of cells counted in four large squares is then multiplied by 500 ($1/200$ dilution) or 250 ($1/100$ dilution).

If a moderate to large number of nucleated red blood cells are present, the white blood cell count can be corrected according to the following formula:

Adjusted WBC count = observed total number of cells counted (WBC and nucleated RBC) ×

$$\frac{100}{100 + \% \text{ of nucleated RBC in blood smear}}$$

For example, if observed total cells = 25,000/cu.mm. and the blood smear shows 25 nucleated red blood cells/100 white blood cells,

the adjusted leukocyte count =

$$25,000 \times \frac{100}{100 + 25} = 200 \times 100 \text{ or } 20,000$$

$$\text{leukocytes/cu.mm.}$$

ELECTRONIC COUNTING OF BLOOD CELLS

Technical progress in hematology in the past decade has flooded the laboratory marketplace with many types of automated instrumentation.[29] Therefore, the prospective purchaser for a clinical laboratory must recognize the criteria that will enable him to make the optimal choice from the perplexing array of products offered. The following considerations are of importance in final instrument selection. Greater detail concerning the entire subject of quality control can be found at the end of this chapter.

NEEDS AND LIMITATIONS OF THE LABORATORY

A thorough review of the systems and workflow of the laboratory should be performed in order to anticipate the impact of the new procedure or instrument. For example, a small laboratory will have needs different from a large one. Or, if the laboratory work plan rotates technologists among all lab departments, then it may be desirable to choose an instrument that is easy to learn and simple to operate. Furthermore, if procedure performance may be interrupted by phone calls or "stat" specimen drawing, then instruments that do not have critical timing steps should be selected. In some institutions, the cost of an instrument may be an important consideration; anticipated volumes of test procedures should be estimated as accurately as possible for cost justification, but also for efficient management of work load.

EVALUATION OF INSTRUMENTS

The evaluation of instruments is time-consuming and, therefore, expensive. Thus, it is wise to eliminate at once instruments that cannot be afforded or used. In addition, it is best to evaluate only those instruments whose manufacturers can offer service on their product. If anything goes wrong with the procedure, will the manufacturer provide technical assistance and replacement of faulty reagents, and will orders be filled rapidly? Finally, the answers to specific questions about downtime, precision, service, and acceptance by technologists should be solicited from laboratories already using the apparatus. Documentation of precision or reproducibility and accuracy is essential.

Precision or Reproducibility

Reproducibility means that approximately the same answer on the same specimen may be obtained day after day, regardless of the person performing the test. Precision studies should be run in both normal and abnormal ranges. An unassayed commercial control can be used for this purpose. These controls should be run once a day for at least 20 days. The mean standard deviation and coefficient of variation can then be calculated. The College of American Pathologists has published some "state of the art" precision guidelines that can be used to determine acceptable coefficients of variation.[18]

Accuracy

Accuracy is very difficult to assess; recovery experiments in chemistry are one way of determining it. It can also be assessed by comparing the test method to a reference method. The reference standard may be derived from a reference laboratory, or it may be an existing standard, and instrument, in the prospective buyer's laboratory. In any case, it is necessary to do at least 40 patient comparisons, covering all ranges of expected clinical results. These determinations should be performed over a period of at least 8 working days. Graph and statistical tests can be very useful in the analysis of the data.

Graph Results. The reference method should be graphed on the x-axis and the test method on the y-axis. This is the simplest and, in most cases, the best way to demonstrate correlation between two methods. If perfect correlation were possible in the clinical laboratory, all results would fall on the 45° angle. However, marked lack of correspondence, in terms of bias and nonlinearity, will usually be readily apparent (Fig. 5-3).

Statistical Analysis. The statistical examination of data can be very helpful in making a decision about an instrument. The following formula may be used:

$$\text{coefficient of variation in per cent} = \frac{\text{standard deviation}}{\text{mean}} \times 100$$

Other factors in the selection of an instrument are the ease with which the test is done, the stability of the reagents, the time taken to perform the test, and the cost per test.

When all the data for all the instruments have been collected, a chart may be compiled that will indicate the instrument that provides the most accurate and reproducible results for the least amount of effort and investment. All data should be retained for future reference.

SEMIAUTOMATED ELECTRONIC BLOOD CELL COUNTERS

There are many types of electronic counting devices at present—Coulter, Fisher, Technicon, Hemac, MK-40, Hycel Counter 500 and 300, and Ultra Logic 800. Basically, in the Coulter Counter (model F_N; model ZBI; model ZF) blood cells are suspended in an electrolyte solution (preferably saline). This solution (a good conductor of electricity) passes through a small orifice that averages 100 μ in diameter. The individual blood cells lower the electrical conductivity of the saline solution in proportion to the size of the cell. Expressed differently, the cells, which are poor conductors, produce resistance to the current and cause a change in the voltage, which is numerically registered by the automating counter. An electronically scaled counter (transistorized models are now available)

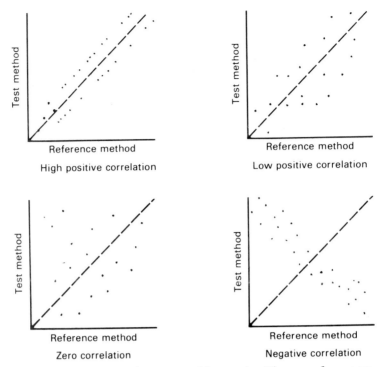

Fig. 5-3. Accuracy can be measured by graphs. There are four representative types that comparative data yield. In each case, the broken line indicates a 45° angle, which is the ideal result. The unit that is plotted on both x and y coordinates is the blood cell count.

records an impulse caused by the impedance change at the orifice. The red blood cell size can be measured by changing the electrical impulse amplitude and by an instrument modification that records the frequency distribution of cells according to size.

In the Coulter method, the automatic counter is turned on and allowed to warm up for several minutes. Two dilutions are made of the blood and a special saline diluting fluid—that is, first 0.02 ml. of oxalated, EDTA, or capillary whole blood is added to 10 ml. of special saline diluting fluid in a 15 ml. glass, capped vial. After the vial is capped, it is inverted several times. This is a 1:500 dilution for the leukocyte count. From this solution, 0.10 ml. is added to 10 ml. of saline diluting fluid in another 15 ml. glass, capped vial. After this vial is capped,

it is inverted. This is a 1:50,000 dilution for the red blood cell count.* The first leukocyte 1:500 dilution is stromatized by adding 0.1 ml. of a special saponin solution (for example, Zaponin) or Cetrimide-citrate solution.[9] Although lysis of the red blood cell takes place in seconds, this solution is allowed to stand for at least 5 to 10 minutes. Normal white blood cells remain intact in this second saponin solution for 2 hours.

A coincident table is used to correct the count because there is a probability of more than one cell simultaneously entering or passing through this 100 μ orifice. This factor is negligible for white blood cell counts, except in rare leukemic diseases in which a white blood cell count of more than 80,000

---

* A flow-through cuvette has recently been described.[9]

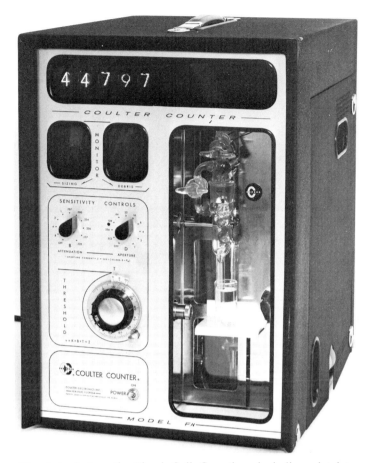

Fig. 5-4. Automatic Blood Cell Counting, including platelets. Coulter Counter Model F_N is fully transistorized and features large, easy-to-read numerical presentation. The unit employs a patented, non-optical scanning principle coupled with a twin monitoring system for dependable accuracy. The scanner measures cell volume, rather than particle shape, dual screens display oscilloscope cell size pattern and presence of any debris in aperture. Addition of Coulter MCV Compter and Hematocrit Accessory units to new or existing Coulter Counters will enable one to perform hematocrit and MCV simultaneously with routine blood cell counts. Model F_N counts cells at rates up to 6000 cells per second—up to 30 samples per hour can be processed with an accuracy of ±1% for RBC and MCV; ±3% for hematocrits and WBC. Numerical presentation of cell count is retained until Coulter Counter is "cleared" in preparation for next sample. Platelet counts can be determined with the same speed and accuracy as RBC and WBC. Other smaller size Coulter automatic blood cell counters are Models ZB1 and ZF. Basic principles for operation are very similar to the F_N. (Courtesy of Coulter Electronics, Inc.)

is reached. The red blood cell count is made by disregarding the last two digits on the digital counter, referring to the correction chart, and multiplying by 100. Because the red blood cell dilution is 1:50,000 and the sample scanned is 0.5 ml., multiplying by 100 equals the red blood cell count in millions (normal = 4 to 6.5 million/cu.mm.).

The white blood cell count is read directly from the digital counter (normal = 4 to 11,000/cu.mm.) because the dilution is 1:500 (Fig. 5-4). For red blood cell counts, the threshold is set at 10 and the aperture current setting (ACS) at 4 or 8. For white blood cell counts one may use the same figures or the threshold may be set at 19 or 20 and the ACS at 5. Coulter Counters should always be calibrated. This involves the use of an aperture current at a level where most cell peaks occupy over half the oscilloscope screen and a threshold level below all cell peaks but above the noise level. This setting must be made for all cell counts. Coulter electronics are linear with respect to function and responding threshold values. The instrument is functioning correctly as long as linearity holds.

Other additions to automated hematology are the Model F_N, ZBI, and ZF and the Model S_R Coulter Counter,[10] which reports seven hematology parameters—red blood cell count, white blood cell count, hemoglobin concentration, hematocrit, mean corpuscular volume, mean corpuscular hemoglobin, and mean corpuscular hemoglobin concentration—utilizing automatic dilution analysis. This instrument is, in reality, six entirely separate counters—three counters each for RBC and WBC. Each count is performed in triplicate with the average of three counts automatically recorded. If one of the results is in disagreement, owing to debris or other difficulties, it is automatically discarded; the average of the remaining two is taken, and the operator is alerted. If two readings disagree, a stop-system alarm is activated. A newly developed hemoglobin method utilizes cyanmethemoglobin and minimizes the effects of debris, reagent density variations, and dirty glassware.*

In the technique, blood is obtained by venipuncture or finger stick and placed in a tube attached to a card print-out. The card print-out has the patient's identification information on it (previously typed and utilizable in the IBM filing and retrieval system). After the morning or afternoon pickup, the blood tubes with attached identification cards are returned to the laboratory and placed on a Lab-Tech type of mixer. When specimens are ready to be run, the caps or stoppers are removed and the blood samples with identification cards attached are submitted to the aspirator pipette tip of the Model S Coulter Counter.† The sample bar or touch control is then pressed, at which time automatic dilution and analysis takes place. The patient identification card is placed into either of the two printers, the machine "remembering" which specimen is drawn up and which card has been submitted for printing. Recording of the data follows automatically within 15 seconds in a remote computer or on the patient card print-out. All results are clearly printed in numerical form with normal values to approximate (Fig. 5-5).

In addition to the advantages just mentioned, the instrument requires only one technologist. No flushing solutions are needed to clear the system as are required in other instruments. In addition, one may run as many samples as necessary without additional resuspension.

In the Fisher Autocytometer, a light beam is scattered by the cell particles suspended in the diluting fluid. These cell par-

---

* The fully transistorized model F_N does not perform hemoglobin determinations. However, this hemoglobin unit and the platelet technique may be added.
† Modification allows blood samples to be introduced at the rate of 3 per minute by means of the batch method. This simply means that each sample is introduced into the machine for counting and sizing, and the machine is reset after each test.

ticles subsequently flow through a narrow chamber where light flashes are recorded as electrical pulses, electronically totaled, and converted to the number of cells per cubic millimeter of original blood.

Advantages. Time is saved, and accuracy is greater. Quality control is possible by use of a standard (stabilized red and white blood cell suspensions). The results may be checked with manual methods and by correlation of results with blood smear examinations, hematocrit, and hemoglobin concentration.

Disadvantages. The Coulter, Fisher, and other counters (and possibly Technicon) are not accurate in white blood cell counts over 100,000/cu.mm. High counts must be diluted 1:2 or 1:10 with saline; the count is multiplied by the dilution factor. Nucleated erythrocytes or very high platelet counts may be counted with leukocytes so that correction must be made if they are observed in the blood film. On the Coulter Model S, the size of the aperture used to count WBCs is 100 μ, whereas the electronic threshold is set to count only those cells over 20 μ in size. In cases of extremely elevated platelet counts, changes occur which could conceivably elevate the WBC count. Therefore, if excessive platelets are observed on the stained blood film (automatic or manual differential counting), it would probably be more accurate to perform the WBC count manually. Rigid and constant standardization is required with daily hemocytometer comparisons. The equipment has a high initial cost, meticulous care is required for operation, and it is occasionally necessary to have an electronics expert available for maintenance of equipment. Error may be caused by improper and inaccurate collection and dilution, dirt, and air bubbles due to vigorous mixing of suspended cells. At least 15 seconds must be allowed to elapse after the suspension has been reshaken and the count made.

The leukocyte count should not be re-

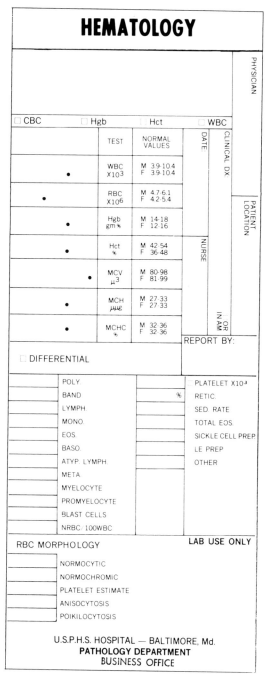

Fig. 5-5. Form on which Coulter Counter Model S records data automatically within 15 seconds. (Courtesy of Coulter Electronics, Inc.)

lied on when the differential smear shows marked lymphocytosis (leukocytosis, chronic lymphocytic leukemia, etc.), due to easy dissolution and breakdown of lymphocytes. That is, when there is marked lymphocytosis, a concomitant increase in smudge cells is seen when these fragile cells are exposed to the rigors of electronic counting machines. Utilization of a careful manual procedure for WBC counts, in these instances, would probably yield a more accurate total WBC count and differential. One might mention here that WBC counts associated with large numbers of blast cells are also best determined manually since electronic counters, especially ones like the Coulter S, enumerate blast and atypical cells on the same basis as any other WBCs.* The orifice of the Coulter and other counters may become plugged; all tubes, caps, and vials should therefore be dry, clean, and fungus- and dust-free. The counting instrument should be checked daily against a background saline count. Results from the Coulter Counter are slightly higher than those using the hemocytometer method. Both should be compared daily; EDTA or Heller-Paul solutions may be used as anticoagulants.

Pseudoleukocytosis (falsely elevated leukocyte counts) as the result of cryoglobulinemia or cryofibrinoginemia has been described.[16, 38] This condition was observed with the Coulter Counter Model S but not with the hemocytometer. Besides counting leukocytes, the Coulter S was counting some particulate material that formed as a result of either the reaction between the cryoglobulin and the fibrinogen, or spontaneous crystallization of the cryoglobulin. The cryoglobulins precipitate out of the solution on cooling and redissolve on warming. Thus, to obtain reliable leukocyte counts with the Coulter S and probably the other automated electronic blood cell counting machines, it has been recommended that blood specimens from cryoglobulinemic subjects be prewarmed to 37°C. However, recently a case was described in which pseudoleukocytosis was

exhibited even when the blood specimen was warmed to 37°C for 1 to 5 hours before being processed through the Coulter S. Further investigation revealed the presence of aggregates of apparently amorphous material (cryoglobulin, cryofibrinogen, or a mixture of the two, perhaps along with complement), which was believed to be responsible for the pseudoleukocytosis.[20] In view of these difficulties, accurate leukocyte counts have been obtained by the manual method and with the Coulter F_N when the lysing agent was added to the counting vial before the preparation of the desired blood dilution. Gulliani and co-workers deem it desirable in such cases to recommend confirmation of leukocyte counts by the manual method if a discrepancy between the Coulter S values and the counts estimated from the peripheral blood scan is discovered. It also is emphasized that cryoglobulins or cryofibrinogen may precipitate out of plasma, even at room temperature; therefore, special care is required in handling the specimens, that is, collecting the blood at 37°C, harvesting the plasma or serum immediately, and maintaining these samples or the blood specimen itself at 37°C until the desired tests are performed.

Hematocrit determinations are not accurate on all occasions, especially when automated hematocrit values are between 30 and 36 (cf. p. 67).

SEMIAUTOMATED HEMATOLOGY INSTRUMENTS

Small laboratories with their problems of relative manual cell counts are able to use semiautomated hematology instruments rather than the larger, completely automated Technicon 8 and semiautomated electronic blood cell counters. These smaller semiautomated instruments include the Clay Adams HA-4, Coulter Model ZF (similar to the F_N model) Fisher Autocytometer II, General Science MK-3$_N$, MK-4, MK-40, and MK 20/90, Hycel Counter

---

* Lewis, L.: Personal communication.

500, and Royco Cell-Crit Model 920-A. The Fisher Autocytometer II employs an electrooptical system for cell counting; the other instruments count by the cell conductivity or resistance methods. Hemoglobin is determined photometrically by the cyanmethemoglobin method in all instruments (the Royco requires its additional 720-A, which also utilizes cyanmethemoglobin methodology for hemoglobin determinations). The Coulter Z_F (with hematocrit accessory), General Science MK-3 and MK-4, and Clay Adams HA-4 calculate hematocrit from the red blood cell count and cell size (MCV). The Royco Cell-Crit Model 920 determines the hematocrit by accumulating the cell volumes of the erythrocytes counted and comparing them to the known volume of the whole blood sample; that is, there is a simultaneous hematocrit digital display on the single readout window, which indicates the count and size of the RBCs. The Fisher Autocytometer II and Hycel Counter 300 do not determine hematocrit; however, by modifying the Hycel HC-500 to the HC-300, such determination may be undertaken.

All small, nonoptic, single-channel, semiautomated hematology cell counters except for the Hycel C-500 and the Royco 920-A, employ a similar principle of electronic cell counting.[21] By means of a constant vacuum source (a mercury manometer), RBCs, WBCs, or platelets in an electrolyte solution are drawn through a small orifice (aperture) located between two electrodes (internal and external). As the cell particles pass through the aperture, they displace an equal volume of electrolyte, which produces a change in current and voltage. The number of such voltage changes per unit of time is proportional to the number of cell particles, and coincidence correction charts are used to adjust counts when more than one particle is counted. The amplitude of each change is proportional to the size (volume) of each cell. Raw cell counts are controlled by a variety of operational adjustments in current flow through the aperture, and by one or more fixed or variable electronic threshold settings to pre-screen desired cell sizes.

Since most instruments are susceptible to electrical interference, they should be grounded and should be inserted in 60-cycle, 115- to 120-volt outlets. Furthermore, they should not be located near instruments, such as most laboratory centrifuges, which have motors with brushes, for electrical arcing is then possible. Electrical interference is also caused by the flickering fluorescent lamps and by any machine or appliance utilizing a 60-cycle motor, for instance, electric clocks. Physical isolation from drafty areas is also desirable, since airborne dust particles may cause other types of interference. However, the disposal of waste from these counters does not affect their location, for their amount of waste is very low.

This verification of function and adjustment for semiautomated hematology instruments requires checking both background counts, several times daily (upon starting, in the morning, and in the afternoon), and also controls, once a day. Since a high background count is often the first sign of interference problems, background counts are done on diluent only or on diluent plus lysing agents, to establish that reagents are free of contaminating particles. Normally, these counts will be lower than 200 particles and, optimally, lower than 100. The isotonic detergents used for cleaning in most systems are as particle-free as the diluents; therefore, it is not necessary to flush the detergent before doing a background count, and, therefore, high background counts should not be blamed on leftover detergent in the system. If interference problems are common, background counts should be repeated more than twice daily. As part of the calibration checks, controls covering both normal and abnormal ranges should be run daily and recorded. Failure of the older vacuum-tube types and of the new solid-state types is usually total. Very little can happen electronically that will give high or low counts; when something in the instrument fails, either the instrument does not count at all or it gives counts so extreme that failure is immediately apparent.

Preventive maintenance is a must to keep these instruments functioning properly, and includes the following procedures: following each series of counts (e.g. Coulter) the glassware part of the system should be flushed with fresh diluent. The stopcock to the aperture of the diluent supply should be opened and fresh diluent allowed to flow into the glassware for about 10 seconds. This process prevents protein buildup on the aperture from lysed RBC debris, following WBC counts. After the counts, the aperture tip should be immersed in either clean diluent or detergent, and it should be filled with and immersed in detergent overnight. This last step is one of the most important preventive measures that can be taken, since it will ensure a clean glassware system free of problems.

In addition, the glassware system should be soaked in isotonic detergent solution at least once daily, either during a slow work period or, even better, overnight if the instrument is not being used. After rinsing the glassware system of protein accumulation, the aperture portion is then placed in a beaker of detergent and the stopcock opened until the detergent fills at least the aperture portion of the glassware (if possible, all of the glassware). With the aperture left immersed in detergent, the instrument should be allowed to soak for as long as possible. It must be remembered that the detergent solutions used with cell counters will not clean a dirty instrument, but with an initially clean instrument, these detergents will maintain cleanliness.

The vacuum pumps used on these instruments require oiling once a week. A drop or two of oil should be applied to the various oil holes on the pump, which will insure almost completely trouble-free operation. Furthermore, if the vacuum trap is inadvertently overflowed and fluid enters the vacuum pump, it is necessary to disconnect corresponding lines and, as much as possible, remove all moisture, to prevent temporary malfunctioning.

The glassware, including the aperture tube, should be disassembled and thoroughly washed (with bleach, if necessary) every 2 weeks. However, such thorough washing need not be done this often if the processes of flushing with fresh diluent and soaking in detergent solution are performed rigorously.

Rubber tubing, leading from the vacuum system to the aperture assembly, and then to the diluent reservoir, should be replaced every 6 months. The frequency of cleaning the mercury manometer is difficult to predict and will depend on both how often the instrument is used and also how clean it is kept. However, as the mercury oxidizes and becomes dark and dirty-looking, it should be cleaned, for the mercury column is responsible for starting and stopping the count. The oxidation of the mercury begins in the top reservoir in contact with the diluent, but it is not deleterious until it progresses to the lower part of the mercury column that activates the start and stop electrodes in the manometer. Eventually, the inner bore of the mercury manometer will get dirty and must be cleaned. In order to be cleaned, the manometer must be emptied and filled with soapy water and allowed to soak for about 30 minutes (this makes cleaning much easier). A vacuum should be used to draw fresh soapy water or dilute nitric acid solution (in stubborn cases) through the manometer, followed by a rinse of distilled water and acetone that causes it to dry completely. Then it should be refilled with new mercury.

In addition to these preventive techniques, it should be kept in mind that if instruments are left on, there is much less wear and tear on electric components. It is wise to leave an instrument on all day and turn it off only for extended periods, such as overnight,[19] even if it is used only a few times daily.

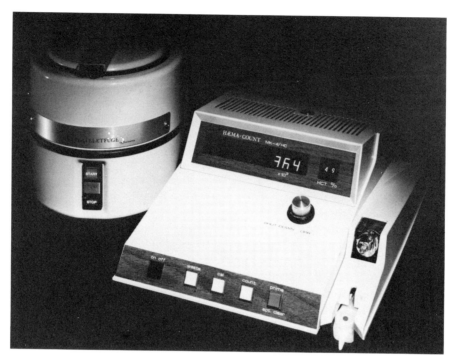

Fig. 5-6. Haema-Count MK 4/HC/plus Plateletfuge. (Courtesy of J. T. Baker Diagnostics)

Besides the small semiautomated Coulter instrument, one might mention pertinent features of some other instruments:

Haema-Count MK-3, MK-40, MK-20/90, and MK-4/4C (Fig. 5-6)

The MK-3 model combines established counting methods for particles and a standard colorimetric method for hemoglobin in a single compact package. A 25-μl. whole blood sample allows the determination of all four parameters—WBCs, RBCs, Hgb, and Hct—in about 2 minutes. A preset, dual-ratio diluter model is supplied with the system. A 1:400 dilution of the sample serves for the simultaneous WBC and Hgb determination after lysing of RBCs and release of Hgb with a stromatolytic reagent. To obtain the other pair of readings, the RBC count and Hct, a 50-μl. portion of the 1:400 diluted sample before lysing is diluted by a second factor of 1:200 for a total 1:80,000 dilution.

An electrical method may be used in counting blood cells. The cells are suspended in an electrolyte that allows current to flow between electrodes placed on opposite sides of a 100 μ. aperture. When a cell passes through the aperture, the current flow is impeded, causing an electrical pulse. These pulses are electrically counted, and the answer displayed on Nixie tubes. The Hct is electrically calculated from the RBC count and the MCV. The MCV depends on the sum of the heights of the counted pulses. This sum is also electrically determined by the instrument. The Hgb is measured by the cyanmethemoglobin method in a colorimeter cell into which the diluted sample flows after leaving the counting chamber. The double-beam colorimeter consists of a tungsten-bulb source, a color glass filter, the sample and air reference cells, and a photoconductive detector. Both the Hgb and Hct determinations are read on a front panel meter scale.

The design of the blood cell counter

hydraulic system differs in two ways from most of the systems which have been available in this country: first, the counting chamber is purged of liquid between counts and primed in a way that is intended to minimize aperture clogging; second, a photoelectric system is used to insure an accurately repeatable volume of suspension for each count. Light source and detector assemblies are located at two positions downstream from the counting chamber. Each detector is positioned at a right angle to the source. When no fluid is present, most of the light bends through the glass tube and strikes the detector. Later, when the electrolyte reaches a source and detector assembly, even more of the light goes directly through the tube, and the detector signal markedly drops. Electronic counting is initiated by the reduced signal from the first detector and is terminated by the reduced signal from the second detector. Use of timing circuits in conjunction with the photovolumetric detectors automatically alerts the operator to potentially invalid counts. If the aperture is partially blocked, the flow will be hindered, and the advancing meniscus will take longer than a preset, control time to reach the second detector. In that case, or if the meniscus advances too rapidly, a warning VERIFY light located above the count readout will flash on.

The instrument also makes recorded counts audible, and their cadence may be used to monitor operation of the system. However, the VERIFY circuit obviates the need for a subjective judgment. The major operating controls are lighted push buttons; several other features assist in correct operation of this instrument. For example, where the sample is inserted, a prime button is pressed to fill the chamber with the new sample and avoid cross-contamination. When this is done, the control corresponding to the last count measured (WBC/Hgb or RBC/Hct is illuminated as a reminder, and it stays lighted until the priming cycle is almost complete.

The hydraulics of the priming action aid in keeping the aperture clear. Then, when either the RBC/Hct or the WBC/Hgb button is pushed, additional fluid from the new sample is drawn into the chamber, and the volumetrically controlled count starts and stops automatically. At the end of the count, the answer remains on the Nixie tube readout with the appropriate scale factor illuminated, and the meter reading of either Hct or Hgb is frozen. Should a minor aperture blockage occur, it may be readily freed by simply removing the aperture and placing it over a compressed air aperture cleaner on the front of the MK-3. The front panel also has a waste-container level warning light.[2]

The Haema-Count MK-40 is a semiautomated three-module system consisting of a diluter-pipetter for preparing cell suspensions, an electrical pump, and an analyzer unit that has an electronic particle detecting aperture tube and a 540-nm. photometer for the measurement of cyanmethemoglobin. It is basically the same instrument as the MK-3, except that the coincidence correction is performed electrically, and certain changes in the rinse and prime have been made.[41]

The MK-4/HC plus Plateletfuge represents the platelet counting modification instrument.

Advantages. For each of these instruments, it takes 2 minutes to perform all four parameters, WBC, RBC, Hgb, and Hct, and uses only 25 μl. whole blood. Its VERIFY and WASTE signals avoid medical technician errors and alert the technologist to the need for cleanup procedures. Also, electronic components with increased reliability have been inserted in newer models of MK-3. It is simpler and less expensive to run than bigger, complex, and more expensive Coulter models. An evaluation study under the auspices of the product evaluation subcommittee of the College of American Pathologists proved its claims.

Disadvantages. The Hct is the least precise channel with respect to the reference method. The Hct adjustment on the Mk-40

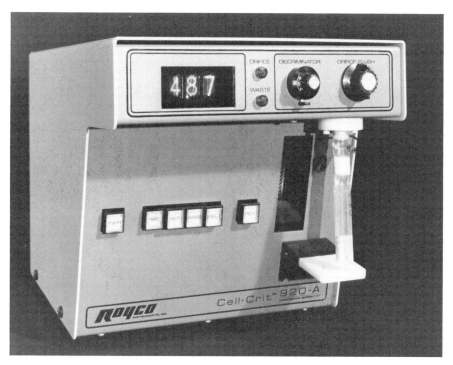

Fig. 5-7. Royco Cell-Crit Model 920-A. This instrument performs RBC, Hct, and WBC counts. (Courtesy of Royco Instruments, Inc.)

was not made to the exact Hct value of the calibrators, but rather to the Hct value that would yield the predetermined Hct to RBC ratio. Thus, the Hct calibration was not affected by a slight variation in successive RBC counts. This reduced the biases of both the Hct value and the calibrated MCV.* The priming plunger might have to be replaced in the MK-3 because of wear of the coating, although the coating in use at present is Teflon S, which may wear better. Also, the rinse and prime system in the MK-40 has been altered. Occasionally, an O-ring might have to be replaced to repair an air leak. Utilization of the 5-gallon container of the isotonic diluent (which lasts

about 1 month) is associated with a marked increase in VERIFY warnings near the end of this period. However, the use of 1-gallon containers might alleviate this difficulty. The use of a cadmium sulfide detector for photometric measurement in the hemoglobin colorimeter may be subject to nonlinearities. However, this tendency would be of concern only to the manufacturer in obtaining a linear calibration, and should never bother a user.

Royco Model 920-A With Model 720-A (Cell-Crit IV System)

The Royco Model 920-A (Fig. 5-7) counts leukocytes in a 1:500 dilution of whole blood plus three drops of lysing reagent, containing Drabkin's reagent, provided by the manufacturer. Erythrocytes and hematocrit measurements are performed in a 1:50,000 dilution in the Isoton using the Royco Model 365 Automatic Dual Dilutor. Hemoglobin measurements

---

* Discrepancies between electrically determined hematocrits (and MCVs) and those determined by centrifugation seem inevitable.[7, 12] The microhematocrit measures cell volume as the RBCs are exposed to the patient's ambient plasma osmolality. The electronic method may allow RBCs to swell or shrink as they adjust to the osmolality of the suspending medium.

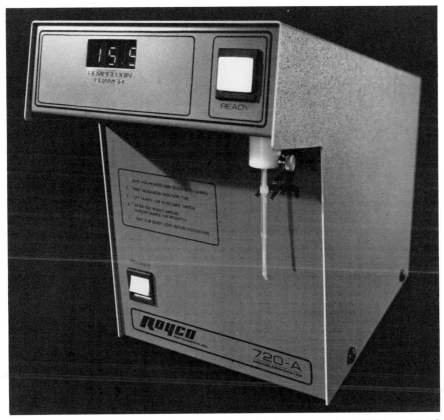

Fig. 5-8. Royco Model 720-A. With the 920-A, this instrument does RBC and WBC counts, HCT, and hemoglobin tests. (Courtesy of Royco Instruments, Inc.)

are done by the cyanmethemoglobin method on the accessory Model 720-A, utilizing the same sample as that for the WBC count. The electronic resistance detection method is used to measure the volume of each individual blood cell as it passes through a counting aperture. There is an internal electrode within the aperture tube, and an external electrode is plated on the outside of the aperture tube. When the count button is depressed, 0.5 ml. of the sample, diluted in an isotonic electrolyte solution, is drawn through a 100 μ. diameter orifice in the aperture tube. The electrical current flows to and from the electrodes, and, therefore, when a blood cell is in the orifice, the electrical resistance to the current flow increases. This change in current is electrically recorded and represents

one RBC. The accumulated total of RBCs is then digitally displayed. The hematocrit is determined by accumulating the cell volumes of the RBCs counted and comparing them to the known volume of the whole blood sample.

Instrument performance is continually monitored during the measurement. A red warning light goes on if a clog occurs in the aspiration system. A green light indicates that the instrument is ready to accept a new sample. RBC, WBC, and Hct are performed and digitally displayed on a single readout window. The Hgb is performed on the Model 720-A (Fig. 5-8), at a 540 nm. wavelength, using a flow-through cuvette with two automatic flush cycles. The reference blank is automatically set, the same sample as for the WBC count is run, with convenient calibration adjusted to the reference cyanmethemoglobin standard. No special cups or reagents are required; the sample is placed under the aspirator probe with a digital result appearing in 3 seconds. The range is for 4 to 24 g. per cent Hgb, with a resolution of 0.1 g. per cent Hgb and a precision of ±0.2 g. per cent Hgb. In all instruments used, the flow system is automatically flushed between samples. When a reverse flush knob is operated, the orifice is cleared of debris. The instrument shuts itself off should the liquid level reach the contact detectors in the waste bottle cap. Emptying the waste bottle restores power.

Calibration is performed with commercial reference material or laboratory assayed blood. It is essential that fresh human blood done by microhematocrit be used for calibration. There is a single discriminator potentiometer knob on the front of the instrument, which sets the discriminator threshold for either RBC or WBC. The RBC or WBC values are "dialed in" to agree with either the package insert of the commercial hematology control or the laboratory assayed material. The hematocrit is calibrated by using clinically assayed material referenced to a spun hematocrit. The hematocrit potentiometer calibrating knob is on the rear panel of the instrument. Coincidence correction is made for either WBC or RBC counts by charts provided by the manufacturer.

Advantages. Saline, not mercury, is used in the manometer, resulting in considerably lessened demands for the attention of the technologist, a need for less skill in instrument operation, and less downtime. Fail-safe controls (indicator lamp system) alert the operator to the existence of problems. Automatic orifice flush removes debris. Operator training is minimal; less than 1 hour of instruction is needed to train the technician. The instrument showed virtually no drift in calibration on a day-to-day basis, and RBCs, WBCs, and Hct could be measured in approximately 1 minute. The instrument is small and compact and requires a minimum of ancillary equipment. The College of American Pathologists Evaluation Subcommittee has verified the technical claims for the instrument, and found no clinically significant bias of results when they are compared to the reference method and the Coulter Model S. Also, the subcommittee noted that the coefficient of variation is within 2 per cent for RBCs, 2 per cent for the Hct, and 3 per cent for WBCs, when 10 replicate counts are performed on a single dilution of a sample in the normal range. Lastly, preventive maintenance requires fewer than 5 minutes per day.

Disadvantages. Two instruments are needed for performing counts for RBC, WBC, Hct, and Hgb. There is a slight bias in the RBC count, which is interpreted as a function of the calibration.

Hematology Analyzer HA/5 and Computer-Assisted Model Ultra-Logic 800

The Hematology Analyzer 5 (Figs. 5-9; 5-11) has two modes of operation, the WBC and Hgb mode and the RBC and Hct mode. The Ultra-Logic 800 Model (Fig. 5-10), which should be used in conjunction with the Analyzer, performs platelet counts and automatically calculates MCV, MCH, and MCHC by computer.

In the 800 Model, the computer power of a conversational microprocessor directs operator input, visualizes threshold position, determines faulty data and procedure, monitors instrument function, signals patient values beyond the expected range, and displays each instruction command or error on an alphanumeric screen. The 800 Model also performs a platelet count from 30 μl. of platelet-rich plasma in less than 1 minute.

For the determination of WBC/Hgb performance by the Hematology Analyzer 5, a diluted whole blood sample is treated with the Lysing and Hemoglobin Reagent to rupture the RBCs and release their hemoglobin. WBCs are counted electronically by passing them through an aperture; hemo-

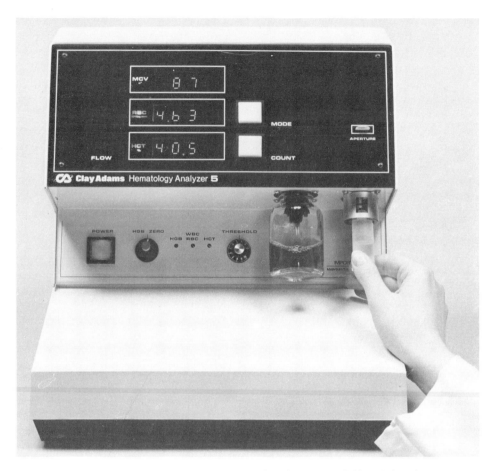

Fig. 5-9. Hematology Analyzer HA/5. (Courtesy of Clay-Adams)

globin concentration is measured optically by a dual-beam colorimeter. In the RBC/ Hct mode, the RBCs are counted elec- tronically, and total cell volume is mea- sured electronically to obtain hematocrit. Samples are drawn from a diluent reservoir into the instrument for a 20-second flow cycle. To ensure a stabilized fluid flow and representative sampling, only the final 10 seconds of the cycle are used for measure- ments. When a fresh reservoir is installed, however, the initial cycle is 30 seconds, the first 20 seconds of which are used for flow stabilization. Thereafter, on subsequent cycles for the same reservoir, timing is 10 seconds purge and 10 seconds counting. Timing cycles are performed automatically.

The Analyzer's flow system is shown in

Figure 5-11. The following description of the Analyzer's operation is based on Figure 5-11, and the numbered paragraphs refer to circled numbers on the figure. Diluted sam- ples are aspirated through the system and into a sump bottle by a vacuum pump. Samples are drawn from the diluent reser- voir through a filter (1) to remove par- ticulate matter that might clog the aperture; into a dip tube (2); through a 90-μ. diameter jewel aperture (3) mounted in a removable slide; through the optical flow cell (4); and into the sump bottle (5), which collects the spent diluted sample.

The sump system is protected from over- flow by two electrodes which project into the sump bottle. When the fluid level in the sump bottle reaches the electrodes, the

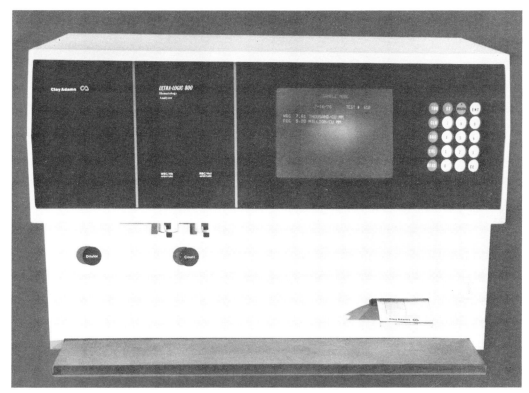

Fig. 5-10. Ultra-Logic 800. (Courtesy of (Clay-Adams)

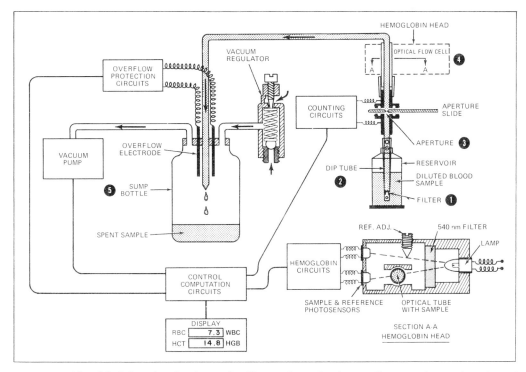

Fig. 5-11. Simplified functional scheme for Hematology Analyzer. (See text for explanation of diagram; Courtesy of Clay-Adams)

pump will not start and operation will not be possible until the bottle is emptied and the electrodes dried.

Vacuum is produced by a vacuum pump, controlled to 55 to 60 torr by a regulator. When the vacuum pump is turned off, a needle valve in the regulator allows air to bleed into the system and fluid flow stops within a few seconds.

The impedance of the aperture is monitored electronically. Air bubbles passing through the aperture or dirt particles clogging the aperture change its impedance and activate a flow interrupt indicator to produce both visual and audible alarms. The visual alarm is a FLOW Indicator light on the front panel of the instrument which lights any time during a count if flow is interrupted. The audible alarm, which operates on the same signal, is bypassed during the purge phase of the count cycle; it is operable only during the last 10 seconds of the count cycle. The volume and sensitivity of the audible alarm may be adjusted with a screwdriver in the back of the instrument. *Note:* Occasionally, the FLOW Interrupt Indicators may flicker on and off sporadically during a count cycle. This is due to their extreme sensitivity and may not be cause for discarding the reading.

Blood cells are poor electrical conductors, while the diluent in which they are suspended is a good conductor. When a blood cell is in the aperture, the electrical resistance across the aperture is increased. This change in resistance is detected by electrodes above and below the aperture. The electrodes are connected to solid-state circuitry, which produces an electrical pulse for each cell passing through the aperture. These pulses are amplified and processed into constant amplitude square waves, each wave having a pulse width which is function of cell velocity through the aperture. The output of the signal processor circuit is then totalized by integration in increments which are converted to proper units on the digital display. The readout indicates RBCs in millions of cells

per cubic millimeter and WBCs in thousands of cells per cubic millimeter.

The measurement of HCT is also a counting process in the Hematology Analyzer. Since hematocrit may be defined as the RBC count multiplied by the MCV, the Analyzer uses the RBC count it has already established to determine HCT. The physical phenomena of the aperture detector result in pulses that have an amplitude proportional to cell volume. In the determination of HCT, each square wave pulse used in counting RBCs is simply multiplied by a factor which is proportional to the cell volume as defined by: $RBC \times MCV = HCT \times 10$. The square wave pulses now of variable amplitude proportional to cell volume are totalized and displayed on the digital readout in the same manner as RBC and WBC.

The Hematology Analyzer automatically corrects cell counts for variations in fluid viscosities and vacuum levels. This is accomplished by weighting each cell pulse as a function of the cell's transient time in the aperture. Changes in aperture area are still important, and, therefore, the aperture must always be kept clean.

The pulse processing circuitry also provides Automatic Coincidence Correction. Depending upon how closely two cells pass through the aperture, they are counted either as two cells, three cells, or one cell (total coincidence condition).

By integrating all output pulses generated by single cells and coincident cells over the total 10-second counting cycle, the Analyzer automatically calculates coincidence-corrected WBC, RBC, and HCT values.

A timer automatically controls aspiration of the sample and synchronizes the counting circuits. The following events occur after depressing the count button: The vacuum pump is turned on to purge the flow system and to establish proper flow conditions. The system automatically performs an initial purge cycle of 20 seconds after installing a reservoir. Thereafter, for that reservoir, the normal purge cycle is 10 seconds. Immediately following the purge cycle, the counting circuits are operated for 10 seconds, during which time approximately 0.25 ml. of sample is aspirated and assayed. The vacuum pump is shut off to stop the flow of sample from the reservoir.

False cell counts can result from very small particles, such as platelets, passing through the aperture and from electrical noise. To avoid them, the Analyzer is provided with a threshold control. Electrical pulses below the selected threshold level setting are not processed, but are excluded from the total count. The threshold level can be varied by adjusting the threshold control on the lower front panel.

There are two internal threshold levels, one for RBCs and one for WBCs. Both levels are simultaneously controlled by a single threshold adjustment. The correct setting of the THRESHOLD Dial for human blood is 2.5. Cell volumes corresponding to this threshold setting are approximately: RBC – 28 cu. μ., WBC – 48 cu. μ., since small cells are excluded from the total count. When the threshold level is lowered, the count will increase, since noise is included in the total count, and the threshold level may be checked or adjusted for any particular sample.

The concentration of hemoglobin is determined by measurement of the light absorption of cyanmethemoglobin produced by reaction of the diluted sample with the Lysing and Hemoglobin Reagent. The lysed and reacted sample is aspirated into an optical flow cell. Light from a tungsten lamp passes through a 540 nm. filter, through the optical flow cell, to a photosensor. The photosensor signal is processed electronically to yield a measure of the light absorption of the reacted sample, which is proportional to the hemoglobin concentration in the blood specimen.

The colorimeter is a double-beam type, with a reference photosensor exposed only to filtered light from the lamp. This reference signal, which is unaffected by hemoglobin concentration in the sample, compensates for variations in output of the lamp due to aging, temperature, and supply voltage.

A special Electronic Reference System is built into the Analyzer which permits the operator to perform instant calibration checks of RBC/HCT and WBC channels and to test the Analyzer's electronic and hydraulic systems for normal operation. This system incorporates an extremely stable pulse generator that develops a train of electronic pulses, simulating the wave forms of blood cells as they would normally be "seen" electronically by the aperture detection device. When the Test Switch on the back panel of the Analyzer is placed in the Electronic CAL or up position, the aperture detection device is bypassed. The pulse generator then provides an accurate electronic reference in the form of prerecorded RBC/HCT and WBC values from which to check and adjust the RBC/HCT and WBC calibration controls. These values are displayed on the digital readouts and calibration of the Analyzer may be established or checked instantly.

When the Test Switch is placed in the APERTURE or down position and the Analyzer is flowing clean counting diluent, the electronic reference pulses are superimposed over the output of the aperture detector. Under these conditions, the Analyzer will recover and display values for RBC and WBC comparable to those displayed in the Electronic CAL mode, indicating normal operation of electronic and hydraulic systems. If this does not occur, it alerts the operator that cleanliness of the system must be checked.

Advantages. The Analyzer is available as a compact instrument selling for approximately $7,000.00+, complete, including analyzer kits, dilutor, and bulb reagents. It is designed to provide precision and accuracy comparable to standard reference methods, based upon validation studies utilizing standard methodologies. The Analyzer possesses automatic coincidence correction, displaying results directly in appropriate units, which saves time and avoids transcription errors. It is easy to operate, maintain, calibrate, and clean. It possesses reliable solid-state circuitry with a 1-year warranty on parts and service. Service is readily available. The Analyzer may be used as a back-up analyzer, since the calibration features allow correlation with other instruments.

Disadvantages. If lipemic specimens have previously been refrigerated, they may clog the aperture. Also, these turbid specimens will cause elevated hemoglobin and WBC values. The RBC and hematocrit results are not reliable if the sample is hemolyzed or is exposed to certain drugs. Also, patients treated with azathioprine and prednisone will have lower WBC counts. If EDTA anticoagulated specimens are kept at room temperature, they must be run within 6 hours; otherwise the RBCs swell, which affects hematocrit values. Also, WBCs are not stable if the specimen is not used within 8 hours of collection at room temperature. A false RBC count may result from cold agglutinins. The instrument must warm up at least 1 hour before performing hematologic determinations.

The Analyzer needs special accessory computer-assistance (Ultra-Logic 800) to calculate platelets and blood indices, which raises the final cost of the complete instrument. False counts will result when the flow through the aperture is interrupted. This may be caused by air bubbles or dirt at the aperture. However, the Flow Interrupt Indicators will be activated and alert the technologist to disregard the reading. Since the WBCs are counted along with the RBCs in the RBC/Hct mode, when there is marked leukocytosis, the technologist may have to correct the RBC count by subtracting the WBC count. With normal blood samples, the WBC count is relatively small and may be ignored. Microcytosis may cause slightly low RBC and Hct readings. The threshold curve should be checked, and a new plateau established when the

MCV is less than 50 cu.μ. In cases of sulfhemoglobinemia, the cyanmethemoglobin method does not represent total hemoglobin, since sulfhemoglobin is not converted to cyanmethemoglobin.

Hycel Counter-500 and -300 (Fig. 5-12)

The Hycel Counter-500 is similar to the electronic blood cell counter already described, for it measures Hgb, WBCs, RBCs, Hct, and, through computer circuitry, MCV. The WBC and RBC counts are obtained through the cell conductivity method of cell detection as they pass through a 100-μ. aperture. Automatic count compensation, based on individual results, is made for cells that pass in coincidence. Hgb accuracy is obtained by utilizing the dual-beam colorimetric method of measurement. This instrument utilizes a 25-μl. sample of either venous or capillary blood.

A detailed analysis of the instrumentation reveals that hemoglobin is determined by cyanmethemoglobin methodology; a 1:400 dilution is made with isotonic buffered saline from a finger-puncture or venous blood sample. Then, with a combination lysing and Hgb reagent that releases the hemoglobin, the cyanmethemoglobin reaction occurs. A 540-nm. light source is used in a dual-beam configuration with one light path through the sample and the other used as a reference. The light transmitted is measured by a pair of photodetectors that, in turn, control the digital display. The WBC count is determined by the cell conductivity method. A precise volume of the same dilution prepared for the Hgb test is automatically drawn through a conductivity chamber, the transducer. Each WBC detected is electronically counted as it passes through a 100-μ. aperture. The circuitry automatically reads out WBCs in thousands per cu. mm. of blood. The RBC count is measured with the same conductivity method as is used for the WBC count. However, a second dilution is made from the Hgb and WBC dilution before the com-

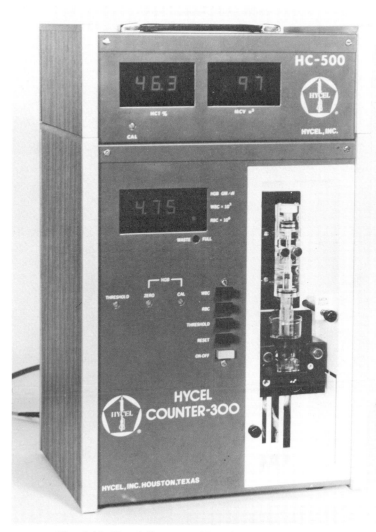

Fig. 5-12. Hycel Counter-300 and HC-500. (Hycel, Inc.)

bination lysing reagent is added, and the total RBC count is read directly in millions per cu. ml. of blood. After this step is completed, there is an instantaneous display of the Hct. This is measured by electronically determining the volume of each RBC counted. The resulting size total of all RBCs counted is an electronic output calibrated to read the Hct percentage on the digital display. Since a large number of RBCs are sampled with coincidence correction, compensation is automatically made for the simultaneous passing of more

than one RBC through the orifice at a time. The MCV is displayed in cu. μ. by the electronic division of the Hct per cent by RBC count in RBCs per cu. mm. of whole blood.

Advantages. Test results for the five parameters are produced in under 2 minutes with a minimum of effort. No special training is necessary for this instrument. Optimal instrument performance may be maintained with minimum technologist service. All elevated readings are automatically corrected for coincidence, and no additional corrections are necessary. The instrument panel contains a flashing alarm signal for clogs, (cleared in seconds by manual back-flush), insufficient solution, waste overflow, or other malfunction (an audible cadence signal indicates normal operation). The threshold level can be adjusted, with no external attachments, for special purposes such as cell-size studies and veterinary use. No manometer and no mercury are used.

Disadvantages. The disadvantages are the same as for the other electronic blood cell counters, for example, lipemic blood, sulf-hemoglobinemia, drugs, and EDTA limitations.

Autocytometer II (Fisher)*

The Autocytometer II, for RBCs, WBCs, and Hgb determination, works on a principle different from the other previously described counters; it is a flow-through hemophotometer. In principle, two opposing light-sensitive cells and an excitor lamp are arranged so that one photocell receives a beam of light transmitted by the sample, and the other is illuminated directly. Filters in both beams provide measurement of only the light of the color absorbed by cyanmethemoglobin. In calibration, the intensity of the reference beam is adjusted in order that the two currents cancel when the constituent measured has a concentration equal to the calibration standard. A higher or lower concentration changes this balance, and a needle is deflected across a scale calibrated to read directly in g. of Hgb per 100 ml. of blood. An auxiliary suction pump allows emptying of the flow-through cuvette.

In actual performance, the artificial "semipermanent" high and low standards are read, set, and checked several times daily, usually before running a series of Hgbs on the instrument. The flow-through cuvette should be removed from the well, after the drain switch has been pressed and the cuvette emptied. When the high and low

standards are placed in the well, they should always face the same direction (this is easily done by placing a dot or line on the standard facing the front of the instrument). The standards are read and checked, and the low and high adjust knobs may be set to the predetermined readings, if necessary. Also the instrument's Hgb calibration should be checked twice each month with a commercial cyanmethemoglobin standard, five dilutions of the commercial standards (5–20 g. Hgb/100 ml.) are prepared using volumetric pipettes. The standardization should be done in the same flow-through cuvette that is to be used routinely. The constricted end of the flow-through cuvette may be stopped by using a short piece of pipe cleaner (which is later easily pushed out). This allows the standard solution to be poured into the cuvette, read, and returned to a tube and later used again, rather than flushed out to waste. The high standard is read, with the high adjust knob used to set the needle on the scale to the assay value. The same is done with the low standard; however, since one adjustment affects the other, reading several times is usually necessary. After the instrument is set on the assay value, the high "artificial" standard supplied with the instrument is read; the noted reading is put on that standard for future reference. The same is done for the low "artificial" standard. If for any reason values are questioned (for example, when running daily controls), the standardization may be checked more simply by using an undiluted assayed cyanmethemoglobin standard. If the reading is not within allowable limits, dilutions may be made and the calibration procedure described above followed.

In the performance of cell counts, the diluted blood sample is placed on the platform of the Autocytometer II, the intake probe is immersed, the switch is set for RBCs or WBCs, and the COUNT button pressed. Hgb determination is run simultaneously with WBC count; seconds later the RBC count results appear.

---

* This instrument's manufacture has recently been discontinued.

As part of preventive maintenance, a concentrated cleaning solution (detergent) is available that should be run through the instrument at the end of the day. The solution is poured into the cuvette and drawn through all tubing by operating the suction pump. It may be left in the tubing overnight; this prevents protein buildup in the tygon tubing that connects different parts of the instrument. In addition, the flow-through cuvette should be removed and thoroughly cleaned every 2 days (or more often according to volume), with a cotton swab but not a stiff-bristle brush; the latter might scratch the cuvette. A detergent solution (such as the one used on all electronic cell counters) is very good for washing. A bleach, also, may be used if a stubborn protein buildup persists. The cuvette should be rinsed well and dried before replacing. In order to ensure a good seal, every 2 days, stopcock grease should be added, sparingly, to the bottom rim of the cuvette where its narrow portion fits into an O-ring. If the seal is not tight, solution may leak around the bottom and into the well. Finally, the two screws on the bottom of the suction pump area should be removed—this will allow access to the pump tubing along which the rollers operate to create suction —and the cuvette should be emptied. This tubing should be inspected for cracks every 2 months (especially if any fluid is noted under the pump) and replaced if necessary. A little stopcock grease smeared on this tubing will prolong life. If the rollers appear to be rolling not exactly along the tubing, an Allen wrench may be used to move them slightly up or down. (This is usually the reason for a screeching noise in the pump).[29]

Advantages. The Autocytometer II was an easy, simple operation with simultaneous determinations of RBC, WBC, and Hgb in less than 1 minute on the digital readout. This instrument has a wide counting range (RBCs up to 9.9 million/cu.mm., WBCs up to 99,000/cu.mm., and Hgb up to 25 g./100 ml.). It is ideal for pediatric work.

Its threshold controls are independent, and a changeover to accommodate an unusual sample can be carried out without affecting the other sample results. Higher WBC count cannot carry over and occasionally may seem abnormally low. Unusually large or small RBCs are detected with the same precision and accuracy as normal-sized RBCs. It is ideal for a veterinary laboratory. All three results are exceptionally repeatable in high or low range. The instrument spots malfunctions immediately; its built-in test unit registers whether counting and readout circuits are functioning properly. Three indicator lights, test switch, and meter (inside cabinet) indicate the source of any electronic malfunction. An integral 300-power dark-field microscope lets one see directly into the counting chamber. One can adjust the optical alignment of the instrument chamber when the microscope is set up. The counting chamber may be checked for contaminating bubbles or cell debris build-up at any time during the counting procedure. Since the "artificial" standards are now marked with values that correspond to actual assayed standard readings, they may be used daily to set and check the instrument.

Disadvantages. The Autocytometer II requires an accessory calculator to compute MCHC, MCV, and MCH. Manually determined Hct may be performed. The failure to press the drain switch and empty the cuvette before removing it will flood the inside of the well and filters, and this will result in high or erratic readings on the instrument until it is completely dry. If one adjustment is moved (in checking high and low standards), this affects the other. Therefore, one must go back and forth several times until both readings are correct and stable. The colored standards supplied with the instrument are so-called "permanent" but may change slightly with age. Variation in instrument components (bulb and electronics) may also cause a long-term drift. In this instrument, the use of the regular tube-type cuvettes should be avoided

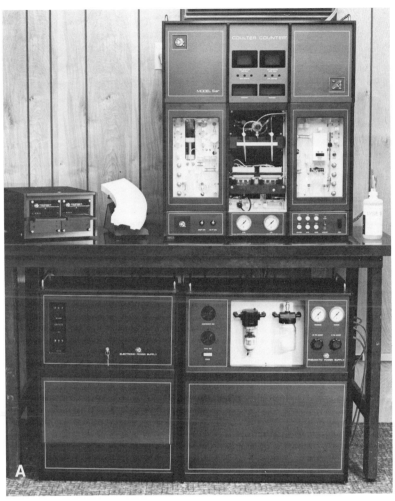

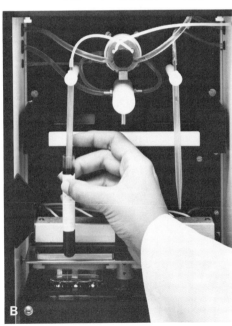

Fig. 5-13. (A) Coulter Counter Model S_{SR}. (B) Close-up of aspirator (Courtesy of Coulter Electronics, Inc.)

since they are not matched to the flow-through cuvette, and may lead to significant errors in reading hemoglobins.

Coulter Counter Model S$_{SR}$

This Coulter Counter Model S$_{SR}$[3] (Fig. 5-13*A* and *B*) is an updated, improved version of the familiar Model S. There are no significant changes in specifications, but there are a number of changes for improved reliability and medical technologist convenience, some of the latter with the objective of minimizing the chance for error. This system may be termed semiautomated, since aspiration of each sample is manually activated, and the cards on which the results are printed are manually inserted.

Following manual activation, aspiration of a whole blood sample is carried out, (Fig. 13*B*), after which the instrument automatically performs counts for RBC and WBC and measures the MCV and the Hgb concentration. The electronic system calculates three parameters from these measurements, HCT, MCH, and MCHC. All seven results are automatically printed on a multicopy report form, which is manually inserted into the instrument printer slot. An alternate aspiration mode is provided for capillary blood samples of 44.7 μl., prediluted in 10 ml. of isotonic solution; a Becton-Dickinson Unopette system is usually used for the required predilution in pediatric cases. Up to three samples per minute may be processed. Each sample cycle takes 40 seconds, but it is practical to aspirate a new sample halfway through each sample cycle.

Cell counting on the Model S$_{SR}$ (and on the Model S) is predicated on the basic Coulter counting technique; that is, electrodes are placed in a conducting, isotonic electrolyte solution on opposite sides of an aperture 100 μm. in diameter, 75 μm. deep. As a blood cell, which is relatively nonconducting, enters the aperture, a marked increase in electrical resistance is produced. This instrument uses a constant current supply so that the conductivity change

causes a voltage pulse, which may then be electronically counted. The size of the generated pulse will increase with the size of the particle; thus, the same system can be used for evaluating the MCV. The Coulter principle is based on electrical conductivity differences between particles and common diluent (Fig. 5-14). Particles act as insulators, diluents as good conductors. The particles suspended in an electrolyte are forced through a small aperture through which an electrical current path has been established. As each particle displaces electrolyte in the aperture, a pulse proportional to the particle volume is produced. Thus a 3-dimensional particle volume response is the basis for all sizing, regardless of position or orientation of the particle in solution.

Since large dilution factors are involved, the method of automating dilution is crucial. In both the S$_{SR}$ and the S, the sample to be diluted (44.7 μl. of, first, whole blood and, next, the diluted blood) is metered by a sampling valve that segments this volume from the larger volume on rotation from one position on the instrument to the other. The diluents (10 ml. of isotonic solution in two cases and 1 ml. of lysing solution in another case) are dispensed by positive displacement devices. The dilution steps are (1) 44.7 μl. blood plus 10 ml. isotonic solution (1:224) yields solution 1; (2) 44.7 μl. solution plus 10 ml. isotonic solution (1:50,000) is the net dilution solution used for RBC and MCV; and (3) 9 ml. of solution 1 plus 1 ml. lysing solution (1:250) is the net dilution solution used for WBC and Hgb.

The Hgb determination utilizes a modified colorimetric cyanmethemoglobin method. During the measurement cycle, isotonic solution is backwashed through the aspirator tube (Fig. 5-13*B*), as it is pivoted to the side for expelling into a waste container, to avoid cross-contamination between samples. The only difference between the standard and microsampling aspiration modes is that, in the latter case, the first dilution step is manually performed

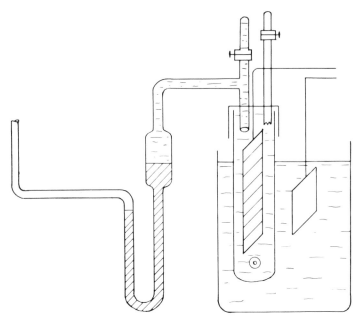

Fig. 5-14. Graphic demonstration of the Coulter principle. There are electrical conductivity differences between particles (blood cells) and common diluent. (Courtesy of Coulter Electronics, Inc.)

before aspiration. A switch activates the applicable aspirator, which bypasses the first automatic dilution. When the normal sampling procedure is used, the time of a separate dilution step is saved, and the possibility of the imprecision of the manual dilution is precluded.

Each of the counting solutions flows through three aperture tubes. Thus, three separate counts are averaged. In addition, to obviate including a false count, which might result from, for example, a partially clogged aperture, the electronic system logic computes the standard deviation for the mean and negates or "votes" out an offender that deviates from the mean by more than 3 standard deviations. If one count is "voted out," the mean of the other two is printed. If none of the three counts for either WBCs or RBCs agrees, the result is printed for that count. In addition, there is a DATA REJECTED indicator for each of the aperture tubes, which is lighted to indicate the rejecting of that tube's count. Immediate attention is needed if there are repeated rejections of the data from any one tube.

The MCV is determined by the heights

of the signals in the RBC aperture tubes. After the MCV is determined from the first tube, the instrument averages the values from the second and third RBC aperture tubes. If the count from either of these has been rejected, the MCV data from that tube will be ignored. Also, if the MCVs from the two chambers deviate significantly from each other, the result will be rejected and no value printed.

Furthermore, correction of the printed WBC and RBC values is made, because two or more cells that are in the aperture at the same time will electronically look like a single large-volume cell. This nonlinear, statistically based correction function is electronically generated and automatically applied. The Hct, MCH, and MCHC are also automatically calculated.

Another factor that directly affects counting precision is the volume of the diluted sample that is counted. The sample solution is drawn through the aperture by a highly regulated vacuum. The vacuum level is both calibrated and monitored by means of a mercury manometer designed for high sensitivity. The precision of the counted volume is also determined by the counting time. The volume is determined by the product of two precisely controlled factors, pressure (vacuum) and time.

Usually, Coulter's modified whole blood hematology control 4C, is used for calibration, and expired blood bank blood is used for a control. Experience has shown that CPD anticoagulant gives more accurate results than ACD, which seems to have less stability. The blood is usually calibrated manually.

As Figure 5-13*A* shows, the total automated system consists of five modules. The focal point is the unit that contains the dilutor, with the analyzer module on top of it. These are usually placed on a table, alongside the printer module. Generally, on the floor nearby are the remaining two modules, the pneumatic supply unit and the electronic power supply unit. Also included with the system are a large number of monitors and medical technologist aids, which facilitate maintenance, cleaning, and service.

Advantages. The Model S_{SR} requires $1/8$ of the service required by the S model although there are only minor automation changes between them. In fact, the service that has been required has generally been accomplished in 2 hours. In addition, the instrument design, the instruction manual, and the training course all enable the medical technologist to service and maintain the instrument with ease. The machine has enhanced precision, especially in its capabilities for pediatric patients and the use of microsamples. The increased precision is also associated with the flow of each of the counting solutions through three aperture tubes. The majority of design changes relate to the pneumatic system, starting with a much quieter compressor than in the Model S. Both the compressor and the printer also have improved reliability; the printer is better primarily because microswitches have been replaced with photosensors. Since the compressor is practically noise-free, it may be left on all day, utilizing a timed turn-off modification if so desired; a

timer automatically shuts down the compressor if a sample has not been aspirated over a 10-minute period, extending the life of the compressor. Initiating the next aspiration automatically restarts the compressor.

Other new features in the S_{SR} are the monitors for both the isotonic solution and the lysing agent. These operate on detection of back-pressure, caused by the presence of fluid at the end of a tube connected to a low air pressure supply. In addition, lights have been added to indicate which aspirating mode is activated. These lights, located above each aspirator, also change color to monitor the stages of the aspirating cycle. Finally, for ease of monitoring, the pressure gauges that are on the pneumatic supply unit of the models are now located at the bottom of the dilutor module. It should be mentioned that these reagent monitors are an important feature of the S_{SR} because they help avoid the occasional waste of a sample because of depleted reagents. The backflushing with diluent, previously described, is new in the S_{SR}. On the Model S, the excess sample was ejected without backwash. The new arrangement has longer periods between cleanout and helps insure the usefulness of stat measurements. In addition, it is now possible to service the dilutor system from the front of the unit instead of requiring access from the sides; the latter can be a nuisance on crowded laboratory benches. Also, many of the plastic fittings have been changed to metal ones requiring less frequent replacement, and more of the fittings are located on the front. Overall, the electronics rarely vary, and the accessibility to the analyzer units (although not perfect) is good and it is easy to change bulbs.

Disadvantages. It is a very, very expensive, semiautomated electronic blood counting machine producing seven hematologic parameters (RBC, WBC, MCV, Hgb, Hct, MCH, and MCHC). Although the system has improved reliability, it is much more difficult to maintain and harder to take apart. For example, the screw latches on

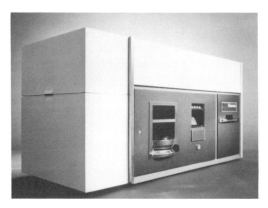

Fig. 5-15. Hemac 630L Laser Hematology Counter. (Courtesy of Ortho Instruments)

the left and right panels (recent reports indicate improvements in the panel latching system of the dilutor module and in glassware clamps) of the dilutor unit are difficult to work. Also, the center section around the aspirators provides little accessibility from the front, necessitating the opening of the left and right panels and reaching in through the sides of the center section. Some users find that service is needed once every 2 to 3 months because of electronic board failures. Although many of the plastic fittings have been changed to metal, some parts are still difficult to grasp or handle, and some of the nylon clamps (recent reports indicate improvements in the panel latching system of the dilutor module and in glassware clamps) on the glassware are excessively stiff, making the expensive glass parts vulnerable to breakage when they are removed for cleaning. The projected aperture images, although brighter than on the S, are still somewhat dim. There still remain the dangers of toxicity and frequent "sloppy" episodes (e.g., the accidental spilling of mercury) associated with mercury usage, since a mercury manometer, designed for high sensitivity, is used.

Hemac 630L Laser Hematology Counter (Ortho Diagnostic Instruments)

The Hemac Laser 630L Hematology Counter (Fig. 5-15) represents an innovation in the field of electronic blood counters; it not only takes advantage of modern electronics but also effectively applies the principles of lasers to blood cell counting. To accomplish this, it utilizes the following three unique characteristics of lasers.

First, a laser beam may be brought to an extremely sharp focus, many times smaller in dimension than any other light source. Second, the spectral band width of a laser beam is extremely narrow, commonly at least 100 to 1000 times narrower than can be resolved by the highest performance research monochromators. This factor is correlated to the first characteristic by basic laws of physics. Third, and related to the spectral band width, it is possible to attain very high energy densities in small areas. However, these densities are not crucial in this counter since a very low-powered Helium-Neon laser is utilized, and the design precludes consideration of this factor.

The physical principle applied in the Hemac is the sharp focus, which is set at 20 μm., comparable to the dimensions of blood cells. Thus, a cell passing the focused laser beam scatters it significantly, and the amount of unscattered light signal reaching the detector depends on the size of the cell. Another innovative feature of this instrument is the flow cell, which creates a fluid aperture for the diluted sample rather than a rigid tunnel. The flow cell looks like an inverted, streamlined funnel. Isotonic fluid flowing into the wide mouth of the funnel serves as a sheath for the narrower sample stream injected at the center. The shape of the funnel and the speed of flow insure laminar flow. As the sheath narrows to 250 μm., the sample is proportionately reduced to 18 μm. in diameter, with no significant mixing between the sheath and the sample.

As each cell passes through the focused laser beam, it attenuates the signal reaching the detector in proportion to its size. An average of about 2,500 red cells per second are counted for 10 seconds, followed by the less diluted sample, for which an average of

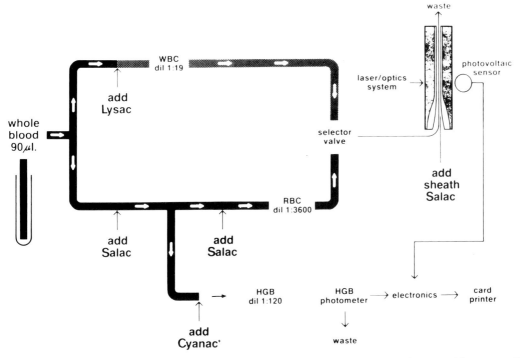

Fig. 5-16. Simplified functional scheme for Hemac 630L Laser Hematology Counter. (Courtesy of Ortho Instruments)

700 WBCs per second are counted, for the same period of time. The hematocrit is electrically determined by integrating the amplitudes of the RBC pulses. The Hgb concentration is automatically determined in an adjunct colorimeter by a cyanmethemoglobin method, which has modified parameters to conform to the 23-second color development time allowed by the testing cycle. The modifications include pH reagent concentration, lysing agent, and blood to reagent ratio.

The laser sources for cell counting is a 1-milliwatt He-Na laser, which exists at 632.8 mm. A silicon photovoltaic cell, which is highly sensitive at this wavelength, is the detector for cell counting. For Hgb, a GaAsP light, emitting dioxide, is the source of 539 nm. radiation, and the detector is a photomultiplier. Before each Hgb determination is made, a blank reagent measurement is automatically made to enhance precision.

When the instrument is turned on, and at the end of every test cycle, the hydraulic system is washed with isotonic solution, and the sampling probe is washed internally and externally and backflushed, to insure virtually no carryover.

In the test procedure, a standard blood tube, containing a sample of 200 μl. or more of whole blood, is placed on a holder in a rotary quadrant at the front of the instrument. Rotating the sample into the instrument automatically pushes the washing system aside, locates the sample under the probe, and initiates the test cycle, which proceeds automatically. The steps (Fig. 5-16), which then occur without further intervention, include the drawing of a 90- to 95-μl. aliquot sample from the sample cup and the discarding of the leading edge. The sample stream is split into WBC, Hgb, and RBC/Hct channels, each of which is diluted according to the test to be performed. Three steps of diluting and mixing increase the precision and homogeneity of the moderately high dilution ratios. The Hgb cell is then blanked with reagent and a portion of the WBC/Hgb sample is directed to the Hgb colorimeter cell. The RBC/Hct solution flows past the laser beam for about 10 seconds, and the RBC count and Hct are recorded electronically. The other parameters (MCV, MCH, and MCHC) are calculated electronically, and all seven parameters are then printed out, after automatic correction for calibration factors. The correction mechanism has lock-knob potentiometers located beneath the top cover of the instrument. Finally, all liquid metering is performed by cam-driven positive displacement pumps. Slide valves are used for splitting and directing the metered fluids precisely to their appointed channels. The entire system is contained in a single bench top unit that is $3\frac{1}{4}$ feet wide (Fig. 5-15).

Advantages. For an instrument with a single counting chamber, the Hemac offers useful levels of remarkable precision. The manufacturer specifies precision to be within 2 per cent for RBCs, 3 per cent for WBCs, 2 per cent for Hgb, and 2.83 per cent for Hct. The working ranges of the Hemac are 0.5 to 8×10^6 RBC per mm.^{3}; 100 to 75,000 WBC/mm.^{3}; 1 to 23 g./dl. for Hgb; and 9 to 65 per cent for Hct.

The Hemac has consistent ease of operation and maintenance, facilitated by an excellent manual. In addition, service is infrequently needed, but when it is, it is highly satisfactory. A calibration is usually run in the morning, followed by a control. The control is repeated early in the afternoon and again just before the evening shift, when a daily check of reagent levels is usually made. The system is usually turned on at least 30 minutes before a sample run in the morning. It takes the medical technologist 15 minutes to complete the startup protocol before running a patient sample.

The entire hydraulic system of the Hemac is enclosed, including the sample probe, which helps maintain cleanliness, the primary safeguard in any cell counting equipment. Hinged covers and removable panels make everything accessible for maintenance; for example, the cams are

located beneath the dispenser pumps and may be kept meticulously clean of grease and leaked reagents; also slide valves are kept greased at all times. All reagents are contained in clear containers beneath a cover on the left side of the instrument. Because reagent consumption is small (i.e., each test consumes 11 ml. of the isotonic solution including wash, 1.6 ml. of the Hgb test reagents, and 0.8 ml. of the lysing solution) and reagent levels are easily visible, no automatic monitoring of reagent level has been incorporated. Also, the lysing solution never runs out because stability requires fresh solution every 5 days. However, the system is frequently run with the top cover raised, because extraneous particles cause visible flashes of scattered laser light, which is helpful in monitoring counts.

A small oscilloscope is included on the front panel for monitoring the shape of the counting pulses. Although the oscilloscope is used only minimally in a system not susceptible to aperture blockage (the aperture is comparable in size to the laser beam, 20 compared to 18 μm.), it can be used on very high counts to distinguish macrocytic from microcytic cells. Also, any blockage that does occur is easy to view directly.

The instrument has a compressor that maintains reagents under pressure. It is quiet and runs only when the pressure is too low.

Status lights are provided; a READY light above the sample indicates when a test may be initiated. Other lighted labels indicate that the Hgb cuvette is filled and the reaction is being read and that the RBC/Hct or WBC count is in process. Results are printed on a standard hematology form.

The dimensions of the Hemac protect against significant coincidence counts. About the only possible cause of a coincidence signal is the passage of two cells that have become stuck together; according to the manufacturer, this is quite rare since the size of the aperture insures that the cells pass the laser beam "single file." An ancillary benefit of this flow cell design permits more modest dilution ratios than normally encountered in other electronic blood cell counters. The dilution ratio is 1:3800 for RBC/Hct, 1:20 for WBC, and 1:60 for Hgb.

Disadvantages. The only limitation of the Hemac noted by many medical technologists is that, at present, there is no means of using capillary blood samples.* The printer will not function in temperatures above 80°F; therefore, this instrument must be in an air-conditioned room. The compressor pressure must not be set above a certain level or the reagent bottles will leak. Occasionally, leaks in lines and leaks in reagent containers occur due to their poor quality. The Hemac lacks the capability to do platelet counts.

A SEMIAUTOMATED DILUTION SYSTEM FOR THE HEMATOLOGY LABORATORY[10]

A substantial portion of the work load in a hematology laboratory involves measurements that are of inherently high precision and accuracy, such as photoelectric hemoglobinometry and electronic cell counting. The potential precision and accuracy often are not achieved because of inadequate dilution techniques. The manual techniques presently in use, however, are both flexible and readily adaptable to the assortment of venipuncture and finger-puncture specimens presented to most hematology laboratories, an asset not afforded by most fully automated systems.

In the laboratory, semiautomated techniques not only have preserved flexibility, but also have increased speed and accuracy. The components of this system are depicted in Figure 5-17.[10] A syringe pump dispenser equipped with a sampling head serves as an automatic dilutor for anticoagulated venous blood. The same dispenser without the sampling head is used to fill test tubes with diluent for use with finger-puncture blood. The finger-puncture samples are collected in capillary tubes designed for this purpose,† which are long enough to be conveniently handled yet have a diameter small enough to make incomplete filling obvious. The tubes fill rapidly and completely by capillarity, and when used with the correct amount of diluent, they are also self-emptying because the diluent extends into the small angular recess formed between the capillary and the wall of the test tube, and thus is available to replace the blood. Because of its higher specific gravity, the blood drains from the bottom of the capillary. The self-emptying action is slow, requiring about 10 minutes, but is uniformly complete by the time that finger-puncture samples picked up on the wards are returned to the laboratory. The sample head, which in combination with the dispenser serves as a dilutor, is a modified microliter syringe.‡ Several other dilutors more recently have become available that can handle sample volumes of 20 μl., any of which presumably would serve equally well in the dilution system, provided they were capable of filling test tubes rapidly and accurately for use with the microcapillaries.

For hemoglobin determinations, 5 ml. of Drabkin's solution in a 13 × 100 mm. tube is employed. A 15 × 125 mm. tube and 5 ml. of saline solution are used for white blood cell determinations. An additional 5 ml. of saline solution plus Cetrimide lysant subsequently is added in the laboratory prior to performing the counts. For red cell counts, which are done only on venous blood, a double dilution technique is used.

---

* A capillary blood sampling system has been developed using a Unopette device and is probably now available. Other changes in the instrument include a new, more reliable retrofillable printer. Also, through an electronics change, hemoglobin linearity has been extended.

† Available as Hemocaps from the Drummond Scientific Company, Broomall, Pa.

‡ The dilutor, consisting of sampling head and dispenser, is available from the National Instrument Company, Baltimore, Md.

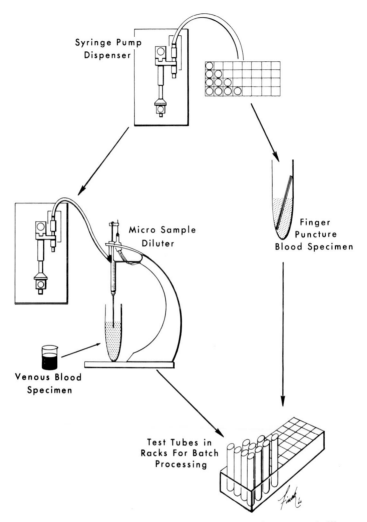

Fig. 5-17. Dilution system. (Bull, B. S.: A semiautomated dilutation system for a hematology laboratory. Bull. Pathol., *8:*13, 1967)

A dilutor is set to draw a sample of 44.6 µl.
and dispense 10 ml. After mixing, the first
dilution is resampled to produce 100 ml. of
a 1:50,000 dilution.

Reproducibility studies of the dilutions
obtained from the microsample dilutor and
from the microcaps have yielded the following coefficients of variation: microcapillaries, 0.9 per cent; Sahli pipettes, 1.2 per
cent; and dilutor, 0.7 per cent.

A major advantage of this system is its
flexibility. Venous blood and finger-puncture samples can be handled in any proportion by varying the use of dilutor and microcaps. Furthermore, the equipment is
disposable, the method considerably faster,
and its results somewhat more precise than
those of using standard hemoglobin pipettes. Its principal advantage, however,
lies in its simplicity, which not only enables
its use to be quickly and easily mastered by
laboratory personnel, but also markedly
decreases the chance of an error due to improper handling of equipment.

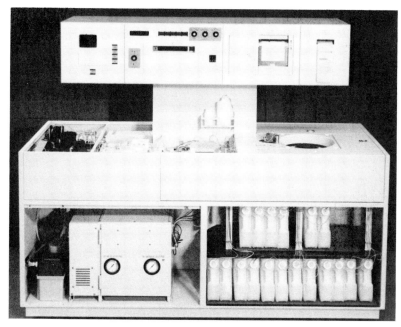

Fig. 5-18. Hemalog D. (Courtesy of Technicon Instruments)

AUTOMATION OF THE LEUKOCYTE DIFFERENTIAL COUNT

The important objectives of differential leukocyte hematologic automation includes the following: an increase in both accuracy and precision through the elimination of manipulations subject to human error and techniques; relief from boredom for specially trained personnel; assistance in handling an increase in test volume; and a reduction in subjective decisions. Several products with a variety of approaches have been developed and have been clinically evaluated. To date, these instruments fit into three categories: flow-through analysis of stained cells (i.e., automatic differential counting of a cell suspension by means of cytochemical reactions—Technicon Hemalog D); computer-image processing (ie., computerized pattern recognition systems for the automatic differential count in a stained slide—Corning LARC, Geometric Data Hematrak, Coulter Differential, Perkin-Elmer Diff 3, and Abbott Differen-

tial Classifier or ADC-500); and automated stage microscope (i.e., automated computerized scanning system that facilitates the differential count on a stained slide by the technologist—Honeywell ACS 1000).

FLOW-THROUGH ANALYSIS OF STAINED CELLS

The Technicon Hemalog D (Figs. 5-18; 5-19) uses the same continuous flow techniques (i.e., air bubble separation of successive samples) that have been used in the Technicon automatic chemistry analyzers. In the system, 0.36 ml. of each whole blood sample (by venipuncture) is mixed with 0.04 ml. EDTA. The resultant 0.4 ml. is then split into three channels. The red blood cells are hemolyzed; the white blood cells in each channel are fixed and reacted with separate cytochemical stains.

The AutoSlide is a self-contained instrument that, when it is attached to the D/90 (a modification of the Hemalog D capable of performing 90 differentials per

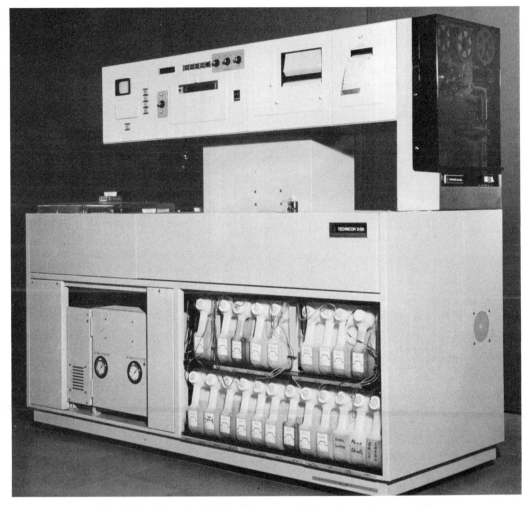

Fig. 5-19. Hemalog D 90. (Courtesy of Technicon Instruments)

hour), will automatically prepare a blood smear (stained and labeled) on a glass slide (Fig. 5-20). Blood is drawn to the AutoSlide module by means of a double-probe assembly on the Hemalog D sampler. The blood is then smeared on a mylar tape, which is dried. The tape then moves through staining and labeling stations. The finished smear is transferred from the tape to a conventional glass slide. Lag-time is 14 minutes, 1 smear per 40 seconds.

A 10,000-cell differential count analyzing one specimen per minute reports all of the normal peripheral blood cell types in both percentage and absolute numbers; in addi-

tion, it reports three other cell categories on the second page of the form. These will be described later.

For detection, classification, and counting, the sample is surrounded by a transparent liquid sheath. The optical properties of both liquids match the erythrocyte stromata, which are not detected by the optical system. In the measurement flow cell, the lamellar flow is constricted to $\frac{1}{5}$ of its entering diameter, reducing the sample stream to 0.05 mm. to minimize coincidence counts and focus errors. The flowing sample never touches the walls of the flow cell, and because the diameter of the sheath is

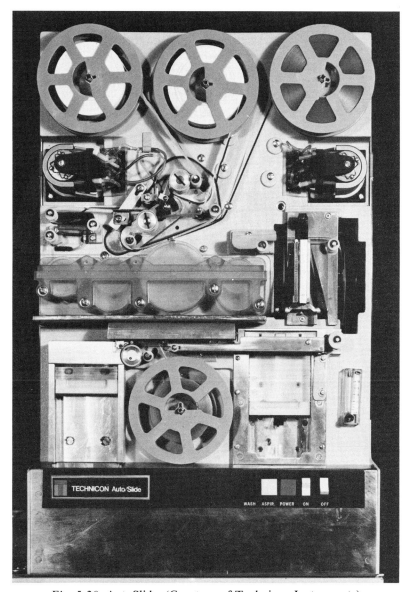

Fig. 5-20. AutoSlide. (Courtesy of Technicon Instruments)

0.25 mm. at the constricted portion, particles up to this size will not clog the cell. All three channels use a common tungsten halogen source. The optical system in each channel focuses the light beam on the constricted portion of the flow cell. For counting cells, a dark-field stop is placed in the beam so that only light scattered outside of the collimated light beam passes around the stop and reaches the detector. In two channels, a beam splitter is placed before the aperture, and the detector in the unstopped beam measures changes in absorption due to the passing particles. In the third channel the beam is also split, but forward scatter is measured in both beams, with filters isolating a different color in each beam. Differential counting and classification of cells in

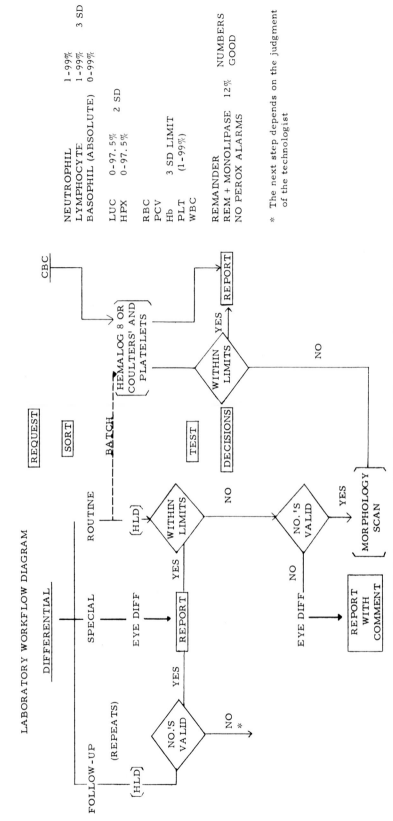

Fig. 5-21. Laboratory workflow diagram. (Courtesy of Technicon Instruments)

each channel depend on the liquid relations among scattering level (particle size), degree of absorption (staining), and spectral characteristics of the scatter or absorption.

The following cytochemical methods and classification approaches are employed:

Monocyte Channel

A brownish red color represents the monocyte stain; it is due to the presence of a specific fluoride-sensitive esterase in cells of the monocyte series. In order to classify a particle as a monocyte, the circuit logic requires: the scatter to exceed a preset threshold, ignoring smaller particles, and the corresponding absorption to be greater than a preset threshold.

Basophil Channel

In the basophil channel, Alcian blue reacts with the heparin in basophil granules, causing them to absorb strongly in the red portion of the spectrum. In this channel the electro-optical system detects the green scatter in the beam and the red scatter in the other. In these two detection currents amplifications are set so that unstained particles show roughly equal scatter signals in both channels. Basophils will exhibit predominantly green scatter because they short-circuit the red light. Preset thresholds count only the green.

Peroxidase Channel

The "remainder" category or data are developed in the peroxidase channel; it is based on differences in staining and size. The horizontal axis on the display screen represents absorption (staining strength) and the vertical axis demonstrates scattering (particle size). The staining differentials are among strongly stained eosinophils, less intensely stained neutrophils, and lymphocytes, which show no peroxidase activity. The two lower absorption thresholds are preset. The other two absorption thresholds are automatically set to track the staining properties of the neutrophils of each sample, and these vary somewhat from sample to sample. In plate 76, the representative neutrophil counted area points by arrow to the large particles between the tracking thresholds as well as the medium sized particles between the fixed absorption thresholds (control box in this plate). Eosinophils with medium sized and smaller particles strongly stained are observed (arrow) in the farthest right box of the center and bottom rows. Lymphocytes are additionally classified in the peroxidase channel where they appear as unstained, medium-sized particles. Platelets, very small unstained particles, or electronic noise appear as signals but are not counted.

Only on the second sheet of the report form are areas of relatively few particles interpreted and counted for neutrophils with very high peroxidase activity (HPX; Fig. 5-21) this is a clue to laboratory personnel. The cells that appear to the left of the fixed low absorption threshold are classified as large unstained cells (LUC). They include atypical lymphocytes and blast cells. The cells between the tracking and extrapolated, fixed low absorption thresholds are lightly stained monocytes and basophils. Counting basophils is a systems check. The difference between the basophil count and the sum of the basophil and monocyte counts obtained in their separate channels is automatically calculated and presented as a remainder category. It is used to determine whether the monocyte staining reaction is atypical; a large remainder demands further investigation. The overall pattern also alerts technicians when there are samples containing neutrophils with low peroxidase staining intensity or samples with low neutrophil density, either or both of which may lead to unreliable automatic tracking thresholds. In addition, this peroxidase channel is also used to accumulate a total white cell count, excluding only pulses that do not cross the lower scatter threshold. This leukocyte count is automatically related to a reference sample white cell count determined by independent reference methods.

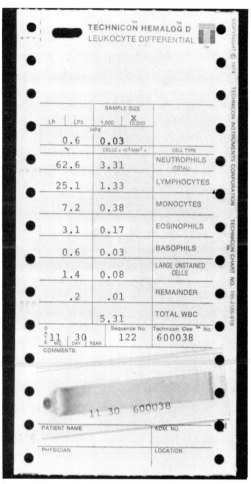

Fig. 5-22. Hemalog D preprinted report form. (Courtesy of Technicon Instruments)

superstructure as are the operating controls, an oscilloscope for monitoring cell counts, a strip chart recorder for monitoring functional operation, a digital printer for the preprinted report tickets, and a test and diagnostic panel. The oscilloscope may be operated to graph patterns, where the y-axis indicates size and the x-axis indicates staining, or to produce pulse height analyses to confirm or adjust the fixed threshold settings. The function recorder shows five channels of information: the rate of cell counting on each of the three flow cells, the neutrophil peak tracking circuit, and the main timing functions. The test and diagnostic panel includes a set of labeled lights that indicate the status of the various functions of the Hemalog D during a test cycle. Also included are a number of malfunction indicators to aid in the diagnosis of problems and to warn of impending supply shortages. A button is provided for testing the bulbs for all indicators.

During a sample run each test channel counts the total number of cells detected; this must normally total 10,000 before the differential count is terminated. If the blood sample is leukopenic—and a total of 10,000 white blood cells cannot be detected during the test interval, a switch selectivity option permits differential counting on a total of 1,000 cells in each channel. From a cold start, the instrument must be on for 20 minutes before calibration, which then takes 10 to 15 minutes. Beyond that, it takes 10 minutes from sample pickup to printout. When a run is completed, there is an automatic system wash cycle. The system may be left in standby—to circulate either water or reagents. To resume testing requires waiting 15 minutes if water has been used but may be immediate if reagents were used. The preprinted report ticket provides three copies of data on pressure-sensitive paper (Fig. 5-22). The hematology technologist need not be present for the run of a sample wheel.

A Polaroid camera is provided for photographing oscilloscope patterns. Many la-

Operation of the Hemalog D

The sample wheel holds 40 blood tubes with a testing rate of one per minute or an effective patient test rate of approximately 50 per hour (which takes into account the controls, primer, and repeats). The sample is mixed by a paddle wheel just prior to aspiration. During the last 6 seconds of each cycle period, there is a wash of the paddle and pickup probe. One can see, in Figures 5-18 and 5-19, that all reagents and the testing console are stored in the base. The electronics and associated components are located along the top of a T-shaped

boratories rerun abnormal samples and photograph the corresponding x-y patterns as an aid in analysis. In addition, options to supplement the Hemalog D include the Technicon IDee system, which generates numbered cards for automatic sample identification, and a computer interface for tie-in with a teletype or with a laboratory computer.

Most owners have initially established a 3 to 4 month testing period, to permit technologists to become familiar with the operation of the Hemalog D and with the nature and interpretation of results. Any skepticism has diminished with experience and with the establishment of a range of normal values specific for each hospital's patient population. Total white blood cell calibration and the problems arising from the absence of a primary standard have been overcome by the establishment of a protocol that uses controls from two commercial sources (other than Technicon).

Pooled human blood is used and is calibrated by counting in triplicate on an electronic aperture-impedance cell counter. The result is used to set the calibration value for the Hemalog D. As an occasional cross-check, the pool is manually counted on a National Bureau of Standards Hemocytometer using N.B.S. calibrated pipettes. Slides are generally prepared for all blood samples; these are scanned and screened as necessary. Leukocytes are usually observed during this evaluation of RBCs. If anything unusual appears, a 100 or 200 — depending on the number of abnormal factors — WBC manual differential is performed. A modified machine capable of 90 differentials per hour is now available, the Hemalog D-90 (Fig. 5-19). The latest model is the HS/90, a collator that combines reports from the Hemalog 8 and D on a single report form (Fig. 5-23).

Advantages. Enhanced precision and reduction in statistical error may be expected from the counting of 10,000 leukocytes in a differential, compared with a 100 or 200 WBC manual differential. The Hemalog D

frequently adds to the information that may be derived from manual slide examination for abnormal blood smear counts. It alerts the technologist to examine the abnormalities in greater detail. That is, the manual counts, which are done on abnormal smears, are far better in detail and accuracy. The Hemalog D avoids the time-consuming task of screening normal hospital populations. Downtime is not too common with good consultative backup telephone service, when it does occur. This device is of value in studying leukopenic counts, especially for patients treated by chemotherapy. The recent development of data collation provides a single report from the Hemalog 8 and the Hemalog D (HS/90).

Disadvantages. The oscilloscope and the printer occasionally need to be replaced. Human error during maintenance might necessitate replacing the sample head and heating bath coil. There may be power supply failures when the board operates under temporary low-line voltage conditions. However, the design of the power supply has recently been improved. The monocyte reagent has been unstable and good for only 1 day. However, a stable monocyte reagent that lasts 6 months has recently been developed. Some technologists believe that the Hemalog D does not save time or work, that it selects too many cases that have to be read manually. It does not provide a permanent record and does not include band counts. Neutrophil percentages tend to be overestimated, whereas lymphocyte and eosinophil percentages tend to be underestimated. Some patients for whom manual techniques assigned normal or high neutrophil and monocyte counts have had low Hemalog D values. Basophil values from the Hemalog D are inaccurate. In a laboratory that examines a high percentage of abnormal hematologic cases, the instrument creates more problems than it solves.* For example, abnormalities owing to immature or unusual cells complicate comparative

---

* Arkin, C. F.: Personal communication, 1975.

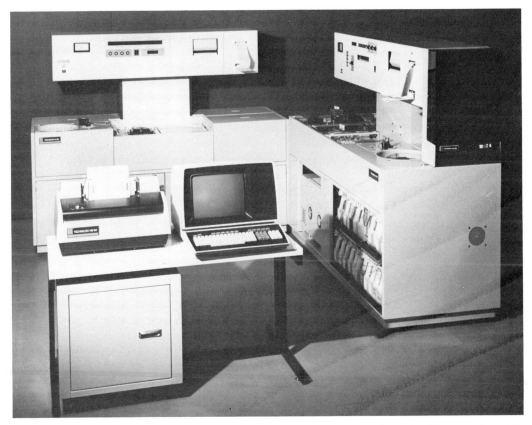

Fig. 5-23. Hemalog Model HS/90, a collator that combines reports from the Hemalog 8 and D (CBC and differential) on a single report form.

classification. The instrument requires dilution for samples having white cell counts above 20,000 per cu. mm. Total agreement was obtained in 72 per cent of the patients and partial agreement in 39 per cent. There were 15 per cent instrument false positive studies and 10 per cent instrument false negatives by the Mayo group. Patients undergoing chemotherapy and having low white cell counts will frequently have an "LR" flag, indicating that the HPX values may not be reliable. However, in these instances, the neutrophil, lymphocyte, and large unstained cell numbers are still valid for monitoring these patients' daily therapy. Elevated peroxidase-activity values have been observed (9.9% compared to a normal range of 0–3.65%). These were found to be due to platelet satellitism, which occurred in Wright-stained smears of EDTA-anticoagulated blood as well as in the effluent of the peroxidase channel. Since all platelets took up the peroxidase stain, the rosette-like clusters of platelets and neutrophils were interpreted to be single, large, intensely stained leukocytes that produced the elevated peroxidase values.[24]

COMPUTER IMAGE PROCESSING

For instruments that process computer images (Corning Larc, Geometric Data Hematrak, Coulter Differential [formerly Perkin-Elmer Diff 3, and Abbott Differential Classifier ADC-500), stained slides are examined in the usual way, by means of a microscope with an oil immersion objective system. Although the optics are unchanged for the automatic systems, motor drives are incorporated for both the focus and the stage; the latter can be moved both horizontally and vertically. For precise positioning, stepping motors that can return to a specific cell location based on digital signals stored in the computer memory are used.

The microscope image is split between the binocular eyepiece and the photoelectric detection system. Filters are used to differentiate three colors, red, yellow, and blue-green; a red filter blocks detection of the erythrocytes. However, by using the binocular microscope, the medical technologist is able to evaluate red cell morphology at some time during the test cycle. The results are entered on the keyboard, which is an integral part of each system. The platelets are simultaneously visually evaluated, and their characteristics are also entered on the keyboard. The photoelectric information obtained is converted to digital signals that the computer can recognize. The microscope stage is automatically scanned for leukocytes, in a regular pattern with a relatively large field. When a white blood cell is detected, the field is automatically narrowed to this white cell. The size, shape, and color characteristics and the variation of transmitted light intensity as a function of position within the small field are stored in the temporary computer memory. (The computer is a Digital Equipment PDP 8M with an additional 8K memory.) It then compares this information with the programmed characteristics for each type of leukocyte and decides which of seven classifications best applies to the cell: segmented neutrophils, band neutrophils, eosinophils, basophils, lymphocytes, monocytes, and those cells that cannot be classified automatically. Cells in the last category (usually less than 5% of the total) are classified by the medical technologist and manually entered in the keyboard. Blood smears that show a very large number of abnormal cells, immature cells, or nucleated red cells are usually removed from the instrument and counted manually.

These flagged cases generally make up about 5 per cent of the patients examined. After each white cell differential has been completed, the results are displayed for review and the technologist may then initiate a printout that includes the percentages of cell types present. Quality control is maintained in various ways in all of the computer image systems. Uusally, the manufacturer provides control slides that have established quality and a confirmed differential. The life span of these slides is limited only by their fading, caused by the repeated application of immersion oil. Periodic cleaning with a solvent may be helpful but may lead to other problems.

Corning LARC Classifier

The LARC is a system consisting of a computerized microscope, a slide spinner, and an automated slide stainer. The computerized microscope classifies leukocytes normally found in the blood (segmented and band neutrophils, eosinophils, basophils, lymphocytes, and monocytes) (Figs. 5-24; 5-25). It flags and automatically relocates atypical and abnormal cells for the technologist to identify. Classification of leukocytes by the LARC is dependent upon criteria similar to those used in morphologic approach (nuclear cytoplasm size, shape, and color). In order to obtain uniform and reproducible counts, the LARC depends upon a blood smear prepared by a slide spinner, which produces a monolayer of blood cells evenly distributed throughout the slide (Figs. 5-26; 5-27; 5-28). In addition, it uses a specially developed Wright's stain applied by an automatic stainer, which produces uniformly standard cell staining characteristics (Fig. 5-29). This approach is usually accurate and precise.

The stained blood smear is inserted onto the microscope stage under an oil immersion lens. One can write directly on the spun, non-frosted slides with a pencil. The LARC automatically identifies and locates each cell encountered until the total number corresponds to the number desired

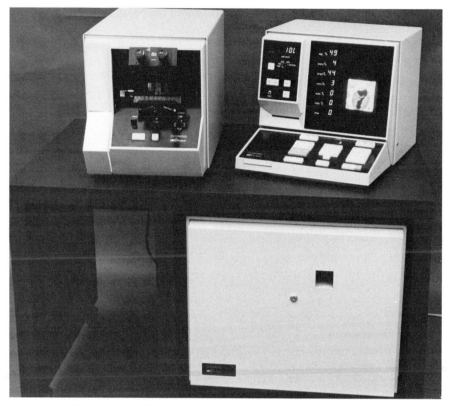

Fig. 5-24. Corning LARC Automatic White Blood Cell Differential Classifier. (Courtesy of Corning Medical)

(usually 100 cells). Cells encountered that the instrument cannot classify are identified as "other" cells. Each cell counted may be manually viewed by the technologist through either the binocular microscope or the television monitor. The slide stage has been designed for automatic relocation of the "other" (abnormal) cells (for identification by the operator) after the completion of a full 100 count of normal cells. The keyboard also permits the technologist to enter comments on red cell morphology and an estimate of platelet numbers. At this point, the printed digital readouts display the results for the normal cells and the number of abnormal cells detected. These atypical, abnormal, or suspect cells may be repeatedly viewed until the slide is removed from the stage. Percentages for each cell type are automatically adjusted for the count, which

then exceeds 100. Selection of normal count totals other than 100 is available through a panel switch. Quality control is usually repeated every four hours.

Advantages. The ability to identify lymphocytes, monocytes, eosinophils, basophils, and total neutrophils is as good as the ability of the medical technologist. Since this ability to differentiate between bands and segments varies considerably among technologists, the instrument's program to differentiate between these two cell types represents a compromise between the extremes of current opinion. Nonetheless, the differentiation provided by the LARC is reproducible. Only rarely will the LARC classify an abnormal or atypical cell as normal; it is at least as accurate and as reproducible as a medical technologist who might be counting an equal number of cells

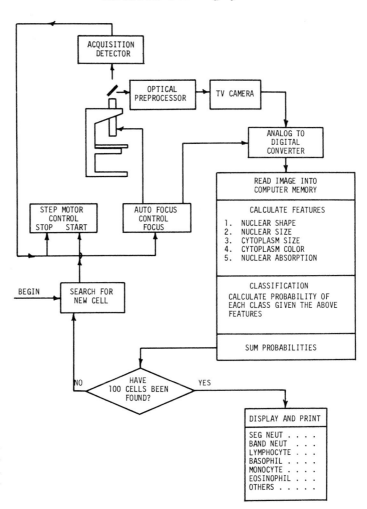

Fig. 5-25. Operational scheme of the LARC Automatic White Blood Cell Differential Classifier. (Courtesy of Corning Medical)

manually. The amount of a technologist's time required to perform a differential count is comparable and frequently better than (by more than double) the manual approach. Although batch testing is not required, when differentials are batched, 25 to 35 specimens can be performed per hour. The time required for each step is as follows: mean slide preparation 0.4 minute (includes time to prepare the smear as well as the usual maintenance and cleaning time); mean staining time 0.1 minute (does not include actual time, 16 minutes, that the slide is in the stainer); mean counting time 2.1 minutes (includes the time of automated cell counting and the manual time required for cell identification and comments); mean clerical time 0.0 minute (the results are automatically printed on a form or fed to an on-line computer). A stat differential may be completed in under 20 minutes.

For most hospital laboratories, cost justification is possible when the number of differentials exceeds 80 per day. The software-based system lends itself readily to improvements, which are likely also to be software-based. The spun slides are quite uniform and, therefore, especially helpful for leukopenic studies. The stain provided with the system produces a more intensely colored stain than with manual method. The convenience of operation enables the technologist to do differentials without having initially to find a WBC. Also, the tech-

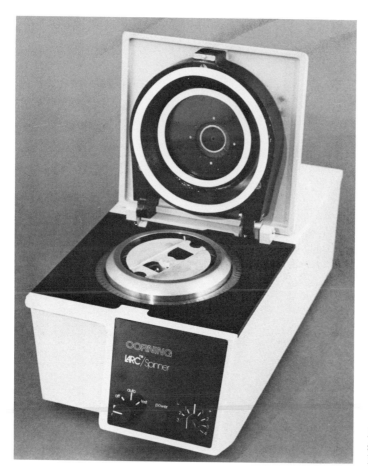

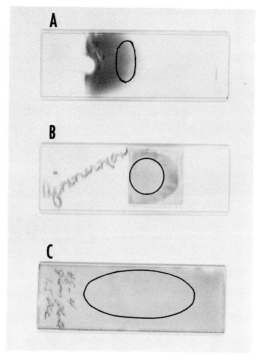

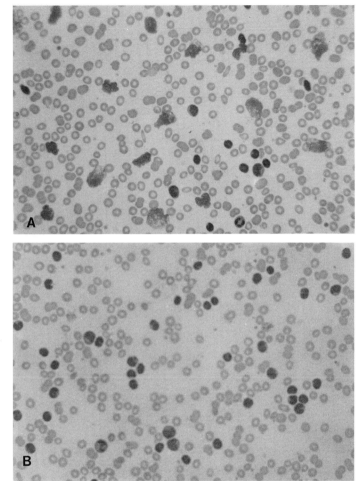

Fig. 5-28. (A) Photomicrograph of a wedged smear made from the blood of a patient with chronic lymphocytic leukemia. Note the smudge cells, formerly very fragile lymphocytes. *(B)* Photomicrograph of a spun smear made from the blood of a patient with chronic lymphocytic leukemia. Note the intact, fragile lymphocytes. (Courtesy of Corning Medical)

nologist need not be present during a scan and therefore may review abnormal or unknown cells upon completion of the differential. Using a single slide for each sample saves money, saves the cost of glass slides. The instrument utilizes a quality control technique in performing automated differential counts. For example, every shift (morning and evening) runs a quality control slide provided by Corning. At each shift, the technologist records the reported cell counts, the number of cells in the review list (a list of the usual, normal WBCs found in every normal differential count), the number of artifacts (objects acquired by the computer, but rejected as cells), and the time required to run the count. Each number is compared to the known values supplied with the slide. In this way, a visible record is available to indicate whether the system is producing reproducible results, shift after shift. The instrument automatically maintains a running average and count of differentials. Therefore, any change in the running average for the hospital (e.g., an outbreak of mononucleosis) indicates a change in the system. This might occur often long before an actual mechanical or electronic failure, and would suggest the necessity for instrument inspection. In this instrument, the technologist also records the number of artifacts. Ninety per cent of the time, this number is less than 20 artifacts per 100-cell differentials. If the num-

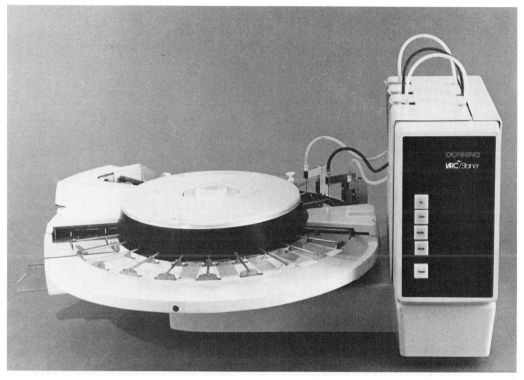

Fig. 5-29. Corning LARC stainer. (Courtesy of Corning Medical)

ber increases on many consecutive slides, it indicates a spinner or stainer problem. In fact, should a large number of artifacts appear on the slide, the slide will be rejected. It is, therefore, impossible to process automatically a poor slide. Usually, the rare, poor slide is due to a blood anomaly. The instrument also rejects slides that have stain characteristics, outside of narrow qualitative limits. If many slides in a batch are rejected, the stainer should be checked. If a differential count shows certain indicative values in combination with numbers of cells in the review list, the slide will automatically be rejected, requiring semiautomatic classification by the technologist. This rejection flags most severe blood problems and saves time by calling attention to abnormal slides. Finally, this instrument constantly monitors the levels of light passing through the microscope. If the intensity changes, the technologist will be immedi-

ately alerted. This precaution makes certain that the instrument is reading properly and that the slides are processed under uniform optical conditions.

Disadvantages. The LARC will not be able to classify about 5 per cent of normal cells, and these cells must be manually classified by the technologist. Also, the LARC occasionally counts a small neutrophil as an eosinophil. The accuracy and reproducibility of the differential count as well as of the normal range are limited by the total number of cells counted. The spinner is a limiting factor because the purchase of a second spinner is required in many cases. Also, a disposable catch basin for the spinner is needed to save cleaning time. It is essential to keep the system in an air conditioned area; it turns off automatically above 78° F (25.5° C). The computer program may be erased on occasion, owing to power line surges.

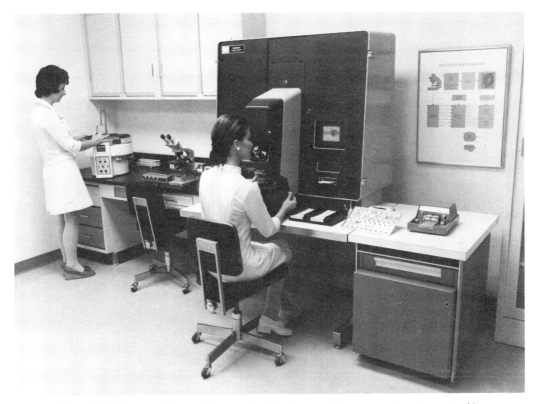

Fig. 5-30. Geometric Data Hematrak. (Courtesy of Geometric Data Hematrak)

Geometric Data Hematrak

The Geometric Data Hematrak is an automated microscope with image analysis of stained smears of blood cells (Fig. 5-30). Although specific slide preparation procedures are recommended by the manufacturer to ensure consistency, the instrument's design is flexible.[5] It can use slides prepared by classical techniques or prepared in any way the laboratory may desire. Either wedge or spun slides may be used. However, an automatic, mechanical slide stainer is available with the system.

In order to obtain speed in the scanning of white blood cells, a two-level computer system for cell identification was designed (Fig. 5-31). The first computer is hard-wired and basically high-speed because it involves no program search or other logic manipulation. The input signal to this first level computer is three million data points relating to density levels for each of three colors at each point resolved by the flying spot scanner (i.e. the recognition technique is performed in a two-step procedure). A processor measures cell parameters from the three-image channels, red, green, and blue. The hard-wired computer reduces these data to only 100 numbers, which serve to characterize the cell. Then, only 100 numbers are fed to the second programmed computer, a Hewlett-Packard 21MX, for logical classification by cell type, a process which takes only 40 milliseconds.

In the test procedure, a stained wedge slide containing a drop of oil is placed on the microscope stage with the feather edge to the left.

Initially, focus is manually adjusted for a neutrophil in order to compensate for stain

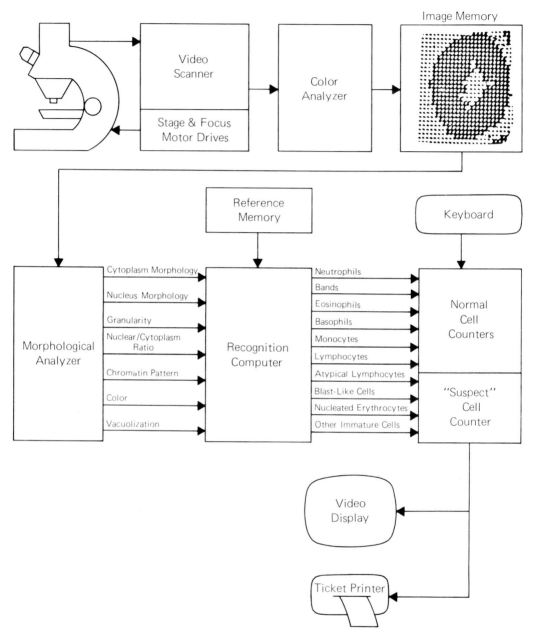

Fig. 5-31. Flow-through pattern of Hematrak, including 2-level computer system. (Geometric Data Hematrak)

variation. The operator then automatically scans (a purchase option) the smear to observe erythrocyte morphology, estimate platelet number, and select an appropriate area of the smear for cell recognition. If abnormal leukocytes are encountered during this pre-screening, the smear is removed from the Hematrak and a visual differential is performed. Abnormal leukocyte recognition falls outside the prime function of the system as a normal cell classifier. If no abnormal leukocytes are seen, the instrument

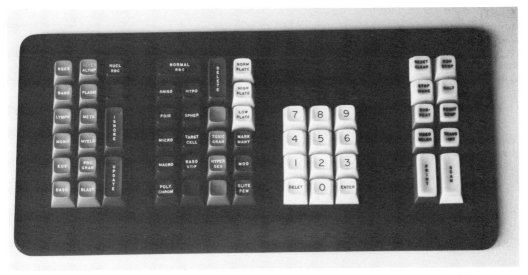

Fig. 5-32. Hematrak keyboard for identifying and entering various WBCs. (Courtesy of Geometric Data Hematrak)

is activated and a preselected number of cells (50–800) are scanned and categorized (Fig. 5-32). The optical resolution of the scanning system is approximately 0.25 μ., and there is an electronic measuring system capable of measurements of about 0.5μ. to 24μ.

This system has the potential to use precise measurement as a recognition parameter, as in the detection of bands in comparison with segmented polymorphs. It also may be useful in the quantification of anisocytosis and poikilocytosis.

Like its emphasis on speed, this system minimizes the dependence on memory and mechanical systems by instantly stopping at each cell it cannot automatically classify, which sounds an operator alert signal. As soon as the technologist identifies the cell and enters it on the keyboard, the Hematrak resumes the automatic scan. The automatic scanning objective is a Zeiss 40 × oil immersion objective. However, the operator may elect to use a 100 × oil immersion objective. Examples of cells that cause a halt are: abnormal leukocytes, nucleated red cells, and degranulated basophils. Atypical lymphocytes are tabulated in a unique

fashion. The total count as well as percentage values are displayed on a CRT for review, and a ticket printout, by means of a keyboard, can then be initiated. An instrument that automatically classifies normal cells without stopping at abnormal cells can be purchased as an optimal mode of operation.

The average sample throughout is between 30 and 50 per hour with a nominal average of 40 per hour, depending, of course, on the technologist and characteristics of the patient population.

There are additional design features in this instrument that contribute to its ability to work with wedge, spun, or nonmachine stained slides; these include automatic focusing for each detected cell, an algorithm that makes classification independent of cell size, and an auto-ranging system that compensates for stain variations and permits working with a range of stain intensity, using intensity levels appropriate to each slide for characterization of its cells.

Advantages. Usually takes only 1 week after installation to begin reporting differential counts with the system. The Hematrak enables a hematology division to handle an increased workload without adding more technologists or fatiguing those already employed. Quality control procedures are followed out each day, and reproducibility is good. Medical technologists have complete control over final differentiation cell decisions, which makes them more critical and helps to standardize and upgrade morphological interpretations. The Hematrak is flexible with regard to slide preparation and staining.

Disadvantages. When the criteria for bands and monocytes are first used, both types tended to be overused by standards that are conservative for most technologists. However, the computer program may be modified to remedy this situation. The system stops for abnormal cells an average of three times on a 100-cell differential count, usually for monocytes or atypical lymphocytes; if there are too many stats, the number of stops increases and manual count may be necessary. A voltage regulator may have to be installed to avoid occasional erratic performance. Deionized water is required for rinsing with the automatic stainer. There is excessive noise from the cooling fan.

Coulter Differential

The Coulter Differential was developed in an attempt to automate the basic differential count without medical technologist attention, on a carrier holding up to 20 slides at the rate of 35 to 40 slides per hour. M. M. Adner has evaluated the instrument by assessing several factors, the speed of the process, the accuracy of the classification, the versatility of the machine, and the relative cost of performing white cell differentials by the instrument or manually.[1]

The instrument is composed of two units, a preprocessor and a minicomputer, and a console unit that contains the microscope, the cell image monitor, the operator keyboard, and the information monitor, which displays the differential count. The dual display system provides a cell picture on one 8 in. color monitor and an alphanumeric display on another, similar monitor. The alphanumeric display can present a large quantity of data and can also accommodate computer program changes that might result from recognition improvement. The Coulter Differential is designed to analyze smears prepared by the spinning method, which produces a monolayer of cells. The spun slide is stained with a modified Wright-Giemsa stain, producing standard cell coloration. The system classifies the preselected number of cells on each slide according to the six most common types, counting the others as "unclassified."

When the stained smear is processed, the cell image is projected by a television camera through an optical path that includes a microscope (Fig. 5-33). The electrical image is processed and presented to the computer as a histogram, a form suitable to describing the various density levels. In order to produce more information for each cell, the cells on the histogram are illuminated by a number of wavelengths of light. The computer extracts information about nuclear and cytoplasmic area and color. These features, plus information related to shape and texture, provide the basis for classification of the leukocytes. The computer stores information on up to 100 slides for subsequent television display or printout and to classify visually the unidentified cells. In order to provide consistency in data acquisition, the instrument features positive bar code slide identification and automatic slide loading, slide oiling and slide focusing. It also has several modes by which the white cells may be analyzed and a mode in which the technologist can scan the slide for red cell morphology and platelet distribution. A grid is provided to aid in cell sizing.

In the manual differential mode, the instrument operates as an automated microscope that oils and focuses the slide automatically, and acquires and displays cells for the technologist to classify. The tech-

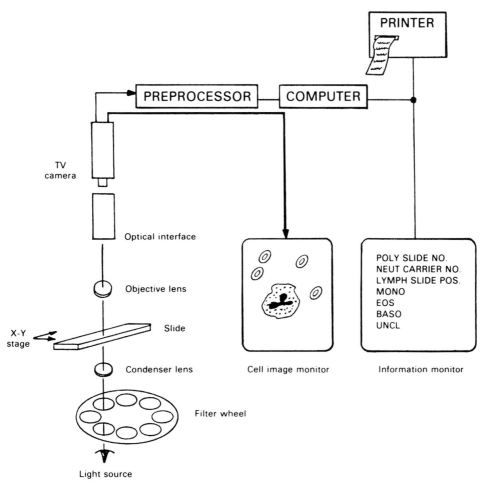

Fig. 5-33. Information processing flow for Coulter Differential. (Courtesy of Coulter Electronics, Inc.)

nologist may also consult the instrument for its system of cell classification.

The automatic differential mode classifies leukocytes by using either a 20-slide carrier or a single slide. Once the carrier has been loaded with up to 20 slides, each with a bar code label, the technologist places the carrier into the unit and initiates operation. The instrument will then remove each slide in turn from the carrier and perform 100, 200, 500, or 1000 white blood cell differentials, attended or unattended by a technologist, and return the slide to the carrier. The x-y coordinates of each unclassified cell, which is usually an abnormal cell, will be stored for later review. When all the slides in the carrier have been processed, the technologist may review the carrier for the unclassified cells. This is relatively simple to do since the computer stores the location of unrecognized cells on each slide and stops only at those cells. Those cells may then be identified by using the binocular of the built-in microscope or the color television display. Red cell morphology and platelet distribution may also be reviewed and evaluated at this time, or a second carrier may be entered, and all parts of the review may be (WBCs, RBCs, and platelets) may be performed at a later time.

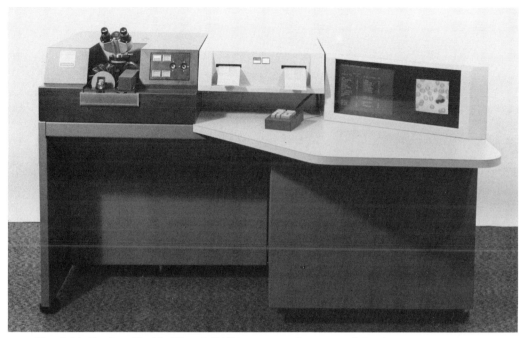

Fig. 5-34. Coulter (Perkin Elmer) Diff 3 system. (Courtesy of Coulter Electronics, Inc.)

At any time during the process, the sequence may be interrupted to analyze a single slide, and then resumed with no loss of information.

An automatic differential may be performed, by using limited visual operation in the find mode. The instrument will locate and project on the monitor a specified cell type while the automatic differential is being performed.

Advantages. The Coulter Differential is an excellent teaching aid and quality control (by monitoring recognition accuracy) because it allows the medical technologist to consult it for its cell classification. Allowing the technologist to leave the instrument unattended while carrier slides are being analyzed will result in more efficient use of technician time and will have an economic impact on the cost of running the hematology division of the laboratory. The multimode design makes it versatile and adaptable to the varying requirements of different laboratories and facilitates rapid, accurate classification of normal cells

and detection of abnormal cells. Since the instrument is a total cell classifier and not just a white blood cell classifier, it has a potential for greater utilization in other types of cell classifying, such as red cell, reticulocytes, Pap smears, and T and B lymphocytes.

Disadvantages. The instrument called 3 to 6 per cent of the normal cells unclassified and had difficulty in detecting some abnormal white blood cells. The time to make a 100 normal white cell count is between 90 and 100 seconds with $2\frac{1}{2}$ minutes for complete slide analysis. Manually, it takes $2\frac{1}{2}$ to 3 minutes per slide in a group of 20 slides. However, the technologist using the Coulter Differential has 30 minutes to perform other lab functions while the autodifferential is being performed. The cost of the Coulter Differential is very high.

Coulter (Perkin-Elmer) Diff 3 System

Automatic analysis and differential counting of white blood cells is at a higher level in the Perkin-Elmer Diff 3, (now

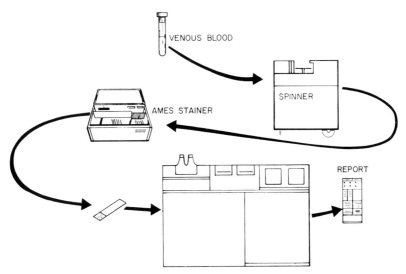

Fig. 5-35. Coulter (Perkin-Elmer) Diff 3 workflow. (Courtesy of Coulter Electronics, Inc.)

called Coulter Diff 3; Fig. 5-34; 5-35), than with other automated instruments, and its design is novel. The instrument automatically performs the total differential count on a spun stained slide and flags only the 10 to 15 per cent of the slides that require review, which is to be done on a laboratory microscope. In the procedure, the substage carrying the blood smear is moved under the objective lenses by automatic traversing and focusing mechanisms and is stopped by the finding and framing computer when a white cell comes into view. The cell image found by the microscope is scanned by a pair of oscillating mirrors at right angles to each other, and the scan is transmitted to a phototube. The cell image is then converted into an electronic signal by a photomultiplier. It may be displayed as a television picture or processed (i.e., quantized and "compressed" by the control computer) for analysis by the special golay logic computer. The computerized image can be displayed, stored in the tape memory, identified as to cell type, and counted (Fig. 5-36). The entire operation may be directed through the teletype keyboard, or it may be done automatically. The auto-

matic differential count includes classification by white cell type into the nine most frequently encountered categories plus other (unclassified cells), an estimate of the white cell count (concentration) in the sample, the number of nucleated red blood cells, the platelet sufficiency, the estimated platelet count (concentration) in the sample, and the red cell morphology. These functions are all automatic on the Diff 3. Unlike the categorization of red cell morphology in the other automatic systems, this instrument quantitatively evaluates erythrocytes according to size (normal, micro- or macro-), color (normal, hypo, chronic, or polychromasic), and shape (normal and poikilocytic). The manual sample throughput with this extent of automation is generally 35 to 40 per hour.

This system is available in two models, one for manual, one-at-a-time slide loading and one for automatic loading from a 14-slide magazine (Fig. 5-37). The magazine loading capability may be added to the manual load system at any time. The instrument includes a specially designed spinner that dilutes the sample. This makes practical the automatic evaluation of red

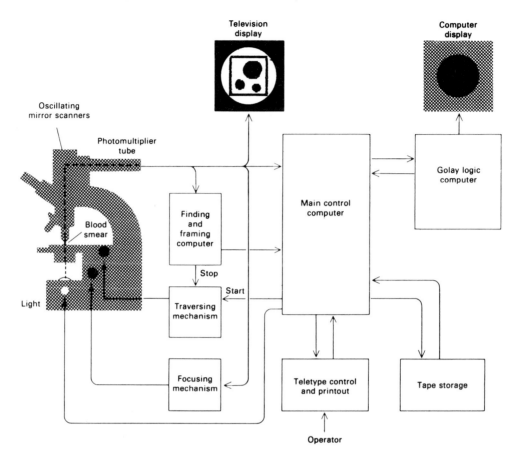

Fig. 5-36. Flow-through processing, analysis, and classification pattern of Coulter Diff 3 system. (Courtesy of Coulter Electronics, Inc.)

cell morphology, by reducing the effects of the variation of viscosity with hematocrit values.

Advantages. The Coulter (Perkin-Elmer) Diff 3 is an effective system of automatic analysis with procedure standardization, improvement over manual cell identification, overall cost reduction, and sufficient flexibility to allow for the addition of new measurements as new understanding of the blood cells develops. This type of cell classification with quantitation provides a complete objective evaluation of red cell morphology, plus the enumeration of giant platelets detected per 100 white cells classified. It may be programmed to perform a number of tasks other than the differential counting of white blood cells, for example, the counting of grains in the emulsions of cell autoradiographs, the location of malarial parasites in red cells, the analysis of human chromosomes, and the identification and counting of reticulated red cells.

Disadvantages. The time to make a 100 normal white cell count is between 90 and 110 seconds; however, the automatic operation without monitoring gives the technologist time to perform other functions in the laboratory. Insufficient comparative information, including information pertaining to technical and instrument difficulties, is available at this time.

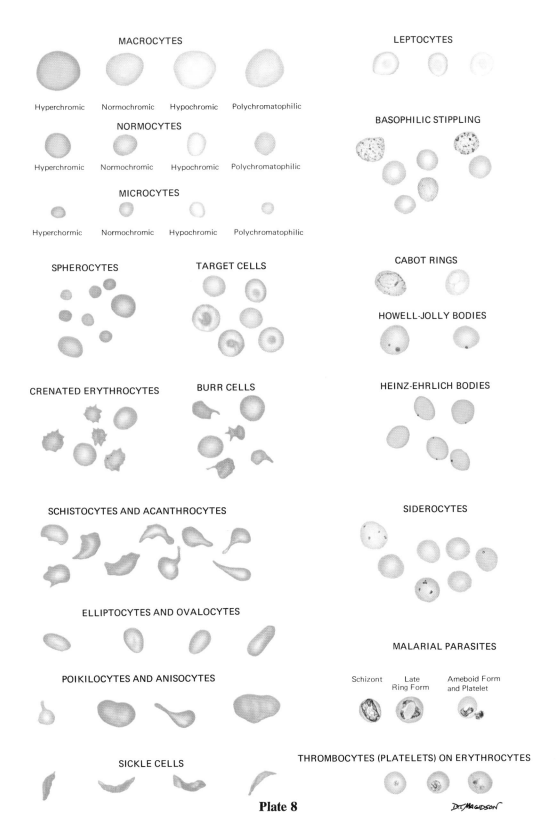

MACROCYTES

Hyperchromic   Normochromic   Hypochromic   Polychromatophilic

NORMOCYTES

Hyperchromic   Normochromic   Hypochromic   Polychromatophilic

MICROCYTES

Hyperchormic   Normochromic   Hypochromic   Polychromatophilic

LEPTOCYTES

BASOPHILIC STIPPLING

SPHEROCYTES

TARGET CELLS

CABOT RINGS

HOWELL-JOLLY BODIES

CRENATED ERYTHROCYTES

BURR CELLS

HEINZ-EHRLICH BODIES

SCHISTOCYTES AND ACANTHROCYTES

SIDEROCYTES

ELLIPTOCYTES AND OVALOCYTES

POIKILOCYTES AND ANISOCYTES

MALARIAL PARASITES

Schizont   Late Ring Form   Ameboid Form and Platelet

SICKLE CELLS

THROMBOCYTES (PLATELETS) ON ERYTHROCYTES

Plate 8

D.T. MAGIDSON

ABNORMAL FORMS OF ERYTHROCYTES, SHOWING VARIATIONS IN SIZE, SHAPE, INCLUSIONS, AND HEMOGLOBIN CONTENT

Plate 9

ERYTHROCYTIC ALTERATIONS AND INCLUSIONS
Peripheral Blood

1. Ovalocytes (elliptocytes) are oval red cells inherited rarely as a simple Mendelian dominant and usually without clinical significance. Occasionally they are associated with hemolysis and may be seen in some macrocytic anemias.

2 & 3. Reticulocytes are light bluish-gray RBCs possessing reticulum visible only by supravital stain (brilliant cresyl blue), i.e., the basophilic material is precipitated into strands, granules or a reticular arrangement.

4 & 6. Schistocytes are irregular red cell fragments which reflect RBC damage and breakdown; anisocytosis refers to variation in RBC size frequently seen in macrocytic, microcytic and hemolytic anemias, especially postsplenectomy.

5. Spherocytosis refers to a rounding of RBCs which have lost their normal biconcave configurations; they are thicker than normal, lack central pallor, and appear smaller and darker than normal cells (often called microspherocytes). Frequently they are associated with congenital or with other types of hemolytic anemias.

7. Siderocytes are RBCs that contain one or more hemosiderin granules demonstrable by Prussian blue stain; when seen with Wright's stain they are called Pappenheimer bodies.

8. Sickle cells (drepanocytes) are bizarre, sickle or crescent-shaped RBCs with tailed, filamentous and spine-like processes.

9. Macrocytes are RBCs with diameters of more than 8.5 μ and are frequently associated with B_{12}, folic acid deficiency, in patients with liver disease and/or reticulocytosis.

10 & 11. Late trophozoites or pre-schizonts or pre-segmenting stages of *Plasmodium vivax* infection are characterized by an increase in size, alteration of shape, protrusion of pseudopodia and deposition of golden-yellow pigment. Late ring (ameboid or trophozoite) stage is characterized by an enlarging RBC with Schüffner's dots (red-staining particles) within the RBC proper and not in the parasite as the golden-yellow granules described above. Ring forms are small, circular structures with pink nucleus and blue cytoplasm with Giemsa stain is used. Pre-schizonts (pS), ameboid (Am).

12. In thick smears the RBC outline is hemolyzed out or destroyed in the staining technic itself.

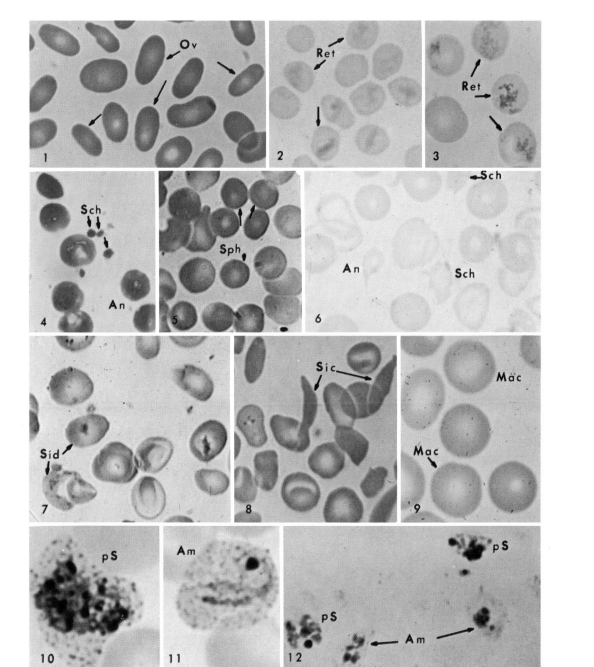

Plate 10

ERYTHROCYTIC ALTERATIONS AND INCLUSIONS
Peripheral Blood

1 & 3. Pappenheimer bodies are hemosiderin granules visible in RBCs stained with Romanowsky stains (e.g. Wright's). When they are stained with Prussian blue stain, the erythrocytes containing them are called siderocytes.

2. Reticulocytes are young erythrocytes containing basophilic material precipitating into strands, granules, or a reticular arrangement, visible when stained with supravital stain (brilliant cresyl blue). It is a property usually directly related to diffuse basophilia or polychromatophilia.

4 & 5. Howell-Jolly bodies are nuclear remnants forming round, dense inclusion bodies situated near the periphery of an RBC; they stain dark blue-black with Wright's stain and are seen in a variety of severe anemias (especially hemolytic disorders), are characteristic of hyposplenism, and are present after splenectomy.

6 & 7. Basophilic stippling (or punctate basophilia as contrasted to diffuse basophilia) are clumped or small aggregates in RBCs of Wright-stained films of patients with lead poisoning or thalassemia and are also seen in conditions associated with accelerated RBC production.

8 & 9. Phase contrast photos of platelets. Platelets stand out as individual round or oval bodies with bluish or purple sheen. On focusing up and down with low power ($\times 100$) microscope objectives, platelets can be seen to have one or more fine processes (pseudopodia).

10 & 11. *Plasmodium falciparum* ring or trophozoite forms are frequently found at the periphery of the RBC; *Plasmodium malariae* forms a rectangular band in the late trophozoite or early schizont form with golden brown pigment in the parasite.

12. Cabot rings are filamentous or thread-like structures that assume bizarre purplish configurations in Wright's stain; they may be artefacts but are associated with disturbances in erythropoiesis (e.g., P.A.).

13 & 14. Heinz bodies are single or multiple refractile granules of precipitated hemoglobin located at the edge of the RBC (seen in supravital stain but not in Wright's stain); they are associated with hemolytic and other RBC injury disorders.

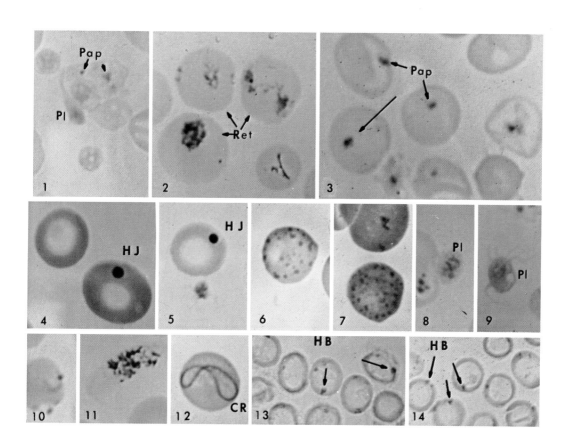

Plate 11

HYPOCHROMIC MICROCYTIC ANEMIA
(Iron Deficiency Anemia)
Peripheral Blood

Anisocyte (An), elliptocyte (El), lymphocyte (L), microcyte (Mic), platelets (Pl), poikilocyte (Poik), ring form RBC (RF), schistocyte (Sch), target cell (Tar).

Diagnostic Features: In this hematologic pattern the hemoglobin content of the erythrocytes is reduced out of proportion to the RBC count and hematocrit levels; it is frequently seen in premature infants, chronic blood loss, pregnancy, hookworm disease, etc., and especially in females. The RBCs show an exaggerated central pallor and a condensed peripheral ring of hemoglobin (these are called ring forms). Microcytosis and poikilocytosis (elongated, elliptical and tear-drop forms) are also seen; occasionally one sees polychromatophilic macrocytes; the reticulocyte percentage is usually reduced; occasionally normoblasts are seen. The WBC count is normal or slightly reduced in number; few multisegmented neutrophils are found; slight absolute granulocytopenia and relative lymphocytosis is observed in long-standing cases; eosinophilia is seen in hookworm disease. Platelets are normal in number and small in size. The serum iron is reduced; the iron binding capacity is elevated.

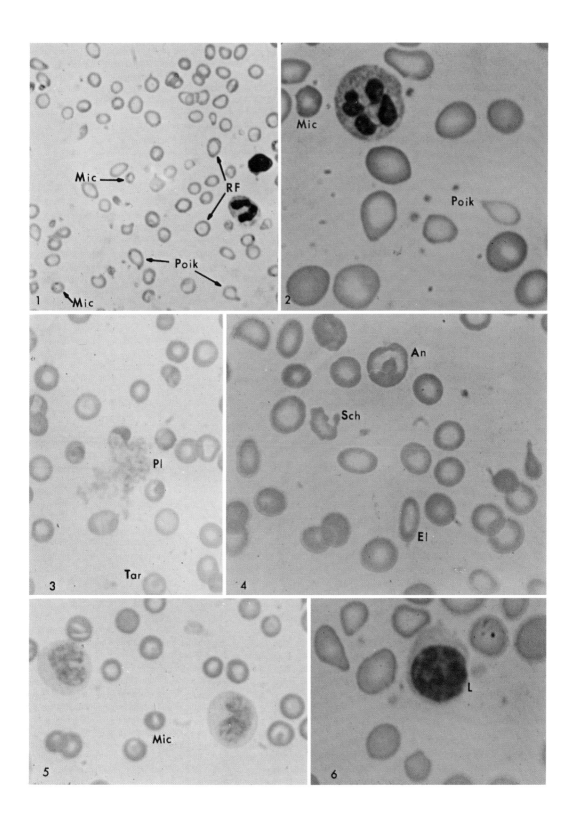

Plate 12

HYPOCHROMIC MICROCYTIC ANEMIA
Bone Marrow

Degenerating (deg), lymphocyte (L), metamyelocyte (mMc), neutrophilic myelocyte (NMc), orthochromic normoblasts (ONb), plasma cell (PC).

Diagnostic Features: There is a relative and absolute increase in the number of normoblasts, especially the small polychromatophilic normoblasts.

After iron therapy there is still greater increase in normoblastic cells (Fig. 3). The bone marrow hemosiderin and siderocytes are virtually absent (Fig. 5): no bluish granular deposits of iron are seen in sections of bone marrow stained with Prussian blue stain (negative Prussian blue test).

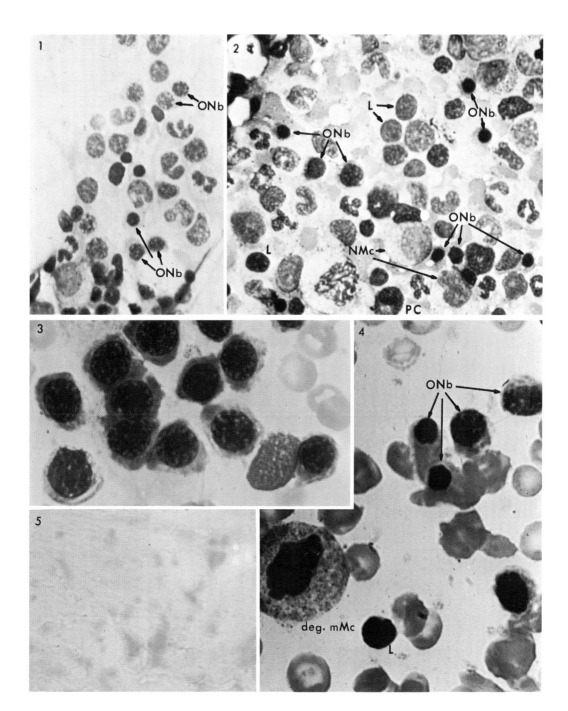

Plate 13

PERNICIOUS ANEMIA
Peripheral Blood

Polymorphonuclear neutrophil (PmN), poikilocyte (Poik), macrocytic RBC (macro), normocyte (norm), elliptocyte (El), anisocyte (An), large platelet (lg. Pl), normal platelet (norm Pl), polychromatophilic RBC (polychr), large neutrophilic myelocyte (lg. NMc), reticulocyte (Ret).

Diagnostic Features: A macrocytic anemia usually characterized by macrocytosis, poikilocytosis, polychromasia, anisocytosis, Howell-Jolly bodies and Cabot rings; leucopenia is also observed with hypersegmentation of polys; occasional giant metamyelocytes, myelocytes and occasionally eosinophilia are seen; thrombocytopenia and bizarre giant platelets are also observed. Also present are histamine achlorhydria, less than 5% excretion of cobalt 57 or 60 vitamin B_{12} in the Schilling test and reduced serum vitamin B_{12} levels. Postvitamin B_{12} treatment (bottom Fig. 7) (i.e., 6 to 48 hours after initiation of therapy) shows increased reticulocytosis.

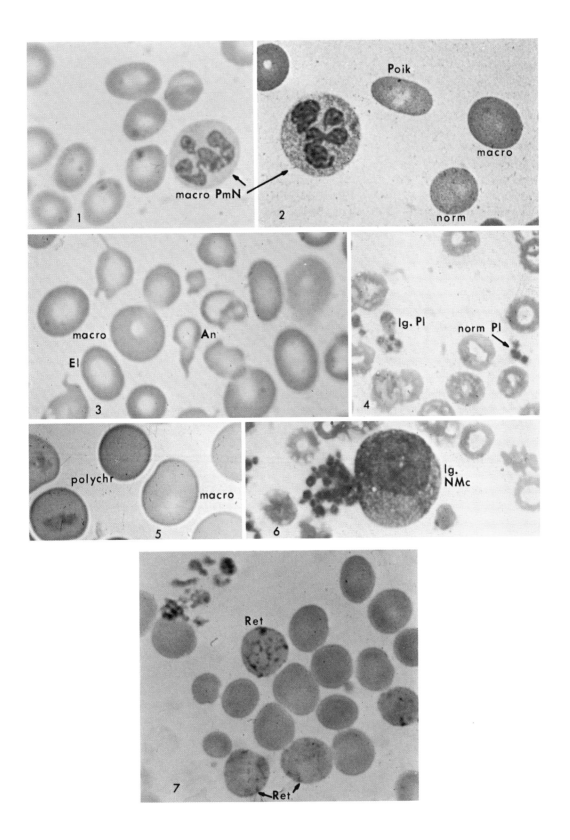

Plate 14

PERNICIOUS ANEMIA
Bone Marrow No. 1

1. Polychromatophilic megaloblasts (arrows) and a megaloblast in anaphase of mitosis. 2 & 4. Polychromatic megaloblasts. 3. Section of femur to show deep red gelatinous (currant jelly) transformation of long bone yellow marrow. 5 & 6. Polymorphonuclear eosinophile. 7. Promyeloblast (prMb), bizarre polymorphonuclear neutrophile and polychromatophilic megaloblast. 8. Orthochromic normoblast (ONb) with Howell-Jolly bodies, orthochromic megaloblast (OMgb) in metaphase mitosis (distorted). 9. Giant eosinophilic myelocyte. 10. Orthochromic megaloblast in late anaphase of mitosis. 11. Large eosinophilic myelocyte (EMc), neutrophilic myelocyte (NMc) and orthochromic megaloblast (OMgb). 12. Polychromatophilic megaloblasts (PcMgb). 13. Polychromatophilic megaloblast and promegaloblast (prMgb). 14. Neutrophilic myelocyte in distorted metaphase mitosis (NMc), doughnut-shaped juvenile (Juy),

eosinophilic myelocyte (EMc), lymphocyte (L).

Diagnostic Features: Thirty to 50 per cent of nucleated RBC series are megaloblasts (nuclei have "scroll-like" or sieve-like appearance and bead-like chromatin strands and parachromatin areas) and promegaloblasts with deeply basophilic cytoplasm; Polychromatophilic and acidophilic megaloblasts are observed in groups of 3 to 6 with many mitoses; giant bizarre metamyelocytes are present with doughnut-shaped nuclei and vacuolated, poorly-stained light blue to basophilic relatively agranular cytoplasm; marrow reticulocytosis, reticulum cells and lymphocytic cells are found; megakaryocytes are reduced and possibly abnormal in pattern. Generally, after vitamin B_{12} therapy, there is disappearance of megaloblasts and enlarged related nucleated red blood cells in the marrow.

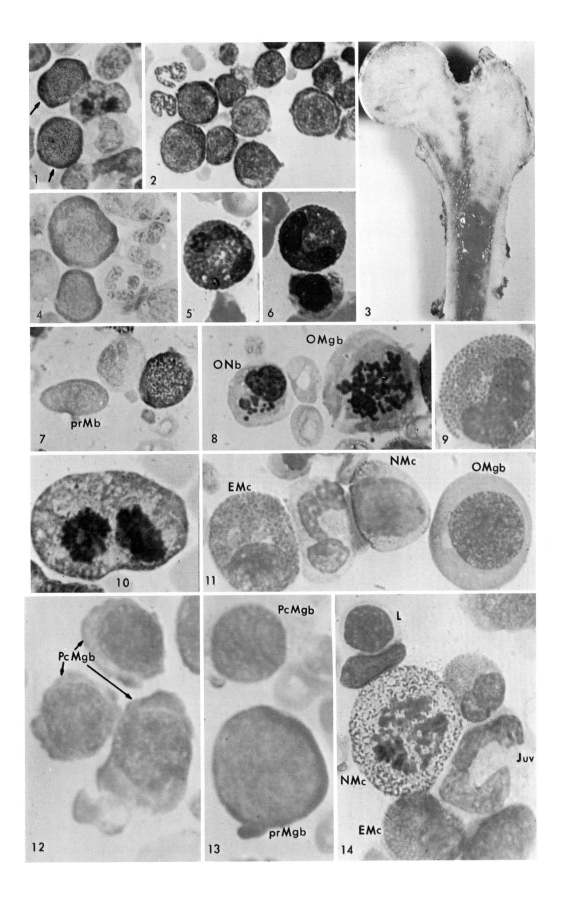

Plate 15

PERNICIOUS ANEMIA
Bone Marrow No. 2

1. Doughnut shaped neutrophilic myelocytes (NMc), polychromatic megaloblasts (PcMgb). 2. Polychromatic megaloblast (mitotic) (PcMgb) and promegaloblast (prMgb). 3. Giant megakaryocytes (Mgk). 4. Promegablasts (prMgb) and megaloblast (Mgb). 5. Macropolycyte (macP), orthochromic normoblast (ONb). 6 & 7. Megaloblasts (Mgb) and pronormoblasts (prNb). 8. After vitamin B_{12} therapy: orthochromic normoblasts (ONb), promyelocyte (prMc), neutrophilic myelocyte (NMc).

Diagnostic Features: See description under Bone Marrow No. 1. After vitamin B_{12} therapy there is a reversion to normocytic-type normoblastic morphology in the bone marrow. The cells that have already matured to a postmitotable stage remain megaloblastic.

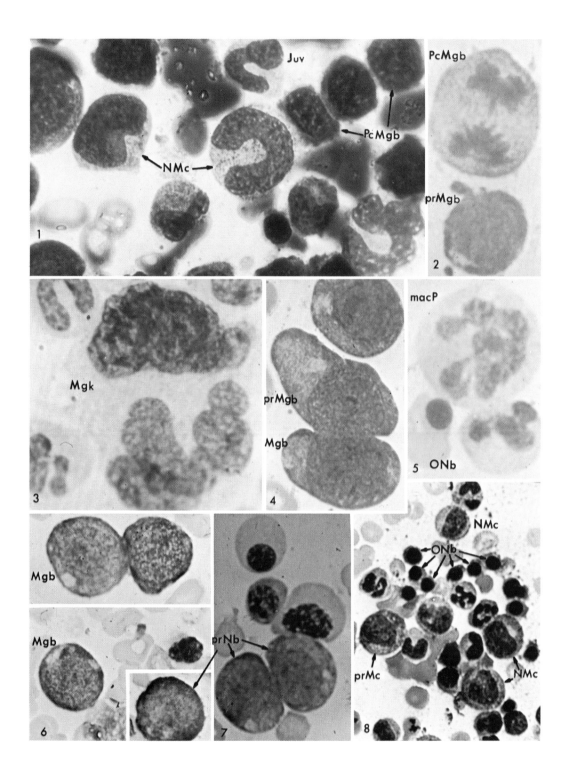

Plate 16

SPRUE, Etc. (MALABSORPTION SYNDROMES)
Peripheral Blood (Top); Bone Marrow (Bottom)

Normal red blood cell (RBC), macrocytic RBC (Mac), microcytic RBC (Mic), Howell-Jolly bodies (HJ), poikilocyte (poik), schistocyte (Sch), lymphocyte (L), burr cell (burr), orthochromic normoblast (ONb), macropolycyte (macP), basophilic megaloblastic normoblast (BMgbNb), polychromic normoblast (PcNb), monocyte (M), basophilic normoblast (BNb), polymorphonuclear neutrophil (PmN), pronormoblast (prNb), megaloblast (Mgb).

Diagnostic Features: This syndrome includes tropical sprue, non-tropical sprue (idiopathic steatorrhea) and celiac disease; also tuberculotic and regional enteritis. These conditions are characterized by impaired absorption of folic acid (most frequently), vitamin B_{12}, etc., with associated increased excretion of fat and excessive loss of calcium in the form of insoluble soaps. Iron deficiency (and, therefore, microcytic RBCs) often is associated with the blood picture. The peripheral blood pattern shows marked anisocytosis, polychromasia and macrocytosis with occasionally hypochromic microcytes. Leukopenia with associated macropolycytosis and giant metamyelocytes with broad tortuous vacuolated nuclei are seen; thrombocytopenia and relative lymphocytosis occasionally occurs. The bone marrow may be pure megaloblastic (like P.A.), especially if the anemia is macrocytic; or the bone marrow may be normoblastic when there is a marked iron deficiency with an associated hypochromic microcytic pattern. When the MCV is normal, the bone marrow pattern is frequently mixed (i.e., megaloblastic and normoblastic).

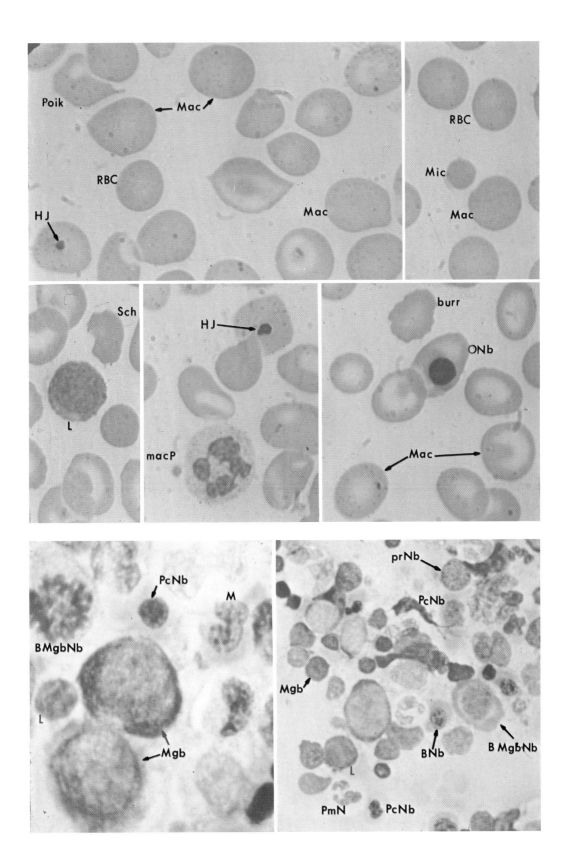

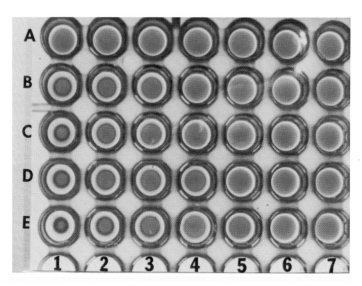

Plate 17

ERYTHROPOIETIN ASSAY

Row A is a primary polycythema vera sera sample with the end point in the 2nd well (first 3 plus). Row B is a secondary polycythema sera with the end point in the 4th well (first 3 plus). Row C is a normal sera sample with the end point in well 5 (first 3 plus). Rows D and E are elevated sera samples from a patient with a kidney tumor and one with sickle cell anemia. The 3 plus end points are in wells 6 and 7.

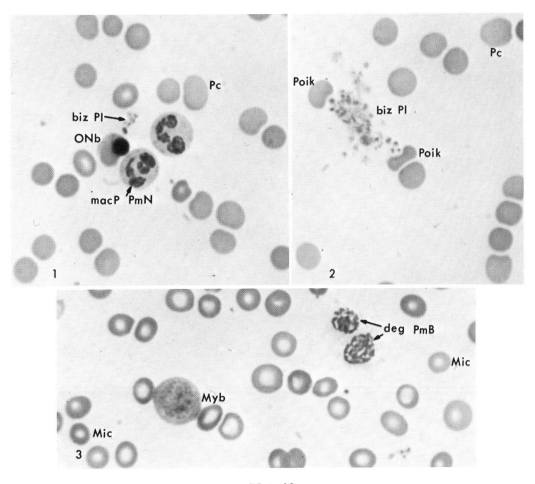

Plate 18

MYELOPHTHISIC (LEUKO-ERYTHROBLASTIC) ANEMIA
Peripheral Blood

Bizarre platelets (biz Pl), orthochromic normoblast (ONb), macropolycytic polymorphonuclear neutrophil (macP PMN), microcyte (Mic), myeloblast (Myb), degenerating polymorphonuclear basophil (deg PmB), poikilocyte (Poik), polychromatic RBC (Pc).

Diagnostic Features: The peripheral blood manifestations may or may not be correlated with the degree of marrow involvement, i.e., the symptom-complex is usually secondary to space-occupying disorders of the bone marrow and the hematologic manifestations are the same regardless of the cause. Typically, a normocytic normochromic anemia is observed with slight decrease in hemoglobin and hematocrit; polychromasia, RBC stippling, roulleaux, reticulocytosis, and normoblasts are also seen. The WBCs may be normal, reduced or more often slightly increased; occasionally a leukemoid pattern may be seen with a small number of myeloblasts, myelocytes, etc., and with a decrease in lymphocytes. The platelets vary in number and qualitative pattern with bizarre, large, and small forms frequently observed.

Plate 19

MYELOPHTHISIC (LEUKO-ERYTHROBLASTIC) ANEMIA
Bone Marrow

Cancer cells (Ca), Gaucher cell (Gc), Niemann-Pick cell (NP), polymorphonuclear neutrophil (PmN), Histoplasma capsulatum (HC).

Diagnostic Features: Bone marrow pattern may be normal, may show increased numbers of lymphocytes and plasma cells, or may contain focal collections of large carcinoma cells, fungi (e.g., Histoplasma capsulatum), and large foam cells containing lipid (e.g., Gaucher's cells and Niemann-Pick cells). These focal "foreign" cells are scattered among normal marrow elements either singly or in small clumps or sheets. Aimed punctures at sites of bone pain or deformity are more likely to produce cells, especially if both aspirates and serial tissue sections (made from marrow particles or clots) are examined.

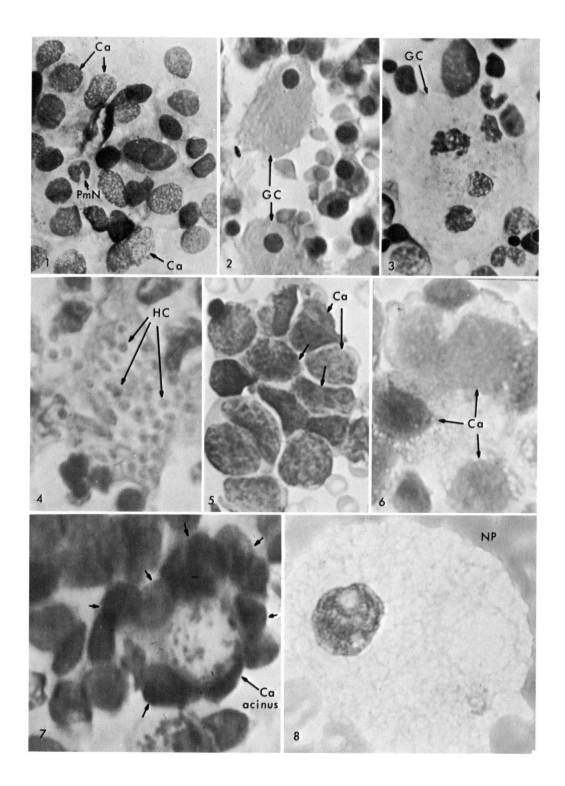

Plate 20

RELATIVE MARROW FAILURE ANEMIA
(Simple Anemias of Chronic Infections and Systemic Diseases)
(Etiologic Agents in Normochromic Microcytic Anemia)
Peripheral Blood

1. Whooping cough (lymphocytosis). Lymphocyte (L). 2. Chronic infection (suppurative osteomyelitis and chronic pyelonephritis). Lymphocyte (L), monocyte (M). 3. Leukemoid reaction. Prolymphocyte (prL). 4. Chronic infection—azure granules [lymphocyte (L)]. 5. Vacuolated cytoplasm (virocyte) monocyte (M). 6. German measles (vacuolated monocyte). Lymphocyte (L), monocyte (M), polymorphonuclear neutrophil (PmN). 7. Periarteritis nodosa (eosinophils). Polymorphonuclear eosinophils (PmE). 8. Kala-azar (mononuclear cell containing *Leishmania donovani*). 9. Chronic infection with toxic granules. Juvenile (Juv). 10 & 11. Toxic granules in lobar pneumonia. 12. Meningococci in monocyte (phagocyte). 13. *Wuchereria bancrofti* lying free in blood.

Diagnostic Features: The peripheral blood is characterized by normocytic anemia with moderate anisocytosis and slight poikilocytosis; occasional polychromatophilia is observed in severe chronic renal disease. The leukocyte pattern, however, depends on the nature of the causative disorder, e.g., monocytosis in tuberculosis, brucellosis and viral infections; polymorphonuclear leukocytosis in acute infections with toxic granule formation; lymphocytosis in typhoid and viral infections —associated with the latter is vacuolation of the cytoplasm (Figs. 5 and 6); eosinophilia is observed in parasitic infections, scarlet fever, periarteritis nodosa, etc.

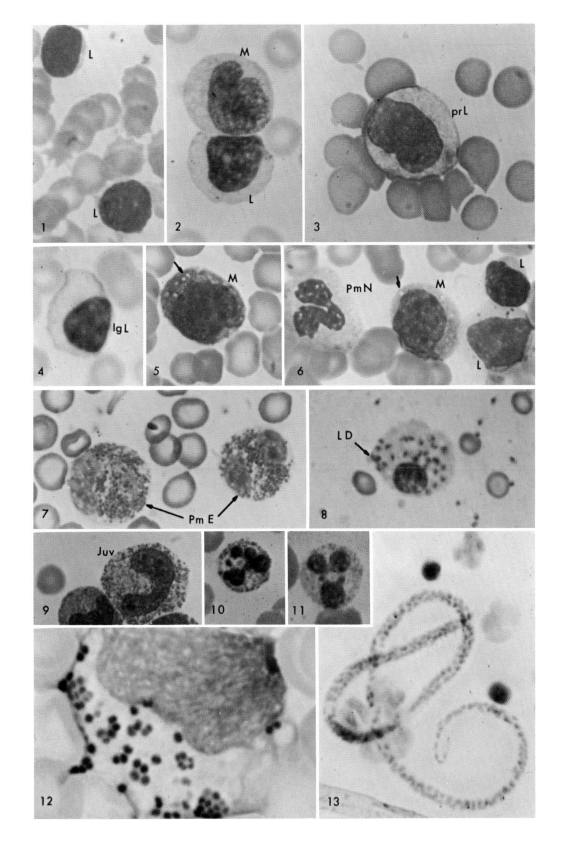

Plate 21

RELATIVE MARROW FAILURE ANEMIA
(Simple Anemias of Chronic Infections and Systemic Diseases)
(Etiologic Agents in Normochromic Microcytic Anemia)
Bone Marrow, Lymph Node, and Spleen Pattern

1. *Histoplasma capsulatum* (HC) in bone marrow. Monocyte (M). 2. Histiocytes (Hist), monocytes (M), and platelets (Pl) in bone marrow. Juvenile (Juv). 3. Histiocytic phagocytosis in bone marrow. Histiocyte (Hist), neutrophilic metamyelocyte (NmMc), polymorphonuclear neutrophil (PmN). 4. *Histoplasma capsulatum* in degenerating monocyte in bone marrow. 5. *Histoplasma capsulatum* (HC) in mononuclear cells in lymph node. 6. Kala-azar, splenic imprint. *Leishmania donovani* (LD) in cytoplasm of mononuclear cells. Lymphocytes (L).

Diagnostic Features: The bone marrow pattern usually shows hyperplasia of the leukocytic elements with an associated qualitative shift to younger normoblast forms (e.g., maturation arrest-like pattern). In renal insufficiency, there is a decrease in the ratio of nucleated RBCs to WBCs due to leukocytic and megakaryocytic hypoplasia rather than to reduction of normoblasts; one also sees a shift to the left of the myeloid cells with an increase in myelocytes, histiocytes, plasma cells, phagocytic cells and eosinophils; karyorrhexis of normoblastic nuclei is also seen.

Imprints can be very useful as an aid in the diagnosis of various bacterial, mycotic and parasitic diseases. Very frequently, one observes the specific infectious agent in the cytoplasm of the monocyte and occasionally in the polymorphonuclear neutrophil. The organism is phagocytosed by the histiocytic or monocytic-type cell and may be destroyed or may proliferate therein, finally disrupting the cell and escaping into the sinusoids of the bone marrow, lymph node or spleen where they are engulfed again by other histiocytes and monocytes. Giemsa and Wright stain may be used on these imprints.

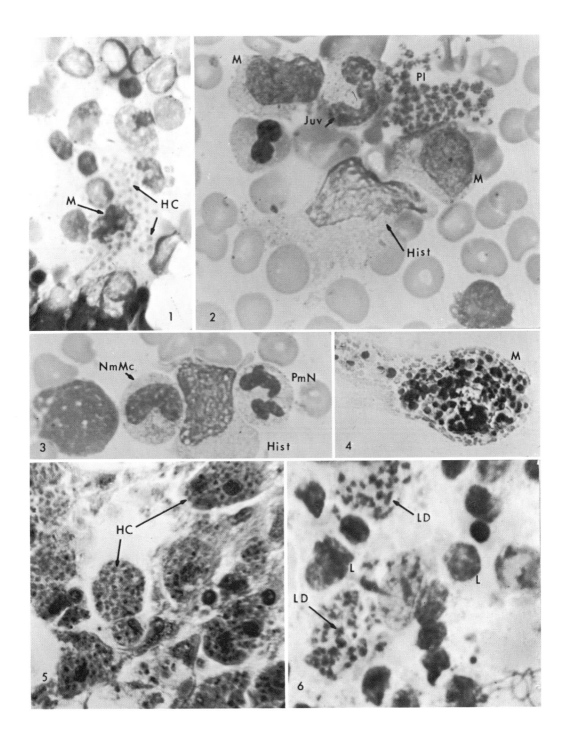

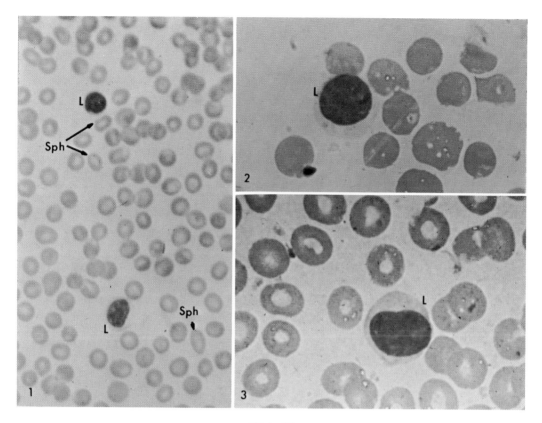

Plate 22

BONE MARROW FAILURE
(Hypoplastic Anemia, Aplastic Anemia, Aregenerative Anemia)
Peripheral Blood

Lymphocytes (L), spheroidal RBCs (Sph).

Diagnostic Features: The peripheral blood is characterized by average total RBC count of less than two million (2,000,000); erythrocytes appear normal, although occasionally anisocytotic and poikilocytotic. There is leukopenia with a lymphocytosis of 70 to 90 per cent; thrombocytopenia is also quite frequently observed. If normoblasts are seen, one also observes occasional immature myeloid cells; in familial cases, a reticulocytosis of six to ten per cent may be seen. If a pure RBC aplasia is present, there is usually no concomitant leukopenia or thrombocytopenia. In patients with bone marrow failure, spheroidal RBCs are frequently observed after many transfusions.

Plate 23 ⟶

BONE MARROW FAILURE
(Hypoplastic Anemia, Aplastic Anemia, Aregenerative Anemia)
Bone Marrow

1 & 2. Hypoplastic to aplastic (reduced) cellular pattern (×100). 3. Marked reduction in myeloid and erythroid cellular content (×430). 4. Hyperplasia, moderate, lymphocytic, myeloid, and erythroid elements (×100). 5. Benzol exposure, normocellular (×970). 8. Section of sternum marrow (yellowish pink instead of normal red color). 9. After 20 transfusions (6+ Iron) (iron represented by Prussian blue particles).

Lymphocyte (L), metamyelocyte (mMc), neutrophilic myelocyte (NMc), orthochromic normoblast (ONb), prolymphocyte (prL), juvenile (Juv), polymorphonuclear neutrophil (PmN).

Diagnostic Features: The marrow is rarely totally acellular, i.e., a nest of marrow cells may be aspirated. The differential count is variable, with a normal, greatly increased, or decreased M:E ratio. There is a relative increase in lymphocytes,

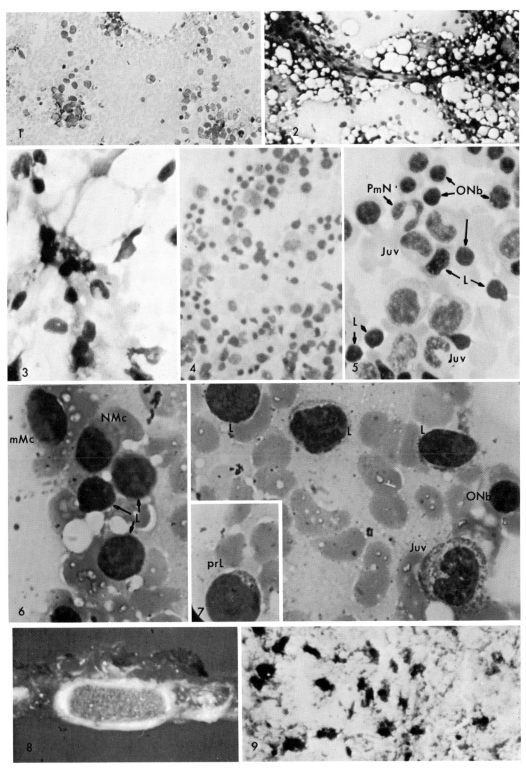

monocytes and plasma cells; megakaryocytes are decreased in number. Normoblast cytoplasm is poorly formed with excessive numbers of large siderotic granules or a bizarre chromatin structure of the nucleus; occasionally one sees an increased number of mast cells. The histologic structure is studied better in fixed tissue sections than in thin bone marrow smears.

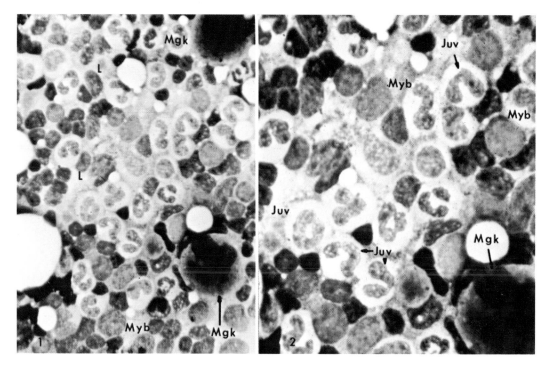

Plate 24

CONGENITAL ERYTHROCYTIC HYPOPLASIA
Bone Marrow

Megakaryocyte (Mgk), lymphocyte (L), myeloblast (Myb), juvenile (Juv).

Diagnostic Features: The marrow is characterized by marked deficiency to almost complete absence of the nucleated precursors of RBCs. Disease is manifest soon after birth; it involves erythropoietic tissue with granulocytes and platelets and their precursors relatively unaffected. If the marrow is hyperplastic, it is believed that, etiologically, the pattern is related to "maturation arrest" at the early to late normoblastic stage.

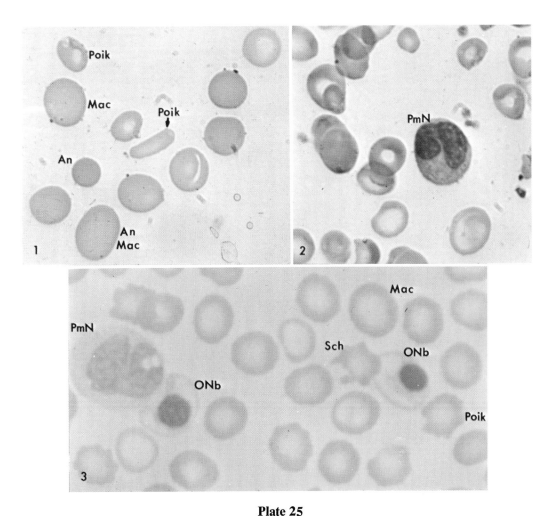

Plate 25

REFRACTORY SIDEROBLASTIC OR SIDEROACHRESTIC ANEMIA
Peripheral Blood

Anisocyte (An), orthochromic normoblast (ONb), poikilocyte (Poik), polymorphonuclear neutrophil (PmN), schistocyte (Sch), macrocyte (Mac).

Diagnostic Features: Hyposegmented poorly granulated PmNs with hypochromia of RBCs and deficiency of hemoglobin in normoblasts. The latter is more pronounced in the peripheral blood of post-splenectomy cases. Also see anisocytosis, poikilocytosis, schistocytosis and monocytosis. The entire clinical pattern is associated with a severe hypochromic microcytic anemia that is refractory to iron and all other types of hematopoietic therapy. The nature of the block in hemoglobin synthesis is not known. Fig. 3—after splenectomy.

Plate 26

REFRACTORY SIDEROBLASTIC OR SIDEROACHRESTIC ANEMIA
Bone Marrow

Basophilic normoblast (BNb), histiocyte (Hist), iron particles (Fe), mitosis (mit), neutrophilic myelocyte (NMc), normoblast (Nb), orthochromic normoblast (ONb), promonocytes (prM), promyelocyte (prMc), sideroblasts (Sb)—ONb and BNb.

Diagnostic Features: Normoblastic hyperplasia with partial "maturation arrest" (megaloblastoid). Cytoplasm of these cells is hypochromic with increased iron found in the perinuclear cytoplasm of the bone marrow normoblasts (called sidero-blasts). There is practically no visible cytoplasmic hemoglobin, but cytoplasmic vacuoles are present in some cases. There is also minimal increase in myeloblasts with associated nuclear-cytoplasmic asynchrony, i.e., persistence of nucleoli in later mature granulocytic forms. 5. Histiocyte surrounded by iron particles revealed by Prussian blue. 6. Nucleated RBC containing black-brown granules of iron stained with Wright's stain. 7. Iron granules stained with Prussian blue, in cytoplasm of sideroblast (orthochromic normoblast).

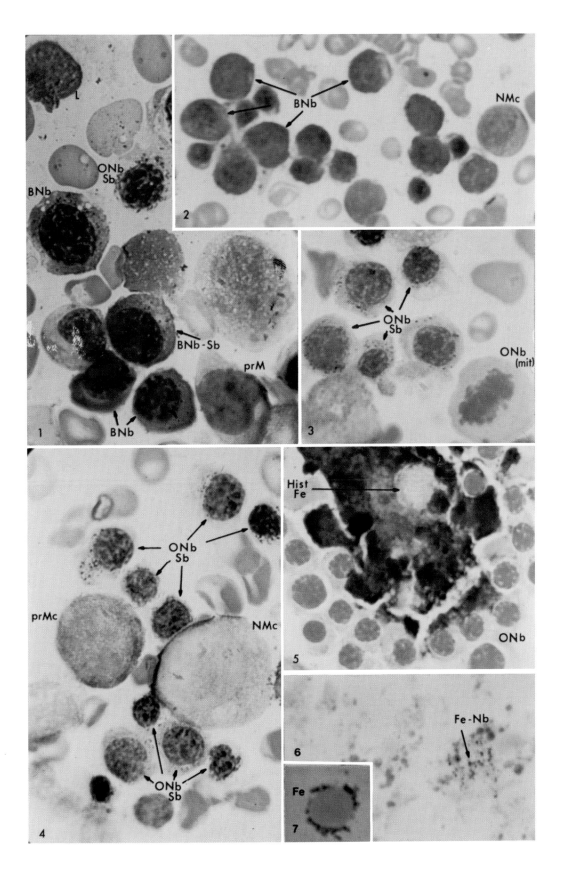

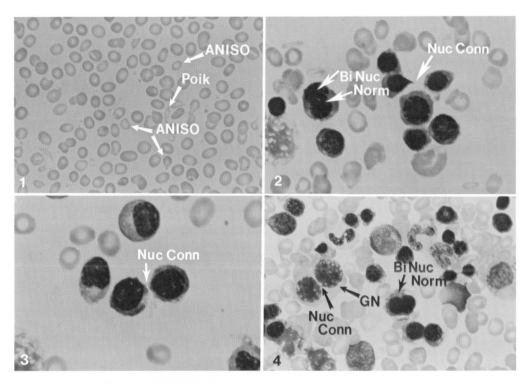

Plate 27

CONGENITAL DYSERYTHROPOIETIC ANEMIA
Peripheral Blood

1. Moderate anisocytosis and poikilocytosis in an associated normocytic anemia (ANISO = aniso-cytosis; Poik = poikilocytosis)

Bone Marrow

2, 3. Multiple (two) nuclei; unknown number of nucleoli plus nuclear chromatin connection (BiNuc Norm = Binucleated normoblast; Nuc Conn = Nuclear chromatin connection)

4. Giant normoblast with nuclear chromatin connection (G N = giant normoblast; BiNuc Norm = binucleate normoblast; Nuc Conn = nuclear chromatin connection; Crookston, J. H., Crookston, M. C., Burnie, K. L., Francorie, W. H., Davis, J. H., and Lewis, S. M.: Hereditary erythroblastic multinuclearity associated with a positive acidified serum test: a type of congenital dyserythropoietic anemia. Br. J. Haematol., *17*:11, 1969)

Congenital dyserythropoietic anemia consists of three types of refractory anemia characterized by multinuclearity, karyorrhexis, and other bizarre nuclear abnormalities of erythrocyte precursors in the bone marrow. There are normoblastosis in marrow, normal reticulocyte count, and elevated indirect serum bilirubin. Type II is known as HEMPAS (hereditary erythroblast multinuclearity with positive acidified serum test). It is characterized by normocytic anemia, variable jaundice, hepatosplenomegaly, anisocytosis, poikilocytosis, and multiple nuclei in later stages of normoblastic development. The acidified serum lysis test is positive in 60 per cent of normal sera. Lysis in those cases appears to be due to an antibody present in normal serum and to a slight increase in the complement sensitivity of the RBCs; that is, cells of HEMPAS patients will be lysed by the serum of many normal donors. Since this lysis is antibody-mediated, absorption of the serum at 0° with washed packed RBCs from the patient markedly reduces the amount of the lysis. No reduction in lysis of PNH cells is seen if serum is absorbed similarly by PNH, normal, or HEMPAS cells.

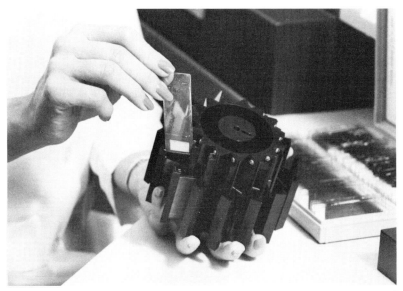

Fig. 5-37. Coulter (Perkin-Elmer) Diff 3 system slide carousel. (Courtesy of Coulter Electronics, Inc.)

AUTOMATED STAGE MICROSCOPE (HONEYWELL ACS 1000)

The automated stage microscope is a computer-based system that automates practically all the steps in the performance of a stained differential count on a microscope stage—except the actual cell classification. The manufacturer's concept is that the process of cell classification requires an inordinate compute capacity, whereas the human brain is both adept and rapid. Thus, the instrument computer (actually a microprocessor) is limited to controlling and automating the visual and mechanical tasks that are slowly or inefficiently handled by the medical technologist. These are the focus scan between cells in a repeatable pattern, the locating of cells and the centering of each in the field, and the relocating of a suspect cell for review after the slide has been removed from the stage. When a cell is automatically located, it is centered in the field and is displayed on a color television monitor with 2500 × magnification, which makes visual examination by the medical technologist easier and less

fatiguing (Fig. 5-38). The same cell may be viewed through the binoculars of the associated microscope at up to 1000 × magnification. The manufacturer claims that these factors enable an increase in sample throughput of 20 to 60 per cent, compared to manually performed differentials. In most hospitals, between 18 and 30 slides per hour may be completed on this instrument, depending on the skills and experience of the medical technologist. Because the computer does not perform pattern recognition, the cost is significantly lower than the previously described instruments. The large magnification color display, together with the associated binocular microscope attachment, makes this system useful for teaching.

This instrument is built around a commercial microscope, in which the focus and stage have been motorized. A display panel is placed to the left of the microscope. During the performance of a white cell count this panel shows the number of cells counted, the number or percentage of each type, and the x and y coordinates of the cell in the field of view. If that cell is atypical or ab-

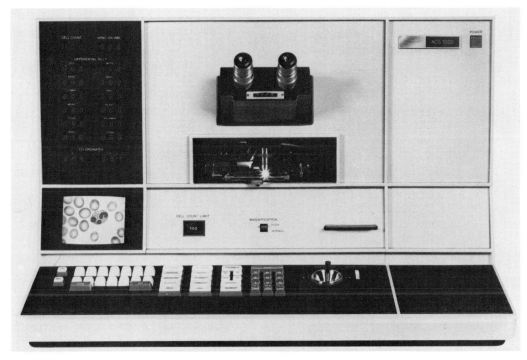

Fig. 5-38. Honeywell ACS 1000. (Courtesy of Honeywell Clinical Instruments)

normal, requiring review by the chief hematology technologist or the pathologist, the technologist may record these coordinates. One of this instrument's primary features, therefore, is that a slide may be removed from the microscope stage and remounted at any time; the recorded x and y coordinates are keyed in, to return to the problem cell. A slide may be repeated, in principle, even at a different location. This capability derives from the use of servo-motors instead of stopper motors, which produces a location resolution of 4 μm. Also, a calibration slide with a "bull's eye" is provided; these are fabricated by a highly reproducible electroplating method that ensures consistency from one system to another. The calibration coordinates are not permanently stored in the computer. Therefore, whenever the system is turned on, the calibration procedure is repeated; it is locked in and stable so long as the power remains on.

Just beneath the display panel to the left of the microscope is the color television

display, which is normally operated at 2500 × magnification. The keyboard extends along the front of the ACS 1000, except for a storage area on the right end. The keys for manually entering the cell's classification are located just beneath the television display. The identification labels of these cell characterization keys are illuminated according to the counting mode selected. In the differential count mode the lighted keys are band and segmented neutrophils, lymphocytes, metamyelocytes, myelocytes, promyelocytes, blasts, and other. When other is selected, the displayed coordinates for that cell are generally recorded on the report form. An additional key available in the differential count mode is used to note a nucleated red blood cell. Entering this information does not add to the total of counted white cells. In the atypical erythrocyte morphology mode, 12 applicable characterization labels are illuminated in addition to two others, for atypical platelet and neutrophil toxic granulation. A reticulocyte counting mode, for which supravitally stained (brilliant cresyl blue) slides are generally required, is also available. For this mode only a reticulocyte key and a key for other are illuminated. Various keys on the keyboard are used to inform the computer of the counting mode selection, operating mode (automatic or manual), entry of date, operator or specimen identification, calibration, mode, and a 0 to 9 numeric keyboard. The last is used to enter identification data, codes for platelet sufficiency and abnormal erythrocyte morphologic variation, and x and y coordinates for reviewing an atypical cell. Also located in the keyboard area are manual focus and stage positioning controls. The ACS 1000 accepts any type of stained slides except those with very thick cover slips.

In the procedure, a portion of the stained slide is placed on the microscope stage, which is manually set for viewing the upper left corner. A drop of oil is then placed on the slide and the technologist enters identification data, if it is desired. The count mode (e.g., differential count) is keyed. Pressing AUTOMATIC CELL FIND initiates a stage scan in a highly repeatable pattern. When a white cell is found, the slide automatically stops with the cell focused in the field of the television monitor and the binocular microscope. As soon as the technologist keys in the identification, the stage scan resumes to locate the next leukocyte, focus and display it; this process generally takes only about 0.3 seconds. When the dialed-in total of white cells is reached (100 or multiples thereof), an audible alarm is sounded, and the running count is automatically converted to percentage.

A fairly recent feature called the Fast Scan Mode displays each cell for a limited length of time, after which the instrument steps ahead automatically to the next cell. The stepping ceases when a 100-cell count is reached. The cell display interval or dwell time may be varied according to 10 different speed settings. The pause may be shortened or lengthened at any time by the medical technologist operating the instrument. This is a convenient method of reviewing previously presented cells, to help maintain a high level of accuracy even at highly increased counting speeds. This review function may also prove valuable in technologist training programs.

The leukocyte differential may be interrupted at any time to record an abnormal erythrocyte morphology or to scan the slide manually for this purpose. Platelet numerical adequacy is normally evaluated at the completion of the differential count, and this information is entered on the keyboard. When the technologist is satisfied with all of the data shown on the illuminated numerical display, he should insert a report ticket in a slot just above the keyboard to initiate printout of all data for that slide.

Although the ACS 1000 does not classify leukocytes, the automatic cell-find circuitry distinguishes between leukocytes and erythrocytes by size and opacity. If the threshold for this discrimination is improperly set, the ACS 1000 will either stop at red blood cells or stain debris, or it will fail to stop at faintly stained leukocytes. Overly frequent stopping will become evident to the technologist. To alert him to instances of passing over some white cells, the system has a "marginal stop indicator." When a leukocyte just barely trips the cell-find circuitry, a red line for each such incident is illuminated along the left edge of the television screen. If the technologist observes these lines frequently and in multiples on a given slide, or if an excessively high number of false stops occurs, the threshold may be adjusted by the technologist. Quality control is accomplished by running a standard slide once every day. This slide is counted, starting at the same coordinates every day, both manually, using the microscope, and automatically. The standard stained slide must be replaced every month because of fading. Also, the threshold setting is checked every morning on a freshly prepared slide.

Advantages. The search function on the

slide is automatically performed, permitting the technologist to concentrate on cell identification, which reduces the time required to perform differentials and reduces medical technologist fatigue.[15] That is, 1½ times as many slides may be processed (from 10–15 slides per hour by manual methods to 15–20 slides per hour by the ACS 1000). There need be less concern with possible bias, compared with manually done slides. There is a natural tie-in with the laboratory computer system. The period of training for each medical technologist is short (e.g., about ½ hour, with the instrument "beeping" at the operator if something is wrong. The original training at the factory takes 2 days for each medical technologist. Technologists have each patient's cumulative report visible, and technologists may be encouraged to practice interpretative hematology. The cell relocation feature works well. Therefore, the instrument is excellent for teaching student technologists or for quickly demonstrating a problem cell to a supervising pathologist. There is practically no downtime, and service has been excellent (1–2 days).

Disadvantages. There is a small discrepancy with monocytes. Initially, on the older machine, this required a service adjustment, but now the medical technologist may make an adjustment on the front panel. It takes time for personnel to learn to overlook the differences in image presentation between the television screen and the microscope field. There are machinery problems, occasionally (e.g. microswitches that serve as cover interlocks malfunction, and there were some early problems with circuit boards and occasional bulb failure). There are occasional logistic problems with the ordering of replacement supplies and parts. The keyboard layout for cell characterization is not the same as the customary manual arrangement. Some medical technologists find it harder than others to adapt to this change. It is difficult to view the television in bright surroundings (the manufacturer has promised a removable shield).

QUALITY CONTROL IN HEMATOLOGY

Although automatic or semiautomatic diluting pipettes and cell counting devices make precision possible in routine hematologic laboratory procedures, they do not eliminate error—that is, a machine performing a leukocyte count cannot tell whether it actually is counting white blood cells, red blood cells, dust particles, fungus spores, or debris. Furthermore, photoelectric hemoglobinometers do not match colors. They merely determine how much light fails to pass through a solution-loaded cuvette; the light may have been absorbed by the colored solution in the cuvette, or it may have been scattered by turbidity or a dirty or scratched cuvette. Finally, if dilutions are made by automatic diluting pipettes, it is easy to overlook the fact that, owing to instrument malfunction (nonreproducible delivery volume), the vial contains too much or too little solution. Therefore, although instrumentation and automation enable one to perform routine hematologic procedures with great accuracy and precision, they do not ensure it. This makes quality control all the more necessary, including its three important components: control of accuracy, control of precision, and detection of random errors.

In hematology, one can define accuracy as the closeness with which the mean value of a series of replicate measurements approaches the true value. Therefore, in order for hematologic results to be accurate a valid universal standard for comparison must be available, every piece of glassware used for quantitative measurements must be calibrated and each instrument used must be calibrated, with frequent rechecking of this calibration.

Although check standards are used to evaluate and partially control precision, they are not the sum of quality control.[14]

In hematology, precision may be defined as the closeness with which the values of a

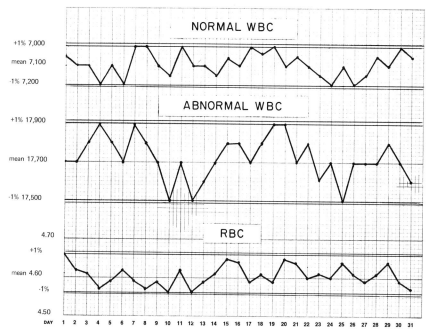

Fig. 5-39. Quality control chart in which reference standards are used.

series of replicate measurements agree with each other. This may be done by repeating the test on a stable check standard once each day, by testing ten or more aliquots of one unknown, or by testing a series of samples in duplicate. From the data thus obtained, statistical analysis may be used to calculate the standard deviation. Many hosptial laboratories perform duplicate red blood cell and white blood cell counts and hemoglobin tests on the first ten specimens each morning and calculate the standard deviation by the method of Youden,[43] and a running graph is kept on these data (Fig. 5-39).

Except for hemoglobin, the check standard method has not been readily available in hematology. However, a stabilized and standardized erythrocyte suspension (Celltrol*) is being used as a control in red blood cell counting and hematocrit determinations, thus probably ensuring the accuracy and precision of these determinations and also of the mean corpuscular constants of

Wintrobe. Celltrol is available in concentrations simulating the normal range of red blood cell count (approximately 4.7 million/cu.mm.) and packed cell volume (approximately 45 per cent), below normal range (approximately 1.6 million/cu.mm. and packed cell volume (approximately 15 per cent). A separate sheet containing the assay value for each lot is enclosed in every shipment. This stabilized red blood cell suspension is stored and used at room temperature. It is resuspended by vigorously shaking the vial until the glass bead therein moves freely for at least 15 seconds and no cells remain on the bottom of the vial. A sample is then withdrawn, and the vial is immediately recapped and firmly closed. This process is repeated each time for successive determinations.

Dorsey states he has used a standard suspension of latex particles as a daily check standard for leukocyte counts on the Coulter Counter.[14] However, there is a coefficient of variation of 2.5 per cent, the latex count does not evaluate the effect of the saponin reagent, and there is difficulty

* Produced by Pfizer.

Table 5-1. Normal Value of Leukocytes

	Range	Average	Average (%)						
			Segmented Neutrophilic Granulocytes	Band Cells	Eosinophils	Basophils	Lympho-cytes	Monocytes Monocytes	Smudge Cells
Adults	5000- 8000/cu.mm.	8400/cu.mm.	56	3	2.7	0.5	34	4	4
Adolescents	4000-13,000/cu.mm.	8400/cu.mm.	53	3	2.5	0.5	37	4.7	4
Infants (10 days to 7 years)	5500-15,500/cu.mm.	10,400/cu.mm.	48	3.0	2.7	0.7	42	4.7	4
Newborn									
1st day	3600-45,000/cu.mm.	15,000	58	10.2	2.0	0.4	24	5.3	
2nd day	5000-13,000/cu.mm.	10,000	52	9.2	2.4	0.5	31	5.8	
3rd–10th day	5000-13,000/cu.mm.	7500	34	5.5	3.1	0.4	48	8.8	

at times in getting uniform stable latex particle suspensions.

There is now available, however, a stable reference control called Leukotrol* for white blood cell counts. It is a suspension of stabilized blood cells standardized for use as a control in manual and electronic white blood cell counting. It is available in concentrations approximating normal range (approximately 7500/cu.mm.) and above normal range (approximately 17,500/ cu.mm.). A separate sheet containing the assay value for each lot is enclosed in every shipment. These suspensions are stored at room temperature and remain stable in the unopened vial for 6 months. Like its erythrocyte suspension counterpart, it serves as a quality control reference for both technique and equipment for the levels of white cell counts most frequently encountered, as well as those of major pathologic significance.

Random errors are detected by utilizing the correlation between quantitatively or qualitatively related tests — that is, when hematologic specimens have a complete blood count. For example, by using mean corpuscular constants and the differential smear, one can check the size and degree of pallor of the red blood cells against the numerical values obtained in the MCH, MCHC, and MCV. Thus, every complete blood count contains its own internal standard. To be specific: If the red blood cell count or hematocrit and hemoglobin tests are repeated whenever the appearance of the erythrocytes is inconsistent with the MCH or MCHC, most random errors will be found and corrected before the report is issued. If one calculates the average MCH for all normal blood specimens each day and records these values on a graph, one should have values near the center of the normal range. Consistently high or low values result from lack of accuracy and suggest the need for recalibration. If one calculates and graphs daily the standard

deviation of values for the MCH, MCHC, and MCV, one can reveal the precision with which routine tests are being done by individual workers or by the entire hematology laboratory. For purposes of quality control, a blood sample is considered normal if it is from an adult and contains 4 million per cu.mm. or more normal appearing red blood cells.

The quality of leukocyte counts can be controlled by use of a standardized white blood cell suspension plus experienced technologists who can learn to make a reasonably accurate estimate of the total instrument or hemacytometer white blood cell count from observation of the differential smear. This is necessary because the automatic cell counter can make huge random errors if hemolysis of red blood cells is incomplete or if the saponin sample has stood too long with resulting loss of fragile leukocytes. If there are too few experienced technologists in the hematology section of the laboratory, the senior technologist in this division should review all differential count reports before they are issued. This same individual should examine the smear if the total white blood cell count is below 5000 or above 25,000, if the lymphocyte count exceeds 40 per cent (adult) or 60 per cent (child), if any abnormal or atypical cells are reported, if any normoblasts are present, or if the platelets (also evaluated routinely) are reported as increased, decreased, or abnormal. A sample quality control chart is shown in Figure 5-38. Normal average values of leukocytes are depicted in Table 5-1.

As electronic blood cell counters have become commonplace in hospital hematology laboratories, vigorous methods of quality control have had to be implemented. Most of the instruments are precalibrated by the manufacturers, and in most labs the preset calibrations are verified by zeroing with blanks before running controls with known values. However, this sytem does not completely check the electronics of the equipment. In some laboratories, a

---

* Produced by Pfizer.

calibration check of automated hematologic instruments is done by running controls and blood samples by other procedures; that is, a manual white count and red count are done twice a week as a tentative evaluation of instrument integrity. These counts are also checked by testing blood samples and controls on a backup instrument. Finally, the results of these instruments are compared with results produced in other hospitals. Every morning, a complete blood count is run on an analyzer using a normal blood sample. This sample is tested at another nearby hospital, and the results are compared. This provides a program of external checks of the lab's hematology instruments. External verification of equipment calibration can also be accomplished by daily testing of control vials. A monthly record of results can then be forwarded to a state association testing group for computation. The results of these quality control tests can then be compared with those of other hospitals using similar equipment.

In the semiautomated laboratory, technologists must be able to check not only their instrument calibration, but their techniques for diluting blood samples as well. In most cases, the dilution techniques can be monitored by comparing the technique routinely used by the lab with another method. An automatic pipette may be compared with several hand dilutions or with another automatic dilutor. In some hospitals, a solution with a known concentration of potassium dichromate is drawn up in the dilutor, and the concentration is calculated on a spectrophotometer. If the concentration is within the accepted limits of error, the lab considers the instrument to be properly calibrated.

With most electronic hematology analyzers and cell counters, each manufacturer recommends a specific technique for checking the preset calibrations. These recommendations should be followed, and if the laboratory has any difficulty, it should contact the instrument manufacturer for assistance.

Still another method for checking the integrity of an instrument is to test the ability of the equipment to reproduce test results. One method is to recheck all abnormal test results from the multitest hematology analyzer. In doing this, one randomly monitors the reproducibility of the instrument by double-checking random patient samples. Another approach to testing reproducibility requires a unit of outdated whole blood from the blood bank. Every day after the controls are run, this blood is run through the instrument several times. All the results must agree, or the instrument is examined for electronic failure. Randomly throughout the day, this same blood is again run to verify reproducibility. Lastly, each patient sample might be accompanied by a card listing previous test results. If any patient's result is drastically changed, the sample is immediately retested.

Each hematology laboratory should also have a routine for cleaning and maintaining instrumentation. Usually, the instrument is rinsed and set at zero, prior to a quality assurance run, which also should be done prior to testing patient samples (since residue from prior testing may be left in lines, and the instrument may not have been rinsed thoroughly after a high white count has been obtained). Every instrument, whether it is a single- or multiparameter hematology analyzer, has a cleaning and maintenance schedule recommended by the manufacturer. These should be followed; any modifications—for example, in technique—should first be checked with the manufacturer. The manufacturer may suggest that accuracy may be improved by increasing the number of times the instrument is rinsed between samples.

THE COMPUTER IN HEMATOLOGY

As part of the trend toward complete automation of the clinical laboratory, computers are rapidly becoming routine in the hematology division. Unfortunately, the knowledge of, and the data supporting the precise functions that computers can and should subserve in the laboratory, lags substantially behind the number of existing and proposed installations.[31] A serious inquiry into this problem requires access to a fully automated hematology laboratory in which the entire software system can be rapidly modified to permit research, parallel processing, and systems progression over extremely short time periods. Accordingly, it would be necessary to be acquainted with the uses of computers in such a hematology laboratory, in order to determine for one's own laboratory the functions useful to computerize (systems analysis) and to be aware of the theoretical concepts that apply to computer systems generally.

The computer systems presently available for hematology laboratories perform a variety of functions. These functions should be analyzed separately by a laboratory director if he is to arrive at the precise set of tasks that he would expect to be assumed by a computer. The tasks are most appropriately identified either by analogy with functions performed by existing machines or by descriptions in the cases where the computer can perform a function that is unique and novel. Among the various identifiable functions performed by a computer are those of: the electric typewriter and the collator, (the worklist generator and the drawlist generator), the filing cabinet, the "baby sitter" for instruments, and the quality control supervisor (procedure panic value alert, specimen panic value alert).

Automated analytic machines (the prime example is the Coulter SR) have enjoyed widespread acceptance in the hematology laboratory for many years. In order to understand what the computer can do in relation to automated hematologic equipment, one must be aware that sophisticated coagulation analyzers have been available for several years, and, very recently, leukocyte differential computers have been introduced. With the advent of the WBC differential machines, total automation of the hematology laboratory is now theoretically possible. If an appropriate selection of these automated devices were to be coupled with an assembly-line transport system and the combination controlled by a computer, then a fully automated hematology laboratory would result. Although no one is likely to build such a laboratory soon, a consideration of just exactly what would take place within its walls is a highly instructive exercise. Such a consideration emphasizes that any approach short of such a total (and highly costly) effort is, perforce, a compromise. It is the extent and rise of such a compromise that renders some laboratory systems useful and assures that others will be disasters. Therefore, an analysis of the daily work-flow (systems analysis) in the hematology laboratory includes a detailed consideration of what each processing step involves and what are the acceptable compromises. It includes an analysis of all the interactions stopping at the actual test performance itself. It also assumes that every laboratory director must acquire some proficiency in the science of systems analysis.

To begin, one should know what the computer in the hematology laboratory should do. In planning a new system or comtemplating the purchase of a system, the director of a hematology laboratory must reconcile his specific needs and requirements. Failure to do this in the formative stages of planning will ensure that the system as finally implemented will conform to the priorities of someone else. The following highly useful concepts are proposed as examples:

The computer system must have as its prime purpose the enhancement of patient care; that is, it must render maximum service to the practicing physician. This necessitates the delivery of the test results to the doctor as efficiently as possible. If approximately 30 per cent of hematology tests (20% from outpatient laboratory) are requisitioned as stat, one can safely say that $1/3$ of the workload is stat. The physician wants the lab results in the same order in which he requested the tests. He may at a later time (if the case is complex or if the volume of laboratory work is large) require a cumulative summary three to four times daily to facilitate trend analysis. Finally, the physician wants results of clinically significant precision at the lowest possible cost to his patient.

The next goal of the computer system is the enhancement of laboratory personnel; it should relieve the professional staff of nonprofessional duties (clerical, etc.). As is well known, it takes a medical technologist approximately 90 seconds to perform an actual average differential. However, if this technologist also has to sort the stained slides and attach them to the corresponding slip, it will take 5 to 7 minutes to do the differential. With a clerk handling the sorting and identifying, approximately 35 differentials per hour can be performed. This is almost as fast as an automated differential analyzer.

Another important goal is the enhancement of test quality and quantity; the system should augment the quality and quantity of work-flow through the laboratory without arbitrarily changing laboratory procedures. The primary determinant is to make sure that the appropriate results are put on the appropriate chart; at this point there is a man-machine interface.

The computer system should test quality; it should maintain a maximum number of quality control checks. This is to say that if the blood indices (MCV, MCH, and MCHC) on the quality control remain stable for a given period of time, one might find in unnecessary to utilize control blood preparations for hemoglobin, RBC, and WBC. A daily stability of indices might possibly lead to the elimination of commercial Hgb, RBC, and WBC quality control preparations.

The computer system should never be bypassed in routine use, but it should be possible to bypass it if the need arose. If there is a delay in the time it takes the computer to answer when a request for laboratory results is made; if a stat order is requested with a need for results more quickly than the computer can generate, and, finally, if there is reporting system inflexibility and the computer is unable to react quickly enough, one might bypass the computer and retreat to a capable manual system.

The computer system should be maximally reliable. Hardware, and software reliability and systems integrity should be satisfactory. In order to be assured of setting up a good software reliability system, one should first contact a medical technologist who has been using one for at least 6 months. The systems integrity is assured when the state license number is placed in the computer before it releases knowledge; also, the clearance code should be changed every 3 to 4 days before it is cleared for use by the medical technologist who will be using it and not for another person.

The computer system should be maximally flexible. It should be able to develop a format for report output, to collect information for management, and to assume control of various test procedure systems.

The computer system should be cost-effective on the hard line. Enough money must be generated and personnel replaced to pay for the system, and finally, it must be able to recover enough previously lost charges to help justify its purchase.

REFERENCES

1. Adner, M. M.: Clinical evaluation of the Coulter differential–education program. Am. Soc. Hematol., [Supple]:13, 1975.
2. Alpert, N. L.: General Science Haema. Count MK-3. Lab World, *24:*32, 1973.
3. ———: Instrument series report No. 36. Lab World, *26:*16, 1975.
4. ———: Hemac Laser Hematology Counter. Lab. World, *26:*16, 1975.
5. ———: Lab. World, *27:*22, 1976.
6. ———: Automatic differential counters. Part 1, Lab World, *27:*16, 1976.
7. Beautyman, W., and Bills, T.: Letter to the editor. N. Engl. J. Med., *293:*45, 1975.
8. Bell, H.: Automation in hematology — recent advances in medical technology (lecture). pp. 1-11. Lawrence, Kansas, University of Kansas, 1966.

9. Bull, B. S.: A flow-through cuvette for the Coulter Counter. Am. J. Clin. Pathol., *47:*107, 1967.

10. ———: A semiautomated dilutation system for a hematology laboratory. Bull. Pathol., *8:*13, 1967.

11. ———: The computer or systems analysis in the hematology laboratory. Education Program. Am. Soc. Hematol., Lecture, 1977.

12. Chanarin, I.: Critical Appraisal of the PCV in quality control in hematology. *In* Lewis, S. M., and Coster, J. F.: pp. 103-110. Academic Press, New York, 1975.

13. D'Angelo, G., and Lacombe, M.: A practical diluent for electronic white cell counts. Am. J. Clin. Pathol., *38:*658, 1962.

14. Dorsey, D. B.: What can quality control do for hematology? J. Am. Soc. Med. Tech., *31:*150, 1965.

15. Education Program Manual. Am. Soc. Hematol., Dec. 5-7, 1975. p. 10

16. Emori, H. W., Bluestone, R., and Goldberg, L. S.: Pseudoleukocytosis associated with cryoglobulinemia. Am. J. Clin. Pathol., *60:*202, 1973.

17. Freundlich, M. H., and Gerarde, H. W.: A new automatic disposable system for blood counts and hemoglobin. Blood, *21:*648, 1963.

18. Gilbert, R. K.: Progress and analytical goals in clinical chemistry. Am. J. Clin. Pathol., *63:*960, 1975.

19. Gottman, A. W., Nosancheck, J. S., and Orr, K.: How to get optimal performance from the Coulter Model S. Lab. Med., *4:*22, 1973.

20. Gulliani, G. L., Hyun, B. H., and Gabaldon, H.: Falsely elevated automated leukocyte counts on cryoglobulinemic and/or cryofibrinogenemic blood samples. Lab. Med., *8:*14, 1977.

21. Hamlin, W. B., Duckworth, J. K., Gilmer, R. R., and Stevens, M. V.: Laboratory instrument maintenance and function verification. College of American Pathologists Manual. Chicago, College of American Pathologists, 1976.

22. Hemalog D Manual, p. 16-26.

23. Larc and Hematrak, p. 22-48 incl. May, 1976.

24. Larson, J. H., and Pierre, R. V.: Platelet satellitism as a cause of abnormal Hemalog D differential results. Am. J. Clin. Pathol., *68:*758, 1977.

25. Maldonado, J. E., and Hanlon, D. G.: Monocytes: A current appraisal. Mayo Clin. Proc., *40:*248, 1965.

26. Mansberg, H. P., Saunders, A. M., and Griner, W.: J. Histochem. Cytochem., *22:*711, 1974.

27. Maughan, W. Z., Bishop, C. R., Pryor, T. A., and Athens, J. W.: Question of cycling of the blood neutrophil concentrations and pitfalls in the statistical analysis of sampled date. Blood, *41:*85, 1973.

28. Moah, J. L., Landry, P. R., Oren, M. E., Sayer, B. L., and Heffner, L. T.: Transient peripheral plasmacytosis. Am. J. Clin. Pathol., *62:*8, 1974.

29. O'Sullivan, M. B., and Dienmann, S.: Evaluation of semi-automated hematology instruments. Education Program. Am. Soc. Hematology, pp. 1-3, Boston, Dec. 4, 1976.

30. O'Sullivan, M. B., and Dienmann, S.: Evaluation of semiautomated hematology instruments. Education Program of American Society of Hematology. pp. 33-34. Dec. 1976.

31. O'Sullivan, M. D., Pierre, R. V., Bull, B. S., and Wang-Peng, J.: The computer in the hematology laboratory. Education program. Am. Soc. Hematol., Dec., 1977, pp. 65-67.

32. Pierre, R. V., and O'Sullivan, M. B.: Evaluation of Hemalog D automated differential leukocyte counter. Mayo Clin. Proc., *49:*870, 1974.

33. Pierre, R. V., et al.: Automation of leukocyte differential count. Education Program. Am. Soc. Hematol., Dec. 5, 1975.

34. Rebuck, J. W., and Crowley, J. H.: A method of studying leukocyte functions in vivo. Ann. N. Y. Acad. Sci., *59:*757, 1955.

35. Rinehart, J. J., Balcerzak, S. P., Sagone, A. L., and LoBuglio, A. F.: Effects of corticosteroids on human monocyte function. J. Clin. Invest., *54:*1337, 1974.

36. Shelley, W. B., and Parnes, H. M.: The absolute basophil count. J.A.M.A., *192:*368, 1965.

37. Swatman. L. E.: How to keep our instruments honest. Medical Lab., *12:*43, 1976.

38. Taft, E. G., et al.: Pseudoleukocytosis due to cryoprotein crystals. Am. J. Clin. Pathol., *60:*669, 1973.

39. Teir, H., and Rytömaa, T.: Elimination of granulocytes in the intestinal tract and its pathological consequences. *In* Bajusz, E., and Jasmin, G., (eds.): Methods and Achievements in Experimental Pathology. vol. I. pp. 639-676. Chicago, Yearbook Medical Publishers, 1966.

40. Weston, W. L., Mandel, M. J., Yeckley, J. A., Krueger, G. G., and Clamen, H. N.: Mechanism of cortisol inhibition of adaptive transfer of tuberculin sensitivity. J. Lab. Clin. Med., *82:*366, 1973.

41. Weisbrot, I. M., and Waldner, D. K.: An evaluation of the Haema-Count MK-40 blood counting system. Am. J. Clin. Pathol., *66:*883, 1976.

42. Yoffey, J. M.: The lymphocyte. Ann. Rev. Med., *15:*125, 1964.

43. Youden, W. J.: Statistical Methods for Chemists. p. 123. New York, Wiley, 1951.

AUDIOVISUAL AIDS*

A Cinematographic Record on Human Peripheral Blood Leukocytes. (1954). Association Films, 600 Grand Avenue, Ridgefield, New Jersey 07657.

Death of a Cell. (1956). E. R. Squibb Film Library, c/o Hammill Studio, 9510 Belmont Avenue, Franklin Park, Illinois 60131.

The Differential Diagnosis of Leukocyte Abnormalities by Morphologic Examination of the Peripheral Blood. [T-2611; The Normal Maturation of Granulocytic Leukocytes (1972). T-2610; Normal Peripheral Blood Leukocytes and the Stress Reaction (1972)]. National Medical Audiovisual Center (Annex), Station K, Atlanta, Georgia 30324.

Dynamics of Phagocytosis: The Interaction Between Group A Streptococci and Human Neutrophils in

---

* Films unless otherwise stated.

Vitro. (1958). Pfizer Laboratories Film Library, 267 W. 25th Street, New York, New York 10001.

Granulocyte Identification. (1973). [35 mm. transparencies, teaching exercise, examination, answer sheet]. American Society of Clinical Pathologists, P.O. Box 12073, Chicago, Illinois 60612.

HL-A Systems (1973). T-2367. National Medical Audiovisual Center (Annex), Station K, Atlanta, Georgia 30324.

Leukocyte Morphology in Healthy and Diseased States. Part 1. Granulocytes and Monocytes. CDC-77-10. Marguerite Candler Ballard, M.D. [28 (35 mm.) transparencies plus handout, 12 pages, and standard audiocassette (lecture)]. Part 2. Lymphocytes and Plasma Cells. CDC-77-11. Marguerite Candler Ballard, M.D. [34 (35 mm.) transparencies plus standard audiocassette (lecture) and handout, 12 pp.]. Communications in Learning, Inc., 2929 Main Street, Buffalo, New York 14214.

Lymphocyte Identification. (1972). [35 mm. transparencies, teaching exercise, examination, answer sheet]. American Society of Clinical Pathologists, P.O. Box 12073, Chicago, Illinois 60612.

Normal and Abnormal Peripheral Blood. [35 mm. transparencies, manual]. A.

Normal and Abnormal Peripheral Blood. Set B1. [35 mm. transparencies, manual]. A.S.H. National Slide Bank, HSLRC T-252 (SB-56), University of Washington, Seattle, Washington 98195.

Normal and Abnormal White Blood Cells in Tissue Culture. (1939). American Cancer Society, 219 E. 42nd Street, New York, New York 10017.

Phagocytosis. Pfizer Laboratories Film Library, 267 W. 25th Street, New York, New York 10001.

Phagocytosis and Degranulation. (1963). Armed Forces Institute of Pathology, Audiovisual Communications Center, Washington, D.C. 20305.

Standardization and Hematology. 247307. [lecture on standard audiocassette plus handout, 1 page]. Communications in Learning, Inc. 2929 Main Street, Buffalo, New York 14214.

White Blood Cell Morphology. 247301. Jean A. Shafer, M. A.. M. T. (A.S.C.P.). [33 (35 mm.) transparencies plus handout, 8 pages, and standard audiocassette (lecture)]. Communications in Learning, Inc. 2929 Main Street, Buffalo, New York 14214.

6 Maturation of Thrombocytes; Preparation of Blood Films and Differential Count

It would be difficult to use the same criteria for thrombocyte maturation that are used for leukocyte maturation, because thrombocytes form by budding from the cytoplasm of megakaryocytes in the bone marrow and, occasionally, in the lungs. According to Marcus and Zucker[2] 3000 to 4000 platelets are produced from a single megakaryocyte. Utilizing fluorescent technique, one can demonstrate the common antigenic structure in human thrombocytes and megakaryocytes, lending support to the concept that platelets are derived from megakaryocytes.[3]

The cytologic characteristics of thrombocytes and their progenitors are briefly described in the following outline, from most to least immature cell (Plate 1):

Megakaryoblast: Smaller than mature megakaryocyte.

Size: 16 to 25 μ.

Nucleus: Lobulated with one or two diploid nuclei; dark purple-blue finely reticulated chromatin. The nucleus:cytoplasm ratio is approximately 9:1.

Nucleoli: Indistinct, two to five.

Cytoplasm: Moderate to reduced in amount: gray-blue with occasional vacuoles.

Promegakaryocyte (basophilic megakaryocyte)

Size: 20 to 45 μ.

Nucleus: Coarse, lobulated purplish chromatin network. The nucleus: cytoplasm ratio is approximately 18:4.

Nucleoli: Hazy, one or two.

Cytoplasm: Slightly polychromatic and purplish with occasional fine azurophilic granules near nucleus.

Megakaryocyte: Largest of all blood cells with pleomorphic uninuclear structure, occasionally with multilobular pattern.

Size: 30 to 90 μ (granular, 30 to 70 μ; platelet-producing, 30 to 90 μ).

Nucleus: Red-purple, coarse, clumped chromatin with multilobular pattern. The nucleus: cytoplasm ratio varies because the nucleus may occupy most of the cell in some cases and may be eccentric and ovoid with a 20:1 ratio in other instances.

Nucleoli: Varies from none to 3 to 5, but so indistinct as to be invisible except those showing intermitotic division in a thin cell.

Cytoplasm: Usually abundant, light purple-blue with local or diffusely distributed azurophilic granules. Frequently shows irregular pseudopodal projections representing platelets in the process of formation.

Thrombocyte (platelet)

Size: 2 to 4 μ.

Nucleus: None.

Nucleoli: None.

Cytoplasm: Total cell is cytoplasm, pale blue, with pink-red azurophilic granules.

PREPARATION OF BLOOD SMEARS (FILMS)

THE WET SMEAR

In the collection of blood and preparation of wet smears, one may utilize either the finger-puncture (capillary blood) or the venipuncture technique (venous blood).

Finger-puncture Technique. (See p. 6 for preparation of patient.) First rub the skin (lobe of ear or end or side of distal phalanx of third or fourth finger) with a piece of dry cotton. Then clean puncture site with 70 per cent alcohol on a cotton pledget; allow to dry. The skin is then made tense, and the needle point or blood lancet is placed on the skin surface. A clean sharp jab, 2 to 3 mm. in depth is then made. The first drop of blood is wiped away with a dry cotton pledget. The next drop will well up freely and naturally. A clean coverslip or clean slide is touched to this drop and the smear made (see below).

Venipuncture Technique. (See pp. 6–8 for description of approach to and preparation of patient and area of venipuncture.) The area of puncture (the median-basilic vein of the antecubital fossa in the bend of the elbow or the prominent vein on the dorsal surface of wrist) is cleaned with an alcohol sponge. A tourniquet is then placed about 2 inches above the puncture site, at which time the patient should open and close his fist a couple of times and then close his fist tightly. The vacutainer containing EDTA or a 5 or 10 cc. regular syringe is used. The limb on which venipuncture is to be performed is grasped with the free hand (usually left) and the left thumb of the technician is placed directly over the vein approximately 1½ inches away from the intended puncture site, and gentle traction is applied. The syringe is placed be-

tween the right thumb and the last three right fingers. With the needle bevel down and the needle placed above and directly in line with the course of the vein, the needle is inserted quickly and steadily under the skin and then into the vein. When the needle has entered the vein lumen, a sense of easy penetration is felt, and blood will flow freely into the syringe.

The amount of blood needed is withdrawn by exerting gentle traction on the plunger. The tourniquet is then released and the syringe and needle combination are removed. Sterile gauze or an alcohol cotton pledget is applied to the entry site, and the patient should apply pressure with his free hand for 3 to 5 minutes to prevent bleeding and hematoma formation. The needle is removed from the syringe, and blood is utilized for various laboratory tests or the tip of the hypodermic needle is gently touched to a coverslip or glass slide, delivering a drop of 1 to 2 mm. in diameter.

The coverslips used should be 22 mm. square and 0.13 to 0.17 mm. thick (No. 0, 1, or 1.5). The No. 2 coverslips are too thick to allow focusing with the oil-immersion objective. The coverslips are washed with detergent and water, followed by plenty of hot water and then distilled or deionized water. They are stored in a closed container of 95 per cent alcohol. Some prefer soaking coverslips in a $K_2Cr_2O_7 \cdot H_2SO_4$ cleaning solution for 4 to 7 hours, followed by washing in hot water and then distilled or deionized water, and finally two complete washings with 95 per cent alcohol and storing. The coverslips may be removed from the alcohol storage solution as needed and polished with a clean dust- and grease-free linen cloth. These dry coverslips may also be stored in a clean dry Petri dish or other clean dry covered container.

General Considerations

As just described, a tiny drop of blood from the finger or ear lobe is placed on a coverslip, which is in turn inverted and gently deposited on a clean, dry glass slide. The entire preparation is then rimmed with petroleum jelly or liquid paraffin. The film is first examined under low power to observe its excellence of preparation; it is then studied under the oil-immersion objective. Wet films enable one to make a quick survey to determine whether more detailed study is necessary. Size, shape (for example, sickling), and color may be noted. Also may be seen the pigment of malarial parasites, motility of spirochetes and trypanosomes, rouleau formation, fibrin quantitation, leukocytic activity, and phagocytic potential. For further study of nuclear and cytoplasmic content, supravital staining can be added to these wet film preparations.

Criteria for good wet preparations include the following: A good blood film should have a smooth even appearance, and be devoid of waves, holes, or ridges. The film should spread out evenly under the weight of the coverslip alone and without pressure. The film should not extend to the edges or to the ends of the slide. In fact, the film should occupy no more than half the slide area. In addition, the leukocytes should be evenly dispersed throughout the film, and the erythrocytes should barely touch but not overlap in at least ten or more low-power fields. Although excellent coverslip films show better distribution of leukocytes, it is difficult to make excellent coverslip films continuously without constant practice. The blood film must be made quickly and inverted onto the glass slide before drying or coagulation of the blood begins. If placed near a radiator or other heating-drying apparatus, the red blood cells may crenate or hemolyze. For best results, supravital stain should be used within 1 hour.

Sources of Error

If a blood drop is too large, the erythrocytes will not lie separately from one another, and their size, shape, and color will not be clearly observed. If pressure is applied to the inverted coverslip, the erythro-

cyte and leukocyte morphology will be disturbed. The motility of the leukocytes also will be disturbed. Delay in inverting the coverslip causes the clotting and drying of the blood. Delay in studying wet film causes the cells to crenate, the morphology to become indistinct, and the motility to cease.

THE DRY SMEAR

In the preparation of dry smears, one may utilize either the slide or coverslip method. In the slide method, slides should be cleaned and prepared just as previously described for coverslips. Also, slides may be purchased already cleaned with rounded "spreading" edges at one end; they must not be touched on any area other than the sides.

After skin puncture, the first drop of blood is wiped away, and the second drop of blood (3 to 4 mm. in diameter) is used. This is placed on one slide by touching the slide to the drop of blood welling up from the finger or ear lobe (do not touch skin), or by allowing one drop of blood to flow from hypodermic needle-syringe when a venipuncture specimen is used. The drop is placed approximately one-quarter of the distance from one end of the slide, which is placed on a flat surface and held down firmly on the opposite end. The narrow edge of a second slide is used to spread the blood or spreader slides may be used; the slide used to spread the blood is held at an angle of approximately 30° from the horizontal. The edge of the spreader slide is moved toward the drop of blood until contact is made within the acute angle formed by the two slides. The drop of blood spreads quickly by capillary action along the edge of the spreader slide. A thin film is then made by moving the spreader slide slowly in the reverse direction so the blood flows behind the edge of the spreader slide (Fig. 6-1).

Variations in the blood film thickness may be made by changing the size of the

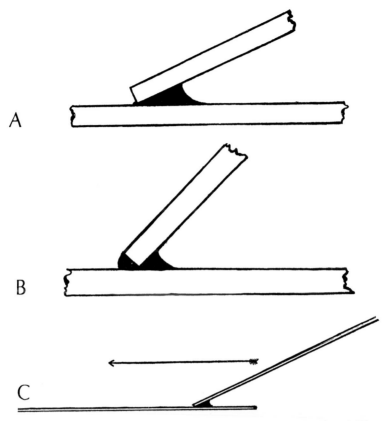

Fig. 6-1. Preparation of dry smear using the slide method. (*A*) The blood collects behind the edge of the spreader slide when the angle between the two slides is small. (*B*) The blood collects in front of the edge of the spreader slide when the angle is too great. (*C*) The slide is moved in the direction indicated to make the blood film. (From Miller, S. E.: Textbook of Clinical Pathology. ed. 7. Baltimore, Williams & Wilkins, 1966)

blood drop, the angle at which the spreader is held, and the speed of spreading. After the slide is dried, the name of the patient and the date are written on the thick end of the blood film. The glass slide with air-dried film is then placed on a flat support (rack in perfectly horizontal position) or on top of a cork stopper. If blood films are made from venous blood, oxalate should not be used as an anticoagulant, because it produces changes in morphologic and staining characteristics. The slide is flooded and completely covered with Wright's stain, and is allowed to stand for 1 minute. This time varies with the batch of Wright's stain used

and is best determined by trial and error. An equal amount of distilled or deionized water, or buffer solution* is added. The mixture of stain and buffer should not be allowed to run off the glass surface. Blow gently on the slide to mix. A green metallic sheen is indicative of proper staining.

After 3 to 6 minutes of stain-buffer mixture standing (each batch of stain must be tested for ideal timing), the stain-buffer

_____

* This is preferably an alkaline buffer with a pH of 6.4 composed of 6.63 g. of anhydrous KH_2PO_4 and 2.56 g. of anhydrous Na_2HPO_4 made up to 1 l. with distilled water. If a pH of 6.7 is desired, 5.13 g. of KH_2PO_4 and 4.12 g. of Na_2HPO_4 are used.

mixture is floated off the glass surface by holding the slides horizontally under gently running tap or distilled water. This prevents contamination of the preparation by precipitate. The film is then washed under running water for a brief period. Excess bluish coloration may be removed by further washing. The finished preparation is then dried thoroughly either by evaporation, by standing the slide on end (not flat on a table), or by blotting gently with filter paper. When it is dry, the stain on the back of the preparation is removed by rubbing with gauze moistened with alcohol.

In the coverslip method, the second drop (2–3 mm. in diameter) of blood is used in the technique just described. The center of a clean coverslip is touched to the blood, not the skin. The coverslip is inverted and placed over a second coverslip crosswise so that the corners form an eight-pointed star. The blood will spread by capillary action between the two surfaces. Two to 4 seconds is allowed to elapse; then the coverslips are drawn apart with a parallel, same-plane sliding motion. The coverslips are not separated by lifting. The coverslips are placed cornerwise in the slit made in a cardboard box or in a horizontal position for air drying on top of a cork stopper fixed to a pan by liquid paraffin. They are stained as previously described. They are quickly mounted by placing the blood side down on a glass slide on which a drop of mounting fluid (Permount) has been placed (Fig. 6-2).

The criteria for a good dry smear include the following considerations: The thin portion of the film should be about 3 cm. long, and the film should not cover the entire surface of the slide or coverslip. However, it should be free of waves, holes, and ridges, and it should have a smooth even appearance (Fig. 6-3). The films should show even dispersion and separation of red cells toward the thin end of the smear with some overlapping of red cells in much of the film. Leukocytes should not be crowded. Slide preparations do not have a uniform distribution of leukocytes, and therefore dif-

ferential white blood cell counts are less accurate using slide preparations than using coverslip preparations.

Sources of Error (Fig. 6-4)

If the smear is made too soon, the film will not cover the entire slide and will be too thick. Any delay in transferring the drop of fresh blood to the coverslip or slide and making the film preparation itself may result in the blood clotting, and it may be difficult to pull the slides apart. Use of a drop of blood more than 2 to 3 mm. in diameter produces too thick a film, and blood will then spread out unevenly and slowly in a thick layer between the two surfaces, and the film will be excessively blue after staining. The use of a spreader slide having a chipped or unpolished end produces uneven films and causes uneven distribution of leukocytes. Use of dirty, dusty, or greasy slides or coverslips causes holes or lines in a finished preparation, imperfect distribution of cells, and improper staining of the cells therein with the precipitation of stain. Blood is usually spread more evenly on one of the coverslips than on the other.

LABELING AND FIXATION OF STAIN

Slides and coverslips can be identified by writing with a soft lead pencil the name of patient, date, doctor, and room number on the thick end of the smear or on the frosted end of the slide. Also, after staining, a paper label with this information can be affixed to the slide. If a definite diagnosis is made, this information is placed on the label, and it is noted whether the blood is peripheral or from bone marrow, or if the blood was taken before or after treatment. Also noted is the type of treatment, if the blood was obtained pre- or post-splenectomy, if a special stain was used, and if the film was counterstained with Wright's stain.

Usually fixation is combined with the staining process because methyl alcohol is

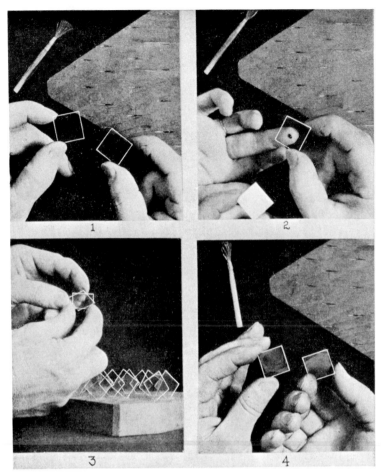

Fig. 6-2. Preparation of blood films by the coverglass method. (*1*) A coverglass is grasped at adjacent corners with the thumb and forefinger of each hand. (*2*) The drop of blood is touched with the coverglass held in the right hand. (*3*) The coverglass carrying the drop of blood is quickly placed over the coverglass held in the left hand. (*4*) The coverglasses are then drawn apart with a sliding motion, care being taken to keep them parallel. The films are allowed to dry in air and are then ready for staining. The drop of blood must be globoid on the fingertip and just large enough to cover the coverglass when properly spread. (Haden, R. L.: Clinical Laboratory Methods. St. Louis, C. V. Mosby, 1929)

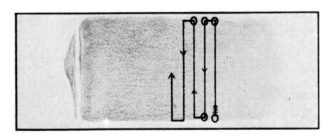

Fig. 6-3. A properly made blood smear. It is margin-free, centrally placed on the slide, and has an adequate thin area. In counting, use the system of crossing shown in the illustration. (Miller, S. E.: Textbook of Clinical Pathology. Ed. 7. Baltimore, Williams & Wilkins, 1966)

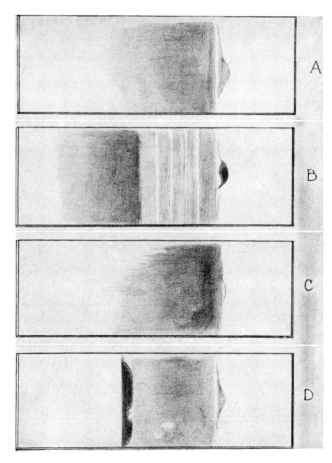

Fig. 6-4. Improperly made blood smears. (*A*) Too short, not margin-free. (*B*) Irregular pressure. (*C*) Too short and thick, jagged ends due to irregular spreading. (*D*) Thick area at end due to spreader hitting supporting finger. (Miller, S. E.: Textbook of Clinical Pathology. Ed. 7. Baltimore, Williams & Wilkins, 1966)

a solvent for Wright's stain, as well as other stains. This process takes place during the first 60 seconds when the undiluted stain is placed on an air-dried slide or coverslip. If methyl alochol is not part of the stain, chemical fixation may be accomplished by using absolute methyl or ethyl alcohol for 1 to 2 minutes. Other fixatives include a 1 per cent solution of formalin in ethyl alcohol, a solution of equal parts of alcohol and ether, and a 1 per cent solution of $HgCl_2$. After using the $HgCl_2$ solution, the excess mercury should be washed out thoroughly with water. Heat fixation is also used for the same indications as chemical fixation. The air-dried film is placed in an oven and the temperature is raised to 150° C, then allowed to cool slowly.

TYPES OF STAIN

Aniline dyes are usually used. *Acidophilic dyes* stain cytoplasm and other structures and are made up of acid dyes such as eosin. Giemsa's stain is a good example, and is best for demonstrating blood parasites and other protozoa. *Basophilic dyes* stain nuclei and certain other blood structures. Hematoxylin and carbol thionin blue are examples. *Polychrome dyes* are usually methyl alcohol solutions of an acid and a basic dye that produce a variety of colors. May-Grünwald-Giemsa stain and Wright's stain are examples. Because Wright's stain is most commonly used and is the most satisfactory stain, its preparation is detailed here.

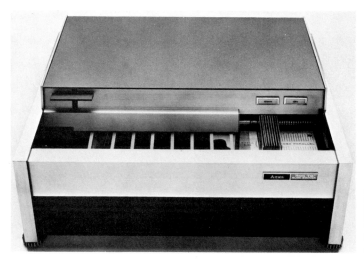

Fig. 6-5. Hema-Tek slide stainer automatically stains blood films with Wright's stain and other stains. (Courtesy of Ames Company)

A powdered Wright stain may be used* that has been certified by the Commission on Staining. It is made by heating alkaline methylene blue with eosin. The end product is thiazine eosinate, a neutral complex dye that is soluble in absolute methyl alcohol. The composition of Wright's stain varies in different batches because it is difficult to control the oxidation of methylene blue, and therefore optimal staining time for each batch must be determined by trial and error. In preparation of the stain, 0.5 g. of the powder is ground in a mortar by slowly adding small amounts of acetone-free, chemically pure absolute methyl alcohol. The supernatant material is poured into a dry bottle. Keep on adding small amounts of methyl alcohol, grinding, and pouring off the supernate into the above dry bottle until all the stain is dissolved and the total measured amount (300 ml.) of alcohol is used. Shake the stain each day for about 2 to 3 weeks; then filter and use. Keep in tightly stoppered, absolutely dry-clean reagent bottles to prevent evaporation and to prevent water vapor from being taken up by the alcohol. A phosphate buffer is made up (see preparations of dry smear slide method, p. 160), or special buffer tablets† may be used together with distilled water. Schleicher's decolorizer (0.5 ml. acetone, 5.0 ml. methyl alcohol, and 100 ml. aq. dest.) may be used, after completion of stain, for 1 to 5 seconds; it is washed off with distilled water.

A recent innovation is the development of a machine that automatically stains blood films with Wright's stain and other stains (Fig. 6-5). Smith Kline and French also has an automatic slide staining machine on the market.

Criteria for the production of good films stained by Wright's method include the following considerations: No precipitated stain should be seen. If precipitated stain is present, it may be due to inadequate washing of the stain at the end of the staining period, unclean slides, failure to hold slides horizontally during washing, drying during the staining period, insufficient filtration of the stain, or dust that has settled on slide or blood film. In a good stain, the film appears pink under gross examination; under the microscope, the erythrocytes are orange or pink rather than green, lemon yellow, or red. The nuclei of the leukocytes are pur-

---

* Produced by the National Aniline Division of Allied Chemical and Dye Corporation, New York.

† Produced by Coleman Instruments, Inc., Maywood, Illinois.

plish blue; neutrophilic granules, reddish to pink-lilac; eosinophilic granules, bright red to orange; and basophilic granules, very dark bluish purple. The basichromatin and oxychromatin of the nuclei are distinctly differentiated; thrombocytes are dark lilac; bacteria are blue and granular. The cytoplasm of lymphocytes stain robin's-egg blue; the cytoplasm of monocytes stains a faint bluish gray tinge; and the cytoplasm of malarial parasites stains sky blue and the chromatin, a purplish red.

Sources of Error

In staining blood films, the following may be sources of error: A poor smear results in a poor stain (too thick, uneven, vacuolated, no thin parts, or a dirty slide). The stain may be too red due to the excessive acidity of the stain, buffer, or water. In this situation the nuclear chromatin is stained pale blue rather than a bright blue, erythrocytes stain bright red rather than pinkish, and eosinophil granules stain brilliant red instead of orange-red. Excessive acidity is usually caused by exposure of the stain or buffer to acid fumes. The problem may be corrected by using a fresh batch of stain or buffer, or both. If tap water is alkaline, it may be used instead of distilled water in washing. If the stain is too pale (especially nuclei, red blood cells, and eosinophilic granules), it is due to excessive washing or understaining. This may be corrected by drecreasing the washing time or increasing the staining time.

The stain may be too basic or blue. When this occurs, the nuclear chromatin is deeply stained and erythrocytes stain blue or green; lymphocytic cytoplasm becomes gray or lavender, neutrophilic granules become overstained and appear larger than normal, and eosinophilic granules become deep gray or blue. These errors are caused by too thick a smear, insufficient washing, too lengthy a staining time, or excessive alkalinity of the stain, buffer, or water. The color may be improved by using less stain or more buffer, or decreasing staining time

or increasing washing time. If the buffer is too alkaline and the preceding procedures do not correct it, the buffer must be remade. The length of the staining time may be affected by the uneven mixing of the buffer, resulting in the formation of sediment; incorrect *p*H of the buffer; and the incorrect storage of stain, in which the stain may be exposed to light and extremes of heat and cold.

CRITICAL EXAMINATION OF THE STAINED SMEAR

The differential count may be defined as a quantitative and qualitative study of the thrombocytes and the numbers of leukocytes of the three types—granulocytes, lymphocytes, and monocytes—plus a consideration of the age and morphologic abnormalities of the red blood cells, white blood cells, and platelets. Another definition sometimes given for the word "differential" is that it represents the percentage distribution of the different types of leukocytes and their qualitative study on a stained blood film. (Plates 3, 4, 5, 6)

Information to be gained from a study of the stained blood smear includes the observation of erythrocytes for the following abnormalities (Plates 8, 9, 10): Variation in size, or *anisocytosis;* after repeated observations it can be ascertained if the average red blood cells are macrocytic (greater than 9 μ), normocytic (7.5 μ), or microcytic (less than 6 μ). The degree of anisocytosis should be estimated and noted as 0 to 4+. Variations in the normal biconcave shape, also called *poikilocytosis,* may be evident, in which the erythrocytes are either spherocytic or ovalocytic, or may show the target cell pattern or sickle cell shape. This observation is of diagnostic significance and should be observed as 0 to 4+. Variation in hemoglobin concentration, whether normochromic or hypochromic, is determined by an estimation of the color intensity of the red blood cells, which in turn may be used to approximate the mean corpuscular hemoglobin concentration and is possibly graded 0 to 4+ (Plate 9).

Erythrocytes may be observed to determine if any abnormal forms are present. *Polychromasia,* or *polychromatophilia,* is characterized by a faint to fairly deep blue tinge of macrocytic cells without the normal pale center. The color is an admixture of residual ribonucleic acid and hemoglobin, and it is mostly found in reticulocytes. *Stippling* or punctate basophilia, refers to the appearance of irregular bluish black granules in red blood cells due to degenerative changes involving ribonucleic acid. It is usually a sign of exposure to lead, but it can also be seen in other anemias. *Cabot's rings* are red or reddish purple, granular, loop-shaped, or form figures of eight. These structures most likely indicate defective regenerative activity. Nucleated red blood cells, or *normoblasts,* when present in the peripheral blood, are indicative of an excessive demand on the blood-forming organs to regenerate erythrocytes. They are therefore an indication of the extent to which the bone marrow reacts to disease. Parasitized red blood cells (most from *Plasmodium* species causing malaria) are characterized by reddish purple *Schüffner's granules* with or without ring forms in macrocytic red blood cells. *Rouleau formation* is a phenomenon of red blood cells characterized by adherence of red blood cells to one another presenting a stack-of-coins appearance. It is seen when the serum contains increased amounts of fibrinogen and globulin. In addition, a reduction in RBC surface charge by neuraminidase has been shown to increase red blood cell aggregation by short molecular chain dextrans. This supports experimental indications that the stability of RBC aggregation depends on a balance between a macromolecular bridging force and an electrostatic repulsive force and that alterations in the RBC surface charge may affect cell aggregation and blood viscosity.[1] It is interesting that the increased agglutinability does not interfere with the normal RBC life span, but may be responsible for occasional vasoocclusive phenomena. *Heinz bodies* are rounded or irregular, deep purple, refractile particles when stained with methyl violet. They are usually situated near the periphery of red blood cells and are demonstrated by brilliant cresyl blue stains as lighter blue bodies. Heinz bodies are suggestive of hemolytic anemia in red blood cells having an unstable glutathione system, when they are exposed to certain drugs or after splenectomy. *Inclusion bodies* in erythrocytes are called siderocytes and are rod to round shaped bodies usually present after splenectomy or in the marrrow of patients with hemolytic anemia of indefinite etiology. They represent red blood cell iron not yet incorporated into hemoglobin (Plate 10).

An estimation of the number of platelets is done on a differential film by first surveying the film under low power, making certain that the platelets are evenly distributed and not clumped in one area of the film. Several oil-dimension fields are then studied, and it is estimated whether the platelets are present in normal, decreased, or increased amounts compared to those in normal blood. Platelets are 2 to 5 μ in diameter and are granular. Observations are also made as to whether the platelets are of correct size and are agranular.

Enumeration of leukocytes can be estimated on a differential film first by the superficial observation of several low-power or oil-immersion fields, to determine whether the quantity of leukocytes is low, normal, or high compared to normal blood. The predominant type of leukocyte and morphologic abnormalities can also be ascertained at this time. The differential count itself is done under the oil-immersion objective without counting the same area twice. A mechanical stage is used, and the slide is moved from left to right, down one vertical field, then right to left, down an adjacent vertical portion of the blood film, and so on. Observations are made in the thin and thick parts of the blood film because the different varieties of white blood cells may be un-

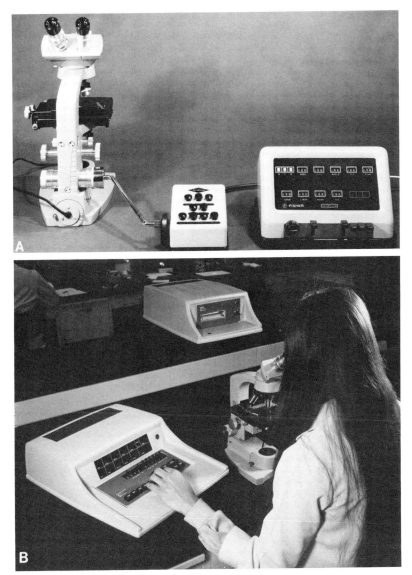

Fig. 6-6. (*A*) Leucodiff Recorder. (Courtesy of Fisher Scientific Co.) (*B*) Leukocyte Entry Module. (Courtesy of T&T Technology)

evenly distributed. Usually, a minimum of 100 cells is counted using a recording blood cell calculator with a separate key for each type of white blood cell. Unclassifiable or unidentifiable white blood cells should be so listed in the differential count. The absolute number for a specific cell type is obtained by multiplying the total white blood cell count by the percentage in the differential count. The relative number is the percentage figure itself.

A recent innovation called the Leucodiff Recorder enables one to register the differential count on a keyboard with the hand that controls the fine focus of the microscope. The count is recorded electrically on a nine-place counter that can be set to show either percentages or actual counts (up to 999) of the Schilling classes. Differential counts are made 30 to 50 per cent faster with an error of less than 0.1 per cent. Other settings on the Leucodiff Recorder give thrombocyte:erythrocyte ratios and reticulocyte:erythrocyte ratios (Fig. 6-6*A*).

A new differential counter and printer is the leukocyte entry module (LEM; Fig. 6-6*B*). This instrument counts up to 10 different cells, for morphology and nucleated RBCs. It will do a complete CBC analysis on one report, which fits any standard Coulter S printer and has been specially preprinted to match the Coulter S printing format. A light key touch enters each count into the LEM, where a running total is instantly registered and displayed. An audible tone signifies when the total count reaches 100, and no additional entries are allowed. The count immediately returns to zero when the CLEAR key is pressed.

Before concluding the discussion of the stained smear, the classification of leukocytes and normal values (normal range = 5000–8000/cu.mm.) should be considered. There are three different approaches to the differential quantitation of leukocytic cells. The most widely used is the Schilling count, a systematic method of counting granulocytic cells in groups according to their sequential developmental stage. In actual cell classification, the younger forms are placed on the left and the more mature forms on the right so that going from left to right there are listed: myeloblasts and promyelocytes (0%); myelocytes (0%); metamyelocytes, young, slightly indented (juvenile cells 0–1%); metamyelocytes, band forms (3–5%); and segmented neutrophils (51–67%). These classifications included with the ordinary differential count constitute the *Schilling hemogram.* The additional portion includes eosinophils (1–4%), basophils (0–1%), lymphocytes (25–33%), and monocytes (2–6%).

Of significance in the Schilling hemogram

is the line that lies in the neutrophilic group between the cells with segmented nucleus and the band cells. An increase in the percentage of cells to the left of this line is the so-called "shift to the left." There are two types of these shifts of clinical significance. The *regenerative* shift to the left is characterized by a high white blood cell count—there is a rapid production of leukocytes in response to an acute need before growth and differentiation are complete, for example, as in acute infections such as appendicitis and acute sepsis. The *degenerative* shift to left is characterized by a low white blood cell count. There is a depression of the leukopoietic centers owing to toxins; this allows neutrophilic development only to a certain stage with irregularities in size and shape appearing subsequently in the peripheral circulation—for example, in tuberculosis and typhoid fever. Simultaneous with this neutrophilic development, the lymphocytes decrease and eosinophils disappear. With increased host resistance and before beginning clinical recovery, the lymphocytes increase again, eosinophils reappear, and there is a sudden rise in monocytes.

The *Arneth count,* another method of quantitative and qualitative classification, is based on the number of lobes possessed by neutrophils. Five groups are listed: one round or indented nucleus (youngest; 5%), two nuclear divisions (35%), three nuclear divisions (41%), four nuclear divisions (17%), and five or more nuclear divisions (oldest cell; 2%). A shift to the left indicates an increase in the younger forms, as in infections, and a shift to the right (older forms increase in percentage) is seen most frequently in pernicious anemia.

Also to be considered in the differential blood film are the filamentous and nonfilamentous forms. Cells that possess segments or lobes connected with a distinct thin chromatin filament are classified as *filamentous cells.* If the nucleus has a thinned-out portion, it is classified as *nonfilamentous.* Nonfilamentous cells include the metamyelocyte, myelocyte, promyelocyte, and myeloblastic forms. In the hemogram, lymphocytes and monocytes are nonfilamentous.

REFERENCES

1. Chen, S., et al.: Acetylneuraminic acid deficiency in erythrocyte membranes: biophysical and biochemical correlates. Blood, *43:*445, 1974.
2. Marcus, A. J., and Zucker, B.: The Physiology of Blood Platelets: Recent Biochemical, Morphologic and Clinical Research. p. 87. New York, Grune & Stratton, 1965.
3. Vasquez, J. J., and Lewis, J. H.: Immunocytochemical studies on platelets: the demonstration of a common antigen in human platelets and megakaryocytes. Blood, *16:*968, 1960.

AUDIOVISUAL AIDS*

Collection of Blood Sample and Preparation of Blood Film. Seminar 303, ASMT Education and Research Fund, Inc., 5555 West Loop South, Bellaire, Texas 77401.

Making and Staining Coverslips. (1962). Film Library Service, U.S. Naval Medical School, National Naval Medical Center, Bethesda, Maryland 20014.

Normal and Abnormal Platelets. E. R. Squibb Film Library, c/o Hammill Studio, 9510 Belmont Avenue, Franklin Park, Illinois 60131.

Preparation of Thick and Thin Blood Films. M-1433. National Medical Audiovisual Center (Annex), Station K, Atlanta, Georgia 30324.

Staining Blood Films for Detection of Malaria Parasites. M-1432. National Medical Audiovisual Center (Annex), Station K, Atlanta, Georgia 30324.

---

* Films unless otherwise stated.

7 Total Eosinophil Count and Cerebrospinal Fluid Count

THE TOTAL EOSINOPHIL COUNT

The exact function of the eosinophil is still unknown. Large numbers are frequently found in the tissues in reaction to foreign protein, in allergic reactions, and in the tissue reaction and peripheral blood pattern of Hodgkin's disease. Recent work reveals an antihistamine activity of these cells.

The significance of an increase in the number of eosinophils (eosinophilia) is indicated by the following list of associated clinical conditions: First, eosinophilia is associated with the recovery phase of most infections during specific parasitic tissue infestations. For example, there is a 50 per cent eosinophilia in trichinosis and high values in echinococcosis, ascariasis, and schistosomiasis. However, there is no eosinophilia with *intestinal* parasitism, such as enterobiasis and amebiasis. Eosinophilia is also seen in scarlet fever, Löffler's syndrome, tropical eosinophilia with associated filiarial infestation, and occasionally, in gonorrhea and Hansen's disease. Second, eosinophilia is associated with allergic diseases, for example, bronchial asthma, urticaria, and drug fever, following hyperimmune serum injection, and, occasionally, malaria.

Third, skin diseases that may be associated with eosinophilia include pemphigus, dermatitis herpetiformis, erythema multiforme, exfoliative dermatitis, dermatitis venenata, pityriasis rubra, mycosis fungoides, and, occasionally, scabies, psoriasis, contact eczema, and prurigo. Fourth, eosinophila may be associated with neoplasias such as metastatic carcinoma, leukemia, Hodgkin's disease, and gastric and pulmonary carcinoma. Fifth, eosinophilia may be familial. Also, it can occur after irradiation. Finally, other disorders associated with eosinophilia include polyarteritis nodosa, pernicious anemia, hypoadrenocorticism, sickle cell anemia, and disorders resulting from certain poisons.

The significance of decreased eosinophils, or eosinopenia, (below 50/cu.mm.) accompanies the following clinical states; hyperactivity of adrenal cortex (Cushing's syndrome), severe infectious granulocytosis, labor, and eclampsia, and it is found after major surgery in patients with good adrenal function and after electric-shock treatment.

Influence of the Adrenal Steroids on the Eosinophil Count

There is also an inverse influence and relationship between the secretion of steroids by the adrenal cortex and the total number of circulating eosinophils. For example, in Cushing's syndrome, hyperadrenocorticism is due to increased cortisol excretion (17-hydroxycorticosteroids) caused by bilateral adrenal hyperplasia, unilateral adrenocortical adenoma, or adrenocortical carcinoma. Therefore, the eosinopenia is absolute. In Addison's disease, destruction of the adrenal cortex causes diminution in the secretion of 17-hydroxycorticosteroids (caused by tuberculosis or other infectious or neoplastic processes), and there is, thus, a normal or an increased absolute eosinophil count.

The Thorn test is, at best, a rough test for adrenocortical function. It is based partially on the fact that intramuscularly injected adrenocorticotropic hormone (ACTH) produces a maximum eosinopenic effect in 4 hours — a decrease of 50 per cent or more in the absolute number of eosinophils in persons with a normal adrenal cortex. The Thorn test is useful as a crude diagnostic test of adrenal cortical function in certain situations: Patients with Addison's disease show no change or a slight decrease in eosinophils (following administration of cortisone they show a normal response, that is, a decrease in eosinophils). It can be used as a test of adrenocortical reserve before surgical procedures. It can be used as a test to distinguish functional hypopituitarism from organic disease of the adrenal cortex.

The mechanism underlying the eosinopenia induced by ACTH and cortisol is unknown; it could possibly be associated with a redistribution phenomenon. That is to say, there could be a blockage of release of eosinophils from the bone marrow; it could be the result of peripheral destruction of eosinophils; or it could be caused by diminished production of eosinophils in the marrow. Also, epinephrin and adrenocortical compounds may act synergistically to produce eosinopenia.

Thorn test:

1. Allow nothing but water after 8 P.M.
2. Perform an eosinophil count in duplicate the next morning (no breakfast). Collect the venous blood in balanced oxalate or EDTA.
3. Inject intramuscularly 25 mg. ACTH; continue the patient on fast for the next 4 hours.
4. Repeat the eosinophil count 4 hours

after ACTH is given intramuscularly (if capillary blood is used, dilute it immediately with eosin-diluting fluid).

Technique

Staining methods for total eosinophil counts are somewhat different from the usual methods used with the Romanowsky stains. The diluting fluids contain acetone, propylene glycol, or urea as the diluent. Dyes have been added to these diluents to stain the cells, and other agents have sometimes been included to cause cells other than eosinophils to rupture. Pilot's solution, which uses propylene glycol as the vehicle, is frequently used. This solution renders the red blood cells relatively nonrefractile and invisible, acts as a vehicle for stains because of its viscosity, and does not evaporate quickly. The Na_2CO_3 in Pilot's solution lyses all white blood cells other than the base-resistant eosinophils; the phloxine stains eosinophil granules red; and the heparin prevents clumping of white blood cells. Pilot's solution contains propylene glycol (50 ml.), distilled water (40 ml.), phloxine (1 per cent aqueous stock solution, 10 ml.), sodium carbonate (10 per cent aqueous stock solution, 1 ml.), and heparin sodium (100 units). The sodium carbonate should be measured carefully, and the solution should be filtered and kept in a well-stoppered bottle. Pilot's solution keeps for 1 month at room temperature.

The final dilution used in the computation of the eosinophil count involves the use of the hemocytometer, the number of chambers used, and the area of chamber used. Blood is drawn to the 1.0 mark in the white blood cell pipette accurately, and blood adhering to the outside of the pipette is wiped away. The diluting fluid is accurately drawn to the 11 mark. This is repeated with a second pipette, and both pipettes are shaken for 2 minutes. The first four drops from each pipette are expelled and discarded. One counting chamber of a *Neubauer* hemocytometer is immediately loaded with each pipette. Fifteen minutes is

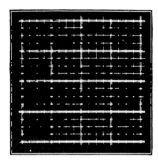

Fig. 7-1. Fuchs-Rosenthal ruled hemocytometer for eosinophil count. (Courtesy of Arthur H. Thomas Co.)

allowed for proper lysis and staining. The chamber is covered during this period with an inverted Petri dish that has a piece of wet filter paper on top. All the eosinophils are counted, under low-power magnification, in all nine large squares in each of the two chambers, within 3 hours. Only the eosinophils can be seen; the granules stain red, but the nuclei do not stain. The initial dilution is 1:10 when all the eosinophils are counted in the two Neubauer chambers. Therefore:

Eosinophils/cu.mm. =

$$\frac{\text{No. of eosiniphils counted} \times 10}{1.8 \text{ (total volume of 2 Neubauer chambers)}}$$

Because of the inherent error of approximately 35 per cent when the Neubauer chamber is used, special types of counting numbers are suggested, for example, the Fuchs-Rosenthal ruling, which consists of sixteen 1 mm. squares bordered by triple lines, with each 1 mm. square subdivided into 16 smaller squares by single lines (Fig. 7-1). Hemocytometers with two Fuchs-Rosenthal rulings, each with a depth of 0.2 mm. (rather than the standard 0.1 mm.) are available. The total volume of each chamber is 3.2 cu.mm., rather than 0.9 mm. as in the standard Neubauer chamber. When all the eosinophils are counted in two Fuchs-Rosenthal chambers and the initial dilution is 1:10,

Eosinophils/cu.mm. =

$$\frac{\text{No. of eosinophils counted} \times 10}{6.4 \text{ (total volume of 2 Fuchs-Rosenthal chambers)}}$$

A Speirs-Levy counting chamber may also be used.

The average normal eosinophil count in normal fasting patients at 8 A.M. is 180/cu.mm. (100 to 300 range). There is a diurnal trend that shows a 20 per cent midmorning decrease below the 8 A.M. level, and a 30 per cent increase above 8 A.M. level at night.

CEREBROSPINAL FLUID

Cerebrospinal fluid is a clear, watery liquid that circulates in the subarachnoid space and ventricles of the brain and spinal cord, and in brain tissue. It is formed by dialysis, ultrafiltration, and secretion from the choroid plexus of the first and second ventricles, or, possibly, from the brain tissues themselves, with the choroid plexus acting as a filter that allows the fluid to enter the ventricles in the brain. From the first and second ventricles, the cerebrospinal fluid goes through the interventricular foramen of Munro to the third ventricle and through the aqueduct of Sylvius to the fourth ventricle. From the fourth ventricle, the cerebrospinal fluid goes through the foramen either of Luschka, or of Magendie, to the subarachnoid space of the brain and cord and thence to the perineural subarachnoid spaces.

Cerebrospinal fluid functions as a mechanical buffer to prevent the brain and spinal cord from being jarred by external trauma; it regulates the volume of the intracranial contents; it acts as a nutrient medium to the central nervous system; and it acts as the excretory channel for the products of nervous tissue metabolism.

Collection

Cerebrospinal fluid is collected by lumbar puncture. This procedure is performed for diagnostic and therapeutic purposes. Diagnostically, lumbar puncture is indicated when symptoms of meningeal irritation are present, as in meningitis, polio, or hemorrhage; when there are focal signs of central nervous system (brain and spinal cord) involvement, such as paralysis and abnormal reflexes; when there are signs of increased intracranial pressure, such as headache, projectile vomiting, convulsions, choked disk, coma, and hemiplegia; and when visualization of the brain or spinal cord by injection of air or dye is desired. Therapeutically, lumbar puncture is indicated for relief of increased intracranial pressure, for the injection of serums, for the introduction of drugs, for spinal anesthesia, and for drainage and irrigation.

In performance of the procedure, the patient usually lies on his side, and fluid is obtained by inserting a 19- or 20-gauge spinal puncture needle through the subarachnoid space, usually in the third or fourth lumbar interspace. For entrance of the needle into this space, the patient is requested to bend his neck forward and to draw up his knees toward his abdomen as far as possible in a position that can be comfortably maintained throughout the procedure. The site for the puncture is found by locating the soft spot between the spinous processes of the third and fourth lumbar vertebrae. This lies on or just above a line joining the crests of the ilia. The sterile spinal needle is inserted at the midline, after previous sterilization of skin (sterile gloves are also used), and the needle is pushed forward with a quick thrust until it reaches the tough spinous ligaments. It is then pushed slowly until sudden cessation of resistance indicates that it has entered the spinal canal. The stylet is then removed; the fluid should flow at once. If fluid does not start flowing out immediately, the needle should be moved a little in or out, or the stylet should be inserted.

The pressure under which the fluid appears should be noted by measuring with a manometer; it should drop slowly from the needle. Occasionally, the patency of the spinal subarachnoid space may be determined using the Queckenstedt test. When the manometer is removed, the first few drops of fluid are discarded because they usually contain some red blood cells, owing to the puncture process. Approximately 3 ml. of fluid is then collected in each of three sterile tubes with screw-cap tops; these are marked 1, 2, and 3. Without replacing the stylet, the needle is quickly withdrawn. Sterile tubes are used because bacteriologic studies are occasionally needed (use tube 1 for this). Anticoagulants are not needed because early coagulation is not common in the diseases in which the cell count is most important. However, the tube that is to be used for the cytologic examination should contain a trace of powdered potassium oxalate.

The fluid should be taken immediately to the laboratory because the leukocyte count must be made within the first half hour after withdrawal. Red blood cells, white blood cells, and tumor cells autolyze quickly in aqueous media; bacteria and fungi die quickly if not transferred to culture media. Virus studies are best done when the fluid is frozen immediately after collection, and spinal fluid sugar quickly becomes reduced and lowered.

Laboratory Studies

It is most essential that cultures of cerebrospinal fluid be made if the patient has meningeal signs, and as a confirmatory and differential diagnostic procedure when organisms are demonstrated in smears. The most specific and desirable method is to allow 1 or 2 ml. of fluid to flow directly from the lumbar puncture needle into a warm culture medium, which is then immediately placed in an incubator at 37° C. If this is not feasible, the fluid can be collected in a sterile tube and sent to the laboratory immediately for prompt inoculation. This is accomplished by pipetting 1 to 2 ml. of fluid directly into a thioglycolate fluid medium, blood agar, and Petragnani's and Sabouraud's medium (the latter two when indicated).

Because frequent contamination of spinal fluid by nonpathogenic organisms occurs and because meningococci viability and growth are tenuous, it is necessary to observe strict bacteriologic technique. Specimens must be examined promptly and must not be chilled or refrigerated before their inoculation into culture media. It is also necessary to examine spinal fluid as promptly as possible (within half an hour) because the sugar level tends to drop rapidly on standing, and the cells tend to degenerate or disintegrate if there is any undue delay before cytologic studies are made. In addition, uniform cell suspensions are difficult to obtain after the cells have settled or fibrin has formed.

A direct smear of undiluted cerebrospinal fluid or centrifuged sediment, stained with Gram's stain and Ziehl-Neelsen carbolfuchsin stain, may at times make immediate diagnosis possible before culture results are obtainable. Gross examination should be made that includes color, transparency, clot formation, presence or absence of blood, and xanthochromia. After bacteriologic and cytologic examinations have been made, it should be noted whether the fluid is colorless (normal) or cloudy, and whether bloody or xanthochromic. If blood is present, the amount of blood in the first tube should be compared with that in the other tubes. A traumatic spinal puncture, caused by the operator in the act of performing the puncture, will result in more blood in the first tube and practically none in the third tube. In addition, the supernatant fluid will be clear, and the specimen will tend to clot. If blood is uniformly present in all three tubes, and the supernatant fluid is yellowish with the absence of a clot, a subarachnoid hemorrhage is indicated, and the yellowish color (xanthochromia) indicates a hemorrhage that occurred 2 to 3 days prior to puncture. If cell counts are made on traumatic bloody fluid, it will be affected by peripheral blood and will not

be diagnostic of the true cytologic condition of the spinal fluid itself. There is approximately one white blood cell for each 700 red blood cells present, if the patient's peripheral blood pattern is within normal range.

Yellowish fluids may also be due to jaundice (bilirubinemia), spinal fluid block, and meningitis; it is also found, when it is associated with a positive indirect van den Bergh test, in the normal spinal fluid of premature infants for 1 to 2 weeks after birth. Clotting due to fibrinogen and a globulin reaction of 2+ or more may also occur in syphilis of the central nervous system (small clots), tuberculous meningitis (web-like clot or pellicle at surface on standing), purulent meningitis (large clot), and in spinal fluid blockage (massive clot formation).

A cloudy or turbid fluid is usually due to a high white blood cell content (mostly polymorphonuclear forms) and is usually associated with bacterial infection of the meninges. An increase in white blood cells in the spinal fluid (more than 10 to 25 cells/cu.mm.) is called *pleocytosis*. Cell counts should be made from the thoroughly mixed third tube of fluid because this tube is less likely to be contaminated by blood from the puncture technique. Although there are methods for estimating bloody spinal fluid leukocyte counts, they are not accurate and are usually not made. However, red blood cell counts are frequently done serially on bloody spinal fluids to serve as a basis for comparison and, thus, to determine the increase or decrease of spinal fluid hemorrhage.[2]

Spinal Fluid Cell Count. The basic principle of the spinal fluid cell count is similar to that of the peripheral blood white blood cell count. A white blood cell counting pipette, improved Neubauer ruled hemacytometer, and a diluting fluid (0.1 g. of crystal violet, 1 ml. of glacial acetic acid, 50 ml. of distilled water, and a few drops of 5 per cent phenol solution) are used. The diluting fluid is drawn up to mark 1 in the white blood cell pipette, and the spinal fluid up to mark 11.

The pipette contents are shaken well and the first two or three drops are discarded. A drop of fluid is then placed on each side of a double counting chamber, and the preparation is allowed to settle as in a white blood cell count. The acetic acid hemolyzes the red blood cells, and the crystal violet stains the white blood cells so that amorphous structures can be distinguished.

All cells within the entire ruled areas on both sides of the counting chamber are counted. The total count obtained when all 18 squares are counted (nine 1 mm. squares on each side) is multiplied by 0.6 to obtain the number of white blood cells per cubic millimeter of undiluted fluid. One may also count five squares (1 sq. mm. each)—that is, four corner squares and the central square on each side—and then total the white blood cells counted. If it is desired, one may multiply the total by 10/9 to correct for dilution.

If a Fuchs-Rosenthal counting chamber is used, the ruled area covers 16 sq. mm. with a 0.2 mm. depth below the cover glass. This makes the total volume 16/5 cu.mm. or 3 1/5 cu.mm. (roughly 3). One proceeds as previously; the counting chamber is charged with spinal fluid (utilizing the white blood cell pipette and diluting fluid). The number of white blood cells in the entire ruled area is totaled and divided by 3; this gives the number of white blood cells in each cu.mm. of spinal fluid.

Normally, one to seven lymphocytes/cu.mm. are found in adults (up to 30 in 1- to 2-week-old infants). Amounts above 10 are considered evidence of pleocytosis. Errors may be due to delay in making the count, failure to mix the fluid thoroughly, and counting spores of *Cryptococcus neoformans*, artifacts, and red blood cells as white blood cells.

Certain diseases cause varying quantities of lymphocytes and polymorphonuclear neutrophils in cerebrospinal fluid. They are: tuberculous meningitis, syphilis of the central nervous system, viral encephalitis, anterior poliomyelitis, and chronic meningitides, all of which are characterized by 25 to 100 lymphocytes/cu.mm. of spinal fluid; and lymphocytic choriomeningitis (without bacteria in spinal fluid), which is usually characterized by 30 to 1500 or more lymphocytes/cu.mm. of spinal fluid, and purulent (acute) meningitis, (meningococcal, pneumococcal, and staphylococcal; cerebral or extradural abscesses and hemorrhage), which is characterized by 100 to 2000 polymorphonuclear leukocytes/cu.mm. of spinal fluid.

If the cerebrospinal fluid is clear or only slightly cloudy, it may be centrifuged and the sediment examined. Because the cells in this fluid are usually poorly preserved, good differential staining is difficult except for lymphocytes, polymorphonuclear leukocytes, large mononuclear leukocytes, and, occasionally, cancer cells.[1]

Smears may be examined using the Papanicolaou technique. Löffler's alkaline methylene blue may be added to the fluid and a moist preparation made of the mixture; that is, add three drops of methylene blue for each milliliter of sediment or straight cerebrospinal fluid. After coverslipping, wait 5 to 15 minutes and examine the concentrated mixture. Use Gram's stain for bacterial differentiation, the Ziehl-Neesen stain for tubercle bacilli from a fibrin web in cerebrospinal fluid, and India ink stain for diagnosis of fluid with lymphocyte-like cells, many of which could be spores of *Cryptococcus neoformans*.

REFERENCES

1. Platt, W. R.: Exfoliative-cell diagnosis of central nervous system lesions. Arch. Neurol. Psychiat., 66:119, 1951.
2. Poser, C. M.: The clinical significance of spinal fluid examination. Am. J. Med. Tech., 25:189, 1959.

8

Pathology of the Erythrocyte Series, Including Abnormal Hemoglobin Syndromes and Indices

The main function of red blood cells is to synthesize, transport, and defend the hemoglobin moieties. In this way the hemoglobin molecules transport oxygen, facilitate carbon dioxide transportation and aid in maintenance of acid-base equilibrium. As soon as the marrow hemohistioblast (hemocytoblast) differentiates into the pronormoblast, hemoglobin synthesis starts (Plates 1, 2). Globin molecules and porphyrin rings form and combine with iron atoms, utilizing enzymes and metabolic substrates and catalysts in the process. From the pronormoblast stage, the nucleated erythrocytes divide by mitosis into basophilic normoblasts, polychromatophilic normoblasts, and finally orthochromic normoblasts. At the same time, hemoglobin, synthesis takes place, associated with a decrease in the cytoplasmic ribonucleic acid (RNA) concentration. By this geometric type of division and multiplication, the acidophilic normoblastic stage with condensed pyknotic nucleus is reached. Approximately 24 hours later the reticulocyte is formed after nuclear extrusion.

Adult erythrocyte maturation occurs after the depletion of cytoplasmic RNA with concomitant hemoglobin formation and iron uptake in the red blood cells. The extrasinusoidal marrow existence of the maturing reticulocyte is completed 1 to 2 days after intravascular reticulocyte diapedesis with the formation of mature erythrocytes and their liberation into the peripheral circulation. After approximately 175 miles travel and 120 days in the bloodstream, erythrocytes are gradually depleted of their total enzymatic content and finally destroyed in the reticuloendothelial system, mostly in the spleen and to a certain extent in the liver and bone marrow. The integral parts of these erythrocytes—the haptoglobins that carry the hemoglobin molecule, including heme and globin, plus other products—are taken up by the reticuloendothelial cells. By a poorly understood process, the hemoglobin splits into three portions—divalent iron, protein (globin), and an iron-free pigment called protoporphyrin, or finally bilirubin. The heme portion, consisting of four pyrrole rings joined to one atom of iron, is responsible for oxygen transport (Fig. 8-1).

The haptoglobins are divided into three types and are associated with the α_2 fraction of gamma globulin; they are therefore elevated in inflammatory states. The ferric protoporphyrin combines with the heme-binding globulin and albumin to form methemalbumin. The protein component—globin—is formed largely from the amino acids of the body depots. These amino acids are obtained from ingested food or protein conservation from disintegration of aging red blood cells. This is consistent with the concept of starvation and protein depletion leading to decreased hemoglobin production. The iron is immediately used in the manufacture of new hemoglobin and red blood cells, and the protein is broken down into amino acids and returned to the body depots to be used for resynthesis.

The breakdown of 1 ml. of erythrocytes liberates approximately 1 mg. of iron and 10 mg. of bilirubin into the bloodstream. Iron is required in the body in amounts of 12 to 15 mg. daily and is taken from three main sources—food, body depots, and aging red blood cells. Food iron is in both ferrous and ferric states. When absorbed ferrous iron leaves the mucosal cells, it is as the ionic ferric form in which it is transported in the plasma of the bloodstream and joined with β_1 globulin to form a ferric compound termed transferrin, siderophilin, or iron-binding protein. How this absorption takes place is not specifically known. The mucosal lining cells of the small intestines contains an iron-free protein known as apoferritin, which combines with the iron to form ferritin. The function accomplished by the buildup of ferritin in the mucosal cells is uncertain. It has been reported that ferritin iron in the epithelial cell is not absorbed but is instead sequestered and prevented from entering the circulation. The iron is lost when the ferritin-containing cells are shed into the intestinal lumen.[28] It is also proposed that the ferritin content of the gastrointestinal mucosal cell differs in normal conditions, iron deficiency, and iron overload.[28]

Other evidence indicates that the active transfer across the cell involves two steps requiring oxidative metabolism—mucosal uptake, and transfer to the serosal surface, or into the plasma.[99, 100] Also, both divalent (ferrous) and trivalent (ferric) iron are taken up at the mucosal surface, but a slower transfer to the serosal surface (or plasma) is relatively specific for ferrous iron (85%). Iron is transported to other parts of the body in both ferric and ferrous forms. The reticuloendothelial cells serve

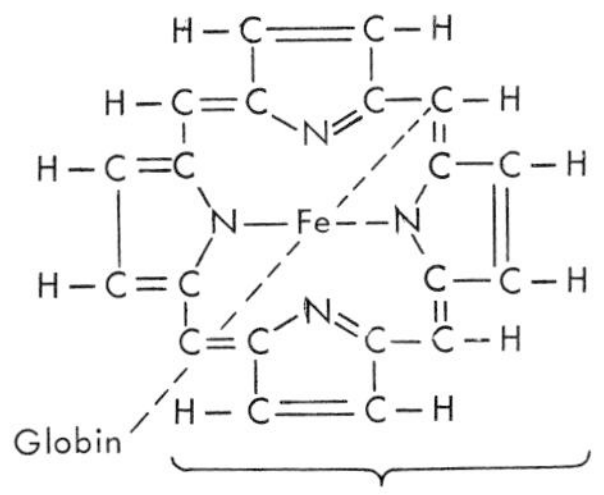

Fig. 8-1. Hemoglobin molecule. The bracketed portion represents heme, which is composed of ferrous iron and protoporphyrin; the latter is composed of four pyrrole rings.

as storage depots of iron in the form of hemosiderin. Myoglobin and cytochromes (iron catalysts) are also prepared from depot iron (total amount of storage iron is approximately 600 mg.). A reduction in available depot iron leads to an immediate increase in the absorption of iron, whereas saturation of iron depots leads to fecal excretion of unchanged iron. Similarly, iron absorption insufficiency is associated with low serum iron, whereas high serum iron indicates interference with red blood cell maturation. Only small amounts of iron are excreted daily—in the urine and bile.

Porphyrin is the complex pigmented portion of heme and, in the form of porphyrin III, is the immediate precursor of heme. It is formed mainly from glycine. Porphyrin I is formed during the synthesis of heme and is excreted as coproporphyrin I in urine, bile, and feces, and is indicative of healthy maturation of red blood cells. An excess of porphyrin I is excreted as coproporphyrin III; therefore when coproporphyrin III is present in excess, it suggests a failure in the synthesis of porphyrin III into hemoglobin, usually caused by toxic heavy metals such as arsenic and lead.

Bilirubin does not participate in hemoglobin metabolism if the liver is functioning correctly. However, the serum bilirubin level is a fairly accurate indicator of the hemolytic process. The chemical formula of bilirubin is similar to that of prophyrin except that the pyrrole ring is open. Bilirubin is transferred from the reticuloendothelial cells to the liver, where it is secreted as a bile pigment into the bile. The yellowish color of the plasma is due to a bilirubin-globulin complex (normally not excreted by the kidney), which is formed in the reticulo-endothelial cells by the removal of hemoglobin iron. In the passage of this complex through the liver, the protein portion is removed and the oxidized pigment (biliverdin) is excreted in the bile.

After concentration in the gallbladder, bilirubin enters the gastrointestinal tract, where putrefactive bacteria convert it into stercobilinogen. A portion is excreted in fecal matter in the oxidized stercobilin form. The rest is reabsorbed into blood, and some of this goes to the liver, where it is reexcreted as bile. The other part is excreted in the urine as urobilinogen and oxidized to urobilin. If the liver is sufficiently diseased, it will be unable to break down the bilirubin in sufficient quantities, and it therefore accumulates in the blood, subsequently imparting a yellowish color to the skin, conjunctivas, and other organs. The same thing happens if the bile ducts leading from the liver are blocked by an intrahepatic or extrahepatic disease.

THE INDICES

The purpose of determining blood indices is to corroborate and correlate the fundamental results obtained in the routine complete blood count—the hematocrit, red blood cell count, and the hemoglobin determination. In this way, the types of anemia may be objectively classified, and red blood cell variations may be specifically studied. Wintrobe accomplished this by using blood indices in which objective quantitative standards were substituted for subjective, inaccurate nonscientific impressions. Definitions, methods of calculation, and normal values for the following indices are important guidelines in the hematology laboratory.

The *color index* (C.I.) is based on the comparison of the mean hemoglobin concentration of a red blood cell with that of a normal red blood cell, which is taken as one. Therefore C.I. =

$$\frac{\text{Hemoglobin \% (gm./100 ml.)} \times 6.9}{\text{RBC count (millions/cu.mm.)} \times 20}$$

The normal range is 0.9 to 1.1. The normal number of red blood cells (100%) is assumed to be 5,000,000 per cu.mm., and the normal hemoglobin is assumed to be 14.5 g. per 100 ml. of blood. The main disadvantage of this index is that the normal red blood cell count is assumed to be 5,000,000, whereas it may vary from 4,000,000 to 6,5000,000 per cu.mm. Also assumed is a normal hemoglobin of 14.5 g. per 100 ml. of blood, whereas it actually may vary from 14 to 15 g. per 100 ml. Consequently, this index gives no true indication of cell size or hemoglobin concentration. Moreover, the normal range is wide (0.9–1.1).

The *volume index* (V.I.) is the ratio of the average volume of erythrocytes in the patient's blood to the average volume of erythrocytes in normal blood. It has replaced the C.I. because it is more consistent in that it does not utilize a so-called normal value in the calculation of the results. V.I. =

$$\frac{\text{Hematocrit} \times 2.3}{\text{RBC count (millions/cu.mm.)} \times 20}, \text{ or}$$

$$\frac{\text{MCV of patient}}{\text{MCV of normal person}}$$

The normal range is 0.9 to 1.1.

The *mean corpuscular hemoglobin* (MCH) indicates the weight of hemoglobin in a single red blood cell in micromicrograms ($\mu\mu$g. or 10^{-12} g.). MCH =

$$\frac{\text{Hemoglobin content in } \mu\mu\text{g./cu. mm.}}{\text{RBC count in millions/cu.mm.}}, \text{ or}$$

$$\frac{\text{Hemoglobin concentration (g./100 ml.)} \times 10}{\text{RBC count (}10^6\text{/cu.mm.)}}, \text{ or}$$

$$\frac{\text{Hemoglobin in g./liter}}{\text{RBC in millions/cu.mm.}}$$

The normal range is 27 to 32 $\mu\mu$g. If an electronic counting device, such as the

Coulter Counter, is not used to make the red blood cell count, the MCH will be somewhat inaccurate. However, because the calculations are made on figures determined by actual count of the blood, it is more accurate than the C.I. in estimating the average hemoglobin content of each blood cell.

The *mean corpuscular hemoglobin concentration* (MCHC) is a term that denotes the average hemoglobin concentration per unit volume (per 100 ml.) of packed red blood cells. This is expressed as a percentage of packed cells as distinct from whole blood. Because the number of red blood cells is not used to calculate the MCHC, it is therefore a poor term to use. Therefore, MCHC =

$$\frac{\text{HGB. concentration (g./100 ml.)} \times 100}{\text{Hematocrit (\%)}}$$

The normal range is 32 to 36 per cent (or g./100 ml. of red blood cells). Because the two most accurate hematological determinations are used in this formula, that is, the hemoglobin and hematocrit, not the variable red blood cell counts (visual determination)—it is most valuable in evaluating therapy. A decreased MCHC, for example, signifies that a unit volume of packed erythrocytes contains less hemoglobin than normal or that hemoglobin has been replaced by erythrocytic stromal material, as in iron deficiency and macrocytic anemias. An increased MCHC usually indicates spherocytosis.

The *saturation index* (S.I.) is a figure denoting the average amount of hemoglobin per unit volume of red blood cells in relation to the normal.

$$\text{S.I.} \times \frac{\text{color index}}{\text{volume index}}$$

The normal range is 0.80 to 1.20. This value presents the same objections as the color index and volume index and therefore is not used much in the estimation of hematological variations.

The *mean corpuscular diameter* (MCD) indicates the average diameter of red blood cells in microns. Most techniques utilize a stained blood film, the most common of which is the Price-Jones method. In this method, direct measurement and direct micrometry are used. Occasionally a diffraction method may be used that requires a halometer. In the more commonly used Price-Jones method, one compares the micrometer eyepiece divisions (calibrated in microns) with the lines in a hemacytometer.[84] This is done by adjusting the microscope tube length so that 50 μ in the eyepiece will exactly coincide with the opposite sides of a small square on the hemacytometer, which are exactly 50 μ apart. After this is done, blood film stained with Wright's stain is examined under the oil-immersion objective using a strong light; the diameters of 100 consecutive red blood cells are examined. Then the slide is moved, another field is examined, and the diameters of another 100 red blood cells are measured. Only the round shaped cells are measured. The average value of these 200 diameters is the mean corpuscular diameter.

The normal range is 6 to 9 μ (average, 7.5 μ). The diameters of abnormal cells vary from 3 to 12 μ. The diameters may be plotted as a curve beginning with 3 μ and increasing by steps of 0.5 μ. The size of the diameters may be plotted on the abscissa and the frequencies on the ordinate. This curve is the Price-Jones curve, and may be compared with a normal Price-Jones curve. In actual hematological, clinical, and hospital practice, an experienced hematologist or technologist can determine an increase or decrease in MCD by microscopic study of a well prepared and stained blood film.

The *mean corpuscular thickness* (MCT) is a hematological value measured in microns. It is indicative of the average volume of a cylinder—that is, the biconcave disk or erythrocyte. Because the thickness of such a disk varies at different points, only the average thickness can be determined so as to obtain data concerning the cell as a whole. This information cannot be obtained by direct measurement but must be calculated by assuming that the erythrocyte has a cylindrical form in which the height represents the average cell thickness with concavities balanced against convexities. The volume of a cylinder = area × height (thickness); therefore, volume = πr^2 (area) × h (height); or

$$h = \frac{Vol.}{\pi r^2}$$

Clinically then, MCT, which is also called MCAT (A for average) =

$$\pi \frac{MCV}{\left(\frac{MCD}{2}\right)^2}$$

The normal range is 1.7 to 2.5 μ (average, 2.0 μ). This determination is only of value to detect spherocytosis, which can usually be done by microscopic study of the stained film. Any error in the MCD determination will greatly magnify the error in MCT.

The *mean corpuscular volume* (MCV) is an index that expresses the volume in cubic microns occupied by an average single red blood cell. Because this index is based on the visual or electronic counting of red blood cells, it is more accurate and therefore of greater value than the volume index.

$$MCV = \frac{Hematocrit\ (\%) \times 10}{Red\ cell\ count\ (10^6/cu.mm.)},\ or$$

$$\frac{Vol.\ of\ packed\ RBC\ in\ ml./liter\ of\ blood}{RBC\ in\ millions/cu.mm.}$$

The normal range is 80 to 100 cu.μ; the average is 87 cu.μ. This determination indicates the average size of the red blood cells; a figure above 100 indicates macrocytosis, and a figure below 80 indicates microcytosis.

Electronic measurement of the MCV meets the requirements for a screening test for many anemias (e.g., Thalassemia trait). The test is rapid, automated, and inexpensive. It definitely excludes the vast majority of normal patients. Since false negative results are very infrequent and the number of false positives is acceptably low, an ab-

normal value for the MCV is a significant finding that demands further investigation.[114]

In conclusion, results from the MCV, MCH, and MCHC require an accuracy of at least ±5 per cent in red blood cell count, hemoglobin, and hematocrit determinations because it is essential to use accurate data to calculate these values. For this purpose, the use of an electronic cell counter, calibrated glassware, precise reagent standards (cyanmethemoglobin), and instrument calibration accuracy are all important. In addition it is useful to compare the appearance of the red blood cell on the stained film with the calculated values, and then compare the calculated values with one another. Thus, very low values for MCH are inconsistent with macrocytosis.

To extend this premise, one might state that macrocytosis revealed by hematologic screening procedures (i.e., an elevated MCV above 115 cu.μm., as performed by a good electronic counter) is a significant abnormality that requires further investigation unless the patient is on medication known to produce this abnormality.[98] The diagnostic yield from following elevated MCV values with Vitamin B_{12} and folate determinations is sufficiently good to allow this to be adopted as a routine procedure in most laboratories.

ABNORMAL ERYTHROCYTIC FORMS

Abnormal Sizes (Plates 8, 9)

Abnormality in size, called anisocytosis, is a common and important erythrocyte morphologic variation. The term *anisocytosis* describes any variation in the size of the erythrocyte outside the normal or normocytic range of 6.2 to 8.2 μ (average, 7.2 μ).

Macrocytosis is a condition in which red blood cells have a diameter greater than 9 μ and frequently have an MCV greater tha 95 to 100 cu.μ. Macrocytic cells can indicate the presence of more hemoglobin than normal. This is found in Vitamin B_{12} and folic acid deficiencies (seen in prenicious anemia and other macrocytic anemias) in the new-born infant, myxedema, and in hemolytic anemias with associated reticulocytosis (frequently polychromatophilic). Further-more, the elevated MCV may prove to be a useful, inexpensive screening test for early liver disease, particularly alcoholic liver disease. Thus, in addition to its function in classifying anemias, measurement of the MCV should be considered a valuable screening test, and significant macrocytosis should be investigated further.

Microcytosis is a condition in which red blood cells have a diameter less than 6 μ and frequently with an MCV of less than 80 to 82 cu.μ. Microcytic cells frequently have less hemoglobin than normal cells, and they are therefore frequently seen in iron defi-ciency anemias and spherocytic and Medi-terranean hemolytic anemias.

Abnormal Erythrocytic Shapes (Plate 9)

Poikilocytosis is a term used to describe the condition in which there are major vari-ations in the shape of the erythrocyte, nor-mally that of a biconcave disk. They in-clude the following:

When the red blood cell thickness is in-creased owing to rounding of the biconcave disk, the cell volume may remain the same or, more commonly, the diameter decreases forming a *spherocyte* or *microspherocyte* with normal hemoglobin saturation. The microspherocyte is smaller but stains deeply and does not have the central pallor seen in hypochromic microcytes and nor-mocytes. The mature spherocytic cell shape itself evidently forms after the re-ticulocyte has matured. This phenomenon of spherocytosis is most commonly seen in congenital and acquired hemolytic anemias, but is occasionally seen in infants, in stored blood, and in patients who have received multiple transfusions. The congenital spherocyte results from an antigen-antibody effect on the surface of the cell. With this decreased deformability there are also alterations in membrane phospholipid (increased cholesterol).[24] Spherocytes have a 14 day life span (normal erythrocytes,

120 days), and they commonly exhibit in-creased fragility in hypotonic saline solu-tions in hereditary spherocytosis and occa-sionally in acquired spherocytosis.

Elliptocytes are red blood cell anomalies frequently inherited as a Mendelian domi-nant in which only a few are seen at birth, the number increasing after 12 days of age. Unstained smears reveal oval to elliptical to baciliform shapes. The phenomenon is seen in healthy persons and occasionally in Mediterranean anemia and in other types.

Target cells, or *Mexican hat cells*, a thin erythrocytes having relatively large di-ameters with apparent central condensation of hemoglobin and adjacent lighter areas resembling the concentric circles of a rifle target. In the wet unstained state these red blood cells appear flatter and are then called *leptocytes* (occasionally platycytes). They occur in various types of hemolytic anemias—sickle cell anemia, hemoglobin C disease, and thalassemia—and also during jaundice and after splenectomy. Cooper and Jandl[25] showed that free cholesterol ac-cumulates in the red cell membrane in ob-structive jaundice and in inhibition of plasma trans-esterase activity; this results in an increase of the surface area and in an increase in the formation of target cells.

Sickle cells, also called *drepanocytes* and *menisocytes*, are elongated red blood cells with sharp double points having crescentic shapes and occasionally U, S, or L shapes with more irregular spine formation occur-ring after exposure to strong reducing agents (sodium metabisulfite) or to reduc-tion in oxygen tension or pH. This poikilo-cytic pattern occurs if the red blood cell contains insoluble hemoglobin S, and this condition occurs in its asymptomatic he-terozygous form as the sickle cell trait and in its homozygous hemolytic form as sickle cell anemia. The Sherman test and elec-trophoretic analysis differentiate between these two forms.

Eccentrocytes are rigid deformed eryth-rocytes caused by an abnormal and ir-reversible intracellular concentration of he-moglobin resulting from dehydration of the

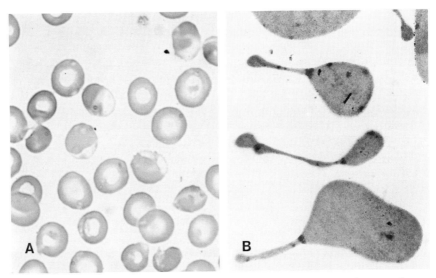

Fig. 8-2. Eccentrocytes. (*A*) These abnormal RBC forms have a dense and contracted area to one side, leaving a thinned out area. (*B*) Cross-section. Sections are perpendicular to the plane of the cell and show mounded hemoglobin and thin portions. (Ham, T. H., et al.: J. Lab. Clin. Med., *82:*900, 1973)

cell with loss of cations and H_2O. These RBCs associated with hemolytic anemia are also observed in patients with G-6-PD deficiency after exposure to oxidant drugs and infection. Susceptibility to the erythrocytic deformity appears to be dependent on the level of G-6-PD in the RBCs (Fig. 8-2).

Crenated erythrocytes possess a crinkled, serrated periphery. They are not clinically diagnostic and merely reflect changes produced by the exposure of red blood cells to dehydration, hypertonic agents, and lytic agents.

Burr cells are erythrocytes that have focal accentuated crenation producing irregular contraction resulting in long spinous processes. Burr cells have been observed in polycythemia due to phenylhydrazine therapy, in renal insufficiency, bleeding gastrointestinal ulcers, malignant neoplasia (especially gastric), acute plumbism, and in naphthaline ingestion.

Ovalocytes are oval shaped red blood cells measuring $7 \times 6 \mu$. They are found in concentration of 90 per cent or more in elliptocytosis, and they may be present in normal blood.

Schistocytes are fragmenting portions of red blood cells derived from "safety-pin" red blood cells having a wedge-shaped disrupted pattern frequently seen in blood smears of severely burned patients. Schistocytes are also seen in thalassemic and elliptocytic hemolytic anemias.

Acanthocytes are spherocytic erythrocytes possessing long needle-like protrusions. They are present in large numbers in homozygous inherited red blood cell states. One example described in the literature is associated with celiac disease and retinitis pigmentosa.

Megaloblasts are nucleated red blood cells found in the bone marrow. They are 15 to 22 μ in diameter and are associated with Vitamin B_{12} and folic acid deficiencies. The cell is larger than its normal counterpart (the basophilic normoblast); the nuclear chromatin is finer, and the cytoplasm is lighter staining and larger in amount.

Abnormal Inclusions (Plate 10)

Erythrocytic abnormal inclusions are cytoplasmic blemishes often indicating disease. These include the following intracellular defects:

Basophilic stippling, or *punctate basophilia,* is a characteristic of polychromatophilic red blood cells in which there are round, fine or coarse bluish-violet or dark blue granules dispersed throughout the cytoplasm. They are seen in chronic anemias, leukemia, Mediterranean anemias, and lead poisoning. The granules are not like the lacy network of reticulocytes, which pattern can only be observed in supravital stains. Jensen and colleagues[68] have shown by electron microscopy that basophilic stippling represents aggregated ribosomes, whereas siderotic granules represent nonheme iron and iron-laden mitochondria.

Howell-Jolly bodies are single or double eccentrically located, small, rounded reddish blue or dark violet (Wright's stain) nuclear remnants frequently found in red blood cells after splenectomy, as well as in other severe anemias. They appear when abnormal mitosis of the orthochromic normoblast occurs, and they represent Fuelgen-positive nonrefractile particles.

Cabot's ring bodies (or just Cabot's rings) are reddish purple, circular or twisted figure-of-eight rings considered to be nuclear remnants of artifacts found after the exposure of the red blood to hemolytic agents. They are seen in lead poisoning, leukemia, pernicious anemia, and hemolytic anemias. They can be differentiated from the *Plasmodium* ring forms found in malaria by their larger size and by the absence of a red chromatin mass.

Siderotic granules are nonhemoglobin, light blue, iron particles that are seen in siderocytic red blood cells after Prussian blue staining. They are associated with some of the developing red blood cells (especially normoblasts and reticulocytes) that do not completely utilize iron in their hemoglobin molecule formation. These granules are frequently seen after splenectomy in anemias associated with impaired hemoglobin formation.

Malarial parasites are sporozoa of the genus *Plasmodium,* four species in type (*P. vivax, P. malariae, P. falciparum,* and *P. ovale*). All these species have the same characteristics in man—they are diagnostic of malaria, inhabit the red blood cells, and they contain hemozoin produced from hemoglobin. The trophozoite, schizont, merozoite, and occasionally gametocyte forms are characteristic for each species. In the red blood cell, the cytoplasm of these parasites is blue, and the nuclear chromatin is red. The trophozoite form must be differentiated from platelets, which are smaller, superimposed on the red blood cell and do not have any ameboid form or hemozoin (Plate 33).

Heinz bodies, sometimes called *Heinz-Ehrlich bodies,* are supravitally stainable, refractile, oval or irregular, purplish inclusion granules produced in certain hemolytic anemias by denaturation and precipitation of hemoglobin. They are located close to the red blood cell membrane. They may be seen in unstained blood smears, and they occur spontaneously in premature newborn infants. They also occur as a result of the introduction of a reversible oxidation-reduction system into the red blood cell—for example, in metabolically hypersusceptible Black patients on antimalarial drugs (pamaquin and primaquine) and polycythemic patients on phenylhydrazine therapy.[37] Heinz bodies may also be associated with methemoglobinemia.

Schüffner's dots are reddish granules frequently found in enlarged erythrocytes parasitized by *Plasmodium vivax.*

VARIATIONS IN HEMOGLOBIN CONTENT AND STAINING PROPERTY

In this category may be included the following phenomena (Plates 8, 9):

Hypochromia is a pattern of increased central pallor in erythrocytes associated with a lack of hemoglobin and caused by impaired hemoglobin synthesis, most commonly from a lack of iron.

Hyperchromia is a term that does not represent a true situation and therefore does not enjoy common use today. In the past, deeply and homogeneously stained, enlarged red cells with a color index greater than one and lacking central pallor were called hyperchromic. However, a macrocyte with a normal hemoglobin concentration contains more hemoglobin than a normocyte only because the cell is larger than normal. Because oversaturation with hemoglobin does not occur, the cell cannot be truly regarded as hyperchromic.

Normochromia is a term used to indicate that the red blood cells contain an amount of hemoglobin equal to the normal level as determined by calculation of the mean corpuscular hemoglobin—that is, the hemoglobin in grams per 1000 ml. of blood divided by the red blood cell in millions per cubic millimeter. It expresses the average hemoglobin content of a single red blood cell in micromicrograms, the normal range being 27 to 32 $\mu\mu$g. and the average being 29.6 $\mu\mu$g. The mean corpuscular hemoglobin concentration (the hemoglobin in g./100 ml. divided by the hematocrit $\times$ 100) yields a normal range of 32 to 38 g. per 100 ml. with an average of 33 g. per 100 ml.; it is the proportion of hemoglobin in the average RBC of blood sample.

Polychromatophilia is a property of the immature erythrocyte or reticulocyte when Wright's stain is applied. The basophilic material gives a diffuse, homogeneous blue color owing to a ribonucleoprotein.[52] Because pure hemoglobin itself stains an orange-red color, combinations of hemoglobin and the basophilic ribonucleoprotein produce color variations of gray-blue to gray-orange-red, a condition called *polychromatophilia* or *polychromasia*.

ANEMIAS

Anemias are a symptom complex characterized by a reduction in red blood cells and hemoglobin values (less than 3,900,000/ cu.mm. in males and 3,200,000/cu.mm. in females, or hemoglobin values less than 10.8 g./100 ml. in males and less than 9.2 g./cu.mm. in females) with associated reduction in the oxygen-carrying capacity of the blood and subsequent hypoxia. Anemia is always a sign of an underlying disease process, and it is never a specific diagnosis. Early findings of anemia involve peripheral blood hemoglobin reduction. Later, there is an associated red blood cell diminution. These findings are reflected in the bone marrow erythroid cytologic pattern—hypoplasia, a normal pattern, or hyperplasia— depending on etiology, duration, and the severity of the anemia.

The symptomatology depends on the severity of the hypoxia, the amount of physical exertion, the duration of the anemic process, and on how much the patient has physiologically compensated for the anemia. For example, a patient at rest with a slowly-developing severe anemia may have practically no symptoms, whereas a strenuously active athlete would develop signs and symptoms, such as pallor, tachycardia, dyspnea on exertion, nervousness, headache, dizziness, cardiac murmurs, weakness, anorexia, nausea, fever, and dyspnea at rest. Finally, if it is severe enough, untreated, and of long enough duration, heart failure and a comatose state would ensue. In addition, a sudden loss of large amounts of blood will produce symptoms in any type of patient, depending on the hemoglobin concentration of the peripheral blood.

ETIOLOGIC CLASSIFICATION[9, 49]

I. Increased loss or destruction of hemoglobin-erythrocyte mass (hyperactive bone marrow).
  A. Anemia resulting from blood loss.
    1. Acute.
      a. External: building blocks (especially iron) not available for reutilization (e.g., trauma).

b. Internal: building blocks (especially iron) subsequently available for reutilization, as in acute gastrointestinal ulceration.

2. Chronic.
   a. External: building blocks (especially iron) not available, as in hemophilia and menses.
   b. Internal; *lungs* — iron not available for reutilization, as in idiopathic pulmonary hemosiderosis; elsewhere as in *gastrointestinal tract,* building blocks (especially iron) available for utilization — e.g., in chronic peptic ulcer.

B. Anemia resulting from excess destruction of red blood cells.
   1. Due to intracorpuscular defects.
      a. Hereditary defects of red blood cells: hereditary spherocytosis, ovalocytosis, thalassemia, stomatocytosis, hereditary nonspherocytic disease, and hemoglobinopathies, such as sickle cell anemia and hemoglobin C disease, etc. Also combinations with other defects, such as primaquine-sensitive hemolytic anemia (glucose-6-phosphate dehydrogenase deficiency), favism, and erythropoietica porphyria.
      b. Acquired defects of red blood cells — e.g., paroxysmal nocturnal hemoglobinuria, thermal injury, and deficiency diseases, such as vitamin B_{12}, folic acid, and iron deficiency.
   2. Due to interaction of intracorpuscular and extracorpuscular abnormalities — e.g., primaquine-sensitive hemolytic anemias, favism, lead poisoning, vitamin B_{12} or folic acid deficiency, and thermal injury.
   3. Due to extracorpuscular abnormalities.
      a. Immune mechanism (antibodies demonstrable) — e.g., naturally occurring immunity (anti-A and anti-B immunity, responsible for most hemolytic transfusion reactions); acquired immunity (Rh factor immunity; subgroup factor immunity); cold agglutinin reaction, as in paroxysmal cold hemoglobinuria; cold hemolysin reaction, as in luetic and nonluetic paroxysmal cold hemoglobinuria; autoimmunity, as in idiopathic acquired hemolytic anemia, secondary or symptomatic acquired hemolytic anemia secondary to leukemia, lymphoma, and disseminated lupus; favism; reaction to drugs such as Fuadin and quinine; and thrombotic thrombocytopenic purpura.
      b. Nonimmune mechanism (no antibody demonstrable) — e.g., infectious agents (RBC parasitism, as in malaria and Oroya fever; bacterial toxins or hemolysins, as in *Clostridium welchii,* hemolytic strep., and bacteroides infections); and chemicals toxic to normal cells (arsine, heavy metals such as lead, naphthalene, phenylhydrazine, oxidant compounds, surface active compounds, and intravenous water).
      c. Unknown mechanisms — e.g., splenomegalic patterns (cirrhoses, Gaucher's disease, splenic vein thrombosis, myeloid metaplasia, and

infection); acute and chronic infections; acute renal disease (hemolytic uremic syndrome); chronic renal disease; malignancy; chronic inflammatory disorders (rheumatic fever); infantile pyknocytosis; and acanthocytosis.

II. Decreased production of hemoglobin-erythrocyte mass (hypoactive bone marrow).

A. Anemia resulting from specific deficiency.

1. Vitamin B_{12} deficiency.

a. Defective diet (rare), low in animal or bacterial products.

b. Deficiency of intrinsic factors—as in pernicious anemia; or as in total and subtotal gastrectomy (associated with deficiency of absorption).

c. Defective absorption (intestinal disease)—as in sprue, regional enteritis, intestinal resection, and blind loop syndrome; or as in fish tapeworm (*Diphyllobothrium latum*) infestation.

d. Deranged metabolism—increased requirement due to thyrotoxicosis, pregnancy, or hemolytic anemias.

2. Folic acid abnormality.

a. Defective diet, low in vegetables and liver.

b. Defective absorption—as in sprue or steatorrhea, or as in intestinal resection and other short circuits of the gastrointestinal tract.

c. Defective utilization—as in scurvy or megaloblastic anemia of infancy; acute alcoholism or liver disease; or due to anticonvulsant drugs or folic acid antagonists.

d. Increased requirement (deranged metabolism)—as in

pregnancy, hemolytic anemia, and malignant neoplasia.

e. Etiology unknown—as in megaloblastic anemia of pregnancy (refractory), intestinal structures, and blind loop syndrome.

3. Vitamin C deficiency.

a. Induced deficiency of folic acid (vitamin C potentiates the hematologic effect of folic acid).

b. Pure dietary vitamin C deficiency(?).

4. Iron deficiency.

a. Increased loss of iron (blood loss).

b. Increased requirements, as in pregnancy or normal growth.

c. Decreased intake due to defective diet or chronic malabsorption.

5. Pyridoxine abnormality.

6. Crude liver factor abnormality.

7. Copper deficiency (?).

8. Protein deficiency or abnormality, as in kwashiorkor or pellagra.

B. Anemia resulting from endocrine abnormality—as in thyroid, pituitary, adrenal, and erythropoietin.

C. Anemia resulting from mechanical interference with marrow function.

1. Inadequate capacity, as in newborn or premature babies.

2. Myelophthisis, as in malignant neoplasia, myelofibrosis, osteopetrosis, and xanthomatosis such as in histiocytosis; and in miliary tuberculosis.

D. Anemia resulting from relative marrow failure, as in infection, renal disease, malignant neoplasia, toxic agents, liver disease, rheumatic fever and rheumatoid arthritis, collagen diseases, and endocrine disorders.

E. Anemia of bone marrow failure,

usually aplastic or hypoplastic—idiopathic more than 50 per cent of this subdivision; congenital or familial pancytopenia, usually in children, e.g., Fanconi syndrome; marrow failure associated with thymic tumors; sideroachrestic or refractory sideroblastic anemia; exposure to ionizing radiation and antimitotic agents; exposure to, or ingestion of, chemicals, such as gold, arsenic, and chloramphenicol, and antimetabolites.

The disadvantage of this etiologic classification is that there is no clear-cut pure subdivision as such—that is, defective erythropoiesis and hemolytic anemias may be concomitant in that the rate of erythrocytic production may be decidedly less than six or seven times the normal rate. Anemias associated with impaired erythrocyte production may be associated with excess hemolysis of erythrocytes. Iron deficiency anemias should include chronic blood loss and should not be classified separately.

MORPHOLOGIC CLASSIFICATION

I. Macrocytic normochromic anemia (MCV = 94 to 160 cu.μ; MCHC = 32 to 36 g./100 ml.)
   A. Bone marrow shows abnormal (megaloblastic) red blood cell maturation. Includes mainly deficiency of vitamin B_{12} or folic acid secondary to gastrointestinal abnormalities, gastrectomy, hepatic disease, or use of anticonvulsant drugs or antimetabolites.
   B. Bone marrow does not show megaloblastic changes, but usually shows normoblastic maturation. Includes chronic liver disease, hypothyroidism, normocytic anemias made temporarily macrocytic because of reticulocytosis, and myelophthisic anemias.
II. Normocytic normochromic anemia (MCV = 80 to 94 cu.μ; MCHC = 32 to 36 g./100 ml.).

A. Sudden blood loss.
B. Hemolytic anemias.
C. Most of the anemias caused principally by impaired production (except deficiencies of vitamin B_{12}, folic acid, and iron); hemoglobinopathies.
III. Microcytic normochromic anemia (MCV = 60 to 80 cu.μ; MCHC = 32 to 36 g./100 ml.).
   A. Atypical "imperfect" blood formation—for example, subacute and chronic inflammatory conditions, toxic drugs and chemicals, malignancy, some endocrine disorders, and splenomegalic extracorpuscular abnormalities.
IV. Microcytic hypochromic anemia (MCV = 60 to 80 cu.μ; MCHC = 20 to 30 g./100 ml.).
   A. Iron deficiency anemia due to blood loss, gastrointestinal absorption difficulties, or excess demand.
   B. Miscellaneous causes, including lead poisoning, thalassemia syndrome, pyridoxine-responsive anemia, or idiopathic hypersideremic anemias.

In the morphologic classification of anemias, if the MCV and MCHC are accurate, the specific diagnosis is almost made, and a preliminary guide to treatment, such as administration of vitamin B_{12}, folic acid, iron, or steroids, and splenectomy is given. Disadvantages are that if the MCV and MCHC are not accurate, then diagnosis and therapy are inaccurate and erroneously carried out. Therefore, a compromise with a simple approach, such as that described in the following section, would be most practical.

PHYSIOLOGIC CLASSIFICATION

Expressed in physiologic terms, anemia can be considered as a reduction in hemoglobin concentration, with its concomitant diminution in the oxygen-carrying capacity of the blood. In terms of plasma volume and red cell mass, anemia may be either dilutional, with associated normal total red cell mass and increased plasma volume (e.g., occasional patients with marked splenomegaly or dysproteinemias) or dehydration-related, with reduced plasma volume masking a true diminution in red cell mass. It is not until the hemoglobin level is much below 10 g. per dl. that symptoms of anemia become apparent. However, a normal hemoglobin concentration may be associated with tissue hypoxia in methemoglobinemia and carbon monoxide poisoning; this is partially related to the left shift of the oxygen dissociation curve, revealing increased oxygen affinity for hemoglobin and leading to impaired oxygen release in the tissue capillaries. An example of this occurs in cigarette smokers with slightly elevated carboxyhemoglobin, who develop angina or secondary polycythemia. In contrast, a decreased affinity for oxygen as mirrored by a right shift of the oxygen dissociation curve is seen in anemic patients. By acting as a compensatory mechanism, this shift enhances delivery of oxygen to tissues. This is brought about largely by a glycolysis intermediate product, 2,3-diphosphoglycerate (2,3-DPG), which combines reversibly with the deoxygenated hemoglobin tetramer, stabilizing it in a configuration having low oxygen affinity. This 2, 3-DPG oxygen affinity effect provides increased oxygen release from hemoglobin in tissue capillaries, while at the same time maintaining essentially normal oxygen uptake by hemoglobin in pulmonary capillaries. Therefore, in most chronic anemias and cardiopulmonary diseases with reduced arterial P_{O_2}, the 2, 3-DPG levels in RBCs are increased and correlate inversely with hemoglobin levels. This is at best a dubious advantage since it may lead to greater desaturation of arterial blood.

The RBC 2, 3-DPG is reduced in acidosis, but it is offset by increased oxygen dissociation with decreased pH (Bohr effect), and oxygen affinity remains within normal limits. Alkali therapy may lead to accelerated increases in pH with temporary shifting of the oxygen dissociation curve to the left. Until the 2, 3-DPG levels return to normal, the oxygen affinity may be very high. The 2, 3-DPG levels of acid-citrate dextrose stored bank blood falls; therefore, fresh blood with normal 2, 3-DPG levels and optimal oxygen delivery may be preferable when massive transfusions are required. However, the usual anticoagulant-blood preservative in use today is CPD (citrate phosphate dextrose), and it maintains normal 2, 3-DPG levels for a 7-day period. Since transfused RBCs in this milieu regenerate to normal 2, 3-DPG levels within 12 to 24 hours, fresh blood is rarely needed.

Through increased cardiac output and redistribution of blood flow to essential organs, the cardiovascular system provides major compensatory mechanisms for anemia. When the hemoglobin level is above 8 g. per dl., cardiac output is normal when the patient is at rest. However when the anemic patient exercises, disproportionate increases in cardiac output occur. Severely anemic patients frequently manifest hyperventilation without much benefit from increased oxygenation. In fact, oxygen release in tissues may occur when respiratory alkalosis causes a shift of the oxygen dissociation curve to the left. If blood transfusions are used in the therapy of severe anemia, the sudden expansion of blood volume may induce pulmonary edema. Therefore, patients with rising venous pressures and questionable cardiac decompensation should have blood transfusions discontinued. In severely anemic cardiac patients, phlebotomy and infusion of packed RBCs can be carried out concomitantly to elevate the hematocrit level without changing the blood volume.

It is necessary to evaluate each anemic patient individually in order to determine whether the etiology of the anemia is blood loss, impaired production of hemoglobin and erythrocytes, or excessive RBC destruction. Impaired erythrocyte production is associated with marrow hypoplasia and a reduced reticulocyte count. Morphologic changes such as fragmented RBCs and spherocytes suggest erythrocytic membrane damage, and when such changes are accompanied by reticulocytosis and marrow erythroid hyperplasia, they indicate compensatory stimulation of RBC production by erythropoietin. RBC life span data may be provided by ^{51}Cr red cell survival studies and hemoglobin synthesis information provided by ^{59}Fe clearance studies to determine plasma iron transport rate.

ANEMIAS DUE TO BLOOD LOSS

Acute posthemorrhagic anemia usually signifies the sudden, rapid loss of large amounts of blood over a short period secondary to perforated peptic ulcer or ectopic pregnancy, or following an internal injury or external laceration. It may also follow ulcerative enterocolitis of various causes, or may accompany the thrombocytopenic diseases (thrombocytopenic purpura, aplastic anemia, or leukemia), hemophilia, and other coagulation defects with or without abnormal blood vessels.

The blood film reveals a normocytic, normochromic pattern with an MCV of 80 to 94 cu.μ and an MCHC of 32 to 36 g. per 100 ml. unless hemorrhage has been marked. There is an associated erythroid hyperplasia in the bone marrow and slight macrocytosis (MCV up to 105 cu.μ) during the fifth to tenth day after hemorrhage with a concomitant period of reticulocytosis. If the blood film is hypochromic, the possibility of previous hemorrhagic exacerbations must be considered. Normoblasts and polychromatophilia appear for 2 to 3 days if severe hemorrhage has occurred.

Red blood cell, hemoglobin, and hematocrit values are at first high due to vasoconstriction and then subnormal for 2 to 3 days due to hemodilution. The white blood cell count ranges from 10,200 to 20,000 (mostly polymorphonuclear leukocytes) with a shift to left (in 2 to 5 hours) in the myeloid series with an occasional meta-myelocyte or myeloblast. The leukocyte count returns to normal in 3 to 4 days. Reticulocytosis occurs 24 to 48 hours later with 5 to 15 per cent values occurring 4 to 7 days after hemorrhage with an occasional normoblast. Platelets are increased and represent the earliest effect, occurring 1 hour after the onset of bleeding, with thrombocytosis up to 1,000,000 per cu.mm. and simultaneous shortening of coagulation time. The serum iron shows a gradual reduction to 60 to 80 μg. per 100 ml. If bleeding into the lumen of the gastrointestinal tract occurs, the BUN rises. If blood passes into body cavities or cysts, the absorbed hemoglobin breakdown product (bilirubin) causes an elevated indirect reaction of serum bilirubin with associated jaundice if sufficiently elevated. Regeneration resulting in a return to normal red blood cell and hematocrit values occurs in 4 to 6 weeks if there is no further bleeding; all other blood values also return to normal (reticulocytosis and leukocytosis persist if bleeding continues).

In *chronic posthemorrhagic anemia,* the blood picture and symptoms are those of iron deficiency anemia described in the following section (Plates 11, 12).

ANEMIAS DUE TO ABNORMAL ERYTHROCYTE PRODUCTION

Iron-deficiency Anemias

Chronic blood loss in adults and rapid growth with inadequate dietary intake in children are the most common causes of hypochromic microcytic anemias associated with iron deficiency (Plates 11, 12). Although different forms vary markedly in the percentages of iron absorbed (dietary phosphates, cereal phytates, and antacid preparations inhibit absorption) iron malabsorption is rarely a major factor. For example, the iron content of meat foods is well absorbed as intact heme, which subsequently appears in the plasma as the ferric ion. Ferritin and hemosiderin (representing reserves of 500–1000 mg. of iron) are present in the reticuloendothelial cells of normal iron-depleted adults. However, a large percentage of females of child-bearing age without anemia may reveal depletion of their iron stores. This is attributed to the excessive blood losses associated with menstruation and pregnancy (see below). In these patients and others with history of chronic bleeding, the mobilization of storage iron precedes development of anemia. After this storage iron is exhausted, the serum iron concentration falls, and the iron-binding capacity (transferrin) increases. Low serum iron is also associated with infectious and inflammatory states. The absence of stainable iron in marrow aspirates and reduced serum ferritin, revealed by radioimmunoassay, are two excellent indicators of iron depleted stores.

A discussion of iron metabolism is helpful in understanding the etiology of iron-deficiency anemias.[103] There are about 4 to 5 g. of iron in the normal adult (70% hemoglobin, 5% myoglobin, 25% in storage depots, and less than 1% in enzymes). The absorption of iron is mainly in the ferrous state; ferric food iron complexes are broken down to ionized ferric iron in the stomach and these ferric ions (Fe^{+++}) are reduced to ferrous ions (Fe^{+}) by ascorbic acid, cysteine, and the -SH groups of proteins in foods. Hydrochloric acid is not essential but helpful. The absorption of ferrous free ions or chelated iron occurs mostly in the duodenum, less in the jejunum, to a small degree in the ileum, and in insignificant amounts from the stomach and colon. The mechanism of absorption is unknown; it is doubtful that the classic ferritin transport mechanism is involved. Furthermore, the control of iron absorption is unknown; the mucosal block mechanism plays a minor role. There is only 5 to 10 per cent absorption of the 12 to 18 mg. intake of iron per day in the average American diet—that is, 0.6 to 1.8 mg. per day is absorbed. In hypochromic anemia, the absorption of dietary iron is greater, but rarely exceeds 20 per cent.

Iron circulates in the plasma in the ferric state bound to β_1 globulin, transferrin, or siderophilin. Transferrin is normally only one-third saturated with iron, and the major target for iron transport is the bone marrow. Release of transferrin-bound iron to red blood cell precursors is an energy-requiring reaction and is unrelated to heme synthesis. The major form of ferric iron (Fe^{+++}) utilization is in combination with protoporphyrin to form heme, which in turn combines with globin to form hemoglobin. Other increments of ferric iron go to enzymes, myoglobin, and storage depots. Utilization of ferric iron is measured by (1) the plasma iron clearance test, in which there is a normal T/2 clearance of 60 to 120 minutes with more rapid clearance seen in increased erythropoiesis and slower clearance in decreased erythropoiesis; and by (2) the radioiron utilization test for hemoglobin formation. Normally, there is less than 75 per cent utilization in 2 weeks. There is greater and more rapid utilization in iron-deficiency anemia and decreased utilization in hypoplastic anemia. Twenty to 25 mg. of iron is utilized to provide the iron in hemoglobin of new red blood cells formed each day. Because absorption provides only 1 mg. of iron each day, the rest (19 to 24 mg.) comes from the reutilization of iron from hemoglobin breakdown or iron stores.

As far as iron storage is concerned, 1 to 1.5 gm. of iron is stored in the normal adult, mostly as ferritin in the liver, spleen, and bone marrow. Ferritin is a combination of a protein (apoferritin) and ferric hydroxide units of up to 23 per cent by weight. It has a typical elution photomicrograph appearance but does not stain with Prussian blue. Hemosiderin, composed of up to 35 per cent iron, is the main storage form in situations of excess iron loads. It has an apoferritin matrix and may be stained blue. Both forms of storage iron are mobilizable for hemoglobin synthesis, and they are completely depleted before hypochromic anemia ensues (Fig. 8-3).

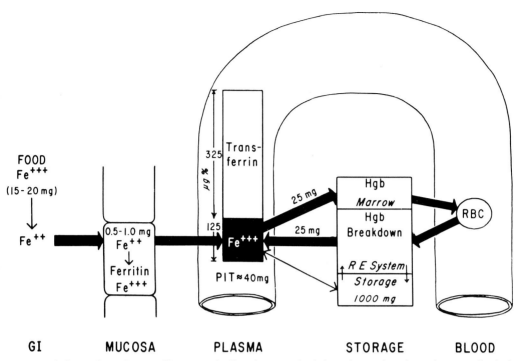

GI   MUCOSA   PLASMA   STORAGE   BLOOD

Fig. 8-3. Schematic pathway of iron metabolism in normal adults. Plasma iron bound to transferrin is the center of activity. Iron released from hemoglobin breakdown is the major source with smaller contributions from the gastrointestinal tract and storage areas. The major pathway of iron is from transferrin to immature red blood cells. With ineffective erythropoiesis, iron is diverted to the liver. (Walsh, J. R., and Mass, R. E.: Hypersiderosis. Resident Physician, *14:*53, 1968)

Recent studies have revealed that serum ferritin values (normal range, 40–70 mg./ ml.; utilizing RIA techniques*) may be used as an index of iron stores. When serum and bone marrow ferritin determinations were made at the time of bone marrow aspiration, a positive correlation was found between serum ferritin levels and bone marrow iron stores, as well as between bone marrow ferritin levels and iron stores. In fact, serum ferritin determinations appear to give an accurate estimation of bone marrow iron stores available for hemoglobin synthesis, thereby providing a reliable guide for iron replacement therapy and reducing the need for repeated bone marrow aspirations. Serum ferritin levels of less than 105 mg. per ml. (20–25 ng./ml.) suggest decreased iron stores, with or without excessive blood loss, and values greater than 120 mg. per ml. indicate adequate or increased iron stores. Preliminary data also suggest that bone marrow ferritin determinations may be useful in quantitating bone marrow iron stores.[101] A patient with a low serum ferritin will have a reticulocyte response when given iron in therapeutic doses—unless there is an additional cause for his anemia.

It is also probable that serum ferritin has a role in the rapid transport of iron originating from destroyed red cells in the reticuloendothelial system (i.e., plasma ferritin releases its iron to hepatocytes, from

* Ramco Laboratories Reaction Kit for Fer-Iron (Serum Ferritin-RIA Test), 3701 Kirby Drive, Suite 490, Houston, Texas 77098.

where it may enter the transferrin pool in the plasma). There is apparently no direct iron exchange between transferrin and ferritin.[138]

Ferritin has a molecular weight of approximately 450,000 daltons, and each molecule of ferritin may accumulate up to about 4,000 atoms of iron. The fully saturated protein consists of over 20 per cent of iron by weight. Ferritin synthesis is induced by iron in almost all tissues. Furthermore, ferritin appears to be a major form in which iron is taken into cells to provide the substrate for the manufacture of hemoglobin. However, not all iron-deficiency states lead to very low levels of serum ferritin (e.g., in some patients with chronic diseases, such as rheumatoid arthritis or neoplasia, iron may be absent from the marrow, but serum ferritin levels will be at the low limit of normal (40–70 ng./ml.).

In iron excretion, the body firmly conserves iron, but does lose it sparingly in the form of cell desquamation from the skin, gastrointestinal tract, genitourinary tract, and in sweat fluid, urine, bile, and other intestinal juices. Blood loss from any source adds to iron excretion loss. The daily excretion value for growing children is approximately 0.6 mg. per day; adult men and postmenopausal women excrete 0.5 to 1.0 mg. per day; menstruating women, 1 to 2 mg. per day. From this it can be seen that menstruating women are in precarious iron balance with absorption barely meeting excretion.

Iron-deficiency anemias due to increased requirements of iron include the following: (1) Menorrhagia is the most common cause, often unrecognized. Normal menstrual blood loss is 35 to 70 ml. per menstrual period. The blood loss can be approximately quantitated by the number and saturation of pads; up to 30 ml. of blood can be absorbed by a pad without soaking through with menorrhagia itself produced when a patient must wear two pads at a time. (2) Anemia can result from repeated pregnancies, which cause a net loss of 300 to 500 mg. iron per pregnancy. Recent experimental clinical data indicate the existence of an anemia of pregnancy characterized by decreased erythropoiesis and normal red cell survival. The decreased urinary erythropoietin levels noted in these patients suggest a possible mechanism for this anemia.[75] (3) Anemia may be caused by frequent blood donations; a donation of 3 pints per year triples the amount of iron that must be absorbed. A similar pattern may be observed in nosocomial anemia. Most adults who are hospitalized 3 to 4 weeks will probably have 500 to 1,000 ml. of blood withdrawn for diagnostic studies, which represent 10 to 20 per cent of their blood volumes. Patients with complex problems who require frequent blood-gas determinations and repeated blood cultures will have much greater blood losses. Thus, it is believed that the use of microtechniques and the elimination of unnecessary studies can reduce the amount of blood loss.[39] (4) Anemia can be caused by hemorrhage—usually from the gastrointestinal tract. Roughly 50 mg. of iron is lost per 100 ml. of blood. Bleeding may be intermittent and may be so little as to be difficult to detect. However, loss of as little blood as 2 ml. per day doubles the amount of iron that must be absorbed to maintain balance. As much as 30 ml. of blood can be lost into the upper gastrointestinal tract without producing a positive stool guaiac reaction.

Iron-deficiency anemias that are associated with a decreased assimilation of iron or a combination of both decreased ingestion and assimilation include the following: (1) Anemia of this sort may be caused by deficient diets—high in cereal content, low in animal protein (kwashiorkor), low in green vegetables, and low in vitamin C, pyridoxine, and possibly copper. At times iron deficiency is accompanied by general complaints that exceed those ordinarily attributable to the degree of anemia. Some experiments have shown lowered activity of heme-containing enzymes in various tissues in iron-deficient animals. Noyes and Green have demonstrated restriction of respiration in the mitochondria of the liver and kidney of iron-deficient rats.[111] Because these organs are vitally dependent on aerobic metabolism, Noyes and Green believe that iron deficiency may be considered a disease of the mitochondria, as well as of the erythron. (2) Anemia may result from defective absorption, such as that found in steatorrhea, hypermotility secondary to diarrhea with resultant inadequate absorption time through the gastrointestinal mucosa, and after either total or partial gastrectomy, in which there is poor iron absorption, associated with meals, that persists as iron deficiency develops.

Poor diet or poor absorption does not cause iron deficiency unless there is growth, repeated pregnancies or blood loss, because normal iron stores and limited iron excretion normally afford protection unless the dietary and absorptive difficulties continue for many years. Therefore, blood loss is usually the cause of iron deficiency anemia in an adult male or a postmenopausal female until malignant neoplasia, infection, or other causes can be proven. However, infants born to iron-deficient mothers and premature infants may be anemic. According to Andelman and Sered, failure to provide exogenous iron in infancy (12 mg. of iron/quart of milk formula) predisposes the preschool child to a poor nutritional status and also to increased morbidity from infection.[4]

To be specific, the risk of iron deficiency is greatest after neonatal iron stores have been depleted and while body growth remains rapid. Recently developed laboratory methods have made it possible to estimate the timing and dose of supplemental iron that is necessary to prevent iron deficiency with greater reliability than ever before. The assay of serum ferritin has been of greatest help, for it reflects differences in iron stores within the physiologic range as well as in states of depletion and overload. Furthermore, the detection of mild iron deficiency has been facilitated by the recognition of normal developmental changes in mean corpuscular red cell volume, serum iron, and transferrin saturation, in addition to the well-known changes in hemoglobin concentration.

In the preterm infant there is virtually no risk of iron-deficiency anemia or even depletion of iron stores during the first 2 months of life. However, after 2 months of age iron stores drop very rapidly, and by 3 months iron-deficiency anemia may be present in infants who have not received iron supplementation. Initiation of supplemental iron (as ferrous sulfate) in a dose of 2 mg. per kg. per day between 2 weeks and 2 months of age in the form of drops or fortified formula should be effective in preventing iron deficiency. Serum ferritin values indicate that a lower dose would not reliably prevent iron-deficiency anemia, and higher doses should be avoided because of the effect of iron on a vitamin E deficiency that can result in hemolytic anemia.

Term infants are most likely to deplete their iron stores after 4 to 6 months of age. However, the maintenance of breast feeding for 5 or more months allows infants to retain larger iron stores at 6 months of age than those fed cows' milk formulas. This protective effect is attributable primarily to the unusually high bioavailability of the relatively small amount of iron in breast milk. Infants absorb about half of this iron or about four times as much as is absorbed from unfortified cows' milk or cows' milk formulas, even though all of these contain similar amounts of iron. Formula-fed infants require supplemental iron after about 4 months of age in the form either of iron-supplemented formula or iron-fortified dry infant cereal.

The extent to which the prevention of iron deficiency has been successful should be monitored by screening for anemia and microcytosis. This is conveniently done between 6 and 9 months in preterm infants and at 1 year of age in term infants.

Diagnosis. Symptoms of anemia include weakness; fatigability; pallor of skin, mucous membranes, and nailbeds; dyspnea on exertion; palpitation, headache, and excessive fatigue.

As iron deficiency develops, there is a decrease in hemoglobin leading to a loss of hemosiderin, an increase in the iron-binding capacity (transferrin), a decrease in serum iron resulting in hypochromia of red blood cells. Manifestations other than those due to anemia also develop—for example, glossitis, stomatitis, dysphagia (Plummer-Vinson syndrome with a weblike structure just below the level of the cricoid cartilage in the esophagus), hypochlorhydria to achlorhydria (in 80% of cases), atrophy of the gastric mucosa with slight gastritis, numbness of the hands and feet, splenomegaly, pearly white sclerae, koilonychia, and occasionally vitiligo, slight dilation of the heart with functional murmurs, slight edema due to hepatomegaly, and a possible deficiency of iron-containing enzymes (cytochromes).

Iron-deficient erythropoiesis is defined as a state in which the supply of iron is inadequate to support optimal erythropoiesis in the developing red cell mass.[52] This may result from depletion of total body iron or from an inadequate supply of plasma iron, which may be due either to a block in the discharge of iron from the reticuloendothelial cell or to the absence of circulating transferrin. The best indication of iron-deficient erythropoiesis in this sense is the percentage of saturation of transferrin (iron-binding capacity). A discrepancy in the sideroblast count from that predicted by the iron supply is a sensitive indication of a block in hemoglobin synthesis.

The laboratory diagnosis of iron-deficiency anemias can be summarized as follows: The blood film shows hypochromia and microcytosis with occasional target cells. The red blood cell count is usually 3,000,000 to 4,000,000 per cu.mm. (may be 5,000,000). The hemoglobin is usually 6 to 10 g. per 100 ml. The Wintrobe constants (blood indices) show an MCV of less than 80 cu.μ, an MCH of 27 $\mu\mu$g., and an MCHC of less than 32 per cent. The leukocyte count is normal or slightly less than normal. The platelet count is usually normal; however, thrombocytosis frequently occurs.[133] Osmotic fragility is normal or decreased.

The serum iron in iron-deficiency anemia is low—less than 60 μg. per 100 ml. The normal value in males is 70 to 200 μg. per 100 ml. and in females is 60 to 160 μg. per 100 ml. In the test, the serum iron is reduced with sodium sulfite and is complexed with buffered 2-2[1] dipyridyl reagent. The resulting pink color is measured after the proteins have been precipitated by heat. Total iron-binding capacity (transferrin) is high—350 μg. per 100 ml. The normal value in both males and females 250 to 400 μg. per 100 ml. In the iron-binding capacity test, ferric iron solution is added to the serum. On shaking with magnesium carbonate, any excess iron not bound to transferrin is absorbed. After centrifuging, an iron determination is carried out on the serum with its iron-saturated transferrin.

The bone marrow pattern in iron-deficiency anemia shows an absence of hemosiderin. The quantitative marrow hemosiderin concentration and the circulating hemoglobin level are the best criteria for determining total body iron. However, the marrow hemosiderin concentration in itself does not indicate the adequacy of iron supply to the marrow. When visualized in the marrow, hemosiderin is bluish due to iron deposits in the reticuloendothelial cell when it is stained with Prussian blue stain, and it appears as brownish iron deposits when stained with the Giemsa stain. Cytologically, bone marrow shows normal or nonspecific normoblastic hyperplasia with the smaller normoblasts having a deficiency of hemoglobin, an irregular shape, and frayed margins. Examination of gastric contents reveals an inconstant histamine-fast achlorhydria (Plates 11, 12).

A new technique measuring the serum ferritin concentration by means of radioimmunoassay has been made available.* This assay gives a quantitative estimate of the amount of iron stores in the body. If it can be shown that it reproduces the results obtained by bone marrow hemosiderin studies, it may prove to be a quick time-saving approach to the quantitative estimation of body iron stores, a superior substitute for serum iron and iron binding capacity studies, and an excellent approach to the identification of iron deficiency in patients on hemodialysis.

Testing for the survival time of red blood cells in iron-deficiency anemia (usually normal), one may use the radioactive ^{51}Cr technique, in which a sample of red blood cells is tagged with ^{51}Cr ($Na_2^{51}CrO4$). The blood is readministered, and the radioactivity is measured on the subsequent withdrawal of the blood. One can also measure the radioactivity that will be found in the feces, if the blood is oozing from a gastrointestinal lesion that may be a source of blood loss. The same technique may also be used to provide a quantitative measure of menstrual loss. The half-life of ^{51}Cr is normally 30 days in this method. As mentioned before, the half-life is normal in this symptom complex. In iron-deficiency anemia the plasma ^{59}Fe clearance is increased — the half-life is less than 1 hour. The serum copper is also elevated (normal level is 68–134 μ g./100 ml.).

In the differential diagnosis of iron-deficiency anemias, only three other types of hypochromic microcytic anemias need be considered: (1) Thalassemia — associated with hepatosplenomegaly, skeletal changes, the presence of many target cells and nucleated red blood cells, elevated bilirubin, elevated serum iron, stainable hemosiderin in bone marrow, increased hemoglobin A_2 and HbgF (fetal), and failure to respond to iron treatment (see p. 225 for further discussion). (2) Pyridoxine-respon-

sive anemias — bone marrow deposits of iron characterize marked hemosiderosis, serum iron is high, and the tryptophan-loading test shows abnormal results. The symptom complex, which responds only to pyridoxine, is also called secondary sideroachrestic anemia or refractory sideroblastic anemia. In addition, those patients with partial or refractory responsiveness to pyridoxine appear to react to a degree to the administration of L-tryptophan.[53] (3) Hereditary hypochromic anemia (also called essential sideroachrestic anemia) consists of a group of anemias in which all or probably part of the same process is involved. One type occurs only in males, and is characterized by marked splenomegaly, normal or high serum iron, and a lack of response to iron treatment. It is also called hereditary iron-loading anemia. Another type is called sideroachrestic anemia characterized by marked hepatosplenomegaly, high serum iron, increased marrow and tissue hemosiderin, and sideroblasts in the bone marrow. Etiologically, the primary defect in hemoglobin synthesis in congenital or acquired sideroblastic anemia is a defect in the heme synthetic pathway, but a nonspecific effect on exogenous hemoglobin synthesis has not been excluded.[155]

Treatment and Response. Two basic concepts in the treatment of iron-deficiency anemia are: the correction of hemoglobin and tissue iron deficiency, and the recognition and correction of the cause of anemia (probably the most important aspect to investigate). Thus, positive results of a fecal guaiac test may indicate the presence of peptic ulcer, hiatus hernia, esophageal varices, gastrointestinal neoplasm, or any other type of neoplasm or parasites in the stools. Therapy consists of exsiccated ($FeSO_4)_2 \cdot 3H_2O$ administered as 0.2 g. tablets four times a day (after meals and at bedtime). Ferrous gluconate may also be given as 0.6 g. tablets four times a day. There is no need for a complex sustained-release preparation or for mixtures with vitamin B_{12}. Either of these two iron prepa-

---

* Ramco Laboratories Reaction Kit for Fer-Iron (Serum Ferritin-RIA Test), 3701 Kirby Drive, Suite 490, Houston, Texas 77098.

rations is usually given with or after meals to minimize gastrointestinal irritation, and the dosage is gradually increased over a 3-day period. Since the absorption of iron occurs selectively with low pH concentration in the proximal part of the small intestines, the use of slow release or enteric control forms may not be effective.

The treatment is continued for at least 2 or 3 months. It is advisable to begin treatment with ferrous sulfate by giving a single dose after the largest meal for a day or two before increasing the daily amount. If the amount given is not well tolerated, it can be reduced to a comfortable level because once the regimen is begun, there is rarely much urgency about completing the restoration of the hemoglobin level. Parenteral iron therapy is rarely needed and usually results in no more rapid recovery from iron-deficiency anemia than if oral preparations are given.[93] A sense of well-being results within 48 to 72 hours after initial therapy, and reticulocytes begin to increase in 5 to 7 days with a peak occurring in 10 to 14 days, returning to normal in 3 weeks. The hemoglobin level begins to increase in 7 to 10 days and continues to increase at the rate of 0.1 to 0.2 g. per 100 ml. per day if the initial hemoglobin is greater than 7.5 g. per 100 ml.; it increases at a rate of 0.2 to 0.3 g. per 100 ml. per day if the initial hemoglobin is less than 7.5 g. per 100 ml. It takes 1 to 2 months for the hemoglobin to return to normal.

Reasons for the failure of iron-deficiency anemia to respond to oral iron are incorrect diagnosis, blood loss is greater than hemoglobin regeneration, failure of the patient to take iron, defective iron absorption, or superimposed infection, inflammation, uremia, or malignant neoplasia depressing iron utilization.

Indications for parenteral iron treatment include inability of patient to tolerate or unwillingness to take oral iron, failure to absorb iron due to regional enteritis, bowel resection, or malabsorption states, and in a patient at the end of pregnancy when iron is to be administered rapidly. In the last instance, an iron-dextran dosage must be given calculated as follows: grams of iron required equals normal hemoglobin in grams less the patient's hemoglobin in grams times 0.255. This formula is infrequently used because it is rarely necessary to give parenteral iron. Also, because of the high cost of parenteral iron, discomfort, toxic reaction in patients, and the possible carcinogenic effects, parenteral iron is rarely prescribed.

ANEMIAS DUE TO DEFICIENCY OF HEMATOPOIETIC FACTORS

Anemias due to deficiencies of hematopoietic factors include those characterized by a slowly progressive macrocytic anemia, leukopenia, and thrombocytopenia; megaloblastic bone marrow patterns; frequent association of oral, gastrointestinal, or neurologic damage; and in most cases hematologic changes following therapy with vitamin B_{12} or folic acid.

Vitamin B_{12} Deficiency

The causes of vitamin B_{12} deficiency (pernicious anemia or P.A.) are listed on page 186 (Plates 13,14,15). An understanding of the causes of B_{12} deficiency is facilitated when one appreciates that B_{12} is a cobalt-containing tetrapyrrole, reddish in color, and is found in meat products from animals that ingest certain bacteria, which in turn synthesize the vitamin. In order for vitamin B_{12} to be absorbed from the diet (extrinsic factor), it must combine with a mucoid substance (intrinsic factor) secreted by the mucosal cells of the gastric fundus. Intrinsic factor is a thermolabile glycoprotein of approximately 50,000 molecular weight that binds strongly to ingested vitamin B_{12}, facilitating its absorption by the ileal mucosal cell receptors. When an excess of vitamin B_{12} is ingested, only a small portion is absorbed if intrinsic factor is absent. From the intestinal wall, vitamin B_{12} goes through the blood in combination with certain proteins and is deposited for the most part in the liver (1 μg. of vitamin B_{12}/g. of liver). It then is released from the liver and is utilized by growing cells in a coenzyme system of nucleoprotein synthesis in bone marrow and other tissues. The average daily adult vitamin B_{12} requirement is approximately 1 μg. with a large reservoir in the liver. It therefore takes a long time for vitamin B_{12} deficiency to manifest itself.

It has been suggested that immunologic processes may cause the atrophy of gastric mucosa frequently observed in patients with pernicious anemia.[145] Circulating antibodies that react with gastric parietal cytoplasm microsomes and later with intrinsic factor have been found in up to 57 per cent and 87 per cent of cases in two series studied.[132] In fact, it has been suggested that several distinct antibodies to gastric juice may be found in the sera of some patients having pernicious anemia. In this respect, pernicious anemia is similar to other autoimmune disorders manifesting several antibody expressions.

Furthermore, there appears to be a high incidence of adult pernicious anemia in association with chronic thyroiditis and myxedema in which autoimmune phenomena have been described and in which thyroid tissue reaction is characterized by marked lymphocytic infiltration, which is also a microscopic characteristic associated with gastric mucosal atrophy of pernicious anemia.[147] Whether autoimmunity is of basic importance in the pathogenesis of atrophic gastritis remains unproved except for strong circumstantial evidence indicating this to be true.[59]

Recent work has shown that all but one of 25 patients with pernicious anemia had an autoimmune process against gastric intrinsic factor, and tests for cell-mediated immunity were positive in 86 per cent of patients. Therefore, this disease complex appears to be a uniform disorder, resulting in all cases from the action of intrinsic factor antibodies either to neutralize intrinsic factor or to suppress its production, and

cell-mediated immunity appears to be at least as important as humoral antibody.[19]

Although attempts to demonstrate intrinsic factor antibodies by immunofluorescence have been unsuccessful, antibodies to gastric parietal cells have been readily shown in a high percentage of pernicious anemia patients.[145] The antigen is found only in the parietal cell cytoplasm of the gastric mucosa, and the parietal cell antibody reacts only with this component.

Because antibody is also found in a high percentage of patients with atrophic gastritis,[2] who may or may not have pernicious anemia, it appears that the frequency of antibody in pernicious anemia is simply a reflection of atrophic gastritis. It is suggested therefore that the parietal-cell immunofluorescent test may prove to be of value as a screening procedure to detect cases of chronic atrophic gastritis at an early asymptomatic stage. It may then be followed up for the development of intrinsic factor deficiency and carcinoma; it is not specific for pernicious anemia.[10] This evidence, however, does not exclude the alternate possibility that immunologic mechanisms play no etiologic part in pernicious anemia and that the circulating antibodies are secondary to injury to the gastric mucosa.

More recent work, however, appears to substantiate the concept that antibody formation is a major etiologic factor in the development of pernicious anemia. Schade and co-workers reported a case of pernicious anemia in which there was an inhibitor of intrinsic factor in the gastric juice.[130] They demonstrated the presence of "precipitating antibody" to intrinsic factor in the gastric juice, and they suggested that such an antibody is the inhibitor that produces vitamin B_{12} malabsorption. An editorial[36] in the same publication raised the possibility that the previously reported intrinsic factor in a case studied by Li and colleagues[88] was in fact the same "precipitable antibody" to intrinsic factor. Li and colleagues[87] then obtained gastric juice from this original patient and found that it did indeed contain measurable amounts of "precipitable antibody" to the intrinsic factor. A report by Carmel and Herbert shows that such an antibody is present in the gastric juice of more than half of all patients with pernicious anemia.[15] These findings support the concept that a vicious circle may be set up in developing pernicious anemia in which "precipitable antibody" further reduces the low residual level of functional intrinsic factor in the gastric secretion, thereby accelerating the development of vitamin B_{12} deficiency.

Li and co-workers mention that they have studied nine patients with coexistent pernicious anemia and vitamin B_{12} malabsorption, and that all nine had "precipitable antibody" in the gastric juice.[87] They believe this lends further support to the concept that such an antibody may have a significant role in the accelerated development of vitamin B_{12} deficiency. Still further support of this concept is their finding that the saliva of some patients with pernicious anemia contains antibody to intrinsic factor precipitable with anti-IGA (immunoglobulin A).

In fact, pernicious anemia shares with other autoimmune diseases several empirical criteria. It is twice as common in women as in men; its frequency increases with age; it is associated with lymphocytic infiltrations at the target organ (the gastric mucosa); it responds occasionally to corticosteroid and other immunosuppressive drugs; it is frequently associated with multiple autoantibodies; and there appears to be a genetic predisposition that is likely to be expressed as an increased frequency of certain antigens of the histocompatibility system of lymphocytes.[19]

Other interesting phenomena associated with pernicious anemia are chromosomal abnormalities-that is, breaks in chromosomes, large swollen chromosomes, and chromosomal deletions with C-21 monosomy in a third of the pernicious anemia cases (such as the Philadelphia chromosome). These chromosome variations disappeared in many of the pernicious anemia cases after treatment.[74] Finally, in 32 patients with preexisting pernicious anemia, gastric carcinoma occurred, twice as frequently in patients having group A blood as in those having group O blood.[50, 55]

Folic Acid Deficiency

Folic acid deficiency (malabsorption syndromes such as sprue) is usually due to the causes listed on page 186 (Plate 16). An understanding of the causes of folic acid deficiency is facilitated when one appreciates that pteroylglutamic acid (PGA), another name for folic acid, occurs in vegetables, is synthesized by bacteria, and is found in the liver. Approximately 1 to 1.5 mg. of folic acid is found in the normal diet; a large amount is destroyed in the cooking process. Folic acid is absorbed in the small intestine, after which it is reduced by liver enzymes to tetrahydrofolic acid. Metabolites include folinic acid, or citrovorum factor. Folic acid and its metabolites appear to act as carbon-transfer agents and as coenzymes in the biosynthesis of nucleoprotein including deoxyribonucleic acid in bone marrow and other tissues. Vitamin E deficiency may also lead to altered nucleic acid metabolism. Because the body does not store folic acid in large amounts or in a stable form, deficiency may occur within 2 to 3 months after a dietary deficiency. Therefore, folic acid deficiency is found in malnourished patients, and because of its rapid turnover in disease complexes, it is associated with gastrointestinal mucosal absorption problems.

Folic acid deficiency may also occur occasionally in the last trimester of pregnancy because of increased requirements associated with an altered metabolism. Patients with cirrhosis of the liver develop folic acid deficiency owing to deficient dietary intake, as well as to improper liver conversion of folic acid to its active metabolites. These same patients (with or without cirrhosis) may also develop problems in thrombokinetics. Folate deficiency may be associated with ineffective thrombopoiesis, defined by an increased platelet-producing capacity of the marrow, without a parallel increase in platelet turnover.[27] In addition, alcohol imbibition affects the platelet economy by depressing megakaryocytopoiesis and decreasing platelet life span, more frequently without than with evidence of increased splenic pooling. Certain drugs, called folic acid antagonists, inhibit the reduction of folic acid by certain enzymes, leading to premegaloblastic arrest. This can be prevented by administering folinic acid to patients receiving these drugs. Folic acid deficiency in infancy occurs in those on dried milk formulas not supplemented with mixed vitamin C and folic acid. In addition, congenital defects in pyrimidine synthesis and folic acid antagonists can produce megaloblastic marrrows by interfering with or altering the production of deoxyribonucleic acid.[17]

Unknown Megaloblastic Deficiencies

There are a variety of causes for unknown megaloblastic deficiencies (miscellaneous and refractory megaloblastic anemias), but nothing has been specifically related to the megaloblastoid marrow pattern; no vitamin B_{12} or folic acid deficiencies are seen. Macrocytosis may or may not be present. This group includes cases with renal insufficiency, infection, neoplastic and leukemic processes, inborn or acquired defects in nucleoprotein metabolism; there are also aplastic and hypoplastic anemias at some phase and erythremic myelosis with or without terminal myelocytic leukemia. One may also see a mixed iron deficiency associated with vitamin B_{12} or folic acid deficiency—for example, in sprue, pregnancy, and pernicious anemia with ulcerated gastrointestinal neoplastic lesions. Occasionally patients with excessive orotic aciduria and a deficiency in their leukocytes of the enzymes orotic acid pyrophosphorylase and orotodylic decarboxylase may develop a megaloblastic anemia.[109] The double enzyme defect is perhaps to be explained on the basis of a deletion of an operator gene.

Occasionally, one sees a symptom-complex called congenital dyserythropoietic anemia, in which there is a congenital refractory anemia with ineffective erythropoiesis and multinucleated normoblasts in the marrow. Differentiation is among macrocytic anemias not responding to folic acid or vitamin B_{12} therapy, primary sideroblastic anemias, atypical thalassemia and atypical hereditary hemolytic anemias.[86]

Clinical Concepts of Anemias Due to Deficiency of Hematopoietic Factors

Classic Pernicious Anemia (P.A.) is a chronic, insidious megaloblastic anemia caused by vitamin B_{12} deficiency. It appears most commonly in persons over 40 years of age, frequently of northern European stock. Twenty per cent of patients have a family history of pernicious anemia. Others have atrophic gastritis, gastric neoplasm (polyps and carcinoma), total gastrectomy, intestinal malabsorption, deranged metabolism due to increased hematopoietic requirements, or defective diet. It is caused by failure of the atrophic fundic gastric mucosa to secrete intrinsic factor in amounts sufficient to enable vitamin B_{12} absorption to take place in the ileum.

Recently, some researchers have demonstrated that vitamin B_{12} deficiency may result in an inability to convert folate to the polyglutamate forms that are needed as active coenzymes. The inability to convert methylmalonate to succinate is associated with vitamin B_{12} deficiency, and it causes an increased urinary excretion of methylmalonate. This finding can be utilized as a sensitive indicator of tissue vitamin B_{12} deficiency. Similarly, methylmalonate accumulation may lead to elevated abnormal lipids in myelin, which in turn, contributes to the neurologic damage associated with vitamin B_{12} deficiency but absent in folate deficiency.

Clinically, there are symptoms related to severe anemia and gastrointestinal and neurologic disturbances. This includes long-standing, progressive fatigability, weakness, pallor, dyspnea, sore anterior tongue and mouth, epigastric discomfort, constipation or diarrhea, symmetrical paresthesias of the toes or fingers progressing to numbness, lack of coordination in walking and the performance of finer tasks, apathy, and psychotic tendencies.

Physically, the patient has a waxy, slightly yellowish pallor; a bulky frame; a beefy red, almost smooth, shiny tongue; tachycardia; and hemic murmurs. Frequently, splenomegaly and occasionally hepatomegaly are associated with pernicious anemia. Other findings include indications of posterolateral spinal cord sclerosis—for example, loss of vibratory and position sense and loss of sensibility to touch in distal extremities, and also occasionally ataxia and positive Romberg test with variable flaccidity and spasticity.

Hematologically, the hemoglobin is very low, as is the red count and hematocrit; there are also associated macrocytosis, anisocytosis, and poikilocytosis. Leukopenia is evident with large macropolycytic (hypersegmented) polymorphonuclear leukocytes and occasional immature leukocytes. If the peripheral blood of a pernicious anemia patient is mixed EDTA and a concentrated buffy coat, stained film is prepared, one will occasionally see DNA-poor, "lacy" open nuclear chromatin megaloblasts. Usually a slight thrombocytopenia is also observed with bizarre platelet forms including giant types. New studies reveal a population of platelets that aggregate more strongly than do the platelets that emerge soon after vitamin B_{12} therapy. However, this may simply reflect a preponderance of young platelets in the blood, and young platelets have more functional capability than older ones.[82] Note the recurrence of the word "giant" in the description of red blood cells, white blood cells, and platelet morphology—an important observation in peripheral blood film studies. However, the total number of all types of cells may be reduced, causing pernicious anemia to be confused with aplastic anemia, subleukemic leukemia, and others (Plate 13).

In pernicious anemia the bone marrow is red, voluminous, and hypercellular, with hyperplasia of all elements, especially the red cell precursors. These precursors do not mature properly because of a disordered synthesis of deoxyribonucleic acid (DNA). This leads to their destruction within the marrow and the subsequent liberation of their heme pigments and elevation of the indirect bilirubin. This disordered cellular metabolism leads to distinctive alterations in all marrow elements, especially the erythrocyte precursors. For example, megaloblast cell formation is characterized by large cell size, bizarre fine nuclear chromatin with intense lumpy basophilic cytoplasm (nucleoli if present are generally very sharply outlined), and occasionally binucleated forms (Plates 14, 15).

Although nuclear maturation is defective, cytoplasmic development and hemoglobin formation proceed normally, resulting in asynchrony in which large cells containing young-looking nuclei and mature orthochromic or eosinophilic cytoplasm. Nucleated red cells may comprise 30 to 50 per cent of all nucleated cells, whereas normally there is one nucleated red blood cell to four myeloid type cells (neutrophils, etc.). Atypical nuclear chromatin and cell enlargement are also found in the granulocyte series with giant metamyelocytes, giant band forms, macropolycytes, and giant megakaryocytes and platelets. Giant epitheloid cells are also found in the oral cavity, gastric washings, and vaginal Papanicolaou smears.

Diagnosis. Diagnosis is further confirmed by the finding of scanty gastric juice volume with associated histamine gastric achlorhydria. Gastrointestinal malabsorption disease, anticonvulsant drug therapy, liver diseases, fad diets, fish tapeworm infestation, and achrestic anemia must be ruled out. If these are excluded, one may measure the vitamin B_{12} serum level by microbiologic assay—the measurement of growth response in *Euglena gracilis* or *Lactobacillus leichmannii*. Also the quantities of bacteria in the small intestine may be measured to further exclude small bowel lesions. Roentgenographic studies of the small intestine should be made to exclude such disorders as diverticula, and a Crosby peroral capsule biopsy of the small intestine should be performed to exclude morphologic alterations. If these disorders are all ruled out, one may then resort to a therapeutic trial test with preceding pretreatment reticulocyte counts as a baseline. After this, one may give 5 μg. of vitamin B_{12} intramuscularly daily.

If the patient has true pernicious anemia, the reticulocyte count increases on the third or fourth day and reaches a peak on the fifth day, then gradually diminishing as the red blood cell and hemoglobin rises to normal. Also the white blood cell and platelet counts come to normal levels together with a change of marrow from a megaloblastic to a normoblastic pattern. If renal insufficiency or infection is present, the marrow response may be inhibited. However, if anemia is severe and the patient has incapacitating symptoms with or without neurologic findings, a megaloblastic bone marrow finding plus Diagnex histamine achlorhydria, a baseline reticulocyte count followed by the therapy outlined below with serial reticulocyte counts will suffice for a basic approach.

To help verify the diagnosis, especially in patients in therapeutic remission who cannot be subjected to a therapeutic trial, the *Schilling test* can be used. This test indicates the presence or absence of gastric intrinsic factor manufactured normally by the gastric mucosa. Oral ^{60}Co-vitamin B_{12}* is given (0.5 to 2.0 μg.) to the pa-

Table 8-1.

	^{60}Co-Vitamin B_{12} Excreted in Urine in 24 hours (in per cent)
Normal patient	7 to 22 (average, 14.2)
P.A. patient	0 to 2.3
P.A. patient with intrinsic factor	3.1 to 30 (average, 9.6)
Achlorhydria (no P.A. symptoms)	2.2 to 29 (average, 11.6)
Total gastric resection	0 to 2.3
Sprue	No excretion

tient. In pernicious anemia, very little of the ^{60}Co-vitamin B_{12} is absorbed; this is determined by measuring the radioactivity of the urine after the patient is given a large, parenteral (intramuscular) flushing dose of nonradioactive (unlabeled) vitamin B_{12}, after which the urine is collected for 24 hours and its radioactivity is measured. This step of the test is designed to cause urinary excretion of much of the stable and radioactive vitamin B_{12} absorbed from the gastrointestinal tract. Because the patient having vitamin B_{12} deficiency caused by intestinal disease may have adequate intrinsic factor but may be unable to absorb the vitamin for other reasons, full confirmation of the diagnosis of pernicious anemia requires a second testing in which ^{60}Co-vitamin B_{12} is given together with an intrinsic factor preparation. In pernicious anemia even in remission, the addition of intrinsic factor increases the absorption of labeled vitamin B_{12}, and the excretion values are normal at this time. In primary intestinal malabsorption, the absorption of labeled vitamin B_{12} does not increase, and the excretion values are less than normal (see Table 8–1 and Fig. 8-4).

The Schilling test should be done after the bone marrow study because during the course of the test, 2000 μg. of vitamin B_{12} is given intramuscularly for flushing. This makes all diagnostic cytologic criteria disappear because megaloblasts mature very rapidly by mitosis.

---

* ^{57}Co may be substituted wherever ^{60}Co is mentioned.

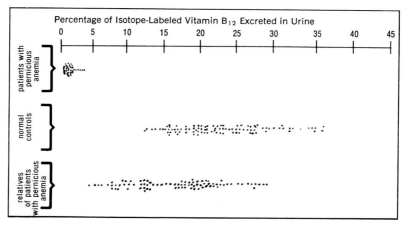

Fig. 8-4. The Schilling test for pernicious anemia. The low vitamin B_{12} excretion rate in patients with pernicious anemia is well below the lower limits of the normal excretion range. The separation of vitamin B_{12} excretion ranges is not as distinct between patients with pernicious anemia and either members of their family or patients with achlorhydria. These are problems in differential diagnosis only when the subjects tested fall within the lowest part of the range. (Courtesy of Ames Company)

A recent diagnostic test of clinical vitamin B_{12} deficiency is the measurement of the serum vitamin B_{12} level using radioisotope dilution and coated charcoal.[79] It makes use of the fact that albumin-coated charcoal adsorbs only free (unbound) vitamin B_{12}. The principle of the method can be summarized as follows: After all the native vitamin B_{12} in the serum sample has been rendered free by heat and acid treatment, a known amount of radioactive vitamin B_{12} is added. Then, by addition of a standardized solution of *hog intrinsic factor* (N.F.), a known amount of the total free vitamin B_{12}, whether cold or hot (radioactive), is bound by the intrinsic factor. This is the so-called *B_{12} biopsy.* When albumin-coated charcoal is added, only the remaining free vitamin B_{12} is absorbed by it, and the supernatant solution, freed of charcoal by centrifugation and containing the same proportion of cold and hot (radioactive) vitamin B_{12}, can be decanted and assayed for radioactivity. A principal control, in which the only difference is that saline solution is substituted for the patient's serum, is similarly run and assayed. From these two de-

terminations, the amount of native vitamin B_{12} originally present in the serum can be calculated by the formula:

B_{12} in $\mu\mu$g./ml. of serum =

$$2 \times \mu\mu\text{g. of }^{57}\text{CoB}_{12}\left(\frac{B}{B_1} - 1\right)$$

where B =

net counts per minute of control tube

and B_1 =

net counts per minute of patient's serum tube
Normal range = 200-1000 $\mu\mu$g.B_{12}/ml.
(B_{12} deficiency = 80-140 $\mu\mu$g.)

The sensitivity range appears to extend from the lowest to the highest vitamin B_{12} values in normal and pathologic serums. The advantage of this test is that results can be arrived at in less than 5 hours for which the *Euglena* assay requires 5 days. Wherever radioactive vitamin B_{12} is used clinically in the diagnosis of megaloblastic anemia, this test should be applied to a serum sample obtained before any therapy is given. Gastric analysis may imply (just as the definitive Schilling test may show) how a defective assimilation of vitamin B_{12} has occurred, but it does not directly demonstrate the existence of deficiency. Moreover, because flushing with a large amount of nonradioactive vitamin B_{12} is used, the Schilling test renders meaningless subsequent analyses of vitamin B_{12} serum levels.

Another recent development that may aid the diagnosis of megaloblastic anemias is the demonstration of markedly elevated carbonic anhydrase activity in erythrocytes in vitamin B_{12} deficiency and probably in folic acid deficiency.[154]

A reduced red blood cell folate level has been found in cases of pernicious anemia. The results of tests that assess folate levels indicate the failure of the synthesis of the folate coenzyme when vitamin B_{12} is deficient. The findings reinforce the view that folate polyglutamate is the active coenzyme. Impaired entry of 5-methylfolate into cells in pernicious anemia is likely to be secondary to failure of polyglutamate synthesis. Failure of formation of RNA in nerve cells probably explains vitamin B_{12} neuropathy. Since it is the exception rather than the rule that most patients with vitamin B_{12} deficiency also show evidence of folate deficiency, the finding that polyglutamate is the active folate coenzyme and vitamin B_{12} is required for its formation provides a more encompassing basis for the explanation of the biochemical and clinical phenomena ensuing from the imbalance of these vitamins.[20]

The treatment consists of daily injections of 100 to 200 μg. of vitamin B_{12} for approximately 1 week and at monthly intervals thereafter for the remainder of the patient's life. After 7 to 10 days of treatment, a marked reticulocytosis is found. This is an excellent way to determine if the therapy is effective. If the hemoglobin is 3 to 4 g. per 100 ml. when the patient is first seen, one transfusion of packed red blood cells should be given slowly. Prognosis is good except when neurologic manifestations are present; these for the most part are irreversible. Also, soon after vitamin B_{12} ther-

apy is instituted, there is excessive availability of platelet factor 3. This may explain the development of arterial and venous thromboses in these patients (i.e., in the course of the "reticulocyte crisis," metabolites capable of inducing platelet aggregation, such as adenosine diphosphate, enter the circulation).[82]

Folic Acid Deficiency. Symptoms of anemia are seen in folic acid deficiency just as they are in pernicious anemia. However, the specific neurologic findings seen in pernicious anemia are absent. Oropharyngeal and intestinal lesions are observed—for example, glossitis, cheilosis, ulcerative stomatitis, pharyngitis, esophagitis with dysphagia, diarrhea, and perirectal ulceration. Peripheral blood and marrow patterns are the same as in pernicious anemia with hyperferremia and hemosiderin in the bone marrow. Diagnosis is made when the findings just mentioned are observed along with blood and marrow findings similar to those in pernicious anemia plus gastric hyperacidity, and oral and intestinal lesions. If achlorhydria is evident, and intestinal malabsorption, hepatic cirrhosis, Dilantin therapy, severe malnutrition, and pregnancy are excluded, then 5 μg. of parenteral vitamin B_{12} will be ineffective, but 0.1 to 0.2 mg. of daily parenteral folic acid will produce clinical and hematologic remission. Dietary folic acid will also accomplish the same end result. Lawrence and Klipstein recommend the routine administration of folic acid supplements to all pregnant women in the last trimester to prevent the occurrence of megaloblastic anemia and its complications (Plate 16).[80]

Recently, it has been demonstrated that certain drugs used therapeutically either impair absorption of folate or produce direct metabolic inhibition of folate. For example, trimethoprim and triamterine are inhibitors of the reductase enzyme necessary to convert folate to metabolically active forms. Primidone, barbiturates, and phenytoin also impair absorption of folate, possibly by inhibition of conjugase, an intestinal enzyme. Conjugase has been found necessary to convert poorly absorbed poly-glutamate forms of dietary folate to the monoglutamate form.

A more prompt diagnosis can be made by the FIGLU test—measurement of the urinary excretion of formiminoglutamic acid, which is a histidine metabolite excreted in large amounts in folic acid deficiency—and by the bacteriologic assay of serum folic acid activity. The sensitivity of the FIGLU method is considerably enhanced by histidine loading prior to urine collection; L-histidine monohydrochloride (15 g. for adults, 100 mg./lb. for children) is given orally to the patient in a fasting state. Food is withheld until 1 hour after administration. The histidine may be administered by mixing it with a suitable fruit juice or water, or it may be given with applesauce. Three hours after administration of the histidine, the patient voids urine, which is then discarded. The urine for the next 5 hours is collected in a bottle containing 1 ml. of concentrated hydrochloric acid and thymol crystals. The volume of urine is measured and a 10 ml. aliquot is used for analysis. The normal concentration of histidine is less than 3 mg. per 100 ml. of urine. Elevated concentrations occur in nutritional folic acid deficiency, idiopathic steatorrhea, and in some cases of congenital hemolytic anemia.

If the administration of vitamin B_{12} causes hematologic response, but folic acid deficiency is still suspected, the therapeutic trial is continued with daily doses of 0.4 mg. of folic acid. With therapy (0.1–0.2 mg.; maximally 5 mg. tablets), full clinical response should occur in 2 to 4 days. However, if the folic acid deficiency is due to dietary deficiency, treatment may be continued for 2 weeks accompanied by a normal diet. In pregnancy, treatment is continued for 2 months after delivery. If symptoms are produced by folic acid antagonists, folinic acid is used, or 100 to 200 mg. of folic acid is given daily. It is also recommended that folic acid (0.1–0.25 mg.

daily) be regularly prescribed in pregnancy —as iron and calcium are.[17]

Diphyllobothrium   Latum   Infestation. Diphyllobothrium latum infestation is diagnosed in the north central United States, where fish tapeworm is endemic. Symptoms are produced because the living parasite competes biologically for the vitamin B_{12} manufactured by the bacteria of the intestinal tract—that is, the tapeworm uses up, or interferes with absorption of, extrinsic factor. It is rare to see achylia gastrica or neurologic findings. The peripheral blood and marrow findings resemble those found in pernicious anemia. Ova from the tapeworm are present in the stools, and anthelmintics are used in treatment.

ANEMIAS DUE TO ABNORMAL BONE MARROW FUNCTION

Anemias due to abnormal bone marrow function (see etiologic classification, p.186) are usually mild but may be severe. The red blood cell size varies, but it is usually normocytic. The causative factor in this type of anemia varies, but it is the most common of all anemias; it may be produced by circulating hemolysins associated with decreased erythroid marrow function—that is, the bone marrow fails to compensate for slightly increased hemolysins without elevated serum bilirubin. There frequently are anorexia and gastrointestinal findings, and therefore one may also see an associated iron, folic acid, or B_{12} deficiency.

Endocrine Abnormalities

Endocrine abnormalities are sometimes etiologically related to bone marrow anemias; during the course of hypothyroidism, hypopituitarism, hypoadrenalism (Addison's disease), and hypogonadism (especially testis), one may observe a slight normocytic anemia. In hypothyroidism (myxedema), a coexistent vitamin B_{12}—intrinsic factor deficiency is frequently seen with associated peripheral macrocytosis, but without marrow megaloblastosis. Occasionally the spleen is mentioned as having a humoral mechanism concerned with the stimulation of the recovery phase in damaged hemopoietic tissue. The kidney and its diseases are also related to red cell formation. The hormone erythropoietin, produced mainly in the kidney (but not exclusively) and probably a glycoprotein, is specifically required for the initiation of differentiation of stem cells into the red blood cell series. It acts in the bone marrow, and no red blood cell formation is possible without it. In a great many clinical conditions in which severe anemia exists, the hormone titer in the plasma and urine may be greatly increased. In advanced renal disease with uremia, underproduction of erythropoietin is related etiologically to the anemia.

A recent erythropoietin assay technique* is a relatively simple screening and quantitation approach that can be performed quickly on multiple samples in any laboratory. It is accurate and economic enough to permit quantitative detection of extremely small differences in serum, urine, or extract in routine use. This test utilizes the principle of hemagglutination—inhibition in which there is binding of the antibody of the ESF, present in the test material or standard, prior to the addition of ESF-sensitized cells. Only the unbound antibody will be free to react with the sensitized cells and provide a particular type of pattern. On Plate 17, Row V is a primary polycythema vera sera sample with the end point in the second well (first 3 plus). Row W is a secondary polycythema sera with the end point in the fourth well (first 3 plus). Well X is a normal sera sample with the end point in well 5 (first 3 plus). Wells Y and Z are elevated sera samples from a patient with a kidney tumor and one with sickle cell anemia. The 3 plus end points are in wells 6 and 7.

Elevated levels are encountered in many anemic patients, in some patients with secondary polycythemia and as a possible early manifestation of kidney transplant rejection. Normal or depressed levels are typically observed in polycythema vera, in the presence of some types of renal disease, and in secondary anemias. The test may also be used as a valuable guide for treatment of patients using androgen drugs. The procedure itself provides definitive results 50 times faster (2–2½ hours each) than bioassay methods.

Gordon and co-workers have produced experimental data from studies on rat kidney tissue that support the hypothesis that erythropoietin behaves like an enzyme to convert erythropoiesis-stimulating factor (ESF) or renal erythropoietic factor (REF), into an active form.[45] This mechanism is analogous to the reninangiotensin system, although renin has chemical properties that are different from the REF. Mechanical interference with marrow function is said to be the cause of some of these anemias. For example, the inadequate capacity of bone marrow in newborn and premature infants is probably rleated to the defective antenatal storage of iron with resultant development of a hypochromic anemia. Early clamping of the umbilical cord may be a related factor. In premature infants, the anemia is probably related to the rapid growth, which places too great a burden on their small and inadequate iron stores.

Myelophthisis

Myelophthisis is another causal factor in this group of anemias. This reduction of the cell-forming function of the marrow is mostly related to foreign, degenerative, neoplastic, or inflammatory products replacing bone marrow functioning elements and space, resulting in a mechanical crowding-out or interference with erythroid bone marrow function. The peripheral blood is

---

* ESF Test Kit, JCL Clinical Research Corporation, Route 6, Strawplains Pike, Knoxville, Tennessee 37914; or Scientific Products, 1430 Waunegan Road, McGraw Park, Illinois 60085.

characterized by polychromasia, reticulocytosis, normoblastosis, a leukocytic shift to the left, marked poikilocytosis, anisocytosis, and slight macrocytosis. This mechanical interference does not hold in all instances because the severity of the anemia does not correlate with the demonstrable bone marrow involvement in many cases[136] (Plates 18, 19).

Relative Marrow Failure

Relative marrow failure anemias are also incorporated in this group, which includes the most common causes of anemia. These are frequently classified as the "simple chronic anemias of infection and systemic disease" (Plates 20, 21). The anemia is usually moderately severe, and has a normal reticulocyte count with frequent fairly normal morphologic pattern. There are usually reduced erythropoietin levels with an inability to compensate for the minimal hemolytic process leading to the concept of relative marrow failure. Furthermore, there are reduced serum iron values associated with the impairment in the release of iron from reticuloendothelial sites of erythrocyte catabolism. However, iron-binding capacity (transferrin) levels are not increased and there is increased storage of reticuloendothelial iron.

Cases due to chronic infection show a degree of anemia that varies with the type, severity, and duration of the infection—for example, in subacute bacterial endocarditis, osteomyelitis, tuberculosis, and rheumatic fever. The anemia resulting from these diseases is usually normocytic and normochromic with diminished reticulocytosis; the hemoglobin is 10 to 11 g. per 100 ml. after 1 to 2 months (lower hemoglobin in acute severe infection). The bone marrow shows a decrease in the proportion of normoblastic cells, some increase in the proportion of immature myeloid cells, and poor hemoglobin production in normoblasts with basophilic or dark polychromatophilic cytoplasm. Both the serum iron and transferrin (iron-binding capacity) decreases within a few days after infection develops. Most workers feel that the combination of low serum iron, decreased transferrin, and high ferritin levels in the serum is characteristic of the anemia of chronic infection and other chronic diseases. If iron is given for treatment of the anemia, it is removed quickly from the bloodstream and deposited in nonmarrow tissues. Whether the increased ferritin synthesis in the reticuloendothelial cells and the resulting trapping of iron in this storage pool has any defense function remains unclear. Hemoglobin synthesis from reticuloendothelial cell phagocytosis of old red blood cells is retarded. Recent work has shown that a neutrophilic and external secretion glycoprotein, lactoferrin, may preferentially draw iron (needed for the synthesis of hemoglobin) from destroyed RBCs rather than from iron stores. The interference of lactoferrin with the metabolism of iron might explain why acute inflammation causes hypochromic anemia (this does not apply in cases of chronic inflammation).[151] Erythropoietin levels are variable; serum copper and red blood cell protoporphyrins are increased. Occasionally red blood cell life is reduced by bacteria induced hemolysins.

Rheumatoid arthritis and other collagen diseases produce a blood picture that is usually similar to that produced by a mild normochromic, normocytic anemia with decreased serum iron and variable transferrin levels. Occasionally, red blood cells are coated with a protein serum factor; red blood cell survival time is usually normal. The anemia usually responds to steroid therapy without treatment of the anemia per se. The hemoglobin levels decrease again after cessation of the steroid treatment. In general, if a severe hypochromic microcytic anemia is found, other etiologic factors must be searched for in addition to rheumatoid arthritis.

Chronic renal disease is usually associated with red blood cell aplasia, in which bone marrow failure and hemolysis both play a part. For example, children with renal insufficiency may develop a hemolytic uremic syndrome together with small contracted red blood cells and thrombocytopenia. Most commonly one sees a normocytic, normochromic anemia, with mild macrocytosis seen in the severely anemic patients. The size and shape of the red blood cells do not vary much until the BUN is 150 mg. per 100 ml. or more, when one begins to see burr cells on the blood films. The severity of the anemia increases as the BUN goes above 70 mg. per 100 ml., and the anemic pattern may be such that the hemoglobin values fall below 5 g. per 100 ml. However, the anemia may develop before significant retention of nitrogenous substance is detectable.

There is an increased rate of hemolysis with shortening (variable) of the erythrocyte survival time in the terminal or predeterminal period. Reticulocytes are decreased except in the hemolytic phase. The bone marrow pattern is usually that of depressed normoblastic proliferation with especially poor hemoglobin formation in the normoblasts (renal insufficiency). Iron-binding capacity is reduced, but the serum iron level is not consistent. Although an extraerythrocytic hemolytic process is seen in some patients with renal insufficiency, there is general agreement that erythropoiesis is impaired so that adequate compensation for decreased red blood cell survival does not occur. The iron is incorporated decreasingly in the red blood cells, and it is stored in the liver and spleen.

The presence and accumulation of a circulating factor inhibits RBC metabolism in some uremic patients. The findings in these patients suggest defective hexose monophosphate shunt activity. Regular hemodialysis with purified water ameliorates the defect in vitro and markedly affects red blood cell survival in vivo, reducing transfusion requirements. The hemolytic agent in tap water was identified as chloramine, a widely used bactericidal agent. The RBC oxidation stress produced by this agent can

readily be estimated by the percentage of methemoglobin in dialyzed patients— which should not be greater than 5 per cent and by the presence of Heinz bodies.[157] In addition, patients with hemodialyzed uremia possess these forms of erythrocytic alteration, that is, burr cells, schistocytes, and "sick" cells (spherocytic RBCs with decreased deformability and difficulty in traversing the splenic microcirculation).[42]

Because the kidneys are the major source of erythropoietin, the concentration of erythropoietin is decreased in acute and chronic renal disease, and probably this factor plays an important role in the lack of bone marrow response to therapeutic agents. Since there is probably an accumulation of toxic metabolites in renal insufficiency cases, chronic hemodialysis therapy is frequently associated with improved erythrocyte production even though therapy may be complicated by folate and iron depletion and the presence of hemolysis associated with toxic components, such as chloramine, in dialysis water baths. Erythropoietin enhancement may be presumed to be the reason for the occasional increased erythrocyte production associated with androgen therapy in patients on hemodialysis. Thus, there may be a reduction in transfusion needs, protecting prospective renal transplant recipients from undue exposure to histocompatibility antigens (HLA, etc.).

Liver disease may play a part in the production of some anemias. However, it is not known exactly what mechanisms are responsible for the anemia associated with liver disease because the anemia itself does not respond to the usual hematopoietic agents but is usually alleviated when liver function improves. Etiologically, the anemia is frequently attributable to many factors, for example, bleeding, folate deficiency, splenic hypersequestration, erythrocytic membrane lipid alterations, and expanded plasma volume (associated with its dilutional effect). Hematologically, the symptom complex has all the characteristics of any type of anemia expressed as such or modified by the superimposed changes of the liver disease anemia. For example, hemoglobin usually varies between 5 and 10 g. per 100 ml. The cells are normocytic to thin macrocytic with leukocytic alterations. Polychromatophilia is seen with a 2 to 5 per cent reticulocytosis. Stippling and target cell formation is also seen.

One may also observe a mild to moderate hemolytic anemia with spur-shaped RBCs in patients suffering severe hepatocellular dysfunction. The first phase of spur cell formation results from the equilibration of the membranes with serum lipoproteins rich in free cholesterol. The second phase depends on circulation through the spleen. Therefore, splenectomy not only reduces the hemolytic rate, but also prevents both nonselective loss of membrane surface area and the remodeling of membrane architecture in vivo. Splenectomy is considered to be a risky surgical procedure in patients in whom hepatocellular function is sufficiently abnormal to cause production of spur cells.[26] Formation of target cells and spur cells is associated with increased RBC membrane uptake of cholesterol from plasma lipoprotein. In fact, excessively high cholesterol:phospholipid ratios in spur cells are associated with loss of membrane plasticity and splenic sequestration.

The bone marrow shows an increase in volume and hypercellularity with macronormoblastic proliferation, and decreased fat. The normoblasts show nuclear chromatin abnormalities with nucleus-cytoplasm asynchrony and abnormal mitoses, as in megaloblastic maturation. However, all stages of maturation are seen with a preponderance of the more mature normoblast forms without leukocytic maturation abnormalities. Osmotic fragility of the erythrocytes is in the range of increased resistance to hypotonic saline, especially after incubation. Hypervolemia is frequently associated with esophageal varices or cyanosis. Occasionally one sees increased fecal and urinary urobilinogen, and the degree of anemia

is roughly parallel to the decreased erythrocyte survival time, the enlarged congested spleen acting as the major source of red blood cell destruction. Although erythroid hyperplasia is present in the marrow, it is not equivalent to the reaction of normal marrow to the same stimulus, and therefore some degree of relative bone marrow failure is present.

Although hemolysis dominates in acute alcoholism, the normal erythroid pattern returns frequently on cessation of alcohol intake, change of diet, bed rest, and folic acid therapy. Although this type of anemia is frequently associated with protein malnutrition and therefore decreased globin synthesis, it is of unknown etiology, usually refractory to therapy, and is exaggerated by hypervolemia and hyperlipemia,[12] with associated erythrocyte destruction and relatively inadequate bone marrow response.

However, a recent finding indicates that these hematopoietic alterations may be direct evidence for the inhibitory action of ethanol on hemoglobin synthesis. The effect may be indicated through inhibition of heme synthesis at a site influenced by pyridoxine. Ethanol may interfere with the mitochondrial function of developing normoblasts in marrow through inhibition of the heme synthetic pathway.[3] Studies in patients with Zieve's syndrome (hemolytic anemia of alcoholic liver disease) reveal evidence for lipid peroxidation. In addition to the expected finding of increased erythrocyte cholesterol in these patients, decreased polyunsaturated fatty acid and decreased RBC and serum vitamin E levels were found. The instability of pyruvate kinase noted in these patients' RBCs was linked theoretically to the alterations of their membranes by a peroxidation mechanism.[44]

Malignant neoplastic disease (nonmyelophthisic) may also produce an anemia that resembles the normocytic, normochromic, or hyperchromic microcytic anemias of infection characterized by decreased erythrocyte production, moder-

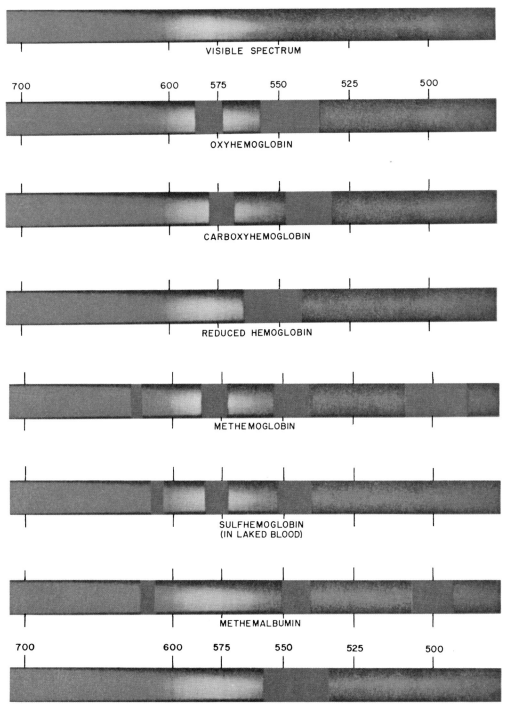

VISIBLE SPECTRUM

700 · 600 · 575 · 550 · 525 · 500

OXYHEMOGLOBIN

CARBOXYHEMOGLOBIN

REDUCED HEMOGLOBIN

METHEMOGLOBIN

SULFHEMOGLOBIN
(IN LAKED BLOOD)

METHEMALBUMIN

700 · 600 · 575 · 550 · 525 · 500

CYANMETHEMOGLOBIN

Plate 28

**VARIOUS HEMOGLOBIN COMPOUNDS VISUALIZED
BY SPECTROSCOPY**

(From *Hematology*. United States Medical School, Bureau of Medicine and Surgery,
Department of the Navy, Washington, D.C.)

Plate 29

SICKLE CELL ANEMIA (DISEASE)
Peripheral Blood

Elliptical RBC (El), Howell-Jolly body (HJ), juvenile (Juv), orthochromic normoblast (ONb), microcytic RBC (Mic), macrocytic RBC (Mac), polychromatic RBC (Pc), target cell (Tar), tactoid or reduced Hgb in RBC (Tac), sickle RBC (Sic), neutrophilic myelocyte (NMc).

Diagnostic Features: This is a marked to severe anemia most commonly observed in Negroid patients. If the blood is stained immediately after an acute crisis, one sees round or oval RBCs, microcytes and macrocytes, elongated and narrow RBCs with rounded or pointed ends, and occasional target cells; nucleated RBCs (normoblasts) occur one to ten per hundred WBCs. Polychromatophilia, basophilic stippling, Howell-Jolly bodies and occasional sickled normoblasts are seen; reticulocytosis

is moderate to marked. Sickle red blood cells may be seen when blood is examined immediately in cover slip preparations; however, maximum sickle effect (bizarre shape with elongated and pointed filaments) occurs in two to six hours. "S" hemoglobin is observed in hemoglobin electrophoresis alone or in combinations. Reduced "S" hemoglobin forms oat, spindle cell or rod-like particles in some cases. High WBC count occurs in crises with myelocytic shift to left; eosinophilia, monocytosis, and erythrophagocytosis also occur. Platelets are increased in number with bizarre forms.

(Below) Electrophoretic patterns of sickle cell disease and variants. AA, normal adult hemoglobin; AS, sickle cell trait hemoglobin; SS, sickle cell disease hemoglobin; SC, sickle cell-hemoglobin C disease.

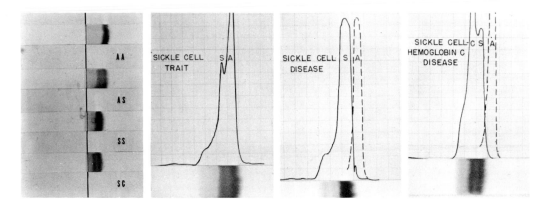

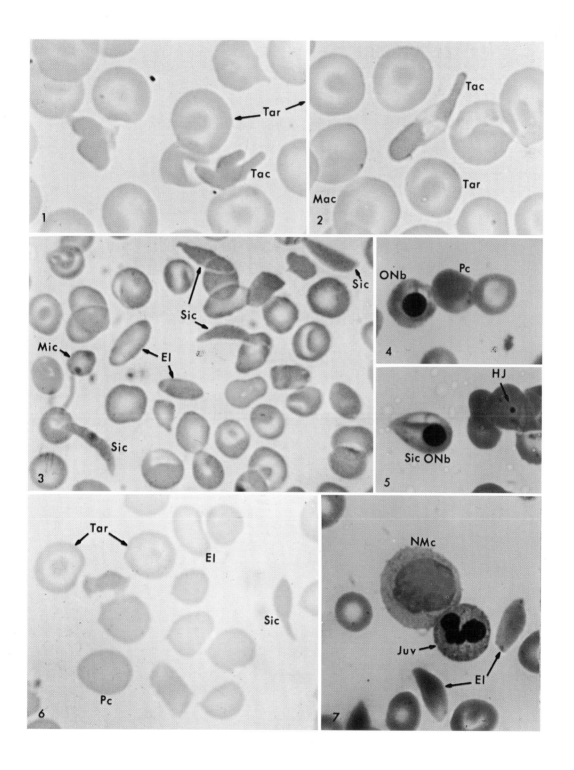

Plate 30

SICKLE CELL ANEMIA (DISEASE)
Bone Marrow

Basophilic normoblast (BNb), juvenile (Juv), orthochromic normoblast (ONb), degenerating (deg), polymorphonuclear eosinophil (PmE), sickled (Sic), neutrophilic metamyelocyte (NmMc).

Diagnostic Features: Grossly the bone marrow is soft, jelly-like, uniformly dark red or purplish-black with 50 to 75 per cent of all nucleated RBCs of the orthochromic or late normoblast type; one also sees polychromatophilic and basophilic normoblasts. There is a marked shift to the left in the myelocytic series, with numerous eosinophils. Increased numbers of megakaryocytes are also observed. Monocytes with erythrophagocytosis, nuclear fragments, and pigment granules are also seen. Occasionally one observes sickled normoblasts and long filamentous RBC cytoplasm.

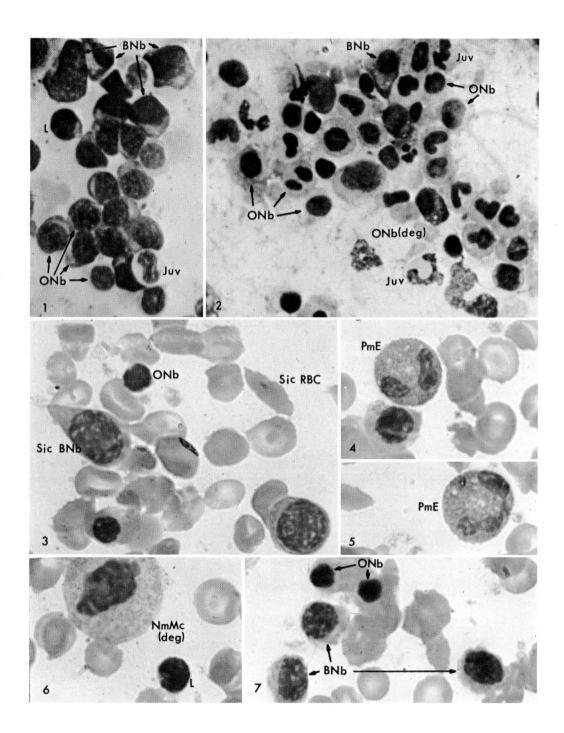

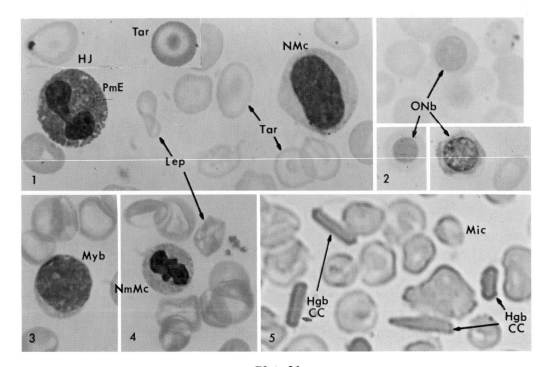

Plate 31

THALASSEMIA MAJOR
Peripheral Blood

Hemoglobin CC (Hgb CC), Howell-Jolly body (HJ), leptocyte with folded edge (Lep), microcyte (Mic), myeloblast (Myb), neutrophilic metamyelocyte (NmMc), microcyte (Mic), neutrophilic myelocyte (NMc), orthochromic normoblast (ONb), polymorphonuclear eosinophil (PmE), target cell (Tar), RBCs containing fetal Hbg (F Hbg), ghost RBCs without Hbg F (gh).

Fig. 6. Betke acid elution. Fetal Hb is acid-resistant and therefore is not eluted from the cells. It stains brilliantly with eosin. All other Hbg is eluted, leaving membrane ghosts. The hematoxylin stains the WBC nuclei and prevents misinterpretation as eosin-positive cells. Some heterozygotes for B-thalassemia have a pattern of irregular staining. Some cells are brightly stained, some pink, and others are ghosts; that is, fetal hemoglobin (Hbg F) is not

eluted from fresh blood slides fixed in 80 per cent ethanol, and afterwards RBCs containing fetal Hbg stain with eosin while those cells without any Hbg F appear as colorless ghosts.

Diagnostic Features: A severe microcytic hypochromic anemia with associated anisocytosis, poikilocytosis, leptocytes with folded or ridged edges, target cells, polychromasia, basophilic stippling and Howell-Jolly bodies (especially after splenectomy). Reticulocytosis and increased numbers of nucleated erythrocytes are also observed. Leukocytosis may be marked with associated increased myeloid cell proliferation including myelocytes and myeloblasts in the peripheral blood; monocytosis and lymphocytosis are seen in infants. Platelet numbers are normal with occasional slight thrombocytosis. Fig. 5 shows hemoglobin CC crystals after splenectomy.

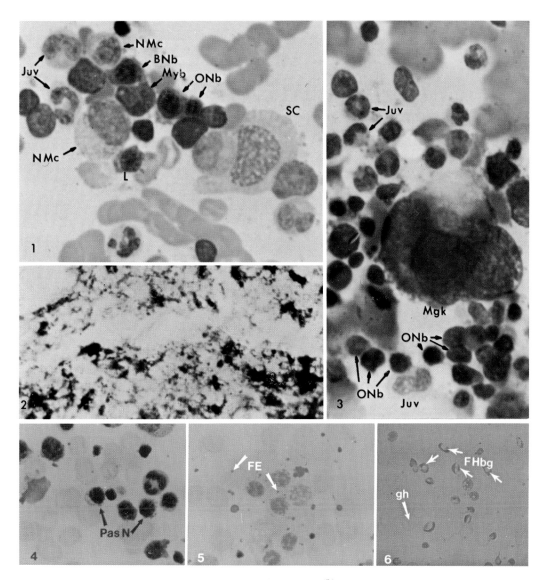

Plate 31 *(Continued)*

THALASSEMIA MAJOR
Bone Marrow

Basophilic normoblast (BNb), juvenile (Juv), lymphocyte (L), megakaryocyte (Mgk), myeloblast (Myb), neutrophilic myelocyte (NMc), orthochromic normoblast (ONb), stem cell (SC), PAS positive normoblast (PAS N), iron granule in cytoplasm of normoblast (Fe).

Diagnostic Features: The bone marrow is hypercellular with increase in all marrow elements, especially in the normoblastic series in which there is impaired hemoglobinization. Stainable marrow iron is increased, i.e., Prussian blue stain reveals marked deposits of blue hemosiderin granules in phagocytes.

Usually there is splenomegaly, and an elevated serum iron and iron-binding capacity; hemoglobin F is usually increased, with rest of hemoglobin electrophoresis normal. Reduced RBC survival time (CR[51]). Fig. 2 shows histiocytes and phagocytes loaded with iron granules (6+), Prussian blue stain ($\times 100$).

Fig. 4. PAS stain. Orange PAS granules in cytoplasm of normoblasts.

Fig. 5. Prussian blue stain. Bluish iron granules in cytoplasm of normoblastic cells (not ringed.)

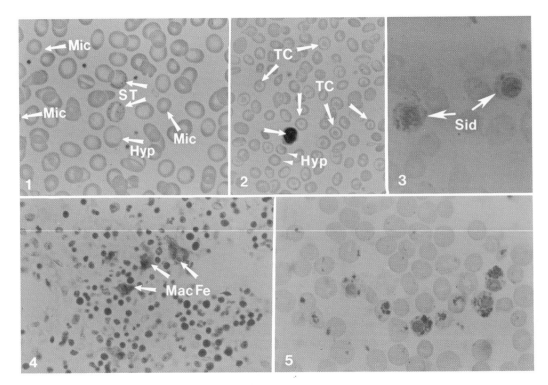

Plate 32

THALASSEMIA MINOR (TRAIT)
Peripheral Blood

Diagnostic Features: 1, 2. Thalassemia minor (trait), the heterozygous state for B-thalassemia, is frequently discovered accidentally; or because hypochromia, target cells, or basophilic stippling was observed in a reactive blood smear; or in the study of a moderate anemia with or without a palpable spleen; or in the study of a family. It may be mistaken for an iron-deficiency anemia occasionally with acute abdominal pain, hemosiderosis, leg ulcer or gallstones, or even thinning of the cortex of long bones and associated osteoporosis. RBCs are leptocytic, microcytic, and normochromic; and there are anisocytosis, poikilocytosis, and the changes mention above. Increased resistance of RBCs in hypotonic saline is also observed; increased HbA_2 with negative to extremely small quantities of HbF. (St = Stippled RBC; Mic = Microcytic RBC; L = lymphocyte; TC = target cell; Hyp = hypochromic cell)

Bone Marrow

3, 4. With Prussian blue stain iron deposition is observed in marrow macrophages but not ringed type. (Mac Fe = Macrophage containing iron; Sid = sideroblast with iron but not ringed)

Plate 33 ——————⟶

HEREDITARY SPHEROCYTOSIS
(Congenital Hemolytic Anemia, Congenital Hemolytic Icterus, Congenital Hemolytic Jaundice)
Peripheral Blood

Basophilic normoblast (BNb), macrocyte (Mac), monocyte (M), microspherocyte (Mic), orthochromic normoblast (ONb), platelet (Pl), poikilocyte (Poik), schistocyte (Sch).

Diagnostic Features: A chronic familial disease characterized by crises of intense anemia, reticulocytosis, splenomegaly, (micro-), spherocytosis (1 & 2), increased osmotic fragility of RBCs and a variable amount of jaundice (elevated indirect bilirubin of serum). Occasional macrocytes, poikilocytes, anisocytes, schistocytes (crisis) and polychromatophilia with variable numbers of normoblasts. The WBC count is normal or slightly increased; leukocytosis with shift to left occurs after a crisis. In the chronic stage, lymphocytes, plasma cells and basophils are increased. Platelets are usually normal in amount.

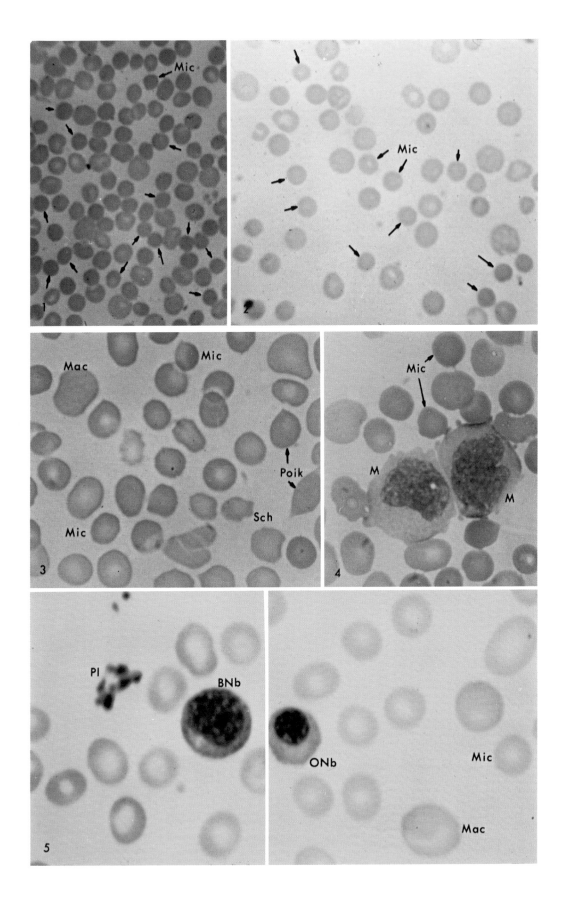

Plate 34

HEREDITARY SPHEROCYTOSIS
(Congenital Hemolytic Anemia, Congenital Hemolytic Icterus, Congenital Hemolytic Jaundice)
Bone Marrow

Basophilic normoblast (BNb), juvenile (Juv), lymphocyte (L) microspherocyte (Mic), mitosis (mit), neutrophilic metamyelocyte (NmMc), orthochromic normoblast (ONb), polymorphonuclear neutrophil (PmN), polymorphonuclear neutrophil with clover-leafing of nuclei due to oxalate crystals (PmN oxal), pronormoblast (PrNb).

Diagnostic Features: Normoblastic hyperplasia (25% to 60%) with many mitoses. Rarely see megaloblasts or abnormal leukocytes.

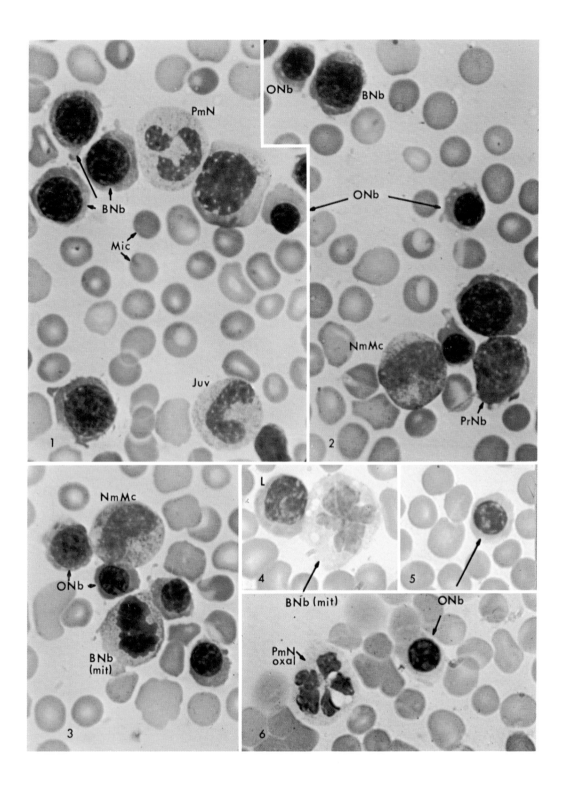

Plate 35

HEMOLYTIC DISEASE OF THE NEWBORN
(Erythroblastosis Fetalis)
Peripheral Blood (Top)

Basophilic normoblast (BNb), eosinophilic myelocyte (EMc), lymphocyte (L), orthochromic normoblast (ONb), orthochromic normoblast, mitosis [ONb (mit)], orthochromic normoblast pyknotic and fragmenting [ONb (pyk)], polychromatophilic RBC (PcRBC), pronormoblast (prNb).

Diagnostic Features: Occurs in newborn with Rh incompatibility and usually with a high maternal titer of anti-Rh agglutinins. Coombs' test of newborn peripheral and cord blood is usually positive with associated icterus of skin, hydrops and elevated serum bilirubin. Large numbers of nucleated RBCs in every stage of maturation, marked RBC polychromatophilia. RBCs with nuclear fragments, reticulocytosis, macrocytosis (spherocytosis frequently observed if due to ABO incompatibility) and also immature forms of granulocytes and lymphocytes are all observed in peripheral and cord blood. Platelets normal to reduced in number. Bone marrow rarely observed; however, there is hyperplasia of all cellular elements, especially the nucleated RBCs.

Cord Blood (Bottom)

3. Coombs' test (slide) showing clumped RBCs (positive). 5. Coombs' test (tube) (positive).

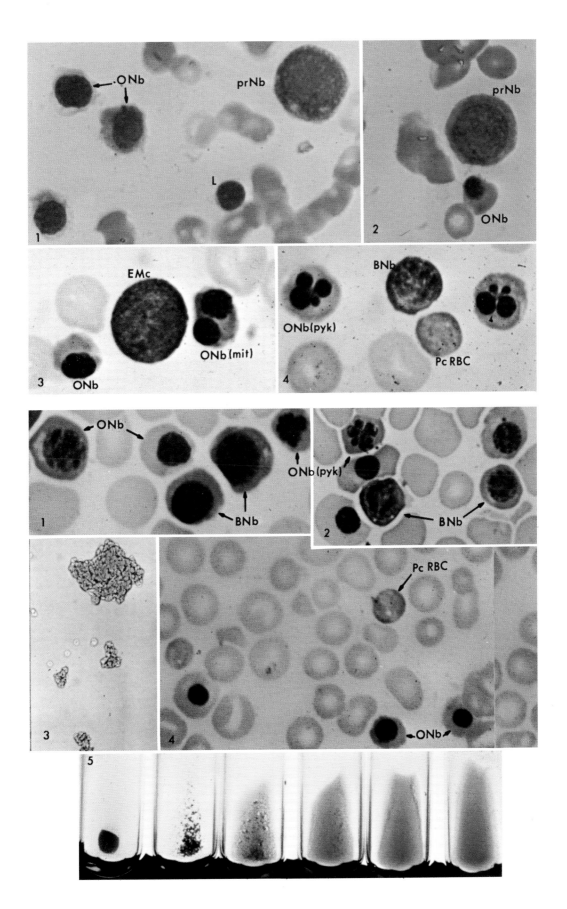

Plate 36

MALARIA PARASITES

Plasmodium Vivax (Tertian)
1—Ring form
2—Ameboid form and Schüffner's dots in the erythrocyte
3, 4 & 5—Ameboid forms
6, 7 & 8—Schizonts
9, 10 & 11—Segmenting stages
12—Liberated merozoites
13 & 14—Microgametocytes
15 & 16—Macrogametocytes

Plasmodium Malariae (Quartan)
17—Ring form
18, 19 & 20—Schizonts
21 & 22—Segmenting stages
23—Microgametocytes
24—Macrogametocytes

Plasmodium Falciparum (Estivo-Autumnal)
25—Ring form
26—Double infection of erythrocyte
27—Ring form with two chromatin dots
28—Triple infection of erythrocyte
29 & 30—Microgametocytes (crescent)
31 & 32—Macrogametocytes (crescent)

Blood Platelets

33, 34, 35 & 36—Blood platelets (Thrombocytes) superimposed upon erythrocytes. These are shown in this plate because they are frequently confused with malaria parasites by the untrained laboratory worker.

Diagnostic Features: Thin as well as thick blood films are examined first with the low power to select a suitable field; then the oil immersion objective is used. Plasmodia are differentiated from other cells and diagnosed on the basis of the blue-stained cytoplasm, the red-stained nucleus or nuclei and the brown to dark brown hematin granules, if present. All stages of development may be found in the peripheral blood in *P. Vivax, P. Ovale* and *P. Malariae* infections. In *P. Falciparum* infections, only ring stages or crescents, or both, are present. The stages of development are diagnosed on the following basis: (1) any plasmodium with more than one nucleus is a schizont of *P. Vivax, P. Ovale* or *P. Malariae* (those of *P. Falciparum* are found only in visceral blood); (2) any Plasmodium which has one nucleus, numerous hematin granules and fills or almost fills the RBC is a gametocyte; (3) any Plasmodium with one nucleus and pseudopods and a few or no hematin granules is a trophozoite; (4) ring stages are morphologically characteristic for Plasmodia, but do not suffice for species identification unless the chromatin has divided. Schizontic rings are very suggestive of *P. Falciparum*.

The three species—(*P. Ovale* is too infrequent to be of importance)—are differentiated on the following basis: (1) Plasmodia in enlarged RBC are *P. Vivax*; (2) Plasmodia in RBC with Schüffner's dots are *P. Vivax*; (3) Plasmodia with more than 12 chromatin masses are *P. Vivax*; (4) Plasmodia with stages older than the ring stage in RBC of normal size are *P. Malariae*; (5) Plasmodia in the band stage are *P. Malariae*; (6) Plasmodia in crescent shapes are *P. Falciparum*; (7) Plasmodia, all of them in the film in the ring stage, are *P. Falciparum*. The species of plasmodia cannot be determined on the basis of a single ring. (After Kracke)

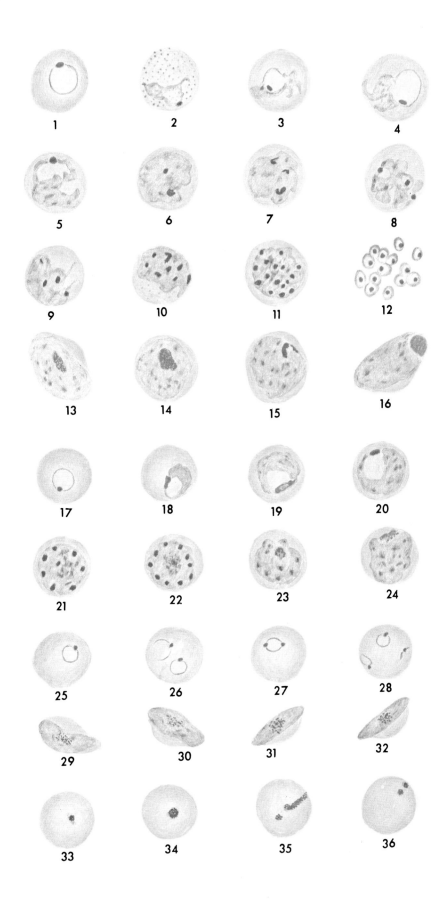

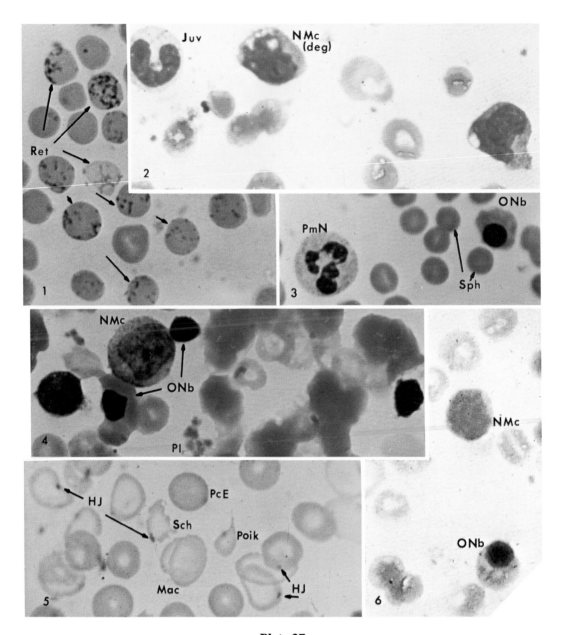

Plate 37

ACQUIRED HEMOLYTIC ANEMIA
Peripheral Blood No. 1

Degenerating (deg), Howell-Jolly bodies (HJ), juvenile (Juv), macrocyte (Mac), neutrophilic myelocyte (NMc), orthochromic normoblast (ONb), platelets (Pl), poikilocyte (Poik), polychromatic erythrocyte (PcE), polymorphonuclear neutrophil (PmN), reticulocyte (Ret), schistocyte (Sch), spherocyte (Sph).

Diagnostic Features: Reticulocytosis (macrocy-tosis), polychromatophilia, anisocytosis, poikilocy-tosis (spherocytosis, schistocytosis), nucleated red blood cells, stippling, thrombocytosis, leukocytosis (neutrophils, myelocytes, metamyelocytes) are all observed. One may also demonstrate the presence of hemolysins (positive direct and indirect Coombs test, etc.), hyperbilirubinemia, and an increase in urine and stool urobilinogen. 5. After splenectomy.

ately increased hemoglobin breakdown, and refractory response to hematopoietic agents. Superimposed complications of blood loss are seen with or without iron depletion, overt hemolysis, and vitamin B_{12} or folic acid deficiency. It is common to see a mild hemolytic anemia with circulating hemolysins, especially in lymphomatous diseases. In fact, an autoimmune process may exist with a positive Coombs test. Rarely, parasitic neoplastic cells may take up vitamin B_{12} or folic acid, leaving the erythrocytes deficient with some hematologic response occurring after specific therapy, cobalt, or androgens.

Diagnostic Summary of Anemias Due to Abnormal Bone Marrow Function

One must first try to determine and evaluate the primary disease, especially looking for chronic blood loss. Blood films usually show a normocytic, normochromic type of anemia with an MCV of approximately 80 cu.μ, an MCHC of approximately 32 per cent, and an MCH of approximately 27 $\mu\mu$g. There is also moderate anisocytosis. Burr cells are seen in cancer patients, and flat target cells are observed in liver disease. The red blood cell count averages 3,000,000 to 4,000,000 per cu.mm.; however, it may be as high as 5,000,000 per cu.mm. Reticulocytes are normal to slightly increased. The hemoglobin averages 8 to 10 g. per 100 ml. The white blood cell and platelet counts are usually normal, but are related to the causative disease.

Serum bilirubin is usually normal unless there is associated hepatic dysfunction. Osmotic fragility shows increased resistance especially in hepatic disease. Serum iron is usually low with the total iron-binding capacity low, especially with chronic infection is present. The erythrocyte survival time is shortened, as demonstrated by the ^{51}Cr-tagged erythrocyte technique, and it is associated with ineffective erythropoiesis. The bone marrow pattern reveals a qualitatively normal pattern with an occasional

decrease in normoblasts. By using Prussian blue stain, the stainable iron (hemosiderin) is seen in the bone marrow in variable amounts. The Coombs test is usually negative, but it is positive if autoimmune hemolysins are present, especially in certain lymphomas. There is no vitamin B_{12} or folic acid deficiency.

Therapeutically, the underlying disease is usually treated. If this is ineffective, blood transfusions are administered when the hemoglobin is in the range of 7 to 8 g. per ml. Renal disease patients are best maintained at a lower hematocrit level of 25 to 30.

Bone Marrow Failure Anemias[49, 90, 104, 153]

The symptom complex of bone marrow failure anemias is commonly called aplastic, hypoplastic, or refractory anemia. The marrow may be normal, aplastic, hypoplastic, or hyperplastic (Plate 23). If there is reduction of all formed elements in the peripheral blood, the disorder is pancytopenia (Plate 22). However, one may only see pure erythrocytic aplasia, anemia, and leukopenia without platelet reduction, or anemia and thrombocytopenia without leukopenia. Occasionally, spontaneous remissions occur with or without treatment by steroids, androgens, or splenectomy, depending on the degree of platelet or white blood cell reduction and related complications.

Etiologically, there are several types of symptom complexes found under the title of bone marrow failure: (1) The idiopathic form tends to occur more commonly in young adults. (2) The congenital hypoplastic or aplastic anemia of Diamond and Blackfan becomes manifest at 2 to 3 months of age and is characterized by severe anemia without reticulocytosis and by mild leukopenia without thrombocytopenia. The bone marrow shows hypoplasia of the erythrocyte series or cessation of development at the large atypical basophilic normoblast stage with large irregular nucleoli (Plate 24). Spontaneous remission occurs in 25 per cent of cases with treatment consisting of steroids and blood transfusions. Recently a case has been described with persistent hypocalcemia and hypoparathyroidism.[144] The Fanconi type of familial aplastic anemia is characterized by pancytopenia with associated growth failure, skeletal anomalies, microcephaly, mental retardation, hypogonadism, nephrosis, glycosuria, amino-aciduria, and skin pigmentation. The bone marrow pattern is that found in aplasia, with early normocellularity or hypercellularity and occasional fibrosis. The spleen is small. A subvariety described by Estren and Dameshek[38] has all these characteristics without somatic and metabolic abnormalities.[38] Pure erythrocyte aplasia or hypoplasia of adults is quite rare, and a good history must be taken to rule out drugs, malignant neoplasia, infection, or renal failure.

(3) Occasionally, an aplastic anemia (suppressed bone marrow activity) associated with thymoma is seen. Thymectomy may afford hematologic remission, and myasthenia gravis may precede the anemia in some cases. New concepts in treatment of pure red cell aplasia (PRCA) include the use of cyclophosphamide therapy of short duration. It is felt that the drug might remove a clone of disordered immunocompetent cells as thymectomy does.[152] (4) Sideroachrestic anemia, or refractory sideroblastic anemia, commonly occurs in patients between the ages of 50 and 75 with a slight preponderance in males. As is described under hypochromic microcytic anemias, the multiple etiologies include a sex-linked hereditary form, lead poisoning, alcoholism, drug toxicity underlying systemic diseases, and an idiopathic group called primary or refractory sideroblastic anemia. The normochromic or hypochromic type of anemia is observed.[8] The hypochromia reflects impaired heme synthesis in the individual erythrocyte, but the bone marrow shows impaired erythropoiesis with associated erythroid hyperplasia. The most prominent feature is the preponderance of normoblasts with nonheme iron granules in the cytoplasm. These cells, called sideroblasts, appear mostly in the bone marrow and are present also in peripheral blood, probably owing to a disturbance in normal release from the marrow. When Prussian blue stain is used, these bluish granules are perinuclear in the normoblasts. In electron microscopic studies, these granules appear to be granular iron-laden mitochondria. These findings suggest a defect of iron utilization in hemoglobin synthesis within erythrocyte precursors with "folate deficiency" megaloblastic-like appearance, but without response to vitamin B_{12} or folic acid therapy (Plates 25, 26).

The myeloid series of cells shows a shift toward immaturity with evidence of nucleus-cytoplasm asynchrony and persistence of nucleoli in later granulocyte forms. One also sees an increased amount of PAS-positive material in developing erythrocytes. The serum iron level is fairly well correlated with the number of coarsely granulated sideroblasts and red blood cell hypochromia. Many observers relate this complex to Di Guglielmo's syndrome with subsequent leukemia development.

Acute myeloblastic leukemia develops in approximately 20 per cent of the idiopathic group. Therefore, some investigators feel that primary sideroblastic anemia probably represents a preleukemic condition characterized by mutation in stem cells rather than an independent block in iron or heme metabolism. Although a true pyridoxine deficiency is rare in the nonalcoholic group, therapy consists in the administration of pyridoxine or pyridoxal phosphate to produce a partial hematologic response in 30 to 40 per cent of cases. In the cases associated with severe alcoholism and abnormal pyridoxine metabolism, approximately 50 per cent will show increased sideroblast formation. These same patients also manifest a folate deficiency attributable to inadequate diet and impaired absorption and inhibition of folate metabolism. The hematologic pattern in the alcoholic with sideroblastic anemia reveals occasional thrombocytopenia and neutropenia, toxic vacuolization of bone marrow cells, transient stomatocytosis and spur cell anemia—all significant abnormalities of RBC membrane lipids.

(5) Antimitotic agents that regularly produce bone marrow failure include ionizing radiation (radiograph, radium, radioactive elements such as ^{32}P, and radiation from nuclear explosions), nitrogen mustards, triethylene melamine, Myeleran, and Urethan. These preparations inhibit mitosis, probably by inhibiting the synthesis of DNA in the nuclei of bone marrow cells. Sequentially, 1 to 3 days after exposure, an increase in the granulocyte count occurs followed by a drop on the fourth or fifth day. On the tenth to fifteenth day, another transient increase occurs. Four to 6 weeks later, the lowest polymorphonuclear neutrophil count is seen. From the sixth week onward, the polymorphonuclear neutrophil percentage increases to normal.

Platelets increase for 1 to 3 days and then decrease to the lowest level between the tenth and fourteenth day, with associated hemorrhagic phenomena due to thrombocytopenia and endothelial capillary damage. After 25 to 35 days, the platelets increase to the normal level. Anemia reaches a level of severity after 20 to 30 days with a depressed reticulocyte count in 1 to 3 days. After 6 to 7 weeks reticulocytosis is evident. The greater the dose of antimitotic agent, the more severe the blood damage is, the more rapidly the blood damage develops, and the more slowly it is repaired. The lymphocyte count returns to normal first, followed by the granulocyte, platelet, and red blood cell counts. In the bone marrow, the normoblasts show pyknosis, and decreased mitosis with diminution in the number of developing red blood cells. The granulocyte and then the megakaryocyte precursors diminish in order with maximal depression after 6 to 7 days. The rate of disappearance is not related to the dose of antimitotic agent administered, but the depression lasts longer with higher doses. The damage may be irreversible, presumably

because of stem cell depletion, or a long period of recovery time is needed. Finally, aplastic anemia may develop.

The anemia itself is due to the long, cumulative effect. The incidence of aplastic anemia in Nagasaki survivors was low compared to the incidence of leukemia development and strictly not related causally to the radiation.[78] However, the incidence of hypoplastic anemia was high in both Hiroshima and Nagasaki survivors.

(6) Chemical agents that produce (occasionally) bone marrow failure include antimetabolites such as 6-mercaptopurine, folic acid antagonists, and benzene-ring drugs and chemicals—for example, chloramphenicol, arsenic preparations, hydantoin derivatives, trinitrotoluene, antithyroid drugs (Tapazole and others), antimicrobial drugs (sulfa, tetracyclines, and streptomycin), antihistamines (Pyribenzamine), insecticides (DDT, lindane, and others), atabrine, antiarthritics (phenylbutazone, gold), transquilizers (promazine derivatives and meprobamate), CCl_4, and hair and aniline dyes. In Sweden, butazones and chloramphenicol were the most common causes of aplastic anemia followed by methyldopa and sulfonamide of hemolytic anemia; dipyrone and antithyroid drugs of agranulocytosis; and oral diuretics and quinine (quinidine) of thrombocytopenia.[13]

Many aspects of how these drugs produce their hematologic effects are left unknown. Although it is known that the antimetabolites interfere with the formation of purines or nucleic acids, only a few patients develop aplastic anemia when treated with the previously mentioned drugs and chemicals. For example, although a high percentage of patients on chloramphenicol have impaired erythropoiesis with frequent vacuolation of bone marrow normoblasts, these changes are frequently reversible.[57] Aplastic anemia however does develop when large doses are used.[134] The development of bone marrow failure is erratic. It can be short- or long-term. Hypersensitivity phenomena are not demonstrated. It is quite possible that aplasia develops in an occasional patient because he has a biochemical deficiency that makes him unable to metabolize the drug or chemical, and he therefore is susceptible to its toxic effects.

(7) Malfunction of the marrow adventitia is not widely recognized as a cause of aplastic anemia. Normally, the production of blood cells can occur only in the marrow; its microcirculation provides a critical ambience. Injury to the microcirculation by some of the factors mentioned above (e.g., immune mechanism or irradiation) can destroy the proliferating marrow. Suppressor lymphocytes have been implicated in the pathogenesis of some cases of aplastic anemia. Experiments have been performed in vitro, in which all lymphocytes were removed from the aspirated marrow of patients with aplastic anemia, whereupon DNA synthesis by other marrow cells resumes and granulocyte proliferation increases. Adding the lymphocytes to normal marrow diminished granulocytic and erythrocytic hemopoiesis.[44a, 51a] The phenomenon has been demonstrated in one-third of adult patients with aplastic anemia as well as in patients with the congenital Diamond-Blackfan anemia. The recovery of a patient with aplastic anemia following cyclophosphamide therapy[7a] has led to the suggestion that the recovery may result from the destruction or depletion of the pathogenic suppressor lymphocytes. When aplastic anemia is a result of suppressor cells or humoral autoimmunity, even a syngeneic transplant is doomed unless the inhibitors are disposed.[128a] Transplantation teams should first identify patients with defective microcirculation.[28a] These patients usually have large volumes of aplastic tissue together with islands of perfectly functioning marrow, in which normal stem cells abound. The stem cells circulate, but they cannot propagate in the defective soil. Crosby feels that bone marrow transplantation carries a "dreadful, unnecessary risk,"[28a] but Storb and co-workers disagree.[141a]

Diagnosis. In anemia due to bone marrow failure, clinical symptoms are characterized by their sudden onset, which occurs when antimitotic, antimetabolite, and ionizing radiation agents are used. Gradual development occurs in cases involving idiopathic and chemical-drug causes. All symptoms depend on the severity of the pancytopenia. When anemia is severe, these oxygen-deficiency symptoms become prominent. In cases with associated agranulocytosis, infections of all types develop. Patients having thrombocytopenia develop bleeding tendencies, which may progress to hemorrhage into any body area. Waxy pallor develops into the bronzing of transfusion hemosiderosis with associated hepatosplenomegaly. If anemia is severe, one may see cardiac dilatation, hemic murmurs, and congestive heart failure.

The blood film shows a normocytic, normochromic anemia with slight macrocytosis and anisocytosis. Poikilocytosis, polyochromasia or basophilic stippling, and normoblasts in the blood are rarely seen. An examination of the red blood cell count shows an average of 500,000 to 3,500,000 per cu.mm. There is a lowering of the absolute number of reticulocytes with occasional episodes of a relative reticulocytosis of 2 to 4 per cent. The white blood cell count usually approximates 2000 to 3000 per cent cu.mm. with a 90 per cent lymphocytosis. Also, deficient granules in polymorphonuclear leukocytes with rare immature forms may be seen. The platelet count is 25,000 to 75,000 per cu.mm. with large and bizarre structures associated with a prolonged bleeding time and an abnormal capillary fragility pattern. Prothrombin consumption and clot retraction times are also prolonged (Plate 22).

Examination of the bone marrow shows a hypoplastic, normal, or hyperplastic pattern. Frequently in cases associated with the intake of benzene-ring drugs, one first sees hyperplasia followed by extensive hypocellularity. Not all marrow elements are involved simultaneously. Frequently there is excessive granulocytic immaturity with hypogranular leukocytes, and differentiating the picture from subleukemic leukemia is difficult. The maturation-arrest pattern in the normal or hyperplastic marrow is probably related to ineffective hematopoiesis plus marrow hyperplasia due to unsuccessful compensation for peripheral erythrocyte and leukocyte reduction. After many transfusions, hemosiderosis develops in the enlarged liver and spleen, with stasis in sinusoids possibly leading to increased erythrocyte breakdown. Rarely is extramedullary hematopoiesis seen in the liver and spleen (Plate 23, 27).

The serum iron is elevated, iron-binding capacity is reduced to 150 to 250 μg. per 100 ml., there is poor utilization of tracer iron for hemoglobin synthesis, and plasma iron turnover is slow. The ^{51}Cr survival measurements reveal a moderately reduced erythrocyte lifespan to a level of 80 to 100 days.

One finds it difficult to differentiate this symptom complex from subleukemic myelocytic leukemia, especially when a full-blown occult leukemia occasionally develops. This group of symptoms is not etiologically related, but possibly predisposes to leukemia development after 5 to 8 years of bone marrow failure. Frequently, one must resort to surgical marrow biopsy to rule out myelofibrosis or myelophthisic changes, especially if marrow smears are indeterminate.

Treatment and Response. The basic principle of therapy is to avoid all contact with an offending agent, if it is known. Other measures include:

1. General supportive care should be taken. All body surfaces and openings should be hygienically cared for. The diet should be well balanced. No antibacterial prophylactic therapy should be used.

2. There should be careful use of fresh blood when the hemoglobin falls below 8 g. per 100 ml. The number of transfusions should be kept to a minimum for the patient's comfort, and to delay hemosiderosis

development and hyperimmune reactions to blood groups, white blood cells, and thrombocytes. There should be careful use of platelet transfusions. That is to say, platelet donors matched for lymphocyte HL-A should be used, since multiple transfusions of platelets from random donors usually result in alloimmunization and refractoriness to additional platelet support. It is believed that the increased use of matched platelets will also help clarify the reason for the differences in immunogenicity and cross-reactivity of HL-A antigens. This knowledge, will in turn, improve techniques of replacement therapy and tissue transplantation.[156]

3. Steroids are used to control platelet deficiency and to help increase the red blood cells and their precursors in marrow and peripheral blood, with a subsequent decrease in transfusion requirements. Diamond feels that corticosteroids inhibit the division of rapidly proliferating cells such as megakaryocytes, erythrocytes, lymphocytes, and eosinophils.[32] He concludes that prolonged corticosteroid treatment affects the bone marrow in such a way that, far from improving bone marrow failures, it may reduce formation of leukocytes, platelets, and red cells.

4. Use of testosterone in conjunction with steroids occasionally bolsters the red blood cell count, especially in children. Anabolic agents appear to have greater erythropoietic activity than testosterone.[129] Androgens are especially beneficial to patients with some residual erythroid activity, and their effect is related to the production of increased erythropoietin and direct stimulation of erythroid precursors.

5. Splenectomy helps if splenomegaly is associated with ^{51}Cr radioactivity measurement over the spleen, indicating a reduced half-life of red blood cells therein and excess splenic versus hepatic participation. One may help reduce the number of transfusions by removing the site of possible splenic marrow depression and hemolysis.

6. Thymectomy is of value in 50 per cent

HL-A Typing

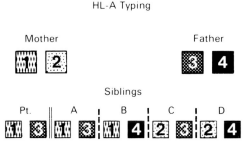

Fig. 8-5. In any family, only four types of HL-A children can result. The chromosome inheritance deduced from the phenotypes show that the HL-A types of all chidren could be accounted for by the two subloci concept. The specificities determined on each chromosome (haplo-types) are inherited as "packets." (Sensenbrenner, L., and Santos, G. W.: Rationale for marrow transplants in human disease. Presented at a symposium of the American Society of Hematology, p. 106, Dec. 4, 1971)

of cases when thymoma and refractory anemia are coassociated.

7. Bone marrow transplantation is one of the most recent advances in the treatment of bone marrow failure (i.e., severe aplastic anemia) and can now be considered the preferred form of treatment. However, there must be a suitable marrow donor, and the patient recipient must meet certain criteria. For example, the Seattle series considers only those patients for transplantation who have: a hypoplastic marrow; a platelet count less than 20,000 per cu.mm.; a granulocyte count less than 500 per cu.mm.; and a corrected reticulocyte count less than 1 per cent, in the presence of anemia.[141a] These provisions seem to pertain to patients who have a very poor prognosis with conventional treatment. However, the occasional patients who have severe aplastic anemia will recover partially or completely, while others with mild aplastic anemia will progress to the severe form of the disease. Although some information (described below) is available on the prognostic parameters of aplastic anemia, more study is needed to identify with certainty those patients who would not survive with conventional treatment.

Patients who have an identical twin or those who are given marrow grafts from HLA-identical siblings (i.e., a histocompatible sibling; Fig. 8-5) have the greatest chances for survival. The HLA antigens are glycoproteins composed of two polypeptide chains that bear the antigenic determinant and are related to the β_2-microglobulin. They are present on the surface of all human nucleated cells and are controlled by a complex genetic locus on chromosome 6, with three segregant series of antigens (HLA-A-SD, HLA-B-SD$_2$, HLA-C-SD$_3$). These antigens form the most complex immunogenetic system identified thus far in man, consisting of more than 40 SD alleles. Additionally, there exist the MLC series (mixed lymphocytic culture) consisting of a major LD and a minor LD locus, as well as the immune response (Ir) genes, which control the specific ability to respond or not respond to a specific immunogen. Detection of the HLA antigens is accomplished by serologic techniques, such as the lymphocyte microcytotoxicity test, which uses antisera to HLA antigens evoked by pregnancy, transfusion, or organ allotransplantation. The MLC determinants are detected by culturing allogenic lymphocytes and assaying radioisotopically their antigenic stimulation and response, as a reflection of the degree of genetic disparity.[126]

In addition to the crucial problems of whether a successful bone marrow transplant will be capable of restoring normal bone marrow function in defective patients, HLA tissue typing and matching of donors and recipients and numerous other complicated problems may arise. These include the presensitization of prospective recipients by previous transfusions, immunosuppression of the recipient, supportive care, and prevention of a fetal graft-host reaction with its secondary disease syndrome (Plate 60). Therefore the basic principle in a bone marrow transplant is the successful transfer of both a lymphoid and hematopoietic system from one person to another.[135]

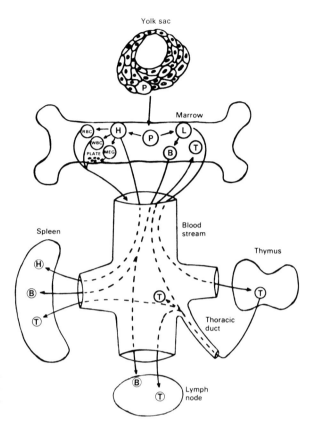

Fig. 8-6. Schematic diagram of the origin and distribution of the cells of the lymphohematopoietic system. (Redrawn after Sensenbrenner, L., and Santos, G. W.: Rationale for marrow transplants in human disease. Presented at a symposium of the American Society of Hematology, p. 106, Dec. 4, 1971)

Early in embryonic life, a group of cells in the yolk sac of mammals migrate to the various marrow areas of the body. Elucidation of the origin and distribution of the cells of the lymphohematopoietic system is shown in Figure 8-6. They are the precursor cells (P cells). P cells are pluripotent cells capable of completely repopulating both the lymphoid and hematopoietic functions. Whether such pluripotent stem cells persist in adult human marrow is an academic question. Operationally they appear still to be there. In the bone marrow cavity the P cells differentiate into either lymphoid cells (L cells) or hematopoietic cells (H cells). The H cells differentiate within the bone marrow cavity into either erythroid, myeloid, or megakaryocytic cells and their progeny. Other H cells migrate from bone marrow by way of the blood stream to other areas, such as the liver or spleen, to take up residence and differentiate to one of the three hematopoietic cell types. The L cells,

on the other hand, may go one of two directions. They may stay in the bone marrow and under the influence of the mammalian counterpart of the chicken's Bursa of Fabricius, become the LB or B cells, that is, those lymphocytes capable of producing a humoral antibody response. These short-lived B lymphocytes may stay in the bone marrow, or they may migrate out to the follicular areas of the lymph nodes or to the spleen. Other L cells leave the bone marrow and migrate to the thymus. There, under its influence, they become the T lymphocytes or L_T cells, which are the long-lived immunologic memory cells responsible primarily for cellular immune reactions, and, in certain instances, they also cooperate with B cells in certain humoral antibody responses. The T cells are found in large numbers in the peripheral blood, bone marrow of some species, thoracic duct lymph, and the paracortical areas of the lymph nodes.

In a bone marrow transplant, all of these various cell types are transplanted, and whether they grow and develop depends to a great extent upon both the humoral and the local cellular environment of the host animal. Thus, with the proper host microenvironment, bone marrow transplantation may be able to repair defects in either or both of the hosts' L or H cells.

The transplantation procedure consists of, first, conditioning the patient with either cyclophosphamide (200 mg./kg.) or total body irradiation (1000 rads) to produce immunosuppression. All the bone marrow obtainable from the anterior and posterior iliac creat areas (approximately 1 L.) of the HLA-compatible donor is then aspirated. To circumvent RBC antigenicity in the donor, 40 units should be subject to plasmapheresis and replaced with AB-negative plasma. Forty vials of Witebsky's substance (group-specific A and B material) should be administered. Afterward, the patient is transfused with the HLA-compatible donor bone marrow at a slow rate of infusion. Finally, skin biopsies every 3 months, liver function studies, and stool counts and volumes should be done routinely, and small doses of immunosuppressive drugs given from time to time.

The prognosis of most aplastic anemia cases is somewhat poor, especially when there is extensive neutropenia and thrombocytopenia, transfusion reactions, and hemosiderosis. The best responses are achieved in patients whose bone marrow show the most nearly normal cellularity prior to therapy. When marrow aplasia is marked, the likelihood of success is poor. The prospects for survival or spontaneous remission are best in patients with comparatively normal or even elevated reticulocyte levels, and reasonably good marrow cellularity. Although most cases are of unknown cause, aplastic anemia in the older adult often is a preliminary phase of myelogenous leukemia. Other causes include drug exposure, chemical intoxication, and infection by various myelopathic viruses.[17]

THE HEMOLYTIC ANEMIAS

The hemolytic anemias, due to decreased erythrocytic survival, are etiologically related to: (1) faulty erythrocyte construction produced by abnormal hemoglobin content or an intrinsic defect of erythrocytes; or (2) effects of an unfavorable environment due to autoimmune diseases, infectious agents, or poisons. Hemolysis may possibly be due to a combination of faulty erythrocyte construction and an unfavorable environment, in the idiopathic variety. Morphologic findings suggesting erythrocyte injury and hemolysis consist of spherocytic RBCs, fragmented erythrocytes (schistocytes), burr cells, and Heinz bodies (denatured hemoglobin aggregates that need a supravital stain such as methyl violet for detection). Macrocytosis and polychromasia on the stained smear indicate the marrow release of young erythrocytes. Increased breakdown of hemoglobin with associated unconjugated hyperbilirubinemia is a frequent concomitant finding; it is usually less than 4 mg. per dl. unless there is associated liver disease. In most hemolytic conditions, reticuloendothelial erythrocyte sequestration is the most common area of destruction. Terminally, the erythrocyte membrane becomes rigid with associated depletion of ATP. Jandl, in an excellent discussion on the pathophysiology of hemolytic anemias, proposes four logical nosologic approaches including cell age factors.[64]

Abnormal Hemoglobin Content

Abnormalities of Hemoglobin Associated with Heme Moiety. (Plate 28) *Carboxyhemoglobin.* Among the abnormalities of the heme moiety is carboxyhemoglobin, which is produced by the union of carbon monoxide (CO) with iron of the heme radical. It is dissociated with difficulty from hemoglobin because it is bound to it with 210 times greater affinity than oxygen. For this reason, hemoglobin carbon monoxide (HbCO) is not available for oxygen transportation by hemoglobin, and tissue anoxia therefore results from this decreased oxygen transportation. Furthermore, even a small percentage of HbCO alters the dissociation curve of normal hemoglobin so that normal hemoglobin also gives up its oxygen less readily. Chief sources of HbCO poisoning are automobiles and instruments that use gasoline. Symptoms do not occur until 26 to 30 per cent blood gas saturation occurs; smaller concentrations cause symptoms in children. These symptoms are headache, dizziness, muscular weakness, and nausea. The symptoms disappear for the most part after 1 to 2 hours of air respiration. Blood with a high concentration of HbCO has a cherry-red color. When clinically suspected, monoxide poisoning can be confirmed by diluting blood, which produces a pink-bluish red color. Spectral absorption produces bands at 576 mμ like those of oxyhemoglobin. (Blood for this should be collected in dry sodium citrate tubes.)

Methemoglobin. Another hemoglobin abnormality associated with the heme moiety is methemoglobin, the presence of which is frequently associated with sulfhemoglobinemia and characterized by cyanosis with severe symptoms consisting of exertional dyspnea, headache, dizziness, euphoria and blurred mental functions. Methemoglobin (MHb) is formed when the ferrous iron in hemoglobin is oxidized to ferric iron, in which it cannot be oxygenated (cannot carry oxygen), but is easily reduced to hemoglobin. When a patient is removed from further exposure to drugs that act as direct and indirect oxidants, a reversion back to hemoglobin is complete within 24 to 48 hours. Methemoglobinemia occurs when there is dysfunction of the specific erythrocyte enzyme system that uses glucose and lactate or when hemoglobin is oxidized at a rate that exceeds the reducing capacity of the system.

Acute or secondary methemoglobinemia reduces oxygen tension and the dissociation curve is altered; therefore, less oxygen is available for hemoglobin transport, resulting in the elevation of blood lactate levels in muscular exertion when methe-

moglobin is present in concentrations of 10 to 50 per cent. Drugs that act as direct oxidants include nitrites, chlorates, quinones, and nitrates in infants ($BiONO_3$ and well water; the nitrates are reduced to nitrites in the gastrointestinal tract). Drugs that act as indirect oxidants are aniline and its derivatives (from aniline-stamped diapers, dyed shoes and blankets, and colored wax crayons), sulfanilamide, Prontosil, sulfathiazole, sulfapyridine, acetanilid, and phenacetin.

Diagnosis is partially made when cyanosis is present without cardiovascular or respiratory disease. Normally one may have 0.06 to 0.24 g. per 100 ml. of methemoglobin in blood. Cyanosis may occur with 0.5 g. per 100 ml. of methemoglobin in blood. If venous blood becomes chocolate brown when shaken with air for 15 minutes, methemoglobinemia should be suspected. The diagnosis is confirmed spectroscopically using a 1:100 aqueous dilution of blood. This will show an absorption band at 635 mμ, which disappears after addition of a few drops of 5 per cent KCN solution. Therapeutically, when the oxidant is removed, methemoglobin will rapidly convert to hemoglobin. If hypoxia is present, a 1 per cent aqueous solution of methylene blue may be used (1 to 2 mg./kg. of body weight) when given over a period of several minutes. The methylene blue solution may be given at hourly intervals if necessary. Heinz bodies are also seen in some of the red blood cells, especially with the ingestion of some chemicals.

Primary or congenital methemoglobinemia is an inborn error of metabolism caused by the failure of the intracellular reducing enzyme system. There are three types. One type is caused by specific deficiency in erythrocyte DPN-linked diaphorase (a recessive trait), which is necessary for the conversion of methemoglobin Fe^{+++} to hemoglobin Fe^{++}. Another type is caused by an abnormality in glutathione metabolism (dominant trait). Recent work by Prins and associates[118] indicates that the erythrocyte depends very little on glutathione for reducing methemoglobin and contradicts the interpretation made by other workers that this variant of congenital methemoglobinemia results from a much smaller deficiency of glutathione. The third type is caused by the presence of many M-type methemoglobins having different spectral properties. These types of methemoglobin are resistant to reduction to hemoglobin by the normal erythrocyte enzymes because of a globin defect. This type of methemoglobinemia is characterized by gray or slate blue cyanosis at birth occasionally with compensatory polycythemia. Venous blood of this type is brown when shaken in air and does not return to normal color (635 mμ, except the M type at 602 to 622 mμ). Treatment is with methylene blue and ascorbic acid, except in the M type.

Sulfhemoglobin is another hemoglobin abnormality associated with the heme moiety. Most clinical findings in sulfhemoglobinemia are similar to those in methemoglobinemia. Sulfhemoglobin is greenish and its exact chemical formula is not known, but it may be produced by the interaction of hydrogen sulfide with oxyhemoglobin. It cannot be oxygenated or reconverted to hemoglobin, it does not alter the erythrocyte life span, and it is lost from the circulation after the red blood cell breaks down (120 days). The concentration in vivo seldom exceeds 10 per cent, and therefore it seldom endangers life. Sulfhemoglobin is produced by some of the compounds that produce methemoglobin; they frequently coexist. The absorption band of sulfhemoglobin is at 618 mμ and is unaffected by the addition of KCN.

Porphyrin. The porphyrins are iron-free pyrrole pigments derived from hemoglobin and constitute the final heme moiety abnormality. The immediate precursors of the heme moiety is porphyrin III and is formed mainly from glycine. Porphyrin I is first formed; this takes no part in hemoglobin formation, but is excreted as coproporphyrin I in the urine, bile, and feces. The small excess of porphyrin III is excreted as coproporphyrin III. Therefore, coproporphyrin I in the urine and feces indicates the healthy maturation of red blood cells, but an excess of coproporphyrin III suggests failure in the synthesis of porphyrin III to hemoglobin. This failure is usually caused by the toxic effects of arsenicals, lead, cinchophen, Sulfonal, and in hemosiderosis. Porphyria is a disease complex characterized by skin lesions sometimes associated with light hypersensitivity. Abdominal colic, psychoses, and neurologic manifestations also occur in some cases. It may be subdivided into two main groups: porphyria erythropoietica and hepatic porphyria.

Porphyria erythropoietica, or congenital porphyria, is an inborn error of metabolism characterized by excessive quantities of porphyrins synthesized in the bone marrow. It is first observed as the Burgundy-red or port-wine staining of diapers by the affected urine, which turns dark on exposure to light. This is also seen in the cutanea tarda symptomatica type of hepatic porphyria and is due to the exessive amounts of preformed uroporphyrin I and to a smaller degree by excessive amounts of preformed coproporphyrin I. Also seen are erythematous, bullous skin lesions, which are exacerbated by light because of photosensitivity due to subcutaneous uroporphyrin. Teeth, nails, and bones have a red to brown to yellowish color (uroporphyrin I).

Hematologically there is a mild, albeit hemolytic, anemia characterized by punctate basophilia, polychromatophilia, normoblastosis, reticulocytosis, shortened erythrocyte life span, and splenomegaly. Fluorescence of bone marrow smears reveals a red color due to prophyrins in the abnormal normoblasts. Destruction of these cells releases porphyrins into the plasma with subsequent uroporphyrinuria. Patients having uroporphyrinuria must be protected from light; they are occasionally helped by splenectomy. No abdominal or neurologic symptoms are seen; porphobilinogen is absent. Laboratory diagnosis is made by testing urine for uroporphyrins (after an extraction process) and detecting a red fluorescence under a Wood lamp (ultraviolet light).

The other type of porphyria is the hepatic type, in which excessive porphyrin and porphyrin precursor production occurs in the liver. Hepatic porphyria may be subdivided into three types: acute intermittent porphyria, porphyria cutanea tarda hereditaria, and porphyria cutanea tarda symptomatica.

Acute intermittent porphyria is characterized clinically in patients 15 to 40 years old by intermittent bouts of abdominal pain with varied neurologic and psychiatric disturbances. The relation between the biochemical disorder and its signs and symptoms is obscure. Many types of porphyrins and their precursors appear in the urine. Most of these urinary porphyrins arise from the precursors after the urine has been passed, and because of this the urine usually darkens on standing. Thus, freshly passed urine in intermittent porphyria and porphyria cutanea tarda hereditaria is colorless because the principal compound excreted is colorless porphobilinogen. On exposure to air, at an acid pH, the porphobilinogen condenses to uroporphyrinogen and is then oxidized to uroporphyrin, causing the urine to darken to a port-wine color. Usually porphobilinogen is identified by its reaction with Ehrlich's aldehyde reagent (p-dimethylaminobenzaldehyde) as modified in the Watson-Schwartz test.[148]

In this test, 2.5 ml. of fresh urine is placed in a test tube, and 2.5 ml. of Ehrlich's reagent is added. The mixture is shaken, and after exactly 15 seconds 5 ml. of saturated sodium acetate is added. Then 5 ml. of chloroform is added, and the test tube is shaken and centrifuged. A positive reaction is indicated by the development of a strong red (or red-purple) color limited to the upper, aqueous phase. If the reaction is strongly positive, it may be differentiated from drugs that give a false positive by spectroscopic examination of the upper aqueous phase (red-purple), which shows a characteristic strong absorption band at 560 mμ. The symptomatic form may be seen as a complication of alcoholic cirrhosis of the liver or as the result of a metabolic defect in the liver. In this case uroporphyrins, not porpholibinogen, are found.

Abnormalities of Hemoglobin Associated with the Globin Moiety. *Characteristics of Various Hemoglobins.* The hemoglobin molecule is composed of two moieties; one is an iron-containing pigment (a ferroporphyrin) called heme (in fact, four hemes are attached to the protein component). Interference with the heme component is seen in the hypochromic microcytic or iron-deficiency anemias and in the macrocytic anemias due to vitamin B_{12} and folic acid deficiencies, and in the anemias in which oxygen transport is interfered with by various chemicals and drugs. The other moiety is a protein called globin. The combination of heme and globin to form hemoglobin has for its chief function the transportation of oxygen.

In the normal adult, there are three physiologic hemoglobins that vary in their globin moiety and that are genetically controlled. The hemoglobin of the fetus differs in many aspects from that of the adult, especially in its increased resistance to alkali denaturation. Later in pregnancy, the adult type of hemoglobin begins to be synthesized. Thus, at birth the newborn infant's blood contains about 80 per cent of the fetal hemoglobin (Hb F) and 20 per cent of the adult type of hemoglobin (Hb A and Hb A$_2$). Fetal hemoglobin decreases until at 6 months of age there is less than 5 per cent left. If there is more than 5 per cent, some abnormality should be suspected. In fact, modest increases in alkali-resistant hemoglobin (Hb F) have been found in adults who have malignant marrow neoplasms, marrow hypoplasia, benign monoclonal gammopathy, and premalignant disorders such as evolving myelomonocytic leukemia. These increases indicate that careful evaluation for serious underlying disease is

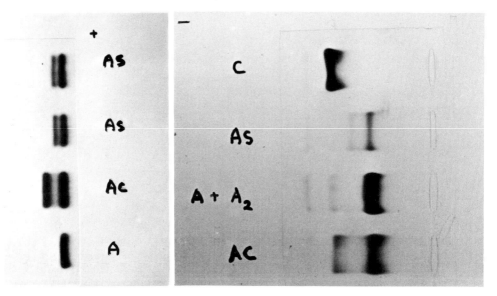

Fig. 8-7. Agar gel hemoglobin electrophoretic patterns. AS = Sickle cell trait. AC = Hemoglobin C trait. A = Normal adult. A + A₂ = Normal adult. C = Hemoglobin C disease.

required in patients with anemia or dysproteinemia and elevated levels of hemoglobin F.[110] In addition, there are several different genes for Hb F, hereditary persistence of fetal hemoglobin (HPFH), with 15 to 20 per cent Hb F found, with electrophoresis, to be evenly distributed (by acid elution) in the erythrocyte of the common type associated with Black people. The distribution is uneven in β-thalassemia trait patients, an important criterion for differential diagnosis.

The change from Hb F (fetal protein) to Hb A and Hb A₂ (adult protein) occurs dynamically at a molecular level. Adult hemoglobin contains four polypeptide chains (2 α and 2 β) and fetal hemoglobin contains two α and two γ chains. These three polypeptide chains are all chemically different. The α chain is associated with both fetal and adult hemoglobin synthesis, whereas the γ chain is part of the fetal hemoglobin molecule and the β chain is part of the adult hemoglobin molecule. The α chain, being needed for both fetal and adult hemoglobins production, remains constant. The γ chains decrease greatly following birth, dropping to an approximate zero level by the time the infant is 6 months old. At the same time the β polypeptide chain of the adult hemoglobin increases. Thus, the α chain gene func-

tions constantly, whereas the γ chain gene production slowly diminishes and the β chain gene production slowly increases. Based on a system of integrated regulator, operator, and structural genes,[58] the switching from fetal to adult hemoglobin production ensures that the adult has adult hemoglobin and the fetus has fetal hemoglobin.[60]

In a number of hematologic abnormalities, quantitative alterations in the relative percentages of these three normal hemoglobins may occur, or quantitative abnormalities of the globin molecule may be found characterized by changes in its amino acid composition (α, β, γ, and σ polypeptide chains). To date, only one amino acid substitution has been found in each of the abnormal hemoglobins. The genetic control of the production of these chains is mediated via autosomal alleles whose precise location on the chromosome is not known.

Hemoglobinopathies fall into four categories: (1) abnormal hemoglobins or mutations that are not associated with pathologic changes or altered physiology but that may be demonstrated on electrophoresis; (2) mutations that produce clinical findings in homozygotes (Hb S, Hb E, and Hb C) and interact with the β-thalassemias (their high frequency in different races is important); (3) mutations that are associated with

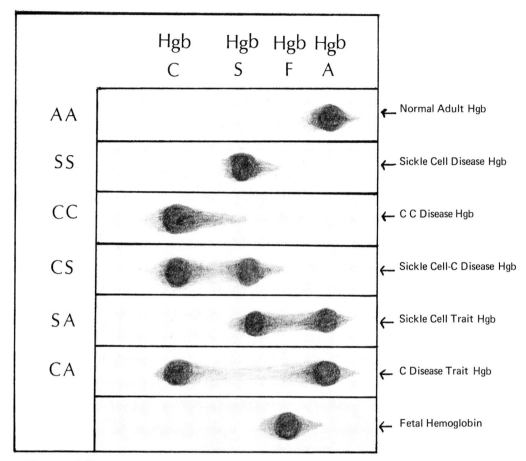

Fig. 8-8. Differential analyses of hemoglobins by electrophoresis. AA—normal adult; SS—sickle cell disease; CC—C disease; CS—sickle cell C disease; SA—sickle cell trait; CA—C disease trait; F—fetal hemoglobin. (Whitby, L. E. H., and Britton, C. J. C.: Disorders of the Blood. ed. 9. London, J. & A. Churchill, 1963)

varying degrees of hemolytic anemias secondary to destabilization of the molecule (Heinz bodies are frequently seen after splenectomy in these cases); (4) mutations in which the molecule's oxygen affinity is altered (i.e., erythrocytosis is associated with a high affinity, which is clinically difficult to distinguish from polycythemia vera and, cyanosis is associated with a grossly low affinity, and anemia with a slightly low affinity). Some of these mutations may not be detectable by electrophoresis.

During the last 10 years, a number of hemoglobin variants have been described, the first of which was hemoglobin S (Hb S), found in sickle cell anemia. The others have been labeled hemoglobin C, hemoglobin D, hemoglobin E, hemoglobin G, hemoglobin H, hemoglobin I, hemoglobin J, and so on, in the order of their discovery. These hemoglobin variants are all permanent and inherited; the differences are in their globin molecules (Figs. 8-7, 8-8).

Disorders in which the presence of a structurally abnormal hemoglobin is considered to play an important pathologic role are referred to as hemoglobinopathies. Disorders involving alterations in the percentages of presumably normal forms of hemoglobin are generally designated by individually descriptive terms—for example, thalassemia. In some hemoglobinopathies, all the hemoglobin is in one abnormal form. In others, two abnormal hemoglobins may be present. In still others, normal and abnormal hemoglobins are found together.

Two forms of each abnormal condition can be differentiated. They differ in severity.

Altered oxygen dissociation curves have recently been described for abnormal hemoglobins. A "left-shift" dissociation curve, resulting in less oxygen available to the tissues, indicates hypoxia. A "right-shift" dissociation curve occurs when an increased red cell mass is accompanied by chronic erythropoietin stimulation. Only mild anemia develops since a normal erythrocyte mass is not required for adequate oxygen delivery to tissues. A hemoglobinopathy should be suspected whenever there is an increased red cell mass without tumors or pulmonary disease.

When both parents transmit the same abnormality to their offspring — when the child receives abnormal genes from both parents — the condition in the child represents the homozygous state. In the case of the sickle cell gene or the thalassemia gene, the homozygous condition is referred to as sickle cell anemia or thalassemia major and is usually more severe than in the heterozygous state. When only one parent transmits an abnormality to his offspring, the child represents the heterozygous state, and one refers to the condition as sickle cell trait or thalassemia minor (thalassemia trait). When one or both parents are heterozygous for one of these diseases, it is likely that the abnormality will occur in the offspring.

In some of these diseases, especially in the homozygous states, the hemoglobin abnormality leads to an increased rate of erythrocyte destruction. The presence of target cells in the peripheral blood is characteristic of most hemoglobinopathies, although it is not specific for them.

Recent observations relating certain minor hemoglobins (A_{1a}, A_{1b}, A_{1c}) with hyperglycemia in animals and man and with certain short-term sequelae of diabetes have suggested an additional relation to diabetes mellitus. Because of its normally high concentration (3–6% of total Hb), Hb A_{1c} has been studied most extensively. It has the same amino acid sequence as Hb A, but additionally has a sodium borohydridereducible hexose at the proposed to be 1 amino, 1 deoxy, fructose. Because circulating RBCs cannot initiate protein synthesis, the production of Hb A_{1c} is a modification of the already synthesized Hb A molecule. The rate of modification appears to depend on the mean circulatory glucose levels to which the RBC is exposed. Hb A_{1c} (and perhaps Hb A_{1b} and Hb A_{1c}) appears to be the index or integrator to the patient's mean blood glucose concentration for the preceding weeks to months. Short-term fluctuations in blood sugar do not influence the measurement of Hb A_{1c}, but changes lasting more than 1 week are reflected in its levels. Periodic evaluation of Hb A_{1c} levels should provide a more objective assessment of carbohydrate control and an improved evaluation of treatment regimens than has previously been possible. Similarly, cholesterol and triglyceride levels in diabetic patients have been shown to be directly related to HB A_{1c} levels.[116]

The following approach will usually lead to an elucidation of a suspected hemoglobinopathy: (1) a full history, including arthralgia, pain crises, and the occurrence of the same symptoms in other family members; (2) a physical examination, including hepatosplenomegaly early in life; (3) a complete blood count, including the study of stained film; (4) blood indices (MCV, MCH, and MCHC, including hematocrit); (5) reticulocyte count and determination of inclusion bodies (hemoglobin H); (6) sickle cell preparation of blood film; (7) solubility determinations for differentiation between hemoglobin S and hemoglobin D; and (8) an osmotic fragility determination, alkaline denaturation tests, paper electrophoresis and chromatography (Figs. 8-7; 8-8).

Hemoglobinopathies in Man. There are several conditions in which normal hemoglobin is replaced by one or two abnormal variants. One of the more common entities is sickle cell anemia (homozygous hemoglobin S disease), which occurs in one of 600 American Blacks as a hereditary, chronic hemolytic process. If it occurs in non-blacks, it is usually due to a combination of Hb S with other hemoglobin abnormalities, the presence of Hb S with thalassemia, or some degree of Black ancestry. Hemoglobin S is present in amounts of 50 to 70 per cent, with 2 to 30 per cent of Hb F on electrophoretic analysis. No Hb A is seen. Finally, a person with a high proportion of African genes is likely to inherit both sickle cell disease and G-6-PD deficiency. The frequency of G-6-PD deficiency appears to be somewhat higher in patients with sickle cell disease than in the general Afro-American population with the usual or unfavorable effect on the clinical pattern.[11]

Hematologically, a normochromic anemia is seen with a normal MCV, MCH, and MCHC (red blood cells may be slightly macrocytic). The red blood cell count averages 2,500,000 per cu.mm.; hemoglobin levels are between 7 and 8 gm. per 100 ml.; mild leukocytosis is observed; and leptocytosis (target cells), polychromasia, occasional sickled red blood cells in direct smear, and occasional normoblasts are seen. Reticulocytosis, erythroid marrow hyperplasia, and shortened erythrocyte survival time also occur (Plates 29, 30).

Sickle cell anemia is characterized by two main clinical features: chronic hemolytic anemia, and episodic painful crises. Although Hb S is freely soluble when oxygenated (the erythrocytes usually appear normal in ordinary blood smears, with occasional to minimal sickling), upon deoxygenation the red blood cells form irregular elongated masses called tactoids, producing the irregular sickle cell shapes.

At equal levels of oxygen saturation, sickling is increased in cells with a high 2,3-DPG content, and reduced in RBCs with a low 2,3-DPG content. Because 2,3-DPG stabilizes the deoxy configuration of hemoglobin, it may favor the aggregation of the hemoglobin S molecule at a specific oxygen maturation level. Therefore, therapy that lowers the RBC 2,3-DPG content may prove beneficial.[66]

Reduced phosphorylation of spectrin has been found in membranes from sickle cells,[54] as has a reorientation of choline phosphatides from inner to outer portions of the membrane. Such changes in phospholipid organization are accompanied by an increased susceptibility to lipid peroxidation.[23]

A quantitative change in shape is directly associated with increased viscosity of the blood, producing the painful crises. The greater mechanical fragility of the red blood cells explains the hemolytic process. It has been suggested that circulating sickled cells are subject to avulsion of their processes by mechanical injury. Such cells may undergo either immediate hemolysis or transformation into spherocytes that are subject to erythrophagocytosis.[67]

The changes in cell shape and the mechanical fragility of the cell cause the flow of blood to be impeded, resulting in anoxia, and they cause an increase in the sickling in vivo. The increase in sickling, in turn, increases the blood viscosity and consequently further decreases the blood flow. This vicious circle leads to localized ischemia and ultimately to infarction. The crises caused by sickled red blood cells producing vascular occlusion affect one or more organs, or the body as a whole. Vascular obstruction is maximal in capillaries. Associated phenomena include vasospasm, loss of fluid into perivascular spaces, hemoconcentration, and fibrin formation. In addition, the vascular wall is damaged by the repeated "logjamming" of small vessels, which facilitates platelet aggregation and fibrin deposition at the site of injury. It is possible that the chronic use of antiplatelet-aggregating agents would reduce the frequency of crises.[125] Recurrent painful and febrile crises with pains in bones, joints, and abdomen plague these patients throughout life. Priapism and regurgitation jaundice are produced by stasis of sickled red blood cells in venous and hepatic sinuses. Diffuse erythrocyte sickling in the body may lead to sudden death. Ischemia, infarction, and necrosis may occur in all organs.

The most common lesions are the hand-foot syndrome in young children,[33] skull changes, gallstones, aseptic necrosis of the femur and humerus, encephalopathies, retinopathies, papillary renal necrosis with hematuria, and infarcts of the spleen (autosplenectomy), intestine, lymph nodes, genital organs, and endocrine glands. Clots are observed in capillaries and veins, but thrombi in larger arteries of the systemic circulation are rare. Pulmonary arterial emboli in the lungs, composed mostly of aggregates of sickled cells, are common. Infarcts of the bone marrow result in fat emboli. In rare instances, there is the alteration in the balance between blood formation and destruction, producing hematologic crises of the aplastic or hemolytic types. Mortality is high in infants and children, with very few patients reaching the 30- to 45-year age group. These patients are resistant to *Plasmodium falciparum* malaria, but are very sensitive to salmonella infection. Furthermore, high concentrations of hemoglobin F appear to protect homozygous sickle cell anemia patients from sickling phenomenon (Fig. 8-14).[115]

Therapy of sickle cell anemia has been quite variable, frustrating nonspecific, and usually dealt only with the complications. Recently chemical inhibitors such as sodium cyanate have been used to increase oxygen affinity (the oxygen dissociation curve shifts to the left), to cross-link hemoglobin into a conformation that cannot aggregate, or to interfere with sickling by steric hindrance. These chemicals must penetrate the cell membrane; otherwise they may alter it and prevent sickling but produce hemolysis. Also, extracorporeal treatment of erythrocytes, perhaps with sodium cyanate, is a very promising new approach. It must be borne in mind, however, that neurotoxicity precludes its routine use. Chronic transfusion therapy may be used to prevent crises, although this is not proved; however, it has been advocated

for use before major surgery, in the last trimester of pregnancy, for leg ulcers, priapism, and other complications. When hypoxia may contribute to massive sickling, exchange transfusions have been attempted. However, there is no evidence that heparin, dextran, oxygen, alkali, transfusion, or intravenous fluids shorten crises, although for each of these treatments there are specific indications. In most cases, painful crises generally improve in a few days to a week regardless of the physician's efforts. Antibiotics are of no use unless infection is present; it is safer to get cultures than to treat empirically.

Sickle cell trait is the variant of sickle cell anemia in which all symptoms are far less severe. Electrophoretically, Hb S makes up less than 50 per cent of the red blood cell; the remainder is Hb A. Under normal conditions, sickling does not occur in the body, and sickling cannot be seen on ordinary blood films unless oxygen tension is reduced by using the sodium metabisulfite method. Clinically, patients having sickle cell trait are well except for occasional episodes of hematuria and side effects of lowered oxygen tension associated with high altitude flying, which may result in splenic infarction and possible other vascular episodes attributable to thrombosis. Also, the specific gravity of the urine is low, and amino-aciduria occurs.

Other Hemoglobinopathies (Fig. 8-14). Disease states caused by abnormal hemoglobins constitute a group of less commonly occurring hemoglobinopathies.[70] In these entities, the disease represents a homozygous state in which the red blood cells contain solely the abnormal hemoglobin. These disease states are associated with a relatively rare, mild, chronic hemolytic anemia resulting in slight fatigue, weakness, occasional intermittent bone and joint pain, mild icterus, and moderate splenomegaly. In Hb C disease, seen in one out of 6000 American Blacks, about 100 per cent of the hemoglobin is Hb C, the rest being Hb F. Hemoglobin C is present in both parents.

The anemia is slightly microcytic and normochromic with 80 per cent or more target cells (leptocytosis). Also occurring are microspherocytosis, crystal-like erythrocyte inclusions that are more numerous after splenectomy, moderate erythroid hyperplasia, and slight reticulocytosis. The survival time of the red blood cell is mildly decreased, and there is a decrease in osmotic fragility.

Charache and Conley believe that the erythrocytes in C-C disease are abnormally rigid, and that decreased solubility in Hb C may be the basic pathophysiologic disorder in C-C disease, leading to the increased rigidity of erythrocytes, microspherocyte production, hemoglobin crystallization, and premature sequestration and destruction of erythrocytes.[21] Disease involving Hb D is similar, but milder. In the trait forms, Hb A combines with Hb C, Hb D, and so on. C trait also has an increase in target cells; the other trait diseases show no target cells to only a few target cells (Plate 31).

Inherited Defects in the Production of Hemoglobin A. Thalassemia Major. Thalassemia major (Cooley's anemia, Mediterranean anemia, hereditary leptocytosis) was the first hemoglobinopathic anemia for which a familial incidence (usually in people of Mediterranean stock) was described. Both parents of patients having thalassemia major must have thalassemia minor; only a few cases have been reported without this arrangement. However, although there is interference in the production of Hb A, there is no abnormal hemoglobin present. It may be said that patients with thalassemia are unable to synthesize normal amounts of Hb A, but are able to produce normal to increased quantities of Hb F or Hb A_2. There are multiple genetic factors with basic biochemical variations involved in the many genetically different forms of thalassemia.

The defects in hemoglobin synthesis may be demonstrated in many ways: (1) There is a reduction in the incorporation of precursors into hemoglobin with both impairment of protoporphyrin synthesis and the partial inability to incorporate iron into protoporphyrin to form heme. (2) There is a partial suppression of the formation of normal α or β chains. There may be synthesis of abnormal α or β chains, the blocking of normal α and β chains linkage, or the operation of an abnormal suppressor mechanism regulating β chain production. In the last instance a defective messenger RNA molecule that blocks the synthetic activity of the cell ribosome is produced so that very few β polypeptide chains are produced. Expressed another way, one might say that the underlying problem in thalassemia is a deficiency or lack of the specific messenger RNA required as a template for globin peptide synthesis, which produces an imbalance in the synthesis of alpha and beta chain subunits of hemoglobin A ($\alpha_2\ \beta_2$). Beta chain synthesis is decidedly suppressed or even absent in homozygous beta thalassemia, leading to the accumulation of excess alpha chains and the subsequent membrane injury and marrow death of maturing RBCs. Thus, there is ineffective erythropoiesis with associated marrow erythroid hyperplasia and subnormal production of viable circulating RBCs. Half-life ^{51}Cr studies of peripheral blood usually demonstrate only moderate shortening. However, patients with severe splenomegaly and high transfusion requirements may be helped by splenectomy. There is a severe compensatory increase in the synthesis of hemoglobin F ($\alpha_2\ \gamma_2$) in homozygotes who have beta thalassemia. The increased levels of hemoglobin A_2 ($\alpha_2\ \Delta_2$) in heterozygotes may be helpful in a diagnosis. Finally, alpha thalassemia is a lethal homozygous state, for there are no mechanisms to compensate for a defect in the synthesis of alpha chains, but heterozygous alpha thalassemia is practically harmless in most instances. (3) There is an increase in the formation of Hb F. (4) The levels of Hb A_2 are elevated.

Clinically, thalassemia major is the expression of homozygosity for an abnormal gene, and it is characterized by onset in infancy and childhood associated with physical retardation in development, prominent frontal bossing, mongoloid facies, icterus, marked hepatosplenomegaly associated with extramedullary hematopoiesis, marked marrow erythroid hyperplasia with associated increased trabeculation and thinned cortices of long bones, and the hair-on-end appearance of the flat skull bones.

In thalassemia major, there is also a hypochromic, microcytic anemia with decreased MCV, MCH, and in many cases a decreased MCHC. Blood films show anisocytosis, poikilocytosis, "safety-pin" forms with schistocytosis, target cells, stippled cells, normoblastosis, (which after splenectomy may be very marked), reticulocytosis, and moderate leukocytosis with a shift to left. Osmotic fragility is decreased, some red blood cells even remain intact when suspended in distilled water. The erythrocyte survival times, using ^{51}Cr, are markedly reduced. Serum iron levels are high, with the marrow iron content normal or high (demonstrated by hemosiderin stain) (Plate 31).

Three major cytochemical abnormalities have been demonstrated in the early normoblasts and minimally in the erythrocytes in thalassemia major: deposition of large amounts of iron-containing material; accumulation of a PAS-positive substance; and the presence of hemoglobin precipitates.[41] Early normoblasts with PAS-positive granules also occur fairly regularly in sideroblastic anemias, Di Guglielmo's syndrome, and iron deficiency anemias. By the alkali denaturation test and electrophoretically, Hb F may be elevated to a level of 90 per cent or more. The values of Hb A_2 are normal.

The measurement of an increased A_2 hemoglobin by cellulose acetate hemoglobin electrophoresis is not accurate and is fraught with dangers of both false-positive and false-negative results. A substantial increase in A_2 hemoglobin is usually between 3.5 to 5.0 per cent. While this is sufficient to indicate impaired β-chain synthesis and β thalassemia, it is not a concentration high enough to be accurately measured by direct densitometry of the cellulose acetate electrophoretic strip. Errors with electrophoresis are mostly false elevations of A_2 that can result in an iatrogenic thalassemia.[159] Therefore, the use of the electronic blood count (hemoglobin, MCV, MCH, and MCHC), microcolumn technique (A_2 hemoglobin), and hemoglobin electrophoresis are recommended for thalessemia screening. Electrophoresis will detect other hemoglobinopathies and a high hemoglobin F. When the MCV is low and the A_2 hemoglobin is borderline, an iron serum and an examination of a peripheral blood smear are recommended. If results are still equivocal, it may be necessary to do family studies and radiochromatography.[56]

The patient's life is shortened because of complicating factors, such as interstitial pancreatic myocardial fibrosis, cardiac dilatation, and hemosiderosis of the liver and skin—all secondary to exogenous iron overload after years of multiple transfusions. Congestive heart failure and cardiac arrhythmias result in death usually before 20 years of age. Hemosiderosis also appears to be reasonably associated with a high dietary intake of iron and a low dietary intake of folic acid.[113] Splenectomized patients are frequently subject to pneumococcal infections, especially if the splenectomy was performed before age 5, when antibody formation is somehow intimately associated with the spleen. This procedure (splenectomy) should only be performed in those patients who manifest thrombocytopenia, leukopenia, or an increasing transfusion requirement. An attempt is made to maintain patients with blood transfusions at the lowest hemoglobin values consonant with their comfort—usually between 7 and 7.5 g. per 100 ml. Hypertransfusion to maintain a normal hemoglobin level leads to normal body growth and prevents bony deformities; however, it does result in increased iron.

Marked urinary excretion of iron can be obtained utilizing desferrioxamine administered subcutaneously by portable pump, and ascorbic acid as agents in iron chelation therapy. Many patients die from cardiac or hepatic failure or hepatoma, even though the removal of excessive iron stores (as much as 20 g. or more) improves the prognosis. Recent work has shown that β thalassemic major erythrocytes have increased susceptibility to lipid peroxidation. Evidence for lipid peroxidation has been demonstrated in vivo by decreases in red cell polyunsaturated fatty acids and in the concentration of serum vitamin E. In several thalassemia patients, oral vitamin E supplement improved red cell survival. Cardiac toxicity may occur with high doses of vitamin C, which mobilizes iron for chelation.[120]

Thalassemia minor, minima, or trait is the heterozygous form of these diseases (Plate 32). Patients are relatively symptomless except for a mild anemia associated with little or no reduction in hemoglobin concentration. Occasionally present are polycythemia and microcytosis and with mild or moderate erythrocyte deformities such as ovalocytosis, poikilocytosis, and leptocytosis. The MCV and MCH are usually decreased; the MCHC may be normal.

Electronic measurement of the MCV (Coulter Counter Model S) has been used to screen for thalassemia trait. Hb A_2 was measured in all subjects with MCVs less than 79 cu.μ to identify those with β-thalassemia. For those with less than 3.5 per cent Hb A_2, a serum iron determination differentiated microcytosis due to iron deficiency. The alpha thalassemia trait can be diagnosed followed family studies. Therefore, consideration of thalassemia whenever microcytosis is detected could be useful in preventing ineffective iron administration.[114] Osmotic fragility is decreased. There is a characteristic elevation in the Hb A_2 fraction, which must be quantified by elution from the cellulose acetate electrophoresis strips and then by spectropho-

tometry in order to be more informative.[158] Occasionally, a Hb F of 5 to 10 per cent is present. Variants of thalassemia may be seen in families with familial microcytosis in which it is difficult to tell whether the disorder is severe thalassemia trait or mild thalassemia major.

Recently, an unusual variant of β-thalassemia trait has been described. People heterozygous for it occasionally exhibit anemia, marked abnormalities in erythrocyte and normoblast morphology, and splenic enlargement. It has been designated inclusion body β-thalassemia trait. The bone marrow material shows large, usually single cytoplasmic inclusions (precipitated α-chains) with methyl violet staining. It is thought that the β-thalassemia mutation distorts the hemoglobin chain synthesis in the erythroid precursors of the heterozygotes, and that this aggravates their clinical course.[141]

Combinations of Thalassemia Minor and Abnormal Heterozygous Hemoglobin. There are a number of combinations of thalassemia minor and abnormal heterozygous hemoglobin possible because either the thalassemia defect or the hemoglobin defect may be present in homozygous or heterozygous forms. Thus, a wide variety of combinations and a multitude of clinical disorders are possible that may in turn suppress the formation of Hb A as effectively as homozygosity for the abnormal hemoglobin gene itself.

Thalassemia-hemoglobin S disease is a disorder that combines the features of sickle cell anemia and thalassemia. Each parent contributes an abnormal gene: for example, the father may contribute the thalassemia gene, and the mother may contribute the Hb S gene. It is possible for one of the parents to transmit both the abnormalities because they are genetically independent. The disorder is clinically characterized by leg ulcers, periodic painful crises, sickling of the red blood cells, marked splenomegaly, hypochromic microcytosis, leptocytosis and stippling. The symptoms may be severe or mild in either member of the complex. In many cases family studies are necessary to confirm the diagnosis.

Thalassemia in combination with Hb C, Hb D, Hb E, Hb G, and Hb H are complexes basically indistinguishable from uncomplicated thalassemias except for the combination of thalassemia and Hb H, which is not found in either parent, although generally one of the parents is a carrier of thalassemia minor. Spherical inclusion bodies, stained with supravital dyes, are suggestive of this combination.

Electrophoresis reveals that Hb H ($\beta 4$) is a fast-moving hemoglobin and is very unstable. The condition results from interaction of α-thalassemia-1 and α-thalassemia-2 or α-thalassemia-1 and Hb Constant Spring (a gene causing an elongated α-chain with a very low rate of synthesis). All the α-thalassemia traits are associated with microcytosis in the neonate and varying amounts of Hb Bart's and are more easily diagnosed at this age than in adults. A mild α-thalassemia gene may be quite common in Blacks and is very common in Arabs. A case of hydrops fetalis associated with Hb H (Barts) has been reported in a Chinese family.[71] The peripheral blood pattern was similar to that in erythroblastosis fetalis plus some erythrocytic sickling and a negative direct Coombs test. A family study revealed that the father was doubly heterozygous for α and β thalassemia trait and his disease was similar in severity to β thalassemia trait.

Laboratory Tests (Fig. 8-14). Laboratory tests used in the diagnosis of hemoglobinopathies depend on the clinical situation. They should include a complete CBC plus indices, a reticulocyte count, a sodium metabisulfite test, and cellulose acetate electrophoresis (see pp. 267, 268). Confirmatory tests include determining Hb S solubility, citrate agar electrophoresis, isopropanol test for instability, and alkali denaturation test. The last is useful in the diagnosis of thalassemia major and thalassemia-hemoglobin S disease. Hb A_2 quantitation should be performed where there is

microcytosis, and the serum iron determination is frequently helpful. An oxygen dissociation curve should be established in instances of erythrocytosis; other special studies may also be necessary. Finally, a family study may be the only way to explore the genetic mixture responsible for a particular syndrome.

The alkali denaturation test utilizes the fact that fetal hemoglobin (Hb F) is less readily denatured and precipitated by alkali than is normal adult hemoglobin (Hb A).

The technique of this test follows:

1. Add 1.6 ml. of N/12 NaOH solution to serologic test tubes and incubate at 20°C for several minutes.

2. Prepare a hemoglobin solution by collecting 5 ml. of venous blood in a balanced oxalate mixture and then washing the drawn off erythrocytes three times with 0.89 per cent NaCl solution. Draw off the saline solution, and add 1.6 volume of distilled water to the washed red blood cells. Mix and add $\frac{1}{5}$ volume of toluene. Shake well for 5 minutes. Centrifuge at 3000 r.p.m. for 30 minutes. Suction off the upper toluene layer and the middle white blood cell sediment layer, and discard. Filter the bottom hemoglobin solution layer. If this layer is not clear, centrifuge and filter again. Add 0.1 ml. of an approximately 10 per cent hemoglobin solution to the incubated NaOH solution and shake for 10 seconds.

3. Exactly 1 minute afterwards, add 3.4 ml. of $(NH_4)_2SO_4 \cdot HCl$ mixture made by adding 2 ml. of N/10 HCl to 800 ml. of 50 per cent $(NH_4)_2SO_4$.

4. Filter through a double layer of filter paper. The percentage of hemoglobin remaining is determined by using a spectrophotometer to measure the optical density (O.D.). The O.D. of the original hemoglobin solution is determined by adding 20 cu.mm. of the hemoglobin solution to 4 ml. of water. Calculation: % Hb F =

$$\frac{\frac{1}{4} \text{ O.D. of filtrate}}{\text{O.D. of original Hgb. solution}} \times 100$$

A pink color in the filtrate indicates an abnormal concentration of Hb F. If the filtrate is colorless, the concentration of Hb F is normal or only slightly increased. Compare this solution with the control. Normally, Hb F (after the first 6 months) is 0 to 5 per cent of the total hemoglobin. When more than 10 per cent of Hb F is present, thalassemia is indicated.

The filter paper electrophoresis of hemolysates is another technique useful in diagnosing hemoglobinopathies (Fig. 8-7).[113] This procedure requires some knowledge of the electric mobilities of proteins, for proteins can be characterized by their rate of migration in an electric field when in solution in a buffer of fixed pH. The rate of migration depends principally on the net electric charge per molecule, the molecular weight, spatial configuration, and the magnitude of the electric field. The net electric charge of a protein molecule is a function of the isoelectric point of the protein and the pH of the solution. The isoelectric point of a protein is the pH at which the net charge per molecule of that protein is zero. At this pH, the protein migrates toward neither the positive nor the negative pole when an electric field is imposed on the solution. However, if the pH of the protein in solution is greater than the isoelectric point of the protein, the protein has a net negative charge per molecule and will move toward the positive pole of the electric field. It is necessary to buffer the pH in order to keep it relatively constant. The use of filter paper as the suspending medium diminishes the degree of diffusion by convection of the proteins being studied (Fig. 8-8).

In the case of human hemoglobins, electrophoretic separation has been found to be best accomplished at a pH greater than the isoelectric points. It is customary to use a pH of 8.6 buffered by a mixture of sodium diethylbarbiturate and diethylbarbituric acid. The magnitude of the electric field depends on the nature of the apparatus actually used. The use of the siliconized glass plate apparatus described by Smith and Conley is quite satisfactory[140] (Fig. 8-7).

In the technique, a vertical line is marked through the center of the paper, and small marks are made about $5/8$ inch apart along the line. The entire paper is wetted in the buffer, and then blotted nearly dry between two pieces of filter paper. Small drops of hemoglobin, approximately 0.003 to 0.005 ml., are added at the small marks at the center line. The center of the paper is placed in the center of the glass plates. The clamps are put on and spaced evenly on both sides of the glass plates. Buffer is added to the glass dishes to exactly the same level. The glass plates are placed between the two dishes and ends of the paper in the buffer. The electrodes are connected to the power supply, which is then turned on. The voltage is adjusted to 350 volts. This should run at room temperature for 10 to 12 hours. At the end of the run, the paper is removed from the plates and dried in an oven at 100°C for 30 minutes.

The various hemoglobins differ in the speed with which they travel in an electric field. Closest to the starting point is Hb B_2, then C, E, E_2, O, S, D, L, T., G, Q, A_1, A_3, M, F, K, J, N, H, and I. Some of these hemoglobins overlap, so that to achieve better separation, starch, agar, or Microzone* electrophoresis or changing pH of the buffer might be tried.

Hemolytic Anemias Resulting from Intrinsic Defects of Erythrocytes

As a group, these hemolytic anemias are characterized by a hereditary defect in the red blood cell (that is, either in the hemoglobin molecule, cell membrane, or stroma). They may also be classified into enzymopathies, membrane defects, and hemoglobinopathies which in some instances are associated with altered oxygen affinity or instability). When normal erythrocytes are transfused into these patients, the survival time is normal but when these erythrocytes are transfused into normal plasma they disappear rapidly from the circulation, usually denoting absence of autoimmune bodies.

---

* Produced by Beckman Instrument Co. — 2500 Harbor Blvd., Fullerton, California.

Spherocytosis (Plates 33, 34). The most common member of this complex is called *hereditary spherocytosis, congenital hemolytic anemia,* or *familial acholuric jaundice.* This disease is found most frequently in Europeans and occasionally in Blacks, the incidence being one in 5000 persons in the northern United States. It is inherited as a Mendelian autosomal disorder and is usually transmitted by an affected parent to half his children. Nearly all patients are heterozygous with regard to the abnormal gene responsible for the condition. It is characterized by the presence of spherocytes or abnormally thick red blood cells in the circulation, but its pathogenesis is not clear. It was formerly thought to be caused by defective utilization of energy from glycolysis in maintaining the lipid structures of the spherocyte during in vitro incubation. However, recent findings indicate that the hemolysis of spherocytic erythrocytes is associated with overwork rather than with a deficiency in energy metabolism.[61]

It is proposed that the primary defect resides in the erythrocyte membrane, which is abnormally permeable to sodium. The heightened influx of sodium stimulates active sodium extrusion from the cell by arousing a usually latent adenosine triphosphatase (ATPase) system. The resulting increased breakdown of ATP provides not only energy for cation transport, but also liberates adenosine diphosphate (ADP) and inorganic phosphate, which in turn stimulates glycolysis. Under optimal conditions, as in the general circulation, these compensatory mechanisms suffice. During metabolic stress, as is believed to occur in the spleen, sodium accumulates intracellularly and irreversible changes in membrane permeability and ultimately hemolysis ensue.

Recently it has been proposed that the basic erythrocytic defect is in the structural protein. This leads to rigidity of the RBCs, splenic entrapment of erythrocytes, and progressive loss of RBC membrane by fragmentation within the splenic pulp. Despite this membrane abnormality, hemolysis is almost completely eliminated by splenectomy.

Clinically, this spherocytotic complex is present from birth, but diagnosis is usually not made until later in life; delay of puberty occurs, especially if splenectomy is not performed during childhood. Other findings are splenomegaly, leg ulcers (which heal after splenectomy), icterus, cholelithiasis in 68 per cent of cases, a radiographic pattern of striation and thickening of the frontal and parietal bones occasionally with tower skull formation, and mild to severe anemia, the latter especially in hemolytic crises.

The laboratory diagnosis should include the following: (1) Instead of the normal biconcave disk shape, the red blood cells assume a spherocytic pattern, frequently microspherocytic in Wright-stained blood films. Rouleau formation of a bizarre type is seen in unstained wet preparations. (2) The peripheral blood pattern shows a moderate to severe hypochromic, microcytic anemia and normoblastosis, especially in the hemolytic crises. The bone marrow pattern during the acute phase shows normoblastic hyperplasia with a reticulocytosis of 5 to 20 per cent. There is also a moderate elevation in the serum bilirubin and urine urobilinogen. (3) There is increased osmotic and mechanical fragility of red blood cells—especially on sterile incubation at 37° C for 24 hours—thus mimicking in vivo splenic sequestration. (4) The automatic electronic erythrocyte osmotic fragility curve (Fragiligraph) may be used (Fig. 8-10). This technique utilizes a micro sample of blood suspended in isotonic saline. This sample is placed in a test cell, formed by dialysing membrane walls, which is in turn placed in distilled water inside the instrument. Dialysis across the membrane continuously reduces the initial salt concentration of the blood suspension causing rupture of the red cells and hemolysis. White light is transmitted through the blood suspension and increases with the increase in the percentage

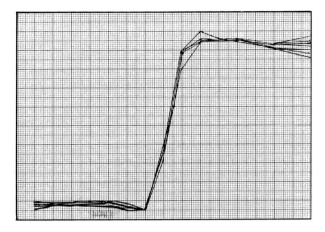

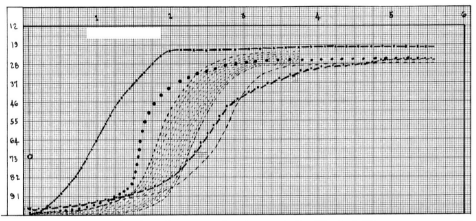

Fig. 8-9. Top—Reproduction of a conventional osmotic fragility test. The curves were obtained by a conventional method. (Dacie, 1956) Bottom—Reading from Fragiligraph.
—.—.—.— Red blood cells made spherical by heating and cooling. (From Carlsen and Comroe)
.... Hereditary sperocytosis after splenectomy.
------------------ Thalassemia minor.
—. .—. .—. .—Blood from a 2 day old child (a single drop was sufficient to repeat the test three times).
Solid area: Range of normal fragility of human erythrocytes.

of hemolysis. Light transmission is monitored continuously and detailed osmotic fragility curves are printed out (Fig. 8-9). (5) There is increased autohemolysis, in which spontaneous lysis of red blood cells occurs in defibrinated blood incubated at 37°C for 48 hours. The percentage of lysis is measured by comparing the serum hemoglobin concentration before and after incubation. The lytic process in these pa-

tients is inhibited by glucose or the slight acidification of blood—a differential point not seen in other types of chronic spherocytosis. The laboratory study of relatives of patients should be carried out because in some cases only incubation fragility tests are abnormal.

When both parents of the patient are hematologically normal according to the foregoing test criteria, a low gene pene-

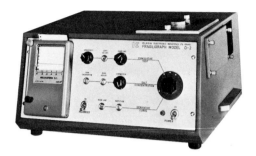

Fig. 8-10. The Fragiligraph, a device that records electronically the osmotic fragility curves of erythrocytes on a graph. (Courtesy of Elron Electronic Industries, Ltd., and distributed by Kalmedic Instruments, Inc., a subsidiary of Kalvex, Inc., New York City)

trance or gene mutation must be suspected. During the last 5 years, the genetic criteria for diagnosis of this disease have been established. An investigation of 180 members of 26 families indicates that not more than four controlled, properly weighted laboratory tests are necessary to diagnose 96 per cent of the affected persons if another family member is known to be affected.[97] These tests include the spherocyte score (0 to 3, depending on the number of technicians who observed spherocytes), the reticulocyte count, and the hemoglobin and bilirubin levels.[96] Because of the therapeutic aids described in the next paragraph, the frequency of the gene in the population is expected to increase over the next several decades.[35]

Therapy consists of cholecystectomy for gallstones, transfusions during crises of severe anemia only, exchange transfusion for hyperbilirubinemia of the newborn, and splenectomy, which is deferred until the patient is at least 2 years old in order to avoid reduction of the immune response and defensive mechanisms against infection. The postsplenectomy period is characterized by retention of the milder type of spherocytosis and usually by the return of the normal erythrocyte life span followed by elevation of the hematocrit and hemoglobin, and reduction of normal reticulocyte count and

serum bilirubin levels. The usually increased postincubation autohemolysis test result remains as such.

Elliptocytosis (Plates 8, 9). Another intrinsic defect of erythrocytes is found in elliptocytic hemolytic anemia, or hereditary ovalocytosis. This disease is present in about one per 2500 of the general population of the United States. The morphologic characteristics of the erythrocyte are inherited as an autosomal Mendelian dominant with marked variation in the hematologic pattern and degree of elliptocytosis in patients so affected. The erythrocyte shape varies from oval to elliptical to bacilliform, and there is very little or no diminution in the number of ovalocytes in affected individuals from the 90 per cent or more figures, regardless of the degree of clinical findings or even in their absence—that is, whether heterozygotic or homozygotic, there is almost complete morphologic involvement of the red blood cell as studied in the blood film. A few ovalocytes are found in normal patients; there are 15 to 25 per cent ovalocytes in hypochromic microcytic anemias, myelosclerosis, and macrocytic anemias. Ovalocytes are seen as "pencil cells" in chronic hemorrhagic anemia.[122]

There is no apparent relationship between the degree of elliptocytosis and the life span of the erythrocytes. Thus, some affected persons have erythrocytes with a normal life span, others are in a compensated hemolytic state, and a minority have overt hemolytic anemia. The rare homozygous state is associated with severe hemolysis. According to Rebuck citing Chevallier, the more oval cells that are present in a patient, the less likely that the patient will suffer from a crippling anemia.[122] Conversely, the more elliptical and bacilliform red blood cells encountered, the more likely that an anemia is present or will develop. Clinically, there is splenomegaly, mild to severe anemia, elliptocytosis, and occasionally microspherocytosis, reticulocytosis, a shortened surivival time of elliptocytes, increased mechanical fragility, normal osmotic fragility, and normoblastic hyperplasia of the bone marrow.

Acanthocytosis (Plate 8). Acanthocytosis is an intrinsic erythrocyte defect in which abnormalities of serum and stromal lipid have been described. It is especially remarkable in that red blood cells in these cases show striking changes in shape and yet little evidence of an increased rate of destruction.[139]

Paroxysmal Nocturnal Hemoglobinuria. Paroxysmal nocturnal hemoglobinuria (PNH), also classified as an anemia due to immune bodies, is an acquired rare chronic hemolytic anemia occurring most often between 30 and 40 years of age. It is associated with an intracorpuscular defect that renders red blood cells more susceptible to hemolysis in an acid medium. In fact it has been demonstrated that reduced glutathione (GSH) produces a corpuscular defect in normal erythrocytes that causes the formation of PNH-like cells indistringuishable from true PNH erythrocytes. The effect is oxidative, ultimately involving the erythrocyte lipid. It is therefore believed that peroxidation of red cell lipid is the underlying corpuscular defect of PNH, which renders the cell susceptible to lysis.[102]

Recent work by Rosse, Dourmashkin, and Humphrey has demonstrated that PNH erythrocytes develop pits on their surface that are demonstrable by electron microscopy.[127] This in turn leads to the immune lysis of the erythrocytes by antibody and complement (Fig. 8-11).

The disease is clinically characterized by continuous intravascular hemolysis with associated hemoglobinemia, metalbuminemia, hemoglobinuria, and hemosiderinuria. Sleep is associated with an increased rate of hemolysis; on arising, the patient's urine is brownish red because hemoglobin is present in large amounts. There is marked loss of body iron in the urine (hemosiderinuria) with some deposition in the renal epithelial cells of the convoluted tubules and loops of Henle. This is mostly compensated for by the increased absorption of dietary iron. There is no increase in marrow or reticuloendothelial hemosiderin unless the patient has had frequent transfusions (eythroid hyperplasia of bone marrow occurs, with occasional cases of bone marrow failure being reported).[119] Hepatosplenomegaly may be moderate; neutropenia and moderate thrombocytopenia with associated thromboses due to severe hemolysis also occur.

The pathogenesis is associated with an abnormality of erythrocyte membrane in PNH patients. The red blood cells are markedly susceptible to hemolysis by certain agents that only rarely affect normal red blood cells—for example, heat-labile lytic factors involving complement, properdin, and Mg^{++} active in a pH between 6.5 and 7.1 hemolyze PNH erythrocytes but not normal erythrocytes. The membrane also appears to be susceptible to lysis by activation of the alternate complement pathway. If there are no visible spherocytes and osmotic fragility is normal, then Ham's acid serum test will usually confirm a diagnosis of PNH. The technique involves acidifying 0.5 ml. of serum by adding 0.05 ml. of 0.2 N HCl. A control is set up using 0.5 ml. unacidified serum. One drop of a 50 per cent suspension of the patient's washed erythrocytes is added to each serum and incubated at 37° C for 1 hour and then centrifuged. In PNH, marked hemolysis occurs after 15 minutes.

A deficiency of erythrocytic cholinesterase activity can also be demonstrated in severe cases of PNH. Erythrocytes in PNH are often hemolyzed by antibodies that agglutinate or coat normal red blood cells but do not hemolyze them. These include isoantibodies, certain autoantibodies, and heterophil antibodies. Furthermore, three populations of RBCs with variations in sensitivity to the hemolytic effect of complement have been delineated; normal PNH RBCs, PNH II RBCs, and PNH III RBCs. Patients with only PNH II

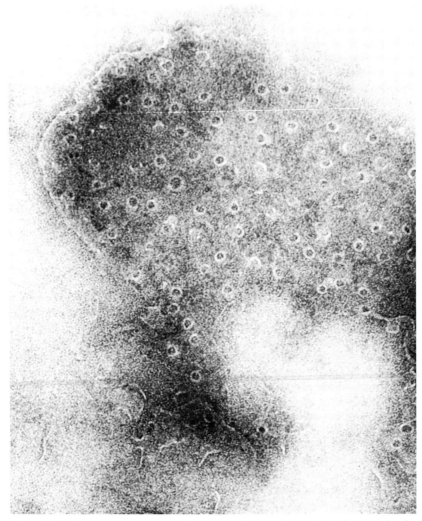

Fig. 8-11. Electron micrograph demonstrating erythrocyte holes or pits in paroxysmal nocturnal hemoglobinuria. (Rosse, W. F., Dourmashkin, R., and Humphrey, J. H.: Immune lysis of normal and paroxysmal nocturnal hemoglobinuria (PNH) red blood cells. III. The membrane defects caused. J. Exp. Med., *123:*969, 1966; *Also in* Dourmashkin, R. R., and Rosse, W. F.: Morphologic changes in the membranes of red blood cells undergoing hemolysis. Am. J. Med., *41:*699, 1966)

or PNH II and I may have the full clinical syndrome of PNH.[128]

Therapy consists of transfusing washed normal erythrocytes during periods of severe anemia. Whole blood should not be used because of the plasma hemolytic component therin. Dicumarol, not heparin, is used for thrombotic episodes plus intermit-tent 6 per cent dextran given intravenously to inhibit hemolysis. Steroid therapy may also inhibit hemolysis. Iron given orally or intravenously may be used for the anemia.

Familial nonspherocytic hemolytic anemia (Fig. 8-12) is a hereditary defect of the erythrocyte. It is of unknown cause, transmitted as a Mendelian dominant by a "weak" gene. Occasionally it may arise from a recessive gene in both parents with associated erythrocyte enzyme deficiencies —for example, deficiencies in glucose-6-phosphate dehydrogenase, glutathione, kinase, and pyruvate.[30] It may imitate hemolytic disease of the newborn. Occasionally, these patients may have an overt, but compensated hemolytic anemia and an associated severe leukocytic G-6-PD deficiency. The latter can lead to impaired leukocytic function and, in some cases, to an increased susceptibility to the infection associated with granulomatous lesions.[47] The hematologic pattern is characterized by small "tails" of fragile cells, normochromic, nomocytic, or macrocytic anemia, reticulocytosis, and erythroid marrow hyperplasia. Osmotic fragility test results are normal. Unlike hereditary spherocytosis, there is no general shift toward increased fragility after incubation. The serum bilirubin and fecal urobilinogen are increased. Also, a rapid turnover of plasma radioactive iron may be seen. Therapy consists of blood transfusions and occasionally steroids. Splenectomy is not considered unless ^{51}Cr tests indicate splenic sequestration of labeled erythrocytes. An excess of hemosiderin deposits in spleen and liver may be observed. This group is also described further in the section idiopathic hemolytic anemias (p. 246).

Stomatocytosis. Stomatocytosis is a hemolytic process in which the membranes of the red cells, called stomatocytes, are metabolically defective, and in which the red cells show a linear unstained area across their center on stained blood films. On wet films, the erythrocytes appear bowl shaped.[89] There is also increased osmotic fragility, increased autohemolysis even with added glucose, increased mechanical fragility, and shortened erythrocyte survival time (^{51}Cr) in the circulation of both patient and recipient. No spherocytes are found.

Other studies have shown that RBCs can undergo disk-sphere transformation with-

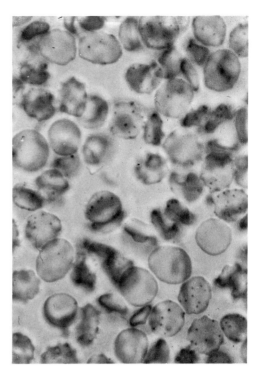

Fig. 8-12. Tetrazolium cytochemical method for identifying G-6-PD activity of individual RBCs: granulated RBCs indicate normal G-6-PD activity; non-granulated RBCs indicate deficient G-6-PD activity.

out change in volume. These changes can be induced in vitro by changes in the pH of the medium or by adding chemicals with an amphophilic molecular structure (detergent type) to the medium. Some workers used low concentrations of these detergent chemicals and concluded that echinocytic and stomatocytic agents are antagonists. Other experiments reveal that RBCs are incapable of resuming their normal discocytic state after having undergone loss of membrane material. These results suggest that echinocytic and stomatocytic agents are noncompetitive inhibitors that act at different sites on the RBC membrane.[18]

An abnormally increased permeability to cations led to the detection of another morphologic RBC variant. The cation pump, in this case, cannot compensate for a K^+ loss that exceeds the Na^+ gain, and the total cation content decreases. Subsequently, cell water decreases, and a population of osmotically resistant, dehydrated RBCs is formed. Morphologically, these "dessicytes" appear to have hemoglobin puddled at the cell periphery and are similar to the "eccentrocytes" seen in dogs treated with oxidant drugs (Fig. 8-16).[43]

The red blood cell membrane consists of a mosaic of macromolecular residues with functional groups that may influence the integrity of the membrane. A rare type of Rh RBC which lacks all Rh-Hr antigens and is called Rh null, is characterized by the dilution of specific lipoprotein sites on the membrane by the action of recessive suppressor (regulator) genes. Consequently, the membrane is defective, and a mild hemolytic anemia develops. In addition, shortened RBC survival, stomatocytosis, increased RBC fragility, mild spherocytosis, and a high reticulocyte count are manifest.

Still another erythrocyte variant is the Bombay defect, characterized by a genetic block in the biosynthesis of ABO blood group substances. This variant is attributed to a homozygous regulator gene that blocks synthesis of the terminal carbohydrate residues specific for A, B, or H. The Bombay erythrocyte membrane remains intact despite this defect and therefore is usually not associated with hemolytic anemia.[83]

Hemolytic Anemias Caused by Unfavorable Environment

Anemias Due to Immune Bodies. The immune body hemolytic anemias are a heterogeneous group of anemias characterized by the alteration of previously normal red blood cells, with the subsequent development of a shortened life span in a random fashion as a result of exposure to hemolytic substances or mechanisms. These anemias are usually detected by a positive antiglobulin test.

Hemolytic Diseases of the Newborn. One of the most common members of hemolytic disease of the newborn is *erythroblastosis fetalis (hemolytic disease of the newborn),* a syndrome that results from the destruction or hemolysis of fetal red blood cells by an antibody produced by the mother against an antigen inherited by the fetus from its father, but not possessed by the mother. The blood group antigens, in their order of frequency and severity, leading to the development of hemolytic disease of the newborn (HDN) are Rh, A and B, K, h, S, s, M, Jk^a, and Fy^a. The mother develops antibodies (most frequently anti-Rh_0), usually during pregnancy and in greatest number during labor, by the passage of fetal red blood cells (most frequently Rh_0-positive) probably through breaks in the placental barrier into the maternal circulation (mother is Rh_0-negative).

The incidence of HDN is only one in 200 births, even though 10 per cent of all newborns are Rh-positive children having Rh-negative mothers. This discrepancy between the expected and observed incidence of HDN occurs because (1) first babies are rarely affected unless the mother has been immunized by previously administered Rh-positive blood or incompatible ABO blood, by a previous miscarriage, or by a heterogenetic antigen such as toxoid or vaccine containing group A substances; (2) not all mothers develop antibodies or develop them in insufficient concentration or not rapidly enough; and (3) it is not known how frequently or in what quantity fetal red blood cells gain access to the maternal circulation. About 0.5 per cent of newborn infants have significant enough anemia and hyperbilirubinemia associated with Rh incompatibility to require treatment. Kell antigens and anti-Kell antibodies also produce clinical HDN in a rare instance with Duffy, Kidd, and M antigens producing isolated, extremely rare cases. One per cent of all babies, including the first baby, have HDN resulting from ABO incompatibility, but only 5 per cent of these are severe enough to require treatment. The mother is usually group O and the baby group A, with the fetuses of group O mothers receiving 16 times the concentration of antibodies that the fetuses of group A or B mothers do.

Red blood cells coated with anti-A or anti-B antibodies are less frequently agglutinable than are those sensitized with anti-Rh and other isoantibodies causing HDN. These decreased (approximately 10 per cent) to negative results in the antiglobulin (Coombs) test are though to be due to the fact that anti-A and anti-B antibodies are not firmly fixed to the A or B agglutinogens of the red blood cells and are therefore easily washed off during the three or four saline washings in the Coombs test. A test for neonatal ABO HDN has been devised by Kaplan and others.[72] It is based on the fact that erythrocyte acetylcholine esterase activity is significantly reduced in this ABO group, whereas infants with Rh HDN have normal erythrocyte cholinesterase activity (70–130 units/mg. of hemoglobin).

Clinically and hematologically, all grades of anemia and sequelae are observed in hemolytic disease of the newborn. In mild cases, the babies are normal at birth having a cord hemoglobin of 15 to 24 g. per 100 ml. and cord bilirubin of 1 to 3 mg. per 100 ml. The Coombs test is weakly to moderately positive (usually negative in ABO cases). Slight reticulocytosis (above 5%), slight normoblastosis, and jaundice may be observed during the first 24 hours. Spherocytosis is seen in ABO cases and is absent in other cases. Usually no treatment is required, but if serial Coombs tests are done in Rh types, one may see a severe development. Most ABO cases are mild (Plate 32).

In severe cases (40% of HDN cases), cord hemoglobin is below 14.5 g. per 100 ml., and cord bilirubin is above 3 mg. per 100 ml. The Coombs test is rapidly and strongly positive; peripheral blood reticulocytosis is above 10 per cent; and peripheral blood normoblastosis of all types is above 10/100 white blood cells. Jaundice develops within the first few hours after birth and deepens rapidly; bilirubin is indirect first and then also direct owing to bile canaliculi obstruction. Hepatosplenomegaly is associated with an increased extramedullary hematopoiesis. Kernicterus develops unless the baby is given exchange transfusions.

In very severe cases, there is usually a history of a previously affected sibling with cord blood hemoglobin less than 10 g. per 100 ml. and cord blood bilirubin up to 8 mg. per 100 ml. Marked reticulocytosis, normoblastosis, and associated thrombocytopenia are often seen with concomitant petechiae. One also frequently sees edematous (hydropic) anemia fetal death in utero with associated pale bulky placenta. This occurs usually during the last 4 weeks of pregnancy. Successive stillbirths, in which the father is homozygous with an Rh-negative mother, are apt to occur earlier each time. Also seen is kernicterus with associated damage due to bilirubin deposition in the cerebral basal ganglia and subsequent signs of permanent brain damage or death. Therapy for infants having the severe form should be given in the form of exchange transfusions as soon as possible (with serum bilirubin levels of approximately 20 mg./100 ml.). These transfusions remove the bilirubin (preventing kernicterus), isoantibodies, and incompatible erythrocytes, and replaces them with compatible plasma and Rh-negative erythrocytes. The exchange is carried out by the alternate withdrawal and infusion of approximately 10 to 20 ml. of fresh heparinized blood. If citrate is used, calcium gluconate should be given intravenously with every 100 ml. of blood. The blood is given through an inlying catheter, usually in the umbilical vein. Recently, phototherapy has been applied to mild bilirubinemia (< 10 mg./dl.). It has reduced the need for exchange in infants with low birth weight and without hemolysis and in term infants with mild hemolysis, and has decreased the necessity for repeated exchange transfusions.[14]

Similarly, attempts have been made to use exchange transfusions in the management of fulminating viral hepatitis. There was no increase in survival and, in fact, probably a worsened prognosis. Much the same occurred when this technique was used to treat defibrination syndrome, severe infection, thrombocytopenia, and leukemia.[124]

Occasionally, intrauterine transfusion of a suspected erythroblastotic fetus—with a history of multiple previous hemolytic disease in newborn fetuses, a rising anti-Rh agglutinin titer, a high amniotic bilirubin, and a reduction of fetal movements—may be attempted according to the method of Liley.[48] The usual type of transfusion is performed if the infant does not have marked hyperbilirubinemia. Early delivery of the fetus may be advisable as a preventive measure in instances when there is a rising anti-Rh agglutinin titer in the last trimester of pregnancy.

Prediction of erythroblastosis fetalis in utero can be accomplished in several ways:

1. The father's Rh subtypes—his genetic capacity to conceive Rh-negative offspring—should be known. If the father is homozygous for the Rh-negative factor, it is almost certain that the fetus will have some degree of hemolytic newborn disease; if the father is heterozygous, there is a 50 per cent chance that any one conceptus will be Rh-negative and thus survive.

2. Rising serum anti-Rh antibody levels are of some assistance in reflecting the possible but not specific severity of fetal disease in utero. This procedure is particularly nonspecific if there have been prior sensitized babies.

3. A more exact estimate of the baby's integrity may be obtained by performing an amniocentesis about the twenty-fourth week, with serial repetition using adequate precautions. Since massive transplacental hemorrhage of 50 ml. of more occurs in 0.25 to 1 per cent of all pregnancies and causes high perinatal mortality and morbidity, fetal red blood cell counting may be used as a routine diagnostic test in the analysis of perinatal death and neonatal morbidity. The maternal blood should be exam-

ined for fetal erythrocytes (Kleinhauer test), after all deliveries, to determine causes of perinatal death, and during the third trimester of pregnancy in every complication associated with fetal bleeding. If blood is aspirated at amniocentesis, the origin of the RBCs should be determined.[150] High or rising concentrations of heme pigment, determined spectroscopically indicate that fetal blood is being destroyed at a rapid rate and that the baby is seriously affected. When this destruction of the blood is extreme and occurs very early, intrauterine fetal transfusion may be advisable; if it occurs later in the pregnancy, early termination of the pregnancy and exchange transfusion may be advisable. A well stocked blood bank, an adequate donor list, skilled technicians on duty at all hours, and trained transfusion teams are necessities.

Recently Cherry and co-workers proposed an examination of the bilirubin and total protein in amniotic fluid in order to give a more accurate indication of danger to the fetus than the current method of measuring amniotic fluid bilirubin content alone provides.[22] In their study, the amniotic fluid of 26 Rh-negative women (having Rh antibodies and immunized) was examined for bilirubin and total protein content. At delivery, cord blood was collected for comparison with predicted levels based on the bilirubin-protein ratio in the amniocentesis specimen. The results revealed that patients with severe erythroblastosis fetalis had a ratio greater than 0.55. Mildly involved or uninvolved infants had a ratio of less than 0.35. In moderate cases, in which infants had ratios between 0.35 and 0.55 and in which studies of amniotic fluid were made in sequence, a rising bilirubin-protein ratio was associated with progression of the disease in utero.

4. Further control of Rh antibody-induced diseases of the newborn has been proposed in an effort to prevent Rh immunization of Rh-negative primiparas by injection of immune gamma globulin after delivery. The purpose of the injection is to

destroy Rh-positive cells in the mother's circulation before the mother's body can build immunologic memory of the foreign cells.[76]

As part of the program, all Rh-negative primiparas are screened at the time of delivery. If an Rh-positive infant is delivered, the complete blood types of the baby and mother are determined, and the mother's blood is examined for the presence of fetal erythrocytes as an indication of transplacental hemorrhage. Arbitrarily, the presence of more than 0.25 ml. of fetal cells is called a large hemorrhage. These patients receive an injection of 5 ml. of purified anti-Rh, 7S gamma globulin, an amount large enough to clear all fetal cells from the maternal circulation. Recent work reveals that 1 ml. of this gamma globulin preparation may be sufficient. In two groups studied none of the 18 women in the treated group were immunized — that is, they did not develop anti-Rh antibodies.

Paroxysmal Nocturnal Hemoglobinuria; Paroxysmal Cold Hemoglobinuria and Hemoglobinuria with Associated Diseases. These acquired hemolytic anemias with demonstrable autoantibodies include those disorders in which a patient's normal red blood cells develop a shortened life span secondary to exposure to hemolytic substances or mechanisms — that is, the development within the body of extracorpuscular hemolytic mechanisms without introducing them from the surrounding environment. (See also p. 233 for PNH.)

Etiologically, the mechanism may be idiopathic (60% of cases are usually in female patients over 50), or it may be part of certain lymphomas (lymphocytic leukemia and lymphosarcoma), lupus erythematosus, carcinomatosis, myelomas, myeloid metaplasia, polyarteritis nodosa, or rheumatoid arthritis. Occasionally, primary atypical pneumonia and infectious mononucleosis may be associated with an acute variety. Paroxysmal cold hemoglobinuria itself is an idiopathic or syphilis-complicated type of autoimmune hemolytic disease (AHD) that

occurs on exposure of the patient to low temperatures. It is characterized by cold hemolysins in the plasma and associated hemoglobinuria. In most instances these autoantibodies are erythrocyte-coating gamma globulins, or (occasionally non-gamma globulins).

Hematologically, there is erythroid (normoblastic) marrow hyperplasia without myeloid or megakaryocytic changes except in certain lymphomatous states. Macrocytosis correlated with reticulocytosis, normoblastosis, poikilocytosis, and Howell-Jolly bodies is observed. Spherocytosis with increased osmotic fragility is frequently seen in the peripheral blood during hemolytic episodes. A reduction in the reticulocyte count indicates impending bone marrow failure. If thrombocytopenia develops, bleeding tendencies may occur. Leukocytosis with a myeloid shift to the left also occurs with occasional leukopenic episodes. Erythrocyte phagocytosis by the reticuloendothelial cells of the marrrow, lymph nodes, spleen, and liver occurs in some instances. Sequestration of erythrocytes in splenic sinusoids may also be seen. Hemosiderotic changes can be correlated with the number of transfusions, severity, and duration of anemia and increased iron absorption.

The tissue cytologic changes associated with carcinoma, myeloma, and sarcoidosis are also present. In most instances, there appears to be a general disturbance in the manufacture of globulin with the associated presence of cryoglobulins, anticomplementary substances, and globulins giving a false positive serologic test for syphilis. Those patients with embolic tumor cells frequently have intramuscular fibrin deposition around these cells, associated with a microangiopathic hemolytic anemia. The anemia possibly represents an imbalance between fibrin formation and fibrinolysis, which would allow the persistence of intravascular microclots.[51] Autoimmune hemolytic disease may also be characterized by specific autoantibodies — for example, anti-B, anti-C, anti-D, anti-c (hr), anti-e (hr"), anti-JK[a], or anti-O[142] — and anti-IgA autoantibodies.[81] These autoantibodies are produced as the result of transfusion immunization secondary to the administration of serologically incompatible red blood cells. The recipient then produces antibodies to the antigens of the foreign red blood cells. Some erythrocyte antigens are highly antigenic — that is, they can stimulate powerful antibody production; others cannot.

If a high titer of strong immune isoantibodies is produced, hemolytic disease will result when incompatible blood is given the second time. Natural isoantibodies may also produce hemolytic disease if red blood cells are given to the recipient that are agglutinated or hemolyzed by the corresponding natural isoantibody (no previous immunization is needed). If incompatible plasma is administered containing a high antibody titer against the erythrocytes of the recipient, hemolysis of the recipient's erythrocytes will occur.

According to Jandl and associates, intravascular hemagglutination renders tissues ischemic, leading to production of spherocytic-producing substances with the subsequent hemolysis of autoantibody-coated erythrocytes.[65] However, because splenectomy is often associated with a reduction in the antibody titer and with lessened globulin-coated erythrocyte destruction, the spleen may be one of the major reticuloendothelial sources of acquired hemolytic disease phenomena. Other reticuloendothelial foci may also be involved when splenectomy itself does not significantly reduce the acquired hemolytic disease phenomena.

Clinically, the underlying disease process (lymphocytic leukemia, lupus erythematosus, and others) may be antedated by hemolytic phenomena and associated autoantibody production long before the primary syndrome manifests itself. An acute self-limiting process is occasionally associated with primary atypical pneumonia and infec-tious mononucleosis. Chills, fever, backache, and the usual manifestations of severe anemia occur with occasional episodes of hemoglobinuria and subsequent hypotension with associated oliguria and uremia. Splenomegaly and mild icterus also occur. Splenectomy and steroid therapy are frequently effective in patients showing RBC hemolysis involving IgG "warm" antibodies; they are of very little benefit in cold agglutinin disease cases. Steroids apparently act by inhibiting macrophagic phagocytosis and by reducing IgG antibody production.

If cryoglobulinemia and severe intravascular hemagglutination occur on exposure of extremities to cold, cyanosis with livid skin, Raynaud's phenomenon, and thrombophlebitis may develop. In primary and secondary hypersplenism, marked splenomegaly without demonstrable autoantibody formation may occur. Drug allergies may be a major cause of so-called idiopathic autoimmune hemolytic anemia. Penicillin may produce it when extremely large doses are administered, particularly in patients with impaired renal function, whose drug levels are elevated.[117] This phenomenon is related to the adsorption of the drug to the erythrocyte, followed by the attachment of an antidrug antibody, and phagocytosis in the reticuloendothelial system. Typically in cases of penicillin-induced hemolysis, there is a positive direct Coombs test. There is a negative indirect Coombs test in the absence of penicillin. Other drugs (e.g., quinidine) plus an antidrug antibody reflect the adsorption of immune complexes to erythrocytes, which activates complement and leads to intravascular hemolysis.

The laboratory diagnosis is distinguished by specific tests used to demonstrate autoantibodies on the patient's red blood cells or in the patient's serum or both (Fig. 8-15):

1. The Coombs test at 37°C (direct antiglobulin test) is used to diagnose the presence of globulins (incomplete antibodies) coating the patient's washed red blood

cells. Several different diagnostic sera should be used, including those reacting with nongamma globulins. These globulins can also be detected by utilizing polyvinyl pyrrolidone, mixtures of normal plasma, or serum with albumin. An indirect Coombs test may also be performed in order to detect autoantibodies in the patient's serum. This is accomplished by demonstrating their capacity to sensitize normal red blood cells for the antiglobulin reaction, to agglutinate and occasionally hemolyze normal red blood cells treated with trypsin or papain, or to agglutinate normal red blood cells suspended in albumin or mixtures of albumin with normal serum or plasma. It has recently been shown that many patients taking certain medications, such as alphamethyldopa and cephalothin, develop a positive Coombs test sometimes with hemolytic anemia.[117]

More investigative work in this division of immunology has emphasized that a positive Coombs antiglobulin test is diagnostic of antibody-mediated hemolytic anemias and is indicative of the presence of either IgG or complement (usually C^3) on the erythrocytic membrane. (Recent evidence suggests that protein-quinone interactions may underlie nonspecific adsorption of IgG to erythrocytes.) This antibody film has very little direct effect on erythrocytic membrane but does render it susceptible to phagocytosis. The surfaces of such phagocytes have been shown to have IgG and C^3 receptors. However, rare intravascular hemolysis as a result of the complete activation of the complement sequence is rare. An essentially normal life span of the RBC may be compatible with the persistent attachment of inactivated complement (C^3d fragment). Clinically, there is excellent correlation between the estimated number of IgG molecules on the erythrocyte membrane surface and the severity of hemolysis; however, there may be poor correlation between the degree of positivity and strength of the Coombs test and the degree of hemolysis.

2. Temperature and pH are important factors in demonstrating autoantibodies—for example, occasionally in primary atypical pneumonia, cold agglutinins may be demonstrated associated with hemolytic anemia. Cold hemolysins are demonstrated by the Donath-Landsteiner test in patients with paroxysmal cold hemoglobinuria and concomitant syphilis. In this test, the patient's serum is mixed with either autologous or normal red blood cells, chilled, then warmed and examined for hemolysis; the Donath-Landsteiner hemolysin is most active at a neutral or slightly alkaline pH (7.0 to 8.0).

3. Agglutination of red blood cells is best noted when blood is drawn into an acid citrate dextrose bottle and tilted, causing a thin layer of blood to flow down the inside of the upper part of the bottle. When the clumping of erythrocytes is due to cold agglutinins, it is most noticeable after refrigeration. When clumping is due to incomplete antibodies (37°C activity), it may persist, even on washing with warm saline solution, and the clumping may interfere with erythrocyte counting, blood typing, and crossmatching.

Therapy consists initially of corticosteroids (prednisone, 10–15 mg. every 6 hours) for 1 to 2 weeks; the dosage is then reduced as the hemolysis subsides. Therapy is discontinued after 6 weeks up to as long as 2 to 3 months. If there is no response or if too large a dose of steroid is needed, splenectomy is advisable with steroids given occasionally, postsplenectomy if hemolysis persists. Other hyperplastic, cystic, and neoplastic processes should be removed if possible. Transfusions of sedimented erythrocytes are preferred if the hemoglobin falls below 5 to 7 g. per 100 ml. or if the hematocrit falls below 15 to 20 per cent. Detailed typing and crossmatching are necessary because of the tendency for immune isoantibodies to develop after transfusion. However, transfusions are, at the best, hazardous in AHD. Hemoglobinemia frequently develops after transfusion, and therefore transfusions should be avoided if at all possible. Administration of heparin, alkylating agents, or antimetabolites may be followed by reduced hemolysis. Syphilis should be treated. Patients with cold agglutinins or hemolysis should avoid low temperatures.

In primary and secondary hypersplenism, steroids are tried but are usually less effective; splenectomy usually is of greater value. However, high-dose steroid therapy will induce a remission in most patients with anti-immune hemolytic anemia, and some patients who respond poorly can be effectively managed by splenectomy. Successful therapy is usually associated with a decrease in Coombs positivity that may occasionally be associated with a concommitant increase in serum antibody.[6] This increase may or may not bear any relationship to the fact that steroids may reduce the number or avidity of IgA receptors in splenic macrophages, which would decrease erythrocyte-receptor interactions and thus increase the survival of sensitized erythrocytes. Decreased sequestration of IgG-sensitized erythrocytes by corticosteroids may be important in inducing remissions in patients with warm antibody hemolytic anemia and may explain the persistently positive antiglobulin test (Coombs) in patients in remission.[5]

In order to determine the degree of splenic reticuloendothelial participation in the hemolytic process, one can measure the accumulated radioactivity in the splenic area after transfusion of ^{51}Cr-tagged donor or autogenous red blood cells. Hypersplenism associated with hepatic cirrhosis is frequently complicated by folic acid deficiency, and therefore treatment of the liver disease and associated malnutrition is considered best by avoiding splenectomy, unless as a last resort.

Hemolytic Anemias Due to Infectious, Physical, and Mechanical Agents. Infectious agents may destroy red blood cells in the following manner: (1) erythrophagocytosis by reticuloendothelial cells of the spleen, lymph nodes, bone marrow, and liver—for example, in subacute bacterial endocarditis; (2) hemolysis associated with spherocytosis and splenic sequestration of erythrocytes—for example, in miliary tuberculosis, infectious hepatitis, infectious mononucleosis, congenital rubella,[121] and psittacosis; (3) hemolysin formation—for example, in β hemolytic streptococcus or *Clostridium welchii* infection—thought to result from the action of lecithinase on erythrocyte stroma; and (4) the infection of red blood cells with the subsequent destruction of parasitized red blood cells—e.g., in *Bartonella* and malarial infection (Plates 36, 38).

Physical agents, such as heat above 51° C, may produce spherocytosis, schistocytes, and hemoglobinuria. Recently, prosthetic materials, used in repair of cardiac valvular defects, have been associated with a shortened erythrocyte life span, hemoglobinemia, hemoglobinuria, and hemosiderinuria. It was concluded that the hemolytic process was due to the mechanical trauma to red blood cells produced either by increased turbulence about the defective prosthetic valve cusp or by the impact of the rigid ball valve against the rigid housing.[31] The hemolytic process has decreased when an elastic silicone valve with a more resilient housing has been used. Iron therapy was formerly thought to be contraindicated because, in many instances, hemosiderosis was already present. However, thoracic surgeons and cardiologists are finding, empirically, that oral iron therapy even in the face of known hemosiderosis may convert a hemolytic state into a preferable compensated hemolytic state in some patients. This suggests that in a hard-pressed reticuloendothelial system or in kidney parenchyma, excessive iron deposits do not necessarily ensure needed available iron for normoblastic use in the marrow.[123]

Hemolytic Anemias Due to Poisons. Hemolysis attributable to toxic agents affects erythrocytes in one of the following ways: (1) In this type of hemolysis, there is formation of defective red blood cells, which are removed by the reticuloendothelial cells of the body, especially the spleen. This is found in lead poisoning and copper intoxication.[95] In reference to the copper intoxication, McIntyre and co-workers have described three patients with Wilson's disease who developed evidence of acute hemolytic episodes.[95] During these attacks, large amounts of copper were excreted in the urine. The sudden release of cooper from the tissues into the blood with a subsequent reduction in erythrocyte glutathione at the onset of the hemolysis (a mechanism analogous to that of enzootic jaundice in sheep) was regarded as the most likely explanation. (2) There is hemolysis of red blood cells associated with methemoglobinemia—for example, from toluene and benzene derivatives such as trinitrotoluene, nitrobenzene, acetanilid, phenacetin, and Promin. (3) There is hemolysis of red blood cells with special susceptibility to certain drugs when a deficiency in the activity of glucose-6-phosphate dehydrogenase (G-6-PD) is present,[16] and when there is a low rate of erythrocytic glutathione synthesis,[118] or when there is reduced glutathione with the subsequent production of oxidant compounds in the body.[112] The drugs most often incriminated are phenylhydrazine, primaquine, pamaquin, para-aminosalicylic acid (PAS), acetanilid, phenacetin, sulfonamides, naphthalene, nitrofurantoin, and the fava bean. Erythrocyte destruction occurs after oxidative denaturation of the hemoglobin and of other parts of the red blood cell that protect the intact erythrocyte membrane. The metabolic defects that result in this type of hemolytic anemia are in the glycolytic cycle, and the resulting deficiencies interfere with the production of proton donors in the form of reduced pyridine nucleotides or high-energy phosphate in the form of adenosine triphosphate (ATP). Glucose-6-phosphate dehydrogenase deficiency limits the availability of reduced triphosphopyridine nucleotide, as well as the enzymatic reactions, such as glutathione reduction, that require this coenzyme as a source of hydrogen. Recent work has revealed the presence of at least 150 variants of G-6-PD. In many of these enzyme instability rather than inhibition appears to be the significant factor in the origin of hemolysis.[69] This enzyme, involved in the hexose monophosphate shunt pathway, is most basically associated with detoxification of H_2O_2 or other forms of activated oxygen within RBCs. Normal cation gradients and membrane plasticity are intimately associated with the ATP that is produced metabolically in the main glycolytic pathway.

This sex-linked inherited enzyme deficiency is found in less than 1 per cent of north Europeans, in 2 to 3 per cent of south Europeans, in 15 per cent of American Blacks (full expression occurs in 10–15% of males and 1–2% of females), and in up to 30 per cent of Sardinians. Reports of new mutants of G-6-PD related to chronic hemolysis contrast with the sporadic hemolysis from the A variant that is typically associated with Black people.

Among the apparently healthy individuals who have been found to have subnormal G-6-PD levels, clinical manifestation of anemia is usually not apparent until a so-called hemolytic drug (see previous partial list, this page) is administered. Usually the patient's older red blood cells are affected first because they have an even lower G-6-PD level. Hemolysis begins 24 to 48 hours after exposure to the drugs previously mentioned. As hemolysis becomes more severe, as much as 30 to 50 per cent of red cell mass may be affected. Physical findings vary depending on the degree of hemolysis. These include jaundice, pallor, and possibly splenomegaly.

Hematologically, polychromasia, reticulocytosis, and normoblastosis are seen. Erythroid marrow hyperplasia with a peripheral normocytic, normochromic anemia in which 40 per cent of erythrocytes contain five or more Heinz-Ehrlich bodies, and hyperbilirubinemia are also observed. Other laboratory findings include minimal spherocyte formation, increased urobilinogen in the urine and feces, normal to slightly increased osmotic fragility, a shortened ^{51}Cr survival time, and an early methemoglobinemia that disappears later (Plates 37, 39).

Remission begins on or about the tenth day with the disappearance of the older erythrocytes.

The diagnosis is made by using wet blood films or supravitally stained (brilliant cresyl blue) blood films and observing multiple refractile coccoid intraerythrocytic granules (Heinz-Ehrlich bodies) representing denatured hemoglobin; by the methemoglobin reduction test, which is based on the inability of G-6-PD-deficient erythrocytes to reduce methemoglobin in the presence of an oxidation-reduction mediator (methylene blue); and by the G-6-PD spot and screening tests described in the following paragraphs. A number of cases of congenital Heinz-Ehrlich body anemia have now been shown to represent hemoglobinopathies in which the abnormal hemoglobin is apparently so unstable as to precipitate spontaneously in vivo. Dacie and co-workers used heating at 50° C to bring out this instability in vitro.[29] It is important to detect this deficiency in blood donors because G-6-PD erythrocytes have only an 80-day life span, and therefore these erythrocytes would be rapidly destroyed and eliminated—especially in recipients undergoing certain drug therapy and in those suffering from severe infection. Furthermore, some cases of neonatal jaundice may be attributed to inherited G-6-PD deficiency, especially among those people with no evidence of immunohematologic incompatibility who live in areas where the abnormal trait is endemic. Studies of families of affected infants have further confirmed the inherited nature of this defect and proved the absence of ABO and Rh incompatibility.[34]

Treatment consists of avoidance of he-

molytic compounds in the care of these infants, careful observation for jaundice, and the treatment of hyperbilirubinemia with exchange transfusions.

The test for G-6-PD is based on the catalysis of the following reaction:

$$\text{Glucose-6-phosphate} \xrightleftharpoons{\text{G-6-PD}}$$

$$\text{6-Phosphogluconolactone} + \text{TPNH}$$

In the test, the reduced triphosphopyridine nucleotide (TPNH) reduces the brilliant cresyl blue dye to a colorless form, leaving visible only the red color of the blood hemolysate. The rate of disappearance of the blue color is followed visually and is proportional to the G-6-PD activity of the red blood cells.*

Other screening tests have been recently reported utilizing different techniques and approaches. Fairbanks[40] has described a method that appears to be simple and practical for large numbers of patients; it approximately doubles the determining of heterozygotes compared to the conventional spectrophotometric method. This technique utilizes specific supravital staining of G-6-PD in individual erythrocytes. It is based on the reduction of 3-(4,5-dimethyl thiazolyl-2)-2,5 diphenyl (MTT) tetrazolium bromide by TPNH to nearly uniform intraerythrocytic formazan granules. Relative G-6-PD activity may be estimated by counting granules in the affected red blood cells. Mosaicism is easily demonstrated in heterozygotes for G-6-PD deficiency. The method is independent of methemoglobin reduction. A microtechnique requires as little as 0.1 ml. of blood. Briefly summarized, it is as follows: (1) The plasma is removed from sedi-

---

* This test procedure is put up in a kit by the Dade Division of Scientific Products Laboratory in Miami, Florida 33152 (P.O. Box 520672). There is also a spot-test kit (No. 860148) produced by California Biochemical Co. (the California Corporation for Biochemical Research), 10933 N. Torrey Pines Road, La Jolla, California 92037. Either one of these tests serves as an excellent screening procedure for the detection of G-6-PD activity.

mented or centrifuged erythrocytes. (2) The erythrocytes are incubated in an $NaNO_2$-saline solution for 20 minutes. (3) They are washed three times in isotonic saline solution. (4) The buffy coat is removed. (5) The erythrocytes are suspended in a substrate medium made up of saline solution, buffer, glucose, Nile blue sulfate, and MTT tetrazolium. This is incubated 45 minutes at 37° C. (6) A wet film is prepared under coverslip, using a drop of resuspended cells from step 5. (7) A 200-cell differential is done, using the scoring system described in original article.

Despite the method's dependence on intact glycolytic and pentose-shunt pathways as sources of G-6-P, TPNH, and ATP, normal results have been found in congenital nonspherocytic hemolytic anemia due to pyruvate kinase deficiency, and in other hemolytic anemias. The method is, then, uniquely sensitive and specific for G-6-PD. It is less tedious than alternative techniques, including the relatively insensitive conventional spectrophotometric assay. More than 300 samples from normal Caucasians, Black men, Black women, and Oriental women have been examined by this and other techniques. The frequency of heterozygotes in 83 Philippine women was found to be 13 per cent. This method is being adapted for the study of enzyme reaction rates and for the study of the effects of metabolic inhibitors on individual intact erythrocytes. Occasional false positives occur, but with modification of the technique it is hoped that this will be eliminated.

Jacob and Jandl have described a one-stage procedure for the detection of G-6-PD deficiency.[62] In the presence of cyanide as a catalase inhibitor, G-6-PD-deficient erythrocytes are rapidly oxidized by the H_2O_2 generated by the coupled oxidation of ascorbate and oxyhemoglobin. The resulting brown hemoglobin pigment appearing in deficient blood suspensions is readily perceived by the naked eye. Blood from Black and Caucasian female heterozygotes, with intermediate or low-normal G-6-PD levels,

was correctly identified as drug-sensitive, as was reticulocyte-rich blood withdrawn during and after primaquine-induced hemolysis. The test is best labeled as a screening test for metabolic hypersusceptibility to oxidative hemolysis. After neonatal life, this is almost always a test for G-6-PD deficiency and has the virtue of detecting heterozygotes and of being dependable during active hemolysis (Plate 38).

(4) Finally, hemolysis attributable to toxic agents may affect erythrocytes by activation of an immune mechanism with subsequent hemolysis in certain drug-susceptible patients—for example, quinidine, sulfa drugs, organic arsenicals, penicillin, Fuadin, and fava bean ingestion.[143] In vitro antibodies can sometimes be demonstrated with associated complement involvement, especially in patients exposed to quinidine and penicillin.

Recent work has proved a more graphic and easily visualized concept of the etiology of drug-induced hemolytic anemias: it has been demonstrated that certain polyene antibiotics (filipin, amphotericin, etc.) are toxic to structures containing cholesterol in their cell walls. This toxicity is manifest by the formation of pits on the surface of these cells, which subsequently leads to lysis of the cells. Rosse and associates have used electron micrograms to demonstrate that in paroxysmal nocturnal hemoglobinuria, erythrocytes, which have a high cholesterol content in their cell membranes, develop these pits (Fig. 8-11), causing immune hemolysis by antibody and complement.[127] It has been further shown that the formation of a single pit results in lysis of the cell (Fig. 8-11).

The erythrocytes of the newborn differ from adult erythrocytes in that they contain more fetal hemoglobin and methemoglobin. There are also marked differences in the activity of many of the glycolytic and nonglycolytic erythrocyte enzymes. In addition, the erythrocytes of the newborn show characteristic membrane variations. These erythrocytes also differ in their osmotic properties, mechanical fragility, and storage characteristics. Cellular energy metabolism also seems to be impaired, and hydrogen peroxide detoxification is limited. These metabolic differences make the cell more vulnerable to a variety of stresses, such as drug exposure and acidosis, and they result in the more rapid appearance of a hemolytic anemia in certain clinical situations. These transient physiologic alterations in erythrocyte metabolism may also contribute to the severity of the anemia owing to an associated congenital defect of erythrocyte metabolism—for example, enzymatic defects of the erythrocyte, erythrocyte morphologic abnormalities, and hemoglobin synthesis defects.

For many years the enzymatic defects have been grouped together as congenital nonspherocytic hemolytic anemias. At present they are identified as resulting from specific distinct enzyme deficiencies.

Idiopathic Hemolytic Anemias; Congenital Nonspherocytic Anemias

One enzyme deficiency described in association with idiopathic (enzyme deficiency) hemolytic anemias is that of *pyruvate kinase*, first documented by Tanaka and co-workers.[143] This deficiency leads to limited production of adenosine triphosphate (ATP) with the secondary effects resulting from its unavailability for reactions critical to cell viability. In addition, the level of 2,3-DPG is markedly elevated due to a block, late in glycolysis. This elevation results in a favorable compensatory shift of the oxygen dissociation curve to the right, which facilitates delivery of oxygen to the tissues. In the process, the red blood cells develop spicules (acanthocytosis) on their surfaces and do not utilize glucose except in the presence of an oxidant drug—for example, primaquine.

In addition, the red blood cells then leak potassium outward at an accelerated rate and attempt to compensate for this cation instability by a temporary increase in the rate of energy-dependent inward pumping.

In this way the combination of deficient glucose consumption and accelerated breakdown of ATP results in rapid cellular loss of ATP. In these patients there is a familial history (northern European and Mexican) with anemia, jaundice and splenomegaly.

However, the possibility that oral contraceptives may exacerbate the anemia of pyruvate kinase deficiency has been raised in a recent report.[73] Also, in a variety of hematologic malignancies not ordinarily associated with hemolytic anemia, secondary deficiencies in pyruvate kinase have frequently been encountered.[1] Marked hypophosphatemia may also develop; pancreatitis or intravenous hyperalimentation may be related to this biochemical abnormality.

Hematologically, the red blood cell may show microcytic, macrocytic, oval, or acanthocytic forms; punctate basophilia; and a 10 to 11 per cent reticulocytosis. Standard osmotic fragility and direct antiglobulin tests (Coombs) are negative; osmotic fragility after incubation may be increased. In any patient with a lifelong hemolytic anemia, especially with persisting jaundice and splenomegaly, in whom spherocytosis or marked poikilocytosis is not evident on a blood film, a diagnosis of pyruvate kinase deficiency should be entertained. The diagnosis may be confirmed by specific assay of the deficient enzyme or by a screening test. Although no certain therapy can be offered, the majority of patients appear to be benefited partially by splenectomy. In some patients, splenectomy has a striking and persisting beneficial effect.

A final note on the survival of the red blood cell might be appropriate at this time in that other enzyme deficiencies in the Embden-Meyerhof cycle have also been suggested as the basis for hemolytic anemia. It is likely that further deficiencies remain to be identified among that group of unidentified types of congenital hemolytic anemia. For example, in addition to glycolytic variations and deficiencies, there are also studies demonstrating hemolytic anemia due to other biochemical defects. Glutathione reductase deficiency has been reported as a cause of hemolytic anemia,[91] and a family with erythrocyte glutathione deficiency has been described in which a mild hemolytic anemia was aggravated by the administration of oxidant drugs.[118]

Such cases support the concept that reduced glutathione is a necessary metabolite for normal erythrocyte viability. It may help protect glycolytic enzymes and proteins with -SH groups, and it also appears to have some bearing on hexokinase activity.[131] It probably also protects the activity of stromal ATPase,[77] which may in turn play a critical part in the maintenance of sodium and potassium balance within the red blood cell.

Valentine and colleagues have shown that hexokinase activity decayed with marked rapidity as erythrocytes aged.[149] More recently, Necheles and colleagues described a partial deficiency of the enzyme glutathione peroxidase as a previously undescribed cause of hyperbilirubinemia in the newborn.[108] They list this enzyme as the last link in a series of enzymes concerned with peroxide detoxication, the others being G-6-PD and glutathione reductase. Assays made of this peroxidase enzyme revealed that the activity of this enzyme, naturally depressed at birth, did not increase with age. In the newborn period, this abnormality (deficiency) is associated with a falling hematocrit, reticulocytosis, and a degree of hyperbilirubinemia that may be sufficiently severe to require exchange transfusion. The hemolytic process appears to be self-limiting, however, because signs of hemolytic disease subside within 2 to 3 months, even though levels of the enzyme remain low. It is therefore assumed that protection of the older person against the deleterious effects of peroxides is due to maturation of the catalase system. Evidence suggests there is an autosomal type of inheritance. A sex-linked mode is ruled out by evidence in one family of a father and male offspring with decreased levels of glutathione peroxidase activity.

Another addition to the pattern of enzyme deficiency and hemolytic anemia is the report of a deficiency of triose phosphate isomerase, another enzyme of the Embden-Myerhof pathway.[137] This enzyme deficiency produces both hemolytic anemia and neurologic damage. Another variant of glucose phosphate isomerase deficiency presents significant numbers of stomatocytes on the peripheral blood smear. Priapism was reported in a 10-year-old boy with this deficiency.[46]

There is also evidence that certain stromal lipids are critical to erythrocyte survival. A number of lipids are included in the membrane structure, and cholesterol is quite important in the maintenance of erythrocyte shape[106] and is necessary for the prevention of autohemolysis on in vitro incubation.[105]

Summary of Criteria for the Diagnosis of a Hemolytic Anemia

Examination of Wright's Stain Peripheral Blood Film. Poikilocytosis, spherocytosis, target cells, polychromasia, anisocytosis, schistocytosis, and an occasional burr cell should make one suspicious of an anemia in which the bone marrow is producing erythrocytes at a greater than normal rate to replenish the deficiency in circulating erythrocytes. This eliminates refractory or aplastic anemia as part of the differential diagnosis. Furthermore, if there is no erythrocyte hypochromia, one may rule out an iron-deficiency anemia unless iron therapy has been given for several weeks, in which case one would not be able to rule out this possibility from the blood film. The absence of giant macropolycytes and bizarre granulocytes, as well as macrocytes or megalocytes, would also allow one to assume with reasonable certainty that a megaloblastic bone marrow was not responsible for the blood picture. Therefore, the most likely possibility would be an anemia associated with increased erythrocyte destruction (hemolytic anemia), especially with the cresyl blue reticulocyte stain showing reticulocytosis.

(Text continues on p. 251.)

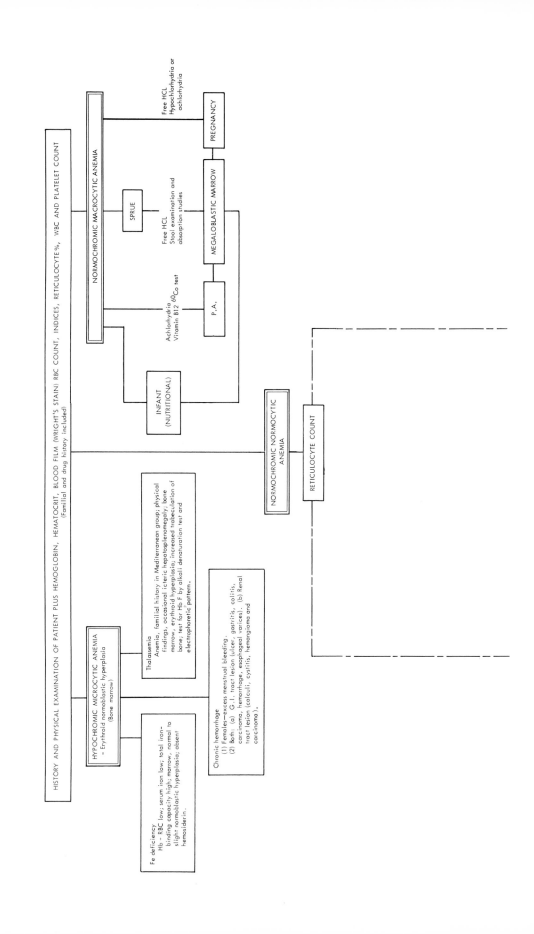

HISTORY AND PHYSICAL EXAMINATION OF PATIENT PLUS HEMOGLOBIN, HEMATOCRIT, BLOOD FILM (WRIGHT'S STAIN) RBC COUNT, INDICES, RETICULOCYTE %, WBC AND PLATELET COUNT
(Familial and drug history included)

NORMOCHROMIC MACROCYTIC ANEMIA

Free HCL
Hypochlorhydria or
achlorhydria

PREGNANCY

SPRUE

Free HCL
Stool examination and
absorption studies

MEGALOBLASTIC MARROW

Achlorhydria
Vitamin B12 60Co test

P. A.

INFANT
(NUTRITIONAL)

NORMOCHROMIC NORMOCYTIC
ANEMIA

RETICULOCYTE COUNT

HYPOCHROMIC MICROCYTIC ANEMIA
- Erythroid normoblastic hyperplasia
(Bone marrow)

Thalassemia
Anemia, familial history in Mediterranean group; physical
findings, occasional icteric hepatosplenomegaly; bone
marrow, erythroid hyperplasia; increased trabeculation of
bone; test for Hb F by alkali denaturation test and
electrophoretic pattern.

Chronic hemorrhage
(1) Females—excess menstrual bleeding.
(2) Both: (a) G.I. tract lesion (ulcer, gastritis, colitis,
carcinoma, hemorrhage, esophageal varices). (b) Renal
tract lesion (calculi, cystitis, hemangioma and
carcinoma).

Fe deficiency
Hb - RBC low; serum iron low; total iron-
binding capacity high; marrow, normal to
slight normoblastic hyperplasia; absent
hemosiderin.

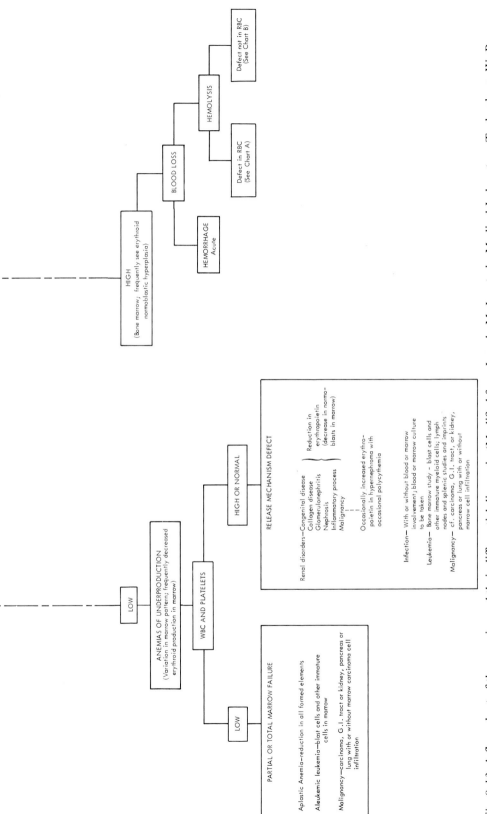

Fig. 8-13. A flow chart of the anemias and their differential diagnosis. (Modified from Lynch, M. J., et al.: Medical Laboratory Technology. W. B. Saunders, Philadelphia, 1963)

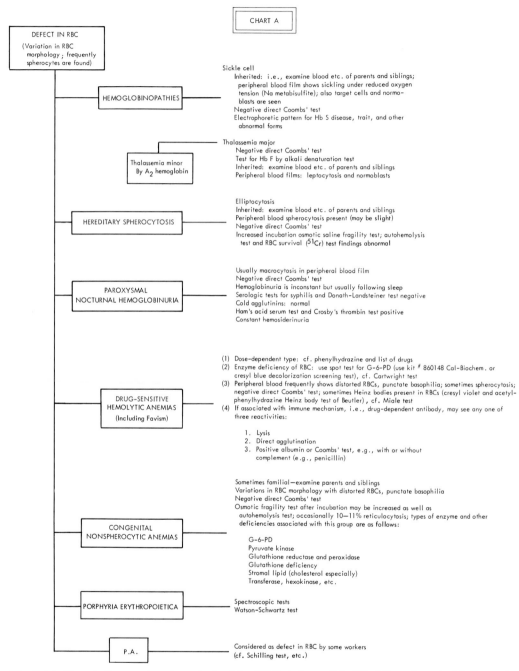

DEFECT IN RBC

(Variation in RBC morphology; frequently spherocytes are found)

HEMOGLOBINOPATHIES

Sickle cell
Inherited: i.e., examine blood etc. of parents and siblings; peripheral blood film shows sickling under reduced oxygen tension (Na metabisulfite); also target cells and normoblasts are seen
Negative direct Coombs' test
Electrophoretic pattern for Hb S disease, trait, and other abnormal forms

Thalassemia minor By A_2 hemoglobin

Thalassemia major
Negative direct Coombs' test
Test for Hb F by alkali denaturation test
Inherited: examine blood etc. of parents and siblings
Peripheral blood films: leptocytosis and normoblasts

HEREDITARY SPHEROCYTOSIS

Elliptocytosis
Inherited: examine blood etc. of parents and siblings
Peripheral blood spherocytosis present (may be slight)
Negative direct Coombs' test
Increased incubation osmotic saline fragility test; autohemolysis test and RBC survival (^{51}Cr) test findings abnormal

PAROXYSMAL NOCTURNAL HEMOGLOBINURIA

Usually macrocytosis in peripheral blood film
Negative direct Coombs' test
Hemoglobinuria is inconstant but usually following sleep
Serologic tests for syphilis and Donath-Landsteiner test negative
Cold agglutinins: normal
Ham's acid serum test and Crosby's thrombin test positive
Constant hemosiderinuria

DRUG-SENSITIVE HEMOLYTIC ANEMIAS (Including Favism)

(1) Dose-dependent type: cf. phenylhydrazine and list of drugs
(2) Enzyme deficiency of RBC: use spot test for G-6-PD (use kit # 860148 Cal-Biochem. or cresyl blue decolorization screening test), cf. Cartwright test
(3) Peripheral blood frequently shows distorted RBCs, punctate basophilia; sometimes spherocytosis; negative direct Coombs' test; sometimes Heinz bodies present in RBCs (cresyl violet and acetyl-phenylhydrazine Heinz body test of Beutler), cf. Miale test
(4) If associated with immune mechanism, i.e., drug-dependent antibody, may see any one of three reactivities:

    1. Lysis
    2. Direct agglutination
    3. Positive albumin or Coombs' test, e.g., with or without complement (e.g., penicillin)

CONGENITAL NONSPHEROCYTIC ANEMIAS

Sometimes familial—examine parents and siblings
Variations in RBC morphology with distorted RBCs, punctate basophilia
Negative direct Coombs' test
Osmotic fragility test after incubation may be increased as well as autohemolysis test; occasionally 10—11% reticulocytosis; types of enzyme and other deficiencies associated with this group are as follows:

    G-6-PD
    Pyruvate kinase
    Glutathione reductase and peroxidase
    Glutathione deficiency
    Stromal lipid (cholesterol especially)
    Transferase, hexokinase, etc.

PORPHYRIA ERYTHROPOIETICA

Spectroscopic tests
Watson-Schwartz test

P.A.

Considered as defect in RBC by some workers
(cf. Schilling test, etc.)

Fig. 8-14. Hemolytic anemias characterized by RBC defects. (Modified from Lynch, M. J., et al.: Medical Laboratory Technology. Philadelphia, W. B. Saunders, 1963)

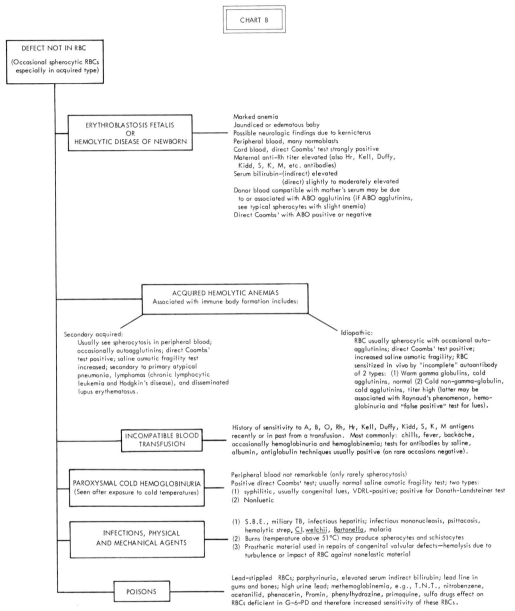

Fig. 8-15. Hemolytic anemias without RBC defect. (Modified from Lynch, M. J., et al.: Medical Laboratory Technology. Philadelphia, W. B. Saunders, 1963)

Laboratory Studies to Confirm Further the Diagnosis of Hemolytic Anemia. The best criteria are the demonstration of an increased concentration of the products of blood destruction in the blood, urine, and stools. An easily measured index is the serum bilirubin, and this should be mostly of the indirect fraction. There should be an elevation in fecal and urine urobilinogen, and in many cases an abnormal erythrocyte fragility, demonstrated by the saline fragility test. The direct Coombs test is positive in many kinds of hemolytic anemias. Free hemoglobin may be demonstrated in the plasma or

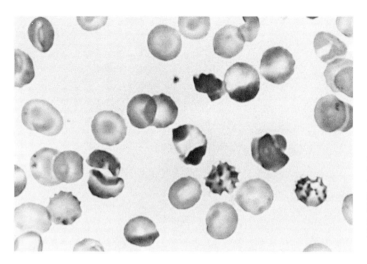

Fig. 8-16. Photomicrograph of peripheral blood of patient with congenital hemolytic anemia characterized by dehydrated red blood cells. (dessicytes; Glader, B. E., et al.: N. Engl. J. Med., *291:*491, 1974)

in the urine, although this is seen in only sudden and extensive hemolytic processes. Determination of the erythrocyte survival time with ^{51}Cr is a very accurate way of detecting and assessing the degree of hemolysis, but it should be remembered that because the bone marrow is capable of producing at such high rate, a clinical anemia will not be present until there is marked shortening of the erythrocyte survival time. Another criterion of a hemolytic anemia is the demonstration of increased erythrocyte production (erythroid normoblastic hyperplasia in bone marrow—the greater the hyperplasia, the greater the degree of hemolytic anemia).

Establishing the Type of Hemolytic Anemia. *Hereditary hemolytic anemias (abnormal hemoglobins).* When the homozygous types of hereditary hemolytic anemia are present, they are usually associated with some morphologic abnormality of red blood cells—that is, elliptical, round, oval, or sickle forms. Heterozygous or trait hemoglobinopathies can be associated with some degree of morphologic abnormality. Thalassemia major shows many target cells and an increased concentration of Hb F, detectable by the use of the alkali denaturation test. Thalassemia minor is also established by finding Hb A in paper and starch block electrophoretic patterns.

Hereditary hemolytic anemias (Erythrocyte enzyme deficiencies). The G-6-PD spot test or the cresyl blue decoloration test is used. Because red blood cells deficient in G-6-PD are most sensitive to hemolysis, it may be more difficult to demonstrate a deficiency during a hemolytic crisis than it would be in a relatively stable period between crises. Pyruvate kinase deficiencies in erythrocytes are usually seen in persons of north Europena stock and occasionally in Mexican families.

Acquired hemolytic anemias usually result from causes outside the red cell, although occasionally the history of a case associated with paroxysms of hemoglobinuria associated with sleep and a positive Ham acid serum test may indicate an intracorpuscular weakness. However, the most common cause is some type of infectious agent—for example, world-wide malaria due to various types of plasmodia or other intraerythrocytic forms, observed especially in thick blood films. Bacteria, especially clostridia, and viruses, particularly infectious mononucleosis, often cause intravascular hemolysis. A positive serologic test for syphilis and a positive Donath-Landsteiner test may be the cause of paroxysmal cold hemoglobinuria in a patient exposed to low temperatures. Also, a high cold agglutinin titer with a negative

Donath-Landsteiner test may be significant of a primary atypical pneumonia associated with the Eaton virus.

Many chemical agents cause hemolysis. Some of these appear to be directly toxic to the red cell, and their effect is directly related to the size of the dose (for example, phenacetin and phenylhydrazine) with Heinz-Ehrlich bodies present, especially in phenylhydrazine toxicity. The hydrocarbons and nitrated hydrocarbons are also toxic agents. With other agents the response is one that is probably either secondary to hypersensitivity or is caused by a latent enzyme deficiency (G-6-PD) within the red blood cell itself; these disorders include sensitivity due to chloroquine, pamaquine, or phenylhydrazine, and favism, with Heinz-Ehrlich bodies also found in these red blood cells on many occasions.

When the hemolysis follows blood transfusion, a transfusion reaction must be considered, and the blood groups of the erythrocytes should be determined. A comparison of the isoagglutinins present in the plasma is made, and the direct and indirect Coombs tests are also performed. If there is jaundice in a newborn, hemolytic disease of the newborn (erythroblastosis fetalis) must be considered with associated Rh, hr, Kell, Duffy, ABO, and other incompatibilities involved. The determination of agglutinin titer, a positive direct Coombs test on cord blood and elevated serum bilirubin in cord blood are part of the diagnostic laboratory work-up. Other secondary hemolytic anemias are those with autoimmune antibodies associated with chronic lymphocytic leukemia, Hodgkin's disease, and disseminated lupus erythematosus (Figs. 8-13–8-16).

REFERENCES

1. Abe, S.: Secondary red cell pyruvate kinase deficiency: I. Study of 30 subjects of malignant hematological disorders. Acta Haematol. Jap., *39:*247, 1976.
2. Adams, J. F., et al.: The histological and secretory changes in the stomach in patients with autoimmunity to gastric parietal cells. Lancet, *1:*401, 1964.
3. Ali, M. A., and Brain, M. C.: Ethanol inhibition of hemoglobin synthesis: in vitro evidence for a heme correctable defect in normal subjects and in alcoholics. J. Haematol., *28:*311, 1974.
4. Andelman, M. B., and Sered, B. R.: Utilization of dietary iron by term infants: a study of 1,048 infants from a low socioeconomic population. Am. J. Dis. Child., *111:*45, 1966.
5. Atkinson, J. P., and Frank, M. M.: Complement-independent clearance of IgG-sensitized erythrocytes: inhibition of cortisone. Blood, *44:*629, 1974.
6. Atkinson, J. P., Schreiber, A. D., and Frank, M. M.: Effect of corticosteroids and splenectomy on immune clearance and destruction of erythrocytes. J. Clin. Invest., *52:*1509, 1973.
7. Bainton, D. F., and Finch, C. A.: Diagnosis of iron deficiency anemia. Am. J. Med., *37:*62, 1964.
7a. Baron, D. T., Griner, P. F., and Klemperer, M. R.: Recovery from aplastic anemia after treatment with cyclophosphamide. N. Engl. J. Med., *295:*1522, 1976.
8. Barry, W. E., and Day, H. J.: Refractory sideroblastic anemia – clinical and hematologic study of 10 cases. Ann. Intern. Med., *61:*1029, 1964.
9. Beeson, P. B., and McDermott, W.: Cecil-Loeb Textbook of Medicine. p. 1072. Philadelphia, W. B. Saunders, 1963.
10. Bernhardt, H., Burkett, L. L., Fields, M. L., and Killian, J.: The diagnostic significance of the parietal cell immunofluorescent test. Ann. Intern. Med., *63:*635, 1965.
11. Beutler, E., Johnson, C., Priors, D., and West, C.: Prevalence of glucose 6-phosphate dehydrogenase deficiency in sickle cell disease. N. Engl. J. Med., *290:*826, 1974.
12. Blass, J. P., and Dean, H. M.: Relation of hyperlipemia to hemolytic anemia in an alcoholic patient. Am. J. Med., *40:*283, 1966.
13. Bottinger, L. E., and Westerholm, B.: Drug-induced blood dyscrasias in Sweden. Br. Med. J., *3:*339, 1973.
14. Brown, A. K., and Showacre, J.: Phototherapy of the neonatal hyperbilirubinemia: Long-term implications. National Institute of Child Health and Human Development. Department of Health, Education and Welfare Publication N. (NIH) 76-1075, 1976.
15. Carmel, R., and Herbert, V.: Presence of "precipitating" or "blocking" antibody to intrinsic factor in gasric juice or serum of nearly all pernicious anemia patients. Clin. Res., *14:*482, 1966.
16. Carson, P. E.: Glucose – 6-phosphate dehydrogenase deficiency in hemolytic anemia. Fed. Proc., *19:*995, 1960.
17. Castle, W. B.: Megaloblastic Anemias; Yearbook of Medicine. pp. 689; 708–709, 1966-67.
18. Chailley, B., Weed, R. I., Leblond, P. F., and Maigne, J.: Echinotic and stomatocytic forms of red cells: their reversibility and convertibility. Nouv. Rev. Fr. Hematol., *13:*71, 1973.
19. Chanarin, I., and James, D.: Humoral and cell-

mediated intrinsic factor antibody in pernicious anemia. Lancet, *1:*1078, 1974.

20. Chanarin, I., Perry, J., and Lumb, M.: Biochemical lesions in vitamin B$_{12}$ deficiency in man. Lancet, *1:*1251, 1974.

21. Charache, S., and Conley, C. L.: Pathogenesis of hemolytic anemia in homozygous hemoglobin C disease (abstract). pp. 22–23. Presented at the annual meeting of the American Society of Hematology, 1966.

22. Cherry, S. H., Kochwa, S., and Rosenfield, R. E.: Ratio test improves fetal diagnosis (in erythroblastosis fetalis). p. 170. Med. World News, Jan. 13, 1967.

23. Chiu, D., Lubin, B., and Shohket, S.: Effect of sickling on the reaction of erythrocytes with 2,4,6-trinitrobenzenesulfonic acid. Fed. Proc., *36:*707, 1977.

24. Cooper, R. A., Ames, E. C., Wiley, J. S., and Shattil, S. J.: Modification of red cell membrane structure by cholesterol-rich lipid dispersions. J. Clin. Invest., *55:*515, 1975.

25. Cooper, R. A., and Jandl, J. H.: Mechanism of target cell formation in jaundice. Clin. Res., *14:*314, 1966.

26. Cooper, R. A., Kimball, D. B., and Durocher, J. R.: Role of spleen in membrane conditioning and hemolysis of spur cells in liver diseases. N. Engl. J. Med., *290:*1279, 1974.

27. Cowan, D. H., and Hines, J. D.: Thrombokinetics in dietary-induced folate deficiency in human subjects. J. Lab. Clin. Med., *81:*577, 1973.

28. Crosby, W. H.: The control of iron balance by the intestinal mucosa. Blood, *22:*441, 1963.

28a.——: Hematology-Contempo. 1977. J.A.M.A., *239:*515, 1978.

29. Dacie, J. V., et al.: Hereditary Heinz body anemias. Br. J. Haematol., *10:*388, 1964.

30. Dacie, J. V., Mollison, P. L., Richardson, N., Selwyn, J. G., and Shapiro, L.: Atypical congenital hemolytic anemia. Q. J. Med., *22:*79, 1953.

31. DeCesare, W., Rath, C., and Hufnagel, C.: Hemolytic anemia of mechanical origin with aortic-valve prostheses. N. Engl. J. Med., *272:*1045, 1965.

32. Diamond, L. K.: Steroids may be harmful in anemia. p. 171. Med. World News, Jan. 13, 1967.

33. Diggs, L. W.: Sickle cell crises. Am. J. Clin. Pathol., *44:*1, 1965.

34. Doxiadis, S. A., Fessas, P., Valaes, T., and Mastrokalos, N.: G6PD deficiency. Lancet, 1:297, 1961.

35. Editorial: Hereditary spherocytosis. J.A.M.A., *193:*954, 1965.

36. Editorial: Intrinsic factor inhibitors, pernicious anemia, and autoimmunity. N. Engl. J. Med., *275:*562, 1966.

37. Emerson, C. P., Ham, T. H., and Castle, W. B.: Hemolytic action of certain organic oxidants derived from sulfanilamide, phenylhydrazine and hydroquinon. J. Clin. Invest., *20:*451, 1941.

38. Estren, S., and Dameshek, W.: Familial hypoplastic anemia of childhood. Am. J. Dis. Child., *73:*671, 1947.

39. Eyster, F., and Bernene, J.: Nosocomial anemia. J.A.M.A., *223:*73, 1973.

40. Fairbanks, V. F.: A tetrazolium stain for quantitative estimation of G6PD in individual erythrocytes and for the identification of weakly expressed heterozygotes for G6PD deficiency. Presented at the annual meeting of the American Society of Hematology, 1966.

41. Fessas, P., and Papayannopoulou, T.: Cytochemical observations on β-thalassemia: I. PAS-positive substance of erythroblasts. Acta Haematol., *34:*1, 1965.

42. Forman, S., Bischel, M., and Hochstein, P.: Erythrocyte deformability in uremic hemodialyzed patients. Ann. Intern. Med., *79:*841, 1973.

43. Glader, B. E., Fortier, N., Albala, M. M., and Nathan, D. G.: Congenital hemolytic anemia associated with dehydrated erythrocytes and increased potassium loss. N. Engl. J. Med., *291:*491, 1974.

44. Goebel, K. M., Goebel, F. D., Schwartz, R., and Schneider, J.: Red cell metabolic and membrane features in hemolytic anemia of alcoholic liver disease (Zieve's syndrome). Br. J. Haematol., *35:*573, 1977.

44a. Good, R. A.: Aplastic anemia: suppressor lymphocytes and hematopoiesis. N. Engl. J. Med., *296:*41, 1977.

45. Gordon, A. S., et al.: Properties of the renal erythropoietic factor (REF) (abstract). Presented at the annual meeting of the American Society of Hematology, 1966.

46. Goulding, F. J.: Priapism caused by glucose phosphate isomerase deficiency. J. Urol.: *116:*819, 1976.

47. Gray, G. R., et al.: Neutrophil dysfunction, chronic granulomatous diseases and nonspherocytic hemolytic anemia caused by complete deficiency of glucose-6-phosphate dehydrogenase. Lancet, 2:530, 1973.

48. Hamilton, E. G., and Pilla, L. A.: Intrauterine transfusion of erythroblastosis fetalis. Mo. Med., *62:*682, 1965.

49. Harris, J. W.: The Red Cell — Production, Metabolism, Destruction: Normal and Abnormal. pp. 115–117; 333–358. Cambridge, Harvard University Press, 1963.

50. Herbert, V., Streiff, L. R., and Sullivan, L. W.: Notes on vitamin B$_{12}$ absorption: autoimmunity and P.A.: Relation of intrinsic factor to blood group substances. Medicine, *43:*679, 1964.

51. Hilgard, P., and Gordon-Smith, E. C.: Microangiopathic hemolytic anemia and experimental tumor cell emboli. Br. J. Haematol., *26:*651, 1974.

51a. Hoffman, R., et al.: Suppression of erythroid-colony formation by lymphocytes from patients with aplastic anemia. N. Engl. J. Med., *296:*10, 1977.

52. Holloway, B. W., and Ripley, S. H.: Nucleic acid content of reticulocytes and its relation to uptake of radioactive leucine in vitro. J. Biol. Chem., *196:*695, 1952.

53. Horrigan, D. L.: Pyridoxine-responsive anemia; influence of tryptophan on pyridoxine responsiveness. Blood, *42:*187, 1973.

54. Hosey, M., and Tao, M.: Altered erythrocyte membrane phosphorylation in sickle cell disease. Nature, *263*:424, 1976.

55. Hoskins, L. C., Loux, H. A., Britten, A., and Zamcheck, N.: Distribution of ABO blood groups in patients with P.A., gastric carcinoma and gastric carcinoma associated with P.A. N. Engl. J. Med., *273*:633, 1965.

56. Huissman, T. H. J., Schroeder, W. A., Brodic, A. N., et al.: Microchromatography of hemoglobins: III. A simplified procedure for the determination of a hemoglobin A_2. J. Lab. Clin. Med., *86*:702, 1975.

57. Ingall, D., Sherman, J. D., Cockburn, M. B., and Klein, R.: Amelioration by ingestion of phenylalanine of toxic effects of chloramphenicol on bone marrow. N. Engl. J. Med., *272*:180, 1965.

58. Ingram, V. M.: The Hemoglobins in Genetics and Evolution. New York, Columbia University Press, 1963.

59. Irvine, W. J.: Immunologic aspects of P.A. N. Engl. J. Med., *273*:432, 1965.

60. Jacob, F., and Monod, J.: Genetic regulatory mechanisms in synthesis of proteins. J. Mol. Biol., *3*:318, 1961.

61. Jacob, H. S., and Jandl, J. H.: Increased cell membrane permeability in pathogenesis of hereditary spherocytosis. J. Clin. Invest., *43*:1704, 1964.

62. ——: A simple visual screening test for glucose-6-phosphate dehydrogenase deficiency employing ascorbate and cyanide. N. Engl. J. Med., *274*:1162, 1966.

63. Jacobs, A., and Wormwood, M.: Ferritin in serum. N. Engl. J. Med., *292*:951, 1975.

64. Jandl, J. H.: The pathophysiology of hemolytic anemias—a foreword. Symposium on disorders of the red cell. Am. J. Med., *41*:657, 1966.

65. Jandl, J. H., Greenberg, M. S., Yonemoto, R. H., and Castle, W. B.: Clinical determination of the sites of red blood cell sequestration in hemolytic anemias. J. Clin. Invest., *35*:842, 1956.

66. Jensen, T. D., Bunn, H. F., Halbas, G., Kan, Y. W., and Nathan, D. G.: Effects of cyanate and 2,3-DPG on sickling: relationship to oxygenation. J. Clin. Invest., *52*:2542, 1973.

67. Jensen, W. N., Bromberg, P. A., and Bessis, M.: Microincision of sickled erythrocytes by a laser beam (abstract). Presented at the annual meeting of the American Society of Hematology, 1966.

68. Jensen, W. N., Moreno, G. D., and Bessis, M. C.: Electron microscopic description of basophilic stippling in red cells. Blood, *25*:933, 1965.

69. Johnson, G. J., Kaplan, M. E., and Beutler, E.: G6PD Long prairie—a new glucose-6-phosphate dehydrogenase mutant exhibiting normal sensitivity to inhibition by NADPH and accompanied by nonspherocytic hemolytic anemia. Blood, *49*:247, 1977.

70. Jonxes, J. H. P., and Huisman, T. H. J.: A Laboratory Manual on Abnormal Hemoglobins. p. 6. Oxford, Blackwell Scientific Publications, 1958.

71. Kan, Y. W., Allen, A., and Lowenstein, L.: Hydrops fetalis with alpha-thalassemia. N. Engl. J. Med., *276*:18, 1967.

72. Kaplan, E., Herz, F., Hsu, K. S., Stevenson, J., and Scheye, E.: Erythrocyte acetylcholinesterase activity in ABO hemolytic disease of the newborn. Pediatrics, *33*:205, 1964.

73. Kendall, A. G., and Charlow, G. F.: Red cell pyruvate kinase deficiency: Adverse effect of oral contraceptives. Acta Haematol., *57*:111, 1977.

74. Kiossoglu, K. A., Mitus, W. J., and Dameshek, W.: Chromosomal aberrations in pernicious anemia—study of 3 cases before and after therapy. Blood, *25*:662, 1965.

75. Kosmin, M., et al.: Decreased erythropoiesis associated with subnormal urinary erythropoietin activity: the anemia of pregnancy (abstract). Presented at the annual meeting of the American Society of Hematology, 1966.

76. Krevans, J. R.: Control of Rh disease: aim of experimental study, J.A.M.A. (Medical News), *193*:37, 1965.

77. Kutscher, H.: Das verhalten der ATPase im intaken erythrozyten bei der oxydation durch glutathion. Folia Haematol., *78*:360, 1961.

78. Lange, R. D., et al.: Refractory anemia occurring in survivors of the atomic bombing of Nagasaki, Japan. Blood, *10*:312, 1955.

79. Lau, K. S., Gottlieb, C., Wasserman, L. R., and Herbert, V.: Measurement of serum vitamin B_{12} level using radioisotope dilution and coated charcoal. Blood, *26*:202, 1965.

80. Lawrence, C., and Klipstein, F. A.: Megaloblastic anemia of pregancy in New York City, Ann. Intern. Med., *66*:25, 1967.

81. Leikola, J., Koistinen, J., Lehtinen, M., and Virolainen, M.: IgA-induced anaphylactic transfusion reactions: report of four cases. Blood, *42*:111, 1973.

82. Levine, P. H.: Qualitative platelet defect in severe vitamin B_{12} deficiency: response, hyperresponse, and thrombosis after vitamin B_{12} therapy. Ann. Intern. Med., *78*:533, 1973.

83. Levine, P., Tripodi, D., Struck, J., Jr., Zmijewski, M., and Pollock, W.: Hemolytic anemia associated with Rh null but not with Bombay blood: hypothesis based on differing antigenic structure. Vox. Sang., *24*:417, 1973.

84. Levinson, S. A., and McFate, R. P.: Clinical Laboratory Diagnosis. ed. 6. p. 735. Philadelphia, Lea & Febiger, 1961.

85. Lewis, M., Lee, G. R., and Haut, A.: The association of hemochromatosis with thalassemia minor. Ann. Intern. Med., *63*:122, 1965.

86. Lewis, S. M., Nelson, D. A., and Pitcher, C. S.: Clinical and ultrastructural aspects of congenital dyserythropoietic anemia type I. Br. J. Haematol., *23*:113, 1972.

87. Li, J. G., Herbert, V., and Carmel, R.: Antibody causing vitamin B_{12} deficiency (correspondence). N. Engl. J. Med., *276*:61, 1967.

88. Li, J. G., Mettier, S. R., Harper, H. A., and McBride, A.: Pernicious anemia due to presence of intrinsic factor inhibitor diagnosed in childhood, with 25-year follow-up. Clin. Res., *7*:90, 1959.

89. Lock, S. P., Smith, R. S., and Hardisty, R. M.: Stomatocytosis: a hereditary red cell anomaly

associated with hemolytic anemia. Br. J. Hematol., *7:*303, 1961.

90. Loeb, V., Moore, C. V., and Dubach, R.: The physiologic evaluation and management of chronic bone marrow failure. Am. J. Med., *15:*499, 1953.

91. Löhr, G. W., and Waller, H. D.: Eine neue enzymopenische hämolytische Anämie mit glutathionreduktase Mangel. Med. Klin., *57:*1521, 1962.

92. Lynch, M. J., et al.: Medical Laboratory Technology. p. 289. Philadelphia, W. B. Saunders, 1963.

93. McCurdy, P. R.: Oral and parenteral iron therapy, a comparison. J.A.M.A., *191:*859, 1965.

94. MacDonald, R. A., Jones, R. S., and Pechet, G. S.: Folic acid deficiency and hemochromatosis. Arch. Pathol., *80:*153, 1965.

95. McIntyre, M., Clink, H. M., Levi, A. J., Cumings, J. N., and Sherlock, S.: Hemolytic anemia in Wilson's disease. N. Engl. J. Med., *276:*439, 1967.

96. MacKenney, A. A., Jr.: Hereditary spherocytosis: clinical family studies. Arch. Intern. Med., *116:*257, 1965.

97. MacKenney, A. A., Jr., Newton, E. M., Kosower, N. S., and Schilling, R. F.: Ascertaining genetic carriers of spherocytosis by statistical analysis of multiple laboratory tests. J. Clin. Invest., *4:*554, 1962.

98. McPhedran, P., Barnes, M. G., Weinstein, J. S., and Robertson, J. S.: Interpretation of electronically determined macrocytosis. Ann. Intern. Med., *78:*677, 1973.

99. Manis, J. G., and Schachter, D.: Active transport of iron by intestine: features of a two-step mechanism. Am. J. Physiol., *203:*73, 1962.

100. Manis, J. G., and Schachter, D.: Active transport of iron by intestine: effects of oral iron and pregnancy. Am. J. Physiol., *203:*81, 1962.

101. Marahmadi, K. S., et al.: Screen ferritin level (determination of iron requirement in hemodialysis patients). J.A.M.A., *238:*601, 1977.

102. Mengel, C. E., Meriwether, D., Ebbert, L., and Kann, H. E., Jr.: Effects of reduced glutathione (GSH) on normal RBCs: Clues to the corpuscular defect in paroxysmal nocturnal hemoglobinuria (PNH) (abstract). Presented at the annual meeting of the American Society of Hematology, 1966.

103. Moore, C. V., et al.: Hematology Notes. Washington University School of Medicine, 1964–65.

104. Movitt, E. R., Mangum, J. F., and Porter, W. R.: Idiopathic bone marrow failure. Am. J. Med., *34:*500, 1963.

105. Murphy, J. R.: Erythrocyte metabolism. III. Relationship of energy metabolism and serum factors to osmotic fragility following incubation. J. Lab. Clin. Med., *60:*86, 1962.

106. ———: Role of cholesterol in determining shape of erythrocytes (abstract). Blood, *24:*838, 1964.

107. Nathan, D. G., Oski, F. A., Sidel, V. W., and Diamond, L. K.: Extreme hemolysis and red-cell distortion in erythrocyte pyruvate kinase deficiency. N. Engl. J. Med., *272:*118, 1965.

108. Necheles, T. F., Boles, T. A., and Allen, D. M.: Erythrocyte glutathione-peroxidase deficiency and hemolytic disease of the newborn (abstract). Presented at the annual meeting of the American Society of Hematology, 1966.

109. Neimann, N., Najean, Y., Scialom, C., Pierson, M., and Bernard, J.: A case of megaloblastic anemia in a child with abnormal orotic acid excretion. Nouv. Rev. Fr. Hematol., *5:*445, 1965.

110. Newman, D. R., Pierre, R. V., and Linman, J. W.: Studies in diagnostic significance of hemoglobin F levels. Mayo Clin. Proc., *48:*199, 1973.

111. Noyes, W. D., and Green, B. C.: Oxygen consumption of iron-deficient mitochondria (abstract). Presented at the annual meeting of the American Society of Hematology, 1966.

112. Oort, M., Loos, J. A., and Prins, H. K.: Hereditary absence of reduced glutathione in erythrocytes. New clinical and biochemical entity? (preliminary communication). Vox Sang., *6:*370, 1961.

113. Page, L. B., and Culver, P. J.: Physiology of the red cell. In Syllabus of Laboratory Examinations in Clinical Diagnosis. pp. 100–101; 126. Cambridge, Harvard University Press, 1960.

114. Pearson, H. A., O'Brien, R. T., and McIntosh, S.: Screening for thalassemia trait by electronic measurement of mean corpuscular volume. N. Engl. J. Med., *288:*351, 1973.

115. Perrene, R. P., Brown, M. J., Clegg, J. B., Weatherall, D. J., and May, A.: Benign sickle cell anemia. Lancet, *2:*1163, 1972.

116. Petersen, C. M., and Jones, R. L.: Minor hemoglobins, diabetic "control" and diseases of postsynthetic protein modification. Ann. Intern Med., *87:*489, 1977.

117. Petz, L. D., and Fudenberg, H. H.: Coombs positive hemolytic anemia caused by penicillin administration. N. Engl. J. Med., *274:*171, 1966.

118. Prins, H. K., Oort, M., Loos, J. A., Zürcher, C., and Beckers, T.: Congenital nonspherocytic hemolytic anemia associated with glutathione deficiency of erythrocytes: hematologic, biochemical and genetic studies. Blood, *27:*145, 1966.

119. Quagliana, J. M., Cartwright, G. E., and Wintrobe, M. M.: Paroxysmal nocturnal hemoglobinuria following drug-induced aplastic anemia. Ann. Intern. Med., *61:*1045, 1052, 1964.

120. Rachmilewitz, E. A., Lubin, B. H., and Shohet, S. B.: Lipid membrane peroxidation in β-thalassemia major. Blood, *46:*495, 1976.

121. Rausen, A. R., Richter, P., Tallal, L., and Cooper, L. Z.: Hematologic effects of intrauterine rubella. J.A.M.A., *199:*75, 1967.

122. Rebuck, J. W.: Critique-hematology check sample No. H-17. (C.C.E.-A.S.C.P.), Oct., 1963.

123. Rebuck, J. W.: Critique-hematology check sample No. H-30 (C.C.E.-A.S.C.P.), Jan., 1967, p. 5.

124. Redeker, A. G., and Yamahiro, H. S.: Controlled trial of exchange transfusion therapy in fulminant hepatitis. Lancet, *1:*3, 1973.

125. Rickles, F. R., and O'Leary, D. S.: Role of coagulation system in pathophysiology of sickle cell disease. Arch. Int. Med. *133:*635, 1974.

126. Ritzmann, S. E.: HLA patterns and disease associations. J.A.M.A., *236:*2305, 1976.

127. Rosse, W. F., Dourmashkin, R., and Humphrey,

J. H.: Immune lysis of normal human and paroxysmal nocturnal hemoglobinuria (PNH) red blood cells. III. The membrane defects caused. J. Exp. Med., *123*:969, 1966.

128. Rosse, W. T., Adams, J. P., and Thorpe, A. M.: Population of cells in paroxysmal nocturnal hemoglobinuria of intermediate sensitivity to complement lysis: Significance and mechanism of increased immune lysis. Br. J. Haematol., *28*:181, 1974.

128a. Royal-Marsden Hospital Bone-Marrow Transplantation Team: Failure of syngeneic bone-marrow graft without preconditioning in posthepatitis marrow aplasia. Lancet, *2*:742, 1977.

129. Sanchez-Medal, L., Gomez-Leal, A., and Duarte-Zapata, L.: Anabolic therapy in aplastic anemia (abstract). Presented at the annual meeting of the American Society of Hematology, 1966.

130. Schade, S. G., Feick, P., Muckerheide, M., and Schilling, R. F.: Occurrence in gastric juice of antibody to a complex of intrinsic factor and vitamin B_{12}. N. Engl. J. Med., *275*:528, 1966.

131. Schench, D., and Rapport, S.: Intrazellulare Regulation der Aktivitat einiger SH-Enzyme durch Glutathion. Folia Haematol., *78*:349, 1961.

132. Schilling, R. F., Muckerheide, M., Jacobs, E., and Abels, J.: Multiple autoantibodies to gastric juice (abstract). Ann. Intern. Med., *62*:1085, 1965.

133. Schloesser, L. L., Kipp, M. A., and Wenzel, F. J.: Thrombocytosis in iron deficiency anemia. J. Lab. Clin. Med., *66*:107, 1965.

134. Scott, J. L., Finegold, S. M., Belken, G. A., and Lawrence, J. S.: A controlled double-blind study of the hematologic toxicity of chloramphenicol. N. Engl. J. Med., *272*:1138, 1965.

135. Sensenbrenner, L., and Santos, G. W.: Rationale for marrow transplants in human disease. Presented at a symposium of the American Society of Hematology, pp. 106-108, Dec. 4, 1971.

136. Shen, S. C., and Homburger, F.: The anemia of cancer patients and its relation to metastases to the bone marrow. J. Lab. Clin. Med., *37*:182, 1951.

137. Shore, N. A., Schneider, A. S., and Valentine, W. N.: Erythrocyte triosephosphate isomerase deficiency (abstract). J. Pediatr., *67*:939, 1965.

138. Siimes, M. A., and Dallman, P. R.: New kinetic role for serum ferritin in iron metabolism. Br. J. Haematol., *28*:7, 1974.

139. Simon, E. R., and Ways, P.: Incubation hemolysis and red cell metabolism in acanthrocytosis. J. Clin. Invest., *43*:1311, 1964.

140. Smith, E. W., and Conley, C. L.: Filter paper electrophoresis of human hemoglobins with special reference to the incidence and clinical significance of hemoglobin. Johns Hopkins Med. J., *93*:94, 1953.

141. Stematoyannopoulos, G., Woodson, R., Rapayannapolous, T., Haywood, D., and Kurachi, S.: Inclusion body β-thalassemia trait: form of β-thalassemia producing clinical manifestations in simple heterozygotes. N. Engl. J. Med., *290*:939, 1974.

141a. Storb, R., et al.: Aplastic anemia treated by allogenic bone marrow transplantation. A report on 49 new cases from Seattle. Blood, *48*:817, 1976.

142. Swisher, S. N.: Immune hemolysis. Ann. Rev. Med., *15*:1, 1964.

143. Tanaka, K. R., Valentine, W. N., and Muva, S.: Pyruvate kinase (PK) deficiency in hereditary nonspherocytic anemia. Blood, *19*:267, 1962.

144. Tartaglia, A. P., Propp, S., Amarose, A. P., Propp, R. P., and Hall, C. A.: Chromosome abnormality and hypocalcemia in congenital erythroid hypoplasia (Blackfan-Diamond syndrome). Am. J. Med., *41*:990, 1966.

145. Taylor, K. B., Roitt, I. M., Doniach, D., Couchman, K. G., and Shapland, C.: Autoimmune phenomena in P.A.: Gastric antibodies. Br. Med. J., *2*:1347, 1962.

146. Thomas, E. D., Fefer, A., Buchner, C. D., and Storb, R.: Current status of bone marrow transplantation for aplastic anemia and acute leukemia. Blood, *49*:671, 1977.

147. Todhope, G. R., and Wilson, G. M.: Deficiency of vitamin B_{12} in hypothyroidism. Lancet, *1*:703, 1962.

148. Townsend, J. D.: An evaluation of a recent modification of the Watson-Schwartz test for porphobilinogen. Ann. Intern. Med., *60*:306, 1964.

149. Valentine, W. N., et al.: Hereditary hemolytic anemia with hexokinase deficiency – role of hexokinase in erythrocyte aging. N. Engl. J. Med., *276*:1, 1967.

150. Van de Putte, I., Renach, M., and Vermylen, C.: Counting fetal erythrocytes as a diagnostic aid in perinatal death and morbidity. Am. J. Obstet. Gynecol., *114*:850, 1972.

151. VanSnick, J. L., Masson, P. L., and Heremans, J. F.: Involvement of lactoferrin in the hyposideremia of acute inflammation. J. Exp. Med., *140*:1068, 1974.

152. Vilan, J., Rhyner, K., and Ganzoni, A. M.: Pure red cell aplasia: successful treatment with cyclophosphamide. Blut, *26*:27, 1973.

153. Vilter, R. W., et al.: Refractory anemia with hyperplastic bone marrow. Blood, *15*:1, 1960.

154. Weatherall, D. J., and McIntyre, P. A.: Developmental and acquired variations in erythrocyte carbonic anhydrase isozymes. Br. J. Haematol., *13*:106, 1967.

155. White, J. M., and Ali, M. A.: Globin synthesis in sideroblastic anemia II: Effect of pyridoxine, delta-aminolevulinic acid and heme, in vitro. Br. J. Haematol., *24*:481, 1973.

156. Yankee, R. A., Graff, K. S., Dowling, R., and Henderson, E. S.: Selection of unrelated compatible platelet donors by lymphocyte HL-A matching. N. Engl. J. Med., *288*:760, 1973.

157. Yawata, Y., Howe, R., and Jacob, H. S.: Abnormal red cell metabolism causing hemolysis in uremia: defect potentiated by tap water hemodialysis. Ann. Intern. Med., *79*:362, 1973.

158. Yawson, G. I., Fessas, A., Boulton, F. E., Huntsman, R. G., and Menzies, I. S.: Estimation of hemoglobin A_2: Is visual assessment reliable? J. Clin. Pathol., *27*:247, 1974.

159. Zaino, E. C.: Iatrogenic β thalassemia. J.A.M.A., *238*:342, 1977.

AUDIOVISUAL AIDS*

Acquired Hemolytic Anemias. [Self-Teaching Slide Review 24]. University of Miami School of Medicine, Department of Internal Medicine (Hematology), Miami, Florida 33136.

Acquired Hemolytic Anemias, Disorders of Iron Metabolism. [Tape 46]. Southern Audio-Visual Exhibition Service, 550 Meridian Avenue, Miami Beach, Florida 33139.

Anemia. (1952). E. R. Squibb Film Library, c/o Hammill Studio, 9510 Belmont Avenue, Franklin Park, Illinois 60131.

An Approach to the Diagnosis of Anemia from the Peripheral Blood Counts and Smear Examination. (1972). *Nomenclature and Definition of Terminology.* T-2497. *Macrocytic Anemia.* T-2498. *Microcytic and Hypochromic Anemias.* T-2510. *Poikilocytosis and Red Cell Inclusions.* T-2511. National Medical Audiovisual Center (Annex), Station K, Atlanta, Georgia 30324.

Blood Banking — Immunohematology: Mechanisms of Action of Red Cell Antibodies. 247604. Frederick J. Koch, M.D. [Standard audiocassette and handout, 21 pp., $14.70]. *Immunohematology: Role of Complement in Blood Banking* [also describes *in vivo* destruction of RBCs]. 247605. Frederick J. Koch, M.D. [standard audiocassette plus handout, 16 pp., $13.70]. Communications in Learning, Inc., 2929 Main Street, Buffalo, New York 14214.

Clinical Applications of Radioisotopes. Robert A. Ackerholt, Ph.D. 247404. [13 (35 mm.) transparencies and standard audiocassette, $29.35]. Communications in Learning, Inc., 2929 Main Street, Buffalo, N.Y. 14214.

Clinical Diagnosis of Anemia. [35 mm. transparencies, manual, audiotape] Set R 1. A.S.H. National Slide Bank, HSLRC T 252 (SB-56), University of Washington, Seattle, Washington 98195.

Clinical Management of Auto-Immune Hematological Disorders. (1958). Audio-Visual Department, Schering Corporation, Bloomfield, New Jersey 07003.

The Combination for Safe Transfusion. Seminars 202, 203. ASMT Education and Research Fund, Inc., 5555 West Loop South, Bellaire, Texas 77401.

The Coombs Test. Part I. Seminar 204. Part II. Seminar 205. ASMT Education and Research Fund, Inc., 5555 West Loop South, Bellaire, Texas 77401.

Cytological Aspects of Immuno-Hematology. International Society for Hematology, James L. Tulles, M.D., 110 Francis Street, Boston, Massachusetts 02215.

Development of the Immune Capacity in the Newborn. (1964). Pfizer Laboratories Film Library, 267 W. 25th Street, New York, New York 10001.

Erythroblastosis Fetalis. (Clinical, Serologic and Pathologic Aspects). T-2021. (1970). National

Medical Audiovisual Center, Station K, Atlanta, Georgia 30324.

Erythroblastosis Fetalis. (Therapy and Prevention). T-2022. (1970). National Medical Audiovisual Center (Annex) Station K, Atlanta, Georgia 30324.

Erythrocytic Stages of Plasmodium Vivax. M-138A. (1954). [4 minutes]. National Medical Audiovisual Center (Annex), Station K, Atlanta, Georgia 30324.

Hemolytic Anemia. [35 mm. transparencies, manual, audiotape]. Set R3. A.S.H. National Slide Bank, HSLRC T 252 (SB-56), University of Washington, Seattle, Washington 98195.

The Hemolytic Syndrome. T-1506. (1969). National Medical Audiovisual Center (Annex), Station K, Atlanta, Georgia 30324.

Hereditary Disorders of RBC. [Tape 45]. Southern Audio-Visual Exhibition Service, 550 Meridian Avenue, Miami Beach, Florida 33139.

Innovations in Transfusion Therapy. (1962). American Association of Blood Banks, 30 N. Michigan, Suite 1619, Chicago, Illinois 60602.

Intrauterine Fetal Transfusions. (1965). [9 minutes]. Abbott Laboratories, Professional Services Department, Abbott Park, North Chicago, Illinois 60064.

Isotopes in the Diagnosis of Anemia. T-1505. (1969). National Medical Audiovisual Center (Annex), (1965). Station K, Atlanta, Georgia 30324.

The Management of Hemolytic Disease of the Newborn. Evanston Hospital, Public Relations Office, 2650 Ridge, Evanston, Illinois 60201.

Megaloblastic Anemias. Seminar 306. ASMT Education and Research Fund, Inc., 5555 West Loop South, Bellaire, Texas 77401.

Megaloblastic Anemias, Acute Leukemias. [Tape 47]. Southern Audio-Visual Exhibition Service, 550 Meridian Avenue, Miami Beach, Florida 33139.

Morphological and Etiological Classification of Anemias. 247701. Barbara L. Stein, M.S., M.T. (ASCP). [19 (35 mm.) transparencies plus handout, 5 pp., and standard audiocassette, $39.05]. Communications in Learning, Inc., 2929 Main Street, Buffalo, N.Y. 14214.

Nutritional Anemias. Part I. Hypochromic Anemia. M-2089-X. Part II. Megaloblastic Anemia. (M-2090-X. National Medical Audiovisual Center (Annex) Station K, Atlanta, Georgia 30324.

Pathogenesis and Management of Hemochromatosis. T-1507. (1969). National Medical Audiovisual Center (Annex), Station K, Atlanta, Georgia 30324.

Pathogenesis of Anemia. T-1504. (1969). National Medical Audiovisual Center (Annex), Station K, Atlanta, Georgia 30324.

Quality Control in Blood Transfusion Service. Seminar 108. ASMT Education and Research Fund, Inc. 5555 West Loop South, Bellaire, Texas 77401.

RBC Production Defects, Granulocyte Production Defects, Myeloproliferative Diseases, Myeloid Metaplasia, Polycythemia, Thrombocythemia. [Self-Teaching Slide Review 23]. University of Miami School of Medicine, Department of Internal Medicine (Hematology), Miami, Florida 33136.

The Rh Factor and Blood Testing Procedures. Ortho Diagnostics, Raritan, New Jersey 18869.

Sickle Cell Disease. Part I. Pathophysiology. Seminar 301. ASMT Education and Research Fund, Inc., 5555 West Loop South, Bellaire, Texas 77401.

---

* Films unless otherwise stated.

9 Reticulocyte Count, Erythrocyte Fragility, and Sickle Cell Studies

RETICULOCYTE COUNT

A discussion of the reticulocyte count should start by defining the reticulocyte as a young, non-nucleated cell of the erythrocyte series that can be recognized only with the use of supravital stains. Normal reticulocyte values are: adults, 0.5 to 1.5 per cent; children, 0.5 to 4.0 per cent; and infants, 2 to 5 per cent. The characteristic differences between reticulocytes and mature erythrocytes are listed in Table 9–1.

In the collection of the blood specimen and the use of anticoagulants, a staining solution should be used that consists of a dye and potassium oxalate diluted in water. The potassium oxalate serves to prevent coagulation and renders the staining solution isotonic. Fresh or oxalated blood may be used. It is usually obtained by sticking a finger and wiping dry with gauze. Blood may be collected on a glass slide or a coverslip and then drawing it into a capillary tube, or leukocyte diluting pipette.

When the young red blood cells are stained with brilliant cresyl blue or other vital dyes that enter the living cell before fixation, the ribonucleoprotein is precipitated, appearing as a blue network or reticulum in the cell, which is therefore called a reticulocyte. This staining characteristic also identifies polychromatophilia. Concerning the chromatophilia, the staining solution may be either brilliant cresyl blue in saline solution or in alcohol with or without Wright's stain as a counterstain, or the new methylene blue N stain* may be used. The basophilic material in the young erythrocyte takes up the supravital stain appearing as a blue-stained reticulum. Multiple linear granules are revealed in young reticulocytes; in old reticulocytes only a few blue granules or scattered blue threads may be found.

Wet Preparation

In utilizing the wet preparation technique, the new methylene blue N solution is used.* One dissolves 0.5 g. of new methylene blue and 1.6 g. of potassium oxalate in distilled water and makes up to 100 ml. of solution, which should be distilled before it is used. Or a solution can be made consisting of sucrose, 8.0 g.; sodium citrate, 0.4 g.; brilliant cresyl blue, 0.3 g.; and distilled water to make 100 ml. of solution. The solution is mixed and shaken to dissolve the ingredients. The solution should stand at room temperature overnight before it is used. It will keep 1 month in a refrigerator. A portion should be filtered every 5 to 7 days through a No. 50 Whatman filter paper.

In this technique, the finger is stuck and wiped dry with gauze. The second drop of capillary blood is drawn up to 0.5 mark in a leukocyte pipette. The new methylene blue

---

* Produced by Burrell Corp., Pittsburgh, Pa.

259

Table 9-1. The Characteristic Differences Between Reticulocytes and Mature Erythrocytes

	Reticulocytes	Mature Erythrocytes
Size	7.5–8.0 μ	7.0 μ
Hypotonic saline	Resistant	Less resistant
Mechanical trauma	Resistant	Less resistant
Phagocytosis	Less likely	More likely
Alcoholic Wright's stain	Nuclear fragments or Cabot's rings	Salmon pink without basophilia
	Diffusely basophilic cells (polychromatophilia); punctate basophilia (stippled cells)	
Supravital stain (aqueous) cresyl blue	Young reticulocytes possess a reticulum of coarse granules. They are also filamentous with plentiful ribonucleoprotein. Older reticulocytes possess ribonucleic acid dots with an associated mitochondrial pattern.	Stains light blue without reticulum or ribonucleic material.

N solution or brilliant cresyl blue solution is drawn up to the 1 mark, or is drawn up into bulb and allowed to stand 15 minutes. A small drop of the solution is expelled on a slide and smeared in the usual manner. Counterstain is not used. The number of reticulated red cells in a total of 1000 red blood cells is determined by examining consecutive fields of the smear under oil immersion. Counting is made easier by placing a screen of stiff paper with a small hole in the center into the eyepiece of the microscope, thus reducing the size of the field. All cells containing blue reticulum filaments or blue granules are counted as reticulocytes.

$$\frac{\text{No. reticulocytes}/1000\ \text{RBC}}{10} =$$

percentage of reticulocytes present.*

Another modification is to mix two drops of blood (fresh or oxalated) and two drops of staining solution on a clean glass slide. The mixture is drawn into a capillary tube and expelled onto a slide several times. The slide is placed in a moist chamber for 10 minutes. An inverted Petri dish with wet filter paper on the top may be used. A small drop of the mixture is placed on a clean coverglass, and thin smears are pulled. The smears are allowed to dry in the air. The coverglass is mounted on a glass slide with a small drop of the immersion oil and the count is made as just described.

Other variations include the utilization of a mixture of blood and staining solution that may be allowed to stand for 10 minutes in capillary pipette, or equal volumes (0.5 to 1 ml.) of blood and staining solution may be added to a small test tube and mixed gently for 10 minutes. In an alternative method a small of staining solution is placed on a coverslip, and the drop is touched to the site of finger-puncture. A small amount of blood is then squeezed into the solution and touched again with the coverslip. The liquid and the cells are mixed lightly on the finger; too much mixing causes the red blood cells to crenate. A coverslip is placed on the slide, and it is rimmed with petroleum jelly. It is allowed to stand 15 minutes before the counting is done. It may be refrigerated 2 to 3 hours if necessary.

---

* This is the usual method of expression. A more clinical approach in the presence of anemia is to express the number of reticulocytes per mm.³ of whole blood. This value is obtained by multiplying the reticulocyte percentage figure by the RBC count per mm.³. In this way a semiquantitative measurement of RBC production is obtained; normally this value is about 90,000 reticulocytes per mm.³ of whole blood.

Dry Preparation

In the dry preparation method, a drop of 1.5 per cent brilliant cresyl blue is placed in 95 per cent alcohol on a coverslip or slide, and it is spread with another slide or coverslip. The film is allowed to dry in air. A large number may be made in advance and stored in a clean dry receptacle. A spread of a small drop of blood is made on top of the dried film of stain. The drying of the blood is retarded by placing the slide or coverslip in a moist chamber. This is allowed to stand for 10 minutes. The slide or coverslip is removed from the moist chamber. The film is allowed to dry in air, and it is counterstained with Wright's stain.

In making a comparison of results of the two preceding techniques, one can say that the moist brilliant cresyl blue preparation is useful in checking the number of thrombocytes in thrombocytopenic states — that is, the platelets can be counted in relation to the erythrocytes and leukocytes. The dry preparation, due to the use of coverslips, technically is more demanding than the slide method. In the test tube method, one can make either a wet preparation or a drop can be added to a glass slide or coverslip and counterstain with Wright's stain. In the dry brilliant cresyl blue slide method, the counts can be made at a later time, whereas in the other wet methods the counts must be made within 1 hour except if refrigerated in the sucrose-citrate method, after which the count can be done 2 to 3 hours later. With the new methylene blue N stain, the reticulum stains a deeper blue and stands out in sharp contrast against the light greenish blue of the red blood cell. Compared with the use of alcoholic solutions of dye, methods employing saline solutions of brilliant cresyl blue may give slightly higher values for reticulocytes because of the prolonged contact with the red blood cells in a wet preparation. One can check the number of reticulocytes in a brilliant cresyl blue preparation by comparing the number of polychromatophilic cells on the Wright's stain preparation. Dry preparations can be left for future reference.

Sources of Error

The sources of error in the techniques just described are listed in the following discussion:

The proportion of blood and staining solution influences the color of the red blood cell. A marked excess of staining solution produces a deep blue color of the red blood cell, obscuring the reticulum. A large excess of blood diminishes the greenish blue coloration of the red blood cells. Equal volumes of blood and staining solution give optimal color contrast. Also, if too large a drop of blood is used on the moist preparation, the preparation becomes too thick, the cells are not well separated, and there is not enough dye in relationship to the cells to stain adequately.

Preparations may fade on storage, but can be restored by fixation in methyl alcohol and restaining with Wright's stain.

Overlapping, rouleau formation, and crenation of red blood cells make an accurate count difficult to achieve. For example, crenated red blood cells should not be confused with reticulocytes because of the refractive, spinelike projections, which do not stain blue with dyes.

Stain precipitated on red blood cells should not be confused with reticulocytes.

Grease on the slides and coverslip prevents even spreading.

Error may result if the blood smear dries before the dye has had time to penetrate the red blood cell and stain the granulofilamentous structures.

Statistical error — greater in low counts than in high ones — is partly due to random distribution of the reticulocytes among the erythrocytes of adults.

Reticulocyte values obtained during the treatment of anemias usually vary directly with the clinical response. For example, in iron-deficiency anemias the peak of reticulocyte response (10%) occurs between

7 and 14 days (usually, on the tenth day). In pernicious anemia, the reticulocyte count rises by the fourth day after treatment is begun, and reaches a maximum on the eighth or ninth day. It usually returns to normal by the end of the second week of treatment. The reticulocyte increase is usually proportional to the severity of the anemia, provided an adequate dose of vitamin B_{12} has been given—for example, red blood cell count of 1,000,000 per cu.mm. is associated with a 40 per cent reticulocyte rise after proper B_{12} therapy. There is also a relative reticulocytosis in cases of thyroid deficiency after therapy with a thyroid extract and after treatment of anemias associated with a vitamin deficiency.

Reticulocytosis occurring without treatment may lead to a diagnosis of hidden bleeding or unrecognized hemolysis. If the reticulocyte count remains low with associated anemia, it usually indicates defective erythrocyte formation in the marrow. In aplastic anemia, a persistent deficiency of reticulocytes suggests a poor prognosis. Aplastic crises during chronic hemolytic anemias are characterized by a drop in the reticulocyte count and usually means marrow failure.

ERYTHROCYTE FRAGILITY

The in vivo and in vitro causes of hemolysis are graphically portrayed in part of the tables on page 248. Most erythrocytes are broken down, lysed, or destroyed in the body because of the following: (1) An introcorpuscular or intrinsic abnormality predisposes them to destruction before their normal 120 day life span is terminated by normal senescence. These are primarily effects of intraerythrocytic enzyme depletions. This pathologic intraerythrocytic intrinsic defect is usually due to a genetic abnormality. Laboratory tests used to diagnose this abnormality are therefore based on methods that reveal this inherited defect. (2) The other main cause of in vivo hemolysis of red blood cells is related to changes in environment of the circulating red blood cells that injure the cells and therefore are the cause of their accelerated breakdown or hemolysis. These are called extracorpuscular, or extrinsic, defects.

In discussing the etiologic factors associated with the hemolysis of red blood cells having intrinsic defects and therefore a shortened life span (for example, hereditary spherocytosis, drug-sensitive erythrocytes, favism, congenital nonspherocytic anemia, paroxysmal nocturnal hemoglobinuria paroxysmal cold hemoglobinuria, elliptocytosis, and the hemoglobinopathies), one must consider the lytic effects of the reticuloendothelial system (mainly the spleen) on abnormal morphologic variants of erythrocytes, such as spherocytosis and sickling, and the subsequent destruction by the splenic lysuns and reticuloendothelial cells in their sinusoids. The sickling process produces a deformed nonflexible erythrocyte, which leads to intracapillary agglutination, sludging and thrombosis. The unknown erythrocytic cell membrane defect in thalassemia causes accelerated intrasplenic reticuloendothelial hemolysis.

Another mechanism associated with shortened erythrocyte life is the increased osmotic fragility of cells having intraerythrocytic defects—that is, intrasplenic depletion of an enzyme concerned with the maintenance of high-energy phosphate bonds—although no direct relationship between in vivo hemolysis and in vitro osmotic fragility can actually be demonstrated.

A third and most recently elaborated concept of the intrinsic defect that causes the hemolysis is the unusual sensitivity of certain types of erythrocytes to certain drugs and fava beans caused by an intrinsic biochemical defect of these red blood cells. This defect manifests itself in the atypical excessive formation of Heinz-Ehrlich bodies when the erythrocyte comes in contact with acetylphenylhydrazine and in the reduced erythrocytic G-6-PD activity demonstrated by incubation of erythrocytes with acetylphenylhydrazine with further reduction in the already reduced erythrocytic glutathione content (see also pp. 242-243). This defect is a hereditary sex-linked deficiency due to a gene on the X chromosome, more commonly affecting senescent erythrocytes.

Also, the lipid abnormality in erythrocytes in paroxysmal nocturnal hemoglobinuria is associated with hemolysis. It is not known, however, whether this aberration is cause or effect.

There are multiple causes of hemolysis associated with extraerythrocytic factors. All types of blood and tissue cells may be involved in the immunologic phenomena observed. Because agglutination frequently precedes hemolysis, but may need complement and therefore may be separate therefrom, and because the process may be an autohemolysis or isohemolysis, two types of antibodies are associated with immunologic phenomena—that is, autoagglutinins or autohemolysins, and isoagglutinins or isohemolysins. The autoantibodies react with the red blood cells of the same group whether in the patient or in another individual. The isoantibodies normally cannot cause the patient's own red blood cells to clump. A hemolytic process due to autoagglutinins may be of the complete (saline erythrocyte agglutinating), usually natural type or it may be of the incomplete (high protein erythrocyte agglutinating), usually immnue type. Depending on the temperature at which they are most active, autoantibodies and isoantibodies may be cold (complete natural, or incomplete immune) or warm (incomplete immune). A hemolytic process due to autohemolysins is usually of the complete cold or complete warm type. Some of these autohemolysins are active at an acid *p*H (acid autohemolysins). This autohemolytic group includes hemolytic processes that are secondary to immunization by antigenic material associated with bacterial infections, primary atypical pneumonia and other virus infections, lymphomatous processes, and disseminated lupus erythematosus.

A hemolytic anemia due to isoagglutinins or isohemolysins is the result of immunization after the transfusion of incompatible blood, or in pregnancy. Erythroblastosus fetalis is more frequently associated with the production of warm, incomplete (immune) Rh antibodies; however, the complete saline ABO antibodies may sometimes be involved.

The hemolytic process produced by autoantibodies and isoantibodies is secondary to damage to the red blood cell and the subsequent shortened life span. When the antibody is a strong hemolytic agent (for example, hemolytic streptococci, *Clostridium welchii*, subacute bacterial endocarditis, military tuberculosis, infectious hepatitis, infectious mononucleosis, and psittacosis or the Donath-Landsteiner hemolysin of paroxysmal cold hemoglobinuria, a massive intravascular hemolysis may be produced directly by the antibody. In paroxysmal cold hemoglobinuria, the antibody is first fixed to the red blood cell at a cold temperature, and hemolysis is then produced when the temperature of the blood is raised to body temperature. Complement is needed for the lytic process, and occasionally hemolysus continues despite a marked deficiency of complement.

Other extracorpuscular causes for erythrocyte hemolysis are those resulting from direct toxic, hemolytic, chemical, or physical damage—for example, severe burns, naphthalene and benzene derivatives, lead and other heavy metal poisons, and prostheses used in valvular repair in congential heart disease. The greater fragility of erythrocyte in valvular repair is due to damage caused by turbulence and nonflexible repair substitutes. Also included in this group are the hemolytic anemias caused by parasitization of erythrocytes by malarial and *Bartonella* organisms with subsequent hemolysis of the intraerythrocytic proliferation of these forms.

In erythrophagocytosis, the red blood cell is first sensitized by autohemolysins or autoagglutinins and then ingested by polymorphonuclear leukocytes, monocytes, and eosinophils. This process can also be produced in vitro by incubating sensitized red blood cells with leukocytes—for example, the LE cell phenomenon in disseminated lupus erythematosus. This process may also take place in the spleen in certain hemolytic anemias and be the reason for the marked reduction of erythrocytes before splenectomy (for example, spherocytosis).

The response of erythrocytes to hypotonic and hypertonic solutions is based on the fundamental concept that the normal biconcave, disk-shaped erythrocyte maintains its morphologic characteristics when circulating in human serum or in 0.85 per cent saline solution (isotonic for erythrocytes). The morphologic status quo of the erythrocyte exists because of the electrolyte ion equilibrium between red blood cells and the saline solution. Because there is no passage of water into or out of erythrocytes suspended in a 0.85 per cent saline solution, the volume and shape of these cells remain unchanged. If these same erythrocytes are placed in a hypotonic saline solution (less than 0.85%), the cells lose ions into the surrounding solution and the cells will then imbibe water, gradually becoming more spherical in shape. Erythrocytes that are more spherical than normal have a reduced capacity to imbibe as much water because the expandable surface available on the cell membrane is less than in normal biconcaved erythrocytes. Smaller volumes of water therefore are required to rupture (hemolyze) such cells. Lysis occurs, depending on the salt concentration and the length of time that the red blood cell has been exposed to the hypotonic environment.

Hypertonic saline solutions (greater than 0.85%) cause the erythrocytes to shrink or become crenated in proportion to the difference in osmotic pressure between cell and fluid. At first, the erythrocyte assumes a crenated disk shape, then that of a crenated sphere. Finally, the crenations disappear, and the red blood cell becomes a

sphere and then a prolytic sphere, which finally hemolyzes to a ghost form with a stromal network.

Means of Demonstrating Increased Erythrocyte Fragility in Vitro

The following methods may be used to demonstrate increased erythrocyte fragility in vitro:

1. Osmotic fragility of freshly drawn blood may be used (see below).

2. Osmotic fragility after incubation at 37° C may be used. Preincubation of blood at 37° C for 24 hours accentuates increased osmotic fragility if it is present and may reveal abnormal osmotic fragility not detectable with the standard test, in which fresh blood is used. After incubation, the technique is the same as that used with fresh blood.

3. The automatic electronic erythrocyte osmotic fragility test (Fragiligraph) may be used (see p. 265).

4. Autohemolysis. When sterile defibrinated blood is incubated at 37° C, various degrees of autohemolysis takes place. Normal red blood cells show a hemolysis of 0 to 0.5 per cent after 24 hours and 0.4 to 3.5 per cent after 48 hours. Autohemolysis is increased in hemolytic disease, and after incubation autohemolysis also indicates increased osmotic fragility, demonstrating that these are closely related processes. In fact, increased osmotic fragility after incubation is seen in some cases of congenital nonspherocytic hemolytic anemia (the osmotic fragility is normal with freshly drawn blood).

5. Mechanical fragility is an indication of increased erythrocyte fragility. This technique is used to estimate the red blood cell resistance to trauma. Injured cells or abnormal cells are more susceptible to trauma. Therefore, mechanical fragility equals grams of hemoglobin liberated by rotation of oxalated or defibrinated blood minus hemoglobin in supernatant saline control divided by grams of hemoglobin liberated by distilled water control minus

the hemoglobin in supernatant saline control. Normal values generally range from 1 to 5 per cent; a normal control is run simultaneously. Mechanical fragility is increased in hereditary spherocytosis, sickle cell anemia, and in some instances of acquired hemolytic anemia.

In the determination of the fragility of erythrocytes, the principles involved in the osmotic fragility of freshly drawn blood are first described. Normally, red blood cells suspended in 0.85 per cent sodium chloride solution undergo no significant changes for several hours, whereas lysis of red blood cells is almost immediate when they are suspended in distilled water. The final end point is somewhat dependent on the relative volume of blood and saline solution, the temperature at which the test is done, and the *p*H of the blood and saline mixture. There are also different methods of reading the end results—that is, visually or colorimetrically.

In the technique, a specific amount of whole blood is added to a definite volume of saline solution. As the salt concentration is progressively reduced below 0.85 per cent (isotonic level), a concentration is reached at which some of the erythrocytes hemolyze; the supernatant watery solution becomes slightly pinkish. This is called initial or *beginning hemolysis*. As the saline concentration is further reduced, a point is reached at which all red blood cells hemolyze. This is called *complete hemolysis*. At this point, the entire solution in this tube is the deepest watery red of all the tubes, and no residue or sediment of red blood cells is visible. A normal control is run simultaneously.

A more accurate determination of osmotic fragility is the Dacie technique, in which volumes of blood and saline are carefully measured and hemolysis is read in a photoelectric colorimeter. When the results are plotted, a sigmoid osmotic fragility curve is obtained; the "tail" ends represent a small number of cells with osmotic fragility either higher or lower than the majority. Incuba-

tion of the blood at 37° C for 24 hours before using the Dacie technique accentuates even more the increased osmotic fragility. In all instances, a normal control is run simultaneously.

Normal hemolysis is first observed with the naked eye at a saline concentration of 0.44 ±0.02 per cent, and is complete at 0.32 ±0.02 per cent. The salt concentrations for initial and complete hemolysis are higher than normal when the cells have an increased osmotic fragility. The initial and complete hemolysis values are lower than normal when the cells have a decreased osmotic fragility, or increased resistance.

Another newer, more accurate, and efficient electronic method for automatically recording osmotic fragility curves of red blood cells in the Fragiligraph osmotic test recorder (Fig. 8-10).* In the technique proper, the microsample of blood is suspended in isotonic saline solution and is placed in a test cell formed by dialysing membrane walls. The test cell is placed in a distilled water bath inside the instrument. Dialysis across the membrane continuously reduces the initial salt concentration of the blood suspension, causing rupture of the red cells and hemolysis. White light is transmitted through the blood suspension and increases with an increase in the percentage of hemolysis. Light transmission is monitored continuously, and detailed osmotic fragility curves are printed out.

In addition to the cumulative curve, a derivative fragility curve (increment hemolysis) can be simultaneously recorded. The derivative curve, normally bell shaped, expresses changes in the rate of hemolysis. It will, therefore, detect multiple cell populations by recording a hump for each population (Fig. 8-9). For correlation with toni-

---

* Manufactured by Elron Electronic Industries, Ltd., and distributed by Kalmedic Instruments, Inc., a subsidiary of Kalvex, Inc., 425 Park Ave., New York City. The Fragiligraph, after modification, can also be used to determine WBC fragility (useful as an aid in the diagnosis of leukemia) and to analyze platelet aggregates.

Table 9-2. Osmotic Fragility in Various Hemolytic Anemias

	Values	
	Initial Hemolysis	Complete Hemolysis
Increased fragility		
Hereditary spherocytosis	0.68 ± 0.14	0.46 ± 0.10
Acquired hemolytic anemia	0.52 ± 0.04	0.42 ± 0.04
Hemolytic disease of newborn (ABO incompatibility)	0.50 ± 0.02	0.40 ± 0.02
Hemolytic disease of newborn (Rh incompatibility)	0.60 ± 0.06	0.40 ± 0.04
Chemical poisons	0.50 ± 0.04	0.40 ± 0.04
Burns	0.50 ± 0.04	0.40 ± 0.04
Normal fragility	0.44 ± 0.02	0.32 ± 0.02
Decreased fragility		
Thalassemia	0.38 ± 0.04	0.20 ± 0.06
Sickle cell anemia	0.36 ± 0.02	0.20 ± 0.04
Polycythemia vera	0.40 ± 0.02	0.28 ± 0.02
Iron-deficiency anemia (occasionally)	0.38 ± 0.02	0.28 ± 0.02

city, a salt concentration curve can also be recorded with either fragility curve. Less than 2 μl. of blood is required for one test, which is normally completed within 5 minutes. The principle of operation of this instrument can also be applied to other particles, such as white blood cells and platelets. Additionally, the Fragiligraph is being used to provide an accurate and practical method for predicting the survival of frozen red blood cells before transfusion.

Effects of Variations in Shape and Size of Erythrocytes on Fragility

Leptocytes. These target cells, which are flatter than normal erythrocytes, are capable of greater expansion, and therefore are more resistance to hypotonic solutions. Platycytes therefore show decreased osmotic fragility (Plate 8).

Spherocytes. These cells are already nearly spherical owing to the antigen-antibody reaction affecting their surface. Minor degrees of swelling will thus cause their rupture and hemolysis. They therefore exhibit an increased osmotic fragility (Plate 9).

Poikilocytes. The two previously mentioned cell types have varying shapes and therefore show varying response to dif-

ferent concentrations of saline solution. Because pernicious anemia shows a marked poikilocytosis that is different from the two just mentioned, the associated osmotic fragility is more representative of the poikilocytic cell type. In this entity, initial hemolysis begins at 0.48 ± 0.04 and ends at 0.36 ± 0.02, indicating occasional ranges of increased fragility, but showing normal osmotic fragility in most cases (Plate 8).

Macrocytes. As in poikilocytes, there are occasional ranges of increased osmotic fragility, but they mostly show normal osmotic fragility (Plate 9).

Microcytes. Because in some cases the apparent diminution in size is due only to the rounding of the normal disk shape, the cell volume remains the same as in the spherocyte; microcytes are occasionally called microspherocytes. These red blood cells show an increased osmotic fragility for the same reasons spherocytes do. However, most microcytes are found in iron-deficiency anemias and because they are accompanied by decreased hemoglobin synthesis, the cells are also hypochromic. These hypochromic microcytes show an initial hemolysis beginning at 0.38 ± 0.02 with a completed hemolysis at 0.28 ± 0.02. This is indicative of decreased osmotic fragility (Plate 11).

Values for the Fragility Test in Various Hemolytic Anemias

An increased and decreased osmotic fragility is seen in the disorders listed in Table 9–2.

SICKLE CELL STUDIES

Principle of Tests

Sickle cell disease is characterized by the presence of hemoglobin S (Hb S) and the ability of the red blood cell to assume a sickled form. Hemoglobin S is the least soluble type of hemoglobin and forms insoluble tactoid crystals (oriented masses of molecules) when exposed to low oxygen tensions. These tactoid crystals together with high viscosity can be observed with the phase microscope. The physicochemical properties of reduced Hb S are believed responsible for the sickling and the resulting capillary thrombosis. Because deoxygenation of low oxygen tension causes erythrocytes with Hb S to sickle, conditions may be produced in the laboratory in which the available oxygen is used up by cellular metabolism in sealed preparations of whole blood while access to oxygen is prevented. The process of deoxygenation may be further enhanced by adding reducing substances (sodium metabisulfite) to the preparation.

Laboratory Diagnosis

Sealed Whole Blood Method. A rubber band is placed around the base of the middle finger and allowed to stay in place for 5 minutes. A finger-puncture is made on the ball of this finger, and a drop of capillary blood is placed on a slide and immediately covered with a coverslip, the edges of which are sealed with petrolatum. The preparation is incubated at room temperature. Readings are made immediately and at hourly intervals for 2 or 3 hours (also after 24 hours, if so desired).

The *advantages* of this technique are as follows: It is a simple test requiring no special, complicated, or expensive equipment. It is easy to interpret the end point by identification of the morphologic pattern of the altered red blood cells. A positive test is diagnostic. Prompt results are obtained with this stasis moist preparation, which may be examined for final specificity at the end of 24 hours, if so desired.

The *disadvantages* of the procedure are as follows: The test does not differentiate between sickle cell anemia, sickle cell trait, or other Hb S syndromes. It does not detect Hb S below a concentration of 7 g. per 100 ml.

Sources of error in the test are as follows: A negative result does not exclude sickle cell anemia because the red blood cells may lose their capacity to sickle before the oxygen has been exhausted. False negative results may occur when the amount of Hb S is too small for detection. False negative results may occur from an admixture of alcohol left on skin, from trapped air under the coverslip, or from inadequate sealing. Distortion of red blood cells caused by ovalocytosis, extreme anisocytosis, and crenation may be confused with sickling pattern.

Method of Reporting. The result is positive if more than 10 per cent of the red blood cells are sickled.

Sodium Metabisulfite Method. Hemoglobin is rapidly converted to reduced hemoglobin by this chemical reducing agent. Aqueous sodium metabisulfite ($Na_2S_2O_5$, 2 g./100 ml.) is made up fresh before use. For convenience, a 200 mg. capsule has been prepared and is available commercially* so that a fresh solution can be made each time by adding the contents of 1 capsule to 10 ml. of water. One or two drops of this 2 per cent solution is added to one drop of capillary or venous blood on a glass slide. After this is mixed, a coverglass is dropped onto the preparation, and the excess blood is expressed by gently pressing the coverglass

---

* From the Aloe Company.

with a piece of filter paper. This produces a preparation thin enough to permit examination of individual cells. Sealing and waiting are not necessary. A control preparation containing a drop of isotonic saline solution in place of the reducing agent should be set up simultaneously. Observations should be made immediately, 15, and 30 minutes after preparation.

The *advantages* of this method are as follows: The results are rapid and reproducible. The test is independent of the rate of metabolism of the leukocytes present in the preparation. A positive test is completely reliable. The control saline solution is useful in differentiating ovalocytosis, crenation, and extreme anisocytosis such as occurs in thalassemia major from the sickling phenomenon. Sickled forms are easily distinguished from crenated cells that are round and have short spinelike projections.

The *disadvantages* of this technique are as follows: It cannot distinguish sickle cell anemia from sickle cell trait or other Hb S syndromes. The presence of Hb S erythrocytes being tested may not be revealed if the concentration of the Hb S is too low for sickling to occur—that is, if the concentration of Hb S is less than 7 g. per 100 ml., sickling does not occur, even in the complete absence of oxygen.

The *sources of error* in this procedure are as follows: The reducing agent is unstable and may be responsible for a false negative result. The reagent deteriorates rapidly at room temperature and should be kept in the refrigerator when not in use. Repetition with a fresh agent is indicated if the test is

negative. False negative results are obtained if the Hb S concentration is less than 7 g. per 100 ml. False negative may be obtained from the admixture of alcohol (left on skin) or from trapped air under the coverslip.

Methods of Reporting. Ten to 100 per cent of the red blood cells assume the sickled form within 15 to 30 minutes when the test is positive.*

There are now available many rapid screening tests for sickle cell pattern, including solubility tests for hemoglobin S, the Murimaya test, and the dithionite tube method. Most of these are commercially prepared and are dependent upon the decreased solubility of deoxygenated hemoglobin S in phosphate buffer solutions. These may be used in laboratories that infrequently test for sickle cell disease; however, a patient should not be considered definitely to have the trait or disease without having been tested by the most reliable primary screening method, electrophoresis on cellulose acetate. This method allows detection of abnormal hemoglobins other than hemoglobin S as well as identification of some of the heterozygous forms of sickle cell disorders. When this technique is used, the solubility test described above may be used to identify the occasional patient who will be found heterozygous for hemoglobin D.

---

* A simplified diagnostic solubility tube test specific for Hb S with results available in 2 to 5 minutes has been described by Diggs, Schorr, Ascari and Reiss. It is commercially available from Ortho Research Foundation, Raritan, N. J.

10 Thrombocytes, Hemostasis, and Blood Coagulation

THROMBOCYTES

When platelets were first discovered, there was much confusion as to their nature and function. In fact, some workers thought that platelets were artifacts. Donne gave the first description of the platelets; he though they were produced from the fatty particles of chyle.[9] Bizzozero studied them in the mesenteric vessels of animals and described their adhesive qualities, their participation in thrombus formation, and their role in blood coagulation.[3] After gradual development of the concept that platelets were cellular particles, in 1910, it was shown that they were produced by megakaryocytes.[35]

The physical properties of platelets are related to the effects of foreign surfaces and the environment in which they find themselves. These properties include the following: (1) Platelets demonstrate adhesiveness or the property of adhering to other particles, surfaces, and occasional bacteria. The adhesiveness of the platelets may be important in hemostasis because they adhere to injured endothelium.[19, 29] This characteristic may be the result of glass-surface negative charge, or it may depend on plasma factors adsorbed onto glass (Hageman factor, thrombin) usually found in calcium-poor medium plus euglobulin. Euglobulin possesses clot-retracting and clot-accelerating properties, and it is reduced during hypersensitivity reactions. (2) Platelets may undergo agglutination, in which they clump, aggregate, and stick together, leading to their ultimate breakdown. (3) Viscous metamorphosis is the formation of large, amorphous, hyaline clumps with loss of platelet identity in the process. This property may be related to agglutination, but it occurs in the presence of calcium ions and a globulin fraction of serum.

DEVELOPMENT OF PLATELETS

The development of thrombocytes (Plate 1) takes place mostly in the bone marrow from primitive totipotential reticulum cells or stem cells (hemohistioblasts). The lung has also been mentioned as a source of megakaryocytes, with platelet development therein. However, some feel that pulmonary megakaryoctyes are effete cells.[13]

The earliest cell is the 25 to 35 μ megakaryoblast, which is a round-oval structure containing one to two nuclei with two to six small, indistinct nucleoli. The cytoplasm has a nucleus-cytoplasm ratio of 10:1, is irregular and basophilic, and occasionally shows blunt extrusions. The next cell in development is larger than the megakaryoblast, and nuclear division to this cell takes place repeatedly leading to the 25 to 50 μ promegakaryocyte, which is irregular, large, coarser than the blast cell, and is lobulated but single. There are zero to two nucleoli; the cytoplasm is moderately baso-philic and contains occasional azurophilic granules.

The next and most common young plate-let progenitor is the megakaryocyte. It measures 40 to 100 μ, and the nucleus is polyploid, extremely pleomorphic, mul-tiform, but usually single with coarse, ir-regularly clumped chromatin. The nucleoli number from zero to many; the cytoplasm is abundant and pale with fine azurophilic granules. Motion pictures of in vitro cul-tures of megakaryocytes show numerous pseudopods forming from the cytoplasm.[31] The pseudopods eventually become fili-form, and the platelets bud off at the ex-tremities.

The normal platelet seen in the blood varies from 2 to 4 μ in diameter and is usu-ally 7 to 8 cu.μ in volume. It is spherical, oval, or rod shaped. The cytoplasm con-tains granules, and occasionally these may become clumped in the center of the plate-let, producing a granulomere-like appear-ance, contrasted to the cytoplasm, or hy-alomere. When the granules are tightly packed, they suggest the appearance of a nucleus,[4] but such a structure has never been demonstrated in a platelet.

Thrombopoiesis may be under humoral control. It has been shown that a heat-stable, ether-soluble fraction of plasma from anemic rabbits will induce an increase in the platelet count of normal rats when administered orally or parenterally.[23] In ad-dition, there is evidence that platelet pro-duction is regulated by the number of circu-lating platelets,[14] and that this regulation is mediated by a humoral mechanism.[30]

Platelet destruction appears most likely to be a random process, suggesting that the platelets are consumed as they are needed.[27] Some workers report that plate-lets disappear from the blood when they become senescent. The lifespan of platelets has not been definitely established, but it appears to be about 9 to 11 days in studies using ^{51}Cr or difluorophosphate ^{32}P as a label.[1]

FUNCTION OF PLATELETS

The functions of platelets include the fol-lowing: (1) Platelets aid in vasocon-striction. Although vasoconstriction may be a primary hemostatic mechanism, it ac-tually may be secondary to the formation of platelet plugs or caps and perhaps also to the poorly defined vascular factor missing in von Willebrand's disease. It has been suggested that vasoconstriction may be en-hanced by an agent released from platelets (for example, serotonin). However, the im-portance of this in hemostatis is now doubted because depletion of serotonin causes no demonstrable defect of hemo-statis. (2) Because two basic reactions must take place for blood to clot—a sufficient amount of active plasma thromboplastin and conversion of prothrombin to thrombin —a diminution in platelets or the presence of abnormal platelets leads to poor or no clot formation. The liberation of platelet factor 3 (thromboplastin-like factor 3) at the site of vessel injury is especially needed for the formation of active plasma throm-boplastin and subsequent fibrin formation. The formation of fibrin also aids in clearing foreign bodies (bacteria and viruses) from the circulation. (3) Chemical factors can be extracted from platelets, each possessing its own special physiologic properties. Among these chemical factors are an-tithrombins, thromboplastin-like substan-ces, catalysts, and histamine. These factors are liberated from platelets at or near the site of vessel injury, and they therefore aid in clot retraction.

A quantitative relationship between the number of platelets and clot retraction is further emphasized when it is remembered that in thrombocytopenic blood there is usually, but not always, poor clot retraction (other factors are fibrinogen concentration and the amount of thrombin available). There appears to be some disputed correla-tion of this process and thromboembolism. Because of the adhesive-agglutination properties of platelets, they are associated

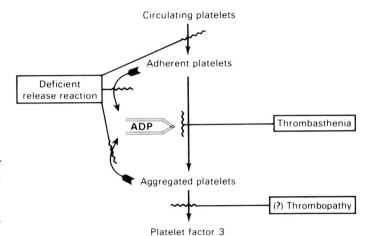

Circulating platelets

Adherent platelets

Deficient
release reaction

ADP

Thrombasthenia

Aggregated platelets

(?) Thrombopathy

Platelet factor 3

Fig. 10-1. Pathophysiology of common diseases of platelet function. (Wintrobe, M. M.: Clinical Hematology. ed. 7. Philadelphia, Lea & Febiger, 1974)

with the formation of thromboembolic phenomena and the adsorption of coagulation factors. It is also possible that clot retraction is in effect a physiologic ligature drawing the edges of the injured vessel together and securing hemostasis.

In summary, one may state that platelet activity is necessary for coagulation to take place. A phospholipid substance is liberated when platelets are lysed or degenerate. This is essential to the second phase of clot formation in that it is essential to thromboplastin generation. Finally, platelet breakdown is brought about by contact with a foreign surface, by thrombin, and possibly the active contact factors in plasma and serum.

Emerging concepts of platelet function are discussed under Bleeding Time Techniques and Platelet Aggregation — Retention Procedures. Figure 10-1 succinctly depicts the pathophysiology of common disorders of platelet function. Indicated are the loci of impairment of platelet adhesion and aggregation processes (solid arrows) and the release reaction (dashed arrows) in the various disorders.[34] Since platelets play a major role in the development of arterial thromboembolic disease, platelet-inhibitor drugs may prevent or modify the course of arterial thromboembolic disease. For example, in valvular heart disease and after installation of prosthetic heart valves, pa-

tients with short platelet survival rates seem to risk developing thromboembolism. Short platelet survival rates may be corrected by high-dose dipyridamole or sulfinpyrazone or by a combination of low-dose dipyridamole and aspirin. In transient cerebral ischemic attacks, there is evidence that platelet emboli arising from platelet thrombi at sites of atherosclerotic plaques in the extracranial arteries have an etiologic relationship with the thrombi. Available data indicate that high-dose sulfinpyrazone or aspirin exert a preventive effect. In coronary artery disease, it is surmised that thrombus formation and platelet deposition with growth and progression of the atherosclerotic plaque may cause myocardial infarction. Aspirin and dipyridamole are considered to be beneficial platelet-inhibitor drugs if they are used before coronary disease becomes severe and clinically symptomatic. Finally, there are recent reports on the beneficial use of thrombolytic agents (e.g., the plasminogen activators, urokinase and streptokinase) in venous thrombosis and embolism.[22]

ENUMERATION OF PLATELETS

The principle of the platelet count is independent of the technique employed. It is based on the readiness with which platelets agglutinate and adhere to a foreign surface, necessitating special precautions during the collection of a blood sample and immediate dilution in an anticoagulant solution. The small size of platelets makes direct counting in a hemocytometer more difficult than other cell counts. In the indirect method, the number of platelets are estimated during the performance of the differential leukocyte count. In the direct method utilizing the counting chamber, capillary or venous blood with an anticoagulant is mixed in an erythrocyte pipette with a diluting fluid. Rapid work is necessary to prevent the clumping of the platelets; other cells may or may not be destroyed depending on the diluting fluid used. Most commonly, the red blood cells are preserved, and the platelets are counted in a hemocytometer.

Platelets are difficult to count because they agglutinate, fragment, and break down readily and quickly. Because of their small size, they are also hard to differentiate from stain, fat, and debris. Another area of difficulty is their affinity for and adherence to glass, and also to any foreign body and particularly to each other. Furthemore, platelets are not evenly dispersed throughout the blood. The unavoidable error is therefore greater than in counting erythrocytes or leukocytes, but it is negligible in practice because only great variations in the total platelet count have any clinical significance.

THE DIRECT METHOD

This method of counting platelets involves the following techniques: (1) the Rees-Ecker method using the light microscope, (2) the Unopette method, (3) the phase-contrast microscopy method, and (4) the electronic counter method, especially the Coulter Counter method.

Rees-Ecker Light-Microscopy Method

In this method, a red blood cell pipette is used to draw the blood up to the 0.5 mark. The diluting fluid is drawn up to the 1.0 mark, and the two are mixed for 3 to 5 minutes. The first several drops are discarded, and two hemocytometer chambers are then filled. These two chambers are covered with a Petri dish containing most filter paper. After 15 minutes the platelets are counted using 10× eyepiece.

The *advantages* of this approach are as follows: Thrombocytes may be counted the same time erythrocytes are. The platelets stand out as highly refractive lilac-blue rounded bodies, $1/5$ to $1/2$ the diameter of the red blood cell. Venous blood gives more reproducible results because it can be collected with a siliconed test tube without loss of platelets due to their adhesiveness to ordinary glass. Also there is no need for the use of petrolatum over the skin for capillary puncture, and therefore minimal contamination with tissue juices occurs.

The *disadvantages* of this method are as follows: The proper adjustment of light is important to distinguish platelets from debris, yeast cells, or precipitated stain. Also, a great deal of experience is needed. If too many or too large extraneous particles are present, the count must be repeated with a new sample of blood and with refiltered diluting fluid, especially if loading the chamber with diluting fluid alone corroborates the suspicion. The diluting fluid may be bad, especially if the red blood cells are hemolyzed owing to formic acid formation from oxidized formaldehyde. Therefore fresh diluting fluid stored in glass-stoppered bottles in the refrigerator should be used. For the sake of accuracy, a comparison should be made with a stained blood smear.

The normal value is 200,000 to 275,000 per cu.mm. $\pm$ 16.3 per cent if two chambers are filled and 250 platelets are counted.

The Unopette Method

The Unopette method, using $K_3 \cdot EDTA$ and ammonium oxalate, is a direct technique for counting leukocytes and platelets. A diluent preserves the platelets as well as they are preserved in the Feissly and Ludin cocaine method.[12] In this method, one avoids the disadvantages of using a nar-

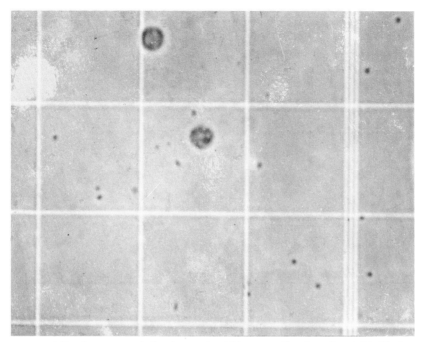

Fig. 10-2. Leukocytes and platelets under 100× magnification after 1:50 dilution of blood in 0.44 per cent ammonium oxalate and 0.22 per cent K$_3$EDTA. (Miescher, P. A., and Gerarde, H. W.: Unopette system in the clinical laboratory. Microchem. J., *9:*340, 1965*)*

cotic, and still the platelets stand out so well in the counting chamber that it is not necessary to use a phase contrast microscope. Furthermore, the use of the Unopette system* makes platelet counting easy, rapid, and reliable, and it also increases the accuracy of counting by eliminating pipetting and by reducing the dilution error to a minimum of less than 2 per cent.[16] The following description of the technique has been adapted from a brochure published by the Becton, Dickinson Company, Rutherford, New Jersey.

The principle of the method is based on the hemolysis of red cells by hypotonicity and complete block of platelet activity by chelating Mg^{++} and Ca^{++} with ethylenediaminetetraacetic acid (EDTA). EDTA as the sole anticoagulant was found to be unsuitable because the platelets had a tend-

ency to adhere to the red cell ghosts. This clumping was completely eliminated by the use of a second anticoagulant, ammonium oxalate. A 1:50 dilution of blood in a diluent containing 0.44 per cent ammonium oxalate and 0.22 per cent K$_3$·EDTA gives a uniform suspension of platelets and leukocytes, and causes complete hemolysis of red cells. This makes it possible to count leukocytes and thrombocytes in the same counting chamber (Fig. 10-2). Staining the leukocytes and platelets is not necessary, but if it is desired it is readily accomplish by adding 3 μl. of a 0.75 per cent solution of crystal violet to the diluent after hemolysis is completed.

In the method, Unopette reservoirs containing 1.225 ml. of a diluent consisting of 0.44 per cent ammonium oxalate and 0.22 per cent of K$_3$·EDTA are used (Fig. 10-3). The diluent reservoir is opened by pushing the plug into the reservoir (Figs. 10-4 and 10-5).

* Produced by Becton, Dickinson & Co., Rutherford, N. J.

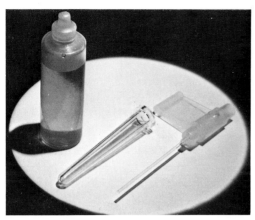

Fig. 10-3. Basic components of the Unopette system are, from left to right: reservoir containing premeasured volume of diluent; polystyrene capillary shield; precision uniform-bore glass capillary fitted into a plastic part that serves as holder, overflow chamber, and handle (*flag*) for capillary. (Miescher, P. A., and Gerarde, H. W.: Unopette system in the clinical laboratory. Microchem. J., *9:*340, 1965)

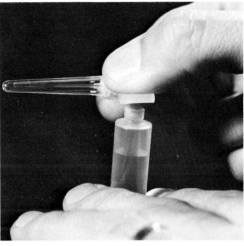

Fig. 10-4. Opening the reservoir containing the diluent. The plug is removed from the reservoir neck. (Miescher, P. A., and Gerarde, H. W.: Unopette system in the clinical laboratory. Microchem. J., *9:*340, 1965)

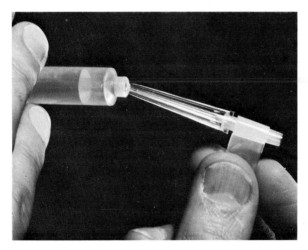

Fig. 10-5. Plug being pushed into reservoir. (Miescher, P. A., and Gerarde, H. W.: Unopette system in the clinical laboratory. Microchem. J., *9:*340, 1965)

Blood was obtained by venipuncture with a B.D. Vacutainer tube containing 0.05 ml. of a 30 per cent solution of $K_3 \cdot EDTA$ (final dilution in 7 ml. of blood, 0.24%). For purposes of comparison, capillary blood was also obtained by fingerpuncture. To guarantee a free flow of blood it is important to introduce the point of the disposable stylet to its full depth into the finger. After the first drop of blood is wiped off, 25 μl. of blood are collected in a calibrated self-filling capillary tube as soon as a large drop of blood is formed again (Fig. 10-6). The blood fills the capillary tube automatically and flow stops when the proper volume of 25 μl. is obtained (Fig. 10-6). Any excess blood is gently wiped off of the exterior of the capillary tube. Blood in the

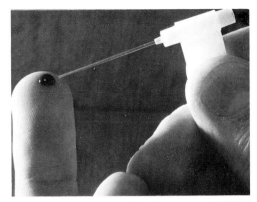

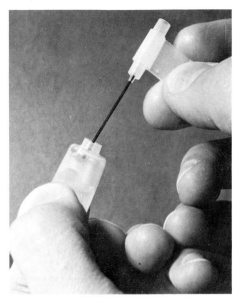

Fig. 10-7. Insertion of capillary containing blood into premeasured diluent in reservoir. (Miescher, P. A., and Gerarde, H. W.: Unopette system in the clinical laboratory. Microchem. J., *9:*340, 1965)

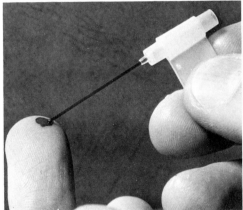

Fig. 10-6. Collection and measurement of capillary blood from fingertip. A, Blood automatically enters the tube on contact. B, Blood flow stops when the tube is filled. (Miescher, P. A., and Gerarde, H. W.: Unopette system in the clinical laboratory. Microchem. J., *9:*340, 1965)

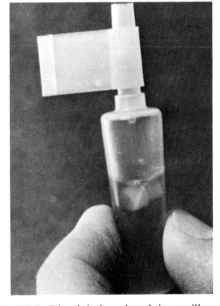

Vacutainer tube is mixed in a rotating mixing device immediately before the capillary tube is filled with 25 μl. of the blood.

To make the dilution, the walls of the Unopette reservoir are squeezed slightly before the capillary holder is fitted into the reservoir opening. When the walls are released, a negative pressure is produced, and blood is drawn from capillary tube into the diluent (Fig. 10-7).

The capillary tube is rinsed with diluent by gently squeezing the reservoir, forcing liquid into the capillary and into the overflow chamber (Fig. 10-8). When the pres-

Fig. 10-8. Blood being rinsed in capillary by diluent forced through capillary into overflow chamber. (Miescher, P. A., and Gerarde, H. W.: Unopette system in the clinical laboratory. Microchem. J., *9:*340, 1965)

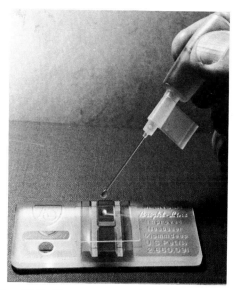

Fig. 10-9. Hemocytometer being charged with diluted blood.

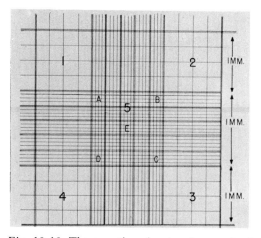

Fig. 10-10. The counting chamber is examined with the high dry objective. The total number of platelets in squares 1 and 3 is recorded. The larger squares are subdivided into 16 smaller squares each. With the high-power objective, only one of the smaller squares is seen at a time.

sure is released, the diluent is again drawn back into the reservoir, and the solution is mixed by gently rolling the reservoir back and forth between the hands for approximately 10 seconds. From 8 to 10 min. is allowed for complete hemolysis to occur. Before the hemocytometer is charged with diluted blood, the plastic reservoir is again

rolled back and forth between the hands for 20 seconds. Shaking should be avoided because it is harmful to both leukocytes and platelets, and it diminishes the counts.

To fill the counting chamber, the micropipette is inserted into the reservoir in the reversed position (Fig. 10-9). The first 2 drops are discarded. A single large drop is required to charge one counting area of the counting chamber. Both counting areas are filled.

The white blood cells are counted first with a $10\times$ objective and a $10\times$ ocular. On each side of the chamber, the four corner squares and the large middle square are counted, each square measuring 1 sq. mm. Leukocytes are thus counted in an area of 10 sq. mm., 0.1 mm. in depth, which contains a volume of 1 μl. of diluted blood. The total count is multiplied by 50 (dilution factor) to obtain the number of leukocytes per microliter of undiluted blood.

After the leukocytes have been counted, the platelets have settled and can be counted without focusing the objective to the various levels in the counting chamber (Fig. 10-10). If only a platelet count is done, the counting chamber is left for 5 min. in order to allow the platelets to settle. A $20\times$ objective may be used in these studies. In one counting area, five of the 25 small squares, each measuring 0.04 sq. mm. of the central large square (four corner and one middle square), are counted. Thus, platelets are counted in an area of 0.2 sq. mm., 0.1 mm. in depth—that is, in a volume of 0.02 μl. of diluted blood. The number obtained is multiplied by 2500 [50 (dilution factor) $\times$50 (aliquot factor)] to obtain the platelet count in 1 μl. of undiluted blood (Fig. 10-11).

There has been available a Unopette system (No. 5806) for use with Coulter Electronic Cell Counters; this includes a self-measuring capillary tube and a reservoir containing premeasured diluent that may be aspirated directly into the instrument. A newer Unopette system (No. 5849) is now available for use on the Coulter Counter. It is designed for laboratories that prefer to use their own diluent, but wish to avoid the hazards of mouth pipetting and the inconvenience of working with loose capillary pipettes. This newer technique utilizes a capillary pipette that has a vented bulb for expulsion and rinsing of the plasma sample. Both models are supplied with plastic sedimentation tubes and racks for preparation of the sample. For those laboratories using the Technicon Autocounter system, there is another Unopette system (No. 5847); that facilitates on-site capillary collection and may also be used with a tube of blood, thus eliminating the need to switch from "macro" to "micro."

The Phase-Contrast Microscopy Method (Brecker-Cronkite)

In the phase-contrast method, blood must be collected properly in two siliconized syringes, using a 20-gauge needle and two siliconized test tubes to avoid platelet clumping. Two mg. of EDTA is placed in one tube together with 2 ml. of blood, and mixed. The tube with the blood is then placed in the refrigerator. The blood is then drawn into one red blood cell pipette to the 1 mark. The diluting fluid (1% ammonium oxalate) is drawn to the 101 mark, and shaken for 3 minutes until sparkling hemolysis is present. The first 4 drops are expelled from the pipette. One chamber is then filled with each pipette, using a No. 1 coverglass. This is repeated with EDTA-blood combination as described previously, but without oxalate. Both sides of a Spencer-Briteline No. 1475 chamber are filled and allowed to sit in a wet house for 15 minutes. All 25 squares (1 sq. mm.) are counted, and the result is multiplied by 1000, which equals the platelets per cubic millimeter. The platelets are counted by phase-contrast microscopy with the light condenser adjusted. They stand out as individual round or black oval bodies with a pink or purple sheen and possess a light halo on a gray background. On focusing up and down, the platelets can be seen to have

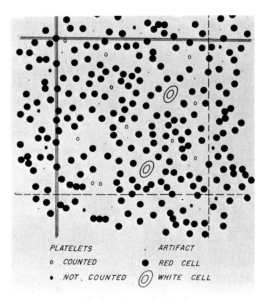

PLATELETS · ARTIFACT
o COUNTED ● RED CELL
• NOT COUNTED ⊚ WHITE CELL

Fig. 10-11. All platelets within the square are counted. Those touching the upper and left boundary lines are not counted. This procedure is followed for all 16 small squares in each large square.

one or more fine processes (Figs. 10-12, 10-13).

Expressed in another way, under high power, the four corner and one central square of the large center square on both sides of the counting chamber are counted. Each side is calculated separately. The volume above each square is 0.004 cu.mm., and the dilution is 1 to 100. Therefore, the number of platelets per cubic millimeter equals the number of cells counted, times the dilution, divided by 0.004, times the number of squares counted, times 5000 or

No. platelets/cu.mm. =
$$\frac{\text{No. cells counted} \times \text{dilution}}{0.004 \times \text{no. squares counted}} \times 5000$$

The *advantages* of this technique are as follows: Crystals, dirt and bacteria, which are confused for platelets, are readily distinguished by their refractivity and absence of pink-purple sheen. This method is more accurate than the Rees-Ecker method. The methods of blood collection reduce the agglutination, fragmentation and disintegra-

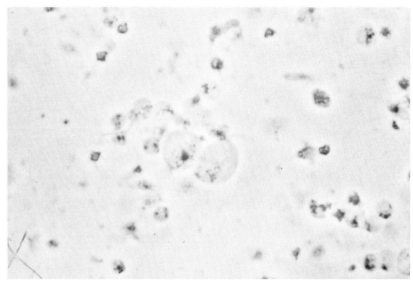

Fig. 10-12. Platelets without pseudopods. Phase contrast photomicrograph at 1350×.

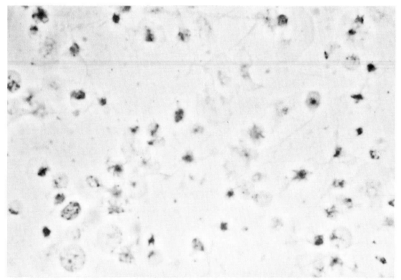

Fig. 10-13. Platelets with pseudopods. Phase contrast photomicrograph at 1350×.

tion. The use of ammonium oxalate as a diluent ensures clearing of the background by hemolysis. The use of phase microscopy overcomes the difficulty of distinguishing platelets from extraneous particles.

The *disadvantages* of this method are as follows: Platelet clumping due to incipient clotting makes counting unreliable. This method requires special, expensive equipment — siliconized glassware — to avoid platelet clumping.

The normal count with this method, in 95 per cent of healthy controls, equals 140,000 to 440,000 per cu.mm.

Automatic Platelet Counters

Coulter Counter Method. In performing direct platelet counts with the Coulter Electronic Particle Counter, the following procedure is used.[7] An aliquot of blood anticoagulated with EDTA is taken up into a small-bore plastic sedimentation tube. The tubes are bent approximately $1/4$ inch from the sealed end, and the double portion of tubing squeezed between the forefinger and thumb. The open end is then dipped below the surface of the blood, and the pressure is gradually released. (Alternatively, the tube may be compressed with a Kelly clamp.) Approximately 0.1 cc. of blood will be aspirated.

The tubes are then inverted and placed open end down in a rack to permit sedimentation. As soon as a plasma layer has formed, it can be diluted. When ready for dilution, the tube is held in the inverted position, and the red cell portion is cut off with scissors. This leaves a portion of tubing containing only platelet-rich plasma.

If sedimentation proceeds too slowly or if the tubes have been permitted to sediment in excess of 90 minutes, an alternate method must be adopted. The cut is made in the center of the red cell portion, and the tubing is placed open end up to sediment. Within 5 minutes, the platelet-rich plasma will pass through the remaining red cells, resuspending the platelets and allowing aspiration to take place directly from the surface.

The three-lambda pipette is then filled with plasma and diluted in 9 ml. of the working potassium oxalate solution, and the pipette is rinsed three times. The solution is gently mixed immediately after dilution and again just before counting. With a Model B Counter, one count is taken with upper and lower thresholds at the appropriate settings. With a Model A or Model F Counter, two counts are necessary — one at the lower threshold setting and another with the threshold set at 10 times the first setting. The difference between these two

Table 10-1. Example Computations

Hematocrit	30%
Machine count	20,000
Plasma platelet count (Chart A)	655,500
Whole blood platelet count $(655,500 \times 0.63$; Chart B$)$	$= 412,965/$cu. mm.

counts is the platelet population. The purpose of the upper threshold setting is to exclude any white or red cell contamination that might occur. The count is corrected using conversion Chart A, which includes both dilution and coincidence corrections and which comes with the instrument. The resultant figure is the plasma platelet count.

In order to obtain a whole-blood platelet count, a factor derived from the hematocrit must be used (Chart B, also is included with the instrument). This factor corrects for repulsion of red cells and platelets in the supernatant plasma. The degree of this concentration is predictable and dependent on the hematocrit (see Table 10–1).

Background counts on the diluent must be kept low in relationship to the number of platelets being counted. Owing to the small size of platelets, care is required to filter solutions adequately and keep them clean and dust-free. Also, the 70 μ aperture used in platelet counting must be kept clean. Generally, for a laboratory doing less than six counts a day, time savings alone may not justify switching from visual to machine counting because of the procedure care involved. However, precision with the Coulter Counter is 4 per cent, whereas visual technique allows only 12 to 16 per cent at best. If the platelet work load is substantial, machine counts are not only more precise, but enable more than 25 counts an hour to be made. The technique may be accelerated and simplified by the purchase of a Coulter Platelet Kit, which contains material for 20 platelet counts.

Autocounter. The Technicon Autocounter yields a rapid (40 samples/hr.) and accurate quantitation of platelets by means of an optical system that generates

System operation

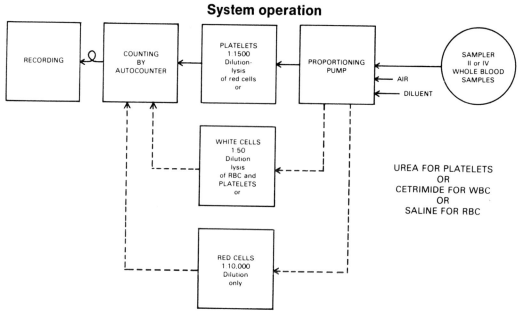

Fig. 10-14. Flow pattern of Technicon Autocounter. (Courtesy of Technicon Co.).

light pulses from the thrombocytes passing through the flow cell. The light pulses are transformed into electrical pulses, amplified, and counted in an electronic system and finally recorded on precalibrated chart paper.

The Autocounter is one of the few platelet counting systems that accepts whole blood samples. Whole blood collected in K_3·EDTA solution is separated and placed in either a Technicon Sampler II (which holds 40 cups of whole blood) or a Sampler IV (with a 40-vacutainer capacity). The contents of the cups or tubes are held in uniform suspension by a rotating mixer. The proportioning pump III then continuously propels separated reagents and samples through the system at precisely determined rates. Samples and reagents are brought together in a manifold under constant physical conditions (Fig. 10-14).

A simple manifold exchange permits the technologist to convert the system from platelet counting to red or white blood cell counting. No coincidence correction factors are required. The aspirated anti-

coagulated whole blood sample is automatically diluted to 1:5000, with a solution of 2M urea, which causes lysis of the RBCs and dissolution of the stromata to the point of optical invisibility. The diluted samples pass from the manifold to the Autocounter module, an electronic device that senses the number of optical distributions per unit of time, created by the passage of platelets and white blood cells through a precise, optically defined volume free from coincidence factors in the ranges used. A single pen recorder accepts analog signals from the Autocounter and presents a continuous tracing of peaks and valleys on linear chart paper that is precalibrated to a range of 0 to 750,000 platelets per mm.[3] The height of each peak is directly proportional to the number of platelets and WBCs in each sample. Comparison with a standard peak provides an accurate platelet or WBC count, reproducible to ±2.5 per cent. Should the recorded number fall below 75,000 platelets per mm.[3], the range may be altered by substituting one pump tube and rerunning the sample with a lower final dilution ratio (1:200). Results on the chart paper may then be read in the 0 to 75,000 platelets per mm.³ range. Two platelet reference controls are available, one for each range. Since the results are linear, single-point standardization is all that either range requires.

Advantages. Extensive operator training and special expertise are not required. Error-ridden manual manipulations are totally eliminated; there is no need for either pipetting and dilution or time-consuming preparation of platelet-rich plasma. No hematocrit correction factor is needed. The instrument has the capability to perform platelet counts on microsamples drawn by finger-puncture techniques.

Disadvantages. With leukemic patients with marked leukocytosis, the platelet count must be corrected by subtraction of the white count from the total platelet and WBC count indicated in the results. When the reported platelet count is in the 100,000 range, a WBC count must be done in case a significant correction is required.

The Hycel Counter 103 (Fig. 10-15) uses either whole blood or platelet-rich plasma, and has precision values for platelet counts of less than 5 per cent CV on whole blood and less than 2 per cent using platelet-rich plasma. Utilizing 20 μl., the instrument performs a platelet count in less than 15 seconds and displays its results digitally in large, easy-to-read figures. A non-mercury manometer system avoids the toxicity and other hazards associated with mercury. Unbreakable 78-μ aperture tubes eliminate downtime, reduce cost, and avoid the inconvenience of glass aperture tubes. A size discrimator may be used for upper and lower platelet values. Audible alarms alert the technologist to any stoppages or overfilled waste bottle; and a reverse flushing mechanism provides for the immediate cleaning of the orifice and automatic coincidence correction. Thus, there are no time-consuming conversion charts.

Royco/TOA Model 910 Microcell Counter can count platelets in a 1:20,000 dilution of

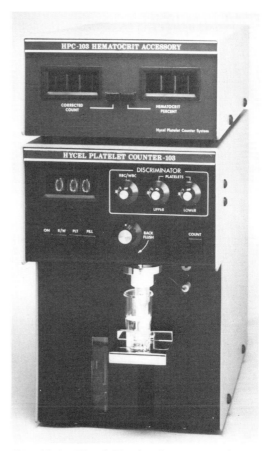

Fig. 10-15. Hycel Platelet Counter, HPC-103. (Courtesy of Hycel Inc.)

whole blood and in a 1:5,000 dilution of platelet-rich plasma in a 14-second period of time. A resistance detection method measures the volume of each blood cell as it passes through a counting aperture. A 100-μ aperture is used for WBCs and RBCs and a 78-μ aperture for platelets. The aperture tube is immersed in a cup containing whole blood diluted with isotonic electrolyte solution. There is an internal electrode within the aperture tube and an external electrode in the solution. When the COUNT button is depressed, 0.1 ml. of the sample is aspirated through the orifice, while the current flows from one electrode to the other. When a blood cell is in the orifice, resis-

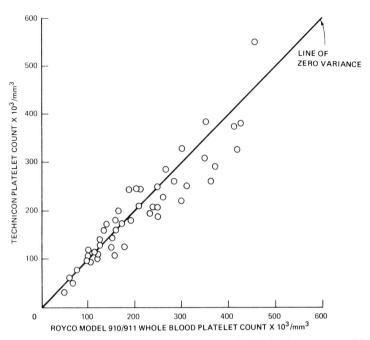

Fig. 10-16. Comparison of Royco whole blood platelet counts with those from Technicon platelet counter. (Courtesy of Royco Instruments Inc.)

tance to the current flow increases. This change in current is electronically recorded as a pulse. The greater the cell volume, the greater the pulse height and width. Pulses generated by RBCs, WBCs, and platelets passing through the orifice are electronically counted and numerically displayed, in terms of counts per mm.[3] of whole blood, to three significant digits. The liquid in the manometer of the Model 910 is isotonic diluent rather than the toxic mercury. Infrared detectors monitor the levels of the isotonic diluent to determine when to start and stop operations. Orifice blockage and waste overfill are signalled by the sounding of an alarm. A reverse flush control is employed to remove debris or clogs in the orifice. Figure 10-16 demonstrates the efficiency and reproducibility of this instrument, compared to the Technicon Platelet Counter.

Haema-Count MK-45 HC uses an electronic rather than a visual method to count platelets. Like a visual count using pol-

arized light, an electronic count senses individual platelets in a diluted and measured sample. The MK-4S utilizes platelet-rich plasma (P.R.P.), because the manufacturers believe that the use of whole blood would require too complex an instrumentation for practical and accurate results (there would be a 100- to 1000-fold excess of RBCs and WBCs). They have recommended the use of a special centrifuge (plateletfuge) to spin down the whole blood specimen, but the similarity in specific gravity of platelets and isolated RBCs and WBCs makes the time and speed of centrifugation critical, and they are selectively controlled. This instrument therefore spins down the whole blood specimen in 3 minutes at a nominal speed of 1715 r.p.m. Rotational (precessional) movement of the numbered sedimentation tube carriers (58 r.p.m.) aids the cellular separation. 1.5 ml. of the P.R.P. is placed in a flask that is placed in the instrument. A metal snorkel is immersed in the flask, and the entire hydraulic system is primed with the sample, which cleanses the aperture, and virtually eliminates cross-contamination between successive samples. Another 1.5 ml. sample is then placed in the instrument and the COUNT button is pressed, which allows a steady stream of sample to flow, first through the cell with its 60-micron aperture in a separately inserted assembly, then past start and stop photovolumetric controls along the volumetric measuring chamber, and finally into the waste container. Power to activate this flow is supplied by a vacuum pump that runs continuously while the instrument is turned on. The pump draws air from the waste container, which creates a vacuum in the hydraulic system. There is an air vent on the cell assembly, just downstream of the aperture, but this vent is closed during a count so that the vacuum can sustain flow through the system. When a count has been completed, the vent opens automatically, and the vacuum is broken. Air admitted through the vent causes liquid remaining in the system to be emptied rapidly into the waste container. In this way, the MK-45 is thoroughly purged of fluid during the interval between counts. When the COUNT button is pressed again, the vent closes automatically, and the cycle begins again. If the SHUT-DOWN/OPR CONTROL is used, the vent remains closed, and fluid flows continuously through the system.

A platelet in the aperture acts as a partial insulator and momentarily raises circuit resistance. The disturbance created by the platelet—a momentary increase in the electric potential—is sensed as an electrical pulse; it is accepted as a single count. Smaller electrical disturbances caused by passage of debris through the aperture are rejected by the threshold circuitry, as are larger disturbances caused by the passage of large particles or stray blood cells in the sample. The high and low thresholds create an "electronic window" capable of discriminating between platelets and particles of other sizes. The sample is diluted 1:4,000, and the count is electronically halved five times, or divided by 32, for presentation in thousands of platelets per cubic millimeter of plasma. Therefore, the volume for a count should be 4000 times 32 divided by 1,000 or 128 cubic microliters.

Advantages.[*] Electronic instrumentation is better than visual. It is more accurate, precise, reliable and also eliminates fatigue and eyestrain. The coefficient of variation is 5 per cent by electronic counting as compared to about 15 per cent by visual methods. Samples to be assayed on this instrument are more dilute than those used for visual counting, but it counts approximately 80 times as many platelets as are counted visually. Nevertheless, it still assays only a measured portion of the total flow through the aperture. Platelets that traverse the aperture before and after the measured portion of the total flow are not recorded. It is necessary to have an accurate count of the platelets in a relatively small but precisely measured sample. Since patients on radiation therapy or chemotherapy frequently have very low platelet counts, this instrument is especially valuable. It is more than four times as precise in the low ranges as visual means. It has a 4 per cent CV, with counts above 150,000 and up to 500,000; 5 per cent CV for day-to-day precision counts between 50,000 to 150,000; and 2.5 CV for precision within 1 day, with a 5-minute determination time.

Disadvantages. The coincidence-corrected count must be converted into per cent volume of whole blood. This additional step plus the need to have a hematocrit performed for each blood specimen prior to performing a platelet count may make a more direct method, the use of whole blood, more desirable than to use P.R.P. Rarely, patients having an abnormally low sedimentation rate may require a re-spin to obtain sufficient platelet-rich plasma.

---

[*] All performance claims have been verified by the College of American Pathologists.

Instrumentation and Morphology. The use of new instrumentation has revealed that platelet contact with collagen at the site of trauma brings about an alteration of the platelet membrane, which initiates an energy-dependent release of cytoplasmic substances. A change in platelet shape, followed by platelet aggregation, leads to the eventual development of a platelet plug at the trauma site. Although many new tests have been developed to evaluate platelet function, thrombocyte counts are still important; platelet-related hemorrhage usually does not occur until values below 20,000 per mm.[3] have been recorded. This lower critical level (compared with previously described values of approximately 100,000 per mm.[3]) can best be attributed to the presence of young megathrombocytes — in their presence, lower platelet counts can be observed without bleeding episodes. These megathrombocytes appear to be effective in clot formation and retraction. However, electronic automatic machine counting does not accurately reveal a true platelet count when these younger and larger platelets are present, and, therefore, machine counts are of limited clinical correlation value. Furthermore, Simplate techniques have improved reproducibility, so that surgical procedures may safely be done with subnormal thrombocyte levels but normal bleeding times.

Although Von Willebrand's disease is associated with a prolonged bleeding time, it is now thought to be directly related to the absence of a plasma component (the Von Willebrand factor), and not to a specific thrombocyte defect. Similarly, the myeloproliferative disorders (chronic granulocytic leukemia, polycythemia vera, essential thrombocythemia, and myeloid metaplasia) are now thought to be associated with enlarged platelets, altered platelet membrane function, and bizarre shapes. Thus, despite a normal or elevated platelet count, the bleeding time may still be prolonged.

Improved, automated instrumentation has illuminated the evaluation of platelet aggregation. Since aggregation is evaluated with differing concentrations of epinephrine, adenosine diphosphate (ADP) and collagen, new instruments can prepare two-wave pattern aggregation curves followed later by partial disaggregation. With proper reproducibility, impaired aggregation, including the absence of the second wave, can be demonstrated in some platelet disorders.

Indirect Method

In this method, a large drop of a 14 per cent $MgSO_4$ solution is placed on skin that has been cleaned and dried. A skin-puncture is made through the liquid, and a drop of the $MgSO_4$-blood mixture is placed on a clean glass slide and a blood film made. Wright's stain is used as in a routine differential count. Platelets are counted at the same time red blood cells are, until at least 1000 red blood cells have been counted. The number of platelets obtained is calculated from the ratio of red blood cells to platelets; the number of red blood cells is obtained from a hemocytometer erythrocyte count done at the same time. One may use brilliant cresyl blue and count reticulocytes at the same time.

The *advantages* of this method are as follows: This involves a simple technique; no expensive apparatus is needed. Red blood cells, white blood cells, platelets, and reticulocytes can be surveyed all at one time. This method offers a good check on the direct method when compared with the history of patient, bleeding time, clot retraction, and the tourniquet test. Some qualitative defects of platelets can be determined with this method — for example, large and bizarrely formed platelets.

The *disadvantages* of this procedure are as follows: It gives a very rough estimate of the total number of platelets because clumping occurs. The red blood cell count must be done separately. A thin film must be made and studied, and the count depends on the distribution of platelets and the red blood cell count. The average of the mean platelet count is higher using brilliant cresyl blue than using Wright's stain.

The normal values are: 140,000 to 350,000 platelets per cu.mm. using Wright's stain, and 500,000 to 1,000,000 platelets per cu.mm. using brilliant cresyl blue.

PHYSIOLOGIC VARIATIONS

The physiologic variations in the number of platelets in the blood indicates the balance between their production and their utilization, loss, or destruction. The level of circulating platelets, although not an absolute measure of the number of available platelets, frequently is a good indicator of platelet deficiency (thrombocytopenia) or an excess of platelet (thrombocytosis or thrombocythemia). The average level equals 250,000 to 350,000 per cu.mm. Qualitative as well as quantitative defects may be present in platelets. The number of platelets increases with an increase in altitude. The number of platelets is higher in winter than in summer. At birth the platelet count averages 150,000 to 300,000 per cu.mm.; at 2 weeks of age, the count averages 175,000 to 350,000 per cu.mm.; at 1 month, 200,000 to 450,000 per cu.mm.; up to 12 years, 250,000 to 450,000 per cu.mm.

PATHOLOGIC VARIATIONS

When the platelet count is below 100,000 per cu.mm., the decrease in platelets may be associated with a tendency toward general bleeding together with prolonged bleeding time with or without petechiae or ecchymoses. The decrease may also be associated with poor clot retraction and diminished prothrombin consumption, becoming more severe as the platelet count decreases. Diseases associated with thrombocytopenia are primary (idiopathic) thrombocytopenic purpura, acute or chronic; and secondary (symptomatic) thrombocytopenic purpura found in blood dyscrasias, infection, intoxications, allergic conditions, and lesions involving the bone marrow.

Increased platelet counts may follow hemorrhage, trauma, a number of infectious diseases, splenectomy, polycythemia, idiopathic thrombocythemia, megakaryocytic or myelogenous leukemia, tuberculosis, and increased counts may be found in any condition in which there is increased megakaryocytic activity.

HEMOSTASIS

Hemostasis is a process by which hemorrhage (spontaneous or induced) ceases. The complete process is associated with the control of bleeding from a traumatized blood vessel and the final cessation of bleeding. Hemostasis is a dynamic, complex mechanism characterized by a multitude of sequential biochemical and physical phenomena, terminating physiologically in the formation of a solid thrombus, or clot, that seals off the injured blood vessel.

Hemorrhage

Hemorrhage is defined as a discharge of blood from its normal vascular channels (arterial, venous, or capillary) into extravascular spaces owing to the loss of continuity in the vessels.

Hemorrhagic manifestations and lesions are generally most prominent on the lower extremities because of increased hypostatic pressure. Petechiae indicate platelet or blood vessel defects. Ecchymoses and hematomas are usually caused by coagulation defects, as well as platelet or blood vessel abnormalities. Hemarthroses are most common in severe coagulation defects, especially in hemophilia. Purpuric lesions are generally asymptomatic except for their cosmetic effects, but if they are characterized by premonitory or late-appearing paresthesias or discomfort, vasculitis and autoerythrocytic sensitization should be considered. These manifestations are somewhat influenced by the quality of perivascular support. Bleeding into solid structures or spaces of limited capacity and compressibility is generally self-limiting because compression of extravasated blood impairs further loss. But because loose subcutaneous and submucosal tissues afford poor support, mucocutaneous signs of bleeding are common in all hemorrhages.

Extravasated blood in a self-limiting cavity in a patient with normal clotting mechanism forms a dark red gelatinous clot, which subsequently undergoes organization and change in color to yellowish red with layering. Finally, organization becomes complete with fibrosis and adhesions between two opposing surfaces. Blood in loose subcutaneous or submucosal tissues is called a hematoma, ecchymosis, or petechia, depending on the size of the hemorrhagic extravasation. The color changes that occur in a bruise are modified by tissue macrophages, which remove pigments from the breakdown of extravasated red blood cells. These colors are, in sequence, dark red-black, blackish green, yellowish green, and finally colorless when completely absorbed and healed.

Causes. Hemorrhage can result from the interruption of vascular continuity due to certain common challenges—for example, menstruation, tooth extractions, tonsillectomy, ulceration in the gastrointestinal tract, surgical procedures, familial history, drug and chemical exposures, trauma (extra- or intravascular), hypertension, platelet deficiencies (qualitative and quantitative), or chemical defects essential to hemostasis. Usually a combination of mechanisms produce the abnormal bleeding.

Factors Governing Hemostasis

Extravascular factors include: the physical effects of adjacent tissue areas—that is, the skin, elastic tissue, and muscle elements that are active in closing off the tear in the lacerated vessels; and the biochemical effects of various components liberated from traumatized tissue that react with the factors in platelets and plasma. This extravascular coagulation process is of some importance in the activation of the intravascular coagulation process of the blood in clinical situations aggravated by trauma and hemorrhage. They include the following clinical entities: purpura senilis and purpura cachectica associated with atrophy of subcutaneous tissue, Cushing's syndrome, Ehlers-Danlos syndrome, epidermolysis bullosa, and pseudoxanthoma elasticum—all associated with fragility and hyperlaxity of the skin or connective tissue.

Vascular factors in the hemostasis are intimately related to the injured vascular structure, which constricts and retracts promptly. Thus, when a blood vessel is damaged, a brief local vasoconstriction occurs, which is rapidly followed by the adhesion of platelets to the wound. If blood escapes from the injured vessel and flows over nearby vessels they also contract. This vasoconstriction may be partly a local reflex and partly humoral—that is, due to histamine or allied substances not necessarily serotonin. Although serotonin is a constituent of platelets and is known to have vasoconstrictive properties, its importance in hemostasis is now doubted because depletion of serotonin causes no demonstrable defect of hemostasis.[17]

A few seconds after the break in the blood vessel occurs in the endothelium, platelets adhere to the margin and stick to the subendothelial collagen fibrils, forming a loose mesh, which reduces the escape of blood. This platelet adherence may be electrostatic with positively charged calcium ions linking the negatively charged platelet and the damaged cell, or platelet adherence may result from the release of adenosine diphosphate (ADP)—a substance that causes rapid platelet clumping with the subendothelial collagen fibrils and to each other. Platelets then release a thromboplastic substance and extrude a retractile or contractile protein (actinomyosin) in a process called viscous metamorphosis. Actinomysin in the presence of glucose and adenosine triphosphate (ATP) draws together the threads of fibrin in a process called clot retraction (hemostatic plug). Thus, the vascular component depends on blood vessels that are structurally and functionally normal.

When a blood vessel structure is abnormal, it is characterized by local or general bleeding involving chiefly skin, mucous membranes, or both. Bleeding, in this group, is not associated with a diminution in the number of thrombocytes or with any known defect of plasma coagulation components. However, these vascular factors do not really form a distinct separation from the other components, especially the extravascular portions. For example, some of the general vascular disorders, such as scurvy and anaphylactoid purpura, are on occasions found associated with a thrombocytopenia. Also qualitative thrombocyte defects (thrombasthenia) may exist even though the platelet count is normal. It is also quite likely that a combination of factors involving vascular endothelium, platelet variations, and hormonal factors produce either increased capillary permeability (abnormal fragility) or poor capillary contractility. Included in this group are vascular abnormalities associated with traumatic injury of vessels, hereditary hemorrhagic telangiectasia and nonthrombocytopenia purpuras—for example, allergic purpuras such as anaphylactoid purpura and Schönlein-Henoch purpura, von Willebrand's disease, hereditary familial purpura simplex, symptomatic purpuras such as those associated with infections, mechanical purpura, orthostatic purpura, and purpura fulminans.

Intravascular factors in hemostasis are mainly those associated with the substances involved in the coagulation of blood. The hemostatic abnormalities in this group are also inseparable and difficult to limit etiologically without also including vascular and extravascular factors. In the main they include those hemorrhagic disease complexes with complicated physicochemical reactions; they involve the factors associated with the ultimate conversion of liquid blood into a firm fibrin clot. In this syndrome (defibrination), there is depletion of Factors II, V, and VIII, and platelets. Hemorrhagic disorders associated with this syndrome are therefore characterized by numerous laboratory abnormalities, fibrinogen deficiency being the predominant factor associated with the liberation of thromboplastic substances into the blood. Although active fibrinolysis accompanies most cases of intravascular coagulation, such coagulation need not precede the fibrinolytic process.

Fibrinolysis is frequently triggered by one or more of the following: (1) obstetric complications, such as abruptio placenta, dead fetus retention, and amniotic fluid embolism; (2) malignancies such as prostatic carcinoma; (3) severe injury or stress situations, such as pulmonary, uterine, pancreatic, or breast surgery, and extensive burns; (4) miscellaneous diseases, such as hepatic disease, hemolytic transfusion reactions, polycythemia vera, and leukemia. (5) Microangiopathic hemolytic anemia pattern is also observed, associated with vasculitis, malignant hypertension, carcinomatosis, and disseminated intravascular coagulation. The erythrocyte fragmentation observed in these and similar disorders is thought to be due to the buffeting of RBCs against fibrin strands in the microvasculature. To be explicit, the hemorrhagic disorders associated with coagulation defects in this group include those associated with deficient blood thromboplastin formation, deficient thrombin formation, defective fibrin formation, increased fibrinolytic activity, and the dysglobulinemias, such as cryoglobulinemia, plasmacytic myeloma, and primary macroglobulinemia (of Waldenström).

The intravascular coagulation syndrome and other bleeding diseases may be difficult to distinguish from fibrinolysis, because the latter eventually depletes supplies of fibrinogen, as well as platelets and Factors II, V, and VIII. However, one can usually see clot dissolution in vitro if fibrinolysis is the predominant factor in the hemorrhagic diathesis. Occasionally, clot lysis occurs so quickly that coagulation may not be visible.

A complex coagulation disorder, resembling disseminated intravascular coagulation (DIC) and related to vitamin K deficiency, is frequently associated with abnormal PTT, PT, thrombocytopenia (secondary to concomitant vitamin deficiency, e.g., folic acid deficiency in malabsorption syndrome), or intercurrent infection. Since the thrombin time is normal, confusion with DIC can usually be avoided. The coagulation mechanism in DIC is activated by the release of tissue factor into the blood. This develops following obstetrical accidents, or after severe trauma, or after leukocytic tissue factor activation by bacterial endotoxin. In some cases, enzymes other than thrombin may lead to the lowering of levels of fibrinogen and other coagulation factors. In addition, platelet production and fibrinogen synthesis may accelerate, in association with intravascular platelet and fibrinogen consumption. Therefore, the turnover rates of platelets and fibrinogen are significantly increased, but blood levels may remain normal.

Therapy for DIC is usually directed toward the underlying disease process. For example, prompt control of gram-negative sepsis with effective antibiotics usually spontaneously and rapidly corrects the coagulation abnormalities. Since heparin is a strong, immediately acting antithrombin agent, therapy with heparin is proposed when circulating thrombin is responsible for the DIC. However, the effectiveness of heparin is, at best, variable, and it has not been tested in controlled studies. Thus, its use is declining. In conditions in which the underlying disease is not responsive, or in which the thrombosis is an important finding, its administration should be attempted cautiously, by continuous I.V. infusion. If increased bleeding occurs, drug therapy should immediately be discontinued.

Waterfall or cascade theory of Breckenridge and Ratnoff graphically demonstrates the process of intravascular coagulation in vivo (blood clotting in vitro is initiated by contact with a foreign surface such as glass).[5] The process of in vivo coagulation is possibly initiated by certain fatty acids or phospholipids liberated from platelets. However, this has not been specifically proven, although microcrystals of sodium urate are definitely associated with experimental initiation of coagulation and are also involved in inflammatory processes.

Several aspects of this proposed waterfall mechanism[8] (Fig. 10-17) should be clarified: (1) Each protein clotting factor shown occurs in plasma in an inactive or precursor form. These inactive proteins are listed on the left side of the waterfall along with their assigned Roman numeral. (2) When clotting is initiated, each clotting factor except fibrinogen is converted to a form possessing enzymatic activity. The activated forms are shown on the right side of the waterfall. (3) The activation of each clotting factor occurs in a stepwise sequence with each newly formed enzyme reacting with its specific substrate and converting it to an active enzyme. The clotting enzyme is thus suggested to be a cascade of proenzyme-enzyme transformations, each enzyme activating the next until the final substrate, fibrinogen, is reached. Each stage represented is fairly well supported by evidence with the exception of the supposed activation of Factor V, which is included for completeness despite lack of information. However, the precise mechanisms by which most of these activation reactions occur are really unknown. In fact, in case of Factors V and VIII, complexes are formed activating coagulation proteins, calcium ions, and phospholipids contributed by the platelets. These complexes, in turn, convert the next factor in the cascade to an active enzyme. Most factors activated in the cascade sys-

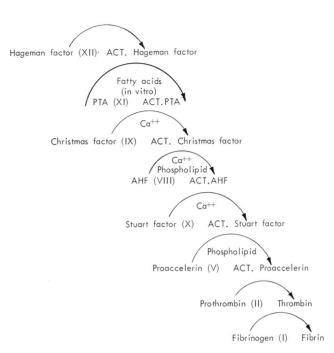

Fig. 10-17. Tentative mechanism for the initiation of blood clotting in mammalian plasma in the intrinsic system. It takes 7 minutes to reach Stuart factor (Factor X). Therefore any deficiency of factors down to the activation of Stuart factor will produce a prolonged coagulation time. (Davie, E. W., and Ratnoff, O. D.: A waterfall sequence for intrinsic blood clotting. Science, *145:*1310, 1964)

tem (e.g., Factors II, VII, IX, X, XI, and XII) have the amino acid serine as their active site. Factor XIII is also activated in the chain, but it is a transamidase rather than a serine protease. A deficiency in any factor, with the exception of Factor XII, the Fletcher factor, and the Fitzgerald factor, may produce abnormal hemostasis and clinical bleeding problems.

In the test tube, this series of reactions is initiated by contact with a surface such as glass and can also be initiated by microcrystals of sodium urate. This reaction, which is the first recognized event in the intrinsic clotting pathway, involves the conversion of Hageman factor to activated Hageman factor possibly accomplished by the unfolding or rearrangement of the Factor XII molecule or by the unmasking of an active catlytic site in the protein. Plasma collected in glassware lined with paraffin, petrolatum, or silicone does not clot and may stay in the fluid state 24 to 48 hours or longer. When this plasma is transferred to ordinary glass containers, it clots in a few minutes. The physiologic mechanism for the activation of Hageman factor (XII) in

vivo is not known, although it presumably involves some enzymatic system with unknown clotting factors.

Once Hageman factor becomes activated, it converts plasma thromboplastin antecedent (PTA) to an activated form. In vitro, this reaction is accelerated by long-chain saturated fatty acids. The next reaction in this sequence is the activation of Christmas factor by activated PTA. In this reaction, activated PTA participates as an enzyme, converting its substrate—Christmas factor—to an activated form. In the reaction, pH of 8.0 is considered best, and divalent metal ions such as Ca^{++} are required. The chemical events that occur during the activation of Christmas factor are unknown.

It has been suggested that activation may involve partial proteolysis of the Christmas factor molecule because partially purified preparations of activated PTA have esterase activity. Once the Christmas factor becomes activated, it interacts with antihemophilic factor (AHF) and Stuart factor in the presence of calicum ions. The final product of the interaction probably corresponds to activated Stuart factor. In the activation of AHF by activated Christmas factor, the latter participates as an enzyme and converts its substrate — antihemophilic factor — to an activated form. The reaction requires calcium ions and phospholipid. Once the AHF is activated, it in turn activates Stuart factor; it also requires calcium ions.

The next event in this series of reactions is the interaction between activated Stuart factor and proaccelerin to form a prothrombin converting principle, activated proaccelerin. This reaction also requires phospholipid. Once proaccelerin becomes activated, it converts prothrombin to thrombin. Thrombin then converts fibrinogen to fibrin by partial proteolysis, which liberates two specific peptides from the N-terminal end of fibrinogen. In the presence of calcium ions and activated fibrin stabilizing factor (Factor XIII), a carbodydrate component and ammonia are released. N-terminal glycine residues disappear and a tough, insoluble fibrin clot is formed. The intrinsic system shown in Figure 10-17 probably overlaps with the extrinsic system at the level of the Stuart factor. In the extrinsic system, tissue thromboplastin and Factor VII act as cofactors and probably are responsible for the activation of Stuart factor and the conversion of prothrombin to thrombin. Consequently, AHF, Christmas factor, PTA, and Hageman factor are bypassed.

COAGULATION

Curiously enough, the main components of the blood (serum, buffy coat, and clot) plus its liquid intravascular and solid clot state after bleeding were known to the Greco-Romans. In 1666, (approximately 2000 years later), Malpighi observed strands of fibers that remained after the washing of a blood clot. In 1845, Buchanan noted that fibrin formed after plasma and fresh serum were intermixed. Schmidt, in 1895, though this was due to an enzyme he

called thrombin. He also theorized that thrombin had a precursor — prothrombin — which required a tissue substance for its activation. In 1877, Hammersten isolated fibrinogen and in 1890, Arthus and Pagis demonstrated the importance of calcium in coagulation by showing the anticoagulant effect of oxalate.

Theories of Blood Coagulation

Morawitz's Theory. In 1905, Morawitz combined all these phenomena into his classic theory of blood coagulation. This theory was an attempt to explain the observation that tissue extracts (thromboplastin) would accelerate the coagulation of blood in the presence of calcium. Thus, according to the theory, in Stage I, prothrombin plus calcium ions plus thromboplastin (tissue) will form thrombin; and in Stage II, fibrinogen plus thrombin will form fibrin.

Howell's theory, on the other hand, proposed the following sequence of events: (1) Prothrombin is inactivated by antiprothrombin (heparin). (2) Thromboplastin neutralizes antiprothrombin and releases prothrombin. (3) Prothrombin plus calcium forms thrombin. (4) Thrombin plus fibrinogen forms fibrin (clot).

Modern Theory. The modern concept of coagulation divides the process into three phases (Fig. 10-18). The various substances involved in coagulation of the blood are called coagulation factors, designated by Roman numerals I to XIII excluding VI. Effective hemostasis itself depends on the integrity of each of these factors (with the possible exception of Factor XII), on the cellular components of the blood, and on the integrity of the blood vessel wall. The basic steps involved in coagulation are the formation of thromboplastin, the conversion of prothrombin to thrombin, and the conversion of fibrinogen to fibrin.

The formation of thromboplastin involves both an intrinsic and extrinsic system. The latter is an artificial system in that it is derived from injured tissues, and as far as is known, there is never a deficiency of

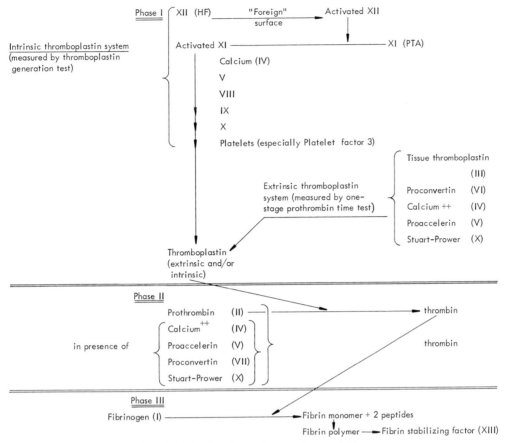

Fig. 10-18. The three phases of coagulation.

extrinsic thromboplastin from injured tissues. In reality therefore, coagulation or hemostatic defects result from a deficiency of the blood substances that react with tissue thromboplastin. In the formation of thromboplastin and the conversion of prothrombin to thrombin, Factor V (proaccelerin) and Factor VIII (Antihemophiliac globulin) are largely consumed and prothrombin (Factor II) is partially consumed; Factor VII (proconvertin or serum prothrombin conversion accelerator), Factor IX (Christmas factor or plasma thromboplastin component), Factor X (Stuart-Prower), Factor XI (plasma thromboplastin antecedent), and Factor XII (Hageman factor) are not consumed and usually remain at stable levels in serum; Factor XIII

is a fibrin-stabilizing factor not normally found in circulating blood.

The enzymatic conversion of fibrinogen to fibrin by the proteolytic enzyme thrombin is the final stage in coagulation. Thrombin is absorbed by the fibrin, an important controlling mechanism, in that thrombin probably has a catalytic action on the entire thromboplastin-activating system.

The plasma fibrinolytic system is responsible for the dissolution of the fibrin clot. The inactive proenzyme plasminogen, normally present in the blood, may become activated to plasmin by various tissue-activator substances. Plasmin is capable of acting on many proteins, including fibrin, fibrinogen, Factor V, and Factor VIII. The system is normally in homeostatic balance, but

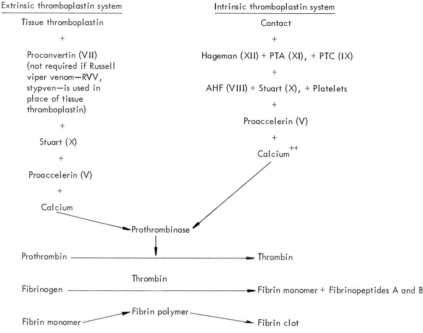

Fig. 10-19. Formation of the fibrin clot. (Gaston, L. W.: The blood clotting factors. N. Engl. J. Med., *270*:236, 1964)

if it becomes disorganized, a severe hemorrhagic disorder may result.

In Phase 1, the main process involved consists of the formation of intrinsic (plasma) thromboplastin—also called thromboplastogenesis. It is initiated by the action of platelets and other factors at a foreign surface. At least eight to ten factors take part in plasma thromboplastin generation: platelets, including platelet factor 3; calcium; Factor V; Factor VIII (AHG); Factor IX (PTC); Factor X (Stuart); Factor XI (PTA); Factor XII (AHF); Factor III; and Factor VII.

Phase 1 (Stage 1) can occur in two separate and distinct ways. Tissue thromboplastin (III), in the presence of plasma Factors V and X and calcium (IV), will activate prothrombin to thrombin. Factor VII is also required and appears to act as a cofactor for tissue thromboplastin (III). Because tissue thromboplastin is not ordinarily found in circulating blood, the system in which it is utilized is called the *extrinsic system*. Phase 1 (Stage 1) can also be accomplished solely by the clotting factors in the blood. Factor VII is not required in this process, but Factors VIII, IX, XI, and XII, and platelets (especially platelet factor 3) are peculiar to this system. Furthermore, Factors V and X and calcium (IV) are necessary here, as well as in the extrinsic system. Because all required components of this system are found in the blood, it is termed the *intrinsic system*.[11]

To those familiar with laboratory tests for coagulopathies, it may readily be apparent that the one-stage prothrombin time (Quick's test) is based on the principle of the extrinsic system, while the thromboplastin generation test of Biggs and Douglas is one that requires the components of the intrinsic system.

The role of surface in the coagulation mechanism is not entirely clear. However, it is generally agreed that when blood comes in contact with a foreign surface, the intrinsic system is initiated. There is good evidence to suggest that the activation of Hageman factor (XII) is the first step in the reactivation and that glass is required in an in vitro system. Furthermore, this effect is less pronounced when blood contacts a nonwettable surface. Thus, the clotting time of normal blood is longer in a silicone-coated tube than in a plain glass tube.

Kim and co-workers showed a correlation between elevated levels of serum cholesterol and blood coagulation factors, with occlusive thrombi developing at a faster rate than in normal animal controls.[20] They also proposed an association of the plasma lipids by means of the coagulation pathway in the production of human vascular disease.

Phase 2 (Stage 2) involves the conversion of prothrombin to thrombin. The reaction is activated by either the intrinsic plasma thromboplastin system or by the extrinsic tissue thromboplastin system. This stage is a pathway through which both thromboplastin systems may act to aid in the initiation of the final step.

Phase 3 (Stage 3) is the only reaction visible to the naked eye. Soluble fibrinogen is polymerized by the previously formed proteolytic enzyme thrombin. An insoluble fibrin clot is the end result of the three-stage system. Fortuitously, the same fibrin clot is the end point of most clotting tests (Fig. 10-19).[15]

A more recent schematic representation depicting new concepts of stable fibrin clot formation is presented in Figure 10-20. It demonstrates the combination of antithrombin III and Heparin inhibiting clotting in at least five steps (Plate 32).[32]

Factors Involved in Coagulation

Definition of each factor involved in each of the three stages, using the international nomenclature and synonyms, plus an elaboration of the origin, physical properties, and role in coagulation of each, seems appropriate at this time.

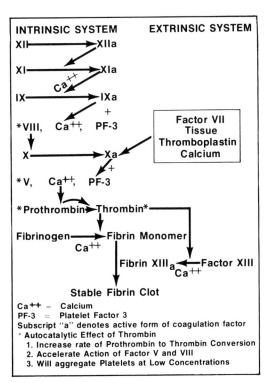

Fig. 10-20. New concepts of stable fibrin clot formation. (Triplett, D. A.: Blood tests proliferate with new knowledge of clotting. Laboratory Management, *15*:40, 1977)

Factor I (fibrinogen) arises from the liver or reticuloendothelial system. Chemically it is a globulin having a molecular weight of approximately 450,000, and it is present in plasma in a mean concentration of 300 mg. per 100 ml. The molecule itself is approximately 20 times as long as it is wide, and it belongs to the keratinomyosin group of fibrillary proteins. It is precipitated from plasma by heating to 56° C, it is adsorbed by Al(OH)₃ and Mg(OH)₂, and it is soluble in saline solution. The molecule is contained in Cohn Fraction I of plasma, and it is separated from Factor VII by bentonite from decalcified plasma. When it is mixed with thrombin, two peptides are split off, leaving a fibrin monomer with subsequent continuous polymerization and depolymerization in the bloodstream. Coagulation end products, produced in the presence of calcium ions and serum, are insoluble in urea — some proof that a fibrin stabilizing factor (Factor XIII) exists in serum.

Fibrinogen itself is increased in inflammatory states, dysproteinemias such as in multiple myeloma and nephrosis, and in pregnancy. Fibrinogen is also associated with an elevated sedimentation rate, in which α and β globulins are altered and albumin is depressed. Fibrinogen is decreased below 100 mg. per 100 ml. when large amounts of tissue thromboplastin appear in the bloodstream, leading to diffuse conversion of fibrinogen to fibrin without local thrombosis. Placental tissue, decidua, and lung tissue have high concentrations of tissue thromboplastin. Fibrinogenopenia is therefore seen in: defibrination of obstetrical complications (as, for example, in missed abortion, retained placenta, and intrauterine fetal death), abruptio placenta, amniotic fluid embolism, and retroplacental hemorrhage; after extensive lung surgery, such as thickened pleura decortication and excision of pulmonary tumors and lung abscesses; incompatible blood transfusions; extensive burns; hepatic cirrhosis; and prostatic cancer (fibrinogenopenia due to the excess production of fibrinolysins). In these clinical states the severity of the hemorrhagic diathesis depends of the degree of fibrinogen deficiency and the extent of associated defects (in platelets, AHF, and Factor V). Congenital fibrinogenopenia is a non-sex-linked recessive trait frequently associated with consanguineous intermarriage. It is manifest at birth by bleeding from the umbilical cord and in later life by excess bleeding from minor cuts, abrasions, or at menstrual periods. Laboratory tests for decreased fibrinogen levels show prolonged whole-blood clotting time, one-stage prothrombin time, thrombin time, and defective clot retraction. The bleeding time, the tourniquet test, and thromboplastin generation tests are all normal.

Factor II (prothrombin) is made in the liver and requires vitamin K as a catalyst. It is also related to Factor VII (SPCA) in that the latter can be converted to prothrombin by the liver. Prothrombin itself is a heat-stable protein of the α_2 globulin type having a molecular weight of approximately 140,000. Prothrombin is present in plasma in a concentration of 0.2 g. per ml. It is precipitated by $(NH_4)_2SO_4$ at 50 per cent saturation and absorbed from oxalated plasma by $BaSO_4$ and $Al(OH)_3$. In the presence of ionized calcium, prothrombin is converted to thrombin by the enzymatic action of thromboplastins from both extrinsic and intrinsic sources. A high concentration of citrate slowly activates prothrombin. It is also one of the factors affected by the common oral anticoagulant drugs and is measured by Quick's test, which is not specific because it is also affected by the levels of Factors I, V, VII, X; and by the two-stage method, which is more specific, accurate, difficult, and time-consuming.

Hypoprothrombinemia is more commonly acquired when vitamin K absorption from the gastrointestinal tract is impaired or its utilization by the liver is interefered with. Because vitamin K is not stored in the body, the alteration of the intestinal flora (synthesizer of most vitamin K) by antibiotics may lead to a reduced prothrombin level. Also because vitamin K is fat-soluble, diseases that lead to the interference of fat absorption may also produce impaired absorption of the vitamin and therefore hypoprothrombinemia, such as in obstructive jaundice and steatorrhea. Severe liver disease (cirrhosis and hepatitis) may also produce the same deficiency because liver cells appear unable to utilize vitamin K sufficiently to make prothrombin in adequate quantity. Anticoagulant drugs (coumarin, Coumadin, and others) in high plasma concentration can also produce hypoprothrombinemia. Factors II, VII, IX, and X are reduced in the newborn but increase with the age of the infant. Congenital hemorrhagic disease of the newborn was formerly thought to be caused by a deficiency of vitamin K or a deficiency of green vegetables in mother's diet with subsequent hypoprothrombinemia of the newborn. However, this theory is not longer tenable, and although vitamin K is given to the pregnant mother before delivery, vitamin K is not necessary for the newborn infant because in large doses it may produce more hemolysis and thus increase any jaundice present.

Factor III (thromboplastin or tissue factor) by which tissue thromboplastin is usually implied (although there is probably a plasma or intrinsic thromboplastin in existence) is a complicated admixture of heat-labile and heat-stable lipoidal protein substance of large molecular weight most commonly obtained from brain, lung, and sometimes other tissue. In the presence of calcium ions, thromboplastin brings about the conversion of prothrombin to thrombin, is prepared commercially, and is used in Quick's test. It is resistant to heating at 60° C, but it retains platelet Factor 3 activity. It requires activation by accessory Factors V, VII, and X in the presence of calcium ions (IV) for optimal conversion of prothrombin (II) to thrombin.

Deficiencies of blood thromboplastin are associated with: a deficiency of Factor VIII (AHG), seen in classic hemophilia and hemophilia A; deficiency of Factor IX (PTC), seen in hemophilia B (Christmas disease), vitamin K deficiencies, and liver disease; deficiency of Factor XI (PTA), seen in hemophilia C; thrombocytopenias; thrombasthenia; vascular hemophilia; circulating inhibitors of stage I — for example, in lupus erythematosus, hemophilia A and B, and in the postpartum period.

Factor IV (calcium) is found in the blood in concentrations of 9 to 11 mg. per 100 ml. and approximately 50 per cent in the ionized state (Ca^{++}). Ionized calcium is necessary to coagulation at different points in the process: in the terminal elaboration or activation of the thromboplastic products of the extrinsic or intrinsic systems with Factor V and Factor X; for the enzymatic conversion of prothrombin to thrombin by active thromboplastin; and in the formation of fibrin. Only minute quantities of Ca^{++} are required in coagulation. Calcium deficiency is therefore quite rare as a cause of coagulopathy, except occasionally after massive transfusions with citrated blood. In some of these transfusions, calcium combines with EDTA, oxalate, citrate, fluoride, and ion exchange resins, and it is therefore not available for coagulation when these ingredients are added to whole blood. In addition, hyperglobulinemia and dysglobulinemia (as in sarcoidosis and myeloma) may cause binding of calcium to abnormal globulins, resulting in a hemostatic defect, even in chemical hypercalcemia.

Factor V (proaccelerin, labile factor, or Ac globulin) is made in the liver. It is a labile, water-soluble globulin that breaks down rapidly, especially in oxalated plasma. It is used up in coagulation and therefore is not found in serum. Factor V is precipitated by $(NH_4)_2SO_4$ at 33 per cent saturation; it is not adsorbed by $BaSO_4$ or $Al(OH)_3$. Factor V is readily inactivated by heating to 58° C and by trypsin or fibrinolysin; it is fairly stable in citrated plasma. This factor is essential to the later phases of thromboplastin formation — that is, the extrinsic and intrinsic thromboplastic products appear to react with Factor V and probably also Factor X in the presence of Ca^{++}.

A congenital deficiency of Factor V results from an autosomal recessive trait that is not sex-linked; it is manifested when the trait is inherited from both parents (homozygosis). The deficiency is characterized by parahemophilia, in which there is a tendency for excessive bleeding from mucous membranes, nosebleed, menorrhagia, and so on. Patients show increased whole-blood clotting time and a prolonged one-stage prothrombin time. Administration of stored oxalated plasma does not correct the defect; however, repeated transfusions of normal plasma or adsorbed normal plasma in small amounts will correct the defect. Acquired Factor V deficiency may occur in severe liver disease (hepatocellular) or from circulating anticoagulants and increased fibrinolysis.

Factor VI is now known as activated Factor V.

Factor VII (proconvertin, stable factor, SPCA or Autoprothrombin I) is present in serum and not destroyed or used up in the coagulation process (Factor V is present in plasma). It is a very stable nondialyzable β globulin, and is undiminished in serum stored for 4 days at 25° to 37° C. Factor VII is destroyed at 56° C within 2½ minutes. It is adsorbed from serum by Al(OH)$_3$ or BaSO$_4$, which can then be eluted from the adsorbent by a sodium citrate solution. Factor VII is further purified by (NH$_4$)$_2$SO$_4$ precipitation, and is present in a concentration of less than 0.07 per cent of serum protein. Factor VII is related to prothrombin, is capable of being converted to prothrombin by the liver, and is therefore subject to the influence of vitamin K, just as prothrombin is. Factor VII is active only in the presence of Factor III. In the body, it activates tissue thromboplastins, and it accelerates production of thrombin from prothrombin. Factor VII is not an essential part of the intrinsic thromboplastin generating process, and it is reduced in concentration by anticoagulant coumarin drugs.

Deficiencies of Factor VII may be congenital or acquired. Congenital deficiencies may be due to an autosomal recessive gene (rare) with hemorrhagic diathesis (skin and mucous membrane) occurring only in the homozygous state, or it may manifest itself as hemorrhagic disease of the newborn associated with bruises, melena, and intracranial hematoma responding to vitamin K treatment of infant or mother before delivery. In the acquired group, Factor VII deficiency is associated with severe liver disease (cirrhosis), vitamin K deficiency, and broad spectrum antibiotic therapy, or it may follow a course of anticoagulant coumarin therapy. It is the earliest factor to be depressed and is characterized clinically by bruising, purpura, and postoperative bleeding and oozing. After the first week of coumarin therapy, Factor VII is not depressed as much as Factor X is. A deficiency of Factor VII produces a prolonged one-stage prothrombin time. Because the half-life of Factor VII is approximately 12 hours, blood or plasma transfusions must be given daily for deficiency. In excessive coumarin treatment, vitamin K restores the Factor VII level to normal in 4 to 6 hours.

Factor VIII (antihemophilic globulin, AHG) is also called antihemophilic factor A (AHF). The clearest data on the site of origin of AHF are those of Langdell and students, which point to the spleen and suggestively to the reticuloendothelial system.[33] That is, the spleen must be regarded as an important organ for the maintenance of AHF under stress, and it serves as a site of formation or storage.

Immunofluorescent studies using a rabbit Antifactor VIII antibody have identified a Factor VIII-related antigen in circulating platelets, bone marrow, megakaryocytes, and endothelial cells lining the blood vessels. Endothelial cell cultures release a Factor VIII antigen that is identical to the normal Factor VIII found in plasma. However, the endothelial cells do not synthesize the portion of the Factor VIII molecule necessary for procoagulant activity. At least two theories are proposed to account for this: The endothelial cell may synthesize an inactive precursor that contains only the antigen and von Willebrand Factor and must be converted at a distant site to produce the procoagulant activity. Or, it may synthesize a molecule that contains the antigen and von Willebrand factor and carries a second molecule that contains the Factor VIII procoagulant activity.[18]

Factor VIII appears to be a globulin or globulin-associated substance contained in Cohn's fraction I and III; it is precipitable by alcohol or acetic acid. It is not removed from plasma by adsorption with Al(OH)$_3$ or BaSO$_4$. The antihemophilic activity of normal plasma is generally lost within 24 hours and is gradually reduced (30–60%) after storage of 3 weeks under blood bank conditions, and is lost more slowly in fresh frozen plasma (50% lost in 1 month, then stable for many months). In addition, there is a rapid loss of antihemophilic activity when frozen plasma is thawed. Most authorities agree that Factor VIII is required for the adequate evolution of plasma thromboplastin and that it makes the clotting of hemophilic blood normal by making a thromboplastic material available in the presence of platelets.[6] Although only 10 per cent of the normal plasma concentration of Factor VIII is necessary to produce a normal amount of thromboplastin, this factor is fully consumed in the coagulation process and readily inactivated by thrombin or fibrinolysin.

A deficiency of Factors VIII, IX, X, or XI gives rise to a deficiency in thromboplastin generation. Factor VIII is deficient in thromboplastin generation. If Factor VIII is deficient, clot formation may occur, but the resultant clot will be soft, jelly-like, and easily dislodged. Poor clot formation is related to defective platelet retraction, which requires more thrombin than is necessary for the development of viscous metamorphosis in platelets. In hemophilia and hemophilia-like states with associated defective thrombin generation, there is also a proportionately defective platelet retraction that in the extrinsic system leads to the formation of a platelet plug. This soft, weak plug is easily dislodged and bleeding begins once again. When bleeding does start again, it is likely to continue because extrinsic tissue thromboplastic factors have been exhausted. Laboratory tests reveal a normal bleeding time, prolonged clotting time of whole blood, reduced thromboplastin generation, and markedly decreased prothrombin conversion (consumption).

Classic hemophilia (hemophilia A) is due to a female sex-linked recessive trait with mutation absent in up to 50 per cent of cases. The female develops the disease in rare homozygous states. Symptom severity is related roughly to the AHF plasma level;

it is severe if AHF level is less than 1 per cent. Pseudohemophilia B (vascular type) is associated with a capillary defect and is not sex-linked. Acquired abnormalities are associated with circulating inhibitors, leading to deficient AHF; increased AHF activity is seen in older patients, especially in coronary heart disease.

Factor IX (plasma thromboplastin component, PTC, Christmas factor, or Antihemophiliac Factor B) is probably a protein necessary for the formation of thromboplastin. It is called Christmas factor from the name of a patient who had the disease, and who was studied in detail by Biggs and associates in 1952. Factor IX is necessary for thromboplastin generation, is present in both serum and plasma, and is not fully consumed during coagulation. It is contained in Cohn fractions III and IV and is absent from Cohn fraction I. It is completely adsorbed by $Al(OH)_3$ and by $BaSO_4$, and it is removed from oxalated plasma by Seitz filtration. Factor IX is very stable when stored at refrigerator temperature and is moderately heat-stable (resistant to heating to 56° C for 10 minutes).

Although this factor is depressed by the coumarin drugs, it is not usually depressed as much as Factors VII and X are. It is thought by some investigators to be the factor involved in most hemorrhagic complications encountered in patients on anticoagulant therapy; other workers believe Factor X to be most frequently involved. Factor IX is activated in the course of the clotting process or by contact of plasma with glass. Clinically its deficiency is seen congenitally (sex-linked and recessive) in hemophilia B or Christmas disease and like Factor VII in association with hemorrhagic disease of newborn. Its deficiency is acquired also like that of Factor VII—in association with vitamin K deficiency, advanced hepatocellular disease, and in prolonged anti-vitamin-K treatment. In the laboratory a deficiency of Factor IX leads to delayed thromboplastin generation and is corrected by adding small amounts of fresh or aged normal plasma or serum, or by the addition of plasma in true hemophilia.

Factor X (Stuart-Prower Factor or Autoprothrombin III), is named after a patient named Stuart. It is a relatively stable factor, being stable in serum at 37° C for 30 minutes at *p*H 6 to 9, but quickly inactivated outside this range. Factor X is not used up in the process of coagulation (i.e., it is found in both plasma and serum and is adsorbed by $Al(OH)_3$ and $BaSO_4$). In its activity it appears to be related to Factor VII. Although it appears that, in the presence of Ca^{++} and Factor V, it forms the final common pathway through which the products of both the extrinsic and intrinsic thromboplastin generating systems work to form the ultimate thromboplastin substances that convert prothrombin to thrombin, its specific nature and locus of activity in coagulation are not definite. That is to say, it is required for intrinsic thromboplastin formation and for prothrombin conversion, but how and where are not specifically known.

Clinically, the deficiency of Factor X is mainly seen in a hereditary disorder due to an incompletely recessive autosomal trait. Other cases of acquired deficiency are usually part of the defect in the "prothrombin complex"—that is, liver disease and vitamin K deficiency. In the laboratory, the blood in Factor X deficiency gives a long PTT and an abnormal thromboplastin generation test. The deficiency is corrected by adding small amounts of normal serum or serum from patients with a deficiency of Factor VII. Factor X or IX deficiency makes up most of the hemorrhagic complications seen in patients on anticoagulant therapy.

Factor XI (plasma thromboplastin antecedent, PTA, or Antihemophiliac Factor C) is stable at room temperature for 2 to 3 weeks; in frozen plasma it is stable for 2 years. It is a β globulin and is partially adsorbed in small amounts from plasma by $Al(OH)_3$ and $BaSO_4$. Factor XI is partly used up in clotting and is therefore present in serum. It appears to be essential to the intrinsic thromboplastin-generating system, and deficiency of the factor is probably inherited as a simple autosomal (not sex-linked) dominant that leads to a mild hemophilia-like state (hemophilia C) following trauma or surgery. In the laboratory, it is characterized by a normal plasma prothrombin time, a long PTT time, and an abnormal thromboplastin generation test. Factor XI is activated by Factor XII and is not affected by the coumarin drugs. Factor XI deficiency is corrected by normal serum, or hemophilia or Christmas disease plasma.

Factor XII (Hageman factor, contact factor, or glass factor) is contained in a stable serum euglobulin fraction precipitated from normal human plasma by acid and by dilution. It is not adsorbed from plasma by $Al(OH)_3$ or $BaSO_4$, but it is adsorbed onto powdered glass, celite, or bentonite. Factor XII is reversibly active by contact with glass and maintained in an inactive state in normal blood by the action of inhibitors. In vitro Factor XII reacts with Factor XI to form an active prothromboplastic substance. A deficiency of Factor XII does not usually produce a hemorrhagic diathesis. Laboratory coagulation studies show prolonged venous clotting time, a long PTT, and an abnormal thromboplastin generation test; the plasma prothrombin time is normal. Clinically, it is transmitted as an autosomal recessive characteristic.

During the last few years a blood coagulation mechanism more complex than the one just described has been delineated. Its prototype is the Fletcher trait, an inherited disorder of blood clotting associated with a prolonged partial thromboplastin time that becomes progressively shortened with incubation of the plasma at body temperature (37° C). It is due to prekallikrein deficiency, a plasma protein precursor of the enzyme, kallikrein, which, in turn, liberates bradykinin from its plasma precursor, kininogen. Kallikrein in time also becomes deficient. Since kallikrein is necessary for the rapid activation of Factor XII, coagulation subsequently becomes slowed. The PTT becomes normal after prolonged incubation of Fletcher trait plasma; this can be elucidated by the slow activation of Factor XII, which occurs even with kallikrein. With the elaboration of this concept, the blood coagulation system mechanism and the kinin-generating plasma system relationships are now reorganized. The Fletcher trait, like Factor XII deficiency, is not associated with a significant bleeding entity, despite the obvious abnormalities of the coagulation mechanism seen in patients with Fletcher trait. The Fletcher trait can be compared to similar entities such as the Flauyeac, Williams, and Fitzgerald traits. These three traits appear to be due to a reduction in one or more of the several forms of plasma kininogen. They have no known enzymatic activity, and their part in the mechanism of coagulation has not been elucidated.

Factor XIII (fibrin stabilizing factor, or FSF or Laki-Lorand factor) is a plasma globulin, activated by thrombin, that participates in clot formation. The function of this factor is to strengthen the clot network; it is closely related to the fibrinogen group. The acquired deficiency is associated with liver disease and fibrinolysis. Chemically Factor XIII is insoluble in urea solution. It acts like an enzyme in that it adds to the loose hydrogen bonds between the polypeptide chains and the much more solid disulfide bridges. Deficiency of Factor XIII produces a severe hemorrhagic disorder with insufficient scar formation. Even minor injuries in these patients produce a very large and extremely thin cicatrix. Losowsky and colleagues have reported three unrelated cases of a congenital deficiency of fibrin-stabilizing factor (FSF) in which the initial presentation was severe bleeding from the umbilical cord during the first days of life.[24] An occasional minor wound, soft tissue, and intracranial bleeding may result. Differentiation from hemophilia is important. Laboratory tests are all normal except the polymerization and formation of a stable fibrin.[2, 10] Estimation of FSF by simple dilution or by an assay method has demonstrated minor abnormalities in apparently unaffected relatives in congenital cases.

A recapitulation of the preceding discussion concerning the characteristics of the factors associated with coagulation is given in Table 10–2, in order to facilitate identification of isolates.

Table 10-2.

Factors Adsorbed by Alumina	Factors Remaining in Plasma after Adsorption
Prothrombin (II)	Fibrinogen (I)
Factor VII	Factor V
Christmas factor (IX)	AHG (VIII)
Factor X	PTA (XI)
	Hageman factor (XII)

Factors Present in Serum

Factor VII
Christmas factor (IX)
Factor X
PTA (XI)
Hageman factor (XII)

Inhibition of Coagulation

Natural Inhibitors. Each step in the process of coagulation probably has its own inhibitor, which controls but does not block the reaction. In this way the uncontrolled spread of thrombus formation is prevented. The term *circulating anticoagulant* is reserved for substances that actively prevent a particular reaction and may give rise to serious hemorrhagic complications. An example of this is antithromboplastin—a lipid inhibitor normally present in the blood—which retards the formation of plasma thromboplastin (intrinsic system) or neutralizes plasma thromboplastin after it is formed. It accomplishes this by binding Factor VIII and probably also Factor IX, making them unavailable for thromboplastin generation. Dissociation of antithromboplastin occurs when platelet Factor III is made available by platelet lysis or by simple dilution of plasma.

Some investigators believe that hemophilia A, hemophilia B, and hemophilia C are caused by an increased amount of antithromboplastic activity, which probably excessively inhibits Factor VIII. This antithromboplastic activity is developed after many transfusions and produces a refractory state in hemophilia from which there is no response to further transfusions. This state is due to the development of an anticoagulant found in the globulin fraction of blood that possibly acts as an antibody against Factor VIII. This anticoagulant is demonstrable by a positive precipitin test in vitro and by the thromboplastin generation test, in which it acts as an antithromboplastin.

Other natural inhibitors occur in women during or following pregnancy. This may be a form of autosensitization and is characterized by a prolonged coagulation time, possibly owing to a fetal-maternal immunization by placental fragments with resultant action against Factor VIII. Excessive antithromboplastic activity is also seen following exposure to ionizing radiation. In connection with certain systemic disease, chiefly those involving alteration in plasma proteins (collagen diseases such as lupus erythematosus, leukemia, neoplasia, cirrhosis, and pemphigus), abnormal globulin may form. This globulin is thought to chelate with some of the normal clotting factors, such as Factor V, to interfere with the conversion of fibrinogen to fibrin and to tie up calcium, causing a functional hypocalcemia. Platelet antibodies (lysins and agglutinins) may cause thrombocytopenic purpura; circulating fibrinolysins may also act as an anticoagulant by lysis of fibrin or of circulating fibrinogen.

The detection and determination of the mode of action of circulating anticoagulant are carried out in the following ways. If normal plasma does not readily correct the clotting defect encountered on the routine testing of the plasma, an inhibitor is indicated rather than a double defect. A circulating inhibitor of coagulation is also suspected if both the adsorbed plasma and serum yield abnormal thromboplastin generation when other reagents in the thromboplastin generation test (platelets and substrate plasma) are normal. This test is very helpful in determining the site of action of an antithromboplastic agent (Phase I). The prothrombin and thrombin times are useful in the analysis of anticoagulant activity in Phase II and III respectively.

Basically, one can suspect anticoagulant action if a small volume of plasma containing inhibitor, when added to normal plasma, causes it to react abnormally. Normally, a small quantity of normal plasma will correct the abnormal clotting test of a factor-deficient plasma, except in fibrinogen deficiency (Factor I), in which equal parts of normal and test plasma may be required to correct a prolonged clotting time.

Inhibitors in Anticoagulant Therapy. Heparin is an inhibitor used in anticoagulant therapy. It prolongs the one-stage prothrombin time irregularly and the whole blood coagulation time regularly. Clotting defects from an excess of heparin are abolished by the addition of small amounts of protamine sulfate or toluidine blue. Dextran, polyvinylpyrrolidone (PVP), and ethylenediaminetetraacetic acid (EDTA) are also inhibitors used in anticoagulant therapy. The hemostatic defect caused by dextran manifests itself by a prolonged bleeding time, presumably resulting from physical adsorption of the large molecule on the platelets and thereby interfering with their function. The delaying effect of EDTA on coagulation is due not only to its chelating action on calcium, but also to its effect on Factor I. The anticoagulant action of PVP appears to be somewhat related to the damage to both endothelium and megakaryocytes and to agglutination of platelets with resulting thrombocytopenia.

Diagnosis of Coagulation Disorders. Hemorrhagic states can be detected or excluded by a complete patient and family history supplemented by certain specific laboratory

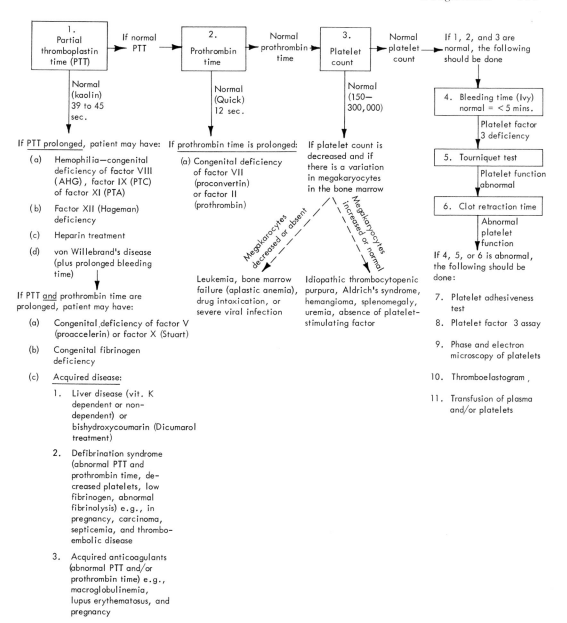

Fig. 10-21. Diagnosis of coagulation disorders. (Lynch, M. J., et al.: Medical Laboratory Technology. Philadelphia, W. B. Saunders, 1963)

procedures. Examinations include: one-stage partial thromboplastin time (PTT), one-stage prothrombin time, direct platelet count, Ivy bleeding time, Rumpel-Leede tourniquet test, and clot retraction time (Fig. 10-21).

The most important single screening test is the detailed history, which when positive, and especially if excessive bleeding has occurred more than once, is diagnostic of a coagulation disorder. The history must include questions concerning blood loss after circumcision, tonsillectomy, adenoidectomy, appendectomy, tooth extraction, or loss of deciduous teeth, as well as gross bleeding or hematoma after injury or operation. It must also include a drug history (e.g., aspirin ingestion 10 days before bleeding episodes) or surgery. Blood loss that requires transfusion or the development of hematoma that persists 12 to 24 hours after any of these procedures is presumptive evidence of a coagulation disorder. A lack of bleeding after major surgery with hemorrhagic complications after minor injury is also significant. Recurrent epistaxis and abnormal menstrual flow should be investigated.

Special commercially prepared PTT kits are available; utilizing these, this test can be performed accurately with minimal training. For all practical purposes, an isolated abnormality in PTT, with an associated normal prothrombin time, is diagnostic of hemophilia. However, the procedure must be carefully performed with an adequate number of controls and replicate determinations. Platelet abnormalities are not disclosed by the PTT or the one-stage prothrombin time. Any deviation of the prothrombin time, however, suggests an abnormality of the prothrombin complex, exact identification of which requires specific assay. Variations from the norm in both PTT and prothrombin time suggest Factor X or Factor V deficiency.

The absence of clot formation or an excessively friable one, indicates hypofibrinogenemia or afibrinogenemia.

An accurate platelet count is essential in investigation of hemostasis—for example, by phase-contrast microscopy or electronic counting. Prolonged bleeding time is usually associated with low platelet count, but it does not in itself indicate a vascular abnormality. Defects in cutaneous hemostasis are related to platelet dysfunction or deficiencies in plasma factors affecting cutaneous bleeding. Usually the tourniquet test is superfluous, especially if the platelet count or bleeding time is abnormal. However, this procedure may be the only sign of a coagulation disorder. If the test is positive, further investigation is indicated even when coagulation dysfunction is evident. Clot retraction is also important to the assessment of platelet function in patients with histories of bleeding and normal platelet counts. Because the Lee-White clotting time test does not accurately detect coagulation dysfunction, it is usually valueless as a screening test. However, Quick does not agree with this statement.[28] He believes that the use of a clean 13 mm. silicone-coated test tube, clean venipuncture, disposable syringes and needles, and use of the original Lee-White technique gives excellent reproducible results.

Many laboratories have suggested panels or profiles, associated with and accompanied by a thorough history of the patient and the patient's family, as one approach to the solution of coagulation problems or as preoperative protective measures. The following list should be of value in achieving these goals, when it is accompanied by a thorough history.

---

*Coagulation Evaluation Profiles**

Easy Bruisability Panel
  Prothrombin time
  APTT
  Platelet adhesiveness
  Platelet aggregation
  Platelet count
  Capillary fragility
  Mielke bleeding time
  Peripheral smear for % megathrombocytes
Qualitative Platelet Disorders Panel
  Platelet count
  Platelet factor 3
  Platelet adhesiveness
  Platelet aggregation
  Mielke bleeding time
  Capillary fragility
  Peripheral smear for % megathrombocytes
Preoperative Coagulation Panel
  Prothrombin time
  APTT
  Platelet Count
  Ivy bleeding time

Thrombotic Tendency Panel
  Antithrombin III activity
  Antithrombin III immunologic
  Factor VIII assay
  Protamine sulfate
  Ethanol gel
  APTT
  Thromboelastograph
Fibrinolysis Panel
  Euglobulin lysis
  Factor VIII assay
  Ethanol gel
  Protamine sulfate
  Staphylococcal clumping
  Thrombo-Wellcotest
  Plasminogen (Immunologic)
Abnormal Bleeding Panel
  Prothrombin time
  APTT
  Platelet count
  Ivy bleeding time
  Thrombin time
  Fibrinogen
  Capillary fragility
Disseminated Intravascular Coagulation Panel
  Prothrombin time
  APTT
  Platelet count
  Fibrinogen
  Thrombin time
  Staphylococcal clumping
  Thrombo-Wellcotest
  Protamine sulfate
  Ethanol gel
Von Willebrand's Panel
  Factor VIII assay
  Factor VIII related antigen Mielke (Simplate)
    bleeding time
  Platelet adhesiveness
  Platelet aggregation
  Platelet count
  APTT
Platelet Antibody Panel
  Clot retraction inhibition
  Platelet agglutination
  Platelet isoantibody screen

---

* Laboratory Bulletin. Memorial Hospital, Muncie, Indiana.

REFERENCES

1. Baldine, M., Costen, N., and Dameshek, W.: The viability of stored human platelets. Blood, *16:*1669, 1960.
2. Beck, E., Duchert, F., and Ernst, M.: The influence of fibrin stabilizing factor on the growth of fi-broblasts in vitro and wound healing. Thromb. Diath. Haemorrh., *6:*485, 1961.
3. Bizzozero, J.: Ueber einem neuen Formbestandtheil des Blutes und dessen Rolle bein der Thrombose und der Blutgerinnung. Arch. Pathol. Anat., *90:*261, 1882.
4. Bowie, E. J. W., Thompson, J. H., and Owen, C. A., Jr.: The blood platelet (including a discussion of the qualitative platelet diseases). Mayo Clin. Proc., *40:*625, 1965.
5. Breckenridge, R. T., and Ratnoff, O. D.: The role of proaccelerin in human blood coagulation. Evidence that proaccelerin is converted to a prothrombin-converting principle by activated Stuart factor. J. Clin. Invest., *44:*302, 1965.
6. Brinkhous, K. M.: Hemophilia-pathophysiologic studies and the evolution of transfusion therapy. Am. J. Clin. Pathol., *41:*342, 1964.
7. Bull, B. S., Schneiderman, M. A., and Brecher, G.: Platelet counts with the Coulter electronic particle counter. Am. J. Clin. Pathol., *44:*678, 1965.
8. Davie, E. W., and Ratnoff, O. D.: A waterfall sequence for intrinsic blood clotting. Science, *145:*1310, 1964.
9. Donne, A.: De L'origine des globules du sang, de leur mode de formation et de leur fin. Acad. Des. Sc., *14:*366, 1842.
10. Duchert, F., Jung, E., and Shmerling, D.: A hitherto undescribed congenital hemorrhagic diathesis probably due to fibrin stabilizing factor deficiency. Thromb. Diath. Haemorrh., *5:*179, 1960.
11. Eichelberger, J. W., Jr.: Laboratory Methods in Blood Coagulation. pp. 10, 11. New York, Hoeber Medical Division (Harper & Row), 1965.
12. Feissly, R., and Ludin, H.: Microscopie par contrastes de phases. Rev. Hémat., *4:*481, 1949.
13. Fidlar, E., and Waters, E. T.: The origin of platelets: their behavior in the heart-lung preparation. J. Exp. Med., *73:*299, 1941.
14. Finch, C. A.: Thrombokinetics. *In* Johnson, S. A., Monte, R. W., Rebuck, J. W., and Horn, R. C., Jr.: Blood Platelets. pp. 629–633. Boston, Little, Brown & Co., 1961.
15. Gaston, L. W.: The blood clotting factors. New Engl. J. Med., *270:*236, 1964.
16. Gerarde, H. W.: The Unopette system in the clinical laboratory. Microchem. J., *9:*340, 1965.
17. Haverback, B. J., Dutcher, T. F., Shore, P. A., Tomick, E. G., Terry, L. L., and Brodie, B. B.: Serotonin changes in platelets and brain induced by small daily doses of reserpine. New Engl. J. Med., *256:*343, 1957.
18. Jaffe, E. A.: Endothelial cells and the biology of Factor VIII. N. Engl. J. Med., *296:*377, 1977.
19. Jenevein, J. E. P., and Weiss, D. L.: Platelet microemboli associated with massive blood transfusion. Am. J. Pathol., *45:*313, 1964.
20. Kim, W. M., et al.: Hyperlipidemia, hypercoagulability and accelerated thrombosis: Studies in congenitally hyperlipidemic rats and in rats and monkeys with induced hyperlipidemia. Blood, *47:*275, 1976.
21. Krivit, W., and White, J. G.: A simplified ap-

proach for the detection of coagulation disorders. Lancet, *85:*381, 1965.

22. Kwaan, H. C.: Thrombolytic therapy. Presented at the Education Program of the American Society of Hematology. San Diego, Dec. 3-4, 1977.

23. Linman, J. W.: Factors controlling hemopoiesis: thrombopoietic and leukopoietic effects of "anemic" plasma. J. Lab. Clin. Med., *59:*262, 1962.

24. Losowsky, M. S., Hall, R., and Goldie, W.: Congenital deficiency of fibrin-stabilizing factor: report of three unrelated cases. Lancet, *2:*156, 1965.

25. Lynch, M. J., Raphael, S. S., Mellor, L. D., Spare, P. D., Hills, P., and Inwood, M. J. H.: Medical Laboratory Technology. p. 350. Philadelphia, W. B. Saunders, 1963.

26. MacFarlane, R. G.: An enzyme cascade in the blood clotting mechanism and its function as a biochemical amplifier. Nature, *202:*498, 1964.

27. Mustard, J. F., Murphy, E. A., Robinson, G. A., Rowsell, H. C., Osge, A., and Crookston, J. H.: Blood platelet survival. Thromb. Diath. Haemorrh., *13* (suppl.)*:*245, 1964.

28. Quick, A. J.: Detection and diagnosis of hemorrhagic states. J.A.M.A., *197:*418, 1966.

29. Slack, J., Seymour, J., McDonald, L., and Love, F.: Lipoprotein-lipase levels and platelet stickiness in patients with ischemic heart disease and in controls, distinguishing those with affected first-degree relative. Lancet, *2:*1033, 1964.

30. Spector, B.: In vivo transfer of a thrombopoietic factor. Proc. Soc. Exp. Biol. Med., *108:*146, 1961.

31. Thiëry, J. P., and Bessis, M.: Mécanisme de la plaquettogénese: étude "in vitro" par la microcinematographie. Rev. Hémat., *11:*162, 1956.

32. Triplett, D. A.: Blood tests proliferate with new knowledge of clotting. Laboratory Management, *15:*40, 1977.

33. Weaver, R. A., Langdell R. D., and Price, R. E.: Antihemophilic factor (AHF) in cross-circulated normal and hemophilic dogs. Am. J. Physiol., *206:*335, 1965.

34. Wintrobe, M. M.: Clinical Hematology. ed. 7, p. 1121. Philadelphia, Lea & Febiger, 1974.

35. Wright, J. H.: The histogenesis of the blood platelets. J. Morphol., *21:*263, 1910.

AUDIOVISUAL AIDS*

Hemostasis: Part I. Laboratory Aspects. Part II. Clinical Aspects. [seminars, slides, and audiotape]. ASMT Education and Research Fund, Inc. 5555 West Loop South, Bellaire, Texas, 77401.

Hemostasis and You. (1976). [35 mm. transparencies, audiotape]. General Diagnostics, Division of Warner-Lambert Company, Morris Plains, New Jersey 07950.

Introduction to Diagnostic Coagulation. 24705. Harry M. Williams. [18 35 mm. transparencies plus handout, 5 pages, and standard audiocassette, $37.60]. Communications in Learning, Inc., 2929 Main Street, Buffalo, New York 14214.

Normal and Abnormal Platelets. E. R. Squibb Film Library, c/o Hammill Studio, 9510 Belmont Avenue, Franklin Park, Illinois 60131.

Ortho Coagulation Seminar Slides. Ortho Pharmaceutical Corporation, Film Division, Raritan, New Jersey 08869.

Platelet Agglutination and Petechial Formation. Boston University, Biology Department, 765 Commonwealth Avenue, Boston, Massachusetts 02159.

_____

* Films unless otherwise stated.

Color Plates   38–55

Plate 38

ACQUIRED HEMOLYTIC ANEMIA
Peripheral Blood No. 2

Diagnostic Features: 1. Spirilla within RBCs in a case of Bartonella fever. This is an acute infectious disease caused by the spirillum of *Bartonella bacilliformis;* it is associated with fever, macrocytic anemia, anisocytosis, poikilocytosis, reticulocytosis, normoblastosis, and leukocytosis. Parasitized RBCs form part of a hemolytic process found to a great extent in the liver and spleen.

2. A case of lead poisoning (plumbism). The lead is stored in the bones, in the marrow, and in RBCs with basophilic stippling. Increased coproporphyrin is demonstrated in the urine, with a diffuse hemolytic erythrocytic process.

3. Malaria is caused by four types of Plasmodia, with variation of the cycle in the RBCs of man. Paroxysms of hemolysis of parasitized RBCs lead to a variegated type of anemia with associated splenomegaly. Diagnosis is made by utilizing thin and thick smears. *Plasmodium falciparum* produces a more severe type of hemolysis involving brain, liver and kidney (blackwater fever). Parasites as ring forms (R) are frequently observed at the periphery of RBCs, frequently with multiple infestation (DR); the gametocyte form (Gam) is crescent-shaped and has a characteristic pattern.

4. The ascorbate screening test for G-6-PD is one of the many tests used to detect an erythrocytic deficiency in glucose-6-phosphate dehydrogenase; RBCs with this deficiency are more susceptible to hemolysis by various drugs (anti-malarials, sulfa drugs, analgesics, antipyretics and nitrofurans). Younger RBCs contain more G-6-PD than older RBCs and are therefore more resistant to hemolysis. G-6-PD deficiency is more common in darkly pigmented racial and ethnic groups; patients with this deficiency are resistant to malaria infestation. Lighter colored suspension (bright red) is from normal patient; the darker suspension (brown) is characteristic of G-6-PD deficiency.

5. Spot test for G-6-PD deficiency (Fairbanks and Beutler) is depicted in three panels, i.e., the upper panel shows the patient's sedimented RBCs, the middle panel demonstrates the elution of hemoglobin in distilled water, and the lower panel reveals little or no color in erythrocytes of G-6-PD deficient patients.

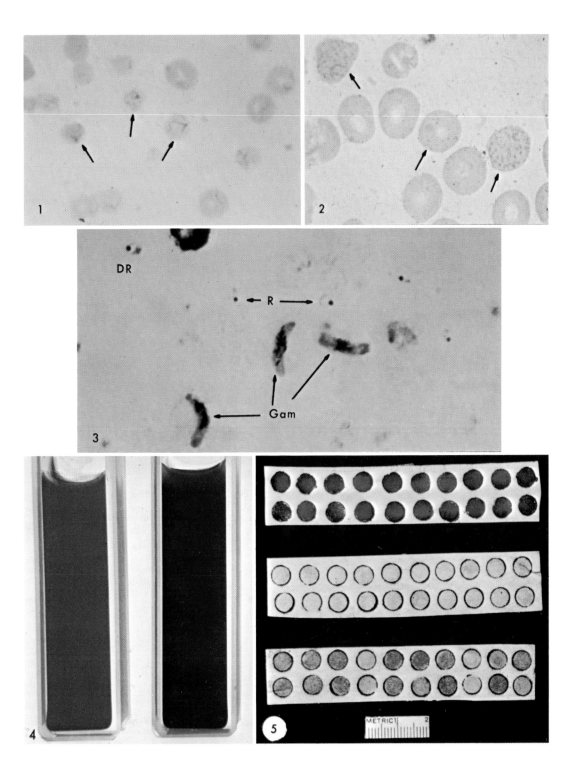

Plate 39

ACQUIRED HEMOLYTIC ANEMIA
Bone Marrow

Juvenile (Juv), lymphocyte (L), monocyte (M), megakaryocyte (Mgk), metamyelocyte (mMc), myeloblast (Myb), neutrophilic myelocyte (NMc), orthochromic normoblast (ONb), polychromatophilic normoblast (PNb), platelet (Pl), prolymphocyte (prL), promyelocyte (prMc), pronormoblast (prNb), stem cell (SC).

Diagnostic Features: Hypercellular marrow with orderly normoblastic erythroid hyperplasia, i.e., approximately 60% (normal is 20%) nucleated RBCs are seen; therefore instead of a normal M:E ratio of 4 or 5:1, the ratio is 1:1 or less. These normoblasts do not usually have the nuclear chromatin scroll work pattern of P.A. and related macrocytic anemias. These are also numerous mitoses. The leukocytic pattern reveals a slight shift to the left of the myelocytic series (myelocytes, metamyelocytes, etc.). Marrow iron content is frequently increased and are visible as bluish particles when Prussian blue stain is used. Other laboratory findings are noted under peripheral blood pattern, e.g. Coombs test, Donath-Landsteiner test for cold hemolysins, serum and urine bilirubin, urine urobilinogen, Cr^{51} RBC survival, serum Fe, etc.

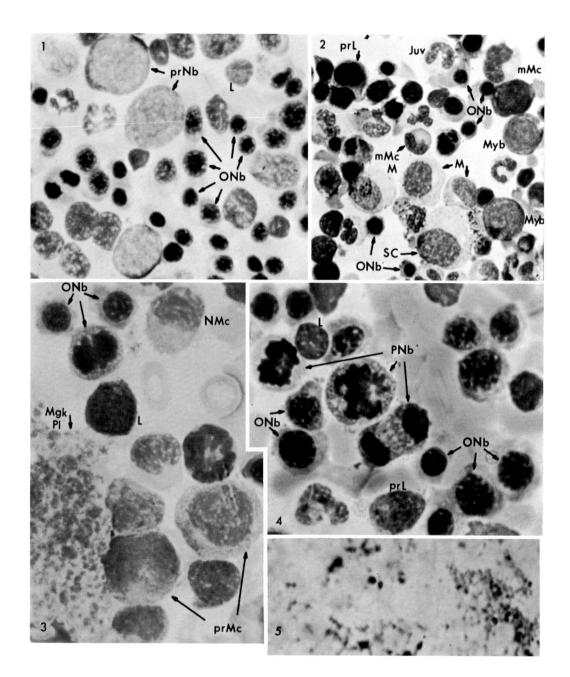

Plate 40

IDIOPATHIC THROMBOCYTOPENIC PURPURA (ITP)
Peripheral Blood

1. Atypical lymphocyte (L). 2. Lymphocyte (L), juvenile (Juv). 3. Deeply stained, bizarre-shaped platelet (Pl). 4. Giant platelet, deeply stained (Pl).

Diagnostic Features: The most noticeable characteristic is the marked reduction in the number of thrombocytes (platelets) and the morphologic changes in those platelets which are present, i.e., giant forms, very small forms, bizarre and deeply stained forms; occasionally, portions of megakaryocytes are seen. The RBCs are usually normocytic; however, if blood loss is long, severe and continuous, a hypochromic microcytic anemia may be present. If blood loss is acute, severe and recent, reticulocytosis, normoblastosis and macrocytosis may be present. The WBC count is usually normal with or without a slight to moderate increase in the number of eosinophils. If the patient has had long-standing bleeding, a slight leukopenia and lymphocytosis may occur with atypical lymphocytes occasionally present; if bleeding is severe, a slight leukocytosis with shift to the left occurs. Also present are prolonged bleeding time, impaired clot retraction, positive capillary fragility test, a shortened serum prothrombin time, elevated serum acid phosphatase and presence of platelet agglutinins on occasions.

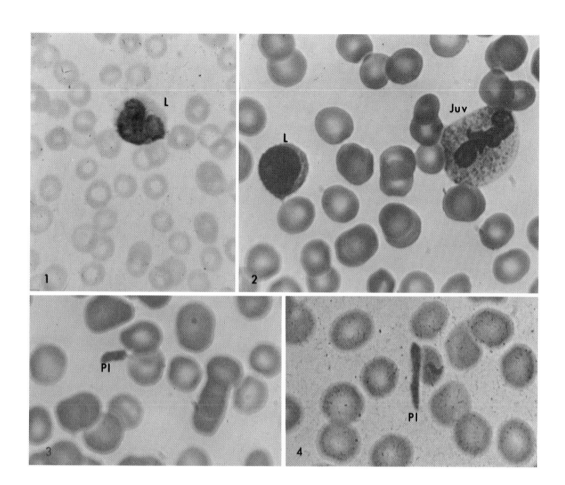

Plate 41

IDIOPATHIC THROMBOCYTOPENIC PURPURA (ITP)
Bone Marrow

Basophilic normoblast (BNb), megakaryoblast (Mgb), megakaryocytes (Mgk), orthochromic normoblast (ONb), polymorphonuclear eosinophil (PmE), vacuole (Vac).

Diagnostic Features: Morphologically, the abnormal marrow findings are limited to reduction in the number of visible platelets separate from or related to megakaryocytes and their progenitors. Megakaryoblasts are seen with single nuclei (Fig. 1) with relatively little or only moderately abundant cytoplasm and few granules; small rounded megakaryocytes (Fig. 1) are characteristic. Also observed are very large megakaryocytes with sharply demarcated borders, with or without nonlobulated nuclei, many vacuoles, few cytoplasmic granules with few to no platelets being formed or pinched off from the cytoplasm. Normoblastic hyperplasia is usually seen, associated with acute severe hemorrhagic episodes; marrow eosinophilia may also be observed.

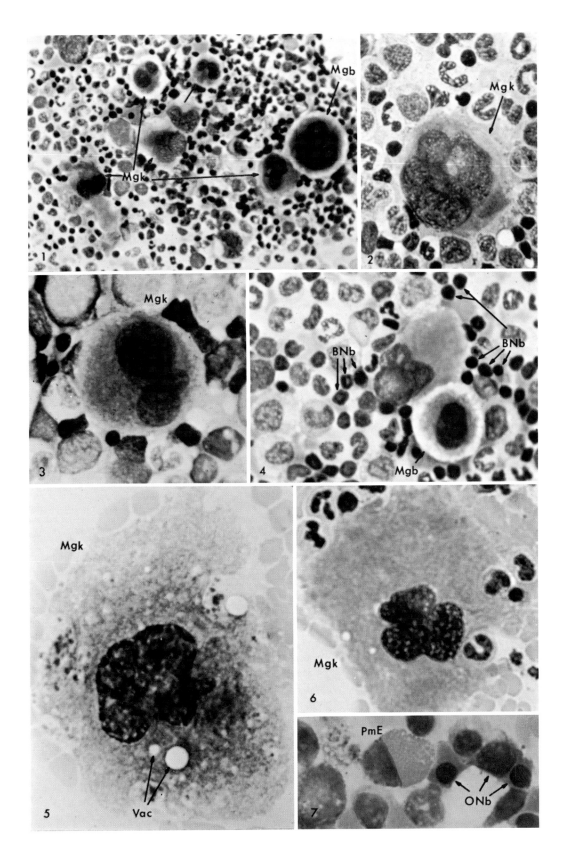

Plate 42

LEUKOCYTIC CYTOLOGIC ABERRATIONS
Diagnostic Features

1, 2, 3, 4, & 9. Chediak-Higashi anomaly. These are atypical cytoplasmic inclusion bodies found in all types of leukocytes. With Wright's stain one observes three to six irregular bluish-green masses; in mononuclear cells they stain bluish-purple (? chromatin); large granules are found in eosinophils.

5 & 6. Döhle-Amato bodies (also called May-Hegglin bodies) represent RNA and most likely reflect an abnormality in cytoplasmic maturation (round to oval inclusions bluish-green in color).

7. Irritation lymphocytes (Türk cells) are hyperchromatic lymphocytes with plasma-cytoid features seen in many infections.

8. Phagocytic histiocyte with engulfed RBC seen in familial lymphohistiocytosis, etc.

10. Endothelial cell with multiple nuclei seen after blood film is made with venipuncture blood.

11. Pelger-Huet anomaly represents a defect in nuclear segmentation of granulocytes. It is most noticeable in neutrophils with band, rod-like or bilobed nuclei. Nuclear chromatin is coarsely clumped. It is inherited as a simple dominant or associated with myxedema, leukemia, etc.

12. L. E. (lupus erythematosus) cells seen most commonly in systemic lupus erythematosus and are most frequently neutrophils that contain a homogeneous structureless inclusion body consisting of nucleoprotein (from lymphocyte nuclei) altered by the L. E. factor (an antinuclear antibody or a gamma globulin) The latter depolymerizes DNA or combines with it and the inclusion body formed is then engulfed by a neutrophil or forms a rosette (an extracellular mass of altered nuclear material surrounded by a group of PmNs). Must be differentiated from nucleophagocytosis by monocytes—the latter consists of nuclear material with a structural pattern and a condensed peripheral chromatin ring.

13. Gaucher cells are atypical histiocytes loaded with cerebrosides (foam cells) found in the bone marrow, liver and spleen of patients with the disease.

14. Clover-leaf nucleus of monocyte caused by prolonged immersion of cells in an oxalate anticoagulant.

15. Virocytes are atypical lymphocytes containing vacuoles and irregular nuclear-cytoplasmic shapes seen in various viral disorders.

16. Leishman-Donovan bodies seen in monocytes of liver, spleen and bone marrow of patients with Kala-azar.

17. Giant neutrophils composed of six to ten lobed PmNs observed as an inherited anomaly.

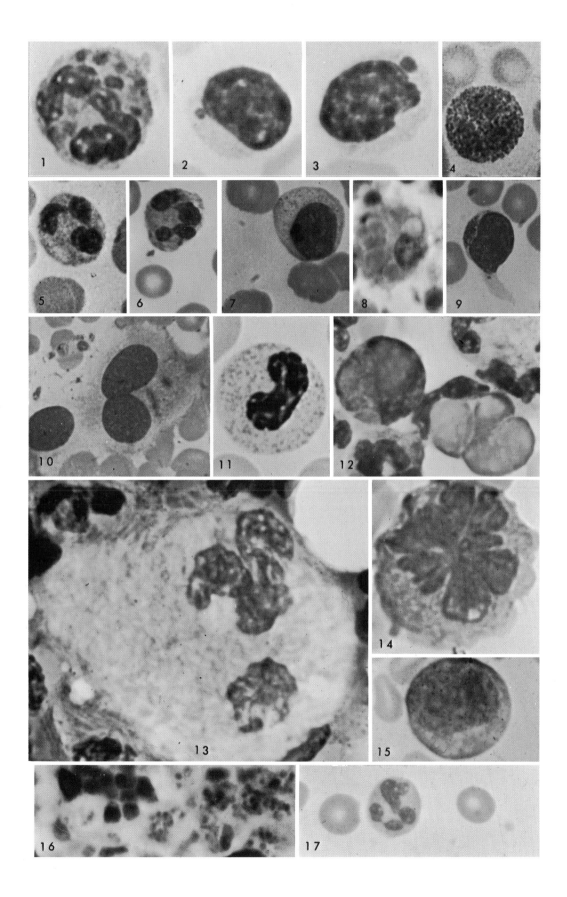

Plate 43

ERYTHROCYTIC AND LEUKOCYTIC CYTOLOGIC PATTERNS
Diagnostic Features

1. Vacuolation in cytoplasm of myelocyte in alcoholic patient. There is depressed bone marrow function (vacuolation of normoblasts and myelocytes, hypoplasia of bone marrow, and thrombocytopenia).

2. Amyloid deposits in bone marrow interstitium characterized by pink-staining homogeneous deposits that take a yellowish-green dichromic birefringence. Other bone marrow and electrophoretic studies are necessary to exclude primary amyloidosis and those secondary to plasma cell dyscrasias (e.g. myeloma, etc.) and chronic diseases (tuberculosis, osteomyelitis, and Hodgkin's disease; (Amy = amyloid).

3. T-cell lymphocyte with sheep RBC rosette formation. These lymphocytes are thymust-dependent, participate in cellular immunity, and compose the majority of lymphocytes in the immediate subcapsular and mantle zone surrounding lymphoid follicles in lymph nodes, as well as in the periarteriolar lymphatic sheaths (white pulp) of the spleen. They form the largest percentage of blood and thoracic-duct lymphocytes, where they are found as long-lived recirculating lymphocytes (TLR = T-lymphocyte rosette).

4, 5, 6. Myelokathexis (chronic idiopathic granulocytopenia) is characterized by the presence of polys with cytoplasmic vacuoles, abnormal nuclei consisting of excessive thinness of filaments connecting the lobes, and chromatin clumping. Bone marrow is hyperplastic with associated hypersegmented and degenerated myeloid forms. There is no response to splenectomy. (TF = thin filament; CC = chromatin clumping; Hyps = hypersegmentation of myeloid forms).

7. Stomatocytes are RBCs with a slot like central pallor giving the surrounding dense area the appearance of a mouth. They are characteristic of a rare hemolytic anemia with associated marked increase in permeability of membrane to sodium and have been described in association with liver disease. When they are examined under a phase-contrast microscope, they are dome-shaped RBCs (St = stomatocyte).

8. Platelet satellitosis is a phenomenon characterized by adherence of platelets (5 to 20) to polys. Its cause is unknown, and it is not related to any specific clinical condition, functional abnormality of the blood, or drugs. All reported cases have been discovered on smears made from EDTA-treated blood. It is usually not seen on smears made from fresh blood, heparin, or in treated blood. It may lead to spurious thrombocytopenia on electronic platelet counting machines. (PS = platelet satellite).

9. Sea-blue histiocyte is a large reticuloendothelial cell (20–60 μm. in diameter) with a single eccentric nucleus containing block chromatin and a single nucleolus. With Wright's stain the cytoplasm contains sea-blue or blue-green granules in varying numbers. These histiocytes also stain with Sudan Black B, other lipid stains, PAS, acid-fast stains, and show autofluorescence. Electron microscopy shows lamellae of lipid molecules. This histiocytic pattern is seen as a primary familial syndrome associated with macular abnormalities, skin manifestations, neurologic and pulmonary findings, hepatosplenomegaly, lymphadenopathy, and thrombocytopenia. The secondary type may be found in patients with ITP, chronic myelogenous leukemia, hyperlipoproteinemia, or other associated diseases (S B H = sea-blue histiocyte; $\times$970).

10, 11. Alder's granules are giant granules that stain darkly (dark blue-black) and are large azurophilic granules in neutrophils in association with other hereditary defects such as gargoylism. This phenomenon is also part of a general metabolic disorder of polysaccharides. The defect may be completely expressed with abnormally prominent granules in granulocytes, monocytes, and lymphocytes or incompletely manifest with only one leukocyte affected. (GAC = giant Alder granules; GG = giant granules; $\times$970).

12. Niemann-Pick cell is a 20 to 100 μm. round, oval, or polyhedral cell found in the bone marrow, whose cytoplasm is filled with clusters of small, round droplets. The nucleus is small, eccentrically placed, and usually one in number. The vacuoles have a faint bluish hue with Wright's stain. The Niemann-Pick cell is a morphologic manifestation of an inborn error of sphingolipid metabolism more commonly observed in Ashkenasic Jews, especially infants, than in other groups. It is associated with central nervous system maldevelopment, hepatosplenomegaly, and lymphadenopathy (Lip Vac = lipid vacuoles; $\times$970).

13. Cold agglutinin disease. Microagglutination of RBCs is first discovered in the counting chamber; it is confirmed by dissolution of clumps upon warming. Cold agglutinin disease is frequently associated with mycoplasma pneumoniae infection and, in some malignancies, with most cold reactive antibodies having specificity for the I-i antigens (MC = micro clumps; $\times$970).

14, 15. Thrombotic thrombocytopenic purpura is associated with disseminated intravascular coagulation (DIC). Peripheral blood shows thrombocytopenia, schistocytes, and nucleated RBCs. Bone marrow shows fibrin thrombus in blood vessel lumen (Sch = schistocyte; Nuc RBC = nucleated RBC; Fib T = fibrin thrombus; VW = vessel wall; $\times$970).

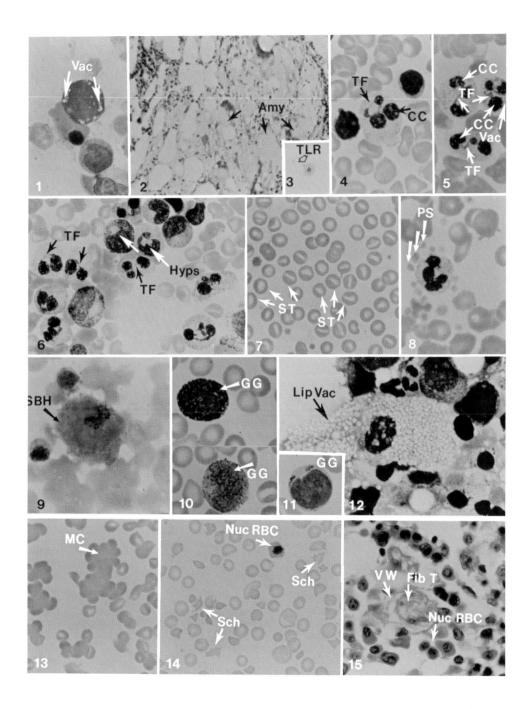

Plate 44

CHEDIAK-HIGASHI SYNDROME
Peripheral Blood

1. Polymorphonuclear neutrophil (PmN) with inclusions. 2. Lymphocyte with inclusion.

Bone Marrow

3. Myelocyte (Mc) with vacuoles (vac.) 4 & 5. Inclusions in a promyelocytes (pMc) and juvenile (Juv).

Diagnostic Features: A familial anomaly of cytoplasmic granulation in various cells of the leukocyte series characterized by anemia, neutropenia with relative lymphocytosis and thrombocytopenia of the peripheral blood in which the neutrophils and lymphocytes show peripherally located pleomorphic inclusions greenish-gray to reddish-orange purple in color resembling toxic granules. Bone marrow cells show anomalous granulation with orange reddish-purple ovoid bodies frequently surrounded by a halo and situated in immature myeloid cells. Clinically there may be consanguinity of parents, albinism traits, abnormal hair and skin pigmentation, photophobia, splenomegaly, hepatomegaly, lymphadenopathy and repeated respiratory and systemic infections with death occurring in childhood.

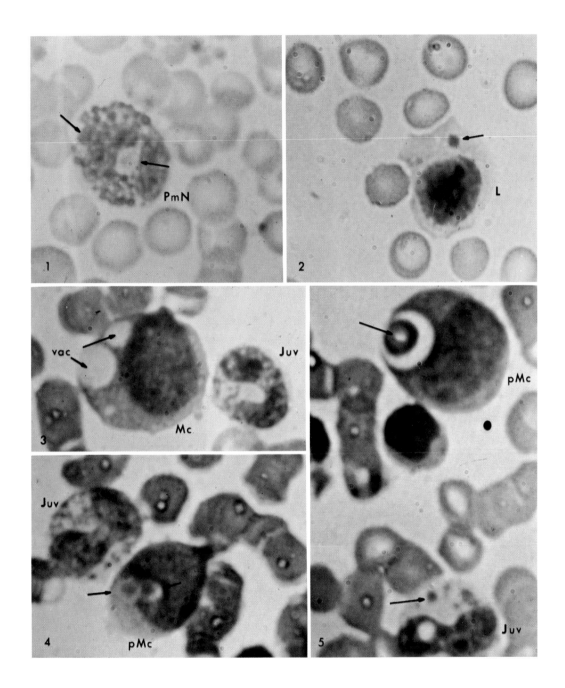

Plate 45

LEUKEMOID REACTION

1. **Infections (Pertussis, Miliary T.B., etc.)**
2. **Intoxications (Severe Burns, Eclampsia, etc.)**
3. **Malignancy with Bone Marrow Metastases (cf. Myelophthisic Anemia, Bone Marrow)**
4. **Severe Hemorrhage with Sudden Hemolysis**

Peripheral Blood

Basophilic normoblast (BNb), juvenile (Juv), lymphocyte (L), monocyte (M), neutrophilic myelocyte (NMc), polymorphonuclear neutrophil (PmN), polymorphonuclear neutrophil with toxic granules [PmN(tox)], promonocyte (prM), promyelocyte (prMc). 6. Stained with peroxidase stain.

Diagnostic Features: Leukemoid reaction is only a descriptive term; it is not a diagnosis or a disease entity. It includes any deviation in total white count, usually leukocytotic (50,000 WBC cu. mm. and above) but may be leukopenic. It signifies the presence of an abundance of mature or usually immature cells in the peripheral blood, i.e., either granulocytic, lymphocytic or monocytic. Commonly there is a shift to immature neutrophilic granulocytes (myelocytes, metamyelocytes, occasionally promyelocytes and rarely myeloblasts). In infants, normoblasts appear in increased numbers in the peripheral blood. Lymphocytic leukemoid reactions characterize such infections as pertussis, acute infectious lymphocytosis and infectious mononucleosis. Tuberculosis of the marrow evokes a monocytic reaction. The peroxidase reaction (Fig. 6) is prominent in members of the granulocytic series. The leukocytic alkaline phosphatase reaction shows high concentration in the myeloid cell series, but it is low in infectious mononucleosis, collagen diseases, pernicious anemia, refractory or hypoplastic anemia and it is usually negligible to absent in leukemic patterns.

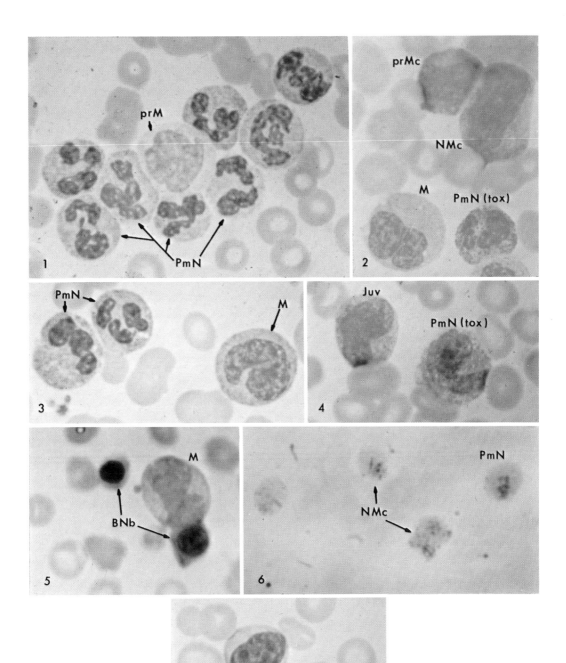

Plate 46

LEUKEMOID REACTION
1. **Infections (Pertussis, Miliary T.B., etc.)**
2. **Intoxications (Severe Burns, Eclampsia, etc.)**
3. **Malignancy with Bone Marrow Metastases (cf. Myelophthisic Anemia, Bone Marrow)**
4. **Severe Hemorrhage with Sudden Hemolysis**

Bone Marrow

Eosinophilic myelocyte (EMc), juvenile (Juv), lymphocyte (L), monocyte (M), myeloblast (Mb), neutrophilic myelocyte (NMc), neutrophilic myelocyte with vacuoles [NMc(vac)], polymorphonuclear neutrophil (PmN), promyelocyte (prMc), stem cell (SC). 5. Alkaline phosphatase stain positive reaction.

Diagnostic Features: In myelocytic leukemoid reactions, there is usually a larger proportion of mature granulocytic type cells (metamyelocytes, juveniles and PmNs); however, the quantitative marrow differential may be very similar to that observed in leukemic processes. Since all transition forms of myeloid cells are observed, there is rarely a "hiatus leukemicus." Also, alkaline phosphatase stain (Fig. 5) is positive and erythroid and megakaryocytic forms are not diminished to any great extent.

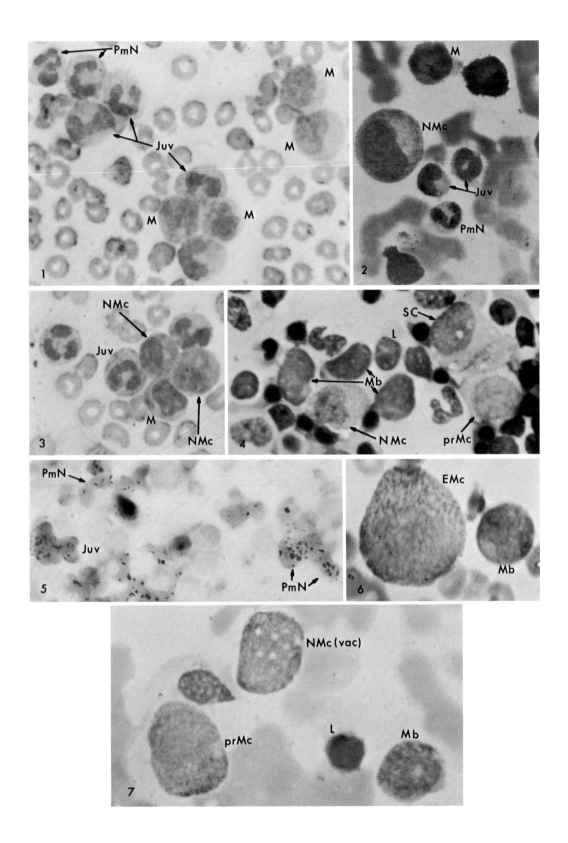

Plate 47

INFECTIOUS MONONUCLEOSIS
Peripheral Blood

Eosinophilic myelocyte (EMc), juvenile (Juv), lymphocyte (L), abnormal forms of lymphocytes [L(I), L(II), L(III)].

Diagnostic Features: A hematologic dyscrasia characterized by an increase in small lymphocytes and monocytes with the presence of characteristic large atypical (mononuclear) lymphocytes in which the eccentric nucleus is oval, kidney-shaped or slightly lobulated, and the basophilic cytoplasm is non-granular (occasionally granular) with irregular cell margins and occasionally pseudopodia-like protrusions. The cytoplasm may also be vacuolated or foamy. The nuclear chromatin forms a coarse network of strands and masses with lack of differentiation from the parachromatin. On the fourth to tenth day there is an elevation to 60 per cent or more of these forms, with occasional myelocytes and stab forms. Type II forms are larger than the usual size in type I; the nucleus is not as condensed; cytoplasm is homogeneous and non-vacuolated; Type III looks like a lymphoblast with sieve chromatin and one or two nucleoli; cytoplasm is vacuolated and basophilic. Mitoses are common and anemia is rare. The blood findings of atypical lymphocytes are observed even after one to two months. Eosinophilia is commonly seen in convalescence. The term "Rieder lymphocyte" usually signifies lymphocytes with indented buttock-shaped nuclei (Fig. 8).

Fig. 5. Downey lymphocyte (type III). Fig. 6. Atypical lymphocyte.

Fig. 9. Atypical lymphocyte type II. Fig. 10. Atypical lymphocyte type I.

Fig. 11. Convalescent picture with abnormal to normal lymphocytes.

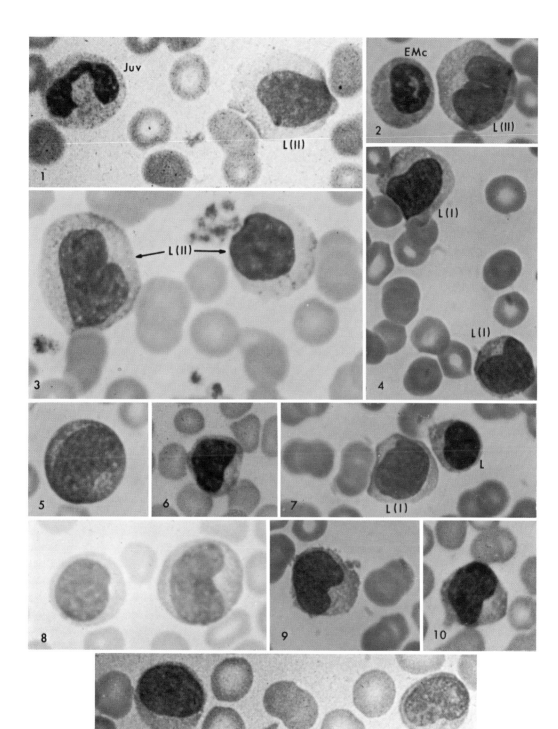

Plate 48

INFECTIOUS MONONUCLEOSIS
Bone Marrow

Abnormal lymphocyte (AbL), juvenile (Juv), lymphocyte (L), neutrophilic myelocyte (NMc), orthochromic normoblast (ONb).

Diagnostic Features: Bone marrow examination is rarely necessary in the diagnosis of this disease. There is a modest increase in the number of myelocytes (left shift); occasionally there is an increase in eosinophilic cells and the presence of reticular and leukocytoid lymphocytes; occasionally granulomata with epithelioid cells are seen. The diagnosis is based upon the clinical picture, the serial serologic reaction (heterophil antibody tube test and now the use of a very efficient slide spot and/or tube test), and a cytologic study of the blood. Acute leukemia is ruled out by the bone marrow pattern. Figs. 6 & 7. Heterophil antibody absorption test of Davidsohn. The upper line of test tubes from one patient's serum shows agglutination of sheep RBCs before absorption by guinea pig kidney antigen; in this set-up the titer is 1:224. The lower row of tubes from the same patient's serum shows agglutination of sheep RBCs after absorption by guinea pig kidney antigen; the titer in this case equals 1:112.

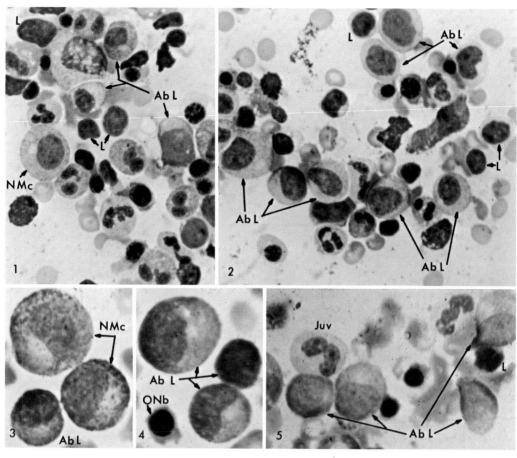

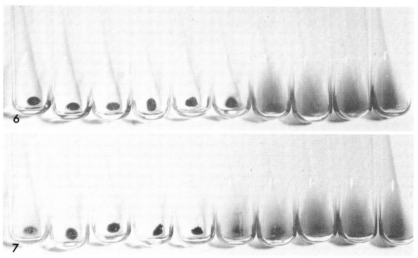

Plate 49
NEUTROPENIA
(Agranulocytosis, Agranulocytic Angina, Malignant Leukopenia)

Peripheral Blood

Lymphocyte (L), degenerating polymorphonuclear eosinophil [PmE(deg)].

Diagnostic Features: The total leukocyte count is usually less than 2,000 WBC/cu. mm.; if more than 4,000 WBC/cu. mm. are present it is usually a secondary type rather than the idiopathic variety. The differential count shows almost complete absence of polymorphonuclear neutrophils. Those which are present contain pyknotic nuclei, vacuolated cytoplasm and poorly stained granules; occasionally Türk irritation type cells are seen.

Although a majority of leukocytes present are lymphocytes, in the acute phase there is usually an absolute decrease in lymphocytes; the monocytes follow the same course as the lymphocytes. Anemia and thrombocytopenia are not present in the acute forms of agranulocytosis; in the chronic forms the hemoglobin and hematocrit may fall concomitantly. When recovery begins, monocytes and myelocytes may be seen increasingly in the peripheral blood.

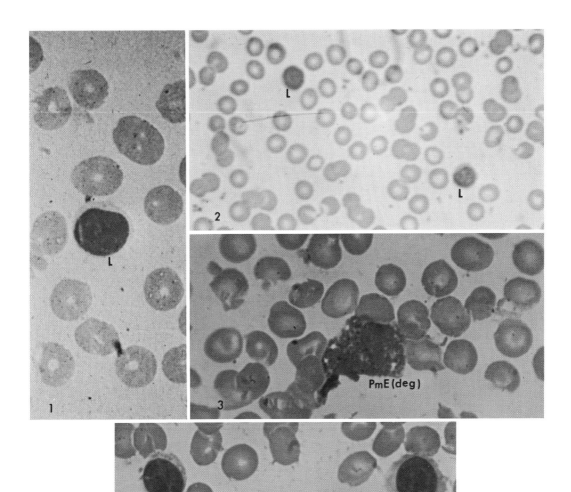

Plate 50

NEUTROPENIA
(Agranulocytosis, Agranulocytic Angina, Malignant Leukopenia)
Bone Marrow

Juvenile (Juv), lymphocyte (L), metamyelocyte (mMc), mitosis (mit), monocyte (M), neutrophilic myelocyte (NMc), orthochromic normoblast (ONb), plasma cell (PC), promyelocyte (prMc).

Diagnostic Features: The granulocytic series is reduced leading to a reduction in the M:E ratio. The myeloid cell type that predominates depends on the duration of action and potency of the offending agent. At first there is a reduction of the PMNs and a shift in the maturation curve to the more immature cell type. With continuation of toxicity the metamyelocytes gradually disappear, then the myelocytes and finally the promyelocytes. Thus the myeloid pattern present at the time of marrow examination varies with the stage and severity of the disease. In the plate (1, 2 & 3), promyelocytes (arrows) and myeloblasts and myelocytes predominate, i.e., so-called "maturation arrest" is seen with diminution to absence of PMNs, metamyelocytes and juveniles. Occasionally there is an increase in plasma cells, lymphocytes and reticulum cells. Erythroid and megakaryocytic cells are apparently normal unless prolonged and chronic toxicity is present.

When the offending agent is removed the marrow pattern gradually reverts to the more mature forms, provided the hematopoietic alterations are in a reversible state; that is, after recovery (Figs. 4 & 5) one sees increased neutrophilic granulopoiesis in the marrow.

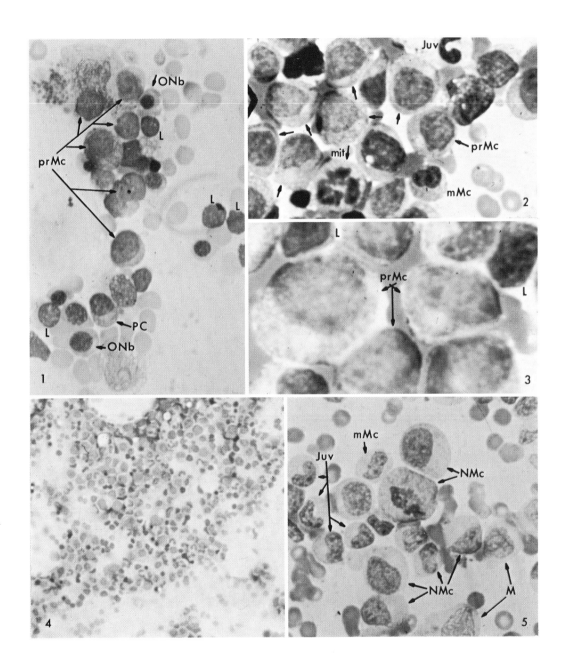

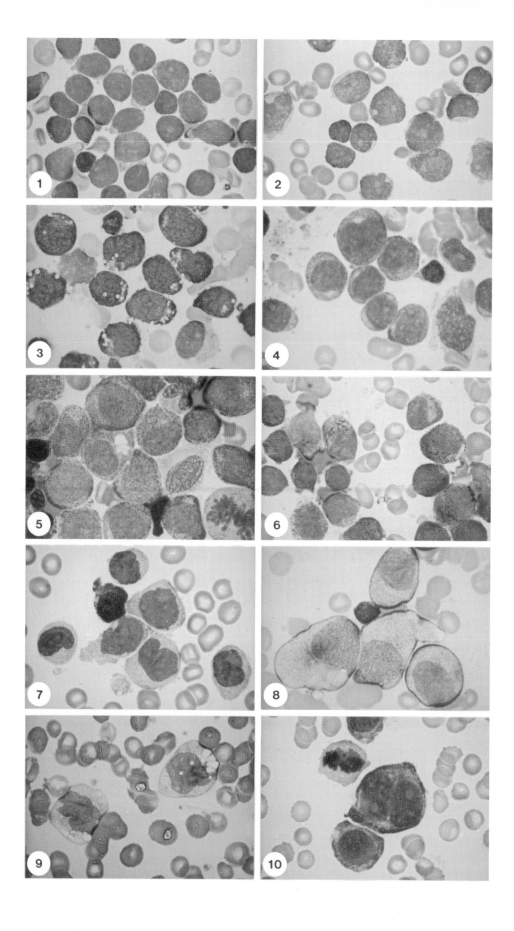

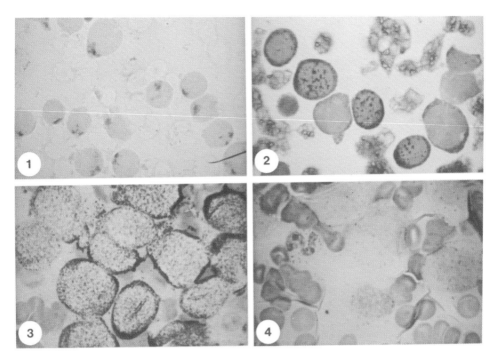

Plate 52

CYTOCHEMICAL REACTIONS IN ACUTE LEUKEMIA

1. Acid phosphatase reaction in acute leukemia. Note the accentuation of the staining reaction in the Golgi apparatus of the cells. This type of reaction is seen in T-cell leukemia. 2. Peroxidase reaction in a case of M1 (acute myeloid leukemia, undifferentiated), which did not show granules or Auer rods. The peroxidase stain is positive, and this is a useful test to separate this entity from the L2 variety of acute leukemia. 3. Naphthol-ASD acetate stain in a case of M5. Note the marked positive reaction in all the cells. 4. Sodium fluoride inhibition of the naphthol-ASD acetate stain. Note that the stain is inhibited in the presence of sodium fluoride, indicative of a monocytic component (either being M4, acute myelomonocytic leukemia or M5, undifferentiated or well-differentiated monocytic leukemia; Gralnick, H. R., et al.: Classification of acute leukemia. Ann. Intern. Med., 87:740, 1977)

←——————— **Plate 51**

MORPHOLOGIC VARIANTS OF ACUTE LEUKEMIA

1. L1: acute lymphocytic leukemia as commonly seen in childhood, homogeneous cell population. 2. L2: acute lymphocytic leukemia more commonly seen in adults, heterogeneous cell population. 3. L3: Burkitt-type cell leukemia. 4. M1: acute myeloid leukemia, without maturation. This form of leukemia must be differentiated from L2 and is done so primarily by the peroxidase stain (*see* Plate 52). 5. M2: acute myeloid leukemia with maturation. This should not be confused with M3 (*see* below); this represents some differentiation into the promyelocyte and myelocyte stages with cells predominantly being blasts and promyelocytes. 6. M3: acute hypergranular promyelocytic leukemia. 7. M4: acute myelomonocytic leukemia; it is important in this variant to recognize that monocytic component may be more predominant in the peripheral blood than it is in the bone marrow. 8. M5: acute monocytic leukemia, poorly differentiated. 9. M5: acute monocytic leukemia, well differentiated. 10. M6: erythroleukemia. (Gralnick, H. R., et al.: Classification of acute leukemia. Ann. Intern. Med., 87:740, 1977)

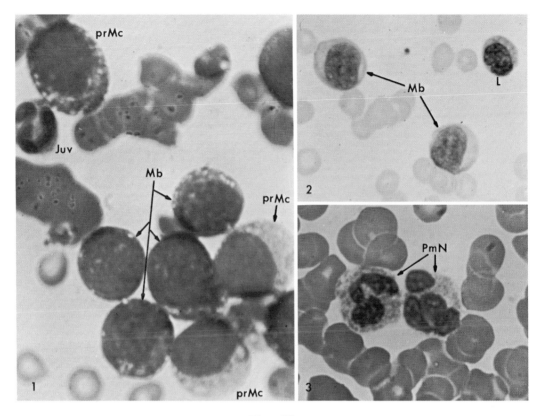

Plate 53

ACUTE GRANULOCYTIC (MYELOID, MYELOBLASTIC, MYELOCYTIC) LEUKEMIA
Peripheral Blood

Juvenile (Juv), lymphocyte (L), myeloblast (Mb), polymorphonuclear neutrophil (PmN), promyelocyte (prMc).

Diagnostic Features: From 30 to 60 per cent of nucleated cells are immature (myeloblasts and undifferentiated myelocytes). The blast cells have round to oval nuclei with fine chromatin, very little to no nuclear membrane condensation, several distinct nucleoli, a rim of blue cytoplasm with few or no granules. The presence of granules is more suggestive of the granulocytic form; however, one may see a pattern of myeloblasts and PmNs with few or no intermediate forms (leukemic hiatus). Mitotic figures may be present as well as Auer bodies (pink, red rod-shaped structures in cytoplasm of myeloblasts).

Plate 54 ⟶

ACUTE GRANULOCYTIC (MYELOID, MYELOBLASTIC, MYELOCYTIC) LEUKEMIA
Bone Marrow

Auer body (AB), juvenile (Juv), lymphoctye (L), myeloblast (Myb), neutrophilic myelocyte (NMc), promyelocyte (prMc).

Diagnostic Features: Marked increase in blast forms with myeloid maturation curve shifted far to the left and the M:E ratio greatly elevated. The smears present a monotonous cytologic uniformity with blast cells constituting 50 per cent or more of all marrow cells. The cell borders of myeloblasts are usually even and smooth, nuclei usually oval with border of basophilic cytoplasm situated to one side of cell. The nuclear membrane is smooth, even and fine with diffuse even nuclear chromatin and prominent nucleoli. Auer bodies (Fig. 1) may be seen in the cytoplasm of myeloblasts. One may see a few promyelocytes and more mature myeloid forms. With peroxidase stain (Fig. 5), granules are observed in the cytoplasm of promyelocytes and myelocytes.

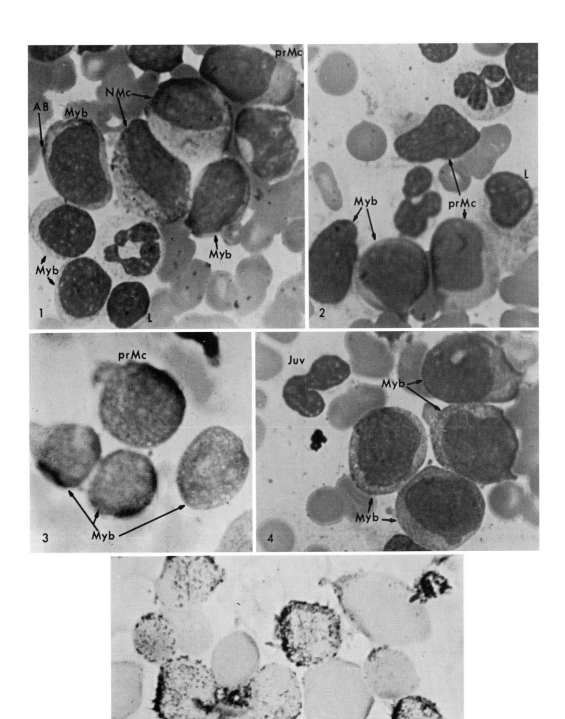

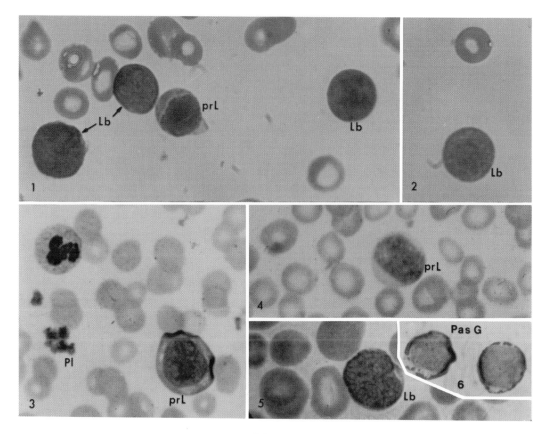

Plate 55

ACUTE LYMPHOCYTIC (LYMPHOBLASTIC) LEUKEMIA
Peripheral Blood

Lymphoblast (Lb), platelet (Pl), prolymphocyte (prL).

Diagnostic Features: This pattern is observed most frequently in children and is associated with pallor, fever, purpura, malaise, lymphadenopathy and splenomegaly. Severe normocytic and normochromic anemia (occasionally macrocytic) with associated thrombocytopenia are frequent, although these findings may be absent early in the disease. The leukocyte count may be low or very high; when the latter, almost all the cells will be lym-phoblasts (10 to 18 micra in diameter, and with an even cell border, oval nucleus, coarse nuclear membrane, mildly coarse chromatin with some condensation, one to two nucleoli, and basophilic cytoplasm without granules). The peroxidase stain is negative. These lymphoblasts are not to be confused with micromyeloblasts which are frequently peroxidase positive and contain granules in the cytoplasm.

6. PAS reaction in lymphoblasts indicates positive granules. (PAS G = PAS granules)

11 Laboratory Diagnosis of Coagulation Defects

History

It is important to follow certain principles in blood specimen collection in order to make an accurate laboratory diagnosis of coagulation defects. For example, if the patient is already hospitalized, the specimens can be obtained immediately. If the patient is to be seen on an outpatient basis, he or she may come directly to the reference laboratory in order that the specimens be drawn and processed immediately. If the patient cannot come to the reference laboratory and if the hospital laboratory cannot do the work required, certain special precautions must be taken to prevent the improper collection and coagulation of specimens. If possible, the pathologist should see the patient. The patient should be questioned about the quantity of bleeding as well as the onset, duration, and type of bleeding. It is also important to know when the bleeding occurs and if there is a family history of bleeding. In the process of history-taking, it is essential to obtain a complete list of whatever medications the patient may be taking currently, as well as of any recent illnesses. It is especially important to find out if the patient is taking aspirin or drugs containing aspirin. It is fairly widely known that aspirin interferes with platelet function and that the effects of aspirin ingestion can last up to a week after ingestion. It is requested that the patient take no aspirin or aspirin-containing drugs for a period of up to 1 week before a complete coagulation profile. It is also important to identify the patient with polycythemia. If the hematocrit is more than 70 per cent, these patients should have their blood drawn in tubes that have 15 to 20 per cent less anticoagulant than normal. These patients have a decreased plasma volume, and spurious results will be obtained unless the ratio of anticoagulant to plasma is lowered.[40]

Preparation

The importance of precaution in the preparation of materials for the laboratory diagnosis of coagulation defects and the necessity of a scrupulously clean collection technique cannot be overemphasized, because in the study of coagulation disorders good technique must be strictly followed. Cleanliness, organization, and attention to details are especially important in this phase of laboratory work because the results obtained will be only as good as the techniques and the persons performing them. For example, it is most important that venous blood be obtained whenever practicable and that all venipunctures be "clean." Any contamination of the blood by tissue juice will hasten the coagulation process, and most probably the blood sample will be clotted before it is removed from the syringe. In infants and small children, capillary blood can be used as a second-best source, especially if venous blood is unobtainable.

Collection Techniques

Before a venipuncture is performed, the tourniquet and the bleeding time tests should be done if they have been requisitioned. Once these tests have been completed, the blood samples are collected by syringe.

To avoid admixture with juices, it is preferable to use the two-syringe technique,[12] withdrawing the blood slowly without allowing frothing to occur. In some areas, only plastic syringes and tubes are used, while in other areas, glass syringes and tubes are used. It is important to use one method consistently when collecting the blood specimens. The vein is entered cleanly with a glass syringe having an 18- or 19-gauge needle. Several milliliters of blood are withdrawn; with the needle remaining in the vein, a silicone-coated syringe is substituted and the desired amount (approximately 20 cc.) of blood is obtained. The needle is then withdrawn from the vein and detached from the syringe, and the blood is immediately and gently distributed as quickly as possible to the following tubes.[10]

1. Four 1 ml. samples are delivered into small (12 × 75 mm.) tubes (2 glass and 2 silicone-coated) previously warmed at 37° C, for the measurement of the whole-blood coagulation time.

2. Three to 4 milliliters of blood is placed in a 12 × 75 mm. tube with inside diameter of 11 mm., containing several glass beads to provide a serum source. The tube should be inverted several times before the blood has firmly clotted.

3. Nine milliliters of blood is citrated by adding the blood to 1 ml. of 3.8 per cent trisodium citrate, already placed in a siliconized centrifuge tube.

4. Two milliliters of blood is delivered into a small tube containing EDTA so that a platelet count can be done, blood films

made, and other routine examinations undertaken. Many laboratories prefer to make the blood film directly from blood taken from the finger. This may then be done at this time.

If venous blood is unobtainable by clean venipuncture, especially from infants or small children, one may utilize the technique recommended by Dormandy and Hardesty[11] as follows: Into a stoppered polyethylene tube 1.8 ml. of buffered citrate-saline solution is delivered. The infant's finger or heel is deeply pricked after thorough warming and, after wiping away the first drop of blood, 0.2 ml. of blood is withdrawn into a pipette that is marked at 0.2 and 0.4 ml. and that already contains 0.2 ml. of the citrate-saline diluent. The blood is then transferred as quickly as possible into the 1.8 ml. of diluent contained in the plastic tube. The suspension of blood can be used quite successfully for a screening PTT test, thromboplastin generation test (Hicks-Pitney type),[22] for estimations of the prothrombin time (prothrombin and proconvertin method of Owren and Aas),[5, 36] or even for assay of antihemophilic factor (VIII).[19] Whole-blood coagulation time measurements carried out on capillary blood, even if free flowing, are less satisfactory and the results are of less diagnostic importance.

At this point, the patient may be released if the testing is done on an outpatient basis; the patient or adult accompanying a child should be advised that depending upon results, further tests may be necessary from new samples. If platelet aggregation is to be done at the same time, another good vein should be used for a clean venipuncture.

Precautions

Precautions to be used in preparation of materials and collection of specimens are that temperature, quality of reagents used, size and nature of vessels and tubes used in the test, glassware care, pipetting, and light sources must be adequately controlled and of the highest order. For example, because pipettes and test tubes should be absolutely clean, new glassware should be soaked in acid-cleaning solution, such as sulfuric acid dichromate, overnight before use. Previously used glassware should be free of any traces of fibrin, thromboplastin, chemicals, or reagents by thorough washing in a detergent followed several rinsings in distilled water. Frequent overnight soaks in acid cleaning solution are advisable. Pipettes with chipped tips or faint gradation markings should be avoided. Test tubes with etched walls or bottoms should never be used in a procedure the results of which depend on the observation of a plasma fibrin end point. Moreover, etched glassware may contain contaminating bits of trapped fibrin or thromboplastin.

It is most important that the pipetting be very accurate because the results of many of the clotting factor assays are based on dilution curves, which are prepared by pipetting amounts of plasma of the order of 0.01 to 0.1 ml. Eyelevel determinations of fluid levels in pipettes plus the use of gauze or lab tissue to wipe away excess fluid from the sides and tip of the pipette are strongly recommended. Fibrin formation is best observed using light from a large microscope lamp fitted with a blue filter. This avoids the inaccurate clot observation and eyestrain associated with natural light, artificial white light, or a white background.

Specimen Handling

The clot tubes are placed immediately into a 37° C water bath for a 2-hour period for monitoring and study of the continuing clot formation, retraction, and possible lysis. The EDTA tube is used for a complete blood count and platelet count. The smear made from the fingerstick is stained with Wright's stain and is studied for platelet morphology as well as for red cell morphology and a differential count.

The citrate tube is centrifuged for 5 minutes with a stopper on at 2,000 r.p.m. The plasma is then placed in three prelabeled tubes. Two of these tubes will contain 1 ml. of plasma each, and the rest of the plasma is placed into the third tube.

The largest amount of plasma is placed on ice and will be used for the testing procedures. The two smaller aliquots will be quick-frozen in a cryostat at −20° C and then placed in a deep-freeze locker for storage. These tubes should be stoppered with cork and paraffin.

The citrate tube that has been placed on ice will be used for an activated partial thromboplastin time (APTT) and prothrombin time (PT). If abnormalities are found in the PT or APTT, appropriate correction studies are performed. Depending upon the results of these correction studies, specific factor assays should be done on the same specimen. The entire procedure can easily be done within a 4-hour time limit.

The best results are achieved when the patient can be studied in the hospital or when the patient can come to the reference laboratory and the assays done within a four-hour period. However, when this is not possible, the plasma must be transported to the reference laboratory.

The same procedure for collecting the plasma in citrated tubes is followed. The citrated plasma is drawn up into small aliquots of 1 ml. of less for immediate transportation to the reference laboratory on dry ice. Quick-freezing of the plasma is required at −20° C. A mechanical freezer is not adequate because slowly freezing the plasma will cause formation of large ice particles that can denature the protein.

When the plasma arrives in the reference laboratory, it should be thawed rapidly in a water bath at 37° C, again to prevent denaturation of protein and fibrinogen. The assays should be run immediately. Slowly freezing and slowly thawing the citrated plasma may cause precipitation of factors I, V, and VIII, as well as of other proteins, resulting in erroneous and erratic results.

Since the effects of freezing and thawing

are still unpredictable, only values in the normal range can be accepted on the specimens. Low or borderline values should not be trusted, but should be confirmed with fresh plasma.

All of these results are reported on a work-sheet that is submitted to the pathologist along with the results of the appropriate assays. The pathologist can then interpret the coagulation studies. Further work may be ordered or the studies may be terminated at this point.

COAGULATION TIME TEST

Technique

When blood is removed from a blood vessel and exposed to a foreign surface, it clots. Any gross alteration in the procoagulants affects the rate of clotting. The procedure of determing coagulation time involves the standard venipuncture technique (two-syringe method); 5 ml. of blood is drawn into a silicone-coated syringe. One milliliter of blood is placed into each of two glass and two silicone-coated tubes (12 × 75 mm.) previously warmed at 37° C. All four tubes are then placed in a water bath set at 37° C. The first glass tube is tilted through a 45° angle every minute until it can be inverted with no flow of blood down the side of the tube. The second glass tube and the silicone-coated tubes are tilted in a similar manner every 3 minutes. Quick[39] believes that the standard Lee-White technique (without the use of three tubes, without tilting, and without temperature alteration) is better as long as silicone-coated tubes are used.

Sources of Error

Sources of error in this method are as follows: Traumatizing or squeezing site of venipuncture or contamination of syringe by tissue juices due to failure in making a clean venipuncture causes error. If a clean venipuncture is not accomplished on the first attempt, another sterile syringe and needle should be used and the venipuncture attempt repeated. An unclean syringe coated with detergent, cleaning solution, irregular silicone particles, and abrasives, can cause error. A disposable needle and syringe should be used if possible. If suction in filling syringe with blood is too vigorous, air bubbles will pass through the blood, which tends to hasten coagulation. If test tubes are irregularly exposed to cleaning solutions or detergents, error may result. Disposable tubes should be used if possible. The use of different types of test tubes with inconstant inside diameters (11 mm. preferred) can cause error. The sizes of the containers must be uniform because blood clots faster in narrow tubes owing to the larger surface of the wall of the container in contact with the blood.

The excessive agitation of the blood due to its overrapid flow from the syringe down the side of the tube tends to hasten coagulation. If the clotting of the blood is measured at room temperature or if there is delay in getting the blood to 37° C water bath, error may result. Temperature markedly influences the speed of coagulation; it is twice as fast at 37° C as it is at 20° C. Body temperature (37° C) is the most desirable temperature because this is the temperature at which coagulation takes place physiologically. Improper, inconstant, and the overenergetic tilting of tubes causes error. Blood clots first at the periphery in contact with the glass container and at the surface exposed to air, where fibrin has formed to support the columns of blood when the tube is completely inverted. The blood clots last in the center of the tube. It is essential, therefore, in reading the end point to tilt the tube gently and always in the same way if standard results are to be obtained.

The importance of standardizing the conditions by which the test is performed cannot be overemphasized. If for any reason the patient's coagulation time must be determined under less than standard conditions, a control sample should be obtained and tested at the same time.

Results

In reporting results, the coagulation time is recorded as the time interval between the appearance of blood in the syringe and the time at which blood no longer flows on complete inversion of the second tube. The clotting time of each type of tube may be averaged or reported separately.

Normal Values. The normal range for the uncoated glass tube is usually 5 to 10 minutes. A clotting time of more than 15 minutes is abnormal. The normal range for the silicone-coated tubes is 25 to 45 minutes with a mean of 30 minutes. A clotting time of less than 20 minutes in the silicone-coated tube may be abnormal or may result from faulty venipuncture. A clotting time beyond 45 minutes in these tubes is definitely abnormal.

Significance of Abnormal Results. Prolongation of the clotting time indicates a severe alteration of the coagulation mechanism. The test itself is primarily one of orientation. The abnormality may be due to (1) a defect in one or more of the stages of clotting; (2) a deficiency of a specific clotting factor, most commonly Factor VIII or Factor IX; (3) the presence of an acquired ciruclating anticoagulant directed against one or more of the clotting factors; and (4) the presence of agents such as heparin used in treating thrombotic disease.

Recently, a new and much more specific, sensitive, and simple assay for measurement of plasma heparin has been developed for use in monitoring both heparin reversal following cardiopulmonary bypass and heparin and miniheparin therapy. It requires only minutes to perform, and, in contrast to existing indirect methods (e.g., coagulation time), it measures heparin levels directly, uses commonly available laboratory equipment, and is uninfluenced by patient variables such as elevated fibrinogen/fibrin degradation products, hypofibrinogenemia, and a decreased amount of antithrombin III. It is a two-stage clotting system that utilizes purified thrombin and a substrate that already contains optimal levels of fibrinogen and antithrombin III. A fibrometer is used to measure the clotting time. The test is especially effective in monitoring heparin therapy, especially low-dose or miniheparin therapy. Before this assay was developed, there had been no test sensitive enough to detect tiny amounts of heparin in the blood, making it difficult to monitor the patient's condition carefully.[14]

BLEEDING TIME TESTS

A small puncture is made through the skin of the earlobe or forearm, and the time during which the puncture bleeds is carefully estimated. The duration of bleeding from a severe capillary depends on the quantity of platelets, the quality of platelets, and the reaction of the blood vessel wall.

Techniques

Three methods used to measure bleeding time are the modified Duke method, the Ivy method, and the standardized simplate test.

In the modified Duke procedure, the area used is 15 to 20 mm. above the rounded fatty portion of the earlobe, which is so richly vascularized that prolonged bleeding may occur in normal persons. A glass slide is held behind the previously warmed ear, and the edge of the ear is quickly pierced with a No. 11 sterile Bard-Parker surgical blade. As the blade passes through the ear it hits the glass slide with a clicking sound. Pressure should not be exerted on the ear to initiate bleeding; the blood should be allowed to fall freely on 4 × 4 gauze sponges.

In the Ivy method, the volar surface of the forearm is cleansed with alcohol and allowed to dry. A blood pressure cuff is placed on the arm above the elbow and inflated to 40 torr. A sterilized area of the forearm without visible superficial veins is selected, the skin is stretched laterally and tautly between the thumb and forefinger, and the alcohol-sterilized skin is punctured twice by means of a No. 11 Bard-Parker surgical blade to a depth of 5 mm. and a width of 2 mm. The edge of a 4 × 4 inch piece of gauze is used to collect the blood by capillary action by gently touching the drop every 30 seconds. This is the method of choice because constant blood pressure is exerted on the vessels, the size and depth of the incisions are uniform, and the arm offers a large enough area for many determinations. The Ivy method also reveals abnormalities not detected by Duke's method.

Standardized Simplate* test measures the overall hemostatic role of platelets in vivo (i.e., platelet plug formation) by determining the duration of bleeding from a standard skin incision while maintaining increased venous pressure. It is especially useful in the systematic evaluation of patients with thrombocytopenia because of its capacity to discriminate between platelets with normal and those with decreased or increased function; that is, platelet plug formation appears to be unimpaired when there are normal platelets with a concentration of 100,000 or more per μl. of blood. Below this level, bleeding increases linearly with decreases in platelet count, according to the following formula:

Bleeding time (in min.) =

$$30.5 - \frac{\text{Platelet count}/\mu l.}{3850}$$

This relationship does not apply when there are less than 20,000 platelets per μl. Disproportionate prolongation reflects platelet dysfunction while bleeding times shorter than predicted indicate platelets with increased hemostatic competence.

The following is the procedure for the simplate method:

(1) Seat the subject with arm supine on a steady support with the volar surface exposed (Fig. 11-1*A*). Select an area of the forearm distal to the anticubital fossa, tak-

ing care to avoid surface veins, scars, and bruises. Cleanse with an alcohol sponge and allow to air-dray at least 30 seconds (Fig. 11-1*B*). If the patient has marked hair, lightly shave the area. Place a sphygmomanometer cuff on the upper arm.

(2) Remove the device from the blister pack (Fig. 11-1*C*), and twist off the white, tear-away tab on the side of the device (Fig. 11-1*D*). Do not push the trigger or touch the blade slot. Inflate the sphygmomanometer cuff to 40 torr. The time between inflation of cuff and incision should be 30 to 60 seconds. Monitor frequently to ensure maintenance of pressure during test procedure.

(3) Place the device firmly on the forearm. Do not press. The incision may be made either parallel or perpendicular to the fold of the elbow.

(4) Depress the trigger and simultaneously start the timer (Fig. 11-1*E*). Remove the device approximately one second after triggering (Fig. 11-1*F*).

(5) At 30 seconds, blot the flow of blood with filter paper (Fig. 11-1*G*). Bring the filter paper close to the incision without touching the edge of the wound. (Do not disturb the platelet plug.) Blot in a similar manner every 30 seconds until blood no longer stains the filter paper (Fig. 11-1*H*). Stop timer.

(6) Remove cuff, clean arm, and apply a bandage across the incision (Fig. 11-1*I*). Advise patient to keep the bandage in place for 24 hours. Record the bleeding time to the nearest 30 seconds. Return the device to the opened blister pack and discard.

The expected range is 2.3 to 9.5 minutes.

Because of the complexity of the primary hemostatic mechanism, the numerous patient-related factors that may affect the bleeding time (age, skin type, skin condition, vascularity, and temperature), and variation in individual techniques, it is recommended that each laboratory establish its own "expected range."

Extreme care should be taken when technologists utilize the simplate method for assay of the bleeding time. For example, if

---

* Manufactured by General Diagnostics, Division of Warner-Lambert Company, Morris Plains, New Jersey 07950.

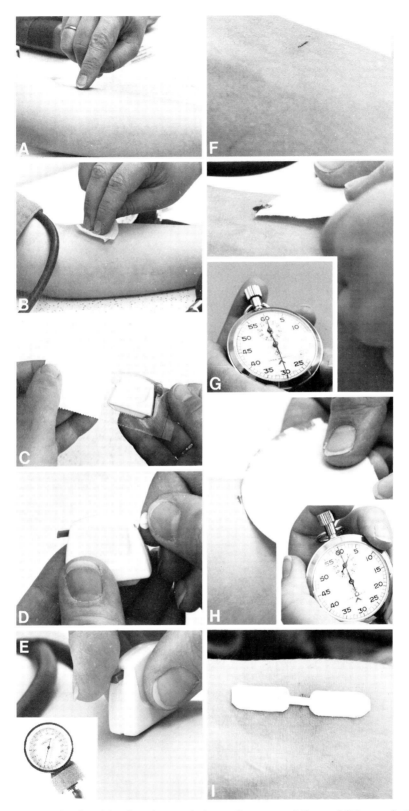

Fig. 11-1. Simplate bleeding time technique (Courtesy of General Diagnostics)

a person puts too much pressure on the blade, the incision will be too deep and the testing time will be falsely prolonged. On the other hand, if a technologist eases his grip on the scalpel blade, the wound will be slight and the bleeding time will be very short. In this case, a bleeding disorder might not be detected. Also, technologists must be very careful not to make the incision over a surface vein. This, too, will falsely prolong the results, and a physician may mistakenly be led to suspect a bleeding disorder that does not exist.

Disposable simplates and scalpel blade holders are now available. Although these kits are more expensive than permanent ones, it is believed that they have solved the difficulties of sterilizing permanent simplates and blades. There are, however, two major drawbacks to the simplate bleeding time. These are the formation of a faint scar on the patient's arm and, rarely, keloid formation. Several laboratories have tried to minimize scar formation by making the incision vertically instead of horizontally. Although the bleeding time might be shorter with the vertical incision, the setting of normal limits for each hospital laboratory utilizing the vertical incision technique would ameliorate the situation. Finally, certain drugs that prevent platelets from functioning normally may interfere with this test. Below are two lists of drugs containing aspirin, the main offender. A patient should be asked whether he or she has taken any of these drugs in the 7 to 10 days prior to testing.

Prescription Drugs That Contain Aspirin

Norgesic
Darvon Compound
Phenaphen
Fiorinal
Percodan
Robaxisal
Robaxisal PH
Zactirin
Daprisal
Edrisal

Over-the-Counter Drugs That Contain Aspirin

Alka-Seltzer
Coricidin
Coricidin-D
Dristan
Novahistine with APC
Super-Anahist
Triaminicin
Anacin
APC
A.S.A. Compound
Ascriptin
Aspergum
Bufferin
CAMA
Capron Capsules
Cope
Counterpain
Derfort/Derfule
Dolor Plus
Ecotrin
Empirin Compound
Excedrin
Liquiprin
Measurin
Midol
P-A-C
Phensal
Sal-Fayne
Stanback
Trigesic
Vanquish

This simplate procedure can be highly sensitive and reproducible once a laboratory staff becomes familiar with it. Technologists should practice it and become aware of the normal limits for their own hospital.

Sources of Error

Sources of error in doing a bleeding time involve the following: (1) Because a needle is used for puncture, the wound cannot be standardized, and the normal range may therefore vary when the puncture is not of standard depth and width. (2) A single prolonged bleeding time does not prove the existence of hemorrhagic disease; a large vessel may have been severed. The puncture should be done twice and the average of the bleeding times taken. (3) Touching the incision will break any fibrin particles, therefore prolonging the bleeding time.

Results

Results from the Duke and Ivy methods may be reported in two ways: The end point is reached when blood no longer drops from the edge of the ear-puncture, or blood no longer exudes from the forearm puncture. Or, the number of drops of blood on the gauze or filter paper is divided by two, and the resulting amount is the bleeding time in minutes.

Normal Values. In the modified Duke method, results between 8 and 10 minutes may be abnormal. Those over 10 minutes are definitely abnormal. In the Ivy method, a bleeding time of less than 5 to 6 minutes is considered normal. The determination should be discontinued if the wound is still bleeding at 15 minutes, and it should be reported if bleeding continues beyond 15 minutes.

Significance of Abnormal Results. Contraction of the capillaries and the small blood vessels is important, and probably blood platelets also play a part by plugging the cut ends of the vessel. Therefore, bleeding time is prolonged in some vessel wall defects and in qualitative or quantitative platelet abnormalities (less than 100,000 platelets/cu.mm.). It is rarely prolonged in plasma factor deficiencies unless the defects are quite severe. It is frequently prolonged in von Willebrand's disease.

CLOT RETRACTION TESTS

Whole blood that clots normally retracts from the sides of the container, resulting in the separation of transparent serum and the contracted blood clot. This reaction is a function of (1) the quantity and quality of intact platelets, (2) the fibrinogen content of the plasma, (3) the ratio of the plasma volume and red cell mass, (4) the activity of a retraction-promoting principle in the serum, and (5) the nature of the surface on which clot retraction is being measured.

Techniques

Comparison of rapid screening and detailed clot retraction techniques reveals the following: In rapid screening, the silicone-coated tubes used in the coagulation time are allowed to remain in the water bath at 37° C until 1 hour after the blood is withdrawn. The tubes are then examined for clot retraction. It is noted whether retraction is from the sides of the tube, the bottom only, or both. If at the end of the hour the clot is not retracted from the wall of the tube, it is gently loosened from the wall by means of a wooden applicator and the extent of retraction is noted – namely, the shrinkage of the clot with expression of serum. Clot retraction is again checked at 2 and 4 hours.

In the detailed clot retraction test 2 ml. of freshly drawn blood (using the standard two-syringe venipuncture technique) is placed in a graduated siliconized centrifuge tube. The tube is closed with a rubber stopper in which is inserted a coiled or twisted glass rod, the lowermost portion of which contains approximately 10 turns and touches the bottom of the tube. The entire tube, including the stopper with glass rod, has been previously warmed to 37° C, and the mixture with blood is placed in a water bath at 37° C; the hematocrit has previously been measured on an aliquot of the blood. The clotting time may be determined by tilting the tube at intervals of 1 minute until it ceases to flow and appears jelled. One hour after clotting has occurred, the stopper and coiled glass are gently pulled up from the serum, thus permitting the hemorrhagic serum to drain to the bottom of the graduated tube while the clot adheres to the glass rod. After another hour, the graduated tube is centrifuged for 15 minutes at a moderate speed and the volume of the serum (without the volume of red blood cells) is recorded.

Sources of Error

Sources of error in these techniques include the following: (1) Inconstant temperature (37° C), unclean glassware, improper siliconization of tubes and syringes, and a faulty venipuncture all can cause error. (2) Mild shaking or jarring of the tube should be avoided because blood having delayed or no retraction may retract when subjected to such treatment. (3) If the hematocrit is high owing to polycythemia or hemoconcentration, the plasma volume and consequently the total amount of fibrinogen is relatively small, and the mass of the red blood cells limits the degree of retraction by the volume that it occupies in the clot. The converse occurs in anemia.

Results

In reporting of results, the degree (slight, moderate, marked) as well as the rate of clot retraction is observed. Separation of the clot from three sides of the tube is considered complete (4+) retraction. Results may be read at 30 minutes, 1 hour, and at the end of 4 hours and 24 hours. If clot retraction is normal and complete, approximately half the total volume is made up of clot and the other half is expressed serum. Clot retraction may be measured semiquantitatively as percentage according to the formula:

$$\frac{\text{Volume of expressed serum} \times 100}{\text{Volume of whole blood}}$$

or quantitatively as the percentage of expressed serum in the total preformed serum:

$$\frac{\text{ml. serum} \times 50}{1 - \text{hematocrit}}$$

The shape and consistency of the clot are also noted and reported.

Normal Values. Normally, retraction of the clot from the sides and bottom of the test tube will have begun by 30 minutes, is appreciable in 1 to 2 hours, is nearly complete by 4 hours, and is definitely completed in 24 hours. Semiquantitatively, 45 to 60 per cent (average 52%) of the serum is expressed from the clot. Quantitatively, 58 to 97 per cent of the serum is expressed from the clot with a mean of 78 per cent. Qualitatively, a normal blood clot after maximal retraction is relatively dry and firm, and it maintains its molded shape after removal from the container in which it was formed. A defective clot is soft and soggy, is readily torn, and after removal flattens out as a shapeless mass from which the serum continues to drain.

Significance of Abnormal Results. Poor clot retraction occurs in thrombocytopenia (platelet count less than 50,000/cu.mm.); in some disorders in which platelets are qualitatively deficient, as von Willebrand's disease; and in disorders due to an increase in red cell mass (polycythemic states). There is a rough, but distinct parallelism between the number of the platelets and the quality of the clot.

Furthermore clot retraction may appear to be increased in severe anemia and extreme hypofibrinogenemia owing to the formation of a small clot as a result of the relative increase in plasma volume.

THE TOURNIQUET TEST

Techniques

Positive Pressure Test. In the positive pressure test, the basic principle involves the venous blood flow in the arm, which is partially obstructed. This produces increased intracapillary pressure with possible subsequent extravasation of blood in the form of petechiae. The pressure and time of application are both standardized; the degree of increased capillary fragility is reflected in the number of petechiae produced in a given area of observation. Although the opposite arm may be used, the first test locus cannot be repeated until 7 to 14 days have elapsed. In the technique, a blood pressure cuff is applied to the upper arm, stabilizing the pressure to a point midway between the systolic and diastolic level for 5 minutes. Fifteen minutes later (after release of the pressure cuff), the forearm, hands, and fingers are examined for petechiae.

Negative Pressure Test. In the negative pressure method, this type of pressure is applied to the skin and indirectly to the extravascular tissues, thus producing extravasation of blood. The number of petechiae produced within a given area provides a measure of capillary permeability — that is, increased fragility or decreased resistance. In the technique, a suction cup of 2 cm. in diameter is applied (lips of the cup having been previously lubricated) to the midportion of the upper arm in close contact with the skin for 1 minute at a pressure of 200 to 250 torr. After release, petechiae within a circle 1 cm. in diameter are counted 5 minutes later.

Sources of Error

Sources of error in these methods include the following: (1) Pressure may vary from patient to patient, depending on the blood pressure. (2) Repetition of the test on same arm before the lapse of 1 week may lead to error. (3) The test should be made more quantitative by utilizing a 5 cm. circle approximately 4 cm. below the bend of the elbow. This gives a standard area for each patient. Even with this technique, the test may be markedly positive, yet only a few of the petechiae may develop within the circle. (4) The negative suction test does not take into account the extreme variability in capillary fragility at different sites. (5) Results may vary owing to the texture, thickness, and temperature of skin.

Results

The results of the test are graded in a rough manner from normal to 4+ as follows: 1+ = few petechiae over the anterior surface of the forearm; 2+ = many petechiae over the anterior surface of the

forearm; 3+ = multiple petechiae over the whole arm and dorsum of the hand; and 4+ = confluent petechiae in all areas of the arm and dorsum of the hand.

Normal Values. In the positive pressure test, a petechial count greater than five to ten is abnormal, indicating increased capillary fragility. The negative pressure test has a normal value of one to two petechiae at 200 torr (medium position of plunger).

Significance of Abnormal Results. The number and size of the petechiae are roughly proportional to the bleeding tendency and possibly to the degree of thrombocytopenia. However, the test may be strongly positive (because of fragile capillaries) with a normal platelet count.

PROTHROMBIN TIME TEST

In this test, blood is mixed with a measured amount of sodium citrate solution, after which the plasma is obtained by centrifugation. In the presence of an excess of tissue thromboplastin (made from rabbit or human embryo brain, then standardized and sold commercially) and an optimal concentration of calcium ions, the normal control plasma and the patient's plasma (if normal) coagulate rapidly. Because it was previously thought that the test indicated the concentration of prothrombin in the blood, it was called the "prothrombin time." It is now recognized, however, that the reaction depends on variables that were unknown when the test was first devised. According to current thinking, the following factors determine the prothrombin time:[31]

$$\text{Prothrombin} \xrightarrow[\substack{\text{Factor V} \\ \text{Factor VII} \\ \text{Factor X}}]{\substack{\text{Thromboplastin} \\ \text{Ca}^{++}}} \text{Thrombin}$$

To measure the prothrombin time, tissue thromboplastin and Ca^{++} are added in optimal concentration, so that the test itself measures the contribution of prothrombin,

Factor V, Factor VII, and Factor X to the generation of prothrombin. Therefore, when one or more of these substances is reduced, the prothrombin time is prolonged. It is generally believed that the reaction is influenced most by the concentration of Factor VII, followed in importance by Factors X and V and prothrombin. Fibrinogen also plays a role in the clotting process; the test end point is indicated by the coagulation of fibrinogen by thrombin. Therefore, the fibrinogen concentration is also critical in the 60 to 100 mg. per 100 ml. range. If the fibrinogen concentration falls below 60 mg. per 100 ml., the following may occur: (1) the prothrombin time is prolonged, probably owing to a reduced fibrinogen concentration (substrate), (2) a small delicate clot may be formed and overlooked, (3) both of the first two reactions might occur, or (4) no clot forms because of such a low fibrinogen concentration.

The prothrombin time may also be prolonged because of very active fibrinolysins. These fibrinolysins not only lyse fibrin but also effectively lyse fibrinogen, thus making the fibrinogen nonreactive to the thrombin action. Thus it is not always possible to say whether a reduced, chemically determined fibrinogen is indeed indicative of hypofibrinogenemia, or whether the low fibrinogen level is due to increased fibrinolytic activity. The prothrombin time will also be prolonged in the presence of the following inhibitors: antithrombins, antithromboplastins, and specific factor inhibitors (for example, anti-Factor V).

Because the prothrombin time test is affected by things other than the prothrombin concentration, it has therefore been suggested that the test be renamed; for example, "accelerated coagulation time" or "thromboplastin time." However, past use in medical literature would tend to cause confusion somewhat like that associated with attempts to rename the components of the erythrocyte series. The prothrombin time of an unknown plasma, expressed as the percentage of the prothrombin time of a control plasma, is known as prothrombin activity.

Techniques

One-Stage Prothrombin Time (Quick's Test). Exactly 4.5 ml. of blood is drawn by clean venipuncture into 0.5 ml. of 3.8 per cent sodium citrate solution (decay of Factors V and VIII is slower in citrate than in 0.1 per cent sodium oxalate). Special evacuated disposable tubes containing a measured amount of sodium citrate are recommended. The blood is mixed well, is immediately centrifuged at 2000 r.p.m. for 10 minutes, and the plasma is removed. The plasma is allowed to equilibrate to 37° C for at least 5 minutes before it is tested. At least one control is run in the same manner. If commercial thromboplastins are used, they are prepared according to the manufacturer's instructions.

A small, empty, clean Pyrex test tube and the empty control tube are placed in a water bath at 37° C. To these empty test tubes (12 × 75 mm.) in the water bath at 37° C, add 0.2 ml. of commercial thromboplastin extract, which contains a calcium chloride-reconstituted suspension. The tubes are allowed to remain in the water bath (37° C) for about 30 seconds. To the calcium suspension, 0.1 ml. of plasma is added quickly by forcibly, but gently, blowing the contents of a 0.2 ml. pipette (splattering onto the walls of the test tube should be avoided). A stopwatch is activated at this time. The tube is gently tilted back and forth in the water bath (at a rate of 40 to 60 tilts per minute) for 10 seconds, the mixture being allowed to flow up and down the wall of the tube. The tube is then removed from the water bath, held in front of a bright light source, and gently tilted back and forth once a second until the clot forms.

As the first appearance of the fibrin clot, the timer is stopped, and the time of clot formation is recorded. The test should be run in duplicate; results should correspond within 0.5 to 1 second. If the results do not correspond a third test should be run. A control test with normal plasma must be run at the same time, and the results for both the control plasma and the patient's plasma should be reported in seconds.

A curve relating the prothrombin time to the prothrombin activity in percentage of normal may be obtained by making various dilutions of plasma in saline solutions and determining the clotting time of the diluted specimen. However, the shape of the curve varies with each batch of thromboplastin and the type of diluent used. If the results are to be expressed in percentage of normal, the dilution curve must be determined for each batch of thromboplastin used and the diluent specified. Therefore, it is susggested that the results be reported in seconds and not as a percentage.

The Prothrombin and Proconvertin Method of Owren and Aas. The plasma is diluted ten times so that the action of inhibitors and the variable concentrations of anticoagulants are minimized. Just as in Quick's test, thromboplastin and calcium are added to the plasma. Prothrombin-free beef plasma (with Factors I and V) is then added. This makes the test more specific for Factor II (prothrombin) and Factor VII because two other variables are added. Some workers believe there is a better correlation between this method and the hemorrhagic state especially in evaluating patients receiving Coumadin drugs.

Two-Stage Prothrombin Method. The first stage is characterized by the conversion of prothrombin into thrombin by the addition of tissue thromboplastin, calcium, and Factors V and VII. In the second stage, the thrombin formed in Stage I is measured by removing samples after varying periods of incubation. The time required for each aliquot to clot a fibrinogen solution is observed. Samples are tested from the incubated mixture until the shortest clotting time, which represents the maximal thrombin yield, has been obtained. This is a specific test for prothrombin, but because of its lack of simplicity and economy, it is used mostly for research and evaluation of atypical clinical syndromes.

Sources of Error

In the Owren-Aas method and the two-stage method, the sources of error include the following: (1) Contamination of speciment with tissue thromboplastin due to lack of clean, free-flowing venipuncture. (2) Exposure of the blood to air bubbles. (3) Delay in adding the blood to anticoagulant. (4) Delay in refrigerating the plasma; Factor V is labile, and the plasma therefore should be refrigerated promptly. (5) Delay in determining prothrombin time; Factor V is labile, and prothrombin time should therefore be done within 1 hour after collection and not later than 4 hours. If plasma is promptly frozen, it may be stored up to 1 week and then thawed.

(6) Poor thromboplastin preparation leads to error; the prothrombin time of normal control plasma should fall between 11 and 16 seconds. Anything greater than 16 seconds is unsatisfactory. According to Miale and Lafond, acceptable thromboplastin should have an activity within a reasonably narrow range, there should be reasonably good reproducibility of replicate determinations on the same plasma, and there should be reasonably good lot-to-lot criteria for the *p*H of the reconstituted product.[32] Therefore an acceptable thromboplastin should possess the following specific criteria: reproducibility of replicate determinations within ±1.0 second from the mean for normal plasma; stability of 1 year at a temperature not exceeding 10° C, plus specified heat lability; a *p*H between 6.8 and 7.6 after reconstitution with distilled water having a *p*H of 6.5 to 7.0; and a prothrombin time for undiluted normal human plasma of no less than 12.0 and no greater than 15.0 seconds; and for a 12.5 per cent saline dilution of normal human plasma, a clotting time from 2.5 to 2.8 times that of the undiluted plasma. (7) Unclean glassware. (8) Too slow discharge of

plasma into test tube may cause error. (9) Too vigorous shaking of tube in water bath may cause the initial delicate fibrin mesh to be broken and therefore not to be detected until more time elapses for further fibrin formation to occur. This would lead to a markedly errouous, prolonged prothrombin time. (10) If the patient is on anticoagulant therapy, such as heparin, the blood must be drawn at least 4 hours after the last injection or the prothrombin time obtained will not be accurate. (11) The use of oxalate instead of citrate as an anticoagulant in the prothrombin time test may cause error. That is, Factors V and VII are more stable in citrated plasma.

Results

The clotting time of the patient's plasma is given in seconds, as is the clotting time of the normal plasma control for that day.

Normal Values. The one-stage prothrombin time varies between 11 and 15 seconds, depending on the thromboplastin used. In the Owren-Aas method, the normal time varies between 30 and 40 seconds. In the two-stage method, the normal level varies between 200 and 400 units per ml. of plasma.

Significance of Abnormal Results. Because these methods are not specific for prothrombin, but are a measure of the entire coagulation process (except for blood thromboplastin formation), a prolonged prothrombin time is seen in deficiencies of prothrombin (Factor II), Factor V, Factor VII, Factor X, fibrinogen (I), in a deficiency of any combination of these factors, or in the inhibition of the second or third stage of clotting. The prothrombin time test is normal in hemophilia (a deficiency of Factors VII, IX, or XI) and in thrombocytopenia. Therefore if the prothrombin time is prolonged, one must test specifically for Factors II, V, VII, and X. The deficiency of Factor I (fibrinogen) may be suspected by the absence of a clot, and a presumptive test for fibrinogen may be performed.

PROTHROMBIN CONSUMPTION TEST (PCT)

As blood coagulates, prothrombin is converted to thrombin by the stoichiometric interaction of the excess amounts of thromboplastin complex present in normal blood. After normal blood or plasma has clotted, thrombin production and prothrombin utilization continue. Practically all (85–95%) the prothrombin is utilized or consumed if the serum is tested 1 hour after the blood or plasma has clotted, leaving relatively little residual prothrombin in the serum. Thus, the prothrombin will have been incompletely consumed, and more than the normal amount will be present in the serum 1 hour after clotting, if there is a deficiency of any factors required for blood or plasma clotting in glass. This occurs even if the blood or plasma itself coagulates within the normal time. Another way of expressing this is to state that the residual prothrombin that is not consumed, and therefore remains in the serum, is measured by supplying fibrinogen to the system and adding tissue thromboplastin and calcium. Normal serum that contains little residual prothrombin clots relatively slowly, whereas serum that contains larger amounts of prothrombin clots rapidly. One measure of the clotting mechanism therefore is the amount of prothrombin remaining in the serum after clotting.

Techniques

In actual practice, serum obtained from blood samples used in the whole-blood coagulation time test can be used in this nonspecific test for the intrinsic thromboplastic system. If this serum is not available, 1 ml. of blood may be placed in each of two clean glass test tubes immediately after a clean venipuncture, without adding anticoagulants. The tubes are then placed in a 37° C water bath and allowed to stand without shaking or testing in any way. One hour after the samples have clotted, these clots are removed, the serum is centrifuged, and the volume is measured. Nine parts of serum is then mixed with one part of 1.1 M sodium citrate solution, which prevents further conversion of prothrombin to thrombin, and the mixture is allowed to incubate for 15 minutes.

Three separate test tubes — one each for serum previously incubated, for commercial thromboplastin-calcium solution, and for serum-sulfate adsorbed plasma (deprothrombinized plasma) — are placed in a 37° C water bath for 5 minutes. Then 0.1 ml. of the citrated serum, 0.1 ml. of barium sulfate-adsorbed plasma, and 0.2 ml. of commercial thromboplastin-calcium solution are placed in a clean test tube. The stopwatch is started immediately. Coagulation time is determined by noting the gross appearance of the thin, weblike strands of fibrin. The procedure is repeated with the second sample. In this way the residual prothrombin in the serum is compared with that found in the patient's plasma.

An attempt was made to increase the sensitivity of the prothrombin consumption test by using silicone coating in the test tubes to minimize surface contact and by prolonging the interval between collection of the blood and determination of the residual Factor II to 3 hours, compared to the 1 hour interval used in the conventional glass technique.[16] This modification gave reproducible residual Factor II determinations, and in 99 per cent of normal subjects the values were consistently below 30 per cent. Also when compared with the 1 hour glass technique, the 3 hour test proved to be sensitive for disclosing deficiencies of certain clotting factors that were not otherwise demonstrable except by specific assays or by thromboplastin generation studies.

Sources of Error

Sources of error in the prothrombin consumption test are as follows: (1) Because barium sulfate-adsorbed plasma is used as a source of fibrinogen and Factor V, they are both used up in the formation of the clot. An error occurs if the adsorbed plasma is not completely deprothrombinized, or prothrombin-free; the prothrombin time should be more than 1 minute. (2) The sources of error associated with the withdrawal of blood for coagulation time determination (p. 308) and those associated with the performance of prothrombin time (p. 317) would cause error in this test. (3) The time intervals given for this test must be adhered to if reproducible results are to be obtained. (4) If the one-stage prothrombin time is abnormal, the normal results cannot be considered as valid.

Results

Normal Values. A serum prothrombin consumption time — the time it takes for a thin weblike strand of fibrin to form — of 28 to 30 seconds or more is normal when a thromboplastin solution that gives a normal plasma prothrombin time of 11 to 15 seconds is used. Values of less than 25 seconds may be considered normal.

Significance of Abnormal Results. As the blood (intrinsic) thromboplastin is generated, it converts residual prothrombin to thrombin, thus using up residual prothrombin. If the generation of intrinsic thromboplastin is delayed because of a deficiency of any one of the factors required in the first stage of coagulation (platelets, Factors V, VIII, IX, X, XI, and XII), then a large amount of prothrombin will remain in the serum; therefore the PCT will be less than 25 to 18 seconds. The test, therefore, is an indirect measurement of thromboplastin generation, and although there are many theoretically valid objections to the test — its nonspecificity, for example — it is simpler than the thromboplastin generation test and is a very useful ancillary test for clinically testing clotting efficiency. For example, it is more sensitive than the whole-blood clotting time. If the PCT is less than 18 seconds, one may add inosithin (soybean substitute for platelet factor 3). If the defect is due to a reduction in thrombocyte numbers, the PCT will come back to normal. However, because the PCT is normal when levels of AHF are 1 per cent of normal, the diagnosis of hemophilia should not be excluded on the basis of a normal PCT alone.

THROMBOPLASTIN GENERATION TEST (TGT)

The combination of adsorbed plasma (deprothrombinized), serum, platelets, and calcium forms a mixture capable of generating a powerful intrinsic thromboplastin. The efficiency of the mixture may be measured according to the ability of the thromboplastin to clot a plasma substrate.

Technique

The technique of this test is as follows:[3] Before setting up the test, the reagents must be prepared. Normal and adsorbed plasma are each diluted $1/5$ with 0.85 per cent NaCl solution and then allowed to stand for at least 10 minutes. The normal and patient serums are each diluted $1/10$ with imidazole (glyoxalin) buffer, and then they are allowed to stand for 1 hour.

A chloroform extract of cephalin (acetone-insoluble brain powder) or Gliddex-O (soybean phosphatide) is diluted $1/100$ with 0.85 per cent NaCl (as platelet substitute). An $M/40$ $CaCl_2$ solution, substrate platelet-poor plasma, and a platelet suspension are also used. The latter two are prepared as follows: 20 ml. of normal whole blood is placed into two silicone-treated 10 ml. graduated centrifuge tubes each containing 1 ml. of 3.8 per cent sodium citrate. This is centrifuged at 1500 r.p.m. for 10 minutes. The plasma containing the platelets is separated into the silicone-coated centrifuge tubes and is centrifuged at 3000 r.p.m. for 15 minutes. The clear supernatant is used as platelet-poor substrate plasma. The platelets deposited in a button at the bottom of tube are fragmented with a wooden applicator stick and washed twice with 0.85 per cent NaCl, after which they are resuspended in 0.85 per cent NaCl at $1/3$ to $1/2$ the original volume of the plasma.

In the method, 0.1 ml. amounts of substrate plasma are placed in Lee-White coagulation tubes in a water bath at 37° C. Into a separate tube, 0.3 ml. of the $1/5$ dilution of normal adsorbed plasma, 0.3 ml. of the $1/10$ dilution of normal serum, 0.3 ml. of the $1/100$ dilution of chloroform extract of brain, or Glidden-O is pipetted. The tube is then placed in a 37° C water bath. Then 0.3 ml. of $M/40$ $CaCl_2$ is added to the mixture, and the stopwatch is started. Agitate with 0.1 m. pipette. At 1 minute 0.1 ml. of the initial mixture is added, and 0.1 ml. of $M/40$ $CaCl_2$ is added to a tube of substrate plasma. The stopwatch is started, and the clot is timed. This procedure is repeated at 1 minute intervals until the minimal clotting time is recorded. It is repeated at 12 minutes to confirm minimal clotting time. The test is repeated, substituting the patient's serum and plasma for normal serum and plasma, and then both the patient's plasma and serum together. The test may be done using a suspension of platelets from the normal control and from the patient; these suspensions are substituted for the brain extract, or Glidden-O. The clotting time versus minutes of incubation may be plotted on a linear graph. Portions of the following six paragraphs have been adapted from J. W. Eichelberger: Laboratory Methods in Blood Coagulation, New York, Hoeber, 1965, pp. 66, 67.

Thromboplastin activity is thought to develop in the intrinsic (blood) system when there are present in the incubation mixture antihemophilic factor, plasma thromboplastin component, plasma thromboplastin antecedent, Factor X, platelets, Factor V, and ionized calcium. The thromboplastin generation test provides a method by which a specific deficiency of one of these factors may be discovered.

Normal plasma treated with $Al(OH)_3$ provides Factor VIII, Factor XI, Factor V, and Factor XII, but does not contain Factor VII, Factor X, or Factor IX. Serum should contain Factor X, Factor VII, Factor XI, Factor IX, and Factor XII. Factor

V and Factor VIII, which are consumed in clotting, are lacking. Factor VII is not essential for the development of thromboplastin activity in the intrinsic system.

If the $Al(OH)_3$-adsorbed plasma, normal serum, and platelets or brain extract are incubated in the presence of $CaCl_2$, there is developed a labile but powerful thromboplastin activity. The efficiency of the thromboplastin activity is then measured by placing aliquots of the incubation mixture in a tube containing a substrate of normal, platelet-free, citrated plasma. Normally coagulation will occur within 10 seconds when thromboplastin activity is fully developed. By serially substituting the patient's serum, $Al(OH)_3$-treated plasma, or platelets in this test, specific deficiencies of the early phase of coagulation may be revealed.

It is important to note that though the substrate plasma contains factors that may be missing from test fractions, the time that would be required for them to react in the substrate tube exceeds the 10-second limit defining normality in this test. The development of thromboplastin activity normally requires 3 to 5 minutes. What is measured when the incubation mixture is transferred to the second tube containing the substrate plasma is the rate of conversion of prothrombin to thrombin and the subsequent conversion of fibrinogen to fibrin.

If the substrate plasma is normal, the end point depends solely on the amount of thromboplastin activity developed during the incubation period. The fibrinogen and prothrombin in the substrate are constant; the potential variables are in the incubation mixture. The variables may then be separated by performing the classic one-stage prothrombin time test.

Comparative dilution to a level 10,000 to 15,000 per cu.mm. of the patient's platelets and a normal control in the thromboplastin generation test are usually necessary before a defect in platelet factor 3 will be detected.

Stated in another way, thromboplastin generation is deficient if plasma from an AHF-deficient hemophiliac is incubated with normal serum and cephalin (or platelets or Gliddex-O), whereas thromboplastin formation is normal if the serum of the AHF-deficient hemophiliac is incubated with normal plasma and cephalin. The same thing is true for Factor V deficiency, although the deficiency can be missed if platelets, which bear adsorbed Factor V on their surfaces, are used instead of cephalin. Factor V deficiency can also be better detected by the TGT if substrate plasma deficient in Factor V is used. In deficiency of PTC or of Stuart factor, it is the serum phase that is abnormal, whereas the plasmas of these patients function normally. If in separate tests a patient's plasma and serum both give abnormal results, it is likely that the patient has a circulating anticoagulant; a dual deficiency of a plasma and serum factor as another, although far less likely, explanation.

If the incubation mixture contains normal plasma and serum, a normal test will result, if the substrate plasma is deficient in any factor except prothrombin and fibrinogen. On the other hand, when the incubation mixture contains either AHF-deficient plasma or PTC-deficient serum, the clotting times of the substrate plasma will be shorter if normal substrate plasma is used than if plasma deficient in AHF or PTC is used. This phenomenon is not specific to AHF or PTC deficiency and is observed whenever an incomplete thromboplastin is added to substrate deficient in the same factor. Failure to recognize this fact led to the postulation of a so-called Bridge anticoagulant in hemophiliacs with AHF and PTC deficiency. This has been shown to be an artifact and not a true anticoagulant. In order to have a negative TGT, residual prothrombin must be present in the serum.

Sources of Error

Sources of error in the thromboplastin generation test are as follows: (1) At times aluminum hydroxide adsorption incompletely removes Factor IX (PTC) from nor-

Table 11-1. Results of Thromboplastin Generation Test on Patients with Various Coagulation Defects*

Incubation Mixture Number	Source of Reagents			Type of Coagulation Defect						
	Al(OH)₃= Adsorbed Alumina Plasma	Serum	Platelet Suspension	Factor VIII	IX Factor	X Factor	V Factor	Factor VII	Thrombas-thenia	Circulating anticoagulants
1	Normal	Normal	Normal	Normal	Normal	Normal	Normal	Normal	Normal	Normal
2	Patient	Normal	Normal	Abnormal	Normal	Normal	Abnormal	Normal	Normal	May be abnormal
3	Normal	Patient	Normal	Normal	Abnormal; corrected only by normal serum	Abnormal	Normal	Normal	Normal	May be abnormal
4	Normal	Normal	Patient	Normal	Normal	Normal	Normal	Normal	Abnormal	Normal
5	Patient	Patient	Patient	Abnormal†	Abnormal†	Abnormal†	Abnormal	Normal	Abnormal†	Abnormal†

* Miale, J. B.: Laboratory Medicine-Hematology, ed. 2, p. 876. St. Louis, C. V. Mosby, 1962.
† Almost always more abnormal than the results from single substitutions.

mal plasma. In tests on patients with mild Factor IX deficiency, this may be a source of difficulty—that is, the amount remaining in the plasma may be enough to correct the defect almost completely. Readsorption of the normal plasma, or use of plasma obtained from patients severely deficient in Factor IX, may obviate this difficulty. (2) Precautions taken in whole blood clotting and prothrombin times must be observed.

Results

Normal Values. The thromboplastin generation test is usually positive when AHF, PTC, or other factors are reduced to less than 20 per cent of normal, although nearly normal results are occasionally recorded when the level is about 10 per cent of normal.[15] Therefore, a value of 8 to 14 seconds, occurring at any time during the test, is evidence of the normal generation of thromboplastin. One run with the three normal reagents is included in all instances in which unknown blood is studied because this gives the control value for 100 per cent generation. To repeat, the greatest usefulness of the TGT is in the study and differentiation of deficiencies of Factors VIII, IX, and X, and in the demonstration and titration of abnormal circulating anticoagulants (Table 11-1).

To summarize: (1) In AHG deficiency, the patient's generation time should be corrected when normal plasma is substituted. (2) In PTC deficiency, the patient's generation time is corrected by substituting normal serum. (3) In PTA deficiency, the patient's generation time is corrected by substituting either normal plasma or normal serum. (4) In Stuart-Prower deficiency, the patient's generation time is corrected by substituting normal serum.

THROMBOPLASTIN SCREENING TEST

A useful variation of the TGT is the thromboplastin screening test of Hicks and Pitney.[22] In this test, diluted citrated plasma is recalcified in the presence of a platelet substrate, and the thromboplastin generation is assayed by adding subsample aliquots of the incubating mixture together with calcium to high-spun, normal plasma (substrate). The clotting time of the substrate is a measure of the thromboplastic activity of the added subsample aliquot.

This procedure is a nonspecific screening test for deficiencies of the thromboplastin generation components. In the actual process, nine parts of blood is added to one part of 3.8 per cent sodium citrate, mixed and centrifuged for 5 minutes at 2000 r.p.m. The plasma is then removed and used within 2 hours after blood collection; it should be refrigerated if it is not tested immediately. One part of the plasma (unknown or normal plasma control) is diluted with nine parts of Owren's veronal buffer solution. This is mixed well, allowed to stand for 1 hour at room temperature, and then tested immediately. For maximum activation, a pipette is placed in diluted plasma while standing.

Technique

In the actual procedure, a tube containing 0.02 M $CaCl_2$ is placed in a 37° C water bath for 2 to 3 minutes. Into each of two (75 × 12 mm.) unsiliconized test tubes is pipetted 0.1 ml. of normal plasma, and this is placed in a 37° C water bath. Into another 75 × 12 mm. test tube 0.2 ml. of prestandardized platelet factor substitute (Cephaloplastin*) is pipetted and allowed to warm at 37° C. To this is added 0.2 ml. of diluted plasma (unknown or control). This is allowed to warm 1 minute, and 0.2 ml. of prewarmed 0.02 ml. $CaCl_2$ is rapidly blown into it. The stopwatch is started, the tube is well shaken and it is returned to the water bath. This is the generation mixture. After adding $CaCl_2$, an applicator stick is placed in the generation mixture.

---

* Produced by Scientific Products Co., Evanston, Illinois.

The clot, which may form in about 2 minutes, is easily withdrawn by removing the stick. At the end of 3 minutes, 0.1 ml. of prewarmed CaCl₂ is pipetted into a tube of normal plasma substrate, and 0.1 ml. of the generation mixture is blown into the tube as rapidly as possible. Simultaneously, a second stopwatch is started, and the formation of the clot is timed. At the end of 5 minutes (on the first watch), 0.1 ml. of prewarmed CaCl₂ is pipetted into a second tube of normal plasma substrate, and as rapidly as possible 0.1 ml. of the generation mixture is blown into the tube. Simultaneously, the second stopwatch is started, and the formation of the clot is timed.

The sources of error in this test are the same as in the thromboplastin generation test.

Results

Normal Values. A normal plasma control should always be run along with an unknown. Normal clotting time is 7 to 12 seconds after a generation time of 5 minutes or less. The difference between the time of a normal and a pathologic plasma is large enough so that slight differences due to technique or reagents are not critical.

Significance of Abnormal Results. This test is a sensitive, quick, and practical way of demonstrating defects of coagulation too small to lead to prolongation of the whole-blood clotting time. It is simpler than, and is at least as sensitive as, the orthodox TGT is in demonstrating the defect in hemophilia and Christmas disease. In fact the test has been observed to be positive in a patient with mild hemophilia and with an AHF level of 38 per cent of normal. Substrate clotting times are also prolonged in PTA (Factor XI) deficiency and in the Hageman trait (Factor XII). Biggs and MacFarlane found it more sensitive than the TGT in detecting PTA and Hageman factor deficiency.[4] To distinguish the latter two conditions, the indirect test of Margolis is very helpful.[28] In it the test plasma is activated with glass, and aliquots are added to normal

intact plasma. This plasma is recalcified in the presence of lysed platelets in siliconed tubes and if the test plasma is deficient in Hageman factor, the clotting time of the intact normal plasma is not shortened as it would be if the test plasma were deficient in PTA (but with a normal complement of Hageman factor).

In the Hicks-Pitney test, normal results may or may not be obtained with the plasma of patients receiving anticoagulants therapeutically. This depends on the extent of the depression of Christmas factor (IX) and Factor X. Abnormal results are obtained in the presence of spontaneously developing anticoagulants. The test is insensitive to thrombocytopenia because the role of platelets in coagulation is by-passed by the addition of the lipoid.

TEST FOR PLATELET FACTOR 3 FUNCTION

Several tests have been described in which the intrinsic thromboplastin generating ability (platelet factor 3 function) of a patient's platelets is compared in thromboplastin-generation tests with that of normal control platelets (properly washed suspensions). For reliable results the platelet suspension should be accurately counted and diluted up to 10,000 to 25,000 per cu.mm. Such tests are time-consuming and suffer from the difficulty of obtaining sufficient platelets from severely thrombocytopenic purpuric patients to carry out the test. These tests may, however, demonstrate a defect, particularly if weak platelets suspensions are used, whereas other tests fail to demonstrate conclusively any abnormality. A convenient and apparently sensitive screening test for platelet function is a comparison of the kaolin recalcification times of a patient's platelet-rich and platelet-poor plasma. A fairly simple platelet thromboplastic function test, although two stages, compares favorably with the orthodox TGT.[6]

Technique

The procedure is a two-stage partial thromboplastin time (PTT) test in which brain residue, normal serum, and a standard suspension of washed platelets are incubated in the presence of added calcium at 37° C. After 15 to 20 minutes, the mixture is tested for thromboplastic activity by adding a subsample with additional calcium to normal citrated plasma. The amount of thromboplastin generated and the rate at which the reaction takes place depend on the quality of the platelets, as well as on plasma factors. Platelet factor 3 is necessary for adequate thromboplastin generation and is measured by using a very dilute suspension of platelets, as in the TGT.

In the test, 0.1 ml. of undiluted serum is added to a button of platelets (citrated plasma from the patient and normal control citrated plasma is collected in siliconized tubes). Platelet counts are carried out on the plasmas and the volumes calculated to contain 200×10^6 platelets. These are pipetted into siliconized tubes and centrifuged at 3000 r.p.m. for 15 minutes. After centrifuging, the supernatant plasma is removed, and the platelet buttons are gently washed in saline solution. This process is repeated, and the washing saline solution is then removed as completely as possible (using blotting paper to mop up saline droplets adhering to the side of the tube) in the siliconized tubes. The platelets are then emulsified in the serum using a wooden swab-stick. One milliliter of brain residue* suspension is then added and after waiting 2 to 3 minutes for the suspension to warm to 37° C in the water bath, 1 ml. of $CaCl_2$ solution (0.025 M) is added. After 15 and 20 minutes of incubation, 0.1 ml. aliquots and 0.1 ml. of calcium chloride are added to 0.1 ml. volumes of normal high-spun citrated plasma in unsiliconized tubes. The clotting times at the two times are usually identical. The test is carried out at the same time with normal platelets.

Results

A calibration graph is prepared by washing a series of dilutions of a suspension of normal platelets so that in the tests the platelet number ranges from 20×10^6 to 200×10^6. The reciprocals of the platelet numbers plotted against substrate clotting times give a straight line. The function of the test platelets can be recorded as a percentage of normal — that is, a 1 per cent suspension gives maximum generation in 9 to 12 seconds in the second or third tube, and a 0.33 per cent suspension gives a minimal clotting time of 16.5 to 18.5 seconds in the fourth or fifth tube.

Thrombocytopathic platelets generate at a slower rate (tube 6, 7 or 8), or maximal generation takes place in the fourth or fifth tube, the minimal clotting time is longer (over 18.5 seconds). The percentage of platelet factor 3 activity is determined from a dilution curve prepared from normal platelets.[12]

Significance of Abnormal Results. The results correlate more closely with bleeding episodes in idiopathic thrombocytopenic purpura than do those from the measurement of platelet numbers; therefore, both a qualitative defect and a quantitative defect are probably suggested in idiopathic thrombocytopenic purpura. About half the patients with uremic bleeding show abnormal in vivo platelet adhesiveness and availability of platelet factor 3. Approximately half the uremic patients without bleeding also show reduced platelet aggregation and clot retraction, Ivy bleeding time, in vivo platelet adhesiveness, and normal platelet factor 3 tests. Therefore, impaired aggregation and adhesiveness suggest an abnormality of the platelet surface, as does the correction of the tests of platelet-coagulant function by mechanical disruption of the platelets. Platelet factor 3 is apparently present, but

---

* A 10 per cent suspension in saline of the residue left after five extractions with chloroform of the acetone-dried human brain is suspended in 0.5 per cent phenol in saline solution. It is kept for 1 month at 20° C.

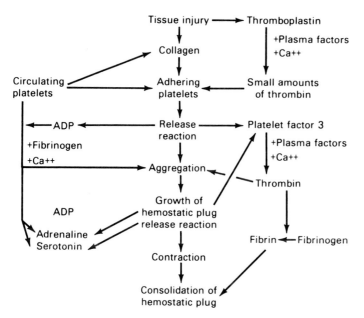

Fig. 11-2. Dynamics of hemostasis. (Luscher, E. F.: Biochemical basis of platelet function. *In* Brinkhous, K. (ed.): The Platelet. International Academy of Pathology monographs. Baltimore, Williams & Wilkens, 1971)

in uremia, contact fails to release it satisfactorily.[8]

PLATELET AGGREGATION AND INSTRUMENTATION

It is well known that platelets participate in hemostasis in both the formation of the primary hemostatic plug and the intrinsic coagulation mechanism. (See Chap. 10 for a discussion of the physical properties, development, function, and physiologic and pathologic variations of platelets and of the factors governing hemostasis.) Platelets adhere to the damaged blood vessel wall, release constituents from their granules, which include platelet factor 3 and adenosine diphosphate (ADP), and then aggregate to form the primary hemostatic plug. Luscher has diagramatically described the dynamics of hemostasis including the role of platelets in Figure 11-2.[26]

Platelet aggregation is clinically significant in the detection and diagnosis of acquired or congenital qualitative or functional platelet defects. The platelet's ability or inability to respond to particular aggregating agents is the basis for differentiating

platelet dysfunctions. For example, adenosine diphosphate is ultimately responsible for platelet aggregation. The term "aggregation" refers to the ability of platelets to stick to one another. Agents other than adenosine diphosphate (i.e., thrombin, epinephrine, collagen, etc.) are able to induce aggregation either alone or by causing the release of endogenous adenosine diphosphate from the platelets.

Primary aggregation, or the first wave of aggregation, is the direct aggregation of platelets by adenosine diphosphate or other aggregating agents. Primary aggregation is accompanied by a shape change and is a reversible process; it is normally followed by secondary aggregation, or the second wave. Secondary aggregation is irreversible and is accompanied by the extrusion of the contents of the granules found in the platelets' cytoplasm.

Platelet aggregation may be observed by use of a platelet aggregometer (Figs. 11-7; 11-8). This is a photo-optical instrument connected to a strip chart recorder. Platelet-rich plasma, which is turbid, is stirred in a cuvette, and the increase of light transmittance, over a platelet-poor standard,

	Platelet Aggregation by ADP	Platelet Aggregation by Epinephrine and Collagen
Thrombasthenia	Abnormal	Abnormal
Thrombopathia or thrombocytopathy	Normal (first phase)	Abnormal
Von Willebrand's disease	Normal	Normal
Non-Steroidal, anti-inflammatory drugs	Normal (first phase)	Abnormal

Fig. 11-3. Aggregation studies on selected platelet function defects. (Courtesy of Bio-Data Corp.)

through the sample is recorded. When an aggregating agent is added to the platelet-rich plasma, the formation of increasingly large platelet aggregates is accompanied by a clearance in the plasma; therefore, the light transmittance through the sample is converted into electronic signals, amplified, and recorded. In other words, more light passes through a suspension of aggregated platelets than through a suspension of non-aggregated platelets. The degree by which platelets aggregate is determined by measuring the resultant decrease in optical density.

METHODOLOGY

Adenosine diphosphate, collagen, and epinephrine are the three most commonly used aggregating agents (Fig. 11-3). These may be obtained in kit form* or may be easily be prepared in the laboratory. ADP induces the biphasic aggregation response; the second phase or irreversible aggregation is caused by the release of endogenous ADP. As Figure 11-4 shows, at high or strong concentrations, only a single broad wave of aggregation will occur.

Epinephrine will also produce a biphasic aggregation response and usually without an intervening lag (Fig. 11-6). The plasma sample should sit undisturbed at room temperature for at least 30 minutes before the

epinephrine is introduced, or an abnormal response may result. Approximately 40 per cent of normal people will exhibit only a primary wave of aggregation with epinephrine. Aggregation with epinephrine is abnormal in conditions that are characterized as release-mechanism failures, for example, thrombopathia. A number of therapeutic agents containing aspirin are known to inhibit platelet aggregation.

Collagen induces only a secondary wave of aggregation, which corresponds to the release reaction of platelets (i.e., the release of endogenous ADP). A typical collagen curve is characterized by a lag period before aggregation begins; platelet swelling may occur at the end of the lag. There is no disaggregation (Fig. 11-6).

Thrombin, as an aggregating agent, induces both a primary and a secondary wave of aggregation. The concentration of the thrombin must be carefully controlled since fibrin formation will occur at higher concentrations. Serotonin will normally produce a wave of aggregation that attains a maximum of 10 to 30 per cent transmittance, which is immediately followed by disaggregation (Fig. 11-5). Maximal aggregation will not be produced if the serotonin concentration is either higher or lower than the optimum. A biphasic response has been reported in a significant number of women. Arachidonic acid is a free fatty acid that induces platelet aggregation and prostaglandin synthesis by the platelet.

* PAR/PAK. Catalog No. 100715. Bio/Data Corp., 3941 Commerce Avenue, Willow Grove, Pa. 19090.

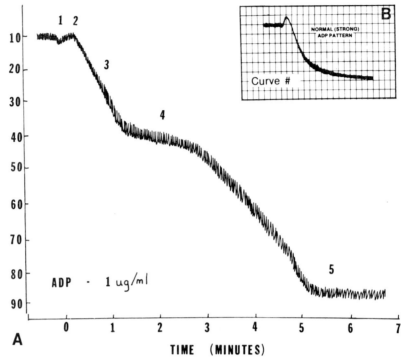

Fig. 11-4. (*A*) Normal changes in per cent transmittance during aggregation. Key: (1) Slight increase due to dilution with aggregating agent. (2) Slight decrease due to platelet swelling or shape change. (3) Progressive increase as platelet aggregates form. (4) Release reaction occurs — begins secondary wave. (5) Maximal aggregation. (*B*) Normal (strong) ADP pattern with single broad wave of aggregation. (Courtesy of Bio-Data Corp.)

Ristocetin is an antibiotic derived from *Nocardia lurida* that induces a biphasic aggregation response, although this is often obscured and appears as a single broad wave. Platelet aggregation with Ristocetin may be reduced or absent in von Willebrand's syndrome, but will correct to normal when normal platelet-poor plasma is added. Abnormal Ristocetin aggregation may occur in several disease states other than von Willebrand's syndrome.

Spontaneous aggregation may occur upon stirring of platelet-rich plasma without the addition of any aggregating agent. This may be indicative of a hypercoagulable state.

A clean, atraumatic venipuncture is recommended in obtaining blood specimens for aggregation studies. Poor venipuncture techniques have been reported to be associated with increased aggregation patterns. Hemolysis must be avoided because red cells contain ADP, which may be released into the plasma. A plastic syringe must be used.

Sodium citrate is the anticoagulant of choice for platelet aggregation specimens. Calcium ions are necessary for aggregation to occur, so the degree of calcium binding, which is dependent on the concentration of the sodium citrate, is critical. A weak concentration of sodium citrate, 0.11 M, has been most commonly used. At this concentration of citrate, free calcium ions will be present in an amount sufficient for aggregation to occur. The 0.11 M sodium citrate should be mixed in a ratio of one part citrate to nine parts whole blood. This ratio may be adjusted to variations of the hematocrit outside the normal range. The blood

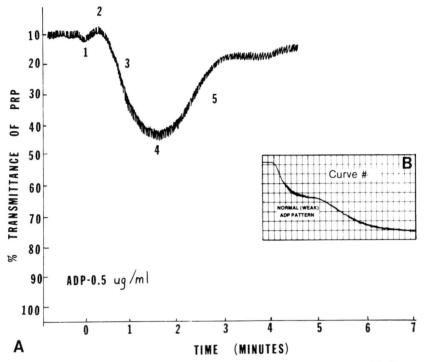

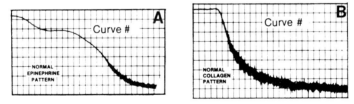

Fig. 11-5. (*A*) Changes in per cent transmittance during aggregation with disaggregation. Key: (1) Slight increase due to dilution with aggregating agent. (2) Slight decrease due to platelet swelling or shape change. (3) Progressive increase as platelet aggregates form. (4) Maximal aggregation occurs. (5) Decrease due to disaggregation. (*B*) Normal (wear) ADP pattern with lag period followed by secondary aggregation. (Courtesy of Bio-Data Corp.)

Fig. 11-6. (*A*) Biphasic aggregation response without intervening lag. (*B*) Typical collagen curve showing lag period before aggregation begins. (Courtesy of Bio-Data Corp.)

sample should be mixed gently with the anticoagulant in a plastic tube.

The blood and plasma preparations for aggregation studies should not come into contact with glass. Plastic or siliconized glass syringes, test tubes, specimen containers and pipettes must be used. Platelets may adhere to glass surfaces and thus affect aggregation results.

Aggregation studies are performed on platelet-rich plasma. To obtain platelet-rich plasma, the blood specimen is centrifuged slowly at room temperature at approximately $100 \times g$ for 10 to 15 minutes. The platelet-rich plasma is removed carefully with a plastic pipette to avoid any red cell contamination. The remaining blood is recentrifuged at approximately $1400 \times g$ for at least ten minutes to obtain platelet-poor plasma. The platelet-rich plasma may be diluted with the platelet-poor plasma to a standard platelet concentration before the test is performed. Lipemic plasmas may cause difficulties in aggregation testing, since the aggregometers operate on a photo-optical principle. It may also be difficult to perform aggregation studies on thrombocytopenic specimens because the difference in the optical density between the platelet-rich and platelet-poor plasmas is so small. Difficulties will be encountered with platelet counts of fewer than 50,000 per ml. of platelet-rich plasma, or 75,000 per ml. of platelet-rich plasma, when epinephrine is used as the aggregating agent.

Variations in the response of platelets to various aggregating agents occur as the time interval increases between venipuncture and plasma preparation, and the performance of the test. When aggregation studies are performed immediately after the sample collection and preparation, the platelets will be less responsive than if stored at room temperature for 1 hour as platelet-rich plasma. After 3 hours, platelet responsiveness to aggregating agents will also decrease. Ideally, platelet aggregation studies should be performed within a maximum of 3 hours following venipuncture.

The platelet-rich plasma used for aggregation tests should be stored at room temperature until immediately before performance of the test, at which time the plasma is warmed to 37° C. Storage of platelet-rich plasma at cold temperatures increases the tendency toward spontaneous aggregation. Storage of platelet-rich plasma at 37° C results in the loss of platelet responsiveness much more quickly than when stored at room temperature. Platelets stored at room temperature are more sensitive to various aggregating agents, especially ADP, but must be warmed to 37° C immediately prior to testing because the release reaction is absent at temperatures below 33° C.

Fibrinogen must be present in the sample for aggregation to occur. In afibrinogenemic specimens, abnormal aggregation patterns will appear, but will normalize upon the addition of exogenous fibrinogen. Other plasma proteins that promote aggregation, but are not required, include gamma globulins, Hageman factor, and Factor V (platelet cofactor 1), which adheres to the surface of the platelet. Potassium ions will also promote aggregation.

Mechanical motion, such as stirring, is necessary to bring the platelets in platelet-rich plasma into contact with each other, thereby permitting aggregation to occur. Aggregation patterns will vary with stirring speed, as well as with the shape and size of the stir bar. The specimen should be at a pH of 6.8 to 8.5 for optimal aggregation results. Generally, no aggregation will occur below a pH of 6.4 or above a pH of 10.0. Changes in the pH of the specimen may be kept to a minimum by keeping the time interval between venipuncture and performance of the test within the recommended limits, infrequent mixing of the sample, and capping the specimen to minimize air contact and loss of carbon dioxide.

A normal, control plasma should be run with each aggregation test performed, primarily as a check of the aggregating agents, and for comparison with the patient's record. The donor should be questioned carefully about drug ingestion, especially the use of aspirin or other drugs that affect platelet function, in the preceding 7 to 10 days. Aspirin inhibits the secondary aggregation induced by ADP and epinephrine, delays and inhibits collagen-induced aggregation, and impairs Ristocetin aggregation. Aspirin will also affect aggregation with arachidonic acid, since aspirin inhibits the enzyme cyclo-oxygenase that is required to convert arachidonic acid, the thromboxane A_2, and other prostaglandins. The patient must also be carefully questioned about a drug history. The effects of such agents may last 7 to 10 days after ingestion. Since aggregation may be dependent on platelet concentration in some aggregometer and coagulation profile instruments, thrombocytopenia may yield poor aggregation patterns.

Qualitative platelet disorders are very common if the many acquired platelet dysfunctional states are included. The following list presents the disorders associated with decreased platelet aggregation:

Hereditary Disorders

Glanzmann's disease
Storage pool defect (decreased content of ADP)
   Chediak Higashi syndrome
   TAR syndrome
   Wiskott Aldrich syndrome
   Hermansky Pudlak syndrome
Inborn errors of metabolism
   Homocystinuria
   Wilson's disease
Connective tissue abnormalities
   Ehlers Danlos syndrome (collagen)
   Pseudoxanthoma elasticum (collagen)
   Osteogenesis imperfecta (collagen)
   Marfan's syndrome
   Constitutional abnormality of collagen (Caen)
Afibrinogenemia
Essential athrombia
Bernard—Soulier (Ristocetin)
von Willebrand's syndrome (Ristocetin)
Swiss cheese platelets
Gray platelet syndrome

Acquired Disorders

Myeloproliferative disorders
   Polycythemia rubra vera
   Myeloid metaplasia
   Hemorrhagic thrombocythemia
   Paroxysmal nocturnal hemoglobinuria
   Di Guglielmo's syndrome
   Chronic myelocytic leukemia
   Acute myelomonocytic leukemia
   Sideroblastic anemias
Immunoproliferative disorders
   Waldenström's macroglobulinemia
   Plasma cell myeloma
Cirrhosis
Uremia
Hypothyroidism (often has decreased Factor VIII levels)
Pernicious anemia
Platelets in idiopathic thrombocytopenic purpura
Drugs (e.g. aspirin, etc.)

Clinical evidence, such as mucosal bleeding or easy bruising, should suggest a qualitative disorder of platelets. It should also be suspected if there is laboratory evidence, such as a prolonged bleeding time in the face of a normal platelet count. In such cases, platelet aggregation studies are usually indicated. A correlation between platelet aggregation and HL-A histocompatibility has also been noted. Family members with negative aggregation were selected as donors, and their platelets were able to provide consistently satisfactory increments in the platelet count of the recipient, who was refractory to random donors. In contrast, platelets from family members who exhibited positive aggregation failed to provide satisfactory increases. These findings suggest that platelet aggregometry may be used to select compatible platelet donors.[45]

Factors That Affect Aggregation Testing

These include:

Time, for example, is important to an accurate aggregation study. The specimen must sit for 30 minutes to an hour before it is tested. It appears that platelets need this amount of time to adjust to their new environment. Yet aggregation must also be completed within 2 to 3 hours after the specimen is drawn, if the study is to be accurate. Beyond this length of time, platelets begin to lose some of their activity.

Centrifugation is also important to the outcome of testing. Speed and duration of spin-down usually depend on the size, diameter, and type of equipment being used. When technologists are preparing platelet-rich plasma and platelet-poor plasma, they must be careful to observe appropriate centrifugation speed and time. They must also allow the centrifuge to stop gradually. Poor spin-down can result in poor sample preparation. Red blood cells, for instance, may still be present in the plasma, and these will interfere with testing.

Certain surface exposures must be avoided. Platelets, for example, will adhere to glass. For this reason, plastic or siliconized glass should be employed in testing. Glass must never be used, since it can affect the ability of platelets to aggregate, and a perfectly healthy patient may appear to have an abnormality.

Drugs such as aspirin, anticoagulants, and nonsteroid, anti-inflammatory agents may interfere with aggregation.

Drugs That Inhibit Platelet Aggregation*

Aminopyrine (Pyramidon)
Aspirin and aspirin containing proprietary drugs
Atromid (clofibrate)
Anturane (sulfinpyrazone)
Dextran
Dextropropoxyphene (doloxene)
Dipyridamole (Persantine)
Furosemide (Lasix)
Glyceryl Guaiacolate
Heparin
Ibufenac (Dytransin)
Ibuprofen (Motrin)
Indomethacin (Indocin)
Imipramine
Meclofenamic acid
Mefenamic acid (ponstan)
Nitrofurantoin (Furadantin)
Paracetamol
Phenothiazines
Phenylbutazone
Volatile general anesthetics

---

* Courtesy Ball Memorial Hospital, Muncie, Indiana.

Technologists should be aware of drug interference, and patients should be questioned about these agents. The patient history should be checked prior to testing for any information about a substance that might alter the ability of platelets to function normally.

Changes in pH also may affect testing. If a sample or reagent is left uncovered, CO_2 may escape from the sample. This causes a change in pH and pH changes affect the ability of platelets to adhere to one another. A loss of CO_2 can be prevented by covering the specimen or reagent with parafilm, placing it in a special incubation chamber, or, if the specimen has been drawn into a syringe, sealing the syringe and removing all air bubbles.

Sample handling, too, is important to the outcome of these assays. Technologists and physicians must watch their technique when they are drawing specimens for these studies. The sample should be drawn into plastic or siliconized syringes or tubes, and mixed gently with the anticoagulant. If it is mishandled and clots or lyses, the test results will be highly inaccurate.

Care must be taken about the amount and type of anticoagulant used. It is recommended that nine parts of blood be drawn into plastic or siliconized syringes or tubes containing one part sodium citrate. The amount of anticoagulant should also be adjusted to the condition of the patient. If the patient is anemic, for example, more anticoagulant should be added, since this patient has more plasma than a normal person.

Reagents, too, play a very important role in aggregation studies. There are a number of reagents commercially available for these tests, and many labs run more than one. Each of these aggregating substances behaves differently, and a laboratory should work with an agent for a period of time to evaluate its effect on platelet function. Some reagents, such as ADP and epinephrine, produce biphasic responses, while collagen produces a monophasic reaction. The curves that a particular reagent elicits will vary from hospital to hospital. Therefore, many experts recommend that reagents be tested in the lab, to familiarize personnel with the specific preparation requirements of the substances, the response of the reagent, and outdating periods for their supplies.

Quality Control. Aggregation studies can provide useful information if the quality control of the lab is good. Personnel must be experienced in this technique. A normal control should be run each day as part of the laboratory quality control program. Results from the normal controls should be plotted each day to show any day-to-day variation in reagents. It is recommended that the test be done frequently, and that an institution devote one full-time experienced and trained person to perform these assays.

PLATELET RETENTION OR ADHESIVENESS TESTING

Glass Bead Platelet Retention Testing

The basic principle in platelet retention or adhesiveness testing is to expose platelets in a blood sample to a glass bead surface, and then measure the number of platelets that are retained by the beads.

One method of platelet retention testing draws the blood sample directly from the patient's arm and passes through a specially prepared glass bead column. The platelet count on this specimen is then compared to the patient's circulating platelet count, and the percentage of platelets retained by the beads is calculated.

Another method of this type of testing draws the blood sample into a syringe, and a Harvard infusion pump is used to pass the blood through the column. This controls the rate at which the sample moves through the glass bead column. The fourth and fifth milliliters are used for platelet counts, and the average of the results from these two counts is then compared to the original platelet count.

The two major difficulties with these procedures are standardization and procurement of supplies. There are only a few companies making the tubing and beads that are necessary for the columns, and once a laboratory receives these supplies, it must standardize its own test. The beads an institution receives are often a size and diameter different from the beads another hospital has obtained. Normal values from laboratory to laboratory may range from 85-per-cent retention to as little as 25-per-cent retention, depending on the supplies and procedures for making the column. The rate of flow over the beads must also be

specific. If the blood flows too quickly, platelet retention will be falsely decreased. Yet if the blood flows too slowly through the column, the platelets will spontaneously adhere to the beads and retention will be falsely increased. Moisture can also affect the glass bead columns and affect the rate of flow. It is, therefore, recommended that the columns be kept in a dessicator when humidity is high.

Borshgervinct Method of Retention Testing

This technique evaluates platelet adhesiveness in vivo. In this procedure a bleeding time is performed, but instead of blotting the blood droplets with filter paper from the wound every 30 seconds, a platelet count is taken from the incision. The platelet count should decrease as the clot forms, in normal patients. If the count does not decrease considerably, there is an abnormality in platelet function. In order to control the depth of the incision and the ease of performing the test, it is suggested that the template bleeding time be used. This controls the incision, and the technologist is free to work out a routine method for performing the assay.[41]

INSTRUMENTATION

Platelet Aggregation Profiler, Model PAP-3

The Profiler manufactured by Bio/ DATA Corp., employs a photo-optical scanning system, a continuous differential amplifier system, and a system for automatic recorder standardization. In operation, two samples of the plasma specimen, one platelet-rich and one platelet-poor, are inserted into the optical test wells. Light emitted from the source is transmitted through each of the samples to photodetectors designed to respond accurately and rapidly to variations in the initial density of the test plasmas as well as to any change in density caused by the aggregation of the platelets. These light signals are fed into a special amplifier system that provides an amplified signal to the chart recorder based

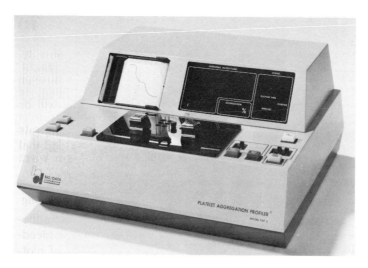

Fig. 11-7. Platelet Aggregation Profiler, Model PAP-3. (Courtesy of Bio-Data Corp.)

upon a continuous differential comparison of the platelet-rich and platelet-poor test specimens. Following this amplification, the electronic signals are fed into a galvanometer-actuated recorder. The recorder is controlled, in part, by specialized circuitry that automatically standardizes the recorder for full-scale deflection, based upon the initial density levels of the test specimens. All manual adjustments or readjustments are eliminated as a result (Fig. 11-7).

Advantages. The Profiler provides a simple push-button method for studying platelet function and platelet capability. Its complete test procedure and instrument operational status are automatically programmed and displayed on an illuminated screen. This provides error-free testing and control in all aggregation studies. It automatically provides a continuous differential comparison of the platelet-rich and platelet-poor plasmas, reducing the time required for instrument set-up, standardization, and restandardization. It automatically standardizes its chart recorder for full-scale deflection, eliminating the need for manual adjustment and readjustment of the baseline.

Disadvantages. Lipemic plasmas may cause difficulty in aggregation testing since

aggregometers operate on a photo-optical principle. It may be difficult to perform aggregation studies on thrombocytopenic specimens because the difference in the optical density between the specimens that are platelet-rich and those that are platelet-poor is very small. Difficulties will be encountered with platelet counts of less than 50,000 per ml. or of less than 75,000 per ml. when epinephrine is used as the aggregating agent. Platelet aggregation studies are highly responsive to storage time. That is, the ideal time for conducting tests is 1 to 3 hours following venepuncture and storage as platelet-rich plasma. Tests using this instrument must be performed frequently and must be performed by one full-time and experienced medical technologist. Finally, results from controls must be plotted each day on a graph to determine if there is a day-to-day variation in reagents.

Chrono-Log Platelet Aggregometer Model 330

The Aggregometer has a simple operating procedure that is screened on the Aggregometer panel (Fig. 11-8). A cuvette containing 0.4 ml. of platelet-poor plasma (PPP) is inserted into the temperature-controlled holder, and a single knob adjustment

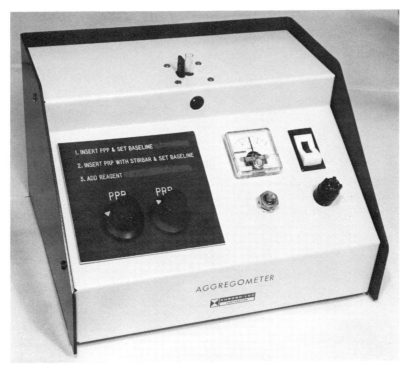

Fig. 11-8. Chrono-Log Aggregometer Model 330. (Courtesy of Chrono-Log Corp.)

sets the PPP baseline to record the 100 per cent aggregation level on the chart. Then, a cuvette containing 0.4 ml. of platelet-rich plasma is inserted, a magnetic stirrer is added, and a single knob adjustment sets the PRP baseline to record the 0 per cent aggregation reading. The aggregating reagent (ADP, epinephrine, collagen, etc.) is added, and the resulting platelet aggregation curve is recorded in the strip chart recorder (Chrono-Log Model 702 Strip Chart Recorder). As the platelets in the plasma aggregate, the solution becomes progressively clearer, causing an increase in light passing through the solution and a continuous positive rise of the recorder pen on the chart. As the platelet aggregates increase in size, they are turned by the stirrer and periodically interrupt the light beam; this produces oscillations in the record roughly proportional to the aggregate size. In this way, the chart record shows the delay (lag period; Fig. 11-9) prior to the start of ag-

gregation, the rate of aggregation, and the amount of aggregation. De-aggregation is clearly indicated by the reversal of the record.

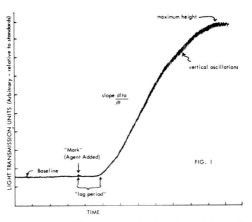

Fig. 11-9. Chart record showing delay (lag period) prior to the start of aggregation, the rate of aggregation, and the amount of aggregation using the Chrono-Log Platelet Aggregometer. (Courtesy of Chrono-Log Corp.)

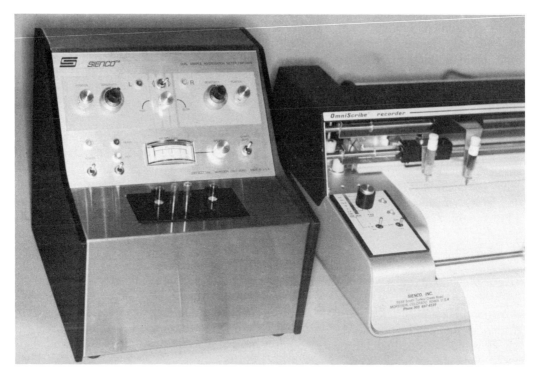

Fig. 11-10. Sienco Dual Sample Aggregometer Model DP-247-D-E. (Courtesy of Sienco, Inc.)

Advantages. Only 0.4 ml. of sample required by the Aggregometer. Its cuvette holder, with proportional controller, accurately and constantly maintains 37° C. The temperature of the cuvette holder is indicated directly on the temperature meter. There is controlled magnetic stirring at 1200 r.p.m. It accommodates a wide range of optical filters (e.g., replaceable optic filters for other tests). Its observation port permits visual examination of sample during test (i.e., viewing the clumping action). It is very sensitive to the optical changes that are used to measure aggregation and also provides the PRP and PPP baselines that are needed to define fully the test and quantitate the results. It uses 5 in. wide chart paper (compared to 3⅛ in. wide paper used by other instruments); this provides increased resolution. With this instrument, it is also possible to use other strip chart recorders if one desires wider displays, since any null-balance recorder can be used. It can add a Differentiator to plot the rate of change of the aggregation curve, as well as the amplitude.

Disadvantages are the same as for the Platelet Aggregation Profiler, described above.

Sienco-Dual Sample Aggregometer Model DP-247-D-E

Figure 11-10 shows an all solid-state instrument with the ability to multiplex. It combines data from its two independent channels onto one strip chart recorder; it permits the simultaneous input on a single pen strip chart recorder of two platelet aggregation curves obtained under identical conditions. The superimposition of the curves facilitates the visual or mathematical assessment of differences in the aggregation pattern.

Operating Instructions. (1) Turn on LINE switch and HEAT switch. (2) Heater block should be at operating temperature, 37.0° C indicated by READY light. (3) Turn stirrer to speed desired (1000 r.p.m. is a common value). (4) Set SENSITIVITY dial to 100 (1 turn out of 10) as a starting point. (5) Depress CHART ZERO button and, with the recorder's own zero control, adjust the 10-millivolt recorder to a convenient zero point a few divisions from the down-scale chart edge. (6) Place cuvette containing platelet-rich plasma and a stirring bar into the left channel. Filters should be in place. Using the left POSITION control, set pen to previously established zero point on recorder (Step (5)).

Coleman cuvettes must be aligned with the etched label pointed toward the filter position. Rotate a cuvette experimentally to observe the optical differences that result. The recommended volume of fluid for use with the 10-mm. cuvettes is 1 cc. (7) Replace the sample with a cuvette containing platelet-poor plasma. Using the SENSITIVITY control, adjust the pen to the desired up-scale position (a cm. or 2 from the edge of the chart is suggested). Plain water is frequently substituted for PPP, although the lack of coloration may result in a reduced chart span when the plasmas are dark-colored. (8) Repeat step 6 for a shift in the zero point. Left channel is now ready to run. (9) Repeat (6), (7), and (8) on the right channel. The PRP setting from step (6) may be offset to avoid coincidental tracings. (10) The instrument is now ready for aggregation determinations. The instrument is very sensitive and will detect ambient illumination if it is directed into the cuvettes. Cover the cuvettes with the light shield provided. (11) To take advantage of the multiplex capabilities of the Sienco Dual Sample Aggregation Meter, the top center switch is moved to the center position. The instrument will then automatically alternate its output signal from the left and right channels in accordance with the rate set by the center knob. Anticlockwise rotation of the rate knob gives short duration down to about 2 seconds per channel, and clockwise

rotation increases the duration for each channel display up to about 80 seconds. Each channel receives equal display time. A figure of about 10 seconds is quite useful for most procedures. For instruments that have the special option of two pairs of output terminals, the left channel is tied at all times to the central pair of binding posts labeled LEFT ONLY, and the multiplex capability is tied to the other pair of binding posts labeled BOTH. Therefore when using two recorders, the left channel may be fed to one recorder, and the second recorder continues to have available to it, at the operator's discretion, right channel or left channel (duplication) or both on multiplex alternation. The manner in which the dual channel output is used has no effect upon the left channel output. (12) Observe good housekeeping. Clean all spills immediately and avoid contaminating the controls with wet hands. Various makes of recorders may have their zero on the right side or on the left side of the chart; therefore, the data presented here refer to UP SCALE (increasing signal), and DOWN SCALE (smaller signal) pen position to avoid confusion.

Advantages. Two samples may be run simultaneously: unknown and standard, unknown and blank, or two unknowns. Two outputs feed into one recorder. Any 10-millivolt recorder may be used. Either channel may be held for continuous recording. It uses standard round or square precision cuvettes. The magnetic stirring is identical for both samples. The rate of stirring is adjustable and indicated on panel meter. Temperature is controlled at 37° C. It has operator-controlled time cycles on multiplex operation and removable filters. It has a life-time solid state light source of optimal wave length and all solid-state circuitry, with very conservative ratings for trouble-free operation. Each channel has individual controls with well-marked ten turn dials that permit rapid set-up. It is very compact, and requires minimum bench space.

Disadvantages are the same as for the Profiler and Chrono-Log (see p. 334).

PARTIAL THROMBOPLASTIN TIME (PTT) TEST

Certain thromboplastins are unable to compensate completely for the defect in the hemophilioid states. These substances are termed *partial thromboplastins.* A partial thromboplastin is more sensitive to a decrease in the hemophilioid plasma factors and gives a prolonged plasma clotting time, whereas a complete (tissue) thromboplastin gives a normal (12–15 sec.) plasma clotting time.

Technique

In the procedure, all reagents, and the fresh, normal, and unknown plasmas are incubated at 37° C, and then 0.1 ml. of normal plasma and 0.1 ml. of the partial thromboplastin (Platelin*, or Thrombofax†) are placed in a clean 75 × 12 mm. test tube. They are mixed and incubated in the water bath at 37° C for 1 minute. Then 0.1 ml. of 0.025 M $CaCl_2$ is added; the reagents are mixed by tapping the tube gently. The timer is started at this time. After 30 seconds, the tube is removed from the water bath and observed for clot formation. The procedure is repeated using the unknown (patient's) plasma. A simple technique for a microcapillary partial thromboplastin test (PTT) has been described, which is quite sensitive and well suited for the detection of coagulation defects.[33] It is especially recommended for preoperative screening in infants and children for the detection of deficiencies of Factors VIII and IX.

Sources of Error

Sources of error in the PTT test are as follows: (1) Plasma must be collected with care, as for the prothrombin time. The plasma should be separated without disturbing the buffy coat. The plasma may be left at room temperature if the test is to be performed within 45 minutes. If not, the plasma may be stored for as long as 4 hours at 4° C. (2) Syringes, test tubes, and pipettes must be thoroughly clean and free of silicone. If possible, a disposable plastic syringe and new test tubes should be used. (3) All components of the test must be measured carefully and delivered into the lower portion of the test tube. (4) Each plasma sample should be tested in triplicate and the values averaged.

Results

The results are reported as follows: After 30 seconds tilt the tube about once every 1 to 2 seconds until the end point, a gel-like fibrin clot, is observed. The timer is stopped the moment gelation occurs.

Normal Values. Normal plasma clots in 60 to 100 seconds, depending on the activity of the partial thromboplastin. The patient's plasma should be compared with the normal plasma—that is, within 10 seconds of the control is normal;[12] greater than 10 seconds, but less than 20 seconds of the control is probably abnormal; greater than 20 seconds of the control is definitely abnormal.

If the unknown plasma is abnormal, mixing studies should be performed for a screening differential diagnosis. Three tubes are labeled *a, b,* and *c.* To each tube is added 0.1 ml. of the partial thromboplastin, and they are placed in the water bath. To tube *a,* is added 0.1 ml. of a 1:1 mixture of normal plasma and patient's plasma, and 0.1 ml. of $CaCl_2$ is added as in the preceding technique. To tube *b,* is added 0.1 ml. of a 1:1 mixture of fresh barium sulfate-adsorbed plasma and patient's plasma, with 0.1 ml. of $CaCl_2$. To tube *c,* is added 0.1 ml. of a 1:1 mixture of a known deficient plasma and patient's plasma, with 0.1 ml. $CaCl_2$, as in technique above.

The results are as follows: (1) If *a* is nor-

---

* Produced by Warner-Chilcott.
† Produced by Ortho Pharmaceutical Co.

mal, an anticoagulant is ruled out. (2) If *b* is normal, Factor VIII deficiency is suggested. (3) If *b* is abnormal, Factor IX deficiency is suggested. (4) If *c* is normal, the plasmas have different deficiencies. (5) If *c* is abnormal, the plasmas have the same deficiency.

Significance of Abnormal Results. The partial thromboplastin time may be defined as the clotting time of recalcified plasma in the presence of a lipid partial thromboplastin rather than in the presence of a complete thromboplastin such as is used in the prothrombin time test. The test is therefore useful as a screening procedure for the detection of a deficiency of any one of the following plasma clotting factors: fibrinogen, prothrombin, Factor V, Factor VIII (AHG), Factor IX (PTC), Factor X (Stuart), Factor XI (PTA), and Factor XII (HF). Therefore, a deficiency of any one of the clotting factors, with the exception of Factor VII and platelets, can be detected with this test. When this test is used in conjunction with the tourniquet test, platelet tests (platelet count, bleeding time, clot retraction), and the prothrombin time, most bleeding disorders can be detected. In addition, many circulating inhibitors (anticoagulants) will also cause prolongation of the partial thromboplastin time.

Related to the PTT is another new coagulation system abnormality, the Passovoy factor deficiency. This autosomal dominant trait is associated with a moderate bleeding diathesia. The only abnormal plasma clotting factor is the PTT.

FIBRINOGEN DETERMINATIONS

CONCENTRATION-DILUTION TEST FOR FIBRINOGEN

Dilutions of citrated plasma are clotted with thrombin. Normally, visible clots form in highly diluted plasma. In fibrinogen deficiency, clots do not form or form in only the higher concentrations of plasma.

Technique

In the test, the patient's plasma and normal plasma are diluted in seven test tubes with normal saline solution from 1:2 to 1:128 dilution utilizing 0.5 ml. volumes. One-tenth milliliter of thrombin (Fibrindex*) diluted 1:2 in saline solution before use is then added to each tube and mixed well in a 37° C water bath and allowed to remain for 15 minutes.

Results

Results are reported as the presence or absence of a clot.

Normal Value. Normally, clots are seen in all dilutions up to 1:128.

Significance of Abnormal Results. In severe hypofibrinogenemia, no clot is found in any dilutions, and in partial states of depletion clots are found in only the first three tubes.

OTHER PRESUMPTIVE OR SCREENING TESTS FOR FIBRINOGEN DEFICIENCY

THROMBIN-FIBRINDEX TEST

In the thrombin-Fibrindex test, thrombin or Fibrindex is used to clot blood. The speed of the reaction and the size of the clot are proportional to the amount of fibrinogen present.

Technique

In the test, 0.1 ml. of bovine topical thrombin† containing 1000 NIH units per ml. or 0.1 ml. Fibrindex (Ortho) may be used plus 1.0 ml. of freshly drawn blood; these are mixed by gently tilting the tube several times.

Results

Results are reported as clot formation, small or large.

---

* Produced by Ortho Pharmaceutical Co.
† Produced by Parke-Davis & Co.

Normal Values. Normal values include the following: (1) In the absence of fibrinogen, no clot forms. This is useful in obstetric emergencies when a defibrination syndrome is suspected. (2) In hypofibrinogenemia, a clot forms that is either small, or of normal size initially, but subsequently decreasing. (3) A firm clot that maintains rigidity after 30 minutes suggests an adequate amount of fibrinogen.

Significance of Abnormal Values. If the blood clots (when it was formerly incoagulable 10–30 min. after withdrawal), it probably means there is a deficiency of one of the factors involved in the first or second stage of coagulation. If the blood does not clot — even after the addition of thrombin — there is a deficiency of fibrinogen or an inhibitor of the third stage of coagulation, such as heparin or some other antithrombin.

CRUDE SCREENING TEST

Another *crude screening test* involves the heating of normal control plasma and the patient's plasma in two separate tubes at 56° C for 5 minutes. The turbidity of the two plasmas is then compared. Less turbidity in the patient's plasma suggests hypofibrinogenemia. The complete lack of turbidity, or a relatively clear plasma solution, indicates afibrinogenemia because fibrinogen is insoluble at 56° C.

RAPID SLIDE TEST

A *simple rapid slide* test based on the agglutination of fibrinogen-coated erythrocytes with latex-antihuman fibrinogen reagent is commercially available (FI test*). Blood specimens with plasma fibrinogen levels of 100 mg. per 100 ml. or less fail to show agglutination. When the plasma fibrinogen level is in the normal range of 250 to 400 mg. per 100 ml., agglutination is apparent.

---

* Produced by Hyland Laboratories.

AUTOMATED BLOOD COAGULATION TESTS AND INSTRUMENTS

Blood coagulation is a process of enzymatic reactions, involving several plasma proteins, lipids, and ions, that transform circulating blood into an insoluble gel through the conversion of soluble fibrinogen to fibrin. Fibrin formation extends, stabilizes, and anchors the evolving thrombus. The coagulation process is a biologic amplification system that enables relatively few molecules of initiator product to activate a series of circulating precursor proteins (proenzymes) by proteolysis, a series that culminates with the explosive production of fibrin-forming thrombin (i.e., an enzyme cascade analogous to a photomultiplier cascade). The efficiency of the entire coagulation system is assessed by measuring the final coagulation substrate concentration (fibrinogen level); extrinsic coagulation (prothrombin time); and intrinsic coagulation (partial thromboplastin time). In addition, the clot solubility test is performed to screen for the presence of factor XIII.

The development of mechanical or optical devices to measure the time of fibrin formation in mixtures of reacting coagulant factors has proceeded with remarkable speed over the past 7 years. Many different types of equipment are now available, some of which are mechanical and some of which are optical. However, all are basically mechanical stopwatches that have the theoretical advantage of removing the variables of various technician skills. Some are multichannel, offering semi- or complete automation in the testing and recording of coagulation times. An evaluation of the overall results obtained from the various types of equipment reveals differences owing to variations in the volumes of plasma utilized or to other added factors (volume is more critical). Certain results point out the limitation of existing techniques. Any attempt to label an instrument as ideal apparatus is limited by the resources and needs of the laboratory, as well as by the available technologist skills and the availability of servicing and spare parts.

In general, the selection of an instrument will depend on the number of tests to be prepared, the types of procedures, and service facilities available. Also, different types of machines may have to be utilized for a specific test (i.e., there may be greater accuracy in one instrument's one-stage prothrombin times than the PTT tests for heparin control that may be done on another type of machine). In addition, the end-point readings of abnormal samples may often result in wide variations among different machines. This necessitates the use of both normal and abnormal range samples to evaluate such instrumentation.

SMALL INSTRUMENTS

Finally, the purchase of automated coagulation instruments should be related, practically speaking, to the size of the hospital. That is, the medical institutions of less than 100 beds should consider the so-called small instruments costing approximately $2,500.00+ The seven most commonly used small instruments are: (1) Clotek (Hyland Laboratories, 3300 Hyland Avenue, Costa Mesa, California 92626); (2) Coagamate – Single Channel (General Diagnostics Division, Warner-Lambert Co., 201 Tabor Road, Morris Plains, New Jersey 07950); (3) Coagulyzer, Jr. (Sherwood Medical Industries, 1831 Olive St., St. Louis, Missouri 63103); (4) Electra-650 (Medical Laboratory Automation, 520 Nuber Avenue, Mount Vernon, New York 10550); (5) Fibrometer (BBL Division, Becton, Dickinson and Co., P.O. Box 243, Cockeysville, Maryland 21030); (6) Sonoclot (Sienco, Inc., Box 108 Star Route, Morrison, Colorado 80465); (7) Coagulation Profiler, Model CP 7 & 8 (Bio/Data Corp., 3941 Commerce Ave., Willow Grove, Pennsylvania 19090).

The basic principle in all of these machines is the change in light transmission associated with thrombin, fibrinogen, and fibrin concentrations. They are all quite small and yet provide a degree of automation in the determination of PT and APTT. Below is a discussion of these instruments.

Clotek

The Clotek tests plasma in a disposable cuvette tube with ball bearing plus reagents; the tube bobs up and down with a magnet holding the fluid and ball bearing in place and out of the light beam. Subsequently a clot forms, the ball becomes enmeshed in the fibrin and is pulled through the light path. This breaks the circuit, stops the timer, and the end-point fibrin concentration is measured. This instrument is no longer made.

Coagamate Single Channel

The Coagamate operates as a photo-optical clot sensing system for the determination of the prothrombin time and activated partial thromboplastin times. This machine (Fig. 11-11) has reached is operating temperature when the decimal point in the time-seconds display is illuminated. The position of the PT-APTT mode switch determines the reagent volume to be delivered and the sensitivity of the clot sensing circuit. Samples, contained in the disposable circular test tray, are placed on the incubation test plate and allowed to reach temperature equilibrium. The index button controls the movements of the sample into testing position. When the test button is pressed, the pump automatically delivers the reagent, which initiates the clotting reaction, and, simultaneously, the electric clock and the air-stirrer circuits are activated. The air stirrer stops after 4 seconds. After a time delay of 8 seconds for the PT test and 20 seconds for the APTT test, the electro-optical sensing circuit is activated. This delay is required to prevent premature end-points caused by turbulence from the reagent delivery and the air-stirring systems. The clot is detected by a rate of change in absorbance that exceeds a

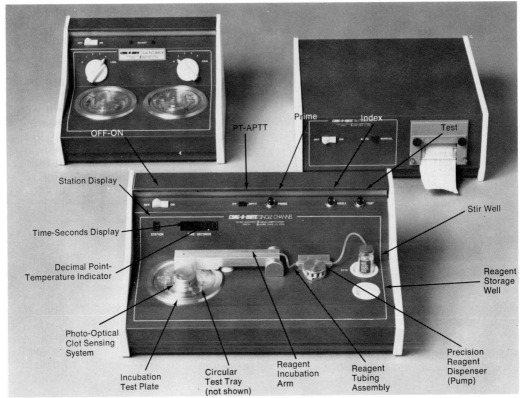

Fig. 11-11. Coagamate Single Channel. (Courtesy of General Diagnostics Division, Warner-Lambert Co.)

predetermined magnitude for a defined period of time. A time delay constant of 1 to 5 seconds is introduced to provide prothrombin times comparable to manual methods.

Figure 11-12 illustrates the basic functional components of the Coagamate and shows their interrelationships. A plastic filter surrounds the light source and provides a uniform light beam through the sample cuvette. A second filter is located in front of the electro-optical sensor. This sensor instantly converts the transmitted light into an electrical signal that is simplified, compared, and conditioned to control the time-display circuit. The circuit is also connected to the time-base generator and four-stage counter. A unique optical waveform simulator is used to calibrate the instrument to close tolerances. The simulator gener-

ates an optical phenomenon that closely duplicates the one produced during a clotting reaction. Each instrument is adjusted individually to ensure optimal response by the optical and electrical systems.

Coagulyzer, Jr.

The Coagulyzer, Jr. is a semi-automated coagulation timer in which clot formation is automatically timed; detection is by means of a photoelectric cell (Fig. 11-13). It contains ten unheated storage wells for plasma, which are located at the top rear portion of the instrument. Control and patient plasmas may also be tested in 20 heated cuvette storage wells; these are located in front of the unheated wells. There are also three heated test tube wells and three heated reagent reservoirs; two of the reservoirs contain a magnetic stirrer. Depres-

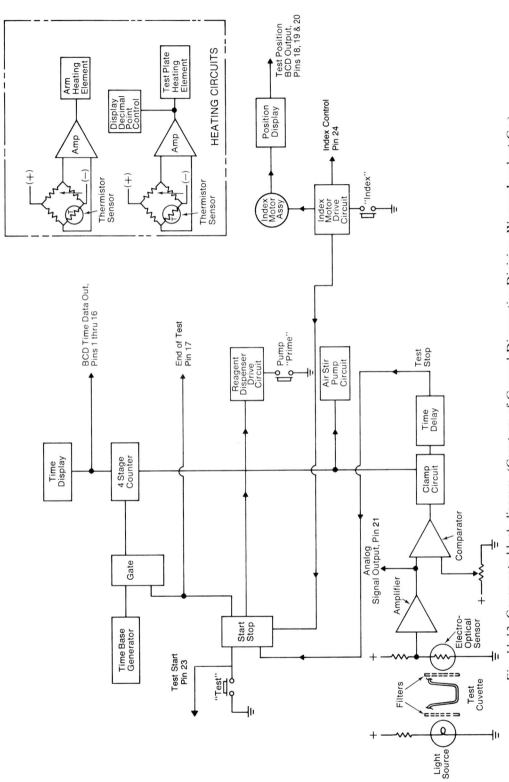

Fig. 11-12. Coagamate block diagram. (Courtesy of General Diagnostics Division, Warner-Lambert Co.)

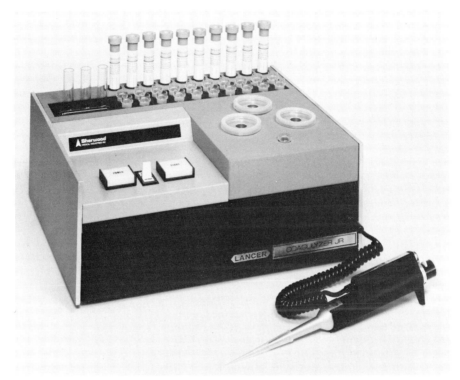

Fig. 11-13. Lancer Coagulyzer Jr. (Courtesy of Sherwood Medical Industries, Inc.)

sion of the power switch turns on the machine. The patient's plasma is placed into the cuvette, which is, in turn, placed in a

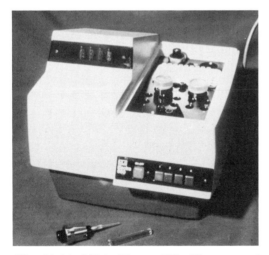

Fig. 11-14. MLA Electra-650. (Courtesy of Medical Laboratory Automation)

test well on the lower front of the machine. At the same time as the reagent is added to the plasma-containing cuvette, the start switch is depressed, which activates the timing mechanism. Care must be taken not to allow too fast a stirring of reagent and plasma, since that might cause a vortex to form. If an automatic pipette is plugged into its jack, as the reagent is pipetted into the test cuvette, the timing mechanism is automatically activated. The digital display shows the registered clotting time; it will return to zero each time the start switch is activated. At the back of the machine is located a reset/light switch; this resets the timer when a false start has been made or when the display is used for timing purposes.

It is best to use only citrated plasmas on the Coagulyzer, Jr., which can be used for the performance of activated partial throm-

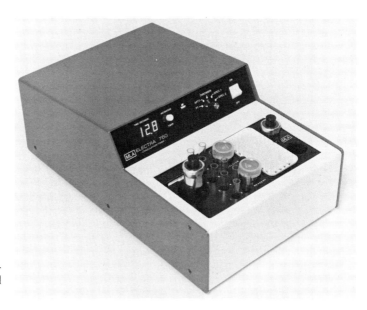

Fig. 11-15. MLA Electra-750. (Courtesy of Medical Laboratory Automation)

boplastin time, prothrombin time, PT and APTT substitution tests, prothrombin consumption Reptilase-R procedures, factor assays, and thromboplastin generation time.

Electra-650

The Electra-650 is a semi-activated blood coagulation timer, in which the clot formation is timed automatically and detected by means of a photocell that reads the change in the optical density as a result of clot formation (Fig. 11-14). A heating system maintains the reagents and plasma samples at 37° C prior to and during the testing. A medical technologist pipettes the reagents and plasma samples, using disposable-tip precision Electra pipettes; both oxalated and citrated plasmas may be used in this instrument. The front of the machine has four mode switches (i.e., No. 1 performs prothrombin times using citrated plasma; No. 2 handles both oxalated and citrated plasma for prothrombin times; No. 3 performs quantitative fibrinogen analyses; and No. 4 does saline dilutions and activated partial prothrombin times).

The Electra-650 will eventually be replaced by the recently developed Electra-750 (Fig. 11-15). Either one appears to be more versatile than the Clotek, the Coagamate, and the Coagulyzer, Jr. Each differs in its combinations of blue buttons and its photo-optical readout. Also, since the reagent-plasma mixtures warm in metal wells, there is a possibility that reagent might be wasted.

Fibrometer

The Fibrometer relies on a stationary and moving electrode that activates a readout counter when fibrin is formed (Fig. 11-16). It is a truly semi-automated instrument that produces accurate and highly reproducible results in the performance of prothrombin times, partial thromboplastin times, and thromboplastin generation times. Technically, it consists of a thermal prep block, an automatic pipette, and a fibrometer component. The prep block and pipette are utilized when moderate-to-large numbers of prothrombin times are determined.

At the beginning of a run, the fibrometer and thermal prep block are turned on and

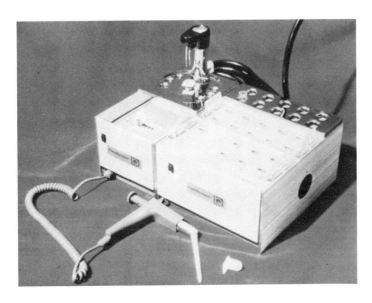

Fig. 11-16. Fibrometer. (Courtesy of BBL Division, Becton, Dickson & Co.)

allowed to warm to 37° C (approximately 10 min.). When this temperature is reached, the indicator light will flash on and remain on as long as 37° C is maintained. The thermal block indicator light alternately goes on and off depending on the heat demand. Disposable coagulation cups are then placed in the plastic tray over the heating wells in the thermal prep block. A disposable fibro-tip is inserted snugly and tightly in the hole in the front end of the automatic pipette; the pipette is plugged into the fibrometer and the pipette switch moved to the OFF position. The plunger of the automatic pipette is then switched to the 0.2 ml. setting. The fibro-tip of the pipette plunger is then completely depressed and placed into a solution of well-mixed thromboplastin-calcium solution; the plunger should be allowed to retract completely. The side of the fibro-tip of the pipette plunger is then placed near the end on the inside top edge of the coagulation cup (in the thermal prep block), but not touching the inside wall of the cup. The plunger is depressed so that the 0.2 ml. of thromboplastin-calcium mixture goes into the coagulation cup. The entire procedure, beginning with the positioning of the fibro-tip pipette plunger in the thromboplastin-cal-

cium (t-c) mixture, is then repeated until the desired number of coagulation cups contain the 0.2 ml. t-c mixture. All are allowed to incubate until they have reached 37° C (2–3 min.). The control and patient plasma is placed into labeled 12 × 75 mm. test tubes and allowed to prewarm in the deep wells of the thermal prep block until they reach 37° C (approximately 3 min.). One of the prewarmed coagulation cups containing 0.2 ml. of the t-c solution is then placed in the reaction well. The plunger of the automatic pipette is turned to the 0.1 ml. setting, and a disposable vibro-tip is inserted into its front end. One-tenth ml. of the prewarmed patient or control plasma is then drawn up by complete depression of the pipette plunger; the pipette switch is then moved to the ON position. The plasma is dropped into the coagulation cup in the reaction well, and as the plunger is depressed, the timing mechanism will automatically begin. The probe arm will drop into position within 1.5 seconds, and the electrode action begins. This action and timing mechanism ceases as soon as a fibrin clot forms in the mixture. The digital readout then records the prothrombin time. The electrodes should be wiped with a clean, lint-free cloth after the probe arm is lifted to its resting position. The timer should be set at 000.0, by depressing the reset button.

It is important to remember that all prothrombin times must be performed in duplicate (prepared on a second fibrometer), and the results should check within 0.5 seconds of each other (unless the result is above 30 sec. and a wider range of variability is acceptable).

The following are advantages in the use of the fibrometer: rigid control of the temperature of the reacting mixture during the test period; convenience of the automatic pipette in delivering reagents and plasma; exceptional accuracy in delivering the desired volume of plasma; increased accuracy due to automatic activation of the instrument when plasma is delivered into the test cup; elimination of variability by automatic end-point readings; and convenience and inexpensiveness of disposable tubes and plastic tubes for the automatic pipette.

However, in order to achieve sensitivity and specificity, the following points should be borne in mind: Falsely shortened results can be eliminated if the electrodes are kept free of lint and debris. Routine 0.2 ml. prothrombin pipettes may be used instead of the automatic pipette. In that case, the fibrometer timer bar must be pressed when 0.1 ml. of plasma is blown into the coagulation cup. The pipette fibro-tip must not get loose (it should be tightened after every 3rd or 4th time) and should be used only one time, except when pipetting the thromboplastin-calcium solution. The Fibrometer on-off switch should be turned to OFF if the timing mechanism is started inadvertently. The unit can be turned back on, then the probe arm replaced in its resting position, and the digital readout reset. Since the fibrometer probe arm is designed for testing a certain volume of solution, the 0.3 ml. vol. probe arm should always be utilized in performance of prothrombin times.

As soon as the plasma has been pipetted and the fibrometer activated, the automatic pipette switch should always be moved to the OFF position. A small amount of solu-tion will remain in the fibro-tip after the plunger on the automatic pipette is depressed; pipette calibration has been adjusted for this.

The following two instruments are new and the details of experience with them are not as yet known.

Sonoclot

The Sonoclot is a relatively simple, yet reliable, continuously recording, bedside, screening instrument that can be used to indicate the general status and kinetics of blood coagulation. It was devised for use by laboratory personnel who do not have specialized training in blood coagulation techniques; very little time and only a few simple manipulations are required to start it, and it can then proceed unattended. The innovations of this instrument make it a strong candidate for numerous situations, such as the operating room and the emergency ward (particularly at night), when blood coagulation information is needed immediately. It can also be utilized to monitor the effect on clotting of various types of anticoagulant replacement therapy and for screening in hospitals that have no special coagulation laboratory.

The instrument works by continuously recording the clotting process (more precisely, fibrin formation). It measures the changes of mechanical impedance (hence, the name impedance machine) imposed on a minute probe that vibrates while it is immersed in a small sample of blood or recalcified plasma (0.04–0.4 ml.). In practice, a disposable solid plastic probe (4.5 mm. diameter) is mounted vertically on a transducer and vibrated axially with an amplitude of less than 1 μm. at a rate of less than 200 Hz. The power input to the transducer is only about 2 μW. The driving frequency and voltage are held constant by a stable oscillator that is coupled to a transducer through a high resistance field. The voltage measured at the transducer is a function of the transducer impedance, which varies with the freedom of movement of the at-

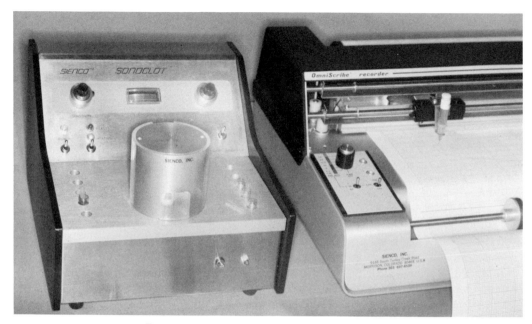

Fig. 11-17. Sonoclot. (Courtesy of Sienco, Inc.)

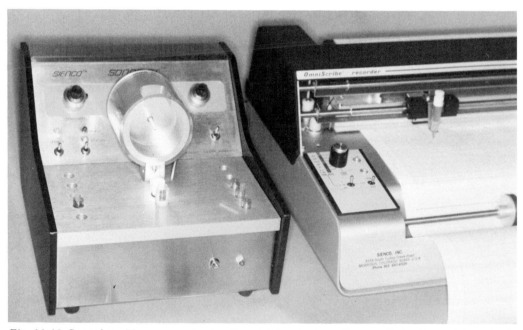

Fig. 11-18. Sonoclot with open sensing head containing the transducer and the disposable probe in the center of the head. (Courtesy of Sienco, Inc.)

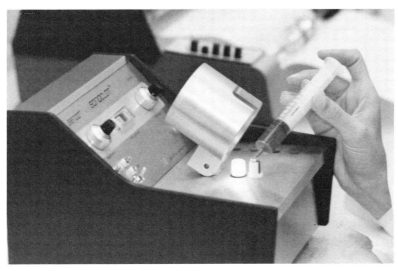

Fig. 11-19. Sonoclot. Blood from second syringe is placed into disposable glass covette, which has been previously fitted into the holder. (Courtesy of Sienco, Inc.)

tached probe. (All this occurs at an extremely small scale of energy and motion.) A clot that is forming increasingly inhibits this freedom of movement, thereby creating an electrical charge of the transducer output, which is amplified. The amplifier output is thus proportional to the changes of the mechanical impedance exerted by the clotting specimen on the probe.

The Sonoclot (Fig. 11-17) consists of a 22 × 25 × 17 cm. impedance machine on the left and a recorder center and timer on the right. The timer shuts off the machine after the preset running time has lapsed. Figure 11-18 shows the open sensing head, which contains the transducer, the disposable probe in the center of the head, the thermostatically (37° C ± 2°) controlled working stage that can hold tubes (the left wells in Fig. 11-18), the extra cuvettes (the right wells in Fig. 11-18), and the control panel behind the head. Also shown is the holder, located in front of the head for the disposable cuvettes, in which the clotting process is monitored.

In the procedure, whole blood is drawn from a clean venipuncture by the two-syringe technique into plastic syringes. The blood from the second syringe is immediately put into the disposable glass cuvette (Fig. 11-19), which has been previously fitted into the holder; the sensing head with the disposable probe is pivoted 90° (thus inserting the probe into the specimen); and the recording is started. With very small amounts of blood (e.g., from the fingertip), microequipment is used. For recording with plasma, double citrated blood (4 parts blood and 1 part 3.8% sodium citrate) is thoroughly mixed in the syringe, spun for 5 minutes at full speed in the international table centrifuge, and 0.4 ml. of the separated plasma is then placed in a siliconized glass cuvette, recalcified with 0.04 ml. 0.5M $CaCl_2$, stirred quickly with a nonsiliconized glass rod, and the recording is started. Since the machine and the recorder are always kept warmed up, these steps require only about 15 seconds; the machine performs unattended until it is shut off by the preset timer.

Normal coagulability is shown in Figure 11-20*A*. The clotting kinetics of the blood or plasma specimen are well reflected by

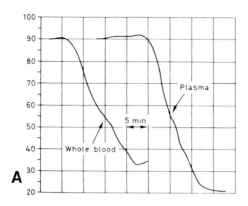

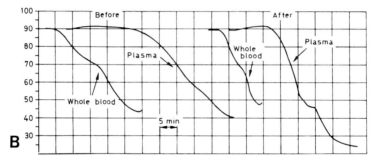

Fig. 11-20. (A) Healthy person. Normocoagulability. *(Left)* whole blood; *(right)* recalcified plasma. The distance between the two heavy vertical lines represents a time interval of 5 min. in this and the following figures. *(B)* Idiopathic thrombocytopenic purpura. Hypocoagulability and its correction by splenectomy. Coagulation curves obtained before splenectomy with platelet count 11,000 (left) and after splenectomy with platelet count 106,000 (right). Note the corrective effect of splenectomy on the initial phase, which becomes shorter, and the slope, which becomes steeper.

the length of the initial phase (the time lag before the curve starts to turn downwards) and by the steepness of the slope of the curve. This is produced by several minutes of a straight recording; then a quickly accelerating downward trend develops, resulting in a steep slope (depending on the clotting tendency), which subsequently becomes level. With whole blood, this leveling off can be followed by an irregular upward trend that indicates clot retraction. This is not observed with recalcified plasma, where the curves remain horizontal after completion of the clotting process, since there is no retraction when siliconized cuvettes are used. With recalcified plasma, the initial straight recording (the early

phase of clotting before measurable fibrin formation occurs) is always somewhat longer than that of the whole blood (Fig. 11-20*A* or normal; Figs. 11-20*B* and *C* or hypocoagulability and Fig. 11-20*D* or hypercoagulability).

Although the Sonoclot is not intended to replace instruments of sophisticated coagulation analyses, it has many advantages over other coagulometers. Whole blood or plasma can be used; the device can be adapted to small (0.05 ml. or less) volumes of blood or plasma; the coagulation process can be observed at all times (specimen is transilluminated); blood or plasma remain practically undisturbed; it produces continuous electrical signals; it writes real time

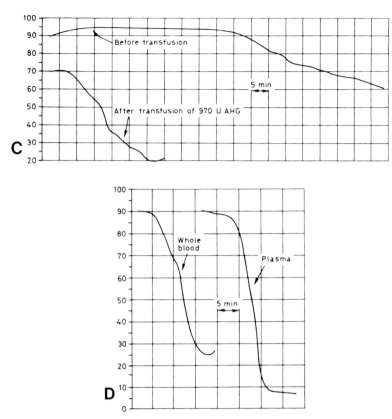

Fig. 11-20. (Continued) (*C*) Hemophilia A. Curve on top: Severe hypo-coagulability before transfusion. Bottom curve: Near normalization 60 min. after transfusion of 970 U antihemophilic globulin. (*D*) Thrombophilia (hereditary). Hypercoagulability. Whole blood (left), and recalcified plasma (right). Note short initial phase and very steep slope of the curves. (Courtesy of Sienco, Inc.)

curves, providing a permanent record; it records long (min. to hrs.) and short (secs.) clotting processes; only disposable elements come in contact with blood or plasma; it is simple, compact, sturdy, and portable, and thermostatically recorded; it is easy to start, runs by itself, and requires little servicing; its sensitivity and characteristics are adjustable to meet specific test requirements; it can be used with most commercial recorders.

Coagulation Profiler (CP-7 & 8)

The Profiler is an integrated semiautomatic system that allows the laboratory to perform routine or in-depth analyses of blood plasma for changes or defects in the coagulation mechanism (e.g., prothrombin time, PTT, thrombin time-quantitative fibrinogen, factor assays, thromboplastin generation test, Russell's viper venom test, prothrombin consumption, and recalcification time). In addition to providing end-point data as a function of time, this instrument provides, automatically, specific data on factor-activity levels in the form of a permanent visual record of the reaction kinetics (i.e., it indicates how the clot is forming). This is important since it is now known that a clot can begin to form in a normal time but in an abnormal manner. This abnormality may result from variations in the fibrinogen-to-fibrin polymeriza-

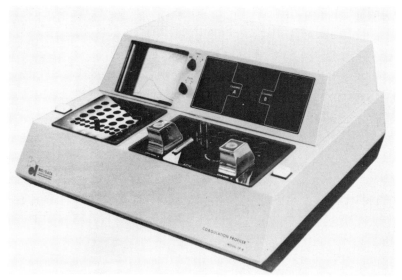

Fig. 11-21. Bio/Data Coagulation Profiler Model CP-8. (Courtesy of Bio-Data Corp.)

tion reaction, which could be overlooked if time is the only element measured.

The Profiler operates on a patented electro-optical principle that measures the rate of change of optical density of the reaction mixture. There are three basic subsystems fully integrated for maximum instrument performance. The first subsystem contains patented electronic circuitry, in which the rate of change of optical density is utilized for the observation and detection of clot formation. Additional processing of the electronic signals by this subsystem provides output data for the kinetic recording of the coagulation process by the second subsystem, which is composed of a galvanometer-actuated recorder and associated simplification and control circuitry. Data supplied to this recorder are displayed on heat-sensitive paper specially gridded to provide rapid analysis of the generated curve. The recording paper is transported at 5 mm. per second, which provides a time base to aid further in curve analysis and also provides a permanent, timed record of each test performed. The third subsystem is composed of various instrument controls and programming that provide instructional and test status information sequentially displayed on the CP-7 & 8.

The advantages of this instrument are as follows: The programmed instructions and instrument status minimize operator-training and reduce the possibility of error in test procedures. It operates with most commercial reagents, including those containing particulate matter, which eliminates the need to change the present reagent system. It operates automatically with either citrated or oxalated plasmas, which eliminates the need to change the existing anticoagulant system. It operates on standard or microvolumes, which reduces reagent cost by 50 per cent and allows the testing of the small volumes of plasma obtained from pediatric patients. It provides quantitative fibrinogen readout with each thrombin test performed, which eliminates the need for additional costly and time-consuming "wet-chemistry" procedures. It detects abnormal factor-activity levels with every PT or PTT test performance, which reduces the possi-

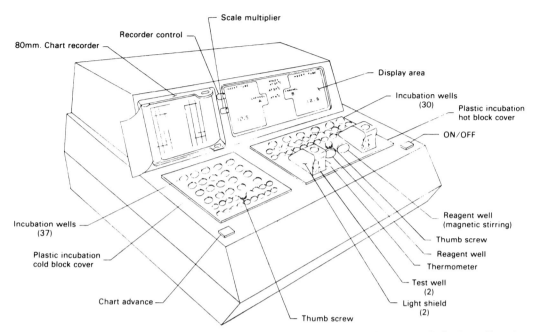

Fig. 11-22. Diagram of Bio/Data Coagulation Profiler Model CP-8. (Courtesy of Bio-Data Corp.)

bility of bleeding emergencies in patients whose PT or PTT may indicate normal time. Utilizing continuous permanent recording of the entire coagulation process enables the laboratory to maintain high quality control standards and also provides a permanent record of the entire coagulation process for future reference. A newer model, the CP-8, possesses dual channel capability and permits PTs and PTTs to be run simultaneously, which reduces the time and personnel required to process daily workloads. Also, an integrated thermoelectric cold block is provided; this can store up to 54 samples at 4° C and allows the laboratory to batch its specimens, thus increasing efficiency by reducing time lost to single-sample analysis (Figs. 11-21; 11-22).

Comparative Survey

A comparative survey of the first five instruments listed above, with the Bio/Data CA-15 as a reference instrument, was completed by Leavell and co-workers of the Mayo Clinic.[25] A brief summary of their findings reveals that there was no significant difference among the machines when PT was analyzed. In the APTT study, the single-channel Coagamate had the best overall precision (coefficient of variation 2–4%), while the Coagamate and the Electra 650 had the best day-to-day reproducibility (coefficient of variation 2–5%). The comparison study indicated good correlation ($r \geq 0.95$) between the reference instrument (Bio/Data CA-15) and the single-channel Coagamate, Electra 650, and Clotek. The correlation for the Coagulyzer Jr. was also quite good ($r = 0.95$), but it could not detect some of the clots detected by the other machines. The Fibrometer showed significantly poorer correlation ($r = 0.87$) when compared with the other instruments.

As far as cost of expendable tests was concerned, the Coagamate cost $0.09 compared to $0.35 for the Clotek. In December 1976, the average cost was, for each of the five instruments, Clotek, $585.00; Fibrometer, $1,295.00; Coagulyzer, Jr., $1,395.00; Coagamate, $1,890.00; and Electra 650, $3,200.00.

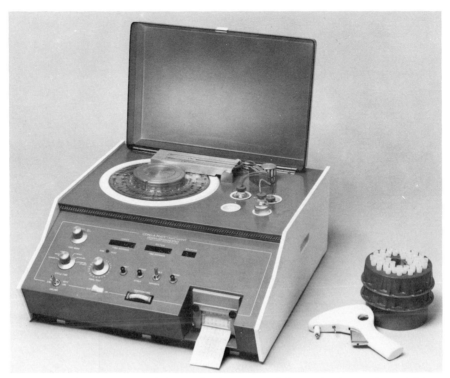

Fig. 11-23. Coagamate Dual Channel. (Courtesy of General Diagnostics Division, Warner-Lambert Co.)

LARGE AUTOMATED BLOOD COAGULATION INSTRUMENTATION

The four most commonly used and evaluated instruments are the following (see Table 11–2):[24] G. D. Coagamate D.C. (General Diagnostics Division, Warner-Lambert Co., 201 Tabor Rd., Morris Plains, New Jersey 07950); MLA-Electra-600 (Medical Laboratory Automation, 520 Nuber Ave., Mount Vernon, New York 10550); Sherwood Lancer Coagulyzer (1831 Olive Street, St. Louis, Missouri 63103); Dade Auto-Fi (Division of American Hospital Supply Corp., P.O. Box 672, Miami, Florida 33152).

Coagamate Dual Channel

The Coagamate Dual Channel is a system quite similar to the previously described single channel model, except that it has the capability of simultaneous measurement of APTT and PT and the option of making each determination in duplicate (Fig. 11-23). Digital readouts are provided for monitoring the measurements in each channel, in addition to the automatic printout of results. The system also provides extraordinary flexibility for purposes of performing other types of coagulation time measurements, such as factor assays and fibrinogen formation.

MLA-Electra-600 and Sherwood Coagulyzer

Since the Electra-600 and the Coagulyzer are basically similar instruments, which sell for about the same price, and automate the determination of coagulation techniques (i.e., their prime applications are for the determination of PT and APTT in laboratories with about 25 or more samples per day) their operating principles will be described as a unit, with the delineation of the differences that distinguish each instrument.

Principle. In general terms, both the

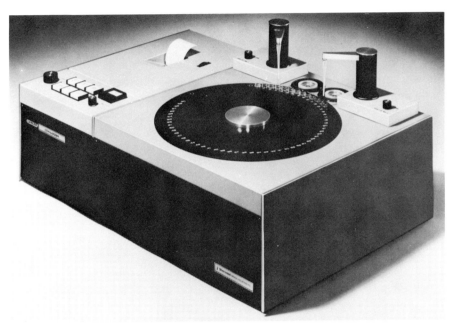

Fig. 11-24. Sherwood Lancer Coagulyzer. (Courtesy of Sherwood Medical Instruments)

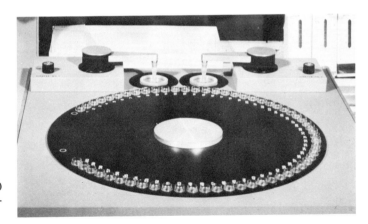

Fig. 11-25. MLA Electra-600 D. (Courtesy of Medical Laboratory Automation)

Coagulyzer and the Electra have automatic turntables for multiple samples, sample and reagent incubators, automatic pipettors for dispensing reagents, a photometric system for detecting clot formation, a clock circuit started by pipetting the activator and stopped by detection of the clot, and a sequential printer for recording answers to the nearest 0.1 second (Figs. 11-24; 11-25). Both instruments are designed to minimize the human variability, thereby enhancing test precision. Also, both systems have features that simplify operation as well as minimize the time per test.

Turntable and Associated Incubation. The turntables occupy the largest portion of the area of each instrument. The capacity is 50 samples on the Electra and 60 on the Coagulyzer.

In the MLA Electra there are two different temperature blocks beneath the sample rack. In the test position and the six stations just before it, the tube fits into a well in a heated block at a temperature of 37° C. The wells ensure good heat exchange between the block and the tube. All samples must proceed through the same seven heated positions prior to testing, resulting in a minimum incubation period of 175 seconds.

Prior to entering the heated region, the samples pass through a U-shaped trough, which is thermoelectrically cooled to below 10° C. This helps prevent thermal degradation of samples, which is more critical for APTT than for PT.

The temperature blocks remain stationary as the turntable rotates from one locked position to the next. Just prior to rotation, pins raise the sample tubes out of their wells in the heated block to facilitate the rotation.

The sample tubes in the Electra are 10 × 75 mm. standard flint glass test tubes with round bottoms.

In the Coagulyzer a single heating block is provided as standard equipment. This is controlled at 37° C ± 0.1° to ensure clot timing within ±0.1° of 37° C. Heating occurs in the six positions prior to testing and in the test position. The minimum time in the heating block is 180 seconds.

The manufacturer contends that keeping a number of samples typical for most institutions at room temperature prior to incubation will not have a clinically significant effect on APTT values. However, to satisfy those who may be concerned, perhaps where laboratory ambient is high, Sherwood has recently introduced an accessary electrothermal cooling rack.

For good thermal contact in the incubator, the sample tubes fit into wells in the block. In both instruments, just prior to rotation of the turntable from one position to the next, the heated block is lowered, leaving the lips of the sample cuvettes resting on the turntable. After the turntable rotates, the block slowly rises until it surrounds the bottoms of the cuvettes and lifts them a short distance.

The sample reaction cuvettes for the Coagulyzer are special polystyrene tubes of truncated conical shape with flat bottoms. The lower section is clear, and the remainder is frosted. A lip is molded in the frosted section. The frosted section is used in the tube detection system, described later, and may be used for recording sample identity. Incidentally, the flat bottom allows placing cuvettes directly on the bench for pipetting samples.

Reagent Storage and Dispensing. The Electra-600 has a single reagent well and associated pipette for dispensing the activator into the sample in the test station. The reagent is kept slightly above the desired reaction temperature. The automatic pipette that dispenses the reagent is peristaltic. The pump tubing and reagent reservoir are an integral assembly, which is intended to be discarded when the cup capacity of reagent for 300 tests has been dispensed. Two color-coded sizes are provided for dispensing either 0.1 or 0.2 ml.

This arrangement limits full automation to single-step procedures. When two-step tests, such as APTT, are performed, the first reagent must be manually pipetted into the sample tubes. The most common coagulation test, PT, is commonly a one-step procedure, although two-step procedures are available.

Because the coagulation reagents are generally suspensions, constant agitation is required. On the Electra this is done by electromechanical shaking of the reagent reservoir during a run.

The Coagulyzer has two reagent reservoirs and associated automatic pipettes. These pipettes are positive-displacement types, with switch-selected volumes of 0.1 or 0.2 ml. Only the reservoir that dispenses into the test station cuvette is heated to 37.5° C. The other pipette dispenses reagent at ambient into the sample just before it enters the incubation block (Fig. 11-26). The reservoirs are disposable. Agitation of both reservoirs is accomplished by magnetic stirrers. Teflon-coated magnetic stir-

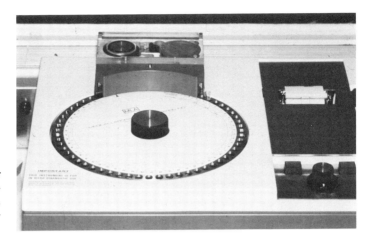

Fig. 11-26. Sherwood Lancer Coagulyzer with reagent reservoirs and incubation block. (Courtesy of Sherwood Medical Instruments)

ring bars are pulled aside during pipetting so that the tip can descend close to the bottom of the reservoir. The loose stirrers must be retrieved when the reservoirs are cleaned or discarded.

Photometric Clot Detection. Both instruments employ the same photometric principle of clot detection, using a tungsten source and a photoconductive detector.

Essentially what is being detected is a decrease in transmitted light due to clot formation. Sherwood does this by measuring the time derivative of the transmission. A value different from zero by a small amount indicates the onset of clot formation. Since different samples and reagents may have widely differing absorption in the visible spectrum, a filter that transmits only the far red and near infrared is placed in the light path. This minimizes the variation in signal level from sample to sample.

MLA applies its patented second-derivative detection system to the Electra. This is said to have a particular advantage when blood samples are collected in a sodium oxalate medium. When the plasma from such a sample is activated, a gradual darkening occurs, unrelated to clotting. This may trigger a first-derivative circuit, but cannot affect a second-derivative system. However, the oxalate medium does not appear to be as commonly employed as citrate, which is free of this darkening.

There are two characteristics of the Electra data processing system that are products of either the second-derivative system or of the electronic design, which may affect clinical results. One is a delay time of 1 second for clot verification, after the clot is initially detected and before the clotting is reported. This tends to lend a positive bias to coagulation times. The second is that each instrument may require "tuning" to the laboratory in which it is installed. This involves an internal lamp-level adjustment appropriate to the reagents and controls in use. A switch beneath the cover enables selection of two sensitivity ranges. A change in reagents or the undertaking of a new procedure may necessitate a change within the instrument. The need for such a procedure is not indicated for the Coagulyzer.

Safety Features. The instruments incorporate a sample cuvette detection system that serves two purposes: prevents dispensing of the reagents when no tube is present, and bypasses the programmed minimum dwell time (e.g., 25 or 30 secs.), and almost immediately steps the turntable to the next position. If the remainder of the turntable is empty, the turntable will continue to step quickly until it reaches its "home" position, where it will be ready to reload for the next batch.

(Text continues on p. 360.)

Table 11–2. Comparative Analysis of Large Automated Coagulating Instrument*

	Coagamate	MLA Electra	Coagulyzer	Auto-Fi
Structural principles	Possesses 2 noncooled and 2 cooled reagent reservoirs (the only one of the 4 possessing these); has 2 concentric circuits that must be synchronized by a set-screw; uses a disposable reaction tray with a variable cycle timer that can be set; has a maximum throughput of 75 prothrombin times/hr. and 24 APTT/hr.	Possesses 7 stations of incubation with a shorter incubation time at each step; reagent reservoir is heated, and medical technologist must personally add second reagent as it passes through reservoir; reagent reservoir can be used for 300 tests; instrument has maximum throughput of 54 prothrombin times/hr. and 27 APTT/hr.	Does not possess timing and tubing parts that can deteriorate as in other instruments; however, does possess a disposable reagent reservoir; has a maximum throughput of 50 prothrombin times/hr. and 26 APTT/hr.	Possesses full automation capable of processing up to 40 samples in single or duplicate sequences for PT, APTT, fibrinogen, or factor assays; values obtained comparable to manual features used in the contrasted systems; utilizes a new concept in end-point detection that is unaffected by sample turbidity or chromogenicity (i.e. filaments move through the sample mixture until fibrin gel formation occurs); clot adheres to filament and passes over a photocell for end-point detection; sample has throughput of 72 prothrombin times/hr., 45 APTT/hr., 72 fibrinogen/hr., 45 extrinsic systems factor assays/hr., and 24 intrinsic factor assays/hr.

	Instrument 1	Instrument 2	Instrument 3	Instrument 4
Prothrombin time coagulation coefficient	0.991	0.986	0.982	0.964
Prothrombin time agreement between duplicates				
Within 0.5 sec.	57.4%	95.9%	95.5%	97.3%
Within 1.0 sec.	90.1%	98.8%	98.5%	98.5%
APTT agreement between duplicates				
Within 0.5 sec.	78.0%	82.0%	87.0%	81.2%
Within 1.0 sec.	95.0%	93.7%	95.5%	95.2%
Technician acceptance	Fair	Good	Good	Good
Computer compatibility (ability to interface)	Difficult	Easy	Easy	Easy
Approximate cost	$11,975.00	$9,200.00	$9,450.00	$17,500.00
Cost of disposable material for 25 tests	$ 2.28	$ 2.47	$ 2.45	$ 5.24
Desirable features	Cool reagent reservoirs	Uses standard test tubes and has good technician acceptance	Large number of samples can be placed on turntables; has good reproducibility and a good pipette system	Uses automatic pipette systems; duplicate determinations can be performed; end results not dependent upon optical factors; end-result reading not affected by hyperlipemic blood.
Undesirable features	Agreement poor at short intervals of 0.5 sec., and only fair technician acceptance; difficult to interface with computer systems; breakdown service poor; rarely affected by hyperlipemic blood	Has only 1 reagent typing system; readings affected by hyperlipemic blood	Small cuvettes; hard to wash; rarely affected by hyperlipemic blood	Complex mechanisms, slower process; has 80 sec. cutoff for APTT; high purchase and operation cost; preadjustments required

Common disadvantages

All photoelectric instruments fail on hyperlipemic blood (except the Auto-Fi); all instruments use an acid-wash that lessens the APTT; elevation above room temperature necessitates correction of fluctuation in results; reagents are not interchangeable on different machines; none of the instruments is fully automated at yet.

* Klee, G. G., Didisheim, P., Johnson, R. J., and Gurre, G. M.: An evaluation of four automated coagulation instruments. Am. J. Clin. Pathol., in press.

Table 11-3. Comparative Analysis of Electra-600 and Lancer Coagulyzer

Feature	Electra-600	Lancer Coagulyzer
Clot detection	Photometric, second derivative	Photometric, first derivative
Automatic pipetting	One reagent	Two reagents
Refrigeration	Standard	Accessory
Adjustments for reagents	May be made if required	Not required
Cuvettes	Standard, glass round bottoms	Special, plastic, flat bottoms
Turntable capacity	50	60

The Electra senses a sample tube with a feeler switch in the test station. In the Coagulyzer, photosensitive systems are used, one at each pipetting station. Light is focused on a detector at the level just below the lip of the cuvette. If a cuvette is present, the frosted section scatters the light, reducing the signal. When no cuvette is present, the signal is a maximum.

Programmed Operation. Programming sets the dwell time appropriate to the minimum acceptable incubation time of the selected test. If the coagulation time is less than the minimum, the turntable uses the minimum time to ensure adequate incubation for all samples. If coagulation takes longer than the minimum, the tube remains in the test station until coagulation occurs. A maximum time is also programmed into the instruments in their automated modes (90 secs. in the Coagulyzer, 150 secs. in the Electra). If coagulation fails to occur in this period, the maximum time will be printed and the table indexed. In the Electra, an alarm switch may set an audible alarm for this case.

Both instruments have preprogrammed modes for PT and APTT tests and a manually programmed mode for special determinations. In addition, the Electra has a mode appropriate for samples with multiple dilutions, which presets the sensitivity for low absorption samples.

Table 11–3 outlines the important distinctions in secondary features between these two instruments.

Advantages of MLA Electra-600. It easily interchanges with the Sherwood Coagulyzer. In comparison with manual instruments, the Electra has permitted a tighter standard deviation and less time to produce each result. Very little training is required to operate the instrument with excellent reliability. Because of its reproducibility and hands-off operation, it enables the medical technologist to tend to other chores during a run. The instrument is easy to operate and to troubleshoot, with adequate dealer service and helpful technical telephone call service. It utilizes solid-state electronics and an extended dynamic range of the detection system.

Disadvantages of MLA Electra-600. Some problems have arisen with the printers. Some of the earlier sample pipettes tended to clog. A redesign has corrected this on later units. Care must be observed to avoid overfilling the reservoirs (i.e., if the reagent spills over, it may cause a short circuit or improper shaking action). Most of the problems that arise in the operation of the instrument are chemically based.

Special Considerations of MLA Electra-600 include these deriving from the controls. With regard to PT controls, duplicates of a high abnormal, a low abnormal, and a normal should be run at the beginning of each shift and every 4 hours. For APTT only one abnormal is available, so two normal controls from different manufacturers are used. No schedule is similar. All controls are reconstituted as they are needed because of limited stability. It has been found desirable, when the controls are included in a run, to put them last. Apparently, the longer equilibrium time that that allows after reconstitution makes possible higher precision. Because of the high volume in some laboratories, it is not customary to change the reagent reservoir and pump tubing every 300 samples (one filling). Instead, the reservoirs are refilled several times, lasting for about 700 patient samples for PT and 500 for APTT. However, this weakens the pump tubing.

Advantages of the SMI Lancer Coagulyzer. It automates the complete APTT procedure. It is very adaptable to special tests (e.g., factor assays). It has great ease of operation and is extremely reliable. Intercomparison studies of this instrument with all of the other instruments in a large, busy laboratory verified that the same normal ranges may be applied in all cases. It possesses a refrigeration accessory and a temperature meter for monitoring the incubator and reservoir.

Disadvantages of the SMI Lancer Coagulyzer. There is false detection of cuvette absence when sample cuvettes are present (due to an out-of-tolerance frosted area on one batch of cuvettes). Hand-operated sample pipettes have had to be replaced a couple of times (spares must be kept on hand).

Special Considerations of the SMI Lancer Coagulyzer. Most laboratories run all samples essentially as stats. They are refrigerated only if there is a delay before running. Three controls are run—a normal and two high abnormals—at the beginning of a day's run. Reagent pipette tips and reagent reservoirs are changed daily. The magnetic stirring bars are retrieved at the end of each day's run. Both the Coagulyzer and the Electra can be used to perform other tests besides PT and APTT (i.e., prothrombin consumption, prothrombin, and proconvertin test, thromboplastin generation test, PT and APTT substitution tests, and factor assay for factors V, VII, VIII, IX, X, XI, and XII).

Auto-Fi Coagulation Instrument

The Auto-Fi is an automated system based on a new method of clot detection (Figs. 11-27, 11-28). It processes up to 40 samples in single or duplicate testing sequences for PT, APTT, fibrinogen, or fac-

tor assays. Push button selection of the test desired automatically adjusts all instrument settings for the test technique.

During the test sequence, the automatic sampling transfer pump aspirates the sample, transfers the sample into the measurement tray well, and returns to the wash station. The sampler tip is then washed two times prior to the next sampling. The measurement tray is processed to the read station during incubation at $37° \pm 0.5$ C. If two reagent techniques are employed, the rear reagent pump adds the first reagent to the sample. Reagent wells are incubated and continuously mixed by elliptical rotation. The front reagent well pump forcibly transfers the initiating reagent at the sampler read station, which starts the timing. Simultaneously, the moving filaments are activated and continue to move through the test mixture until fibrin-gel formation occurs, causing the clot to adhere to the filaments. The filament effectively drags some of the clotted material onto a light beam, causing a drop in the signal as it passes over the photocell for end-point detection. The printer then records the test result in 0.1 second increments.

Immediately after completion of the test, the fibrin clot is transported to the waste receptacle; the filament is then collected on the take-up reel, and the instrument advances to the next sequence.

Sample cup positions are identified to the printer and monitored for an empty position, for the automatic completion of the run when the last sample is processed. Prior to and during a run, the instrument status is automatically monitored to verify the presence of a sample cup in the carousel, the programming of the sample and reagent pumps to deliver the correct volumes for the test selected, that measurement trays are in position, and that filaments have tension to the take-up reel.

The proper functioning of the electrical circuits that control the temperature in the carousel refrigeration, in the heaters at reagent reservoirs, and in the read station is

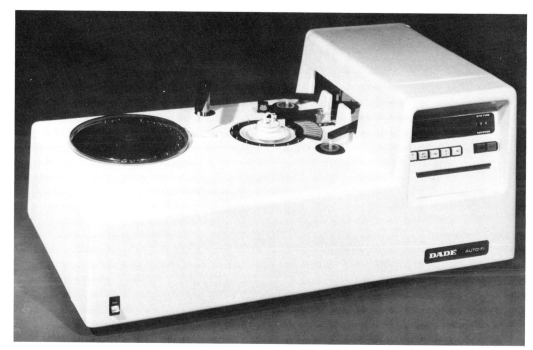

Fig. 11-27. Auto-Fi. (Courtesy of American Hospital Supply Corp.)

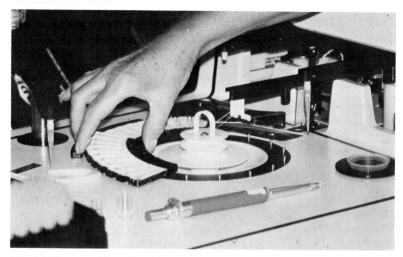

Fig. 11-28. Auto-Fi monitoring presence of sample cup in carousel and positioning of measurement trays. (Courtesy of American Hospital Supply Corp.)

automatically monitored. (These circuits should be supplemented by an external temperature gauge.) During a test run, if instrument status requirements are maintained, a special character is noted on the printout.

Advantages. This method is claimed to preclude any problems owing turbidity or chromogenicity. It yields values comparable to classic manual techniques. It accommodates $12\frac{1}{2}$ per cent on the prothrombin activity-dilution curve and detects up to 1:40 dilutions of normal plasma for fibrinogen assay. It has fixed incubation times and uniform activation to support precision. Degradation is reduced since samples are refrigerated prior to testing. It uses disposable items that come in contact with patient samples. The technologist need only use a single push button to select the test, without complicated adjustments. An auxiliary panel allows operation in manual mode for out-of-range samples and permits manual over-ride at nearly every test stage. The repeated wash of the sampler tip between samplings minimizes cross-contamination. Sample-throughput rates are PT, 72 per hour; APTT, 45 per hour; fibrinogen, 72 per hour; extrinsic systems factor assays, 45 per hour; and intrinsic factor assays, 24 per hour.

ASSOCIATED INSTRUMENTATION

Automatic Recording of Clot Lysis

In spite of decades of considerable evidence suggesting an important role for the blood fibrinolysin system in both health and disease, large-scale attempts to test and evaluate this far-reaching concept continue to be impeded by the technological difficulties of routine performance of fibrinolytic assays.[44] Without a simple, comparatively inexpensive instrument for measuring and recording fibrinolytic activity automatically, extensive field studies have been scarce and clinicians have been reluctant to adopt fibrinolytic tests as a matter of routine.

Fibrinolytic activity is determined by measuring the time needed for a blood, plasma, or fibrin clot to dissolve completely. Thus, it is important that the actual end-point of lysis be ascertained. Most laboratories use visual determination of the lysis end-point by the time-honored "rising-bubble" method. This method not only requires the undivided and often quite prolonged attention of a trained person, but is subject to errors in human judgment. Different observers frequently obtain divergent results for the same test.

Efforts to eliminate continuous observation by registering lysis end-points automatically have not yet produced an instrument capable of meeting the broad range of existing and anticipated needs. Present or proposed methods based on time-phase photography, isotope labeling, release of incoporated dyes, or photoelectric registration of transparency changes, as well as the more recent attempt to record clot lysis thermometrically, are too involved technically, too limited in scope and capacity, and too expensive for routine use in large-scale investigations. Thromboelastography, as a lysis-recording method, records the lysis of only those fibrin strands that attach to the probing stainless steel cylinder. Consequently, it merely records the beginning of clot lysis but not its end-point.

A lysis-detecting unit appears to be the instrument needed for the automatic determination and recording of clot lysis end-points. Its straightforward design, dependable performance, and optimally unlimited capacity fill the urgent need for "relatively inexpensive automated procedures for establishing"[44] coagulant fibrinolytic profiles to detect hypercoagulation and thrombotic tendency.

Figure 11-29 (*A* and *B*) illustrates an elapsed-time recording unit. A rectangular aluminum block (AB) contains 12 cylindrical channels (Ch) arranged in parallel to ac-

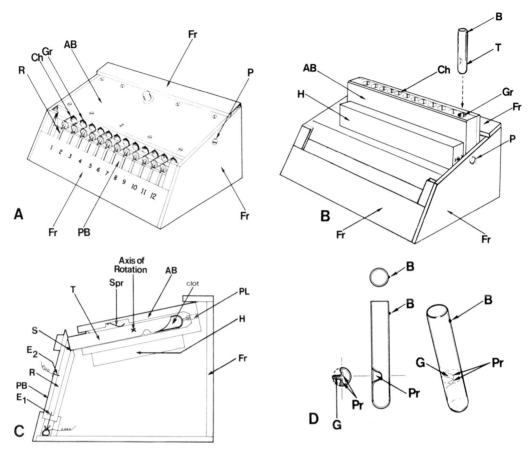

Fig. 11-29. Automatic clot lysis recording instrument. (*A*) Lysis-detecting unit in operating position. (*B*) Lysis-detecting unit, showing aluminum block and attached heating unit in tilted-up position. (*C*) Cross-section of lysis-detecting unit. (*D*) Schematic representation of modified test tube. (Courtesy of Nathan Back, D. Sc., Department of Biochemical Pharmacology, State University of New York School of Pharmacy, Buffalo)

commodate 12 clot-containing glass test tubes (T) of modified design. A thermostatically controlled heating unit (H) attached to the aluminum block serves to maintain the unit at a selected constant temperature, usually 37° C. Both the aluminum block and appended heating unit are suspended in a rectangular frame (Fr) by means of pivots (P), allowing them to be tilted about their longitudinal axis.

Ordinary 10- × 75-mm. glass test tubes are modified as shown in Figure 11-29D. Most important is the raising of two parallel protuberances (Pr) inside the tube and about 1 inch from its bottom, so as to form

a narrow gate (G). This narrow gate permits the passage of fluid formed upon clot lysis, but retains the nonliquefied material in the bottom of the tube when it is tilted to 10 degrees below horizontal. The only other change is the attachment of a small glass bead (B) at the outside of the test tube near its mouth and diametrically opposite the gate. This glass bead engages into a groove (Figs. 11-29A, D; Gr), in order to secure the correct alignment of the tubes within the heated aluminum block.

Figure 11-29C shows further details of the positioning of the test tubes (T) within the heated aluminum block (AB). A leaf spring (Spr) protruding from above presses the tubes downward, whereas a spring-loaded nylon plunger (Pl) at the rear acts as an elastic backstop.

As shown in Figure 11-29*A*, a removable rectangular block of transparent plastic (PB) contains 12 narrow cylindrical receptacles (R) aligned with and closely adjoined to the mouths of the downwardly tilted test tubes. Further details regarding these receptacles and their spatial relationship to the test tubes are depicted in Figure 11-29*D*. As can be seen, the upper face of the plastic block (PB) is slanted and appropriately milled to provide a tight-fitting seat (S) for the mouth of each individual test tube. Each receptacle (R) is equipped with two level-sensing electrodes (E_1 and E_2); one placed in the bottom and the other a measured distance higher up. Each pair of electrodes is connected to one of 12 sensitive relays housed in the elapsed-time recording unit.

When each of the relays is in the "open" position, it energizes a resettable digital timer when a toggle switch in the circuit is turned on. Operation of this switch permits each timer to be started separately the moment a clot has formed. Pilot lights indicate that the timers are running and when counting stops at the completion of clot lysis.

Lysis fluid draining from the test tubes gradually accumulates in the receptacles, making contact first with the lower and, upon completed lysis, also with the upper electrode. At that point, the fluid, acting as a conductor between both electrodes, trips a relay in the elapsed-time recording unit, placing it in the "closed" position. As a result, the pilot light goes out and the digital timer stops, thus indicating, for immediate or later inspection, the elapsed time between clot formation and completed lysis.*

---

* A film of fluid is always retained in the test tubes. For this reason slightly less fluid than the volume originally added needs to accumulate in the receptacles to make contact with the upper electrodes.

It seems that this is an instrument capable of automatically determining and registering the lysis end-points of as many as 12 clots prepared from whole blood, plasma, or fibrin. Experimental data show that the instrument records lysis times ranging from a few minutes to several hours, with reproducible accuracy under a variety of circumstances. The results recorded by the instrument closely match those of parallel tests obtained by an experienced medical technologist, on the basis of the rising-bubble method. Clot syneresis does not interfere with the performance of the instrument, since the fluid extruded by that process is far too small in volume to bridge the two electrodes in the receptacles.

Colysagraph Blood Plasma Analyzer

The Colysagraph, manufactured by Damon/IEC Division, is a photoelectric instrument for measuring and recording the changes in optical density that accompany the following (Fig. 11-30): conversion of fibrinogen to fibrin; lysis of fibrin clots; retraction of fibrin clots; and aggregation of platelets and other particles. Therefore, it can record changes in the amount and clotting ability of circulating fibrinogen, alterations in antithrombin activity, disorders of platelet aggregation, and variations in fibrinolytic activity. It combines the advantages of both analog and digital reporting by measuring the complete kinetics of clotting, with time end-points and amplitude of curves permanently recorded for collection, classification, and retrieval of data (i.e., the technologist no longer has to rely on gross viewing of clot formation or on a single digital printout).

The reagent is injected into the sample cuvette, which produces an instantaneous chart drive from an automatically set time and amplitude zero. If the reaction extends beyond the scale, the instrument resets to zero to provide an amplitude sum. A manual zero balance for plasma density compensation or for the repeating of the test with a different baseline is also provided.

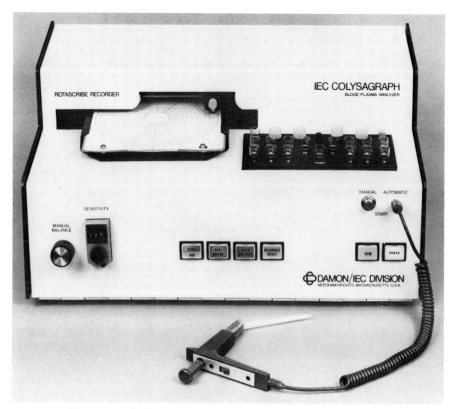

Fig. 11-30. Colysagraph. (Courtesy of Damon/IEC Division)

This instrument tests for the following co-agulation parameters: thrombin clotting time, Russell's viper venom clotting time, plasma lysis time, euglobulin lysis time, antithrombin III assay, generation tests (thromboplastin generation time, Hicks-Pitney modification and thrombin generation time), prothrombin time, prothrombin consumption time, partial thromboplastin time, activated PTT, and recalcified plasma clotting time. It also performs platelet aggregation tests (platelets, ADP, collagen, epinephrine, RBCs and antiserum, and latex particles—labeled or unlabeled—by antigen or antiserum) and any test in which fibrinogen is converted to fibrin or in which another indicator substance alters its optical density (e.g., tests for circulating anticoagulants and inhibitors, tests for neutralization and inhibition, and tests for sensitivity or resistance and assay of he-

parin, streptokinase, urokinase, and pit viper venom).

Advantages. There are no reagent restrictions. Any commercially available reagent may be used. It has an automatic baseline zero. It uses coagulation and aggregation modes and electronic baseline damping in the aggregation mode. A procedure manual is provided for coagulation, lysis, and aggregation tests. It has magnetic stirring (1200 r.p.m.) for aggregation tests and disposable stir bars. It has an expanded sensitivity-range selection for low fibrinogen and aggregation curves. It has high optical quality; keyed cuvettes eliminate density inconsistencies. There is a small specimen requirements, 0.1 to 0.2 ml. for most tests.

Disadvantages. The Analyzer contains only one test well, and, therefore, only one test at a time can be performed, a drawback for a busy laboratory.

PLASMA THROMBIN TIME TEST

Thrombin coagulates plasma and the clotting time of plasma thrombin is dependent on the strength of the thrombin, the concentration of the fibrinogen in the plasma, and the presence of any antithrombin substances such as heparin, and the temperature.

Technique

In the test, the powdered, dried thrombin is dissolved with normal saline solution so that 0.1 ml. of the thrombin solution clots 0.1 ml. of normal plasma in 12 to 15 seconds in a 37° C water bath. (The timer is started immediately at the addition of the thrombin solution, when the clot formation is being timed.) The procedure is repeated, using the patient's plasma. If 0.2 ml. of thrombin solution (incubated at 37° C for 30 secs. prior to adding 0.1 ml. normal plasma) is used, the clotting time of the normal plasma will be 15 to 20 seconds.

Results

The results are reported as clot formation in the test tube.

Significance of Abnormal Results. Prolongation of the plasma time occurs when there is a deficiency of fibrinogen or an inhibitor of the thrombin-fibrinogen reaction, such as heparin, antithrombin, and products of fibrinogenolysis is present. The test is sometimes abnormal in liver disease, and occasionally the plasma of a newborn has a prolonged thrombin time. A normal thrombin time may be observed in patients known to be undergoing heparin therapy. Presumably this is caused by a low concentration of heparin in the patient's plasma, which may be detectable when a lower concentration of thrombin is used.

SCREENING TEST FOR FIBRINOLYSIS

The fibrinolytic activity of a patient's plasma may be semiquantitatively measured by adding the test plasma to normal plasma, clotting the mixture, and observing the clot for zones of lysis.

Technique

In the test, six tubes are labeled 1 to 6, and a mixture of normal and patient's plasma is prepared as follows:

Tube	Normal plasma (ml.)	Patient's plasma (ml.)
1	1.0	0
2	0.8	0.2
3	0.6	0.4
4	0.4	0.6
5	0.2	0.8
6	0	1.0

The plasmas are mixed by inverting the tubes several times, and 0.1 ml. of topical thrombin (10 μg./ml.) is added to each tube. The plasmas are again mixed by gentle inversion, and the tubes are placed in a 37° C water bath. The tubes should be examined hourly for zones of lysis and if necessary allowed to incubate overnight.

Results

Tubes 1 and 6 are the normal and patient's plasma control tubes. Clots of normal plasma usually do not undergo any lysis, and the clots in all the tubes therefore should appear solid and well formed. These should be regarded as negative results. In the presence of a lysin, zones of lysis are observed. An approximate percentage of lysis may be determined by calculating the concentration of the patient's plasma in the tubes.

Significance of Abnormal Results. The manner of initiation of fibrinolytic activity is still poorly understood.[37] It has long been known, for instance, that serum demonstrates increased fibrinolytic activity after exercise, major surgery, stress such as pregnancy, anoxia, and the administration of certain pyrogens, apparently via a blood activator. In addition, it has recently been demonstrated that contraceptive hormones (progestogen, estrogen, and a combination of these, norethindrone with mestranol) produced minimal changes on selected parameters of the blood coagulation and plasma fibrinolytic system of normal women, except for the increase of fibrinogen level in postmenopausal women.[7]

Individually, progesteron and estrogen had little effect, whereas the combination caused changes in 14 of 27 parameters studied. Changes were significant only when treatment had continued for some weeks. After discontinuation, establishment of normal values for some parameters was delayed. Blood coagulation was slightly enhanced. The fibrinogen concentration remained unchanged. Spontaneous fibrinolytic activity increased, and plasminogen levels decreased. Inhibition of urokinase did not increase. In contrast to the coagulation changes, during hormone treatment the fibrinolytic system did not reproduce the changes occurring during pregnancy. The recent observation that coagulation Factor XII (Hageman) initiates both the clotting and the fibrinolytic processes upon surface activation throws further light on this mechanism.[23] It is indeed conceivable that as clotting starts, its antagonist reaction — fibrinolysis — also begins, maintaining in this way the homeostatic balance.

The recently observed association between clotting, fibrinolysis, and the plasma kinins,[13] with the Hageman factor possibly playing an important role, lends further support to the concept of its participation in initiating fibrinolysis. Moreover, it has been recently observed that thrombin may activate plasminogen directly.[14] This suggests another pathway through which fibrinolysis may become active as a consequence of coagulation.

STYPVEN COAGULATION TIME TEST

Russell's viper venom, active in high dilutions, has thromboplastic activity when added to recalcified plasma. Concentrated solutions exhibit inhibitory activity. The thromboplastic action of Stypven* is dependent on platelets, phospholipid, prothrombin, and Factor V. Factor VII does not affect the reaction. Therefore, the test is a useful measure of prothrombin plus Factor V when it is performed on platelet-poor nonlipemic plasma.

Technique

In the test, blood from a fasting patient is withdrawn cleanly into a silicone-coated syringe. Then 4.5 ml. of blood is added to 0.5 ml. of 0.1 M sodium oxalate in a silicone-coated centrifuge tube. The blood and oxalate are mixed and centrifuged at 3000 r.p.m. for 30 minutes. The platelet-poor plasma is then aspirated. All reagents are warmed in a 37° C water bath, and 0.1 ml. plasma and 0.1 ml. of dilute venom (1:10,000 dilution with distilled water) are then placed in a test tube. One-tenth milliliter of 0.02 M $CaCl_2$ is blown in, and the stopwatch is started. The time at which the clotting takes place is recorded as in the one-stage prothrombin time test.

Results

Normal Values. Normal values are the same as those obtained with tissue thromboplastin.

Significance of Abnormal Results. The Stypven coagulation time is prolonged by the deficiency of prothrombin, Factor V, and Factor X. In Factor X deficiency, the prothrombin time (with tissue thromboplastin) and the venom time are both prolonged. In Factor VII deficiency, the venom time is normal.

DETECTION OF A CIRCULATING ANTICOAGULANT

Abnormal laboratory results obtained on a combination of coagulation tests (bleeding time, clotting time, prothrombin time, thromboplastin generation, and others)

---

* Produced by Burroughs Wellcome & Co., Inc., Tuckahoe, N. Y.

may be an indication of a circulating anticoagulant.[12] The inhibitor may be directed against one or more specific clotting factors, the formation of blood (intrinsic) thromboplastin, the action of tissue (extrinsic) thromboplastin, or the action of thrombin.

A circulating anticoagulant can be demonstrated by determining the effect of the addition of the patient's whole blood (or plasma) on the clotting time of normal blood. A prolongation of the clotting time of the normal blood by the addition of the patient's blood suggests the presence of an anticoagulant. Conversely, correction of the abnormal clotting time of the patient's blood in the presence of normal blood rules out an inhibitor and suggests a clotting factor deficiency.

Technique

In the test, at least 5 ml. of blood is collected simultaneously from both the patient and also from a normal control, using silicone-coated syringes. The blood is immediately transferred to the precooled siliconized tubes (15 × 150 mm.). Using silicone-coated pipettes, a mixture of normal blood and the patient's blood is prepared in glass tubes (13 × 100 mm.) in the following proportions:

Tube	Normal blood (ml.)	Patient's blood (ml.)
1	1.0	0
2	0.7	0.3
3	0.5	0.5
4	0.3	0.7
5	0.1	0.9
6	0	1.0

The tubes are gently tilted several times to ensure complete mixing of the samples; they are immediately placed in the water bath. The tubes are examined at 1 minute intervals, and the coagulation times are recorded. The coagulation times of each tube depend on whether the unknown blood contains a circulating anticoagulant or is deficient in a coagulation factor. Ex-

Table 11-4. Whole-Blood Coagulation Times for Circulating Anticoagulant

Tube	1	2	3	4	5	6
Factor deficiency	−	−	−	−	±	+
Anticoagulant	−	+	+	+	+	+

+ = abnormal; − = normal; ± = may be normal or abnormal

pected results of whole-blood coagulation times in a screening test for circulating anticoagulant are demonstrable in Table 11–4.

Recent workers have demonstrated that immunosuppressive agents (azathioprine and mercaptopurine) may be effective in helping to control hemorrhagic disorders characterized by an endogenous circulating anticoagulant.[17] This coagulation inhibitor is antagonistic to the action of Factor VIII; it occurs relatively frequently and results in a significant mortality. Spontaneous development occurs in otherwise healthy persons; it is also seen in patients with hemophilia, postpartum patients, etc. The ratio of males to females is 2:1, excluding pregnancy and hemophilia cases. An autoimmune process has been suspected as the cause, but the exact mechanism remains to be elucidated. Treatment with adrenocorticoids has been only partially effective.

All cases have shown abnormal prothrombin consumption, a long clotting time, a long PTT, a positive test for circulating anticoagulant, a low Factor VIII assay, inhibitory activity to added Factor VIII, a normal prothrombin time, and a normal assay of all other coagulation factors. After therapy with azathioprine (two courses of 7 days each) or mercaptopurine (150 mg./day), clotting values returned to normal except for minimal prolongation of the partial thromboplastin time.

SUMMARY

Numerous assays for specific clotting factors have been described. These methods commonly involve the addition of

(*Text continues on p. 372.*)

Table 11-5. Hemostatic Factor Deficiencies and Related Laboratory Findings.[9]

Test	Tourniquet Test	Clotting Time	Clot Retraction	Platelet Count	Bleeding Time	Prothrombin Consumption	Prothrombin Time	Partial Thromboplastin Time	Hicks Pitney (TGT)	TGT
Normal	Less than 5 petechiae	5-10 min.	Complete 24 hours	150,000-400,000	3 minutes or less	Greater than 15 seconds	12.0 seconds	40-80 seconds	7-12 seconds	7-12 seconds
Antihemophilic globulin (VIII), mild	—	Normal to prolonged	Normal	Normal	Normal	Normal or abnormal	Normal	Abnormal	Abnormal	Abnormal, corrected by plasma
Antihemophilic globulin (VIII), severe	—	Prolonged	Normal	Normal	Normal	Abnormal	Normal	Abnormal	Abnormal	Abnormal, corrected by plasma
Plasma thromboplastin component (IX), mild	—	Normal to prolonged	Normal	Normal	Normal	Normal or abnormal	Normal	Abnormal	Abnormal	Abnormal, corrected by serum
Plasma thromboplastin component (IX), severe	—	Prolonged	Normal	Normal	Normal	Abnormal	Normal	Abnormal	Abnormal	Abnormal, corrected by serum
Plasma thromboplastin antecedent (XI)	—	Normal	Normal	Normal	Normal	Normal	Normal	Abnormal	Abnormal	Abnormal, corrected by plasma and serum
Hageman trait (XII)	—	Prolonged	Normal	Normal	Normal	Normal	Normal	Abnormal	Abnormal	Abnormal, corrected by plasma and serum

Pseudohemophilia A (von Willebrand's disease)	±	Normal	Normal	Normal	Normal or prolonged	Normal	Normal	Normal	Normal	Normal
Pseudohemophilia B	rarely —	Normal or prolonged	Normal	Normal	Prolonged	Abnormal	Normal	Abnormal	Abnormal	Abnormal, corrected by plasma
Thrombocytopenia	+	Normal	Abnormal	Decreased	Normal or prolonged	Abnormal	Normal	Normal	Normal	Abnormal, corrected by normal platelets
Stuart-Prower factor (X)	—	Normal or prolonged	Normal	Normal	Normal or prolonged	Abnormal	Abnormal	Abnormal	Abnormal	Abnormal, corrected by serum
Factor V	—	Normal or prolonged	Normal	Normal	Normal or prolonged	—	Abnormal	Abnormal	—	—
Factor VII	—	Normal	Normal	Normal	Normal or prolonged	Normal	Abnormal	Normal	Normal	—
Prothrombin (II)	—	Normal or prolonged	Normal	Normal	Normal or prolonged	—	Abnormal	Abnormal	—	—
Fibrinogen (I)	—	Prolonged	Abnormal	Normal	Prolonged	—	Abnormal	—	—	—

various dilutions of the plasma being tested to a substrate plasma that is deficient in one factor only, all other factors being present. The degree to which the prolonged clotting time of the substrate plasma is shortened by the diluted test plasma is compared to a normal control plasma, the results usually being expressed as a percentage of normal. For assays of Factors I, II, V, and VII, the prothrombin time method is usually used. For assay of AHF, PTC, PTA, and Hageman factor, methods using the PTT, the prothrombin consumption test, recalcification time,[34] the kaolin-PTT,[38] or the thromboplastin generation test have been described.

The prothrombin time, the recalcification time, and PTT are called one-stage methods because the incubation mixture and the final clot are in the same tube. On the other hand, the method using the TGT is called a two-stage assay. One-stage assays, properly employed, give results comparable to the two-stage methods. For reliable results in the assay of AHF, PTC, PTA and Hageman factor, attention to contact activation is essential; this area has been carefully studied by Waaler.[43]

Ideally, the substrate plasma should be congenitally deficient in one factor, and such a plasma, deficient in AHF or PTC, is readily obtained. For assay of prothrombin, Factor V, and Factor X, reliable assay methods, employing substrate plasmas artificially depleted of a single factor are available.[2, 18, 43] A different approach to the solution of problems of blood coagulation has recently been proposed by Mann.[27] He believes that some coagulation defects are due to inhibitor substance firmly bound to coagulation factors, rather than to the lack of specific coagulation factors. Accordingly, Mann believes that it is not necessary to postulate a specific coagulation factor to explain each different observed abnormality of coagulation.

Although most of the clotting factors are found to have a relatively small variation in the normal population, AHF differs in that levels of healthy persons may range from 50 to 200 per cent of normal. AHF levels may be markedly increased in normal subjects and patients with mild hemophilia by exercise, epinephrine, and pregnancy. This fact should be borne in mind in the selection of normal controls for AHF assays. Other coagulation factors whose levels rise significantly with pregnancy are Factors I, VII, IX, and X.

In order to understand the clinical events associated with coagulation defects, the following must be appreciated. To begin with, hemostasis in a wound starts with vasoconstriction and platelet adherence to the injured tissue, thus releasing tissue thromboplastin for the quick activation of an extrinsic system of clotting factors. The extrinsic system is supported by an intrinsic clotting system that is slower acting and on which hemostasis principally depends thereafter until the wound is healed. The junction point of the two systems is the activation of Factor V, which converts prothrombin to thrombin in the presence of calcium. In the extrinsic system, this requires only tissue thromboplastin and Factors VII and X. On the other hand, in the intrinsic system a "cascade" initiated by the glass activation of Factor XII involves several factors that are individually missing in hereditary bleeding disorders, before the junction point is reached. This distinction between the two types of systems is helpful in understanding the clinical events as they occur.

A summary of hemostatic factor deficiencies and their related laboratory findings is given in Table 11–5.

REFERENCES

1. Alpert, N. L., Automated blood coagulation timers. Lab. World, 25:30, 1974.
1a. Bick, R. L., Dukes, M. L., Wilson, W. L., and Fekete, L. F.: Simple assay for plasma heparin. Presented at a meeting of the American Society of Clinical Pathologists. Las Vegas, 1977.

2. Bachmann, F., Duchert, F., and Kohler, F.: Stuart-Prower factor assay and its clinical significance. Thromb. Diath. Haemorrh., *2*:24, 1958.

3. Biggs, R., and Douglas, A. S.: The thromboplastin generation test. J. Clin. Pathol., *6*:23, 1953.

4. Biggs, R., and Macfarlane, R. G.: Hemophilia and related conditions: survey of 187 cases. Br. J. Haematol., *4*:1, 1958.

5. Biggs, R., and Macfarlane, R. G.: Human Blood Coagulation and its Disorders. ed. 3, p. 385. Oxford, Blackwell Scientific Publications, 1962.

6. Bonnin, J. A., and Cheney, K.: The PTF test. An improved method for the estimation of platelet thromboplastic function. Br. J. Haematol., *7*:512, 1961.

7. Brakman, P., Albrechtsen, O. K., and Astrup, T.: Blood coagulation, fibrinolysis and contraceptive hormones. J.A.M.A., *199*:69, 1967.

8. Castaldi, P. A., Rozenberg, M. C., and Stewart, J. H.: The bleeding disorder of uremia: a qualitative platelet defect. Lancet, *2*:66, 1966.

9. Coagulation Procedures—Scientific Products. pp. 30, 31, Dade, 1965.

10. Dacie, J. V., and Lewis, S. M.: Practical Hematology. ed. 3, p. 210. New York, Grune & Stratton, 1963.

11. Dormandy, K. M., and Hardisty, R. M.: Coagulation tests on capillary blood—a screening procedure for use in small children. J. Clin. Pathol., *14*:543, 1961.

12. Eichelberger, J. W.: Laboratory Methods in Blood Coagulation. pp. 13; 41; 66; 67. New York, Hoeber Medical Division (Harper & Row), 1965.

13. Eisen, V.: Fibrinolysis and formation of biologically active polypeptides. Br. Med. Bull., *20*:205, 1964.

14. Engel, R., Pechet, L., and Alexander, B.: Activation of trypsinogen and plasminogen by thrombin. Fed. Proc., *22*:561, 1963.

15. Gaston, L. W.: The blood clotting factors. N. Engl. J. Med., *270*:290, 1964.

16. Goldstein, C., Pechet, L., and Alexander, B.: Three hour prothrombin consumption test in siliconized glass. Am. J. Clin. Pathol., *46*:48, 1966.

17. Goldstein, M. A., Sherman, L., and Shore, H. S.: Circulating anticoagulant (anti-Factor VIII) treated with immunosuppressive drugs (abstract). Presented at the 9th Annual Meeting, American Society of Hematology, 1966; also in Medical News Section, J.A.M.A., *199*:26, 1967.

18. Goldstein, R., LeBolloc'h, A., Alexander, B., and Zonderman, E.: Preparation and properties of prothrombin. J. Biol. Chem., *234*:2857, 1959.

19. Hardisty, R. M., and Macpherson, J. C.: A one-stage factor VIII (antihemophilic globulin) assay and its use on venous and capillary plasma. Thromb. Diath. Haemorrh., *7*:215, 1962.

20. Harrower, H. W., and Brook, D. L.: An instrument for the study of blood coagulation and lysis. Ann. Surg., *160*:870, 1964.

21. Harrower, H. W., and Brook, D. L.: Clinical application of coagulographic studies. Am. J. Clin. Pathol., *47*:190, 1967.

22. Hicks, N. D., and Pitney, W. R.: Rapid screening test for disorders of thromboplastin generation. Br. J. Haematol., *3*:227, 1957.

23. Iatridis, S. G., and Ferguson, J. H.: Active Hageman Factor: plasma lysokinase of human fibrinolytic system. J. Clin. Invest., *41*:1277, 1962.

24. Klee, G. G., Didisheim, P., Johnson, R. J., and Gurre, G. M.: An evaluation of four automated coagulation instruments. Am. J. Clin. Pathol., in press.

25. Leavelle, D. E., Beckala, H. R., and Didisheim, P.: A comparison of five manually operated coagulation instruments. Am. J. Clin. Pathol., *70*:71, 1978.

26. Luscher, E. F.: Biochemical basis of platelet function. *In* Brinkhous, K. (ed.): The Platelet. International Academy of Pathology Monograph. Baltimore, Williams & Wilkins, 1971.

27. Mann, F. D.: Further evidence for a simpler view of the coagulation of blood. Am. J. Clin. Pathol., *46*:612, 1966.

28. Margolis, J.: Initiation of blood coagulation by glass and related surfaces. J. Physiol., *137*:95, 1957.

29. Miale, J. B.: Laboratory Medicine-Hematology. ed. 2, p. 876. St. Louis, C. V. Mosby, 1962.

30. Miale, J. B.: The Fibrometer system for routine coagulation tests. Am. J. Clin. Pathol., *43*:475, 1965.

31. Miale, J. B.: Determinants of prothrombin time. Bull. Pathol., *7*:167, 1966.

32. Miale, J. B., and Lafond, D. J.: 1963 prothrombin time test survey, College of American Pathologists, Standard committee, subcommittee on coagulation. Am. J. Clin. Pathol., *47*:40, 1967.

33. Mochir-Fatemi, F., and Leikin, S.: An evaluation of a capillary micro partial thromboplastin test in hemophiliac disorders. Am. J. Clin. Pathol., *47*:91, 1967.

34. Nilsson, I. M., Blombäch, M., and Von Franchen, I.: On inherited autosomal hemorrhagic diathesis with antihemophilic globulin (AHG) deficiency and prolonged bleeding time. Acta Med. Scand., *159*:35, 1957.

35. Nygaard, K. K.: Hemorrhagic Diseases; Photoelectric Study of Blood Coagulability. p. 320. St. Louis, C. V. Mosby, 1941.

36. Owren, P. A., and Aas, K.: The control of dicumarol therapy and the quantitative determination of prothrombin and proconvertin. Scand. J. Clin. Lab. Invest., *3*:201, 1951.

37. Pechet, L.: Fibrinolysis. N. Engl. J. Med., *273*:965, 1965.

38. Proctor, R. R., and Rapaport, S. I.: Partial thromboplastin time with kaolin. Am. J. Clin. Pathol., *36*:212, 1961.

39. Quick, A. J.: Detection and diagnosis of hemorrhagic states. J.A.M.A., *197*:418, 1966.

40. Starr, A. J., Schmidt, P. J., Dade, D.: Proper handling of specimens for coagulation studies. Laboratory Medicine, 8:26, 1977.

41. Swatman, L. E.: Platelets: Should you do qualitative screens. Medical Lab. Bulletin, 8:23, 1976.

42. Von Kaulla, K. N.: Chemistry of Thrombolysis:

Human Fibrinolytic Enzymes. Springfield, Charles C Thomas, 1963.

43. Waaler, B. A.: Contact activation in intrinsic blood clotting system. Scand. J. Clin. Lab. Invest., *11* (Supple. 37):1, 1959.

44. Wilkens, H. J., and Back, N.: New instrument for automatic recording of clot lysis. Am. J. Clin. Pathol., *66:*124, 1976.

45. Wu, K. K., Hoak, J. C., Thompson, J. S., and Koepke, J. A.: Use of platelet aggregometry in selection of compatible platelet donors. N. Engl. J. Med., *292;*130, 1975.

AUDIVISUAL AIDS*

Determining Prothrombin Activity. Warner-Lambert Film Department, 201 Tabor Road, Morris Plains, New Jersey 07950.

Prothrombin Time Test: Clinical and Laboratory Aspects. Seminar No. 300. ASMT Education and Research Fund, Inc., 5555 West Loop South, Bellaire, Texas 77401.

_____

* Films unless otherwise stated.

12 *Coagulation Disorders*

ABNORMALITIES IN PHASE I OF COAGULATION (THROMBOPLASTOGENESIS)

THROMBOCYTOPENIC STATES

Quantitative platelet deficiency, or thrombocytopenia, is one of the most common causes of hemorrhagic diatheses. It is characterized, clinically, by petechiae and ecchymoses of the skin and mucous membranes. These may develop in superficial injuries or in an apparently intact mucosa. Whenever one observes bleeding tendencies in a patient, one not only must think of the failure of vascular or platelet factors of hemostasis, but also most consider a deficiency of coagulation agents, the presence of anticoagulants, and the activation of fibrinolysis.

Clinically, bleeding due to platelet deficiency differs from that observed in disorders of plasma clotting factors. Coagulopathies are characterized by larger hemorrhages into skin, muscle and joints, whereas thrombocytopenic bleeding usually results in petechiae of the skin and mucous membranes and a tendency to internal (cerebral and gastrointestinal), menorrhagic, nose, gum, and tongue bleeding. Furthermore, the petechiae are more numerous over dependent parts because of increased venous pressure, and they may be confluent leading to larger ecchymoses with petechiae present around the margins.

Etiologic Classification

In order better to understand the thrombocytopenias, the following etiologic classification is given as a practical guide from both a clinical and a laboratory diagnostic standpoint.

I. Amegakaryocytic disorders, or those due to decreased platelet production.
  A. Congenital disorders.
    1. Hypoplastic anemia (e.g., Fanconi's syndrome), characterized by sex-linked skeletal abnormalities and associated hypoplasia of all three cell lines.
    2. Hypoplastic thrombocytopenia, possibly due to a lack of a circulating megakaryocytic-ripening factor; also, for example, May-Hegglin anomaly with faulty maturation of platelets and granulocytes, and with basophilic inclusions in the white blood cells.
    3. Acute leukemia (at birth, poor prognosis).
    4. Sepsis (may be due to impaired thrombocytopoiesis), congenital syphilis, other infections, viral diseases (e.g., cytomegalic inclusion disease).
  B. Acquired disorders.
    1. Nutritional deficiency (megaloblastic anemias, scurvy, iron deficiency, etc.).
    2. Depression of bone marrow activity by drugs, radiation, oncolytic agents, severe viral infections (chicken pox, mumps, measles, infectious mononucleosis), severe bacterial infections, possibly uremia (with

or without marrow hypoplasia), and idiopathic disorders.

3. Replacement of bone marrow, as in leukemia, carcinoma, sarcoma, lymphoma, granuloma, lipoidosis, sclerosis, fibrosis.

II. Megakaryocytic disorders (increased platelet destruction or decreased megakaryocytic platelet production; normal lifespan of platelets is 8 to 10 days).

A. Congenital disorders.

1. Children of nonthrombocytopenic mothers.

a. Idiopathic thrombocytopenic purpura (ITP), rare at birth. During the last 5 to 10 years, some families have been investigated whose members have thrombocyte counts ranging from 42,000 to 82,000 mm.[3] and in whom normal and megathrombocytes have been observed. Normal and shortened platelet life spans have been detected with ^{51}Cr as a tag. No ultrastructural abnormalities have been found. Since platelet aggregation may be abnormal and bleeding time prolonged, thrombocytopenic patients with a positive family history should not have a splenectomy (it is not helpful).

b. Platelet-type material, as in fetal incompatibility.

c. Disorders associated with erythroblastosis fetalis.

d. Aldrich's syndrome in baby boys (eczema, diarrhea, increased susceptibility to chronic infection, and decreased platelets; transmitted as a sex-linked recessive character).

e. Viral infection in mother especially early in pregnancy (especially measles). Widespread petechiae and thrombocytopenia have been observed in newborn infants born to mother who had had rubella during pregnancy. This was recently reported by Bayer and co-workers in 11 newborn infants in which the rubella virus was isolated from ten cases in which platelet agglutinins were found in all the infants tested.[7] Autopsy findings were those of multisystem disease with intravascular coagulation, especially in liver and kidneys. According to others, it is possible that the virus had a greater tendency to affect the megakaryocytes in the bone marrow, or to affect the circulating platelets, causing their destruction or alteration and leading to their removal from the bloodstream.[24] According to Bayer and co-workers, an alteration of platelets by the rubella virus might have caused them to become antigenic, leading to antibody production and an autoimmune mechanism for thrombocytopenia.[7]

2. Children of thrombocytopenic mothers.

a. Transplacental transfer of platelet agglutinins from mother to fetus.[28, 46]

b. Drug thrombocytopenia, due to transfer of drug and platelet-destructive factor through placenta.

B. Acquired disorders.

1. Hypersplenic thrombocytopenia, usually with splenomegaly or possibly because of excessive sequestration of cells due to:

a. Chronic infections (malaria, syphilis, kala-azar, brucellosis, tuberculosis, histoplasmosis, viremia). May be due in part to inhibition of activity of megakaryocytes despite the adequacy of their numbers. Viruses and bacteria appear to be capable of inducing acute depletion of circulating platelets—that is, platelets adhere to one another and to the endothelium when living microorganisms are introduced into the bloodstream. The degree of thrombocytopenic purpura is partially responsible for hemorrhagic manifestations. Use of dextran (6% in saline) in a dosage of 500 mg. per kg. of body weight every 3 days leads to apparent recovery.[45]

b. Portal hypertension (cirrhosis, cavernous portal vein).

c. Splenic vein thrombosis.

d. Lipoidosis (Gaucher's disease and allied syndromes).

e. Nonspecific hyperplasia.

f. Sarcoidosis.

g. Tumors and cysts of spleen.

h. Rheumatoid diseases (Felty's syndrome, *lupus erythematosus*)

i. Lymphomas, myeloid metaplasia, and so forth.

2. Stagnation of blood flow due to extensive hemangioma with "helmet cell" anemia,[51] congestive heart failure, or hypothermia.

3. Massive blood loss and replacement with bank blood, which is frequently platelet-poor diluting the patient's platelets (for example, exchange transfusion in infancy).

Platelets may also be diluted by posttransfusion purpura, an acute severe thrombocytopenic state that appear about 1 week after transfusion of a blood product. It is mediated by an isoantibody, usually directed against the platelet P1-A1 antigen. However, platelets with and without the Pl-Al antigen are destroyed.

The diagnosis is presumed when thrombocytopenia occurs 7 to 10 days after the blood transfusion. Other coagulation studies are normal, and the bone marrow shows abundant megakaryocytes. Several methods are available to demonstrate the presence of the antiplatelet antibody. Platelet-poor plasma from some patients has induced spontaneous aggregation of Pl-Al-positive platelets. Platelet-poor plasma from others, when it is incubated with Pl-Al-positive platelets, has inhibited the normal response to ADP. The most sensitive method appears to be ^{51}Cr release from PNH platelets.[1]

Gradual recovery from PTP occurs in 1 to 6 weeks, and corticosteroids do not appear to alter the course of the disease. Exchange transfusion has been associated with a more rapid recovery, but has often been accompanied by severe transfusion reactions. Plasmapheresis has been shown to decrease antibody titer, to increase platelet count, and not to be associated with transfusion reactions.[26]

4. Accelerated intravascular coagulation, due to obstetric accidents, amniotic fluid embolism, placenta previa, and other causes. More commonly bleeding in this group is due to afibrinogenemia.

5. Thrombotic thrombocytopenia, frequently in females. Platelets are decreased; clots form with fibrin but not with platelets. Heart, brain, spleen, lymph nodes, and adrenals are involved; it is treated with steroids and heparin. It is of unknown etiology, is uniformly fatal and is characterized by fever, hemolytic anemia, thrombocytopenic purpura, migratory transient central nervous system signs and symptoms, and renal involvement. Acute, chronic, and relapsing forms are found. Microscopically, vasculitis is observed in which fibrin and entrapped red blood cells and platelets are seen. Occlusions occur in terminal arterioles and capillaries, most prominently in the myocardium, adrenal capsular zone, renal cortex, pancreas, and gray matter of brain. Doubt exists whether it represents an autoimmune mechanism.

6. Onyalai, which is seen in Bantus, in males more than females. It is characterized by idiopathic hemorrhagic bullae of the mucosa and purpura, with spontaneous recovery.

7. Viremia; bacteremia. In viremia, abnormal megakaryocyte forms are seen in the marrow of patients with dengue fever with associated thrombocytopenic purpura and early suppression of megakaryocytopoiesis. It is also seen in 65 per cent of infants with rubella.

8. Incompatible transfusion reactions; the degree of thrombocytopenic purpura is seldom of sufficient severity to induce bleeding.

9. Drug-induced thrombocytopenia, which is due to an immunologic mechanism, may be brought about by quinidine, ristocetin, Sedormid, and certain other drugs, chemicals, and foods. This type of thrombocytopenia is produced in three ways—by bone marrow depression (megakaryocytes), destruction of platelets in the

blood, and by immunologic reaction. The most common type is bone marrow depression by antimetabolic agents and chloramphenicol; in very low doses these drugs interfere with attachment of enzymes to ribosomes, and subsequently interference with protein synthesis occurs. In the bone marrow, destruction of megakaryocytes or its precursors takes place. Treatment is withdrawal of the drug. When platelet destruction occurs in the blood, Spontin or ristocetin produces thrombocytopenic purpura on the first trial of therapy. Complement is not needed in this destructive system, and less than 50 mg. of the drug per kilogram of body weight produces thrombocytopenic purpura. With lower dosages, one may reuse the drug, and no thrombocytopenic purpura will be produced. There is no effect on the bone marrow. However, new laboratory tests, which define the mechanism of platelet destruction in ITP, have revealed that complement becomes bound to the membranes of platelets that have been in contact with idiopathic thrombocytopenic purpura (ITP) plasma. This demonstration of an abnormal protein coating of ITP platelets is consistent with the presence of platelet destruction taking place, in many instances, by sequestration in the reticuloendothelial system (spleen). It is also possible that a similar pathogenesis is associated with the thrombocytopenia seen in systemic lupus erythematosus (SLE) and other collagen-vascular diseases. Therefore, the technique of surface monitoring of ^{51}Cr-labeled platelet sequestration in the spleen deserves further attention and consideration for a role in the selection of patients for splenectomy. The immunologic or hypersensitivity concept appears to be related to certain chemotherapeutic and antibiotic drugs, anticonvulsants, tranquilizers, and sedatives. Thrombocytopenic purpura occurs any time after the first week of drug administration and is associated with lethargy, pruritus, chills, fever, bleeding, and ulcers in the mouth. The peripheral blood shows thrombocytopenic purpura in 1 to 3

hours, and the bone marrow shows a relative decrease in mature megakaryocytes with platelet formation. The patient's serum gives a positive complement-fixation test and a platelet agglutination test associated with the inhibition of clot retraction (2 ml. of patient's freely shed blood plus saline control, and 2 ml. of patient's freely shed blood plus drug solution).

No clot retraction occurs in the tube with the offending drug, Ackroyd believes that the hapten theory* is most applicable here, involving the attachment of drug to the cell itself with subsequent coating of the platelets with antibody and platelet destruction.[2] Shulman believes that the antigen-antibody complex adsorbs nonspecifically on platelets, leading to thrombocytopenic purpura and platelet destruction.[58] What determines to which drug the antibody adheres is not known. Therapy consists of removing the drug; recovery occurs in 7 to 14 days if the patient can survive the thrombocytopenic purpura. Steroids are also used satisfactorily. A rebound thrombocytosis may follow, and if the patient is not re-exposed to the drug, the antibody gradually disappears from the patient's plasma over a period of several months. It returns again within a few days if re-exposure takes place. This differs from bone marrow aplasia due to marrow toxins.

A most important drug, digitoxin, has recently been implicated in a thrombocytopenic purpura based on a sensitivity specific for digitoxin, the drug being bound to the gamma globulin fraction of the serum. In vitro studies have demonstrated a digitoxin-reacting antibody. The platelet factor 3 assay is specific for digitoxin sensitivity, gives the earliest indication of the cause, and permits selection of a safe substitute digitalis preparation.[66]

Reported cases of thrombocytopenia associated with drug use have increased

---

* A hapten is a small antigenic molecule that, by itself, cannot produce antibodies, but when it is combined with other moieties, it can form antibodies.

markedly with the routine use of automated instrumentation and associated routine thrombocyte counting. Consequently, a theory has developed in which drug and antibody combinations are joined to the platelet membrane to produce coated platelet sequestration in the reticuloendothelial system (spleen). However, this does not explain the thrombocytopenia associated with thrombotic thrombocytopenic purpura. Dipyridamole and heparin have been somewhat therapeutically successful in those cases, which suggest that TTP is probably an endothelial disorder. But no therapy aside from massive steroid use and splenectomy has been advocated.

10. Idiopathic thrombocytopenic purpura (ITP).

a. Without demonstrable antibodies or plasma platelet-destructive factor. These include cases of platelet deficiency related to alcohol and chlorathiazide bone marrow suppression. Automated platelet counters in routine CBC testing have been especially helpful in identifying ethanol related cases and in indicating the need to change to less toxic diuretics with a lower incidence of related thrombocytopenia. Therapy during the period of withdrawal is directed toward correcting the folate deficiency, associated with the alcoholism, that may accompany platelet deficiency.

b. With demonstrable antibodies or plasma platelet-destructive factor.

11. Associated with tumors other than splenic tumors and not invading bone marrow—for example, carcinoma of the lung, uterine tumors, bowel tumors—possibly involving an immunologic mechanism.

12. Postpartum thrombocytopenic purpura.

Idiopathic Thrombocytopenic Purpura (ITP)

ITP is most common in young children (especially females less than 15 yrs. of age) and in premenopausal women; however it may be seen in any age group (Table 12–1; Plates 40, 41). In the acute form, one sees sudden severe bleeding from nose or gums or extensive petechial and ecchymotic areas, menorrhagia or metrorrhagia, gastrointestinal hemorrhage, hematuria, pulmonary hemorrhage resembling circumscribed consolidation by radiographs, intracerebral hemorrhage, and ophthalmic (vitreous or retinal) hemorrhage. The hemorrhagic diathesis occurs most frequently in the order just mentioned, persisting until death with intensity, and usually lessening with advancing age. The spleen is rarely palpable.

Exacerbations are often precipitated by (1) infections; for example, in infancy and childhood an upper respiratory infection frequently antedates the onset of thrombocytopenic purpura. The child may be convalescent or fully recovered from rubella, varicella, or mumps when purpura abruptly appears.[6, 8] (2) Pregnancy; if an autoimmune process is at work, the spleen apparently removes platelets modified by the antiplatelet antibodies produced. These antibodies cross the placenta, and the patient gives birth to a thrombocytopenic infant even if her purpura is in remission following splenectomy. If no antibodies are produced, the pregnant patient may be purpuric and give birth to a normal infant. Also, the mother may be immunized to fetal platelets as in Rh isoimmunization, and although normal herself, give birth to a thrombocytopenic purpura infant. Exacerbations of ITP are also caused by (3) postpartum reactions 1 to 2 months after delivery, lasting a few weeks or months, and recurring after subsequent pregnancies; (4) puberty; (5) menopause; (6) chronic lymphocytic leukemia and disseminated systemic lupus erythematosus; (7) drugs such as Sedormid, quinidine, sulfa drugs and ristocetin; and (8) hypersplenism.

According to Shulman and colleagues, the unresponsiveness of splenectomized subjects to both ITP plasma and isoantibodies suggests that the role of the spleen

*Table 12–1. Laboratory Diagnostic Characteristics of Idiopathic Thrombocytopenic Purpura**

Laboratory Diagnostic Characteristics	Acute ITP	Chronic ITP
Peripheral blood		
Platelet count	5,000–20,000/cu. mm.	40,000–200,000/cu. mm.
Platelet morphology	Normal platelets	Larger, bizarre platelets
Eosinophilia	Often (child)	0
Lymphocytes	Often (child)	0
Anemia	Normochromic with associated reticulocytosis	Normochromic with associated reticulocytosis (if active bleeding into urinary tract or GI tract)
Leukocytes	Leukocytosis with associated increase in granulocytic forms	Same if purpura is excessive
Platelet agglutinins	Platelet agglutinins rare	Platelet agglutinins in 50% of cases
Bone marrow	Normoblastic and myeloid hyperplasia	Hyperplasia not present unless active bleeding
Megakaryocytes	Normal number, small agranular, vacuoles, degenerative forms, immature forms; no platelets formed	Increased numbers, normal size, granularity reduced; mature in granularity reduced; mature in construction; fewer platelets formed from megakaryocytes
Eosinophils	Often present	0
Effect of plasma from ITP patient	Rare effect (fall in platelets)	Drop in platelets (60% of cases)
Platelet survival time	Very short (1–6 hrs.)	Short (12–24 hrs.)
Bleeding time	Prolonged	Prolonged
Coagulation time	Normal	Normal
Clot retraction	Poor to absent	Poor to absent
Tourniquet test (capillary fragility test)	Positive	Positive
Prothrombin consumption test	Abnormal (indicates impaired thromboplastin formation)	Abnormal

* See Plates 40 and 41.

was to remove sensitized platelets selectively from the circulation.[58] The ITP factor could be adsorbed from ITP plasma by platelets and was found in the 7S gamma globulin fraction of serum. The proposal that ITP is an immune disorder is thus substantiated by the observations that the ITP factor reacts with autologous platelets, appears to be species specific, is adsorbed by platelets, and is in the 7S gamma globulin fraction of plasma (certain ITP patient plasma has platelet-sequestering properties).

The measurement of platelet-bound antibody (or complexes) appears to be more useful in the evaluation of immune thrombocytopenia than other diagnostic procedures. The measurement of platelet-associated IgG (PA IgG) in ITP and related disorders, using either the complement lysis inhibition assay or the Fab-antiFab assay, has been reported. Positive results are obtained, essentially, in all patients with significant thrombocytopenia, and correlate with the patient's clinical status. PA IgG values normalize immediately after splenectomy, if a remission occurs, but may become abnormal several weeks after surgery, in spite of a continued clinical response. This probably reflects ongoing, compensated platelet destruction. In acute childhood ITP and immune, complex-induced thrombocytopenia, PA IgG values are higher than expected for a platelet count, which suggests a different mechanism of destruction.[31]

For drug-induced immune thrombocytopenia, several serum assays, including complement fixation ^{51}Cr release and platelet factor 3 release techniques, are useful.

[51]Cr-platelet kinetic studies show that all patients with ITP and other types of autoimmune thrombocytopenia have markedly shortened platelet survival times ($T\frac{1}{2}$ 0.1–30 hrs.; normal $T\frac{1}{2}$ 100–120 hrs.), and normal or only slightly subnormal platelet recoveries at T_0 (40–80%); normal (60–80%). About 75 per cent of patients have splenic platelet sequestration only, and 25 per cent have splenic and hepatic sequestration. Although initially sites of platelet sequestration were thought to be useful in predicting response to splenectomy, recent data show no significant differences in response rates from presplenectomy sequestration patterns; both groups had an 85 to 90 per cent complete remission rate 2 years later.[17, 54]

Aster has demonstrated the existence of a reservoir or pool of platelets in the spleen, roughly proportional to the size of the organ.[5] Thus, the spleen may divert the circulating platelets to cause a significant thrombocytopenia. This work also clearly demonstrates the exchangeability of platelets between the splenic and the general systemic pools. Penny and co-workers also showed a sizable pool of platelets in the spleen, which is in dynamic equilibrium with circulating platelets, a certain constant ratio being maintained in each patient.[48]

Idiopathic thrombocytopenic purpura (ITP) of childhood is generally an acute, self-limited disorder with peak incidence between the ages of 2 to 5 years, characterized by peripheral thrombocytopenia concomitant with increased platelet production, and a decrease in platelet life span. In more than 50 per cent of children, the ITP is postviral, while in the remaining children no preceding viral infection can be documented. Most patients with childhood ITP (80–90%), make an uneventful recovery,

with a return of the platelet count to normal in approximately 3 weeks, ranging from 3 days to 6 months. The term chronic ITP is reserved for those children in whom thrombocytopenia has persisted for from 6 to 12 months. Although an insidious onset without preceding viral illness, a low IgA value, or ITP in a child over 10 years of age all point to impending chronicity, there is no definitive test, to date, that distinguishes the acute self-limited form of this disorder from the chronic variety. Recent evidence raises the possibility that chronic childhood ITP may occur in families with underlying cellular or humoral immunologic defects, and that these abnormalities may be associated with a familial haplotype. Studies on additional groups of children with chronic ITP appear warranted.

However, the role of the humoral immune system in childhood ITP has been explored, and a significant increase in platelet-associated IgG in both the acute and chronic forms of this disorder has been documented. The spleen and bone marrow have been shown to be sites of production of the platelet-binding IgG. These findings, along with the discovery of a complement-fixing platelet antibody in approximately 50 per cent of children with ITP, point to an immune-mediated thrombolytic state as the basis for the disorder.[40]

Treatment. Complete bed rest and protection from trauma are prerequisites to specific therapies. If the adult patient is bleeding acutely, 60 mg. of prednisone is used daily, tapering to 30 mg. with the relief of active purpura. If platelet elevation returns, the dose is tapered early. If platelets again fall, steroid therapy is reinstituted. A second remission is obtained in many cases. However, if after a second 3-week trial of steroids in adults there is no remission of platelet rise or purpuric manifestations, preparations for splenectomy should be made. The main effect of steroids is to delay splenectomy 3 to 6 weeks in order to stabilize platelet counts. In addition, sustained high-dosage prednisone therapy may, paradoxically, lead to a thrombocytopenia effect, and adults with ITP rarely have spontaneous remissions. Splenectomy is, therefore, often necessary if there is severe ITP in the adult and usually within 1 to 3 months after diagnosis. Splenectomy is usually associated with prolonged complete remission. It is most frequently undertaken when the bone marrow shows megakaryocytes, when splenomegaly does not respond to treatment for underlying disease, when steroids are contraindicated (as in infection and tuberculosis), or when steroids have proved ineffective in ITP and in occasional instances of lupus erythematosus. Immunosuppressive therapy with cytotoxic drugs should generally not be used until the patient has had the benefit of splenectomy; this is particularly the case for younger patients since these drugs may have serious, adverse effects. Vincristine now seems to be drug of choice for patients with autoimmune thrombocytopenia who do not respond to splenectomy, who relapse after an initial good response to splenectomy, or in whom the risk of splenectomy is too high. Seventy-eighty per cent of patients with refractory autoimmune thrombocytopenia will show a significant increase in platelet count when they are treated with vincristine. Vincristine appears to be more effective, less toxic, and is more readily tolerated by most patients than autoimmune thrombocytopenia.[53, 61]

Controversy exists regarding the use of steroid therapy in the management of acute childhood ITP. The major cause of mortality and morbidity in this disorder is intracranial hemorrhage, with the risk of this complication varying from 0 to 2 per cent. Hemorrhage is generally reported during the first few days of the acute illness. Proponents of steroid therapy, therefore, administer the drug for the initial 2 to 3 weeks of the illness (i.e., the "risk period"). However, the claim is unsubstantiated, for no attempt has been made to document the incidence of intracranial hemorrhage or other major bleeding manifestations in controlled and steroid-treated groups. Steroid therapy may alter the bleeding time and prevent various endothelial changes induced by thrombocytopenia in the experimental animal. In children there is evidence relating to an early beneficial effect of steroid therapy on capillary resistance and platelet count.[43, 67]

Fresh whole blood, collected into plastic equipment with EDTA as anticoagulant, is given to tide the patient over an acute episode of thrombocytopenia. (If the patient requires more than 5 to 6 L. of blood, begin using fresh blood, that is, 2–3 hrs. old. Do not use vacuum method of giving blood, which causes the formation of small clots during bubbling.) Because platelet transfusions contain antigens and isoimmunization usually develops over a period of weeks, they are only given if the clinical status of the patient is poor. Survival of transfused platelets may be impaired or prevented by intravascular coagulation, sepsis, splenomegaly, autoantibodies (ITB), or alloantibodies.

Platelets are highly immunogenic, and the most important resulting antibodies are directed against HLA antigens. Patients whose alloimmunization has made them refractory to platelets from random donors may have normal survival if HLA-compatible platelets are provided. It will usually be necessary to obtain these from a very limited number of donors by plateletpheresis. Patients may eventually become refractory to HLA-identical platelets, which suggests that other antigen systems may also play a role. Evidence has been presented that leukocyte-poor platelet concentrates may result in improved platelet survival in the immunized recipient,[32] but this remains to be confirmed. Discrepancies may be related to differences in the degree of leukocyte contamination of the original and recentrifuged platelet concentrates.

Recently, the use of lymphocyte HL-A-typed platelet donors has reduced these immune complex complications, and the recipients have accepted the platelet support. One caution should be mentioned in the acceptance of platelet donors; platelets from donors taking approximately 600 mg. of aspirin 36 hours before donation achieve effective hemostasis in thrombocytogenic recipients, but those from donors taking aspirin between 12 hours and 1 hour before donation fail to correct the bleeding time or pattern of platelet aggregation. If a lymphocyte HL-A-typed platelet donor has taken aspirin within 36 hours of donation, the platelets should be pooled, before infusion, with those from another lymphocyte HL-A typed platelet donor who has not recently taken aspirin.[60] If thrombocytopenic patients are facing situations in which bleeding may be a complication of the procedure, as in surgery, or situations in which platelets may be further depressed by treatment, as in massive chemotherapy, approximately $3/4$ of these patients respond promptly to splenectomy. In 75 per cent of these, the remission lasts more than 10 years, (same for systemic lupus erythematosus).[23]

THROMBOCYTOPATHY (THROMBOCYTASTHENIA)

Classification of Qualitative Platelet Diseases

I. Thrombocytopathy (deficient or ineffective platelet factor 3).[66]
  A. Deficient thrombocytopathy.
    1. Congenital.
    2. Acquired (liver disease, uremia, scurvy).
  B. Functional thrombocytopathy.
    1. Congenital.
    2. Acquired (macroglobulinemia, systemic lupus erythematosus).
    3. Plasmatic type.
    4. Ehlers-Danlos syndrome. Using electron microscopy, Kashiwagi and associates showed that the hemorrhagic diathesis associated with this syndrome is probably related to the fact that these patients'

platelets are aggregated, have blunted edges, and show osmiophilic retention.[35] This abnormal ultrastructure differs markedly from that of normal platelets, which usually occur singly and have pronounced dendritic processes. Other tests revealed normal plasma clotting time, abnormal prothrombin consumption time, and defective TGT in two out of three cases. It was suggested that this thrombocytopathy indicated a normal content but a suboptimal release of platelet factor 3.

II. Thrombasthenia (diminished clot retraction) — Glanzmann's thrombasthenia.

III. Defective platelet aggregation (von Willebrand's disease).

IV. Compound platelet defects.
  A. Thrombocytopathic hemophilia A (thrombocytopathy plus the deficiency of Factor VIII).
  B. Thrombocytopathic hemophilia B (thrombocytopathy plus the deficiency of Factor IX).
  C. Thrombocytopathic thrombasthenia (thrombocytopathy and thrombasthenia).
  D. Thrombasthenic hemophilia (thrombasthenia plus the deficiency of Factor VIII).

Secondary thrombocytosis may be distinguished from essential thrombocythemia by platelet aggregation studies, especially those with epinephrine. In secondary thrombocytosis, the bleeding time and platelet aggregation are always normal. Uremic states and the use of certain drugs (e.g., aspirin, phenylbutazone, and indomethacin) often interfere with aggregation studies. For example, the ingestion of acetylsalicylic acid is associated with irreversible inhibition of platelet aggregation, which may persist for the life cycle of the thrombocyte. Other analgesics produce a short-lived platelet aggregation abnormality and are considered reversible. Aspirin produces acetylation of the platelet membrane and, thereby, interferes with aggregation by impairing the release of ADP. Although the bleeding time may be lengthened by ingestion of acetylsalecytic acid, and lead to serious blood loss in hemophiliacs, in most people, the bleeding time remains within the normal range.

Clinical Findings in Thrombocytopathic States

The two main types of thrombocytopathy (Glanzmann's and von Willebrand's) are characterized by qualitative platelet defects. Clinically, both types are characterized by a purpuric type of bleeding with superficial hemorrhages into the skin, oozing from mucous membranes, easy bruising, and excessive bleeding from small cuts and abrasions.

Laboratory Findings

Glanzmann Type. This qualitative platelet defect is hereditary, transmission of which is suggested to be recessive-autosomal in character. It is difficult to distinguish it from vascular pseudohemophilia. Adenosine triphosphate (ATP) is required for clot retraction, and defective glycolysis with impaired ATP generation has been demonstrated in patients. The platelets contain adequate clot-promoting material (platelet factor 3). However, they exhibit impaired adhesiveness, abnormal clot retraction, a lack of aggregation in blood smears, and a predominance of the round type of platelet in electron micrographs—that is, the normal "spread" and dendritic forms.[59] Other laboratory findings include increased capillary fragility (positive tourniquet test) and normal results from the prothrombin consumption test, with a normal or prolonged bleeding time.

Von Willebrand Type. Von Willebrand's disease is characterized by an autosomal-dominant mode of inheritance; the platelets are almost the size of erythrocytes, and the granulation is more diffuse and finer than normal. The megakaryocytes have a similar atypical granulation. Although intermittent thrombocytopenia is frequently found, bleeding occurs without relationship to platelet levels because of the basic associated, qualitative defects. Although clot retraction is normal, there is concomitant prolonged bleeding time, increased capillary fragility, abnormal prothrombin consumption, abnormal thromboplastin generation test, reduced plasma level of Factor VIII (antihemophilic factor), and reduced in vivo platelet adhesiveness.[59] The disorder is frequently seen equally in males and females; menorrhagia is a frequent manifestation. Occasionally this syndrome may be called vascular hemophilia or pseudohemophilia B.

It is now known that platelets from normal patients are aggregated in vitro by the antibiotic ristocetin, whereas platelets in von Willebrand's (V.W.) disease are not aggregated by ristocetin. Normal Factor VIII plasma, containing Factor VIII_{VWF}, will restore platelet aggregation in the V.W. patient. Although Factor VIII_{VWF} is normal in patients with Hemophilia A, in patients with V.W. disease it is reduced in direct proportion to the diminution of Factor VIII_{AHF} and Factor VIII_{AGN}. Thus, V.W. disease appears to result from a failure in the manufacture of the Factor VIII complex, rather than from the synthesis of some abnormal forms. Ristocetin-induced platelet aggregation is now used as a diagnostic test for V.W. disease.

Experimentally, an aorta denuded of endothelium is exposed to flowing blood, and the attachment of platelets to the subendothelial portion is evaluated. The results obtained reveal that platelets in V.W. disease become attached in smaller numbers than normally. However, the platelets that do attach are able to aggregate additional platelets in a normal manner. Collagen and V.W. platelets aggregate normally; however, the substernal area of the aorta to which platelets attach is probably not collagen, and its identity is not known at this time. Therefore, it may be that a hemostatic defect explains this failure of platelets to react with the subendothelial vascular components. Furthermore, the reduced retention of platelets in glass bead filters (adhesiveness test) may also indicate a pathogenetically important phenomenon.

Therapeutically, blood from patients with V.W. disease responds to intravenously administered normal plasma or to Factor VIII concentrates by developing an increase in Factor VIII$_{AHF}$ and a reduction in the prolonged bleeding time. This increase in Factor VIII$_{AHF}$ is far greater than that which could be accounted for by the concentration of Factor VIII$_{AHF}$ in the administered plasma or Factor VIII concentrate. In addition, Factor VIII$_{AHF}$ activity is elevated over a longer period of time than would be expected from studies of Factor VIII half-life in patients with classical hemophilia. On the other hand, the plasma level of Factor VIII$_{AGN}$ attains the level predicted for the original material and disappears more rapidly than Factor VIII$_{AHF}$. The bleeding time correction is also short-lived. Although therapy may require replacement of plasma components (e.g., cryoprecipitate) to correct the prolonged bleeding time, hemostasis is usually satisfactorily improved when the Factor VIII level is raised to effective hemostatic levels (i.e., usually more than 25% of normal). Bleeding control ultimately determines the adequacy of therapy.

THROMBOCYTHEMIA

Thrombocythemia is frequently associated with a marked myeloproliferative tendency—that is, platelet counts above 1,000,000 per cu.mm., bleeding tendency, concomitant polycythemia vera, chronic myelocytic leukemia, or myelofibrosis with myeloid metaplasia. It is also seen after splenectomy, trauma, fractures (neck of femur), and surgery. It is occasionally associated with acute rheumatic fever, suppurative infections, asphyxiation, acute hemorrhage, Hodgkin's disease, metastatic carcinoma,[38] hyperadrenalism, and hyposplenism. Patients with continuing hemolysis show the most striking persistence of thrombocytosis after splenectomy because of two factors: the enlarged splenic pool has been removed, and the total volume of active marrow is increased.[16]

Clinically, there is a hemorrhagic tendency (mucocutaneous and gastrointestinal), often spontaneous, posttraumatic bleeding, splenomegaly with distension of cords by thrombotic masses, and extramedullary hematopoiesis that is restricted to megakaryocytic foci. Hemophilioid features, such as deep muscle hematomas, and hemarthroses are also observed, as are frequent thrombotic phenomena (venous and arterial) with hemorrhagic infarcts. Removal of the spleen is contraindicated and may be followed by serious vascular occlusion. The disease is often a premonitor of leukemia or polycythemia. It is thought by some that the hemorrhagic tendency is associated with a defect in platelet or plasma factors; in some cases it is characterized by ischemia and vascular injury secondary to capillary thrombosis, as in sickle cell anemia and thrombotic thrombocytopenic purpura.

The laboratory findings include platelet counts of over 1,000,000 per cu.mm. (platelets are qualitatively normal). Thromboplastin genesis is interfered with, and therefore the abnormal thromboplastin generation test is due to the inhibitory effect of a high platelet concentration on the generation of plasma thromboplastin. Also seen is a decrease in fibrinogen and activation of fibrinolytic enzymes. Therapy consists of ^{32}P and possibly alkylating agents. These two chemotherapeutic agents reduce the platelet count by suppressing bone marrow megakaryocytes. Thrombocyte levels may also be reduced by plastic blood bag plasmapheresis, plateletpheresis, or continuous blood cell flow centrifuge, which also leads to acute control of bleeding. Drugs such as salicylates or dipyridamole, by altering platelet aggregation, cause improvement in vascular complications. However, an approach that reduces thrombocyte count is preferred because of the risk of hemorrhage associated with the drug therapy.

FACTOR VIII
DEFICIENCY – HEMOPHILIA

Etiology

The functional concentration of AHF in the blood is directly related to the severity of hemophilia observed, the plasma abnormality itself being observed almost exclusively in males. It is transmitted by a sex-linked recessive gene in female carriers who usually do not have symptoms of the disease, but who may have sons with manifestations, sons without disease, normal daughters, or carrier daughters. Although so-called sporadic cases are observed, apparently occurring as the result of spontaneous mutation, one must exclude unrecognized mild familial incidence, unrecognized carrier females in several generations, and illegitimacy. Present data suggest that the heteropyknotic chromatin or nuclear sex chromatin represents a single X chromosome, tightly coiled and functionally inactive. Thus only one X chromosome is thought to function per cell. On a random basis, in any line of cells in a female (XX), it is believed that there is a determination at an early age as to which of the two X chromosomes will furnish the heteropyknotic chromatin.

According to Brinkhous, normal plasma collected from time to time under standard conditions from a single subject has a relatively constant level of AHF – that is, a steady state exists representing a balance between the synthesis and utilization of AHF.[13] Furthermore, the synthesis of AHF requires both the proper genetic information and properly functioning cells or tissues in which it is manufactured. The clearest data on the site of origin of AHF are those of Weaver and colleagues, which point to the spleen and suggestively to the reticuloendothelial system.[64] Thus, the spleen must be regarded as an important organ for the maintenance of AHF under stress in that it serves as a site of formation or storage.

In the past 10 years, the understanding of hemophilia has become much more complicated. At present, three types of hemophilia have been identified, hemophilia A (Factor VIII or AHF deficiency), hemophilia B (Factor IX, PTC or Christmas factor deficiency) and hemophilia C (Factor XI or P.T.A. deficiency). The first two are X-linked, hemophilia C is not. Somewhat confusing are several nonbleeding states in which laboratory tests suggest hemophilia; these include deficiencies of Factor XII (Hageman factor), Fletcher factor (prekallikrein), and contact activation cofactor (Fitzgerald factor or high MW kininogen).

More confusing still is a second disease characterized by a deficiency of Factor VIII but inherited autosomally, unlike hemophilia A. This second Factor VIII deficiency state is von Willebrand's disease (see p. 384). Characteristically, the patient with hemophilia has in his plasma a Factor VIII molecule antigenically that lacks clotting ability. The patient with von Willebrand's disease usually lacks even the antigenic molecule. Unfortunately, from the standpoint of diagnosis, variants of both hemophilia A and von Willebrand's disease that blur the distinction between the two diseases have been described. The signs and symptoms of a hemophilia A patient are strictly a function of the amount of Factor VIII in his plasma (i.e., mild hemophilia occurs in patients with levels of Factor VIII above 5%). There is little tendency toward spontaneous bleeding, but the patient may still bleed seriously if he is traumatized or subjected to surgical procedures. If the Factor VIII level is as high as 10 per cent of normal, the tendency to bleed may be so mild that the disease may be unsuspected for years and perhaps always. Obviously, it is important to identify the type of hemophilia and the level of the deficient factor in order to plan with the patient and his family a way of life as close to normal as possible.

Determination of Factor VIII concentrations is based on the extent to which an unknown sample corrects the abnormality in a plasma with a known deficiency. The Factor VIII level is then assumed to be proportional to the concentration of the deficient factor in the sample. Normal ranges of Factor VIII in the plasma vary from 50 to 100 per cent of normal, depending on the exact method employed.[37]

Clinical Findings

Defective clotting may be present at birth, and serious or fatal hemorrhage may occur in the neonatal period, often following circumcision. In infancy, one may observe a minor injury leading to soft tissue hematomas. Later, in childhood, joint hemorrhages occur that are limited by the joint space with increasing deformity, limitation of motion, and joint fusion occasionally resulting from these hemarthroses. Some patients are minimally affected; others are severely crippled by joint deformities; death may occur from hemorrhage. Soft tissue hematomas may dissect, subsequently becoming firm calcified masses, or they may produce contractures, as in claw hand. Bleeding from tongue, pharynx, or neck may interfere with swallowing or breathing. Retroperitoneal hemorrhage may simulate appendicitis or compression of the common bile duct with obstructive jaundice. Hematuria and ureteral colic occasionally coexist; gastrointestinal hemorrhage; hemorrhage after tooth extraction or tonsillectomy may be severe; subdural hematomas rarely occur.

A small wound, such as a needle puncture, usually stops its bleeding promptly. This is because the extrinsic coagulation system, which does not require the missing antihemophilic globulin (Factor VIII), is activated by the thromboplastin released by the injured tissue cells. However, if the clot occluding the small wound is detached, bleeding may begin and is often prolonged because it cannot be controlled by the defective intrinsic coagulation system. Presumably disturbance of other clots might be the result of fibrinolysis, which might be preventable by epsilon-amino-caproic acid

(EACA). In dental extractions, the all-important procedure in hemophilia is to keep the primary clot, formed by the tissue thromboplastin, intact and in place in the tooth socket, until healing can begin. For this reason, EACA was used in addition to the usual prosthetic devices by Reid and coworkers for a day before and 3 to 5 days after 31 dental extractions.[52] There was no need for transfusions or plasma fractions to assist the adequate hemostasis that resulted.

Laboratory Findings

In hemophilic blood, there is a block in the conversion of prothrombin; the basic defect is a lack of available thromboplastin related either to the plasma, or cells and platelets. In 1947, it was demonstrated that normal plasma contained the factor that normalizes the clotting of hemophilic blood by making a thromboplastic material available in the presence of blood platelets.[15]

The coagulation time of whole blood and of recalcified oxalated plasma is significantly prolonged in marked deficiency of Factor VIII, but may be borderline in moderate deficiencies and normal in patients having a minor inherited defect. In addition, the partial thromboplastin time is prolonged (over 100–120 secs.). The prothrombin time (Quick's one-stage method) is normal — that is, when thromboplastin and calcium are added to plasma, the thromboplastin supplies what is lacking (prothrombin, accelerator factor, and fibrinogen being normal in hemophiliac plasma). Bleeding time is normal; blood vessels retract and contract normally; the platelets are normal and tissue thromboplastin is present.

Classic hemophilia A (Factor VIII deficiency) and Von Willebrand's (V.W.) disease are both associated with a reduction in the functional level of Factor VIII. However, most of the plasma of a patient with hemophilia A contains material that will react with an antibody produced in white rabbits immunized with partially purified human Factor VIII (which is also called "cross-reacting material"). Physiologic and biochemical factors in hemophilia A and Von Willebrand's disease have been revealed by these observations. For example, a glycoprotein found in normal plasma with a molecular weight of 1 to 2 million corrects the abnormal coagulation of hemophilic plasma (procoagulant activity of Factor VIII$_{AHF}$), the abnormally functioning platelet activity from patients with Von Willebrand's disease (procoagulant activity of Factor VIII$_{VWF}$), and forms a precipitate, with rabbit antibodies, to Factor VIII (procoagulant activity Factor VIII$_{AGN}$) (for antigen). Hemophilia A patients have high to normal levels of Factor VIII$_{VWF}$ and Factor VIII$_{AGN}$, but have reduced levels of Factor VIII$_{AHF}$. Other work has produced evidence that the term "Factor VIII" (high molecular-weight plasma component) can be broken down into two components, a lower molecular-weight substance (one that has Factor VIII$_{AHF}$) and a larger component with Factors VIII$_{AGN}$ and Factor VIII$_{VWF}$. Therefore, hemophilia A (a heterogenous disorder) may indicate either failure to synthesize Factor VIII$_{AHF}$ or synthesis of a defective Factor VIII$_{AHF}$. Almost all patients with classical hemophilia have plasma components that will react with Factor VIII rabbit antibody; however, only about 10 per cent of these patients have components that will cross-react with human Factor VIII antibody. This is indicative of the variations in the affinity of the abnormal Factor VIII molecule for antibodies of different origins. These findings have been applied to the detection of female hemophilia A carriers; hemophilia A patients manifest rare immunologically reactive but functionally inactive Factor VIII. Female carriers possess one X chromosome that directs manufacture of normal Factor VIII and an X chromosome that directs synthesis of antigenically intact Factor VIII$_{AGN}$ and functionally inactive or absent Factor VIII$_{AHF}$. Clinical studies have corroborated these findings. At least 90 per cent of obligatory female carriers possess twice as much Factor VIII$_{AGN}$ as Factor VIII$_{AHF}$. However, one must bear in mind certain cautions; some carriers cannot be detected by this technique and some people who are not carriers may have a positive test.

Treatment

The modern treatment of Factor VIII disease is either cryoprecipitate or more highly fractionated products. Fresh frozen plasma is now rarely used because of the complications of hypervolemia. Factor IX concentrates also contain Factors II, VII, and X (the prothrombin complex). Thus, they can be used for other factor deficiency states, as well as in emergencies for patients with severe liver disease or coumadin overdose. The half-life of Factor IX is approximately 24 hours. The half-life of Factor VIII is 12 hours. Replacement therapy now offers the possibility to make hemophiliac patients normal hemostatically.

For most minor bleeding manifestations, 3 days' minimal therapy is suggested, usually 10 to 15 units of purified Factor VIII per kg. body weight. Specifically, this includes uncomplicated hemarthroses, hematomas in noncritical areas, hematuria, dressing changes, arthrocentesis, and removal of sutures and drains. With cryoprecipitate, no loading dose is required, and the maintenance dose advised is approximately 1.25 to 1.75 bags for every 10 kg. body weight every 12 hours for 2 to 4 days. For therapy of major bleeding, which includes hematomas in critical locations, traumatic injuries, multiple tooth extractions and major surgery, a loading dose of 3.5 bags of cryoprecipitate with a maintenance dose of 1.75 bags per 10 kg. body weight every 8 hours for 1 to 2 days and every 12 hours thereafter is recommended, if the Factor VIII blood level does not fall below 25 per cent for any length of time. Therapy is usually continued for 10 to 14 days, followed by half doses for 4 days. Following tooth extractions, therapy for 5 to 7 days is usually sufficient.[65] It is important that the patient response be monitored by serial PTTs.

The discovery of cryoprecipitate and the marked reduction in volume, and the appearance of multiple fractionated products, have increased the number of multiply transfused patients. However, only with time will the complications of therapy begin to be observed. For example, to date, multiple liver-function abnormalities are being seen. The data for this are just beginning to be collected, and it appears that almost 70 per cent of patients with hemophilia have abnormal liver function (elevations of SGOT and SGPT). Only a few patients have had liver biopsies, and cirrhosis has been found in a few cases. In addition, splenomegaly is found in 30 per cent of patients.* Whether the abnormal liver function is due to frequent exposure to virus (such as hepatitis, CMV, etc.) or antigen-antibody complex disease remains unclear. However, it is important that these patients be observed for the incidence of liver disease and its etiology, so that it can either be eliminated or treated. Unfortunately, there are no good control groups. It is now well known that there are multiple types of hepatitis that transfusion therapy exposes to patients. Hepatitis B antigen (i.e., the Australian antigen) is frequent in hemophiliacs (15%). However, the antibody titer is significantly elevated in a much larger per cent of hemophiliacs. The same is true for hepatitis in Factor IX patients, both in the United States and abroad. The findings of elevated Australian antibody in a large number of hemophiliacs probably means exposure to hepatitis virus, but whether or not this is related to the abnormal liver functions is still unclear.

During therapy with cryoprecipitate (mostly Factor VIII), antibodies to coagulation factors develop. They usually act as specific inhibitors; they inactivate a single factor and produce a clinical and laboratory pattern resembling a hereditary coagulation disorder (hemophilia, etc.). Antibodies to Factor VIII are the most commonly found specific inhibitors and are known to occur in 6 to 22 per cent of hemophilia A patients, especially in those with severe manifestations of Factor VIII deficiency.

The PTT test is used to monitor the development of these inhibitors; after the priming cryoprecipitate transfusion, the PTT is reduced to near normal values. Thereafter, with maintenance cryoprecipitate transfusions, the PTT is kept at or below the 100-second level, with cessation of hemorrhage. By mixing equal parts of the transfused patient's plasma with the normal plasma, the PTT becomes a test for inhibitors that may develop as an undesirable side effect during the course of therapy. If the PTT continues to be within the control range, the indication is that a high titer of inhibitor has not developed and that the patient's hemostatic defect may be corrected by transfusions. This implies that thrombin is being formed at the bleeding site, and is important not only for fibrin formation but also for the formation of the platelet agglutinates, or the white (hemostatic) thrombus.

Most patients who have Factor VIII specific inhibitors (antibodies) develop a rapid elevation in the antibody titer when cryoprecipitate continues to be infused. Therefore, in these instances, continuation of Factor VIII replacement therapy should be avoided if at all possible. Treatment of this complication centers around therapy combining immunosuppressive drugs and massive doses of cryoprecipitate.[30]

Factor VIII concentrates are derived from large pools of plasma and, thus, contain anti-A and anti-B antibodies that cannot be totally removed during processing. Despite their low titer, large infusions of Factor VIII can produce hemolysis in patients with type A, AB, or B blood. This does not seem to be true for Factor IX concentrates. Because of the hemolytic potential of concentrates, all patients receiving large amounts of Factor VIII should be

---

* Levine, P. H.: Personal communication.

studied for signs of hemolysis, a decrease in haptoglobin and a quantitative Coomb's test. The development of a positive Coomb's test is variable. Hemolysis can be massive, and require transfusion. It is important to recognize it so that the appropriate transfusion can be given. Type O blood should be used. No patient with type O blood has ever had a product-induced hemolytic episode. In all cases of hemolysis, the withdrawal of Factor VIII concentrates leads to eventual cessation of hemolysis.[4]

Recently, self-therapy of hemophilia has been used in an effort to minimize the long-term disabilities secondary to the consequence of joint and muscle disease. Therefore, at this time, immediate correction of each hemorrhagic episode remains the most practical therapeutic method of minimizing the development and progression of the musculoskeletal deformities. Home therapy allows application of such therapy at "aura" of hemorrhage long before the development of physical findings. This kind of program greatly increases work and school attendance and performance, minimizes hospital and doctor contact, and decreases the consumption of plasma products as well as the expense. It has recently been demonstrated that there is clear-cut evidence of decreased development or progression of hemophilic arthropathy, in proportion to the intensity of therapy. Further, the intensity of therapy is not correlated with either inhibitor-antibody development or liver-function abnormalities.

Teaching patients to infuse antihemophilic factor is not a panacea for hemophilia. Self-therapy encourages the patient to be independent, and clearly allows subtle lesions to develop, with absence of physician supervision. Also, many patients fail to treat themselves intensively, due to discernible emotional, financial, vocational, or other problems. All patients on home therapy must be seen in formal comprehensive-care clinics, preferably at least biannually. The minimum staffing for such clinics must

be experts in hematology, pediatrics, orthopedics, dentistry, physical therapy, nursing, and social services. Other services, such as genetic counseling, psychiatry, and vocational rehabilitation, should be available to those who need them. When self-therapy is regarded as only one necessary aspect of comprehensive hemophilia care, and when patients are treated by a team with whom they develop long-term rapport, the results are strikingly good.[39]

FACTOR IX OR PTC DEFICIENCY (CHRISTMAS DISEASE OR HEMOPHILIA B)

Etiology

Classic hemophilia was once considered to be a single disease, until cross-mixing of plasma of some patients with so-called "hemophilia" (Christmas disease) revealed mutual correction of the prolonged clotting time, and cross-transfusions led to cessation of bleeding in both recipients (hemophilia and Christmas disease). Hemophilia B is now considered to be due to hereditary deficiency of beta thromboplastin or plasma thromboplastin component—a stable protein factor not utilized during coagulation and not destroyed by aging. The PTC factor is an important part of the intrinsic (plasma) thromboplastin generating system, in which it influences the amount rather than the rate of thromboplastin formation. PTC is also believed to be depressed by coumarin drugs.

Clinical Findings

This disorder is usually indistinguishable from, but milder than, hemophilia with a 1:10 relationship. However, it can be just as severe, with associated joint and soft tissue hemorrhages. First described in an English family named Christmas, it is transmitted by a sex-linked recessive gene. It reveals itself in half the sons; half the daughters of a carrier mother become carriers and may show bleeding tendencies.

Also, about half the mothers of affected patients show a decrease in Factor IX activity.

Laboratory Diagnosis

As can be surmised from the foregoing discussion, a defect of PTC (Factor IX) leads to delayed thromboplastin generation and is correctable by the addition of small amounts of either fresh or aged normal plasma or serum, but not by adsorbed plasma or serum. The defect is also corrected by adding very small amounts of plasma from classic hemophilia patients or plasma from PTA-deficient patients. Other laboratory findings include a normal platelet count, bleeding time, and capillary fragility. The coagulation time is usually abnormal, the recalcified plasma time is usually abnormal, the clot retraction and prothrombin time are normal, and the partial thromboplastin time is abnormal.

New work has revealed that the heterogeneity of Factor IX deficiency is even more complicated than that of classic hemophilia. The concentration of cross-reacting material in the plasma ranges from normal to intermediate to zero levels, with some patients showing abnormalities in the one-stage prothrombin time performed with ox-brain thromboplastin (hemophilia B_M). In addition, a variant has been reported in which Factor IX activity increases with the patient's age (hemophilia B Leyden).

Treatment

Since there is a rapid initial disappearance of Factor IX from the circulation and a low initial recovery of Factor IX in the body, loading doses of stored, outdated citrated plasma, or plasma after removal of cryoprecipitate or purified prothrombin complex, are suggested even when minor bleeding occurs. These contain therapeutic amounts of Factor VII, prothrombin, Factor IX, and Factor X. When Factor IX levels reach 25 per cent or more, effective hemostasis can usually be achieved. These concentrates are also thought to contain activated coagulation factors and, therefore,

may be thrombogenic, especially in liver disease patients. Using the list of minor bleeding etiologies provided for hemophilia A therapy, one can recommend a loading dose of 30 ml. of citrated plasma per kg. body weight, followed by a maintenance dose of 7 ml. of citrated plasma per kg. body weight every 12 hours for 2 to 4 days. When purified prothrombin complex is used, the loading dose suggested is the same, and the maintenance dose in 10 U. per kg. every 12 hours for 1 to 4 days. When major bleeding occurs (see the list under hemophilia A therapy), it is often difficult to attain hemostatic levels with plasma alone; therefore, a loading dose of purified prothrombin complex (60 U./kg. body weight) and a maintenance dose of 10 U. per kg. body weight should be given every 12 hours.[65]

INCREASED ANTITHROMBOPLASTIC ACTIVITY

Etiology

Antithromboplastin is a lipid inhibitor normally present in blood; it binds Factors VIII and IX, making them unavailable for thromboplastin generation—that is, it retards the formation of plasma thromboplastin or neutralizes it after it is formed.[41] Before thromboplastin itself can be formed, dissociation of the factor-inhibitor conjugate must occur. The dissociation process takes place when platelet lysis makes platelet factor 3 available, or it occurs spontaneously on a glass surface and can be produced by simple plasma dilution. It is thought that this is one of the mechanisms by which normal blood clotting is controlled. For example, it is felt by some workers that hemophilia is due to an excess of inhibitor rather than to a reduction in AHF.

Mechanism of Antithromboplastin Activity

Some poorly understood bleeding conditions are caused by a defect associated with an increased amount of antithromboplastic activity (hemophilia-like ones). For example, the anticoagulant activity appears to neutralize the thromboplastin precursor in some cases, and thromboplastin appears to be neutralized in other cases. It is not known whether these two types of activity are caused by one or more antithromboplastic substances — for example, heparin inhibits thromboplastin formation and neutralizes formed thromboplastin.

Examples of hemorrhagic entities related to and apparently associated with antithromboplastic activity are as follows: (1) Some hemophiliacs who have been transfused several times become refractory to subsequent transfusions. In these cases, excessive antithromboplastin can be demonstrated that possibly inhibits AHF. This is thought to be an anticoagulant found in the globulin fraction, because a positive precipitin reaction is noted when the two are combined in vitro. The thromboplastin generation test reveals this anticoagulant to be an antithromboplastin, which implies that the "bridge effect" is not longer tenable — that is, poorer thromboplastin generation occurs when the substrate itself is deficient in one of the thromboplastic factors. (2) Hemorrhagic disease occurring in females and associated with childbirth reflects antithromboplastic activity that resides in an anticoagulant and that may act against AHF. Fetomaternal immunization by placental fragments may be the cause of the antibody development. (3) Following exposure to ionizing radiation, there is excessive antithromboplastic activity plus thrombocytopenia and antithrombic activity. This activity occurs in concentrations of 200 to 250 per cent of normal 12 to 30 days after exposure, depending on the dosage. The antithromboplastic activity probably also acts against AHF. (4) Elderly patients (56 to 82 years) with tuberculosis, syphilis, stovarsol treatment, pemphigus, and nephritis arising de novo are subject to this disorder.

ABNORMALITIES IN PHASE II OF COAGULATION (THROMBIN FORMATION)

DEFICIENCY OF PROTHROMBIN AND ASSOCIATED FACTORS

Hypoprothrombinemia and substances required for rapid conversion of prothrombin to thrombin are frequent causes of bleeding. This reduction in Factor II is most frequently due to a vitamin K deficiency and is also associated with reduced concentration of other vitamin-K-dependent clotting factors (as is well known, vitamin K is synthesized by bacteria of the intestinal tract).

Recently, the literature has described several molecular abnormalities of prothrombin (e.g., prothrombins San Juan, Pardua, Cordeza, and Barcelona). These are rare abnormalities and are characterized by production of an immunologically reactive and functionally atypical prothrombin subtype.

Congenital Etiology

Hereditary prothrombin deficiencies and deficiencies of the prothrombin accelerators are rare. Familial hypoprothrombinemia is almost unknown; vitamin K is not effective in treating this condition.

Parahemophilia, or Owren's disease, is a congenital or hereditary defect occurring in both males and females with symptoms and signs similar to hemophilia. It is caused by a deficiency of proaccelerin (Factor V). Quick's one-stage prothrombin time is prolonged; the partial thromboplastin time is also abnormal. The deficiency is corrected by fresh normal and adsorbed plasma. A test for Factor V deficiency in a patient with a prolonged clotting time, in the presence of tissue thromboplastin and calcium, begins with the storage of normal plasma at 4 to 6° C for 2 days. At this time, Factor V activity will be partially destroyed, and the coagulation time of the plasma will be longer than 40 seconds. The plasma factor is then frozen and stored until used. To test, add 0.01 ml. of patient's plasma to 0.09 ml. of plasma deficient in Factor V. After mixing and incubating, thromboplastin and calcium are added. If the clotting time of the mixture is significantly decreased (20 secs. or less) it is proof that the patient's plasma contains Factor V. If the mixture's clotting time is prolonged, the patient's plasma does not contain Factor V.

Factor VII deficiency disease (congenital hypoconvertinemia) is associated with abnormal bleeding after trauma. Ecchymoses, epistaxis, and abnormal menstrual bleeding are common. In the laboratory, it is associated with an abnormal prothrombin time and is corrected by viper venom and by serum. The deficiency may be treated with bank blood, with serum, or with fresh whole blood or plasma.

The inheritance of Factor X deficiency disease, which is rare, appears to be controlled by an incompletely recessive autosomal gene; carriers (heterozygotes) may display mild bleeding tendencies. This factor, together with Factor V in the presence of calcium ions, forms the final pathway through which the products of both the extrinsic and intrinsic thromboplastin-generating system work to form the ultimate thromboplastins that convert prothrombin to thrombin. The blood of Factor-X-deficient persons gives an abnormal TGT, the defect being correctable by the addition of small amounts of normal serum or of serum deficient in Factor VII.

Acquired Etiology

Bleeding phenomena observed are cutaneous ecchymoses, and nasal, bladder, gastrointestinal, postoperative, and intracranial bleeding. Hypoprothrombinemia (Factor II deficiency) occurs when something interferes with the production of vitamin K. Because vitamin K is synthesized by bacteria in the intestinal tract, the prolonged oral administration of antibacterial agents may interfere with this synthesis and subsequently lead to vitamin K or prothrombin deficiency. In the first several days of life before intestinal flora have become established, hemorrhagic disease of the newborn may result from an inadequate supply of vitamin K. It can be corrected by the injection of 5 mg. of menadione sodium bisulfate (vitamin K_3).

Vitamin K is fat-soluble and requires bile for its absorption. In jaundice associated with biliary obstruction, bile is missing in the intestinal tract and therefore vitamin K is not absorbed, leading to a decrease of blood prothrombin (hypoprothrombinemia) with possible subsequent hemorrhagic phenomena. Therefore, vitamin K should always be given preoperatively in these cases because anesthesia, surgical shock, anoxemia, decreased food intake, blood loss and the loss of clotting components in the fibrinous exudate may lead to severe depletion of prothrombin after surgery, even though there are no hemorrhagic findings preoperatively and even though the prothrombin time is normal preoperatively. Furthermore, in patients with biliary fistula, although there is no jaundice, there is insufficient vitamin K absorption because of the loss of bile from the intestinal tract. Therefore vitamin K given orally together with bile salts, or the parenteral administration of vitamin K, will supply the factor necessary for prothrombin formation.

In chronic gastrointestinal disorders (chronic ulcerative colitis, sprue and other malabsorption syndromes, and chronic bacillary dysentery), or in short-circuiting gastrointestinal operations or intestinal fistulas, there may also be inadequate vitamin K absorption and subsequent bleeding phenomena. Parenterally given vitamin K overcomes this.

In severe liver disease associated with cirrhosis, severe hepatitis, carcinomatosis, or hepatotoxic chemicals, the liver is unable to form prothrombin or prothrombin conversion accelerators, even in the presence of adequate vitamin K. Patients therefore have hypoprothrombinemia and bleeding tendencies. Also in liver disease, there is an associated fibrinogen, Factor VII, and platelet deficiency. Treatment is with blood or plasma. (Vitamin K has no effect unless there is an associated vitamin K deficiency.)

Various coumarin derivatives used in thromboembolic disease therapy (dicumarol, Tromexan, and warfarin) behave as competitive antagonists of vitamin K and impair the synthesis of prothrombin and Factor VII. Because response to coumarin therapy varies in different patients, one must test daily for prothrombin activity with the prothrombin time test until the dosage has been stabilized. In addition, if prothrombin activity is affected in a previously controlled patient when a sedative or tranquilizer is added to the regimen, the possibility of stimulation of the microsomal metabolizing enzymes by this drug should be suspected.[29]

The coagulation defects produced by these agents fail to respond rapidly to menadione infection (naphthoquinone with potent vitamin K activity). Instead vitamin K_1 (phytonadione, 50 mg.) given intravenously is promptly effective. Salicylates have an effect similar to coumarin drugs because of their similarity in chemical structure. Also, following propylthiouracil treatment for thyroid disease, one sees a similar effect. Therapy for these disorders, except coumarin drug toxicity and severe liver disease, includes the use of vitamin K orally or intravenously plus blood transfusions on occasions.

Recent biochemical studies have delineated the prothrombin that is abnormally induced by vitamin K deficiency or therapy with sodium warfarin; it is an anti-vitamin K anticoagulant. There is a severe deficiency in the coagulant activity of Factor VII, Factor IX, Factor X, and prothrombin in the plasma of patients treated with warfarin. However, when immunologic tests are performed, each of these factors is usually present in normal quantities. Therefore, an immunologically reactive, functionally inactive form of each factor is present in the plasma. The immunologically reactive form of prothrombin is not activated by physiological systems (e.g., those using tissue thromboplastin); however, nonphysiologic activators such as certain snake venoms coactivate prothrombin. This suggests a molecule of limited abnormality.

A comparison has been made between the properties of the abnormal prothrombin in animals treated with vitamin K antagonists and the properties of normal prothrombin, in order to delineate the molecular abnormality and the mechanism of action of vitamin K. The characteristic of calcium-normal prothrombin binding is associated with a specific locus in the molecule that contains several residues of gamma-carboxyglutamic acid. This amino acid produces acidic quantities at this locus of the prothrombin molecule and is directly related to the process of calcium binding. In order for the gamma-carboxyl group to be added enzymatically to the glutamic acid residues in the liver's prothrombin precursor, vitamin K must be present. When it is not, the prothrombin precursor is liberated into the circulation as the immunologically reactive, functionally inactive prothrombin of vitamin K deficiency. Improper calcium binding occurs when gamma-carboxyglutamic acid residues are not present; this leads to an inability of calcium activation by the tissue thromboplastin system. Since snake venoms do not require calcium as a cofactor, abnormal prothrombin can be activated.

Acquired parahemophilia (Owren's disease or Factor V deficiency) may occur in association with severe liver disease, septicemia, leukemia, and other malignant neoplasias. It is not reduced in coumarin-treated patients, and the deficiency is not corrected by vitamin K treatment. The biologic half-life of Factor V is short, and its effectiveness after transfusion does not exceed 4 to 12 hours. Therefore, one must treat these patients with fresh blood transfusions.

Acquired Factor VII deficiency (SPCA disease or acquired hypoconvertinemia) may be seen in the immediate neonatal period, in patients treated with coumarin drugs, in liver disease, in vitamin K deficiency states, and in malignant neoplasias. Patients with this deficiency tend to bleed excessively. If patients with this deficiency are operated on without preoperative vitmain K, serious postoperative bleeding and oozing may occur. Patients with severe liver disease will not be helped by vitamin K, preoperatively. Laboratory diagnosis reveals prolonged one-stage prothrombin time; the addition of small amounts of normal serum will correct the defect shown by this test. Because the half-life of Factor VII is probably the most short-lived of all the clotting factors (less than 3 hrs.), fresh blood must be given immediately and often.

Stuart-Prower factor (X) deficiency (acquired) is associated with a stable factor formed in the liver and dependent on vitamin K for production. It is depressed by coumarin drugs and is adsorbed from plasma by barium sulfate. It is associated with a prolonged one-stage prothrombin time test, and its deficiency is not corrected by viper venom.

EXCESSIVE ANTITHROMBIC ACTIVITY

This property of plasma can produce a prolonged one-stage (Quick) prothrombin time and clinical evidence of abnormal bleeding. Heparin-like anticoagulants have produced most of the clinical cases of hemophilia-like disease described in the literature, but a specific anticoagulant has not been accurately identified. They appear to be complex proteins usually with the properties of gamma globulin, and they most often interfere with the early stage of coagulation. For example, one type appearing in hemophiliacs specifically inactivates AHF;

another similar one occurs in the plasma of women following pregnancy, producing a hemophilia-like disorder. Previously healthy patients or ones who have had a chronic disease also have developed a hemorrhagic disease attributable to an anticoagulant. Some patients with systemic lupus erythematosus have a circulating anticoagulant that interferes with the conversion of prothrombin to thrombin. These antithrombic substances may disappear spontaneously, or sometimes after many months or years. This occurs in about 10 per cent of all patients with systemic lupus erythematosus (SLE). Although it is not clear exactly how the SLE anticoagulant behaves, it is especially effective in inhibiting the activated partial thromboplastin time. In addition, patients with SLE demonstrate anticoagulant activity against other steps in the coagulation sequence, with decreased prothrombin activity levels found in some. There are no clinical signs of low prothrombin levels, and it is not known how prothrombin deficiency is produced in these patients; however, it is thought not to be due to circulating anticoagulant. On the other hand, serious bleeding may occur if severe thrombocytopenia and qualitative platelet abnormalities or prothrombin deficiency are present. The coagulation process is restored to normal after corticosteroid therapy. Bleeding manifestations associated with dysproteinemias (for example, multiple myeloma) are not clearly related to retarded clotting.

Laboratory Diagnosis

The laboratory measurement of antithrombic materials consists of two types of tests: those based on the clot-retarding effect of heparin measure heparin cofactor activity; those that depend on a determination of the degree of thrombin neutralization measure "natural" plasma and serum antithrombin.

Therapy for these conditions is quite difficult because the anticoagulant effect of the

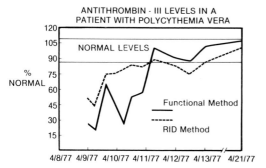

Fig. 12-1. Results of tests on patient with poly-cythemia vera who was unresponsive to heparin therapy. On 4/10/77 chromogenic substrate tests show that the *functional* antithrombin III level was low, although *total* antithrombin was normal—a problem undetected in standard RID tests. (Montgomery, B.: Automated test measures functional antithrombin coagulation enzymes. J.A.M.A. *238:*1005, 1977)

patient's plasma does not allow trans-fusions to correct the clotting defect.

In the past 3 years, thrombosis research has increasingly focused on the check and balance system of enzymes that activate and inhibit coagulation. This has been directed especially at the excessive coagu-lation associated with certain drugs and many malignant neoplastic and septicemic states. Four substances are often con-sidered key coagulation inhibitors: anti-thrombin III, alpha-antitrypsin, alpha$_2$-macroglobulin, and C$_1$-inhibitor. Of these, the heparin cofactor, antithrombin III, is of primary importance. Brinkhous and co-workers first reported a "factor" in plasma that acts with heparin to prevent the forma-tion of thrombin.[14] Additional studies have recognized this factor as antithrombin III, and have showed that, in the presence of heparin, it neutralizes thrombin and other serine proteases; that is, the anticoagulant action of heparin in normal blood is me-diated by activation of antithrombin III, which also inhibits the active coagulant en-zymes, Factors XII a, XI a, IX a, Xa, and thrombin. Therefore, deficiency of an-tithrombin III tends to lead to hyper-coagulation and a failure to respond to

heparin therapy. Minard and Petersen have reported that AT III measurements have potential value in interpreting throm-boembolic disease, in evaluating patients with disseminated intravascular coagula-tion (DIC), in selecting candidates for hep-arin therapy, and as a screening test to iden-tify women on birth control medication who might risk thrombosis.[42]

Several methods have been developed for measuring AT III; the most sensitive technique appears to be the radioim-munodiffusion assay. It measures the amount of AT III present in a blood sam-ple; however, it does not indicate its bio-logic or functional activity. In patients who are about to undergo surgery and who have family histories of thrombotic disease, it is important to determine not only total AT III levels, but also functional AT III levels. That is, it is possible for the total AT III level to be normal, while the functional level is depressed (Fig. 12-1). If this func-tional antithrombin level is low, heparin therapy will be ineffectual.

Two functional tests, one by Von Hamill and one by Howie, have been used in the past.[33, 63] A new test by Bick and Fekete is now available using purified thrombin and fibrinogen.[9] This technique eliminates a problem encountered in other tests, that of obtaining artificially high levels of AT III in patients with DIC, due to the use of rela-tively low dilutions (1:2, 1:4, 1:8) of plasma samples in the presence of elevated levels of fibrin (ogen) degradation products (FDP). These elevated levels inhibit the low concentrations of thrombin used to defibrinate the plasma for assay. In the test, the plasma sample is mixed with a thrombin-like enzyme, ancrod (snake venom), at a final concentration of 0.67 μ. per ml., and the resulting defibrinated plasma is diluted 1:20, 1:30, and 1:60, with heparinized veronal buffer for assay.

The assay itself involves the precisely timed incubation of the prepared plasma dilutions with a precise amount of purified thrombin, The solution is added to purified

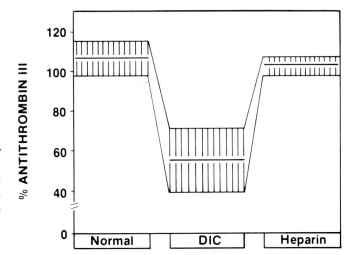

Fig. 12-1. Plasma levels of antithrombin III (mean values with their 95% confidence limits) in 21 normal, 7 chronic D.I.C., and 3 heparin-treated subjects, (Thrombo screen Antithrombin-III Bioassay Kit. Pacific Bio-Medical Corporation)

fibrinogen and the time required for clot formation is measured in a Fibrometer Coagulation Timer (BBL). AT III levels are computed from a prepared standard curve that is linear between 0 and 150 per cent. The normal range is 88 to 126 per cent (Fig. 12-2).

This technique* correlates well with the radioimmunodiffusion assay. In assays with a series of 13 patients with a confirmed acute or chronic DIC, all but one demonstrated low levels of AT III. The test also provides a reliable means of monitoring the heparin therapy. In another series of assays of 20 patients with solid malignancies, abnormally low levels of AT III were found in patients with liver involvement and normal AT III levels in the patients without liver involvement (another possible use of the assay). If it appears that a patient may have a hypercoagulable condition, and if there is some question whether the patient should be on anticoagulants, finding a low AT III level could be an indication for anticoagulant therapy or aggressive therapy of the underlying disease. In addition, if there is any suggestion of thrombotic disorders in the histories of patients on oral contraceptives and who have unusually low AT III levels, the medication should be stopped and mini-heparin therapy, for a brief period of time, should be considered.

Thrombosis, a pathologic manifestation associated with abnormalities of the blood vessel wall, qualitative and quantitative irregularities, blood coagulation components, and atypical platelet physiology still has inexplicable etiology and pathogenesis. Nevertheless, there have been significant advances in the understanding of prevention and therapy. As has been mentioned, heparin is a strong antithrombic enzyme (antithrombin) that is inhibited by a reaction involving antithrombin III, a plasma protein cofactor. In fact, it has been shown that heparin and antithrombin III work together in the inhibition of other blood coagulation enzymes including activated Factor X. Factor X is thoroughly inhibited by much lower concentrations of heparin-antithrombin III than is thrombin. Some researchers believe that activated Factor X may indeed be the primary site of coagulation inhibition by heparin, rather than the present theory that advocates "minidose" heparin in the prevention of thrombophlebitis and pulmonary embolism. The first study indicated that the occurrence of postoperative venous thrombosis was markedly reduced when subcutaneous hep-

---

* Thrombo Screen Antithrombin-III, Bio Assay Kit. Pacific Bio-Medical Corporation, P.O. Box 4719, Walnut Creek, California 94596.

arin was given 2 hours postoperatively in doses of 5000 units and then every 12 hours postoperatively. Pulmonary embolism, myocardial infarction, and venous thrombosis were markedly reduced in a "minidose" medical and postoperative heparin regimen of every 8 hours. There was associated slight prolongation of the PTT.

Another antithrombotic agent that has received much attention is aspirin, with its effect on platelet function and the pathogenesis of thrombosis, especially coronary thrombosis. In fact, many physicians now prescribe 10 gr. of aspirin (ASA) daily as a preventative in the development of coronary thrombosis, even though controlled clinical trials of antithrombocyte agents have produced conflicting results.

Other studies in preventing postoperative thrombophlebitis and pulmonary embolism using other antiplatelet agents such as dextran, dipyridamole, sulfinpyrazone, or aspirin have shown variable results. Arterially, the use of these drugs has been associated with good results in the prevention of transient ischemic attacks or myocardial infarction. The frequency of thrombotic complications in patients with prosthetic heart valves has been markedly reduced when combined dipyridamole and warfarin therapy is used.

ABNORMALITIES IN PHASE III OF COAGULATION (DEFIBRINATION SYNDROME OR CONSUMPTIVE COAGULOPATHIES)

FIBRINOGEN DEFICIENCY

Afibrinogenemia or hypofibrinogenemia is a rare symptom complex in that degrees of fibrinogen deficiency sufficient to cause abnormal bleeding rarely occur. This occurs because of retarded production of fibrinogen and more often as a result of rapid utilization or destruction of fibrinogen. Fibrinogen concentrations below 60 to 100 mg. per 100 ml. are clinically significant and

are associated with bleeding tendencies. There are two types, congenital and acquired.

Dysfibrinogenemia is a term now used to signify molecular fibrinogen abnormalities; they are usually diagnosed by a prolonged thrombin time or prothrombin time. Using the criteria of coagulability, one may see that fibrinogen levels are much lower than the levels estimated by immunologic or gravimetric methods. Hypofibrinogenemia results from a more than normally rapid rate of metabolism of abnormal fibrinogens (e.g., fibrinogen Philadelphia), but when the fibrinogen level is measured chemically or immunologically, it is usually within normal range. There are three steps in the conversion of fibrinogen to fibrin; (1) the release of fibrinopeptides A and B by thrombin, thus converting fibrinogen to fibrin monomer; (2) the formation of the fibrin clot by the aggregation of fibrin monomers; and (3) the formation of the insoluble fibrin clot by cross-linking the molecules of the fibrin monomer clot by activated Factor XIII. Fibrinopeptide release or fibrin monomer aggregation is abnormal in most instances of dysfibrinogenemia. The acquired defect due to fibrin degradation products in DIC, or due to the paraproteins associated with macroglobulinemia or multiple myeloma, may be related to abnormal fibrin monomer aggregation. Also, hepatoma patients may produce abnormal fibrinogens that subsequently lead to the production of hypofibrinogenemia; which appears to be due to the use of fibrinogen in cases of DIC rather than to defective fibrinogen production or manufacture of an abnormal type of fibrinogen.

Etiology

Congenital. This rare type is due to failure of fibrinogen production and is an anomaly dependent on a rare recessive mutant gene. Patients are born with either a marked decrease in fibrinogen or a complete absence of it. The platelet levels and vascular mechanisms are normal. Even though their blood lacks coagulability and is associated with an extremely long clotting time with defective clot formation, these patients may live for years until they begin to have recurrent episodes of severe hemorrhage following trauma. Most of the inherited disorders of prothrombin and fibrinogen have been associated with the manufacture of abnormal molecules. The molecules are now named for the place of their discovery as the Hemoglobinopathy Convention suggested.

Acquired. Clinically, patients are usually hypofibrinogenemic; they have episodes of excess bleeding from surgical wounds, bleeding through gauze packs, spontaneous bleeding from mucous membranes, bleeding from needle puncture wounds, cutaneous ecchymoses, and general bleeding. Severe uterine hemorrhage may occur in patients with associated complications of pregnancy, including premature separation of the placenta, induced abortion, retroplacental hematoma, prolonged retention of a dead fetus, toxemia, and amniotic fluid embolism. Associated with these, there is infusion of products of placental and fetal origin into the maternal circulation, possibly secondary to the pressures of uterine contractions. Intravascular coagulation and disseminated fibrin emboli are produced by these circulating substances. The available fibrinogen in the plasma of these patients is converted into fibrin faster than it is formed, resulting in severe fibrinogen deficiency. Thus, the coagulation defect appears to result from excessive utilization of fibrinogen, most likely by intravascular defibrination.

According to Miale, it is more likely that, in most instances, the apparent defibrination is caused by a sudden increase in fibrinolytic activity.[41] When there is prolonged retention of a dead fetus, owing to the secondary terminal effects of Rh and ABO incompatibilities, the sudden uptake of large amounts of antigen into the circulation of a sensitized mother may be an additional factor in producing shocklike states.

Intravascular coagulation occurring at the time of delivery may play a part in the postpartum syndrome of pituitary necrosis, cortical renal necrosis, and aseptic necrosis of the head of the femur.

The reduction in fibrinogen with its associated hemorrhage may also follow the transfusion of incompatible blood, lysis of which liberates into the blood thromboplastic substances that in turn defibrinate the plasma. This defibrination syndrome is also associated with neoplasms involving bone (for example, metastatic carcinoma of prostate), leukemia, and metastatic carcinoma from stomach, lung, pancreas, and gallbladder. These may lead to a massive depletion of platelets, clottable fibrinogen, and other coagulation Factors (V and VIII). Abnormal bleeding in patients with neoplasms, particularly multiple myeloma and metastatic carcinoma of the prostate, is occasionally associated with a qualitative abnormality of fibrinogen (cryofibrinogen).

Hypofibrinogenemia has also been seen after major operations and in association with extensive venous thrombosis, suggesting that the fibrinogen may be depleted by its excessive utilization. Thus, the fibrinogen is converted to fibrin, which may be deposited locally at the site of tissue damage or throughout the circulation. Finally, transient hypofibrinogenemia may be seen at the onset of purpura fulminans with associated sudden gangrene symmetrically affecting peripheral or superficial areas of the body. Also deficiency of fibrinogen and certain other proteins involved in coagulation may result from excessive proteolytic activity of plasma.

In summary, Rosner and Ritz have listed the following possible mechanisms for fibrinogen deficiency[55]: (1) impaired utilization due to polymerization of fibrinogen; (2) defective production due to liver disease; (3) increased destruction due to increased fibrinolytic activity; (4) increased utilization due to intravascular coagulation initiated by (a) the release of a thromboplastic substance from the placenta, decidua, amnion, lung or other organs, tumor tissue, bacteria, snake bites, or (b) massive fibrin deposition at the site of nests of tumor cells, large vascular spaces, hemangiomas, retroplacental hemorrhage, and areas of trauma.

Laboratory Diagnosis

The diagnosis of afibrinogenemia or hypofibrinogenemia may be made by utilizing any of the following tests.

1. The coagulation time is prolonged. In this test, blood obtained by venipuncture is divided between a dry test tube and one with oxalate. Presumptive hypofibrinogenemic diagnosis is made when the blood fails to clot in the tube without an anticoagulant. This may be confirmed by adding 1 to 2 drops of thrombin. If no clot is formed, no fibrinogen is present.

2. In the fibrinogen determination (screening test)* failure of a clot to form or a very poor clot formation usually indicates fibrinogen concentration below 60 to 100 mg. per 100 ml.

3. In the clot observation test (or formation of small clot), a 5 ml. sample of blood is placed in a 15 ml. test tube. The tube is agitated gently four or five times. The clotting mechanism is defective if no clot forms within 6 minutes, if a clot forms but shatters if shaken a few times after standing half an hour, or if the clot retracts to less than 35 to 45 per cent of the total volume of specimen.

4. In the dilute whole blood clot lysis time (Fearnsley), 0.2 ml. of fresh citrated blood is clotted in 1.8 ml. of phosphate buffer (pH 7.4) containing 2 NIH units of thrombin previously cooled in an ice bath and kept at this temperature for 15 minutes after the addition of the blood. The hypofibrinogenemic or afibrinogenemic syndrome is probable if the blood fails to clot when thrombin is added. Diagnosis is confirmed if the subsequent addition of normal plasma produces a clot that undergoes lysis after incubation at 37° C. The normal range is 2

to 7 hours. The phosphate buffer solution (pH 7.4) is prepared by adding 9.47 g. of Na_2HPO_4 per liter of distilled H_2O to 3.02 g. of KH_2PO_4 per 250 ml. of distilled water.

5. In the fibrinogen qualitative test, 0.2 ml. of bovine thrombin (100 units/ml.) is added to 0.5 ml. of patient's plasma in a test tube at 37° C. In the presence of a normal fibrinogen concentration, turbid solidification should occur almost immediately. In significant fibrinogenopenia, a thin translucent gel or a delicate network of fibrin strands appears.

Treatment

If the defibrination syndrome is due to intravascular coagulation with a rapid increased consumption of fibrinogen and a decreased activity of Factors II, V, and VIII, treatment consists of the intravenous administration of lyophilized human fibrinogen (Cutter) and the transfusion of fresh whole blood or plasma. In premature separation of the placenta or retained dead fetus, fibrinogen promptly returns to normal after the uterus has been emptied. Administration of estrogens to patients with carcinoma of the prostate is often followed by rapid restoration to normal of the plasma fibrinogen. Epsilon-amino-caproic acid (EACA) is given if defibrination is due to increased plasma fibrinolytic activity. Its use is questioned by some researchers. Platelet transfusions and heparin may also help. Heparin (i.e., continuous I.V. infusion starting with at least 10,000–20,000 units/day and increasing judiciously, as needed) is indicated if there is fibrinogenopenia and thrombocytopenia without fibrinolysis.[62] Heparin should not be used in DIC unless the bleeding is unmanageable by replacement therapy.

EXCESSIVE FIBRINOLYSIS

The fibrinolytic system acts as an antagonist to the clotting system; thus blood coagulation produces and fibrinolysis dissolves fibrin. Although this statement seems dog-

---

* Produced by Hyland Laboratories.

Color Plates   56–74

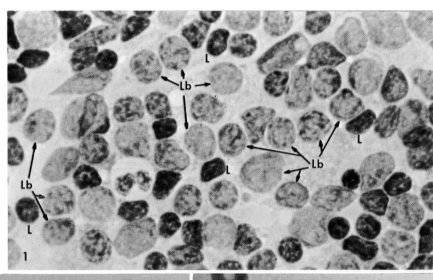

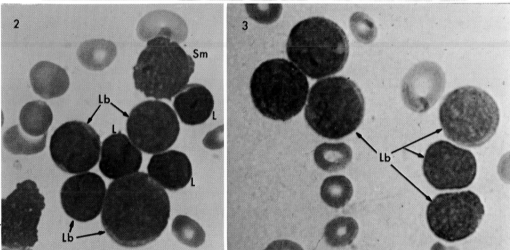

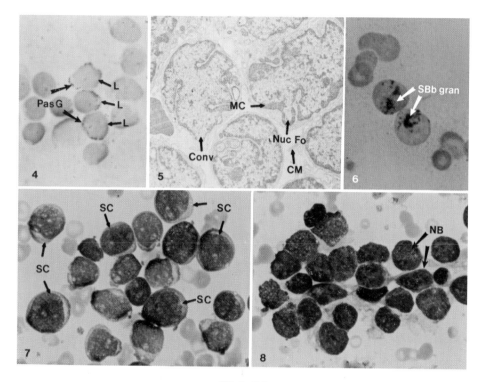

Plate 56

ACUTE LYMPHOCYTIC (LYMPHOBLASTIC) LEUKEMIA
Bone Marrow

Lymphocyte (L), lymphoblast (Lb), smudge cell (Sm), Nuclear folding (Nuc Fo), cytoplasmic microfilaments (CM), convolutions (Conv), marginated chromatin (MC), Sudan Black B granules (SBb gran), stem cell (SC), neuroblasts (NB), Pas granules (PasG).

Diagnostic Features: Here one sees massive infiltration with lymphoblasts and replacement of normal marrow elements, i.e., decreased normoblasts, myeloblasts, myelocytes, metamyelocytes, PmNs, megakaryocytes and platelets. One also frequently sees 20 to 30 per cent prolymphocytes and lymphocytes; the peroxidase stain is negative.

4. PAS stain demonstrates acute lymphoblastic cell crisis in chronic leukemia. Blast cells contain granular block-like PAS positivity without a diffuse background (×970).

5. Electron micrograph of acute lymphoblastic leukemia shows typical primitive blast cells with nuclear folding and convolutions with cytoplasmic microfilaments without significant number of lysosomal granules (almost absent), sparse cytoplasm, and marginated chromatin.

6. Sudan Black B stain demonstrates acute micromyeloblastic leukemia. Strong positivity in two leukemic cells (×970).

7. Acute undifferentiated (stem) cell leukemia in bone marrow, a term used by some as a synonym for acute lymphoblastic leukemia. With Wright's stain differentiation is quite difficult, if at all possible.

8. Metastatic neuroblastoma. Immature cells resembling lymphoblasts but forming a syncytium (×970).

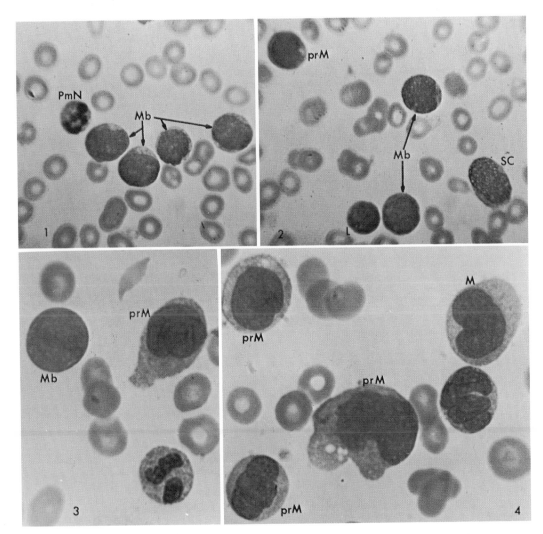

Plate 57

ACUTE MONOCYTIC (MONOBLASTIC) LEUKEMIA
Peripheral Blood

Lymphocyte (L), monocyte (M), monoblast (Mb), polymorphonuclear neutrophil (PmN), promonocyte (prM), stem cell (SC).

Diagnostic Features: Total leukocyte counts vary (below 4,000 cu. mm. and up to and above 100,000 per cu. mm.). Monoblasts usually dominate the picture. They are approximately 12 to 20 micra in total diameter with irregular, frequently indented, kidney-shaped and lobular borders. The nuclei are usually centrally placed, the nuclear membrane is fine and delicate, the nuclear chromatin is fine and reticular; nucleoli (2 to 5) may or may not be prominent. The cytoplasm is grayish blue and may contain many very fine dust-like, reddish granules. Reaction to peroxidase stain is variable ($\pm$). Many promonocytes and monocytes are present. Auer bodies may be present in the cytoplasm of monoblasts. RBCs are usually normocytic and normochromic but in myelomonocytic type (Naegeli), marked anisocytosis and poikilocytosis are present. Nucleated red blood cells also may be present.

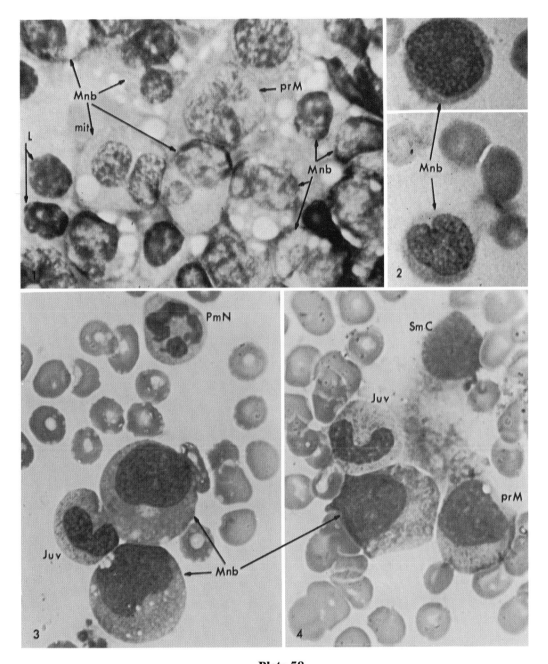

Plate 58

ACUTE MONOCYTIC (MONOBLASTIC) LEUKEMIA
Bone Marrow

Juvenile (Juv), lymphocyte (L), mitosis (mit), monoblast (Mnb), polymorphonuclear neutrophil (PmN), promonocyte (prM), smudge cell (SmC).

Diagnostic Features: The morphologic pattern is the same as the peripheral blood pattern of acute monocytic leukemia. In addition, megakaryocytes and platelets are reduced. Blast cells are primitive and undifferentiated. One almost sees a "hiatus leukemicus" in the above pattern on many occasions. In Fig. 3, phagocytosis of a juvenile can be seen.

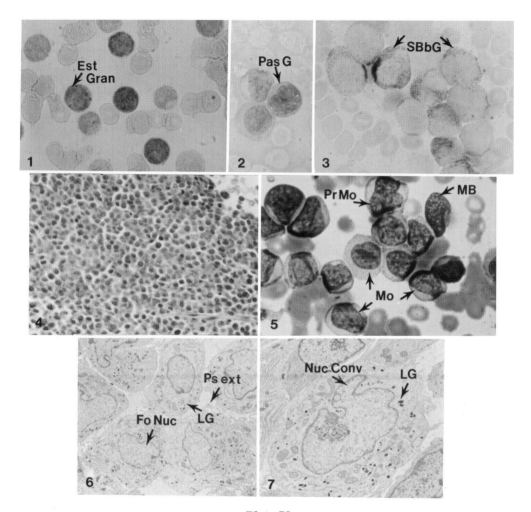

Plate 59

ACUTE MYELOMONOCYTIC LEUKEMIA

In this variant of monocytic leukemia there is invasion of the bone marrow by highly motile promonocytes. The nucleus of many of the cells is folded, and nuclear chromatin is fine but reticulated. Irregular abundant cytoplasmic borders with pseudopodial extensions with or without granules. Peripheral blood contains more monocytic type cells. 4. Marrow shows solid infiltration. 6. and 7. Electron micrographs of promonocytes. (Est Gran = esterase granules in monocyte; PAS G = PAS granules in cytoplasm of monocytes; SBbG = Sudan Black B granules in cytoplasm of monocytoid cells; Mo = Monocyte; Pr Mo = promonocyte; MB = monoblast; LG = lysosomal granules in E. M.; Ps ext = pseudopodial extension in E. M.; Nuc Conv = Nuclear convolution in E. M.; Fo Nuc = Nuclear folding.

Plate 60 *(Plates on following two pages)*

BONE MARROW TRANSPLANTATION THERAPY FOR
ACUTE LEUKEMIA PATIENTS
Recovery
Similar Pattern After Therapy for Aplastic Anemia

1. Myelofibrotic marrow in patient prior to transplantation. Absence of hematopoietic foci with fibrillar replacement throughout. (MF = marrow fibrosis)

2. Marrow recovery in myelofibrotic patient after bone marrow transplantation from HLA-, MLC-, and ABO-compatible matched donor. (HF = hematopoietic foci)

3. Skin pattern. Myelofibrosis patient treated with interferon with disappearance of graft versus host reaction in dermis of skin.

4. Acute lymphoblastic leukemia marrow in male patient. Absence of hematopoietic foci with lymphoblastic and lymphocytic replacement throughout. (L = Lymphocytic cells)

5. Bone marrow pattern in post-bone-marrow transplantation in acute lymphoblastic anemia male patient. No leukemic cells present. Only female cells from donor are present (8-year-old HLA-identical sister).

6. Post-bone-marrow transplantation marrow pattern in acute lymphoblastic leukemia male patient after marrow transplant from HLA-identical brother. No leukemic cells seen. (HF = hematopoietic foci)

7. Lymph node atrophy pattern. Post-cytoxan immunosuppressive therapy in acute lymphoblastic leukemia patient. Beginning repopulation by small lymphocytes of possible donor origin. (LF = lymphoid foci)

8. Recovery bone marrow in acute myelogenous leukemia patient. Donor selected by karyotype analysis. (HF = hematopoietic foci)

Graft versus Host Reaction

9. Post-bone-marrow transplantation (24 days) erythematous maculopapular rash. (Patient had severe combined immune deficiency disease.)

10. Bronzing parchment-like skin (severe exfoliative dermatitis), 5 months post-bone-marrow transplantation.

11. Skin showing florid graft versus host reaction, consisting of marked edema in dermis with associated leukemic cell infiltration.

12. Atrophic bone marrow with lymphoid foci but no hematopoietic foci. This was in a patient with acute myelogenous leukemia, who received a bone marrow transplant from his sister, who differed by one histocompatible allele.

13. Fibrotic marrow in post-marrow transplant (acute myelogenous leukemia patient).

14. Acute myelogenous leukemia patient after cytoxan immunosuppressive therapy and bone marrow transplantation from HLA-identical brother. Graft versus host reaction consisted of severe liver necrosis with almost complete loss of liver cell architecture. All that remains in many areas is a bare outline of supportive reticulin network.

15. Graft versus host reaction in myelofibrosis patient post-bone-marrow transplantation. There is marked interstitial pneumonitis with marked thickening of the alveolar walls.

16. Developing lymphoid atrophy in splenic architecture of acute myelogenous leukemia with graft versus host reaction.

Bone marrow transplantation is being used in many ways and for many different reasons. For example, in patients suffering from overwhelming malignant disease, massive whole-body irradiation and cytotoxic drug therapy are being used. This combination produces almost fatal marrow aplasia. Therefore, attempts have been made to use bone marrow transplantation to allow the use of higher radiation and chemotherapeutic doses. In some cases, autogenic marrow has been removed from the patient before treatment and, after suitable preservation, has been returned to the patient when and if severe marrow aplasia develops. In other cases, allogenic marrow has been used, partly because autogeneous marrow was unsuitable, as in the case of patients with leukemia, and partly in the hope that immunocompetent cells in the transplanted marrow would react with, and possibly destroy, the malignant cells present in the recipient.

Bone marrow is obtained by inserting large-bore needles into the marrow cavities of the iliac bones. Aspiration may yield as much as 1×10^{10} nucleated cells. These are given to the recipient intravenously.

Success following allotransplantation of bone marrow is complicated by the development of graft-versus-host (GVH) disease in the recipients. This produces a variety of gastrointestinal symptoms (anorexia, vomiting, and diarrhea); which may be followed by exfoliative dermatitis, anemia, and hepatic necrosis. The patient may then develop overwhelming viral or mycotic infection. The lymphoid tissues of the body become aplastic, and there is depression of immunoglobulin production. Attempts have been made to reduce the incidence and severity of GVH by giving drugs such as cyclophosphamide and antithymocyte globulin. The mortality rate of this procedure is about 35 per cent at 1 year in aplastic anemia patients who receive bone marrow transplants from a HLA-matched sibling donor. At 2 years, only 40 to 50 per cent of patients are alive and are hematologically normal or nearly normal. In addition, bone marrow transplantation is extremely demanding and carries high risks unless it is performed at special centers. Nevertheless, it appears to be a logical therapeutic alternative in older acute leukemic patients and in some patients with idiopathic severe aplastic anemia, both of whom have a grim prognosis.

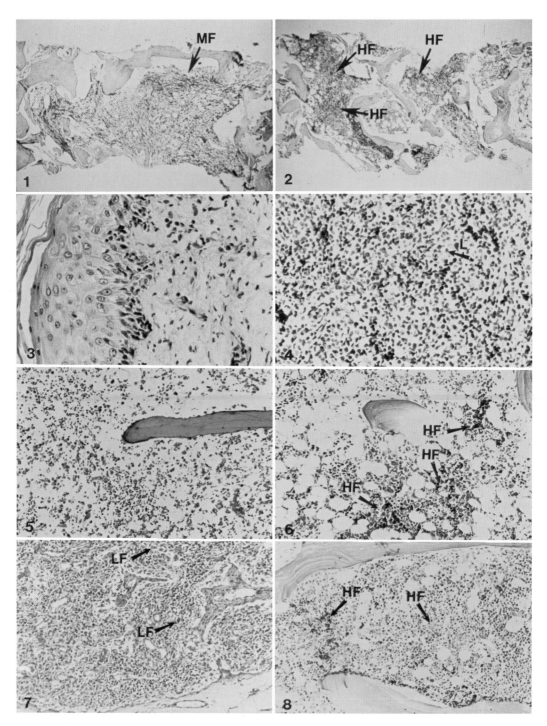

Plate 60

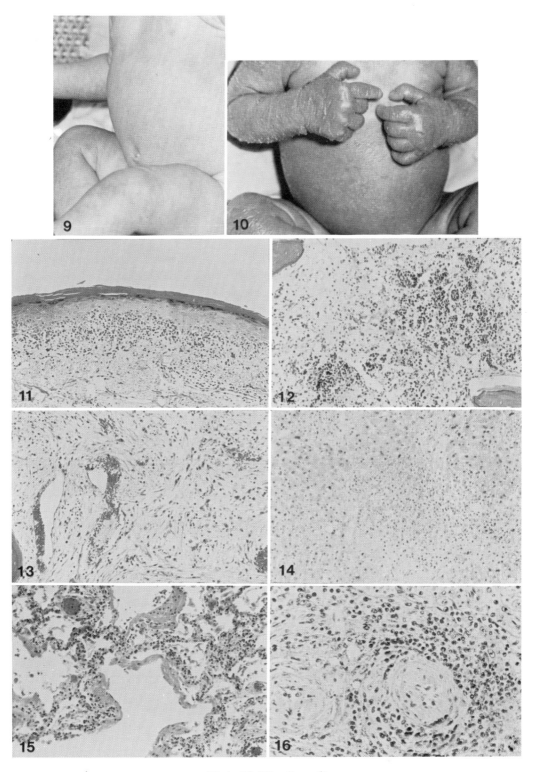

Plate 60 *(Continued)*

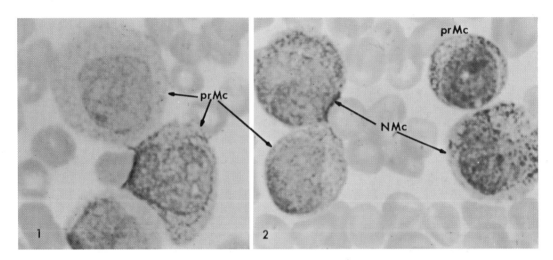

Plate 61

ACUTE PROMYELOCYTIC (PROGRANULOCYTIC) LEUKEMIA
Peripheral Blood

Neutrophilic myelocyte (NMc), promyelocyte (prMc).

Diagnostic Features: The morphologic characteristic of this blood dyscrasia is similar to other acute leukemias in that immature myeloid cells are observed in the peripheral blood. However, in this symptom complex, a variant of acute myeloblastic leukemia, there are many promyelocytes, severe bleeding tendency and low fibrinogen levels in the peripheral blood.

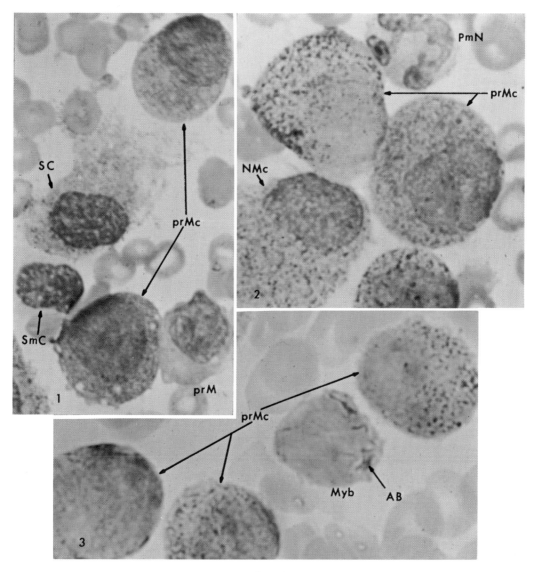

Plate 62

ACUTE PROMYELOCYTIC (PROGRANULOCYTIC) LEUKEMIA
Bone Marrow

Auer bodies (AB), myeloblast (Myb), neutrophilic myelocyte (NMc), polymorphonuclear neutrophil (PmN), promonocyte (prM), promyelocyte (prMc), smudge cell (SmC), stem cell (SC).

Diagnostic Features: Myeloid hyperplasia is seen with promyelocytes predominating the marrow pattern, suggesting a type of maturation "arrest," i.e., a diminution in metamyelocytic, juvenile and polymorphonuclear forms in the marrow.

Plate 63

CHRONIC LYMPHOCYTIC (LYMPHATIC, LYMPHOID) LEUKEMIA
Peripheral Blood

Lymphocyte (L), mitotic pattern in lymphocyte L(mit), lymphoblast (Lb), prolymphocyte (prL), smudge cell (SmC).

Diagnostic Features: Early in the disease the RBCs are normocytic and normochromic. If hemolysins develop (this occurs in 10% of the cases), the RBCs show characteristics of overt hemolytic anemia (polychromasia, nucleated RBCs, reticulocytosis and abnormal osmotic behavior); occasionally immature granulocytes are seen. WBC count is between 20,000 to 200,000 per cu. mm. (a relative and absolute lymphocytosis). Mature small lymphocytes predominate; they differ from normal lymphocytes in having larger and denser clumps of chromatin and accentuation of parachromatin; occasionally medium and large lymphocytes (prolymphocytes) are seen. At first there is a relative neutropenia, then absolute neutropenia. Platelets are in adequate numbers at first, then thrombocytopenia develops. Occasionally one sees large lymphocytes (lymphoblast-like) called "Rieder-type" with a lobulated pattern (Fig. 7). The peroxidase stain is negative.

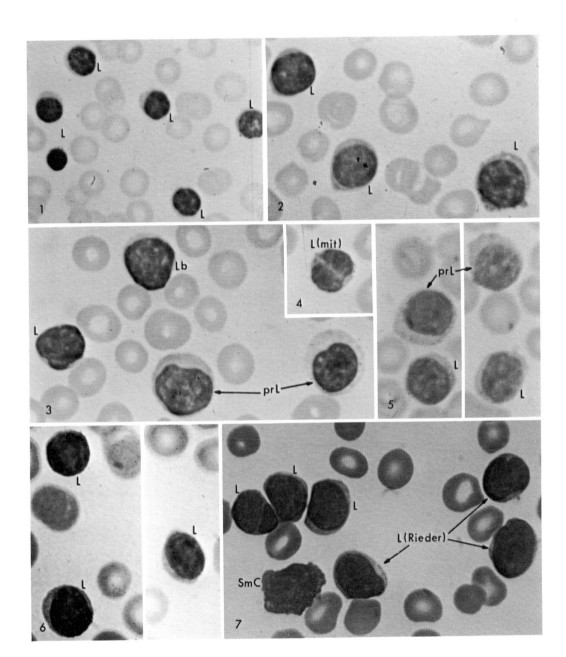

Plate 64

CHRONIC LYMPHOCYTIC (LYMPHATIC, LYMPHOID) LEUKEMIA
Bone Marrow

Lymphocyte (L), Rieder type of lymphocyte [L (Rieder)], mitosis (mit), monocyte (M), metamyelocyte (mMc), neutrophilic myelocyte (NMc), orthochromic normoblast (ONb), prolymphocyte (prL), promyelocyte (prMc), polymorphonuclear neutrophil (PmN).

Diagnostic Features: Initially there are increased numbers of mature small lymphocytes without depression of the normal erythroid and myeloid ele-ments. Later on, 50 per cent or more of the marrow cells are lymphocytes. Finally, the hypercellular marrow consists almost wholly of small to medium-sized mature lymphocytes with replacement of normal erythroid, megakaryocytic and granulocytic elements. If hemolytic phenomena are present, the marrow pattern consists of lymphocytes and nucleated RBCs. Grossly, the red marrow assumes a greyish-pink hue (Fig. 1).

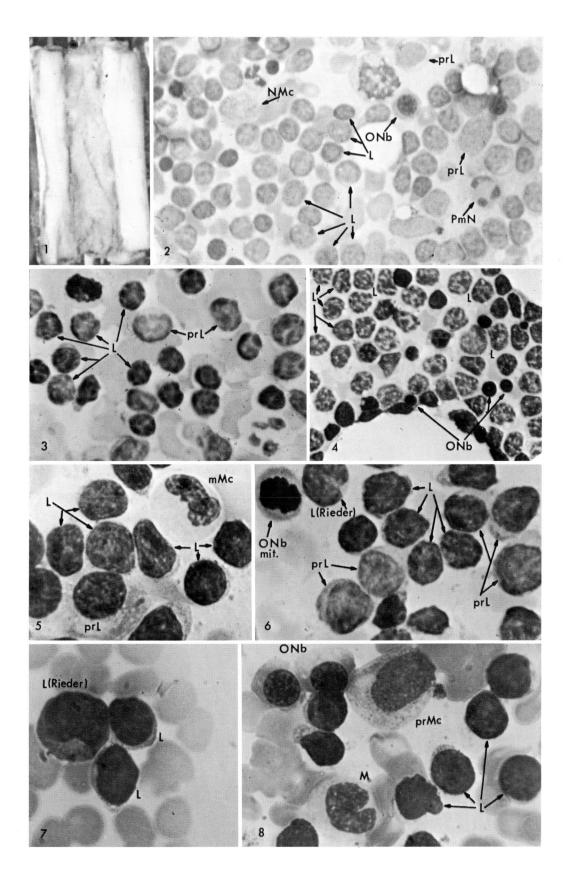

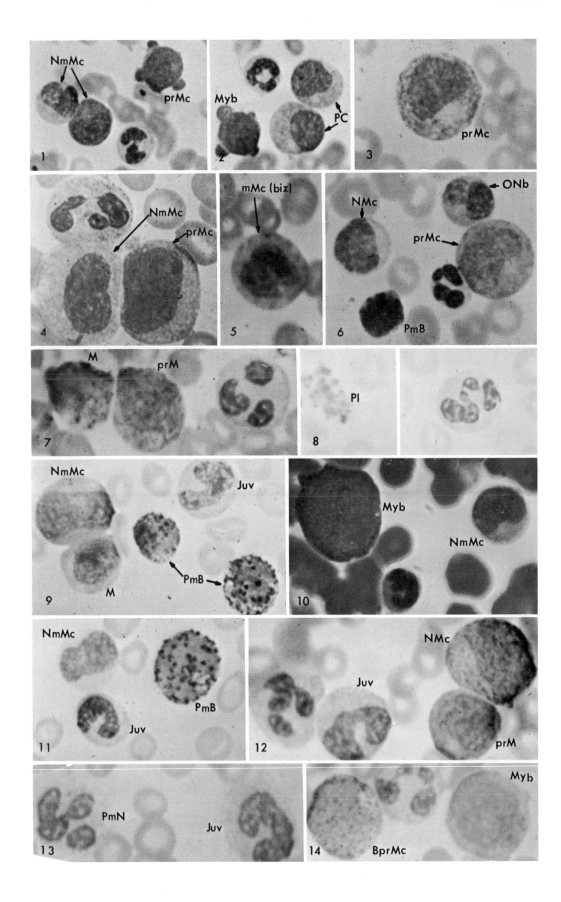

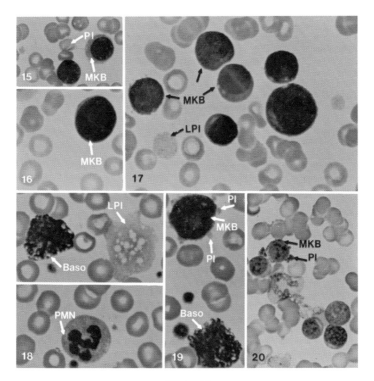

Plate 65

CHRONIC GRANULOCYTIC (MYELOID, MYELOCYTIC, MYELOGENOUS) LEUKEMIA
Peripheral Blood

Basophilic promyelocyte (BprMc), juvenile (Juv), monocyte (M), metamyelocyte, bizarre [mMc(biz)], myeloblast (Myb), neutrophilic metamyelocyte (NmMc), neutrophilic myelocyte (NMc), orthochromic normoblast (ONb), plasma cell (PC), platelet (Pl), polymorphonuclear basophil (PmB), polymorphonuclear neutrophil (PmN), promonocyte (prM), promyelocyte (prMc), megakaryoblast (MKB), platelet (Pl), large platelet (LPl), basophil (Baso), poly (PMN). (×970).

Diagnostic Features: The WBC counts vary from 100,000 to 300,000 per cu. mm. with relative to absolute increase in PmNs. All stages of myeloid series cells are present, including small numbers of myeloblasts and promyelocytes, the latter cells increasing with advanced disease. Alkaline phos-

phatase stain is subnormal to negative. Thrombocytosis occurs early; thrombocytopenia, late. Occasionally large and atypical platelet forms with fragments of megakaryocytes are sometimes seen. The RBCs shows slight polychromasia with associated anisocytosis; if hemolysins are present one may see nucleated RBCs, basophilic stippling, and reticulocytosis.

15–19. Megakaryoblast with attached platelet. Nuclei have rounded shape and when single lobed range in size from 10 to 21 μm. They are dark staining and have smooth, glossy surface. These are seen in the peripheral blood in cases of myelogenous leukemia and signify a poor prognosis and the onset of myelofibrosis.

20. Megakaryoblast with attached PAS positive cytoplasm and platelet.

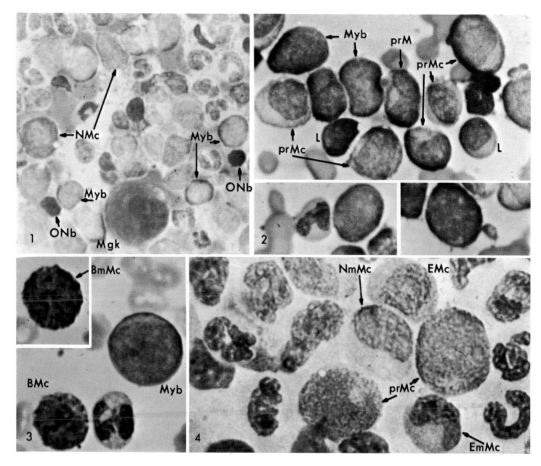

Plate 66

CHRONIC GRANULOCYTIC (MYELOID, MYELOCYTIC, MYELOGENOUS) LEUKEMIA
Bone Marrow

Basophilic metamyelocytes (BmMc), basophilic myelocyte (BMc), eosinophilic myelocyte (EMc), eosinophilic metamyelocyte (EmMc), juvenile (Juv), lymphocyte (L), large lymphocyte (lg L), megakaryocyte (Mgk), myeloblast (Myb), neutrophilic myelocyte (NMc), neutrophilic metamyelocyte (NmMc), orthochromic normoblast (ONb), polymorphonuclear neutrophil (PmN), promonocyte (prM), promyelocyte (prMc), sea-blue histiocyte (SBH), reticulum cell (RC).

Diagnostic Features: A hyperplastic, hypercellular granulocytic marrow is seen; at first myelocytes or metamyelocytes and later on promyelocytes and myeloblasts combined are found, indicating disor-

derly proliferation and maturation. Megakaryocytes are increased at first, later depressed with reduced numbers of platelets. Erythropoiesis is decreased with reduction in the quantity of nucleated RBCs. Ph[1] (Philadelphia) chromosomes are demonstrated in most cases (cf. Chap. 16).

9. Sea-blue histiocyte. Found in primary familial and secondary associated syndromes. In the latter, it may be due to overloading the normal enzyme system or due to a mild enzymatic deficiency. It is seen frequently post-splenectomy with or without preceding steroid therapy and in patients with ITP, chronic myelogenous leukemia, hyperlipoproteinemia, and so forth. ($\times$970).

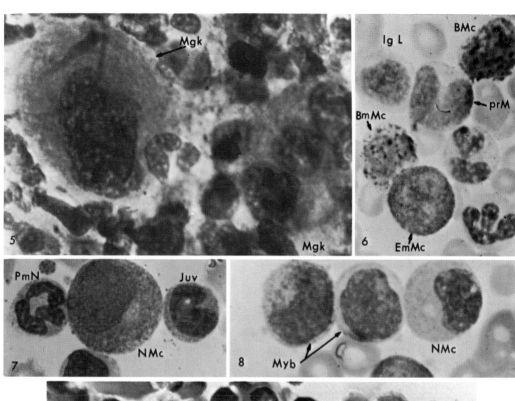

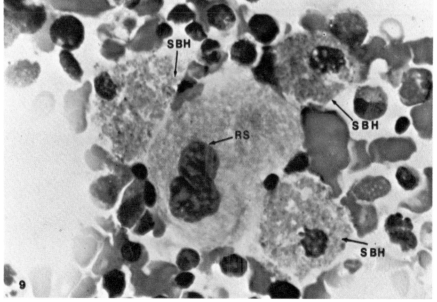

Plate 67

CHRONIC MONOCYTIC LEUKEMIA
Peripheral Blood

Atypical (atyp), Auer body (AB), basophilic myelocyte (BMc), lymphocyte (L), monocyte (M), monoblast (Mnb), polymorphonuclear neutrophil (PmN), promonocyte (prM).

Diagnostic Features: Varying shapes are observed in approximately 60 per cent of monocytes and promonocytes, and occasionally in monoblasts. Mature forms have irregular nuclei with very fine reticular chromatin; nucleus is lacier than normal monocytes and may appear to be folded or segmented; nucleoli are inconspicuous. The cytoplasm of these cells is greyish-blue, with innumerable very fine and a few coarse dust-like, reddish-lilac granules. Cell boundaries of monocytes and even oc- casionally promonocytes are irregular, with serrated borders due to extrusion of short granule-free pseudopodia. Monoblasts have nucleoli with few or no granules in the basophilic cytoplasm. Promonocytes are similar to monoblasts, but usually without nucleoli and occasionally having fine pinkish granules. Auer bodies (pinkish, rod-like structure—Figs. 1, 3) may be present in the cytoplasm. Some believe that there are two types of chronic monocytic leukemia: (1) Naegeli type, with moderate to large numbers of myelocytes together with monocytes; (2) Schilling type, in which mostly monocytes with large lacy chromatin bizarre nuclei and irregular cell borders are observed.

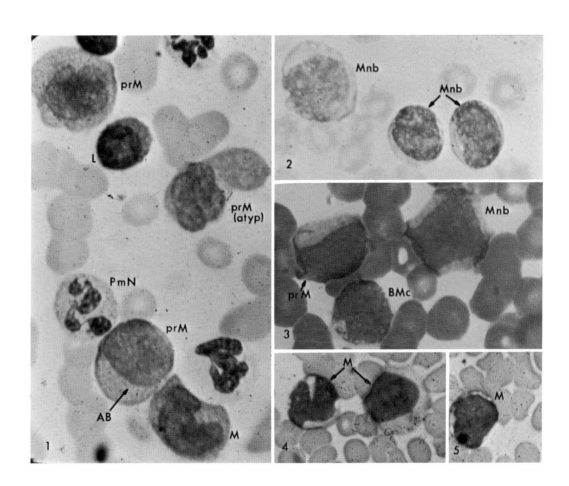

Plate 68

CHRONIC MONOCYTIC LEUKEMIA
Bone Marrow

Histiocyte (Hist), juvenile (Juv), lymphocyte (L), monocyte (M), monoblast (Mnb), neutrophilic myelocyte (NMc), orthochromic normoblast (ONb), promonocyte (prM), promyelocyte (prMc).

Diagnostic Features: The descriptive morphologic pattern is the same as the peripheral blood, with more immature promonocytic and monoblastic forms observed. Figs. 1 & 3. Schilling type. Figs. 4 & 5. Naegeli type.

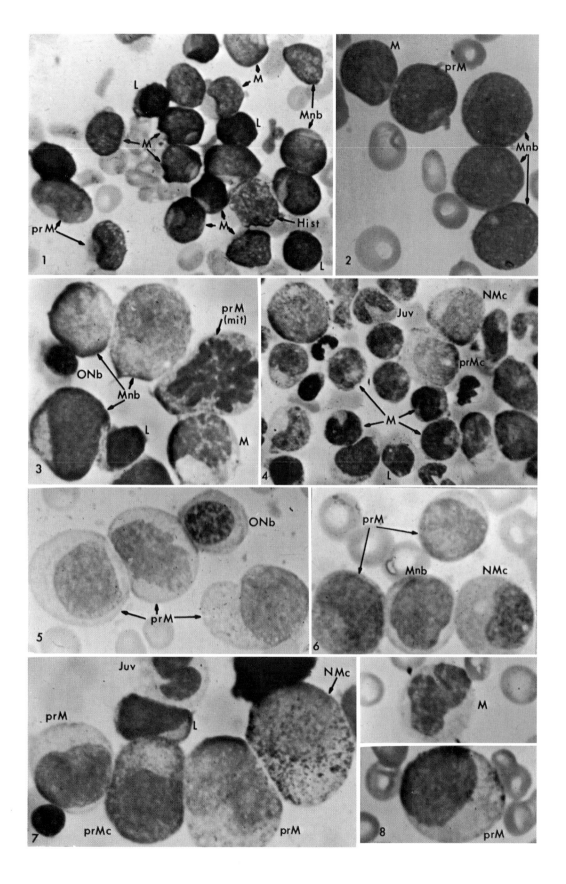

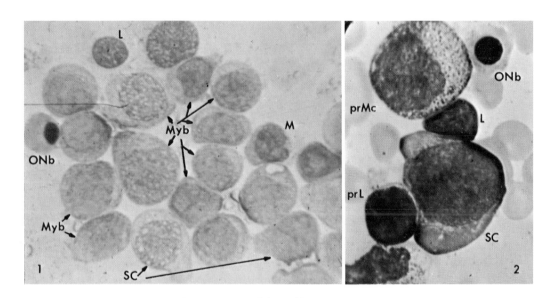

Plate 69

SUBLEUKEMIC LEUKEMIA
Bone Marrow

Lymphocyte (L), monocyte (M), myeloblast (Myb), orthrochromic normoblast (ONb), prolymphocyte (prL), promyelocyte (prMc), stem cell (SC).

Diagnostic Features: Characterized by a leukemic process with a circulating leukocyte count of less than 15,000 per cu. mm., but with 'blasts, promyelocytes, myelocytes, prolymphocytes or promonocyte forms in the peripheral blood. This can be differentiated from the aleukemic form if one examines the buffy coat of the peripheral blood.

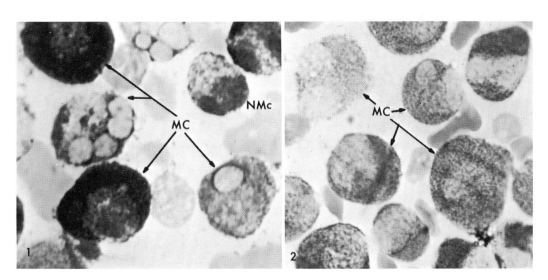

Plate 70

SYSTEMIC MAST CELL DISEASE (SYSTEMIC MASTOCYTOSIS)
Bone Marrow

Mast cell (MC), neutrophilic myelocyte (NMc).

Diagnostic Features: This is characterized by recurrent headaches, flushing of skin, migratory bone pain and occasionally hepatomegaly and splenomegaly with or without skin lesions. Cytologically, the mast cells are derived from reticuloendothelial cells and are round, large, 15 to 40 micra in diameter, with spherical nuclei (7 to 10 micra) and dense chromatin; the nuclei are eccentric in location and occasionally are obscured by granules;

they occasionally have 1 to 2 large nucleoli, cytoplasm is pale, vacuolated and backed with basophilic granules. There is also an associated erythrophagocytosis (Fig. 1). Mast cells differ from basophilic leukocytes in that the latter are smaller, have a lobulated nucleus and arise in the bone marrow; basophil granules are few in number and irregularly distributed; it is rare to see basophilia in systemic mast cell disease.

Plate 71

ACUTE AND CHRONIC ERYTHREMIC MYELOSIS
(Erythroleukemia or DiGuglielmo's Disease)
Peripheral Blood

Basophilic normoblast (BNb), degenerating cell (Deg), juvenile (Juv), lymphocyte (L), monoblast (Mnb), myeloblast (Myb), neutrophilic myelocyte (NMc), orthochromic normoblast (ONb), pronormoblast (prNb), polychromatic normoblast (pcNb), polymorphonuclear neutrophil (PmN), promonocyte (prM).

Diagnostic Features: In this blood dyscrasia one observes leukemic proliferation involving both the erythrocytic and granulocytic precursors. Some feel that the term is inappropriate and that this entity should be called "myelomymonocytic leukemia." The acute form is characterized by atypical normoblasts, some multilobed nuclei and altered nuclear-cytoplasmic ratios. Occasionally myelocytes and myeloblasts are seen. The chronic form is usually associated with an increased reticulocytosis. Hepatosplenomegaly and thrombocytopenia varies. Some believe that acute and chronic erythremic myelosis and erythroleukemias are all separate disorders, with the latter having more myeloid proliferation.

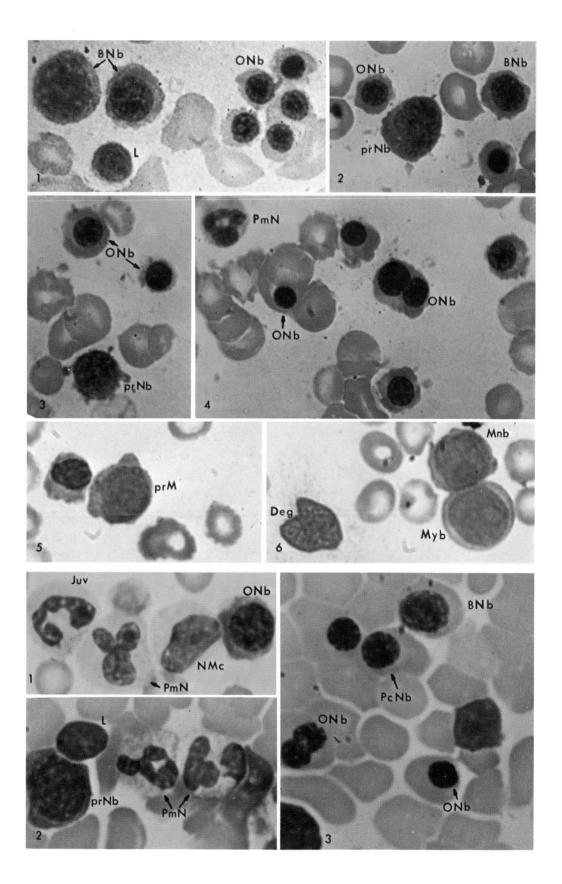

Plate 72

ACUTE AND CHRONIC ERYTHREMIC MYELOSIS
(Erythroleukemia or DiGuglielmo's Disease)
Bone Marrow

Basophilic normoblast (BNb), degenerating cell (deg), Littoral cell (Littoral C), lymphocyte (L), monocyte (M), myeloblast (Myb), orthochromic normoblast (ONb), promonocyte (prM), promyelocyte (prMc), pronormoblast (prNb), ringed sideroblast (RSb), megakaryocyte (MKy), PAS positive (PAS pos), smudge (Sm), orthochromic normoblast (ONb), juvenile (Juv), neutrophilic myelocyte (NMc), binucleate orthochromic normoblast (Binuc ONb).

Diagnostic Features: This is characterized by the presence of basophilic forms of normoblasts and early pronormoblasts, especially in the acute form.

PAS positive granules may be found in the cytoplasm of some pronormoblasts. The chronic form contains more orthochromic normoblastic forms. Immature myeloid forms (myeloblasts and promyelocytes) are also observed in varying quantities.

5. Ringed sideroblasts showing positive Prussian blue (iron) granules in rim of cytoplasm of orthochromic normoblast sideroblast.

6. PAS positive megakaryocytes show reddish deposits in platelet cytoplasm.

7. PAS positive orthochromic normoblasts (cytoplasm).

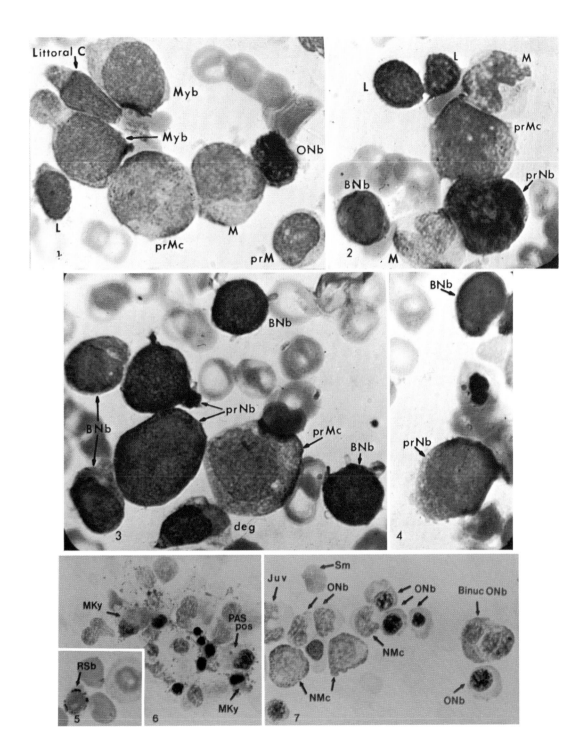

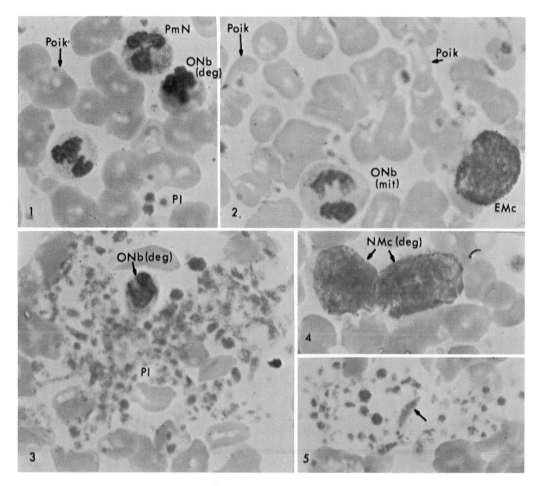

Plate 73

MYELOFIBROSIS WITH MYELOID METAPLASIA
(Agnogenic Myeloid Metaplasia)
Peripheral Blood

Eosinophilic myelocyte (EMc), mitosis (mit), degenerating neutrophilic myelocyte [NMc(deg)], degenerating orthochromic normoblast [ONb(deg)], poikilocyte (Poik), platelets (Pl), polymorphonuclear neutrophil (PmN).

Diagnostic Features: In this blood dyscrasia one sees minimal to moderate normocytic normochromic anemia, increased polychromasia, occasional nucleated red blood cells, and a slight reticulocytosis (especially in patients with superimposed hemolysis). There is also marked anisocytosis and poikilocytosis, e.g., tailed, tear-drop, comma and other bizarrely-shaped cells. Moderate leukocytosis with relative and absolute granulocytic cell increase is also observed; small numbers of immature cells are seen (e.g. promyelocytes, myelocytes and occasionally myeloblasts). Leukocyte alkaline phosphatase granules are normal in quantity except they appear to be increased in patients with a polycythemic pattern. Platelets are markedly increased with associated bizarre large forms with pale chromosomere (arrow in Fig. 5) and hyalomere; occasionally megakaryocytic fragments and even megakaryoblasts are seen in the peripheral blood.

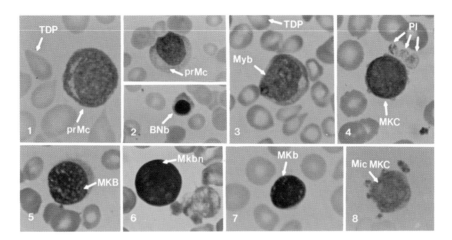

Plate 74

MYELOFIBROSIS WITH MYELOID METAPLASIA
(Agnogenic Myeloid Metaplasia; Acute Megakaryocytic Myelosis)
Peripheral Blood

Myelofibrosis is now considered to be part of a symptom-complex called myeloproliferative syndrome and has various names, such as agnogenic myeloid metaplasia, acute megakaryocytic myelosis, megakaryocytic splenomegaly, and myelosclerosis with myeloid metaplasia. It is characterized by abnormal proliferation of myeloid, erythroid, and other hematopoietic precursors plus anemia, marrow fibrosis, and hepatosplenic myeloid metaplasia. It may manifest itself as a variant of chronic granulocytic leukemia or terminate in such. Hematologically, as this plate reveals, there are various erythroid variations (teardrop RBCs), giant platelets, myeloid precursors, and megakaryocytic cells of all types. (prMc = promyelocyte; TDP = teardrop RBC; BNb = basophilic normoblast; Myg = myeloblast; MKCN = megakaryocytic nucleus; MKb = megakaryoblast; Mic MKC = micromegakaryocyte; Pl = platelet)

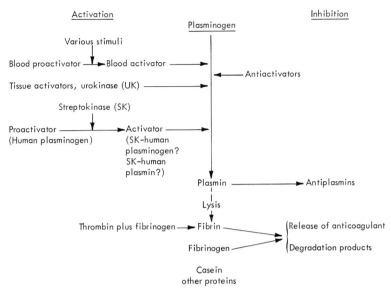

Fig. 12-3. Pechet's proposed simplified scheme of fibrinolysis. (Pechet, L.: Fibrinolysis. N. Engl. J. Med., *273:*966, 1965)

matic and simple, it serves a practical purpose because the initiation of fibrinolytic activity is still poorly understood. Plasminogen, normally present in plasma, may be activated under many different conditions so that proteolysis of fibrinogen and other plasma proteins occurs. The rate of lysis is usually not great enough to produce hypofibrinogenemia or the tendency to bleed. Hemorrhagic disorders directly due to intravascular proteolysis, and therefore increased fibrinolytic activity, have been infrequently found after major surgery, exercise, stress, anoxia, or the administration of certain pyrogens—apparently caused by a blood activator. For example, intravenous administration of streptokinase, a potent activator of plasminogen, may cause abnormal bleeding.

Some workers have shown that Factor XII initiates both the clotting and the fibrinolytic processes upon surface activation.[34] It is therefore possible that as clotting starts, its antagonistic reaction, fibrinolysis, also begins, thus maintaining a state of homeostatic balance. Thus, although the products of lysis of fibrinogen

appear to inhibit coagulation, excessive fibrinolysis initiates the hemorrhagic manifestations. Further support to the concept that Factor XII initiates fibrinolysis comes from recent observations concerning the association of clotting, fibrinolysis, and plasma kinins.[25] Moreover, Brackman and co-workers have observed that thrombin may activate plasminogen directly, suggesting another pathway through which fibrinolysis may become active as a consequence of coagulation.[12] Pechet has proposed a simplified scheme of fibrinolysis (Fig. 12-3).[47] Koller has depicted the antagonism of the coagulation sequence by fibrinolysis and its therapy (Fig. 12-4).[36]

Laboratory Diagnosis

1. In the plasma euglobulin clot lysis test 1 ml. of plasma is added to 9 ml. of Milstone solution (10 volumes of water containing 0.32 volumes of 1% acetic acid added to 1 volume of plasma).[57] This is centrifuged and the supernatant is removed. The precipitate is resuspended in 0.5 ml. of 0.01 M veronal buffer. This is clotted with 0.5 ml. of thrombin and placed in a 37° C

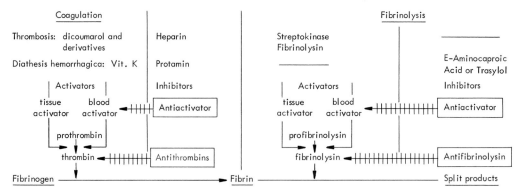

Fig. 12-4. Antagonism of the coagulation sequence by fibrinolysis and its therapy. (Koller, F.: Clinical and genetic aspects of coagulopathies. Ann. Intern. Med., *62:*744, 1965)

water bath. The time for complete lysis is then recorded.

This technique has been found to be very sensitive for assaying small amounts of fibrinolytic activity in plasma. Because in fibrinolytic assays the activity is a direct function of the reciprocal of the lysis time, a logarithmic plot of the lysis time versus units of activity gives a linear relationship. Utilizing such a plot and arbitrarily assigning an activity of 1 unit to a lysis time of 30 minutes, lysis times observed with this technique are converted into units of fibrinolytic activity. All lysis times greater than 300 minutes are referred to as less than 0.1 unit. Most specimens from normal adults lyse in 6 to 24 hours; however, shorter or longer lysis times are not unusual.

2. In the test for significant fibrinolysis, to each of four ($^{11}/_{12}$ mm.) tubes is added 1 ml. of glyoxalin buffer (680 mg. of glyoxalin is dissolved in 50 ml. of distilled water, and 2.5 volumes of this solution is mixed with about 1.86 volumes of 0.1 normal HCl.[56] The mixture is adjusted to *p*H 7.4 and made up to 10 volumes with distilled water.) To the first tube, 0.5 ml. of patient's plasma is added, and so on to give trebling dilutions of plasma—that is, $^1/_3$, $^1/_9$, $^1/_{27}$, and $^1/_{81}$. This procedure is repeated with trebling dilutions of citrated plasma in a solution (1 mg./ml.) of epsilonaminocaproic acid (EACA) in saline solution or glyoxalin buffer. The

procedure is repeated in a third row of tubes using a normal control plasma. Each dilution is placed in a water bath at 37° C for 3 minutes, and then all tubes are clotted with 0.1 ml. of undiluted calcium-free thrombin. This is mixed well, and the tubes are examined for evidence of lysis after 15, 30, and 60 minutes. The test is designed to detect violent lysis and to indicate the true level of fibrinogen in the presence of this phenomenon. The EACA inhibits lytic activity, thus revealing whether an apparent absence of fibrinogen represents a true depletion or is due to clots lysing as they form. Excessive lysis is considered to be present if the fibrinogen titer is two dilutions lower with buffer than with EACA in 30 minutes, or if all the clots in the tests with buffer lyse in 60 minutes. Normal plasma used as a control must be tested in a similar way because some batches of human thrombin have been found to contain fibrinolytic activator.

Treatment

In excessive fibrinolysis, the following approaches are used.

1. Urokinase, a physiologic activator of plasminogen normally present in urine, may be responsible for the rapid dissolution of clots formed in the urinary tract. For this reason EACA, an inhibitor of the activation of plasminogen, has been used to

lessen bleeding following prostatectomy. Other clinical trials have led to enthusiastic descriptions of the dramatic control of bleeding from fibrinolysis in disseminated carcinoma of the prostate, leukemia, cirrhosis of the liver, and in extracorporeal cardiopulmonary bypass. Successful treatment of pathologic fibrinolysis after resuscitation from cardiac arrest has also been achieved, and the fibrinolytic state induced by administration of streptokinase and other activators of plasminogen has been reversed. Control of bleeding from irradiation cystitis and carcinoma of the bladder has also been effected.[22]

A dose of EACA is 4 to 6 g. (40–60 ml, of a 10% solution) given intravenously over a period of about 15 minutes. An additional gram per hour may subsequently be given by intravenous drip if further treatment is required. EACA should be given only if active fibrinolysis can be demonstrated and is associated with abnormal bleeding. Because EACA inhibits lysis, any blood clot forming after this drug has been given will probably organize into fibrous tissue. If, therefore, there is free blood in any duct or cavity, such as the ureter and pleural cavity, the dangers of fibrous organization must be set against the risk of leaving the fibrinolytic process untreated. Therefore, EACA should be given only if the severity of bleeding outweighs the potential hazards of the drug. The indiscriminate use of the drug in desperation in a nonspecific "hemostatic cocktail" is not recommended.

2. Bleeding associated with excessive fibrinolysis may be general but is most severe at the site of a surgical wound. Treatment in these cases consists of whole fresh blood transfusions and of concentrates of fibrinogen (5–6 gm. reconstituted in a total of 400 ml. distilled water).

3. Plasminogen inhibitors may be helpful.

4. If there is doubt that fibrinolysis is primary or secondary to DIC, the patient should first be treated for DIC with heparin. Antifibrinolytic therapy can fatally aggravate DIC if heparin is not used first. If evidence of fibrinolysis continues to appear in a heparinized patient, antifibrinolytic therapy may be started with 5 g. EACA (I.V. over 1 hour or PO in a single dose) followed by 1 g. per hour for 8 hours. No more than 30 g. should be given in a day.

INHIBITION OF FIBRIN FORMATION BY DYSPROTEINEMIA

Hemorrhagic manifestations related in part to interference with the thrombin-fibrinogen reaction and subsequent delay in blood clotting are occasionally observed in some patients with atypical globulins, as in cryoglobulinemia, Waldenström's macroglobulinemia, and plasma cell myeloma. Associated vascular weakness and platelet deficiencies may also occur. A gelatinous nonretractile clot without normal fibrin strands forms even when the thrombocyte level is within the normal range. There is also marked prolongation of the coagulation time when thrombin is added to a patient's plasma containing these atypical globulins. However, the thrombin time becomes normal when the plasma is diluted. Further proof of the clot-delaying effect of the atypical globulins is seen when normal and abnormal plasmas are mixed. Other irregularities observed in these dysproteinemic plasmas are the prolongation of Quick's one-stage prothrombin time test due to the atypical globulin acting like an antithrombin, and the unpredictable prothrombin consumption tests due to difficulties in obtaining serum because of the gelatinous nature of the blood clots of these patients.

INCREASE IN CIRCULATING ANTICOAGULANTS

Circulating anticoagulants interfere with thromboplastin activity development and therefore are associated with coagulation factor deficiency findings of this type.

Treatment is made even more difficult when one must treat this complication as well as the original hemorrhagic defect. If these anticoagulants develop during pregnancy, they may last for a long time and be associated with a bleeding tendency. Other diseases also associated with circulating anticoagulants are chronic glomerulonephritis, tuberculous lymphadenopathy, syphilis, and collagen diseases. The main laboratory test showing abnormal findings in this clinical complex is the thromboplastin generation test. When the patient's serum or adsorbed plasma is substituted in the incubation mixture, there is a diminution of thromboplastin activity. If one uses 50 per cent normal and 50 per cent patient's adsorbed plasma with normal serum in the incubation mixture, the thromboplastin activity is diminished. This allows identification of presence of a circulating anticoagulant because any genetic defect that would be confused with it would have been corrected by the addition of 50 per cent normal adsorbed plasma. In order to differentiate heparin-like compounds from circulating anticoagulants, protamine sulfate or toluidine blue must be added to the plasma. This neutralizes the heparin-like compounds and leaves the circulating anticoagulants uninvolved.

These circulating anticoagulant substances are said to interfere with the process of thromboplastin activity in the intrinsic system and possibly also with the action of formed thromboplastin. Because circulating anticoagulants are part of the gamma globulin plasma fraction, they are thought to be the result of some immunologic mechanism, especially because they are found in patients who have had multiple transfusions, pregnancy, or diseases of hypersensitivity such as systemic lupus erythematosus. They are relatively stable to heat and cold—for example, 0 to 4° C for long periods. Circulating anticoagulants in the order of frequency against Factors VIII, IX, V, and VII have been described. If they interfere with

thromboplastin activity itself or even with Factor V or VII, the one-stage prothrombin time is prolonged. Treatment consists of large transfusions with fresh blood, occasional adrenocortical steroids, and Factor VIII concentrates if the disorder is due to circulating anticoagulants against Factor VIII. Protamine sulfate and toluidine blue are of help occasionally if the problem is due to heparin-like compounds.

STUDY AND DIAGNOSIS OF PATIENTS WITH HEMORRHAGIC DISEASE

It is apparent from the foregoing discussions that pathologic bleeding may be the result of an almost limitless number of disorders, many of which are not associated with abnormalities of the coagulation mechanism. Accurate diagnosis is essential for the intelligent and effective treatment of a hemorrhagic disorder.[19]

As is obvious, the most common difficulty is differentiating the normal from the abnormal. The efficiency of the normal hemostatic mechanism has already been emphasized, but it is also evident that normal persons do bleed after injury. A large number of apparently normal women note ecchymoses in the skin from time to time and report that they bruise easily. Slight bleeding from the gums when brushing the teeth has been experienced occasionally by many healthy persons without other evidence of a hemorrhagic disorder. Epistaxis occurring after vigorous exertion or minor trauma is not rare in otherwise healthy children. A certain amount of bleeding, sometimes a considerable amount, may follow tooth extraction or tonsillectomy in normal persons. Because denuded surfaces may be left exposed, these operative procedures are more often followed by bleeding than are major surgical procedures in which close approximation of tissues is achieved.

Faced with the problem of a hemorrhagic disease, the physician may tend to rely on the results of an elaborate array of complex laboratory tests of blood clotting and all too often assign an unwarranted significance to a questionable or slightly abnormal result. In most instances of abnormal bleeding, the substantial clues are provided by examination of the patient and by careful analysis of his history, although appropriately chosen laboratory tests may be essential to pinpoint the diagnosis.

In the following section a scheme is suggested for the investigation of a patient suspected of suffering from a hemorrhagic disorder:[10]

I. Symptomatology
   A. Is a hemorrhagic state present?
Points in favor of a hemorrhagic state:
   1. Hemorrhages from different parts of the body.
   2. Abnormal bleeding since early childhood or for many years.
   3. A similar state occurring in blood relatives (obtain as complete a family tree as possible).
   4. Localized bleeding, such as from the nose, gastrointestinal tract, respiratory tract, or urinary tract, without a demonstrable organic lesion.
   5. Hemorrhage into joints or large hemorrhage into deep tissues without history of severe trauma.
   6. If the patient has needed a blood transfusion after dental extraction or tonsillectomy (patients who have had many dental extractions and removal of tonsils and adenoids without excessive hemorrhage have no congenital deficiency of AHF).
   7. Hemorrhage for more than 24 hours after an operation on the nose or throat.
   8. Hemorrhage from the gums for more than 48 hours after dental extraction may be significant, although the commonest causes of this state are local trauma and sepsis.

   B. If the history suggests the presence of a hemorrhagic state: Is it likely to be a coagulation defect or a capillary or platelet defect?

   1. In favor of a coagulation defect.
      a. Abnormal bleeding not limited to the skin and mucosae.
      b. Abnormal bleeding usually related to trauma, as in hemarthrosis, deep hematoma, and slow persistent oozing from skin or mucosae.
   2. In favor of a capillary or a platelet defect.
      a. Spontaneous petechiae or ecchymoses in the skin.
      b. Spontaneous bleeding from the mucosae.
      c. The obvious presence of a disease known to be associated with a platelet deficiency or a capillary defect, such as leukemia, carcinomatosis, drug toxicity, and thrombocytopenic purpura.

Defects in blood coagulation and capillary or platelet abnormalities may occur simultaneously in the same patient. For example, some patients with a capillary defect of von Willebrand type have an associated deficiency of AHF.

   C. If a coagulation defect is present, is it hereditary? The history may determine this point.
   1. Hemophilia (Factor VIII deficiency) and Christmas disease (Factor IX deficiency) are inherited as sex-linked recessive characters (female hemophiliacs are extremely rare).
   2. Congenital Factor V and Factor VII deficiencies are inherited as non-sex-linked dominant characters—both males and females suffer from this disorder.
   3. Congenital deficiency of fibrinogen (Factor I), which usually occurs as a result of cousin intermarriage, is probably inherited as a non-sex-linked recessive character—both males and females suffer from this disorder.
   4. Stuart-Prower factor (X) deficiency is inherited as a highly penetrant and incompletely recessive autosomal characteristic.

Even when a negative family history is

elicited, if a hemorrhagic state has existed from early childhood, it is likely to be passed on to subsequent generations.

D. The occurrence of acquired coagulation defects (a negative family history associated with the onset of a hemorrhagic state in late childhood or adult life favor acquired defects). These may be due to the following:

1. Deficiency of plasma factors.

a. Factor V deficiency may occur in liver disease, following massive blood transfusions, postoperatively in carcinomatosis, in acute infections, or as a congenital deficiency.

b. Factor VII deficiency follows tryatment with coumarin drugs. It is also found in vitamin K deficiency and in newborn infants, and it may occur in obstructive jaundice and steatorrhea, or as a congenital deficiency.

c. Stuart-Prower factor (X) deficiency occurs after therapy with coumarin drugs. The level of the factor drops only after several days of this treatment. Such a deficiency may be congenital.

d. Prothrombin deficiency (II) occurs in liver disease, treatment with coumarin drugs, vitamin K deficiencrn infants, and rarely as an isolated condition.

e. Fibrinogen (I) deficiency may be due to deficient production, as in some cases of general malignant neoplasia such as carcinomatosis and leukemia, general infections, such as tuberculosis and syphilis, malabsorption syndrome, and liver disease.

f. Combined deficiencies are not uncommon. Thus, prothrombin Factor II, factor VII, Stuart-Prower factor (X) and Christmas factor (IX) are reduced by coumarin drugs. Factors VII and IX may be reduced together, as may factors V and VIII.

2. Circulating anticoagulants. Some are idiopathic and others are associated with the so-called collagen diseases and infections such as tuberculosis. They may be stimulated by blood transfusion or pregnancy. They may diminish human thromboplastin formation and utilization, or their activity may resemble that of heparin, especially after irradiation and other antimitotic therapy.

3. Defibrination. Apart from deficient production, fibrinogen deficiency may be caused by rapid utilization of fibrinogen as a consequence of extensive clotting of blood in vivo, or as a result of fibrinolysis in the circulation in association with pregnancy, pulmonary surgery, thyroidectomy, prostatic disease (especially malignant), liver disease, leukemia, and blood transfusion reactions.

4. Dysproteinemias. Abnormal hemorrhage may be due to idiopathic hyperglobulinemia, macroglobulinemia, or cryoglobulinemia.

II. A suggested method of procedure:[21]

A. Complete blood count including erythrocytes, hematocrit, leukocytes, and hemoglobin, and the inspection and study of a blood film, using Wright's stain.

B. Platelet count, using the phase-contrast technique or the electronic counter technique.

C. Whole-blood coagulation time, clot retraction test, bleeding time, and capillary fragility test.

In most instances, it should be possible, by this stage of clinical investigation, to have decided whether the patient is suffering from a coagulation, or a platelet or vascular defect. The personal history, with information such as symptoms and drug ingestion, and family history, and the clinical findings may also be of help in deciding to which category the patient belongs. If a coagulation defect is suspected, proceed as follows:

D. Screening thromboplastin-generation test (Hicks-Pitney) or partial thromboplastin time test (PTT).

E. One-stage prothrombin time test by the Quick or P and P method (prothrombin and proconvertin).

F. Prothrombin consumption test on serum from the whole-blood coagulation time test.

If all the preceding tests give normal results, a major defect in the hemostatic mechanism is unlikely. If however, an abnormal result is obtained, proceed as follows:

G. Thromboplastin-generation test. This should enable a diagnosis of hemophilia or Christmas disease (Factor IX deficiency). If the disorder is hemophilia, an AHF assay is useful.

H. Tests for circulating anticoagulants. Try the effect of adding normal plasma to the patient's plasma in the thromboplastin generation test. Carry out other tests for circulating anticoagulants and for heparin-like substances.

I. If the one-stage prothrombin time is prolonged, carry out the following:

1. Qualitative tests for Factors V and VII.

2. A one-stage test using Russell's viper venom.

3. Two-stage ef prothrombin.

If the diagnosis is still obscure, consider the question of contact factor (XI or XII) deficiencies, hypofibrinogenemia, and fibrinolysis. Carry out:

J. Contact activation tests.

K. Estimation of plasma fibrinogen.

L. Tests for abnormal fibrinolysis and thrombin-fibrinogen reaction.

If a platelet or capillary defect is suspected, proceed as follows:

M. Measurement of clot retraction.

N. Tests for platelet function, in thromboplastin generation and other tests.

O. Tests for platelet antibodies.[44] Screening for autoimmune or induced platelet antibodies can be easily carried out by a method in which regular rather than silicone-treated glassware is used. In this procedure, 7 ml. of fresh O negative Versenated (EDTA) blood is centrifuged at 1000 r.p.m. for 10 minutes. The platelet-rich plasma is withdrawn and recentrifuged at 2400 r.p.m. for another 10 minutes. The supernatant is discarded, leaving a platelet button. The platelets are washed three times in 0.85 per cent saline solution, and they are then suspended in 2 ml. of saline solution by gentle inversion for 5 minutes. Parafilm is used to cover the tube. This is centrifuged at 500 r.p.m. for 5 minutes to remove large platelet clumps. This platelet suspension should be used immediately. A fasting blood specimen is obtained and allowed to undergo firm clot retraction. The serum is centrifuged for 10 minutes at 3000 r.p.m. to remove the remaining platelets. Then 0.2 ml. of test serum is incubated with 0.2 ml. of platelet suspension for 1 hour at 37° C. At the same time, a control is run using 0.2 ml. of 0.85 per cent saline solution and 0.2 ml. of platelet suspension. Platelet counts are performed on the control and patient specimens. A decrease of platelets of 50 per cent or more in the patient specimen as compared to the saline solution control is a significant decrease, and suggests the presence of platelet antibodies.

P. A sternal marrow aspiration study may occasionally help in the diagnosis of a hemorrhagic state.

Summary

If the results of the preceding tests down to *F* are normal, then the investigation can generally be stopped unless there is clear evidence that the patient has bled unduly in the past. In the absence of such a history (with normal screening test results), it can be predicted with a fair measure of confidence that the patient is unlikely to bleed severely if his hemostatic mechanism is put to the test, say by surgery. If there is a history of excessive bleeding, which is sometimes difficult to ascertain, the patient should be investigated further, even if the screening tests give normal results, although the expectation of an abnormality being demonstrable is not high. Perhaps the most practical thing to do is to investigate the patient on several different occasions.

Where screening tests give abnormal results, the patient should naturally be investigated first along the lines suggested by the results of the preliminary tests. Most patients who complain of an undue tendency to bleed suffer from a chronic illness, and there is no particular hurry in carrying out the appropriate investigations, which should proceed step by step. At or just before parturition, the defibrination syndrome may necessitate an emergency state. Five tests are carried out concurrently: the platelet count, one-stage prothrombin time, rapid determination of fibrinogen, modified Hicks-Pitney screening TGT, and a thrombin clotting time designed to test for fibrinogenolysis and to detect the presence of heparin.

REFERENCES

1. Abramson, N., Eisenberg, P. D., and Aster, R. H.: Post-transfusion purpura: immunologic aspects and therapy. N. Engl. J. Med., *291*:1163, 1974.
2. Ackroyd, J. F.: Allergic purpura, including purpura due to foods, drugs, and infections. Am. J. Med., *14*:605, 1953.
3. Ahlberg, A., and Dormandy, K.: Clotting factors prevent hemophopathy. Medical Tribune, pp. 1, 14, Oct. 10, 1966.
4. Aledart, L. M.: Hemophilia: the impact of replacement therapy. Presented at the Education Program of the American Society of Hematology. San Diego, Dec. 3-4, 1977.
5. Aster, R. H.: Splenic platelet pooling as cause of "hypersplenic" thrombocytopenia. Trans. Assoc. Am. Physicians, *78*:362, 1965.
6. Banatvala, J. E., Horstmann, D. M., Payne, M. C., and Gluck, L.: Rubella syndrome and thrombocytopenic purpura in newborn infants: clinical and virologic observations. N. Engl. J. Med., *273*:474, 1965.
7. Bayer, W. L., Sherman, F. E., Michaels, R. H., Szeto, I. L. F., and Lewis, J. H.: Purpura in congenital and acquired rubella. N. Engl. J. Med., *273*:1362, 1965.
8. Bentegeat, J., Verger, P., Marc, Y., and Nouaille-Degorce, P.: Viral etiology of acute thrombopenic purpuras of childhood. Ann. Pediatr., *41*:372, 1965.
9. Bick, R. L., Kovacs, I., and Fekete, L. F.: A new two-stage functional assay for antithrombin III (heparin cofactor). Clinical and laboratory evaluation. Thrombosis Research, *8*:745, 1976.
10. Blackburn, E. K.: Investigation of hemorrhagic states with special reference to defects of coagulation of blood. Broadsheet No. 31 (new series). Association of Clinical Pathologists (England), April, 1961.
11. Bowie, E. J. W., Thompson, J. H., and Owen, C. A., Jr.: The blood platelet (including a discussion of the qualitative platelet diseases). Mayo Clin. Proc., *40*:625, 1965.
12. Brackman, P., Klug, P., and Astrup, T.: Fibrinolytic activity of thrombin preparations. Thromb. Diath. Haemorrh., *11*:234, 1964.
13. Brinkhouse, K. M.: Hemophilia-pathophysiologic studies and the evolution of transfusion therapy. Am. J. Clin. Pathol., *41*:342, 1964.
14. Brinkhous, K. M., Smith, H. P., and Seegers, W. H.: Inhibition of blood clotting. An unidentified substance which acts in conjunction with heparin to prevent the conversion of prothrombin into thrombin. Am. J. Physiol., *125*:683, 1939.
15. Brinkhous, R. M.: Clotting defect in hemophilia: deficiency in a plasma factor required for platelet utilization. Proc. Soc. Exp. Biol. Med., *66*:117, 1947.
16. Castle, W. B.: Spleen and Reticulo-Endothelial System. Yearbook of Medicine. p. 725. Chicago, Year Book Publishers, 1966-67.
17. Cimo, P. L., Pisciotta, A. V., Desai, R. G., Pino, J. L., and Asher, R. H.: Detection of drug-dependent antibodies by the ^{51}Cr lysis test: documentation of immune thrombocytopenia induced by diphenylhydantoin, dizepam, and sulfisoxazole. American Journal of Hematology, *2*:65, 1977.
18. Cohen, P., and Gardner, F. H.: Thrombocytopenic effect of sustained high-dosage prednisone therapy in thrombocytopenic purpura. N. Engl. J. Med., *25*:611, 1961.
19. Conley, C. L.: Management of hemorrhagic diseases. J.A.M.A., *181*:985, 1962.
20. Corley, C. C., Lessner, H. E., and Larsen, W. E.: Azathioprine therapy of "autoimmune" diseases. Am. J. Med., *41*:404, 1966.
21. Dacie, J. V., and Lewis, S. M.: Practical Hematology. ed 3. pp. 260, 261, 263. New York, Grune & Stratton, 1963.
22. Editorial: Epsilon aminocaproic acid. N. Engl. J. Med., *273*:336, 1965.
23. Editorial: Platelet transfusions. N. Engl. J. Med., *274*:351, 1966.
24. Editorial: Purpura in German measles. N. Engl. J. Med., *273*:1390, 1965.
25. Eisen, V.: Fibrinolysis and formation of biologically active polypeptides. Brit. M. Bull., *20*:205, 1964.
26. Eisenberg, P. D., and Abramson, N.: Post-transfusion purpura revisited. N. Engl. J. Med., *296*:515, 1977.
27. Friedman, L. L., Bowie, E. J. W., Thompson, J. H., Brown, A. L., and Owen, C. A.: Familial Glanzmann's thrombasthenia. Mayo Clin. Proc., *39*:908, 1964.
28. Goldsmith, K. L. G., Jenkins, W. J., Muchlow, E. S., and Normand, I. C. S.: Significance of platelet

antibodies in neonatal thrombocytopenic purpura affecting a pair of siblings. J. Clin. Pathol., *18:*462, 1965.

29. Goss, J. E., and Dickhous, D. W.: Increased bishydroxycoumarin requirements in patients receiving phenobarbital. N. Engl. J. Med., 273:1094, 1965.
30. Green, D.: Suppression of an antibody to factor VIII by a combination of factor VIII and cyclophosphamide. Br. J. Haematol., *37:*381, 1971.
31. Hedge, U. M., Gordon-Smith, E. C., and Worlledge, S.: Platelet antibodies in thrombocytopenic patients. Br. J. Haematol., *35:*113, 1977.
32. Herzig, R. H., *et. al.:* Correction of poor platelet transfusion responses with leukocyte-poor HLA-matched platelet concentrates. Blood, *46:*743, 1975.
33. Howie, P. W., Prentice, C. R. W., and McNicol, G. P.: A method of antithrombin estimation using plasma defibrinated with ancrod. Br. J. Haematol., *25:*101, 1973.
34. Iatridis, S. G., and Ferguson, J. H.: Active Hageman factor: plasma lysokinase of human fibrinolytic system. J. Clin. Invest., *41:*1277, 1962.
35. Kashiwagi, H. J. M., Riddle, J. M., Abraham, J. P., and Frame, B.: Functional and ultrastructural abnormalities of platelets in Ehlers-Danlos syndrome. Ann. Intern. Med., *63:*249, 1965.
36. Koller, F.: Clinical and genetic aspects of coagulopathies. Ann. Intern. Med., *62:*744, 1965.
37. Leslie, J., and Ingram, G. I. C.: The diagnosis of long-standing bleeding disorders. Semin. Hematol., *8:*140, 1971.
38. Levin, J., and Conley, C. L.: Thrombocytosis associated with malignant disease. Arch. Intern. Med., *114:*497, 1964.
39. Levine, P. H.: The self-therapy of hemophilia: benefits and deficits. Presented at the Education Program of the American Society of Hematology. San Diego, Dec. 3-4, 1977.
40. McClure, P. D.: Idiopathic thrombocytopenia purpura in children. Should corticosteroids be given? Am. J. Dis. Child, *131:*357, 1977.
41. Miale, J. B.: Laboratory Medicine-Hematology. ed. 2. pp. 729–731. St. Louis, C. V. Mosby, 1962.
42. Minard, B., and Petersen, C. A.: Comparison of functional and immunologic antithrombin III values. Presented at the ASCP/CAP Interim Meeting. Dallas, 1976.
43. Mueller-Eckhardt, C.: Idiopathic thrombocytopenia purpura: clinical and immunological considerations. Seminars in Thrombosis and Hemostasis, *3:*125, 1977.
44. Osterberg, M. M.: Detection of platelet antibodies in serum-flor-ocular. (Florida Div. ASMT.), *13:*6, 1965.
45. Patterson, J. H., Pierce, R. B., Amerson, J. R., and Watkins, W. L.: Dextran therapy of purpura fulminans. N. Engl. J. Med., *273:*734, 1965.
46. Pearson, H. A., Shulman, N. R., Marder, Y. J., and Cone, T. E., Jr.: Isoimmune neonatal thrombocytopenic purpura, clinical and therapeutic considerations. Blood, *23:*154, 1964.
47. Pechet, L.: Fibrinolysis. N. Engl. J. Med., *273:*966, 1965.

48. Penny, R., Rozenberg, M. C., and Firkin, B. G.: Splenic platelet pool. Blood, *27:*1, 1966.
49. Poller, L., and More, J. R. S.: A study of naphthionin in the management of the bleeding defect in patients with thrombocytopenia. J. Clin. Pathol., *17:*680, 1964.
50. Pool, J. G., and Shannon, A. E.: Production of high-potency concentrates of antihemophilic globulin in a closed-bag system. N. Engl. J. Med., *273:*1443, 1965.
51. Propp, R. P., and Scharfman, W. B.: Hemangioma-thrombocytopenia syndrome associated with microangiopathic hemolytic anemia. Blood, *28:*623, 1966.
52. Reid, W. O., Lucas, O. N., Francesco, J., Geisler, P. H., and Erslev, A. J.: The use of epsilon-aminocaproic acid in the management of dental extractions in the hemophiliac. Am. J. Med. Sci., *248:*82, 1964.
53. Ries, C. A.: Vincristine for treatment of refractory autoimmune thrombocytopenia. N. Engl. J. Med., *295:*1136, 1976.
54. Ries, C. A.: Platelet kinetics in autoimmune thrombocytopenia: relation between splenic platelet sequestration and response to splenectomy. Ann. Intern. Med., *86:*194, 1977.
55. Rosner, F., and Ritz, N. D.: The defibrination syndrome. Arch. Intern. Med., *177:*17, 1966.
56. Sharp, A. A., and Eggleston, M. J.: Hematology and the extracorporeal circulation. J. Clin. Pathol., *16:*551, 1963.
57. Sherry, S., Lindenmeyer, R. L., Fletcher, A. P., and Alkjaersig, N.: Studies on enhanced fibrinolytic activity in man. J. Clin. Invest., *38:*810, 1959.
58. Shulman, N. R., Marder, V. J., and Weinrach, R. S.: Comparison of immunologic and idiopathic thrombocytopenia. Trans. Assoc. Am. Physicians, *77:*65, 1964.
59. Strauss, H. S., and Bloom, G. E.: Von Willebrand's disease. N. Engl. J. Med., *273:*171, 1965.
60. Stuart, M. J., Murphy, S., Oski, F. A., Evans, A. E., Donaldson, M. H., and Gardner, F. H.: Platelet function in recipients of platelets from donors ingesting aspirin. N. Engl. J. Med., *287:*1105, 1972.
61. Varlin, M., Laros, R. K., and Penner, J. A.: Treatment of refractory thrombocytopenia purpura with cyclophosphamide. American Journal of Hematology, *1:*97, 1976.
62. Van Dam, J., Hensen, A., Loeliger, E. A., and Leeksma, C. H. W.: Defibrination syndrome treated with heparin. Ned. Tijdschr. Geneeskol., *109:*894, 1965.
63. Von Kaulla, E., and Von Kaulla, K. M.: Deficiency of antithrombin III activity associated with hereditary thrombosis tendency. J. Med. (Basel), *3:*349, 1972.
64. Weaver, R. A., Langdell, R. D., and Price, R. E.: Antihemophilic factor (AHF) in cross-circulated normal and hemophilic dogs. Am. J. Physiol., *206:*335, 1965.
65. Wintrobe, M. M., *et. al.:* Clinical Hematology. ed. 7, pp. 1187–1189. Philadelphia, Lea & Febiger, 1974.

66. Young, R. C., Nachman, R. L., and Horowitz, H. I.: Thrombocytopenia due to digitoxin. Am. J. Med., *41*:605, 1966.
67. Zuelzer, W. W., and Lusher, J. M.: Childhood idiopathic thrombocytopenia purpura: to treat or not to treat. Am. J. Dis. Child., *131*:360, 1977.

AUDIOVISUAL AIDS*

An Approach to the Diagnosis of Bleeding Disorders. Set H1. [35 mm. transparencies, audiotape, manual]. A.S.H. National Slide Bank, HSLRC T-252 (SB-56) University of Washington, Seattle, Washington, 98195.

The Bleeding Diseases. 26. MedCom Series. E. J. Walter Bowie, M.A., B.M., Bch., M.S., and Charles A. Owen, Jr., M.D. [100 color (35 mm.) transparencies plus descriptive booklet, $65.00]. MedCom, Inc., 2 Hammerskjold Plaza, New York, New York 10017.

Blood Component Therapy—Platelets for Transfusion. University of Miami School of Medicine, Department of Internal Medicine (Hematology), Miami, Florida 33136.

Essential Thrombocythemia, RBC Production Defects, WBC (Granulocytic) Production Defects, Polycythemia and Myeloid Metaplasia. Tape 44. Southern Audio-Visual Exhibition Service, 550 Meridian Avenue, Miami Beach, Florida 33139.

Hemolytic Transfusion Reactions. T-1497. (1968). National Medical Audiovisual Center (Annex), Station K, Atlanta, Georgia 30324.

Hemophilia. Set H2. [35 mm. transparencies, audiotape, manual]. A.S.H. National Slide Bank, HSLRC T-252 (SB-56), University of Washington, Seattle, Washington 98195.

Innovations in Transfusion Therapy. (1962). Fenwall Laboratories, 6301 Lincoln Avenue, Morton Grove, Illinois 60053.

Introduction to Modern Transfusion Therapy. T-2016. (1970). National Medical Audiovisual Center (Annex) Station K, Atlanta, Georgia 30324.

Technique of Platelet Transfusion. OM-1284. (1966). National Medical Audiovisual Center (Annex), Station K, Atlanta, Georgia 30324.

That Blood May Flow. Becton-Dickinson Co., Inc., Film Service Department, Rutherford, New Jersey 07070.

Why Johnny Bleeds—Collaborative Diagnosis of a Hematologic Problem. (1960). ASMT Education and Research Fund, Inc., 5555 West Loop South, Bellaire, Texas 77401.

---

* Films unless otherwise stated.

13 Pathology of Leukocyte (White Blood Cell) Series

REVIEW OF MATURATION OF LEUKOCYTES*

Although the earlier writers' descriptions and discussions of cell origin pointed out in great detail the existence of three developmental schools of thought — *unitarian* or monophyletic, *dualist,* and *trinitarian* or polyphyletic — the last is the most commonly held concept. That is, there is a division of the reticuloendothelial system into reticulum and endothelium with a parent hemohistioblast developing into a hemocytoblast, with the latter producing a parent blast for each type of blood cell (Plate 1). Some feel that erythrocytes come from a specific blast derived from endothelial cells. One must acknowledge that the number and specificity of blast forms between reticulum cells and definitive cell types are really unknown. In fact, many investigators regard the lymphocyte as being multipotentially capable of transforming into any other type of blood cell according to need or as a type-specific cell with a specific function of antibody formation. Others feel that lymphocytes must be converted into plasma cells before antibodies can be made.[44]†

It must be understood that immature cells — blasts, promyelocytes, promonocytes, prolymphocytes, pronormoblasts, and promegakaryocytes — do not develop in sudden abrupt transformations but by gradual transition, and that all cells present in the bone marrow and peripheral blood therefore do not conform exactly to one type of cell or another. Also because a cell is composed of nucleus, nucleolus, cytoplasm, and cytoplasmic granules, each part undergoes change. Normally, these changes occur at the same time and in parallel fashion in the cells of each series. This is called synchronism. A different rate of maturation for the nucleus and cytoplasm is called asynchronism. The reference cell is the erythrocyte, having a mean diameter of 7.0μ. Erythrocyte maturation is somewhat different from that of cells of the granulocyte series in that the most immature cell (pronormoblast) contains no hemoglobin. Gradually a little hemoglobin appears until finally the acidophilic normoblast contains a standard and maximal amount of hemoglobin. After this stage, the nucleus is no longer necessary for cell metabolism, and nucleolysis or extrusion results in the mature erythrocyte. Their average life span is 100 to 120 days (Ashby method); 55 to 75 days with an average of 60 days (^{51}Cr method).

A simple guide is available for identification and differentiation of certain leukocytes in reference to determining the age of the cells of the granulocyte series.[130] These maturation characteristics are (1) Blast cells usually have a large nucleus ($^3/_4$ to $^7/_8$

---

* See also discussion on morphologic details, page 83.

† Trentin[191] concludes, from his experiments, that the concept of a "wandering hematopoietic stem cell" is much more logical, i.e., in the proper milieu this pluripotential cell may give rise to lymphoid-type clones, etc. Ebbe[57] also accepts a pluripotential stem cell concept. She feels that this type cell develops into a committed stem cell, with cellular proliferation occurring at the level of the committed stem cell, e.g., into 3 recognizable types of megakaryocytes.

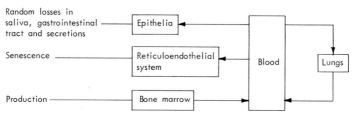

Fig. 13-1. Pattern of white blood cell loss from peripheral blood.

of cell area), and there are no granules in the small amount of basophilic cytoplasm. (2) As the cells become older, the cytoplasm becomes less basophilic (contains less RNA; the deeper blue the cytoplasm, the younger the cell), except the plasma cell. (3) As the cells become older, nucleoli (RNA) disappear, and the nuclear chromatin becomes heavier (DNA). The darker the nucleus stain, the heavier the chromatin is. (4) As the cells become older, they become smaller, except the megakaryocyte. (5) There are four different types of colored granules seen with Wright's stain — neutrophilic, basophilic, eosinophilic, and azurophilic. These granules become less prominent and smaller as the cells become older. (6) Changes in shape occur with two or more lobulations connected by nuclear membrane filaments.

The physiology, function, life span, and turnover rates of leukocytes are data requiring more precise, specific information than is presently known. However, certain knowledge is available. For example, white blood cells are known to participate in host resistance to infection and in repair processes. Granulocytes contain phagocytin, lysozyme, and lactic acid as antibacterial agents. Phagocytosis of bacteria may be affected by opsonins, or no antibodies may be necessary. For example, surface phagocytosis may take place with associated partial degranulation (decrease in the number of granules).

Whereas red blood cells remain in the peripheral blood until their life span is over, white blood cells are carried from the bone marrow and other tissues of origin, and after 6 to 11 days are distributed to the blood and thence to other tissues, where they perform their functions. The life span of the granulocyte is 7 to 10 hours (leukocytes tagged with radioactive diisopropyl fluorophosphate). During the development of the leukocyte series, mitosis occurs at the myeloblast, promyelocyte, and myelocyte stages before completion of maturation. A granulocytic marrow storage pool is approximately 25 times greater than the circulating leukocyte pool. Approximately half the peripheral blood granulocytes freely circulate over a 9 hour transit time.[44] The rest collect in capillaries as a marginated pool potentially available to peripheral blood after stimulation of epinephrine, exercise, and so on. In the tissues, the polymorphonuclear leukocytes remained for an indefinite period and rarely re-enter the peripheral blood in large numbers. Some polymorphonuclear leukocytes break down in the liver, spleen, and lymph nodes, and some are lost in body secretions. However, lymphocytes appear to recirculate and have a life span of about 100 to 200 days.

Observations have been made of the movement of labeled cells through the successive stages of bands, segmented neutrophils, and their appearance in the peripheral blood after a degree of maturity is reached, which permits cells to penetrate through the sinusoidal endothelium. Cells are lost from the peripheral blood in two ways — random loss and senescence (Fig. 13-1). In the overall life cycle of the granulocyte, all evidence to date points to a unidirectional flow out of the bone marrow parenchyma. The regulation of release of marrow cells in normal and pathologic states appears to be related to the degree of cell maturation, marrow pore size, and the presence of a chemical attractant. The development of deformability, motility, and surface receptors for chemoattractants at late stages of granulocytic development allows egress of cells through the marrow sinusoid wall. This process can be modulated by humoral agents that enhance directed movement of cells and may also increase marrow pore size (Fig. 13-2). Like normal myeloblasts and progranulocytes, leukemic blast cells may not respond to chemoattractants because of an inability to migrate and deform but rather because of an absence of surface receptors.

In addition, the degree of cell maturation and marrow pore size has been proposed to interact to influence the rate of cell egress. The rate of marrow granulocyte egress was highly correlated with barrier pore diameter, the morphologic age of cells, and the presence of a chemical attractant. More mature granulocytes appear able to traverse easily and immature WBCs (myeloblasts, progranulocytes, and leukemic blast cells) appear unable to deform sufficiently and migrate.[72,4] Finally, the granulocytes circulate in the peripheral blood in a closed circuit with all cells making repetitive transits through the lungs, which may play some part in the fine regulation of their concentration in the blood.[111, 162, 207]

Although erythropoietin appears to be a specific factor that induces stem cells to become erythropoietic precursors with their subsequent maturation, a granulopoietin has not yet been identified.[46]

Review of Normal White Blood Cell Values for Adults

The normal number of total white blood cells in the peripheral blood equals 5000 to 10,000 per cu.mm. (average 7500/cu.mm.). The proportion or concentration of the various types of leukocytes in the peripheral blood is shown in Table 13–1.

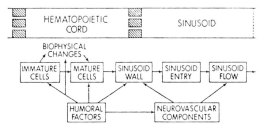

Fig. 13-2. A schematic diagram of the possible factors involved in controlling release of marrow granulocytes. The central relationship of the hematopoietic cord to the sinusoid is shown. In the hematopoietic cord maturation of cells adapts them for egress. The number of maturing cells and the rate of maturation may be governed in part by humoral factors (granulopoietins) and chalones (granulosuppresins). The marrow barrier or sinusoid wall also appears to be a dynamic structure, and its porosity may be influenced by humoral agents, as well as cell crowding, particularly by rigid leukemic blast cells The role of modulation of sinusoidal delivery has not been defined, although evidence of extensive neurovascular networks suggests the possibility of neural or humoral control of sinusoidal flow into the efferent circulation of bone. The latter may be particularly important for erythrocyte delivery. (Giordano, G. F. and Lichtman, M. A.: Marrow cell egress: central interaction of barrier pore size and cell maturation. J. Clin. Invest., *52:*1154, 1973)

LEUKOCYTOSIS

Leukocytosis may be defined as an elevation of the total number of leukocytes above the upper normal range of 10,000 per cu.mm., or a relative increase in neutrophils above 70 to 80 per cent. Because there is such a wide latitude between the low and high normal leukocyte count and in the ranges between which different types of leukocytes are considered to show normal variation, the relative numerical values, which are those expressed in percentages of the patient's actual total leukocyte count, are of limited value and in fact are frequently misinterpreted. The use of absolute values prevents this, and it is therefore essential to be familiar with the absolute val-

Table 13-1. Various Types of Leukocytes in Peripheral Blood

Cell Types	Range (%)	Average (Relative) (%)	Range (Absolute No.)	Average (Absolute No. in cu. mm.)
PMN band	0–5	3	0–500	250
PMN segs	50–70	60	2500–7000	4500
PME segs	1–5	3	50–500	200
PMB segs	0–1	0.5	0–100	40
Lymphocytes	20–40	30	1000–4000	3000
Monocytes	1–6	4	50–600	300

ues of the different types of leukocytes per cubic millimeter of blood. One may calculate the absolute values from the total leukocyte count and the percentage:

Absolute number or value =

$$\frac{\text{Total number of leukocytes/cu.mm.}}{100}$$

$\times$ % of cell type

Physiologic Leukocytosis

The physiologic type of leukocytosis is due to causes unrelated to disease complexes or injurious agents. Usually there are no stab cells in the peripheral blood or any other type indicating a shift to the left. Also there is no decrease or disappearance in eosiniphils or monocytes, as occurs in infectious states. This type of leukocytosis is most closely related to the neutrophilic leukocytosis associated with a sympathomimetic response that is accompanied by the emptying of origin vascular depots and accelerated blood flow. Included in the sympathomimetic leukocytosis responses are those etiologically related to excitement, nausea and vomiting, emotional upsets, pain, exercise (spleen, liver, lungs) adrenalin injection (postsplenectomy and splenic contraction), anesthesia, labor of pregnancy, acute anoxia, massage and cold showers, dehydration (also includes eosinophils, basophils, lymphocytes, and monocytes), hemoconcentration, newborn, sunlight, and eteveted temperature.

Pathologic Leukocytosis

Pathologic leukocytosis is due to infections, hypersensitivity states, anoxia associated with or without drugs and poisons, loss or destruction of erythrocytes, degenerative states (diabetic acidosis, eclampsia, gout, uremia), and tumors involving peripheral blood, marrow, serous cavities, the gastrointestinal tract, and liver. The cell type involved is intimately associated with the etiologic agent—for example, the eosinophilia of allergic and hypersensitivity states; the lymphocytosis of infectious mononucleosis, typhoid fever, and brucellosis; and the monocytosis of Hodgkin's disease, leukemia, and tuberculosis. An increase in immature leukocytes and a corresponding increase in segmented forms is known as a shift to the left, which occurs in infections and leukemias. An increase in mature hypersegmented polymorphonuclear leukocytes is called a shift to the right, as in pernicious anemia and chronic morphine addiction. In early chronic granulocytic leukemia, one sees both a shift to the left and a shift to the right.

Neutrophilic Leukocytosis

Etiology. The increase in the number of white blood cells shows not only an increase in neutrophils, but also a variable increase in band forms and occasionally a leukemoid reaction. This neutrophilia may occur in acute infection within a few hours, or with chronic infection, either general or local. If the infection results from pyogenic bacteria, the absence of polymorphonuclear leukocytes suggests an erroneous diagnosis or bone marrow failure. For example, in acute severe pulmonary infections, the absence or decrease in neutrophilic polymorphonuclear leukocytes suggests a viral instead of pneumococcal etiology. However, if pneumococci are found in the sputum or blood culture, then neutropenia or a decreased neutrophilia suggests either overwhelming infection or toxic depression of bone marrow and possibly a poor prognosis.

Other systemic infections may be preceded by a transient early leukopenia, particularly if the infection is overwhelming. Thus, severe tissue destruction causes the available leukocytes to be rapidly used up, with the leukopenia persisting until the marrow can meet the demand. Local infections—for example, appendicitis, otitis media, salpingitis, and mastoiditis caused by streptococci, staphylococci, and pneumococci—produce an effect on the total leukocyte count; this effect is decreased with the organization of a limiting pyogenic membrane. Not all infections are associated with neutrophilic leukocytosis; some organisms depress the marrow, especially its granulocyte-producing or marrow-releasing capacity, with resulting leukopenia and neutropenia. Examples are typhoid, paratyphoid, salmonella, brucellosis, tuberculosis, viruses, malaria, and other metazoan agents, except when complicated by a secondary pyogenic infection.

The response, therefore, of leukocytes in different stages of the same infectious process is continually changing. Significant information may be obtained by serial observation of the total number of leukocytes, the distribution of major cell types, the maturity of the cells, the signs of degeneration in individual cells, and the changes that occur in successive hematologic examinations.

Favorable peripheral blood signs in an infectious process are: a drop of total leukocyte count and number of polymorphonuclear neutrophils, a disappearance of a shift to left, an increase in number of monocytes (except in the tuberculosis, where decreased monocytes and increased young leukocytes and lymphocytes are favorable), an increase in eosinophils when decreased or absent during the height of disease, an increase in lymphocytes, and the disappearance of toxic granulation.

Unfavorable infectious disease peripheral blood signs are: the marked or slight increase in total leukocyte count associated with a marked shift to the left at the height of the disease, the failure of eosiniphils to reappear in the end stages of infectious disease when absent before, an absolute reduction of lymphocytes, and an excess of cells having toxic granules.

After the ingestion of certain toxic agents—for example, digitalis, lead, mercury, illuminating gas (CO) and $KClO_3$—there is a neutrophilia possibly secondary to a leukocyte-promoting factor attracting neutrophils from the marrrow, or a substance (anoxia, etc.) specifically stimulating the marrow may cause it. After the injection of an insect venom, such as that of a black widow spider, bees, and wasps, or after the injection of a foreign protein, there is usually a leukopenia followed by a neutrophilia leukocytosis. This may be caused by injury to leukocytes by the foreign protein resulting in the release of a pyrogenic substance from the leukocytes, thus causing fever and leukocytosis. Also uremia, gout, and diabetic acidosis produce neutrophilia. In eclampsia, the leukocytosis may be due to convulsions with increased muscular activity. The acute granulocytosis associated with paroxysmal tachycardia or convulsions may be the contribution of a shift of neutrophilic leukocytes from the marginal endothelial-adherent area of blood vessels to the central circulating blood stream area, rather than an increase in overall granulocytic pool size.[8]

Tissue necrosis from any cause—for example, infarction, trauma, thermal burns, surgical procedures without infection, necrosis of tumor tissue, and after turpentine injection—may produce neutrophilic leukocytosis. The absorption of denatured proteins, as in burns, or other types of circulating proteins, may be etiologically related to granulocyte release from the marrow or to the characteristic release of leukocyte-promoting factor due to tissue destruction.

Acute hemorrhage into the peritoneal cavity, or the pleural or subdural space produces extensive leukocytosis. Acute hemorrhage, and acute hemolytic anemia (after rapid hemolysis, hemolytic crises of hemolytic anemia, or hemolytic transfusion reactions) all produce a sudden demand on the bone marrow to deliver leukocytes, probably secondary to leukopoietin production. In such cases, the earliest peripheral blood pattern may show neutrophilic leukocytosis with an occasional true leukemoid pattern.

Myeloproliferative disorders — myelofibrosis with myeloid metaplasia and myelocytic leukemia, polycythemia vera, thrombocythemia, and DiGuglielmo's syndrome — are neoplastic proliferations of cells of the myeloid system associated with marked erythrocyte or platelet hyperplasia. In these conditions, there may also by striking neutrophilia. Occasionally granulocytosis is associated with primary and metastatic tumors, in which cases a leukemoid pattern, occasionally with marked neutrophilia and eosinophilia, occurs. Metastatic tumors involving the bone marrow may demonstrate an irritative effect with many immature leukocytes appearing in the peripheral blood and the bone marrow. In most cases of polycythemia vera, there is an absolute increase in all leukocyte forms, including neutrophils. Factors that stimulate the increased proliferation of red blood cells and platelets (polycythemia and thrombocythemia, respectively) also stimulate the neutrophilic leukocytes.

Abnormal Inclusions and Abnormal Forms in Granulocytes (Plate 42)

Toxic granules are large, dark purple granules that may fill and replace the entire neutrophil cytoplasmic area. They are associated with many extensive infections and in drug reactions with fever. In contrast with the dark blue basophil cell granules, toxic granules are smaller, darker, and more variable in number. Döhle's inclusion bodies are 1 to 2 μ small, round, and sometimes irregular; they are found, together with nuclear pyknosis and vacuolated cytoplasmic areas, in the cytoplasm of neutrophils associated with severe infection, burns, pregnancy,[1] scarlet fever, and in some cases of thrombocytopenic purpura. They are associated with cell immaturity and possibly increased granulopoiesis. Amato bodies are said to be the same as Döhle's inclusion bodies and together with abnormal fibrillar material are seen in the neutrophils in leukemia under the electron microscope.

In the Chediak-Higashi syndrome, one finds giant Döhle-like cytoplasmic peroxidase-positive granules, and cytoplasmic inclusions in neutrophils and monocytes. Their inflammatory response, phagocytic ability, and motility are normal. In the neutrophils these bodies appear as irregular slate green masses. They are considered giant lysosomes under electron microscopy. In lymphocytes and monocytes, they appear as bright orange-red spherical inclusions with large vacuoles in monocytes, erythrocyte-like inclusions in neutrophils, and giant eosiniphilic granules in eosinophils. The condition is invariably fatal, is seen in infants, and is inherited as a non-sex-linked Mendelian recessive. The disorder is associated with a decreased resistance to infections but with normal immune response. It is characterized by hepatosplenomegaly, lymphadenopathy, albinism, photophobia, and the manifestations of lymphomas, including leukemia (Plate 44).

Neutrophils having rodlike or dumbbell shaped nuclei but without segmentation or lobulation are also found. This disorder is transmitted by a non-sex-linked dominant gene and is seen partially or completely in many members of the same family. This nuclear phenomenon is called the Pelger-

Huet anomaly and is observed mainly among Orientals, but it is also found in Holland, Germany, and Switzerland. Affected neutrophils are occasionally mistaken for unsegmented granulocytic forms. However, they still have defensive and phagocytic properties, and therefore patients so affected are not predisposed to infections. Alder's anomaly is a constitutional heavy azurophilic granulation occurring in all leukocytes of an affected individual.

Eosinophilic Leukocytosis (Plate 3)

At birth, 300 to 400 eosinophils per cu.mm. are seen; at 8 years and over, an average value of 200 eosinophils per cu.mm. is found. Eosinophilic leukocytosis is said to occur when there is an increase above 400 to 500 per cu.mm. The exact function of eosinophils is unknown, although they are characteristically found in large numbers in the tissues in reaction to foreign protein, in allergic reactions, in parasitic infestations, and in lymphomas such as in Hodgkin's disease. The eosinophil is a phagocytic, sluggishly motile cell with iron and phospholipids incorporated in its granule chemical moiety.

Etiology. A high percentage of eosinophils is seen in the acute phases of allergic disorders—for example, in the blood and sputum of patients with bronchial asthma, in malaria, urticaria, angioneurotic edema, drug fever (liver extract and penicillin), erythema multiforme, and after administration of hyperimmume serum. Immediately after the first introduction of the antigen into the host, there is no eosinophilia because these cells are not intimately related to antigen-antibody reaction and subsequent antibody formation. Histamine, an amine chemotactically related to the eosinophil response, is liberated at the antigen-antibody reaction site with subsequent infiltration of the site with large chunky orange granules. In chronic skin diseases such as pemphigus and dermatitis herpetiformis, one frequently observes the highest and

most constant eosinophilia. However, such eosinophilia may also occur with scabies, psoriasis, eczema, and prurigo. Thus, there is both a local skin eosinophilic infiltration and a systemic marrow and peripheral eosinophilia whenever there is a severe enough dermatologic condition.

Local and systemic eosinophilia is marked when larval forms of parasites invade tissues and encyst in the host's tissues such as in muscle, lung, liver, skin, and intestinal mucosa. An example is trichinosis associated with ingestion of meat containing the encysted larva of trichinella spiralis (40–60% of eosinophilia at the height of response). In visceral larva migrans associated with infestation of the larval stage of dog roundworm (*Toxocara canis*) or cat roundworm (*Toxocara cati*), there is an associated Löffler's military pneumonitis, leukocytosis and 20 to 50 per cent eosinophilia. Infestations of roundworm (*Ascaris lumbricoides*), hookworm (*Necator americanus*), pinworm (*Enterobius vermicularis*), whipworm (*Trichuris trichiura*), beef tapeworm (*Taenia saginata*), and pork tapeworm (*Taenia solium*) all produce a slight to moderate eosinophilia. Hematopoietic disorders such as Hodgkin's disease, and granulocytic and eosinophilic leukemia are associated with eosinophilia. Their cause is undetermined. Eosinophilic cells may also be increased in some cases of infectious mononucleosis, pernicious anemia, and sickle cell anemia.

In various miscellaneous disorders, an increase in eosinophils may be found. For example, in scarlet fever on the sixth day after the rash appears, there may be a 5 to 10 per cent eosinophilia. In periarteritis nodosa, metastatic carcinoma, during convalescence from infectious bacterial disease, in tropical eosinophilia (? filarial), and in Löffler's syndrome due to inhalants or to blood-borne antigen, eosinophila may be observed. Familial eosinophilia, possibly genetically associated with an allergic state or due to a common parasitic infestation is occasionally observed.

Basophilic Leukocytosis (Plate 3)

The basophil rarely enters into clinical thinking, because it is usually absent from the ordinary routine differential count (0–2% or 50/cu.mm.). However, determination of the absolute basophil count can provide significant information.[179] Shelley's report describes a new technique for the absolute basophil count that gives reproducible counts coupled with excellent visualization of cell morphology. Basophilia is found in association with myxedema, colitis, polycythemia vera, sometimes with chronic hemolytic anemia, myeloid leukemia and after splenectomy, as well as in the sensitized individual. A count of over 50 per cu.mm. is often a sign of allergic sensitization, whereas a count below 20 per cu.mm. regularly accompanies allergic reactions.

Lymphocytosis (Plate 4)

From birth to 2 years of age, there are 5500 to 6300 lymphocytes per cu.mm. of blood; from 4 years to 12 years, there are 4500 to 3000 lymphocytes per cu.mm.; from 14 years up to adulthood, there are approximately 2500 to 2900 lymphocytes per cu.mm. Therefore lymphocytosis develops when the number of leukocytes exceeds 9000 per cu.mm. in infants and young children; exceeds 7000 per cu.mm. in older children, and exceeds 4000 per cu.mm. in adults. Physiologically the lymphocyte is motile and may possibly convert to tissue macrophages and plasma cells.[162] Although some workers feel that these cells play a role in immune mechanisms, this is not too well defined. Although there is evidence that some lymphocytes are short-lived, Norman and co-workers have established that probably most lymphocytes have a half life of 100 to 300 days.[134] Earlier studies gave misleading results because it was not fully appreciated that lymphocytes recirculate between blood and lymphatic tissue.

In contrast to the fleeting hours of the granulocyte (8 to 10 days), the lymphocyte may well need a long life to preserve a long memory for immunologic events. In fact, a lymphocyte foot appendage described by McFarland and Heilman[120] may play a part in lymphocyte interactions in normal and pathologic states; the passage of instructive material between lymphocytes could provide a possible means of sustaining antibody-forming capacity without the persistence of antigens in tissue; finally the lymphocyte probably plays a part in transplantation immunology and the graft versus host reactions. In fact the use of an antilymphocyte serum (ALS) is now creating widespread interest as an immunosuppressive agent. Woodruff quoted by Gowans[76] has shown that ALS is effective in prolonging the survival of homografts in experimental animals and therefore may turn out to be most powerful and the safest immunosuppressive agent yet devised for controlling the homograft reaction.

Etiology. Infectious mononucleosis, measles (especially German measles), and infectious hepatitis are acute viral diseases characterized by marked lymphocytosis. Chronic nonviral infectious states such as brucellosis, typhoid fever, syphilis, and tuberculosis may also be associated with lymphocytosis. Pertussis is especially characterized by lymphocytosis; recovery from acute pyogenic infections may also be associated with this cellular reaction. Thyrotoxicosis (10% of cases have splenomegaly) may be associated with either an absolute or relative lymphocytosis.

In giant follicular lymphoma, lymphocytic lymphosarcoma, leukosarcoma, and chronic lymphocytic leukemia, there may be a relative or absolute lymphocytosis. In Hodgkin's disease, lymphocytes are usually decreased. According to Dimitrov, lymphocytes obtained from patients with lymphoproliferative disorders possess metabolic patterns that are not only quantitatively and qualitatively different from normal lymphocytes but also are distinct for each particular leukemic disease.[51]

Monocytosis (Plates 5, 20, 21, 42)

Monocytes are phagocytic, actively motile cells whose increase is not diagnostic of any specific disease. An average of 500 per cu.mm. is seen in children and 300 per cu.mm. in adults. An increase above 750 per cu.mm. in children and 440 per cu.mm. in adults indicates monocytosis, although some workers accept 500 cells as a reasonable dividing line between a normal and elevated monocyte count.

Etiology. Although one may see an increase in monocytes in the peripheral blood in many longstanding chronic infections, especially those involving the reticuloendothelial system, an absolute increase occurs most commonly in exacerbation, extension, and reactivation of tuberculous infections. In most instances, it is indicative of an unfavorable turn in the tuberculous infection. In fact the lymphocyte:monocyte ratio is normally 2.9, and a level under 1.0 is most unfavorable. Similarly, monocytes are increased in cases of subacute bacterial endocarditis, brucellosis, rickettsial infections such as typhus and Rocky Mountain spotted fever, in syphilis, typhoid fever, and lobar pneumonia (resolution phase). It is also high in Hodgkin's disease, tetrachlorethylene poisoning, Gaucher's disease, and other reticuloendothelial diseases. After exposure to heat, injection of epinephrine, sarcoidosis, the recovery phase of agranulocytosis, and in chronic granulocytopenias of childhood, phagocytosis of erythrocytes and leukocytes by monocytes may be observed in the blood smear.

Parasitic infections or infestations, most commonly malaria, kala-azar, and trypanosomiasis, are also associated with monocytosis. Monocytosis is also observed in preleukemias;[122] patients with cytopenia may have an associated monocytosis appearing for some time before typical leukemic features develop. Acute myelocytic leukemia itself is the most common terminus of preleukemia, but monocytic leukemia has also developed after the preleukemic state. Previous retrospective studies have suggested that as many as one-third of patients will exhibit a preleukemic phase and that it may be characterized by a refractory anemia with or without associated leukopenia and thrombocytopenia.[17, 170]

THE LYMPHOCYTE AND IMMUNOPATHOLOGY

During the past 15 years, the role of lymphocytes in the immune system and indirectly in association with certain neoplasias has been suspected and possibly specifically identified. It is important, at this point, to recognize that these concepts are in areas of current experimental and clinical investigation and, with the accumulation of newer data, many statements will require modification and reinterpretation. Among the first developments in the study of the lymphoid system, Chase demonstrated that delayed hypersensitivity was transferable by cells, but not by serum.[34] Early evidence in favor of lymphocyte system specialization was demonstrated by morphologic studies indicating distinction between two cell types, small lymphocytes that predominate in delayed hypersensitivity and all graft rejections,[77] and plasma cells that produce antibody.[41] Further impetus to these studies was provided by Glick and associates who found that removal of a gut-associated lymphoid organ, the bursa of Fabricus of the chicken, resulted in depression of antibody production.[73]

Understanding the significance of the bursa (B) cells came with the simultaneous observations by Martinez and colleagues[124] and Miller,[127] who demonstrated that the removal of another lymphoid organ, the thymus, affected an apparently different immunologic phenomenon, that involved in transplantation immunity. In these experiments, mice that had undergone neonatal thymectomy showed a prolongation of skin allograft survival; similar results were reported in rabbits and in chickens.[75, 199]

*Table 13-2. Anatomical Location of T- and B-Lymphocytes**

	T-Cells	B-Cells
Peripheral blood	60–80%	20–30%
Thoracic duct	85–90%	10–15%
Lymph nodes	Paracortical regions	Germinal centers
		Subscapular region
		Medullary cords
Spleen	Periarteriolar sheaths	Germinal centers
		Periphery of periarteriolar sheaths
		Red pulp

* Boggs, D. R., and Winkelstein, A.: White Cell Manual. Ed. 3, p. 40. Philadelphia, F. A. Davis, 1975.

Therefore, it became apparent that in the chicken (postthymectomy and postbursectomy), two major lymphoid subpopulations were detectable: (1) thymectomy experiments revealed that thymus-derived lymphocytes (T-cells) are largely responsible for delayed allergy and allograft rejection,[96] and (2) bursectomy experiments revealed that bursal-derived (B) cells are necessary for formation of germinal centers, formation of plasma cells, and immuno-globulin (Ig) production (Table 13-2).[42]

Additional understanding of B-cell differentiation was provided by the demonstration that the bursa, but not the thymus, contains lymphocytes with high-density Ig.[118, 155] It is these surface and intracytoplasmic, Ig-bearing (B) cells that are postulated to be precursors of Ig-secreting plasma cells (Plate 1).

Immunoglobulin on and Within B-Lymphocytes

Ig is detectable on the cell surface of a lymphoid-type cell by means of fluorescein-conjugated anti-immunoglobulin sera.[198] The percentage of cells with high-density surface Ig varies with the animal species and lymphoid organ, with a trend toward high values in germinal center-containing regions and low values in thymus-dependent areas of spleen and lymph node and in peripheral blood (Fig. 13-3). Much interest and controversy has centered around the function of the high-density Ig on the surface of B-lymphocytes. Most models of B-cell differentiation propose that Ig acts as an antigen receptor and that the interaction of antigen with specific Ig receptors results in B-cell activation with cellular proliferation and maturation. Because of the interrelationship of B-lymphocytes and plasma cells, the question is thus raised whether the Ig secreted by the plasma cell is identical to the Ig on the B-cell surface. The answer does not appear to be a simple one and must embrace several observations[102] (1) more than one class of Ig (e.g., IgM and IgD) may be present as a single cell type; (2) antibody responses to most antigens result in a switch from IgM to IgG synthesis during the period of observation; and (3) cells with membrane-bound Ig of one class may contain Ig of another class in their cytoplasm.[198] Also, structural differences between surface-associated and serum (secretory) immunoglobulins have been reported.[36]

Finally, one must bear in mind the possibilities that T cells may or may not possess surface immunoglobulin. If it is present, surface Ig might be involved in antigen recognition on T-cells, as is thought to be the case on B-cells. Highly-sensitive techniques (e.g., radioiodination and autoradiography) have demonstrated surface Ig on thymus cells.[198] However, the possibility that much or all of this Ig is absorbed has not been excluded.

Hematopoietic Cell Differentiation

Because of some of these discoveries, there has been some reconsideration of some of the phases of hematopoietic cell differentiation. Figure 13-4 reveals that in mammals hematopoietic cell precursors (stem cells) are first demonstrable in the yolk sac and the fetal liver.[125] Further differentiation and migration is thought to occur in the bone marrow, because it has been observed that human and mouse bone

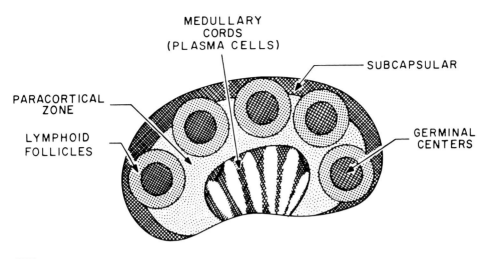

MEDULLARY
CORDS
(PLASMA CELLS)

SUBCAPSULAR

PARACORTICAL
ZONE

LYMPHOID
FOLLICLES

GERMINAL
CENTERS

THYMUS DEPENDENT AREAS

THYMUS INDEPENDENT AREAS

Fig. 13-3. Development of immune system. Anatomical location of T- and B-cells in lymph node. T-cells are found in the thymic dependent areas (paracortical zone) while B-lymphocytes and plasma cells populate the thymic independent areas (germinal centers, subcapsular zones, and medullary cords). The predominant cell type in the lymphoid areas surrounding germinal centers has not been fully established. (Boggs, D. R., and Winkelstein, A.: White Cell Manual. ed. 3. Philadelphia, F. A. Davis, 1975)

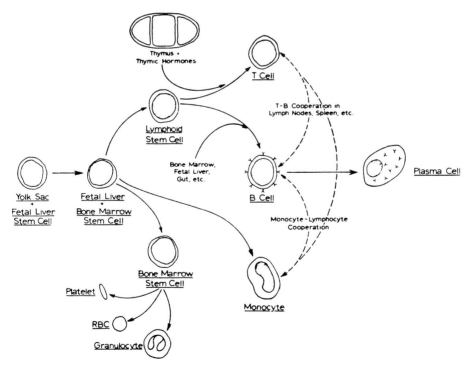

Fig. 13-4. Model of human hematopoietic cell differentiation. (Kersey, I. H., and Gajl-Peczalska, K. J.: T and B lymphocytes in humans. Am. J. Pathol., *81:*446, 1975)

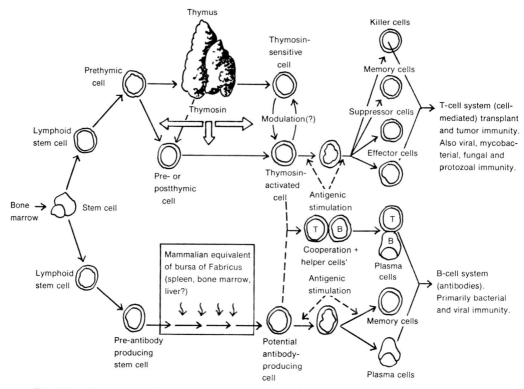

Fig. 13-5. Maturation of the immune system. (Medical News. J.A.M.A., *237*:431, 1977)

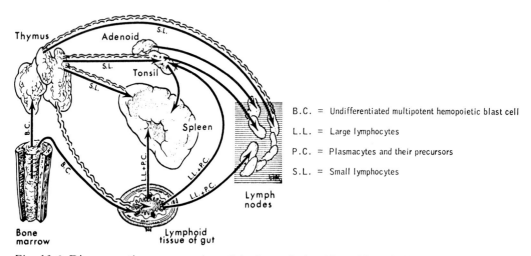

B.C. = Undifferentiated multipotent hemopoietic blast cell

L.L. = Large lymphocytes

P.C. = Plasmacytes and their precursors

S.L. = Small lymphocytes

Fig. 13-6. Diagrammatic representation of the interrelationships of lymphoid tissues concerned in immunity. Solid lines represent cell migrations; double-wave line indicates humoral effects. (Raphael, S. S.: Lynch's Medical Laboratory Technology. ed. 3. Philadelphia, W. B. Saunders, 1976)

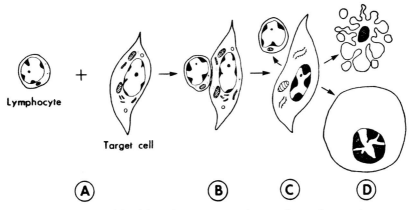

Lymphocyte

Target cell

(A) (B) (C) (D)

Fig. 13-7. The sensitized lymphocyte recognizes and attaches to the target cell by a still not clearly defined "recognition" mechanism (*A, B*). This step requires Ca^{2+} and Mg^{2+} and is not especially temperature-dependent. Evidence presented indicates that the lymphocyte discharges lymphotoxin, which may be higher in concentration in the narrow space between the two cells (*B*). Alternately, the lymphocyte may apply the lymphokine directly to the target-cell surface, where it binds to receptors. The next phase of cytolysis is temperature-dependent and may proceed without the continuous presence of the lymphocyte (*C*). The target cell lyses either by fragmentation or swelling and rupture (*D*). Whether these two lytic processes are due to differences in target cells or to differences in the effector mechanism (e.g., two separate cytotoxins) is unknown. (Rosenace, W. and Tsoukas, C. D.: Lymphotoxin, a review and analysis. Am. J. Pathol., *84:*580, 1976)

marrow can reconstitute erythroid, myeloid, and lymphoid elements.[125] Additional differentiation of bone marrow stem cells may result in the generation of lymphoid cells and monocytes and in the development of a precursor of myeloid, erythroid, and platelet elements. The putative lymphoid stem cell has not been isolated and identified, although chromosomal marker studies suggest a common origin for the two lines of differentiation.[125] T-cell differentiation is known to occur within the thymus and under the influence of thymic hormones.[198] Fully differentiated T-lymphocytes are known to be present in lymph nodes, spleen, and peripheral blood (Figs. 13-5; 13-6).

The effector functions of T-cells include the following: (1) the direct-contact killing by cytotoxin elaborated by sensitized lymphocytes. The cytotoxin binds to target-cell receptors, triggering events that progress to final cytolysis. (2) The production of short-range effector macromolecules (collectively known as lymphokines, of which more than 20 are detectable). The mechanism by which this intriguing lymphokine kills cells is for the most part unknown. Morphologic changes in target cells preceding their lysis would suggest injury to the cell membrane. The cytotoxin may be singular or double (lymphotoxin); other lymphokines may include macrophage migration inhibiting factor. (3) The production of antigen-specific and antigen-nonspecific molecules that cooperate with B-lymphocytes in antibody responses (Fig. 13-7). Finally, Rosenace intimates that lymphotoxin has an important function in lymphocyte-mediated cell destruction.[163]

B-Cell Differentiation in Humans. Many observations have revealed the existence of a distinct line of differentiation in humans involving B-lymphocytes and plasma cells. Studies using conjugated anti-Ig sera showed that a subpopulation of lympho-

Table 13-3. Markers of Human Peripheral Blood Mononuclear Cells*

	B-Cells	T-Cells	Mono-cytes
Surface Ig	+	—	—
Human B-lymphocyte antigen (HBLA)	+	—	—
Sheep erythrocyte receptors (E rosette)	—	+	—
Human T-lymphocyte antigen (HTLA)	—	+	—
Fc receptors (aggregated IgG or EA rosette)	+	—	+
Complement receptors (EAC rosette)	+	—	+

* Kersey, J. H., and Gajl-Peczalska, K. J.: T and B lymphocytes in humans. Am. J. Pathol., *81*: 446, 1975.

cytes contains intracytoplasmic Ig, surface Ig, or both. Also, newborns bear predominantly δ and μ heavy chains and adults, μ or γ heavy chains. The percentage of human lymphocytes with membrane-associated Ig varies with the anatomic site, that is, thymus (1–2%), tonsil (30–60%), and peripheral blood (10–30%), using fluorescence-conjugated anti-Ig sera.[198]

Furthermore, B-cell differentiation usually occurs in multiple sites, such as fetal liver, bone marrow, and gut-associated lymphoid tissue. B-cells are usually defined as those possessing high-density surface Ig (Table 13–3).

Receptors for Immunoglobulin and Complement on Human B-Lymphocytes. A second marker is present on the surface of most human lymphocytes with high-density Ig (i.e., B) lymphocytes; this marker is the receptor that binds immunoglobulin.[49] This receptor does not appear to bind free Ig, but rather binds complex or aggregated Ig and only Ig of certain γ-type subclasses (Fig. 13-8). This receptor, which binds the Fc portion of IgG, is not restricted to B-lymphocytes but is found also on macrophages, granulocytes, and tissue cells of diverse origins, including epithelial cells. Current evidence indicates that the Fc receptor is present in humans on the surface of the same population of lymphocytes as those that bear membrane Ig. The functional role of the Fc receptor remains conjectural (Table 13-4).

Receptors for components of complement are found on a subpopulation of

Table 13-4. Surface Markers of Human Lymphocytes*

Marker	Cell Distribution	Assay Procedure
Surface immunoglobulin: IgM, IgD, IgG, IgA	B-cells	Immunofluorescence
Complement receptors: CR$_1$, CR$_2$	B-cells, K-cells	Rosette assay
IgG Fc receptors	B-cells, K-cells, and suppressor T-cells	Fluorescence or rosette assay
IgM Fc receptors	helper T-cells	Rosette assay
Erythrocyte receptors		Rosette assay
Sheep	T-cells, K-cells	
Mouse	B-cells	
Monkey	B-cells, K-cells	
Surface antigens		Immunofluorescence or cytotoxic assay
Ia antigens	B-cells, K-cells	
T-cell antigens	T-cells	

* Ross, G. D.: Surface Markers of B and T Cells. Arch. Pathol., *101*:337, 1977. Copyright, 1977, American Medical Association.

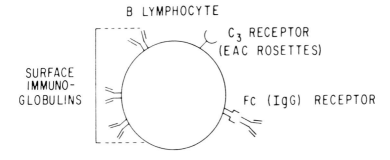

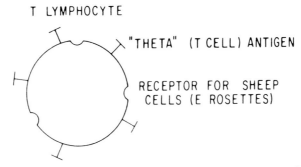

Fig. 13-8. Diagrammatic representation of surface membrane features of B- and T-lymphocytes. (Boggs, D. R., and Winkelstein, A.: White Cell Manual. ed. 3. Philadelphia, F. A. Davis, 1975)

human lymphocytes. At least two complement component receptors are present, that for $C3_b$ and that for $C3_d$ (the inactivated form of $C3_b$).[113, 165] Most lymphocytes with complement receptors also bear high-density surface Ig. However, a few of the complement receptor-bearing lymphocytes (CRL) do not have surface Ig; complement receptors are also present on nonlymphoid cells (e.g., granulocytes and monocytes). Human CRLs are generally detected in assays using heterologous RBCs sensitized with antibody and complement in a rosette assay. The percentage of CRLs in human peripheral blood generally ranges between 11 and 23. The role of complement receptors on lymphocytes remains unknown, although several functions have been suggested; the receptors may focus antigen-antibody-complement complexes in the an-

tigen-processing areas such as germinal centers, and complement receptors may be involved in B-cell activation, perhaps directly or by binding other complement receptor-bearing cells (e.g., macrophages).

T-Cell Differentiation. Current evidence indicates that in most species (including humans), T-lymphocytes represent a specialized subpopulation. As indicated in Figure 13-4, these cells are thought to develop from a common lymphoid stem cell, under the influence of the thymus and thymic hormones. While much T-cell differentiation occurs within the thymus, especially in fetal life and in infancy, expanders of the thymus-derived lymphocytes (i.e., thymosin and thymopoietin) probably also act outside the thymus.[79]

A major development in the study of human lymphocytes was the demonstration

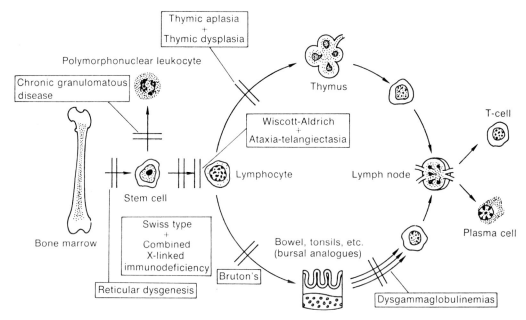

Fig. 13-9. Demonstration of immunocyte development by way of cell-mediated (thymic) and humoral (bursal analogues, e.g., bowel, tonsils, etc.) pathways. Double vertical bars signify proposed defect sites in immunocyte maturation. (Raphael, S. S. Lynch's Medical Laboratory Technology. ed. 3. Philadelphia, W. B. Saunders, 1976)

that a subpopulation of human lymphocytes binds nonsensitized sheep RBCs. In human peripheral blood, the number of lymphocytes that binds sheep RBCs is found to vary from 25 to 80 per cent, depending on conditions of incubation. It is significant that the cells that bind sheep RBCs are distinct from cells that carry surface Ig, and that 95 to 98 per cent of thymocytes bind sheep RBCs.[97, 205] The sheep RBC-binding assay, also known as the T-rosette assay, has been very useful in the evaluation of human T-lymphocytes in normal and pathologic states.

Human T-lymphocytes also are detectable using heterologous absorbed antithymocyte sera. In several laboratories, antisera prepared in this manner will detect a lymphoid subpopulation that corresponds closely to the T-rosette forming population. The antigens detected by the antisera are generally known as human T-lymphocyte antigen (HTLA).[104, 183]

B- and T-Cells in Immunodeficiency Diseases

The various human immunodeficiency syndromes have provided significant insights into immunologic function (Fig. 13-9). Figure 13-9 shows that boys with X-linked (Bruton's) agammaglobulinemia have normal cell-mediated (T-cell-dependent) immunity but generally have very few B-lymphocytes. Other patients with an autosomal recessive form of B-cell deficiency have surface Ig-bearing but no Ig-secreting lymphocytes. In both groups, serum Ig levels are exceedingly low, and patients have clinical problems with encapsulated organisms (e.g., *Haemophilus influenzae*, *Pseudomonas aeruginosa*, and *Diplococcus pneumoniae*).[15]

A syndrome of isolated T-cell deficiency is observed in patients with failure of third–fourth pharyngeal pouch development and is known as DiGeorge's syndrome. It results in defective facial development, tetany due to absent parathyroids, and thymic aplasia. Patients with this disorder characteristically have difficulty with viral infections, fungal infections, and nonencapsulated bacterial.[15] They have a marked increase in B-lymphocytes but few sheep RBC rosette-forming (T) lymphocytes are detectable.[69]

The vast majority of congenital immunologic disorders involve both the T- and B-cell systems and are thus known as combined-system immunodeficiency syndrome. Patients with these disorders have an increased susceptibility to infections of varying types, as well as an increased risk of development of lymphoreticular malignancies. In varying degrees, they tend to have hypogammaglobulinemia, lymphopenia, and decreased numbers and function of T- and B-lymphocytes. Diseases in this group include (1) an infantile form, severe combined immunodeficiency; (2) childhood diseases, that is, Wiskott-Aldrich syndrome (a sex-linked recessive syndrome that includes eczema, thrombocytopenia, recurrent infections with predisposition to development of lymphoproliferative disorders, and marked clinical improvement in some patients following administration of transfer factor); and ataxia-telangiectasia (an autosomal recessive-trait syndrome characterized by cerebellar ataxia, cutaneous telangiectasia, immunologic deficiencies associated with decreased IgA and IgE, and recurrent sinopulmonary infections and abnormal lymphocyte function with increased susceptibility to developing lymphoma); and (3) adult diseases (e.g., late onset or variable immunodeficiency).[15]

Studies in vitro have been used to define defects in patients with impaired antibody synthesis. Some hypogammaglobulinemic patients were found to produce antibodies in vitro after stimulation with pokeweed mitogen; others did not respond.[204] In some instances, mixing cells of hypogammaglobulinemic patients with normal cells resulted in the suppression of Ig synthesis

by the normal cells; some of these people were therefore suspected of producing increased numbers of lymphocytes that suppress activity of antibody-producing cells in vivo.[195]

It is possible that autoimmune disorders may also be the result of defective T- and B-lymphocyte regulation. For example, one study reveals that the majority of myasthenia gravis patients treated in a NIH study possessed an abnormal γ-globulin that binds to and presumably blocks the acetylcholine receptor.[157] The postulated abnormal γ-globulin produced by B-cells of lymphoid tissue seems partially related to an abnormality of the thymus. It is also of interest that patients with systemic lupus erythematosus often have hypergammaglobulinemia, and they were shown to have decreased numbers of T-lymphocytes in many instances.[201]

Secondary Immunodeficient Syndromes

Secondary immunodeficient syndromes may be classified into non-neoplastic and neoplastic.

Non-Neoplastic includes the following syndromes: (1) those associated with hematopoietic deficiency in which the marrow is not producing enough cells or those cells that are produced have some deficiency in phagocytosis (e.g., chronic granulomatosus disease, reticular dysgenesis, and marrow replacement such as tumor metastasis, spleen, and myelosclerosis); (2) those associated with protein-losing states in which the loss of protein is greater than that being anabolized (e.g., protein-losing enteropathy, malnutrition, and nephrotic syndrome); (3) deficiencies of complement factors C_3 and C_5 have been associated with significance in resistance to infections; (4) renal failure patients and those with diabetes are known to have increased susceptibility to infectious disease; (5) those natural immune responses reduced intentionally before, during, and after transplantation surgery.

Since the process of immune body formation is accompanied by cell proliferation, the following agents are used to depress cell generation in cancer therapy.

Cortisone and adrenocorticotrophic hormones help to stabilize polymorphonuclear lysosome membranes when they are used as immunosuppressive agents. When the membranes are ruptured, lysosomes release enzymes that are part of the inflammatory response. Other unknown factors are probably associated with the immunosuppressive action of these steroid preparations.

Irradiation is of little importance in clinical immunosuppression, but it is of more significance in cancer therapy, by breaking DNA linkage or by causing DNA cross-linkages, especially in dividing cells; it may inhibit viable cell proliferation.

Drugs, such as cyclophosphamide, busulfan (Myloeran), and mechlorethamine (nitrogen mustard), act by forming links across the DNA helix or by rupturing it. In this way, they prevent the passage of accurate information to mRNA as well as disorganize correct DNA replication.

Antimetabolites, such as 6-mercaptopurine and 5-fluororacil, are able to enter the DNA base (by substituting for the purine or pyrimidine base) and thus upset the genetic code. Concomitantly, they act as anti-inflammatory agents.

Antilymphocytic serum (ALS) is used in immunosuprressive modalities and is usually prepared by immunizing animals against human lymphocytes. The antibodies formed (antilymphocyte type) are absorbed out, and the IgG fraction alone is used in therapy. Certain immune complex reactions such as anaphylactic serum sickness may occur from these fractions; these may be reduced by using the ALS together with chemical immunosuppressives. However, the major effect of ALS is apparently directed against thymic lymphocytes and, therefore, against cell-mediated immune responses.

Neoplastic diseases involve the im-munogenetic system. Patients with neoplasms of varying types are known to have abnormalities of T- and B-lymphocyte function.[106] In these patients, the role of immunologic abnormalities in the development of the malignancy remains unknown, since primary and secondary deficiencies cannot be easily separated. However, since there are many patients on the drugs described above for cancer therapy who develop primary or drug-induced immunodeficiency syndromes, a unique opportunity for study is provided. For example, patients with many of the inherited immunodeficiency syndromes and those with the drug-induced immunodeficiency associated with renal transplantation have a 35- to 100-fold increased risk of development of malignancy.[93, 105] The data from both groups indicate that these patients develop the more common malignancies with only a slightly increased frequency. The increased rate of cancer development is largely accounted for by the high risk of lymphoreticular malignancy, including lymphocytic leukemia and solid lymphoreticular neoplasms. The pathogenetic mechanisms responsible for development of lymphoid neoplasms in a defective lymphoid system are undoubtedly complex, but may include increased malignant transformation of genetically defective lymphoid cells, increased cellular proliferation due to chronic antigenic stimulation with various bacteria, and enhanced infection with exogenous and endogenous oncogenic viruses.

Surface Marker Evaluation of Human Lymphoid Neoplasms

Studies of lymphoreticular solid neoplasms and leukemias have been greatly aided by the development of surface marker analysis of tumors. Morphologic and functional assays are brought together for the first time in the evaluation of tumors of the plasma cell line. Development of electrophoretic analyses permitted the observation that plasma cell tumors (plasmacytomas emerging into multiple or plasma cell myeloma) secreted Ig of a single class in the majority of instances.[140] With the development of methods for evaluation of surface Ig, a number of investigators demonstrated that many cases of chronic lymphocytic leukemias (CLL) carried surface Ig and these were of apparent B-cell origin.[146, 203] Thus, it appears that B-type lymphocytes or their offspring can develop into a group of malignancies in which the major manifestations are associated with the altered manufacture of immunoglobulins. These protein moieties have been categorized as follows: (1) failure to produce a sufficient amount of normal humoral antibodies to protect the patient from environmental pathogens, (2) an excess production of a single homogeneous immunoglobulin or a portion of the immunoglobulin molecule (monoclonal gammopathy), and (3), occasionally, the development of autoantibodies.

It is now believed that most cases of CLL carry surface Ig, which in the majority of cases is monoclonal with respect to Ig class, although more than one heavy chain is sometimes demonstrable. Most of the surface Ig-bearing cases of CLL also have complement receptors; a few have complement receptors alone.[165, 180] In a few instances, CLL cells form sheep erythrocyte rosettes and are probably of T-cell origin.[177]

When solid lymphoreticular malignancies (lymphomas) occur in adults, they carry monoclonal surface Ig and are therefore of B-cell origin in most instances, according to studies from several laboratories.[2, 70, 186] These solid neoplasms are either diffuse or nodular, but in both instances most of the lymphomas carry surface Ig or complement receptors.[68] It is of interest that some cases that morphologically appear as "histiocytic or reticulum cell" lymphomas are found to have B-surface markers.

Childhood lymphomas, on the other hand, are most often devoid of surface Ig and complement receptors but instead bear a T-cell marker (i.e., sheep erythrocyte receptors).[100, 103] When acute lymphoblastic leukemias occur in children, they have the same T-marker in about 25 per cent of cases.[24, 178] An additional 25 to 50 per cent of cases of acute lymphoblastic leukemia are found to lack sheep RBC receptors but carry the human thymic lymphocyte antigen (HLTA).[35]

Therefore, these data and the rapidly growing body of knowledge demonstrating the high frequency of T and B leukemias and lymphomas indicate that, for example, malignancies involving lymphoid subpopulations are very age-dependent; adult lymphocytic leukemias are often chronic and involve B-cells; childhood lymphocytic leukemias are often acute and involve T-cells. These findings merely corroborate the observations that in early childhood, the thymus is large and an extremely active organ during the development of the immune system. In older patients, the thymus is a less active organ. A comparison may be drawn between T-cell and B-cell leukemias and lymphomas in man and mice. In the mouse, lymphomas induced by viruses involve the thymus-derived cells[98A] and those induced chemically in certain strains of mice involve B lymphocytes.[84] From these experimental findings, it is easy to postulate that chronic lymphocytic leukemias of older patients, usually involving B-cells, may often be chemically induced, whereas acute lymphoblastic leukemias of childhood, usually involving T-lymphocytes, may often be owing to viral agents. In addition, cells with detectable surface markers are not identified in many cases of acute lymphoblastic leukemia, since the sum of lymphocytes with T- or B-markers, or both, generally is somewhat less than 100 per cent (80–90%) in the peripheral blood of normal patients. The 10 to 20 per cent of cells not detected have been called "null" or "stem" cells; the latter suggests that these cells are precursors of T- and B-cells. Finally, it has been noted that a small percentage of normal human lymphocytes carry surface markers characteristic of both

T- and B-lymphocytes.[48] Similarly, dual T- and B-lymphocyte surface markers have been noted in a few lymphomas and leukemias.*

Nevertheless, there still remain many questions relating to the fundamental aspects of T- and B-lymphocyte function, as well as to pathologic events in the lymphoid system. In all probability, the following answers will be found in the very near future: the nature of the antigen receptor(s) on T-lymphocytes, the role of surface Ig as either an active or passive participant in B-lymphocyte activation, the role of Fc and complement receptors on B- and T-lymphocytes, and the molecular interaction involved in the T- and B-lymphocyte collaborative responses.[102] Additionally, questions have arisen concerning the pathologic adaptation of human T- and B-lymphocytes: the possible role of regulator or suppressor lymphocytes in the development of immunodeficiency, autoimmune, and neoplastic lymphoid diseases; the molecule basis of the defects in a variety of immunodeficiency diseases; the role of T- and B-lymphocytes in surveillance against malignancy, both within the lymphoid system and throughout the rest of the human body; and, finally, the need for a more detailed study of lymphocytes and lymphocyte subpopulations.[102]

TECHNIQUES FOR THE IDENTIFICATION, ISOLATION, AND QUANTITATION OF B- AND T-LYMPHOCYTES FROM HUMAN PERIPHERAL BLOOD

It is obvious that the object of studying cell (especially lymphocyte) surface markers is to define cells with different functions; it would also seem wise to study as many as possible in the same cell populations. In addition, some markers may be properties of both B and T populations, or

may define other populations. The use of markers has also shown that subpopulation of cells occur within B and T categories. The current practical definition of B cells is the possession of readily demonstrable surface membrane Ig, (frequently referred to as SmIg). SmIg is a product synthesized by the cell that carries it and is to be distinguished from external Ig that has become attached to the lymphocyte cell membrane. Very immature B-lymphocyte cells and mature plasma cells may lack SmIg. In relation to the mature cells, other cell markers should be considered; most cells that form rosettes with sheep RBCs (E rosettes) lack SmIg and are considered to be T-cells. Finally, a few lymphocytes carry both T- and B-markers or completely lack either marker. Before a marker is used as a criterion of B- and T-cells, the following should be established:[200] (1) the expression of the marker on B, T, or other cell populations or subpopulations should be determined; (2) the marker system should be titratable to a plateau or saturation point that delineates a distinct population or subpopulation. (3) under unusual conditions such as rapid proliferation, there may be differences in the expression of markers. If possible, the expression of the marker on normal B- and T-cells under similar conditions should be verified.

Evidence concerning the relationship of cell markers to B- and T-cells has already been presented; however, Table 13–5 indicates that some markers are not found exclusively in lymphoid cells.

As Table 13–5 shows, the major practical difficulty is introduced by monocytes, which may carry cytophilic IgG, bind aggregated IgG, and form EA and EAC rosettes. Methods for identification and removal of monocytes in lymphocyte preparations are discussed later. The reporting of marker studies on peripheral blood lymphocytes should be expressed both as a percentage of total lymphocytes and as the number per mm.[3] of blood, because an increased percentage alone could

---

* Kersey, J. H., and Gajl-Peczalska, K. J.: Personal communication.

be due to an increase in the cell population carrying the marker, or to a decrease in other populations.

Table 13-5. *Markers of Human Peripheral Blood Mononuclear Cells**

	B-Cells	T-Cells	Monocytes
SmIg	+	−	−
E rosette	−	+	−
EA-ox	+	−	+
EA-hu	−	−	+
EAC	+	−	+
Agg-IgG	+	−	+
EBV	+	−	−

* WHO/IARG Sponsored Workshop on Human B and T Cells: Identification, enumeration and isolation of B and T lymphocytes from human peripheral blood. Scand. J. Immunol., *3*:521, 1974.
1. Surface IgG is readily demonstrable on monocytes.
2. Not all B cells are EAC+.
3. A small proportion (1–3%) of cells have been found in healthy patients with the following characterization: E+ EAC+; E+ SmIg+; E+ AggIgG+; and E+ EA-ox+. A similar proportion of cells has been found which react with neither of these pairs of markers.
4. In addition to B and T cells, a third population of lymphoid cells has been described. These are: EA-hu+, EAC+, Agg-IgG±, SmIg−, and E−. This pattern of reactivity resembles that of phagocytic monocytes.

LYMPHOCYTE ISOLATION FOR QUANTITATION OF T- AND B-CELLS

Numerous methods have been reported for quantitating T- and B-cells; however, the Ficoll-Hypaque technique is most widely used. In selecting a procedure, the following point must be considered, no separation technique has a yield greater than 90 per cent; therefore, there may be selective loss of particular lymphocyte subpopulations. To avoid this, no attempt should be made to remove monocytes from mononuclear cell preparations. If an adherence method is used, B- and T-cell ratios will usually favor T-cells. The Ficol technique, however, may result in a higher proportion of monocytes and preferential loss of T cells, which is inversely related to the yield. In practice, yields of greater than

70 per cent appear to give genuine B- to T-cell ratios. In some disease processes, the isolation of lymphoid cells of abnormal physical properties may require modification of the separation procedure. However, most monocytes may be readily distinguished from B- and T-lymphocytes by their general morphology, by phagocytic capacity, and by endogenous enzymatic activity (e.g. peroxidase).[153]

The phagocytic activity method uses latex particles (1 μm. diameter), which are added to the cells in the presence of 50 per cent fetal calf serum at 37° C for 30 to 60 minutes. Whether all nonphagocytic monocytes show specific enzymatic activity remains to be established.

COLLECTION OF BLOOD SPECIMENS

Collect 20 ml. of blood into two 10 ml. heparin preservative free (green top) vacutainers. (EDTA may also be used, but defibrination should be avoided due to possible cell loss). Mix the specimen well. Determine total and differential white cell count.

GRADIENT CENTRIFUGATION SEPARATION AND ISOLATION OF MONONUCLEAR CELLS (MOSTLY LYMPHOCYTES)

Materials

(1) *Ficoll 400* (code No. 74001, approximately $14.00/100 g. with an inert high molecular weight > 400,000 polymer of sucrose and epichlorhydrin supplied in a spray dried powder from Pharmacia Fine Chemicals, Inc., 800 Centennial Ave., Piscataway, New Jersey 08854) and

(2) *Hypaque* (Hypaque sodium 50% (a brand of diatrizoate sodium injection, U.S.P., sterile, aqueous). Ficoll-Hypaque solution (24 parts 9% Ficoll and 10 parts 34% Hypaque to give a density of 1.08 g./ml.) is prepared as follows:

Solution A. Dilute 90 g. Ficoll spraydried powder to 1000 ml. with double distilled water. Shake vigorously until dissolved.

Solution B. Dilute 283.3 ml. of 50 per cent Hypaque sodium to 416.7 ml. with double distilled water. Invert gently several times.

Add solution B to solution A. Filter through a 0.45 micron millipore filter and store at 4° C. Bring to room temperature before use.

(3) *SBSSA* (Seligman's balanced salt solution). Dissolve the following in 2000 ml. of distilled water:

NaCl	61.2 g.
KCl	1.6 g.
NaCo$_2$CH$_3$ (Na acetate)	12.0 g.
NaH$_2$PO$_4$	0.4 g.
KH$_2$PO$_4$	0.8 g.
NaHCo$_3$	3.6 g.
Dextrose	8.0 g.
Ascorbic acid	0.024 g.
EDTA	4.0 g.
Bovine serum albumin	10.0 g.

This is a 4× concentrated solution with *p*H of usually 6.7 but not controlled. Filter through an 0.45 μ millipore filter and store at 4° C. To use, add 1 part of the above 4× concentrated SBSSA solution to 3 parts of distilled water. Bring to room temperature before use.

(4) *SBSS solution for rosettes*. Prepare as SBSSA solution, but omit EDTA and albumin.

(5) *Hanks and Fetal Calf Serum*.

No. 614 HI Calf Serum—heat inactivated; approximately $35.75/500 ml.

No. 402 (HBSS; Hanks balanced salt solution); approximately $6.00/500 ml. GIBCO, 3175 Staley Road, Grand Island, New York 14072.

(6) *Latex*.

No. 3102-56 Bacto-Latex 0.81 5 ml/bottle; Difco Laboratories, Detroit, Michigan.

(7) *Fluorescent Antisera*.

No. C-520 High Fluorescein to Protein Ratio (F/P)—conjugated antisera to polyvalent immunoglobulins; approximately $48.00/2 ml. vial. (F/P ratio usu-

ally 2.8-4.0; however, these antisera should be individually checked for specificity, titrated by serial dilution in SBSSA and reacted with lymphocytes from several donors to determine optimal working titer with minimum background fluorescence.)

(8) *50 ml. Polycarbonate Tube*.

No. 245, Sorvall, Newton, Connecticut)

Technique of Gradient Separation of Lymphocytes

1. Pour each tube of 10 ml. blood collected as above into a 50 ml. polycarbonate tube (Yields may occasionally be less when very large tubes—approximately 50–100 ml.—are used. Therefore, it may be preferable to use smaller replicate tubes).

2. Add 23 ml. SBSSA, rinsing the blood tube with the SBSSA. Mix well, but gently.

3. Using the pump, layer underneath with 10 ml. Ficoll-Hypaque. This will fill it to the top.

4. Spin at 400 × G for 25 minutes.

5. Using the pump, remove the layer of lymphocytes at the upper interphase of the Ficoll-Hypaque into a 50 ml. Polycarbonate tube. Fill up the tube with SBSSA.

6. Spin at 300 × G for 10 minutes.

7. Pour off the supernatant.

8. Resuspend the cells by hitting the tube against your hand. Lyse the red cells by adding 9 ml. of distilled water with swirling and then add 2.9 ml. of 3.5 per cent NaCl within 10 seconds.

9. Spin at 200 × G for 10 minutes. Pour off the supernatant and resuspend.

10. Add 6 ml. of a 1:200 dilution of latex particles in HBSS with 20 per cent fetal calf serum. Incubate in a 37° C water bath for 45 minutes.

11. Wash twice in SBSSA at 200 × G for 10 minutes.

12. Resuspend cells and add 3 ml. of SBSSA and do a Coulter count.

Interpretation

Demonstration of E (T-Cell) Rosettes. 1. Put 1.5 × 10^6 cells from the lymphocyte preparation into a 12 × 75 plastic tube.

2. Dilute with SBSS for rosettes and spin at 200 × G for 10 minutes.

3. Pour off the supernatant and resuspend the pellet.

4. Add 0.1 ml. human-type AB serum or fetal calf serum that has been heat-inactivated at 56° C for 30 minutes and absorbed with equal volumes of packed sheep red blood cells for 30 minutes at 37° C and 30 minutes at 4° C.

5. Add 0.1 ml. of a 2 per cent suspension of washed sheep cells in Hanks' Balanced Salt Solution.

6. Mix, incubate for 5 minutes in a 37° C water bath.

7. Centrifuge for 5 minutes at 200 × G.

8. Incubate for 60 minutes at 4° C. in an ice bath.

9. Very gently resuspend the cell button by rocking the tube.

10. Make a wet mount and read 400 lymphocytes. Express as per cent rosettes and absolute number per mm³.

Quality Control. The E rosette test is generally used as a marker for T-lymphocytes. Several varieties of the E test have been used, and it is thought likely that the marked divergence of published results is probably owing to technical differences and criteria for positive rosettes. The following points were considered to be of particular importance:

The use of sheep red cells (SRBC), stored in Alsever's solution at 4° C for not more than 2 weeks, was recommended. Commercially available RBCs and cells from individual animals or pooled from several animals were found to be satisfactory.

A SRBC to lymphocyte ratio of above 50:1 appears necessary, and 100:1 is recommended.

The reaction should be carried out in round (not conical) plastic or siliconized glass tubes, and the cells can be suspended in a variety of balanced salt solutions (e.g., Hank's, Earle's saline). When rosette tests are being used on a larger scale for preparative purposes, the proportion of rosettes obtained should be checked against a smaller test aliquot.

The presence of protein in the medium increases the stability of the rosettes. Ten per cent human AB serum or 25 per cent fetal calf serum has been used. The sera should be heat-inactivated and absorbed with SRBC, preferably at 37° C and 4° C. If human serum is used, care must be taken to exclude the presence of antilymphocyte antibodies that may partially or totally inhibit the rosette reaction. Some laboratories have found that neuraminidase pretreatment of SRBC (2 units/ml., 37° C, 30 mintes) obviates the need for serum and may provide more stable rosettes.

Reproducible results have been obtained using a 5-minute incubation at 37° C, followed by centrifugation at 200 G for 5 minutes and incubation at 4° C overnight. It appears, however, that the period of incubation in the cell may be shortened to 1 to 2 hours. A method using centrifugation and incubation at room temperature for 1 hour has been suggested, but has not been successful in all laboratories. It is recommended that the different methods be compared and the technique giving the best reproducibility and the highest number of positive cells be adopted.

The final resuspension of rosettes for enumeration should not be too vigorous. Sufficient agitation to resuspend the pellets into single cells and rosettes can be achieved by gently tapping with a finger, carefully pipetting through a wide-bore Pasteur pipette, or slow mechanical rotation. Medical technologists should compare these procedures to determine which gives the most reliable results.

Since dead T-cells do not form E rosettes, cell viability should be assessed by trypan blue or other vital dye.

The number of red blood cells attached to individual lymphocytes varies. Under optimal conditions, the great majority of T-cells from normal donors bind three or more red blood cells, and the number of lymphocytes binding one or two red blood cells is small. Since this latter group may be increased in some patients, it is recommended that rosettes with three or more red blood cells and those with one or two red blood cells be recorded separately.

Rosettes may be enumerated either in suspension or in fixed and stained preparations. Cytocentrifugation may produce changes in the apparent proportion of rosette-forming cells, and is not recommended.

A modified, rapid E rosette test has been described to identify active E rosettes.[206] These are a minority of the total T-cells. Their proportion may be reduced in disease, even if the total number of E rosette cells is normal. The significance of the active E rosette test remains to be established.

Technique for Staining Lymphocytes for Surface Immunoglobulin

1. Place 1.0 to 1.5 × 10⁶ cells from the lymphocyte preparation into 12 × 75 plastic tubes.

2. Fill the tubes with SBSSA and spin at 200 × G for 10 minutes. Pour off the supernatant, removing as much as possible.

3. Place 0.1 ml. of the properly diluted fluorescent anti-immunoglobulin over the cell button and gently resuspend the cells. (The antiserum should be titered to determine the best dilution.)

4. Place the tubes in a 4° C refrigerator for 30 to 60 minutes. The tubes should be tightly capped to prevent evaporation.

5. Wash the cells three times using SBSSA for the first two and PBS with 0.05 per cent NaAzide for the last wash. All washes are 10 minutes at 200 × G.

6. After the last wash, pour off all the supernatant and resuspend the cells. Seal tubes until ready to read.

7. Set the fluorescent microscope for fluorescein (preferably Zeiss microscope with red suppressor BG-23, FITC reflector, and FITC exciter and barrier filters).

8. Make a wet mount and read with 100×-immersion oil-phase.

9. First count the total cells in the field and then the number of fluorescent cells,

checking that each positive cell is a lymphocyte. Positive cells are those having at least three distinct fluorescent dots. Be sure to look at the entire cell surface by continual focusing. Count 200 lymphocytes.

10. Per cent S-Ig positive lymphocytes equals number of fluorescent lymphocytes divided by total lymphocytes.

Technique for EAC (B-Cell) Rosettes

EAC Preparation. 1. Wash sheep RBCs three times with SBSS.

2. Resuspend to a 5 per cent suspension in SBSS.

3. Add 0.5 ml. of the SRBC to 0.5 ml. of sheep hemolysin (diluted 1:50 in SBSS). The hemolysin is 1:2 in glycerol when received; therefore, the final dilution is 1:100. The hemolysin is obtained from GIBCO (see p. 432).

4. Incubate at 37° C (water bath) for 30 minutes.

5. Wash once with SBSS (this can be done in a serofuge for 35 seconds).

6. Resuspend the cells to 0.5 ml. in SBSS.

7. Add 0.5 ml. of a 1:5 dilution of mouse serum in SBSS. Mouse serum should be stored in 0.1 ml. aliquots at 80° C.

8. Incubate at 37° C (water bath) for 30 minutes.

9. Wash 3 times in SBSS (35 seconds in a serofuge).

10. Resuspend in 0.5 ml. SBSS.

B-Cell Assay. 1. Put 4.5 × 10⁶ cells from the lymphocyte preparation into a plastic 12 × 75 tube, fill the tube with SBSS and centrifuge for 10 minutes at 200 × G.

2. Pour off the supernatant and resuspend the pellet. Add 0.4 ml. SBSS.

3. Add 0,1 ml. of the EAC suspension.

4. Incubate at 37° C for 30 minutes on a wheel rotating at 20 r.p.m. Keep on the rotator until each is read.

5. Make a wet mount and count 400 lymphocytes. Express as per cent rosettes and absolute number per mm³.

The binding of RBCs sensitized with

IgM antibody and complement (C), as used above, detects lymphocytes carrying C receptors.[165]

Quality Control. As a source of RBCs, the ox RBCs appear to be the most satisfactory, since they show little agglutinability after sensitization and do not bind spontaneously to human T-cells. Sheep RBCs can also be used as in the above technique, but controls are needed to exclude the formation of E rosettes. Human RBCs should be avoided since they themselves carry C_3 receptors. Commercially available RBCs can be used for up to 3 weeks following collection if they are stored at 4° C. The use of RBCs from a single animal may give more consistent results. IgM antibody is required, since IgG antibody-coated RBCs may bind to lymphocyte Fc receptors. Commercially available 19S anti-RBC preparations appear to be suitable. The agglutination activity of the antibody preparation should be titrated and half the minimum agglutinating dose used for sensitization for 15 minutes at room temperature. Fresh serum from C_5-deficient mice is the most common source of complement for this test. EAC prepared in this way can be used over a period of 6 days. R_3 human serum or purified human C components can also be used. Fresh serum from normal mice (as in the above technique) can be used, but these EAC preparations cannot be used after 2 days. In fact, for satisfactory results, it is necessary to collect mouse blood on ice, and separate serum within the first 3 hours. Each complement source should be adsorbed with the relevant RBCs before use. The activity of the complement source should be titrated by enumerating the number of EAC rosettes in a given lymphocyte suspension, using EAC prepared with increasing amounts of complement.

The ratio of EAC to lymphocytes should be between 20:1 and 100:1. Incubation is carried out for 15 minutes with continuous mixing. If SRBC are used, it is necessary to incubate at 37° C to prevent the formation of E rosettes, whereas incubation at 4° C can be used with ox RBCs. Controls using E and EA preparations should be included. The reading should be performed under phase contrast and in the presence of 0.5 per cent toluidine blue to visualize nucleated RBCs. Lymphocytes with three or more EAC are considered positive.

The mean value of EAC-positive lymphocytes in peripheral blood of healthy adults was 15.4 per cent, in a range of 10.0 to 19.0 per cent. Similar values were obtained when lymphocytes were tested for the presence of either C_{3b} or C_{3d} receptors.[164] Since monocytes also form EAC rosettes, the procedures listed above should be used to identify these cells.

Successful attempts to produce antisera specifically reactive with either B- or T-cells have been reported. It is evident, however, that such antisera are at present difficult to prepare; problems arose with some of the techniques, with the methods for absorption, with tests for specificity, and with tests for B- and T-cell identification.

Heparin Procedure

Since studies of human lymphocytes often require large amounts of pure cells, it is essential to have a method in which one obtains a good yield without discrete contamination by other cells or which provides pure lymphocytes in maximum amounts. A new procedure for purification of lymphocytes suggests a possible solution to the problem (Fig. 13-10).

Technique. Heparinized blood (10 units of heparin/ml. blood) is obtained by a standard aseptic technique.

Leukocytes and platelets are counted and percentages of lymphocytes determined. Ten-milliliter fractions of blood are then filtered through 12-ml. plastic syringes, fitted with 21-gauge needles and containing 8 ml. of 0.3-mm. glass beads, prewashed twice with phosphate-buffered saline solution (PBS, *p*H 7.35). The blood filtrates are collected in 10-ml. plastic syringes fitted with 25-gauge needles plugged

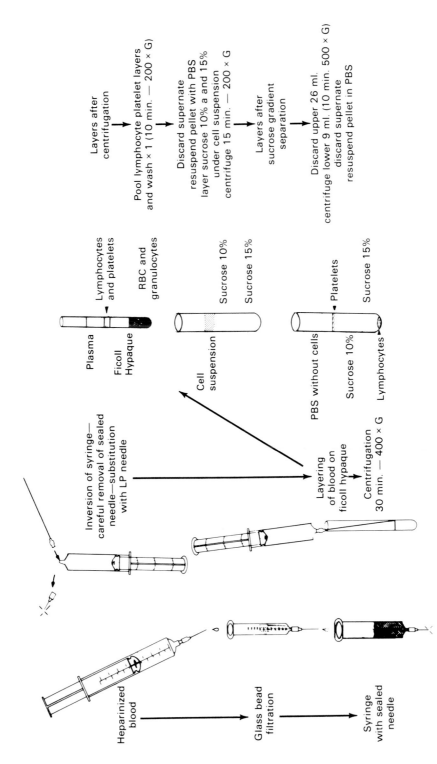

Fig. 13-10. An improved method for purification of lymphocytes. (Carpentieri, U., Thorpe, L., and Sordahl, L. A.: An improved method for purification of lymphocytes. Am. J. Clin. Pathol., *68:*763, 1977)

with Seal-Ease.* The glass-bead columns are washed with an amount of PBS sufficient to fill the underlying syringes with diluted blood to a total volume of 20 ml. The sealed 25-gauge needles are then replaced by 20-gauge, 2.5-inch lumbar puncture needles and the 10-ml. fractions of diluted blood are carefully layered onto 5 ml. of freshly prepared Ficoll-Hypaque solution in 1.6 × 12.5-cm. 18-ml. glass centrifuge tubes. The Ficoll-Hypaque solution is prepared dissolving 9 g. Ficoll (MW 400,000)† in 50 ml. distilled water and adding 30 ml. Hypaque (50% sodium diatrizoate; MW 635.9);** distilled water is gradually added until a final specific gravity of the solution at room temperature of 1.080 is obtained. The tubes are immediately centrifuged at 400 × G for 30 minutes in a swinging-bucket centrifuge. The layers from each tube containing lymphocytes and platelets are carefully removed, pooled into two 2.5 × 12-cm. 50-ml. graduated glass tubes, and washed once with PBS by centrifuging 10 minutes at 200 × G. The cell pellets are resuspended in 5 ml. PBS and a discontinuous gradient of 10 per cent sucrose (20 ml.) and 15 per cent sucrose (10 ml.) is carefully layered in this order under the cell suspensions with 21-gauge, 3.5-inch lumbar puncture needles. The tubes are centrifuged at 200 × G for 15 minutes in a swinging-bucket centrifuge, avoiding sudden changes of speed. The top layer (26 ml.) of supernatant is then removed and the remaining material (9 ml.) centrifuged at 500 × G for 5 minutes. The supernatant is discarded and the resulting pellet resuspended in 5 ml. PBS. Fractions are taken for determinations of cell count, cell viability, and smears. Cellular morphology is checked with light and electron microscopy. Cellular viability is determined by the standard trypan blue and erythrocin B dye exclusion methods. T- and B-lymphocytes

are identified and responsiveness of T-cells to mitogens is assessed. The entire procedure is carried out at room temperature, using clean siliconized, but not sterile, glassware.

Quality Control. This method provides a feasible approach to obtaining sufficient numbers of purified and viable lymphocytes from small volumes of circulating human blood. Pooling of blood from a group of donors and culturing of lymphocytes from a single donor are alternate procedures but introduce variables that might invalidate subsequent studies. Compared with others, this method offers many advantages: smaller initial blood sample, higher yield, higher percentage of intact lymphocytes, extreme purity of the final suspension, shorter time of preparation. These advantages are particularly evident when a limited amount of blood is available, as when blood is obtained from children, and a large amount of cells is necessary for subsequent biochemical studies.

The chief advantages are the drastic reduction of transfers with consequent cell loss, and the use of discontinuous sucrose gradient, which completes the purification only partially achieved with glass-bead column filtration and Ficoll-Hypaque gradient separation.

Lymphocyte losses are distributed among glass-bead columns, Ficoll-Hypaque solution, and sucrose gradient. Only the loss on Ficoll-Hypaque is related to technical skill in cell harvesting and is, therefore, further reducible without compromising the purity of preparation.

The intactness of the lymphocytes, the results obtained in identification of B- and T-lymphocytes, and the T-cell responsiveness to mitogens prove that one is dealing with intact viable cells.

The good preservation of the B cell:T cell ratio suggests that this method may precede the separation of B- and T-lymphocytes when a pure preparation is needed. The slightly greater loss of B-cells does not interfere with the final quantitative result.

---

* Clay Adams, Parsippany, New Jersey, 07054.
† Sigma Chemical Co., St. Louis, Missouri.
** Winthrop Laboratories, New York, New York.

VANDERBILT UNIVERSITY
MEDICAL CENTER FORM-1-1537 REV. 11/75
NASHVILLE, TENNESSEE 37232-PHONE: 322-2682
IMMUNOPATHOLOGY LABORATORY
WILLIAM H. HARTMANN, M.D., DIRECTOR OF LABORATORIES

CODES

S = SERUM

C = CALL LAB
FOR DIRECTIONS
EXT. 2682

NUMBER TO LEFT
OF TEST INDICATES
ml OF BLOOD
NEEDED.

TEST PRINTED IN
RED REQUIRE
SCHEDULING WITH
LABORATORY

DATE
OF
SERV.

PT.

UNIT #

- ☐ OUT-PATIENT-O
- ☐ IN-PATIENT-I
- ☐ PRIVATE OUT-PATIENT-P
- ☐ EMERGENCY ROOM-E
- ☐ NON-PATIENT-N
- ☐ OTHER-Z

BUDGET NUMBER

REQ. CLINIC | REQ. PHYSICIAN

CONTRACTING AGENCY

ACCIDENT RELATED ☐ YES ☐ NO | WORKMEN'S COMP. ☐ YES ☐ NO

DATE SAMPLE COLLECTED			TIME	
MO.	DAY	YEAR		A.M. P.M

CLINICAL INFORMATION TO BE COMPLETED BY REQUESTING PHYSICIAN

SPECIMEN: Please Note Source

Previous Immunopathology Work-up

☐ YES (YEAR? _____) ☐ NO

Diagnosis: _____

Present Admission Data: PCV _____ Platelets _____
WBC _____ Lymph _____ EOS _____
Bone Marrow Abnormalities: _____

Adenopathy: _____
Hepatosplenomegaly: _____

Chief Diagnosis: _____

Major Clinic Problem: _____

Information desired from these tests:

REQUESTING PHYSICIAN | SEND REPORT TO

X			RESULTS	X			RESULTS
		IMMUNOGLOBULIN STUDIES				**IMMUNOLOGIC TYPING STUDIES**	
	1-S	IMMUNOELECTROPHORESIS			C	B + T CELL TYPING	
	24 HR.	URINE IMMUNOELECTROPHORESIS			C	TISSUE FLUORESCENCE	
	C	CRYOGLOBULIN QUANT.					
	C	CRYOGLOBULIN EVALUATION					
	1-S	IgG (770-1130 mg/dl)					
	1-S	IgA (80-200 mg/dl)				**IMMUNOLOGIC FUNCTIONS STUDIES**	
	1-S.	IgM (90-170 mg/dl)			C	MITOGENIC LYMPHOCYTE STIM.	
	1-S	IgD (0-30 mg/dl)			C	MACROPHAGE INHIBITION FACTOR	
	1-S	IgE (< 100 u/ml)			C	MIXED LYMPHOCYTE CULTURE	
		COMPLEMENT					
	1-S	CH50: COMPLEMENT ACTIVITY (> 150 UNITS)					
	1-S	C-3, QUANT. (120-185 mg/dl)				**MISCELLANEOUS**	
	1-S	C-4, QUANT. (14-51 mg/dl)			1-S	ANA	
	1-S	C-5, QUANT. (9-13 mg/dl)			1-S	ANA TITER	
					1-S	ANTI-DNA	
		OTHER			1-S	MURAMIDASE	
					10ml	URINE MURAMIDASE	
					5-S	RAST	

☐ ADDITIONAL RESULTS TO FOLLOW

INTERPRETATION

REPORTED BY:

PATHOLOGIST | DATE

CHART COPY

Fig. 13-11. Laboratory form depicting immunologic studies to be performed in the diagnosis of immunoglobulin disorders. (Courtesy of William H. Hartmann, M.D.)

CLINICAL USE OF B- AND T-CELL TYPING[189]

Classification of Lymphocytosis of Unknown Etiology

T- and B-cell typing can be of considerable diagnostic value in differentiating benign and malignant lymphocytosis (Fig. 13-11). A markedly increased percentage of B-cells associated with a high absolute lymphocyte count is suggestive of a lymphoproliferative disorder. Typing of cell surface immunoglobin for the heavy-chain class and light-chain type in this case can provide evidence of malignant proliferation of a single clone. Almost all patients with chronic lymphocytic leukemia or non-Hodgkin's lymphoma with involvement of the blood show a monoclonal pattern of surface immunoglobulin with the same light chain expressed on the majority of lymphocytes. IgM and IgD are found singly or together on the surfaces of most of these malignant cells, and both immunoglobulin classes are thought to share the same variable region when they are present on the same cell as detected by anti-idiotype antiserum. A normal or decreased percentage of B-cells with a polyclonal pattern of surface immunoglobulin is good evidence that there is no involvement of the blood with a malignant lymphoproliferative process. However, rare T-cell leukemias or lymphomas have been reported.

Diagnosis of Immunodeficiency Diseases

Assays for T- and B-cells can be an adjunct in the diagnosis of congenital agammaglobulinemia (Bruton's disease) in childhood. All cases of Bruton's disease have been associated with an absence or marked reduction of the percentage of B-cells in the peripheral blood. A normal percentage of B-cells associated with hypogammaglobulinemia indicates an acquired disease process.

Congenital absence of the thymus (DiGeorge's syndrome) can be documented by the lack of T-cells in the blood and a high percentage of B-cells. This diagnostic adjunct can be particularly useful in infants with hypocalcemia and doubtful thymic shadow on chest radiograph.

Monitoring of Immunosuppression in Transplant Recipients

Serial quantitation of percentage and of absolute number of E-RFC in the peripheral blood of recipients of renal or heart transplants has been reported to be beneficial in predicting early rejection crises. A sharp rise in the absolute number and percentage of E-RFC during the first several weeks following transplantation frequently heralds the onset of graft rejection. This information can be useful in altering immunosuppressive drug therapy, and in assessing the outcome of therapeutic changes.

Aid in the Diagnosis of Hodgkin's Disease

Recent evident suggests that rosette formation of circulating T-cells in untreated Hodgkin's disease is inhibited by serum factors found in Hodgkin's disease. However, rosette formation of target cells from normal subjects and patients with carcinoma or non-Hodgkin's lymphoma is not inhibited by the serum. In order to demonstrate this inhibition, the Ficoll-purified peripheral blood lymphocytes must first be incubated in tissue culture medium and fetal calf serum in order to reverse alterations in the surfaces of freshly drawn cells. The incubated cells are subsequently cultured in the presence of Hodgkin's disease serum and the percentage reduction of E-RFC is determined. Differences in target cell sensitivities to these inhibitory serum factors provide the basis for a diagnostic test for Hodgkin's disease.

LEUKOPENIA

Leukopenia may be defined as a reduction of the total number of leukocytes below 4000 to 4500 per cu.mm. In most situations, this decrease is due to a marked decrease in the number of cells of the granulocyte series. Occasionally there is a balanced leukocyte reduction with the differential count remaining essentially normal. One may see leukopenias as low as 1500 to 2000 per cu.mm. without unusually subsequent extensive repeated infections, if the polymorphonuclear forms constitute 15 to 20 per cent or more of the cells. Septicemia, and mucous membrane and skin involvement are observed more often when the total neutrophil count becomes lowered below 10 per cent. It is difficult to evaluate the pathogenesis of leukopenia; different combinations of factors are involved in different situations.

An aid in understanding leukopenias is to realize that the leukopoiesis of polymorphonuclear cells exists in three divisions—the marrow, the circulating blood, and the body tissues. The bone marrow, besides being the production locus, is also a storage reserve containing at any one time a greater number of mature or nearly mature cells than those in the peripheral blood. Normally, circulating leukocytes are found on their way from their production site to the extravascular tissues. The peripheral blood concentration represents a balance dependent on the following rates: production, marrow release, migration from vascular to extravascular tissues, and peripheral destruction. Because leukocytes occasionally may be unevenly sequestered in capillary beds, the total leukocyte count in an extremity does not necessarily compare with the leukocyte count in visceral areas. Therefore, leukopenic states reflect the many combinations associated with changes in the varied factors responsible for normal leukocyte balance.

Etiology

Although no direct specific etiologic proof is available, it is thought that the leukopenias produced in infections by typhoid and paratyphoid bacteria, certain viruses, and by malarial parasites result from inhibition of leukopoiesis. Other bacterial infections that cause leukopenia are brucellosis and tularemia. Occasionally agents that induce overwhelming leukocytosis produce secondary leukopenia. Specific viral leukopenic agents are those of influenza, measles, dengue fever, infectious hepatitis, rubella, and psittacosis. Rickettsial causes include Rocky Mountain spotted fever, typhus, scrub typhus, and rickettsialpox. Protozoal leukopenic agents besides malaria include relapsing fever and kala-azar. Leukopenia also occurs in vitamin B_{12} deficiency and folic acid deficiency, in sprue and other chronic inanition states that probably have a metabolic basis —for example, animal experiments in which the giving of folic acid helps to correct the leukopenia produced by a protein-deficient diet.

Following the anaphylactic shock associated with the injection of foreign protein, such as typhoid vaccine, there is a rouleaux formation of erythrocytes with peripheral margination and redistribution of leukocytes from the large vessels to their aggregation in the capillaries of the lung, spleen, and other organs, which may then lead to the production of temporary leukopenia. Peripheral capillary positioning of leukocytes is also seen after the injection of gelatin, globulin, or fibrinogen. An autoantibody called a *leukoagglutinin* may also be a factor in the leukocytic redistribution seen in some newborn infants (antibody from mother) and in some allergic states in which the circulating granulocytes shift to certain body areas involved in the allergic reaction.

In pernicious anemia and related macrocytic anemias, the leukopenia is related to a deficiency of vitamin B_{12}. In aleukemic leukemia, there is leukopenia of the peripheral blood with large numbers of leukemic cells in the bone marrow and other tissues. In agranulocytic angina, the leukopenia is associated with the menstrual cycle and with certain antidysmenorrheic drugs acting on the bone marrow. A reduction in leukocyte count is also observed in splenic dysfunction and in almost any condition associated with splenomegaly, either as a leukopenia or in combination with anemia or thrombocytopenia—for example, in chronic congestive splenomegaly, Gaucher's disease, Felty's syndrome (with associated rheumatoid arthritis), and in primary splenic neutropenia. Leukopenia is also seen in disseminated lupus erythematosus, paroxysmal nocturnal hemoglobinuria (possibly associated with the increased destruction of leukocytes by the same factors causing hemolysis of red blood cells), cyclic or periodic leukopenia, chronic hypoplastic neutropenia, familial leukopenia, and transitory neonatal leukopenia. Also a reduction in the total leukocytes is observed in diseases previously involving the bone marrow or interfering with its normal function—for example, aplastic and hypoplastic anemias, and aleukemic leukemia, and occasionally myelosclerosis, myelofibrosis, and lymphosarcomatous marrow replacement.

Leukopenia may also be seen in patients exposed to leukotoxic agents in industry or in their environment. Most cases, however, follow the therapeutic action of certain drugs—for example, cytotoxic nitrogen mustard and its analogous, alkylating drugs such as Myleran, Demicolchin, and urethan, and a wide variety of antimetabolites including 6-mercaptopurine and folic acid antagonists such as Aminopterin and A-methopterin. In some cases, the leukopenia appears to be associated with individual sensitivity or immunologic reactions associated with the use of the drug, such as anticonvulsants (Mesantoin and Tridione), antimicrobials (chloramphenicol,[16] arsenobenzol, and sulfa drugs), antithyroid agents (thiouracil, propylthiouracil and Tapazole), sedatives and analgesics (Sedormid and amidopyrine), the phenothiazine antihistamines, the antidiabetic drugs (tolbutamide, chlorpropamide, and carbutamide), and antiarthritic agents (gold preparations and phenylbutazone). Other occasional offenders of this endless list are chlorpromazine, amphetamine, procaine amide, Atabrine, pyribenzamine, Diamox, and various antimicrobial drugs. Exposure to benzol, certain industrial chemicals, solvents, insecticides, and sprays may produce leukopenia due to marrow depression.

Marrow depression and leukopenia also occur from exposure to certain physical agents—for example, from radiographs and other sources of external ionizing radiation, and from therapeutic use of radioactive material such as [32]P.

Neutropenia

Specific reduction of neutrophilic granulocytes below 1500 per cu.mm. in children and below 1800 per cu.mm. in adults is caused by the peripheral distribution of abnormally great numbers of polymorphonuclear cells, as seen in infections by the salmonellae, in which there is mild, early leukocytosis followed by neutropenia with relative and absolute lymphocytosis and occasionally monocytosis. Typhoid fever is associated with focal necrosis, hyperplasia of reticuloendothelial elements, and subsequent neutropenia. Measles is associated with a leukocytosis during the incubation period, and neutropenia occurs after the rash appears. Rubella is characterized by neutropenia and lymphopenia seen at the beginning of the disease and followed by a lymphocytosis and plasmacytosis. In hepatotoxic diseases one sees a neutropenia. Acute radiation sickness is associated with an initial transient neutrophilic leukocytosis followed during the second week by leukopenia and neutropenia. When the bone marrow is injured by cytotoxic agents or radiographs or impaired by inadequate nutrition, diminished production is usually considered a major etiologic factor.

Lau, Brody, and Beizer[112] observed that neutropenic bone marrow from patients with peripheral neutropenia, once removed from the body, is capable of normal sequential growth in duplicate suspension cultures (autologous or homologous plasma) and is not inherently defective. The ability of neutropenic plasmas to accelerate maturation of normal bone marrow implies that they contain a component that influences the kinetics of the complex granulocytic maturation cycle. The observations (paired) imply that leukopenia in these patients is the result of the inappropriate removal of circulating neutrophils, which distorts a normal feedback mechanism regulating leukopoiesis.

An inherited, sex-linked defect of neutrophils called chronic granulomatous disease of childhood is associated with chronic, frequently fatal infections with catalase positive bacteria (i.e., capable of destroying H_2O_2). Degranulation, chemotaxis, and recognition are within normal range. Hexose monophosphate shunt activity, increased oxygen consumption, and hydrogen peroxide generation usually accompany normal phagocytosis; in chronic granulomatous disease one observes blunting or absence of these responses. The important metabolic defect is thought to be due to failure of the neutrophils to generate H_2O_2 and perhaps superoxide, since organisms that are catalase-negative, and therefore produce H_2O_2, are normally destroyed in chronic granulomatous disease (CGD). Other similar, bacterial-killing, acquired defects have also been described.

Primary splenic neutropenia is characterized by hypersplenism, which produces a selective nonspecific granulocyte lysis, or splenic inhibition of marrow production of granulocytes, or reticulum cell hyperplasia. In idiopathic hypersplenism and those states of splenic overactivity associated with other diseases, the bone marrow is normally cellular or hyperplastic with a concomitant reduction in mature granulocytes. Malabsorption syndrome and agammaglobulinemia may also be associated with neutropenia. Cyclic or periodic leukopenia is associated with a regular, recurrent reduction or disappearance of neutrophils over a period of years, and this is characterized by average cycles of 21 days associ-ated with malaria, signs of other infections, or idiopathic. Animal experimentation suggests a fluctuation of peripheral blood neutrophils as secondary to fluctuation in rates of cell production, with an associated defect of early precursor cells restored by allogenic marrow transplantation.[80] Defects of precursor cells are acquired and are accompanied by antineutrophil antibodies, with resultant neutropenia produced by accelerated neutrophil destruction at unknown rates, a pace increased production cannot equal.

Chronic hypoplastic neutropenia reveals a hypoplasia of granulocytic precursor cells in the marrow. In familial leukopenia or neutropenia, one observes an inherited, moderately dominant blood dyscrasia, associated with diminished neutrophil production, having apparently adequate quantities of neutrophils (500–1500/ul.) to avoid life-threatening infection. It is difficult to distinguish this dyscrasia from congenital chronic benign neutropenia; however, the chronic benign neutropenia is not inherited and is usually associated with a lower percentage of neutrophils than the familial form. The etiology of the latter is unknown. Transitory neonatal neutropenia is associated with maternal isoimmunization, which may be produced by fetal leukocyte antigens similar to the erythrocyte antigens in erythroblastosis fetalis. Foreign protein reactions are characterized by temporary sequestration of neutrophils in the splanchnic capillary beds. In some instances of neutropenia secondary to the previously mentioned drugs and chemicals, immune phenomena resulting in agglutination and destruction of white blood cells is a causative factor (e.g., amidopyrine and associated agranulocytic angina). In other cases, steroids may interfere with migration of granulocytes into the inflammatory site.[7]

Therapy of neutropenia consists of removal of the offending agent, and the use of antimicrobial agents. Splenectomy aids neutropenia associated with splenic dysfunction. In pernicious anemia and other nutritional disorders, the administration of vitamin B_{12}, folic acid, and other dietary factors is of help.

Lymphopenia

An absolute decrease in lymphocytes below 1400 per cu.mm. in children and below 1000 per cu.mm. in adults occurs after acute irradiation or the administration of alkylating agents; in terminal renal failure with or without leukopenia, in active tuberculosis; in acute pyogenic infections with marked right shift in polymorphonuclear cells; in infants with hypogammaglobulinemia associated with elevated temperature, diarrhea, and an increase in the frequency of episodes of infection; in disseminated lupus erythematosus; in Hodgkin's sarcoma and lymphosarcoma; and following administration of adrenocortical hormones with associated lymphocytolysis and lymphopenia in the presence of a normal intact adrenal cortex.

Eosinopenia

An absolute decrease in eosinophils below 50 to 100 per cu.mm. occurs after stress situations—for example in shock and 4 to 6 hours after major surgery, severe burns, blood loss, and also after electric shock, eclampsia, labor, and severe infections—with return to normal on recovery. Eosinopenia is also observed in Cushing's syndrome and after administration of cortisone-like preparations or ACTH in the presence of a normally functioning intact adrenal cortex. The eosinopenia just described is thought to be due either to a redistribution change caused by the blocking of eosinophil release from the bone marrow, to peripheral destruction of eosinophils, or to a reduction in marrow eosinophil production.

Basopenia

An absolute decrease in basophils below 20 per cu.mm. occurs in hyperthyroidism, pituitary basophilism (Cushing's syndrome), and in stress reactions. It may also follow prolonged steroid therapy or the immediate allergic reaction itself.[179] In the course of many infections, both the basophils and eosinophils disappear during the period of leukocytosis and neutrophilia, and they reappear during the recovery of the patient.

LEUKEMOID REACTIONS

These are varied syndromes characterized by morphologic hematologic changes in peripheral blood that resemble those of leukemia (Plates 45, 46). In this group, one may observe leukocyte counts as high as 20,000 to 25,000 per cu.mm. with occasional moderate or minimal cell immaturity. Whereas lymphocytic and myelocytic leukemoid patterns are fairly common, monocytic ones are uncommon. If the total leukocyte count is low, normal, or reduced, immature leukocytes must be seen for the pattern to be classified as leukemoid. Small numbers of blast cells may also be found. In infectious and toxic states, toxic granulation and granulocytic vacuolation are common. Frequently, one sees a preponderance of nucleated erythrocytes compared to leukocytes. A reduction in the erythrocyte and platelet count does not occur unless the primary disease itself is responsible for such. Bone marrow changes are nonspecific with hyperplasia of the myeloid elements and a shift to the left in the myelocytic form with or without toxic changes in the granulocyte series. Red blood cells and megakaryocytic cell types may be normal, stimulated, or depressed, depending on the etiology. In the lymphocytic leukemoid reactions, bone marrow lymphocytes may be increased without the almost complete lymphocytic replacement of normal marrow that occurs in lymphocytic leukemia.

Etiology

Infections such as pneumonia, tuberculosis, meningococcal meningitis, and diphtheria are also associated with myelocytic or granulocytic leukemoid reactions. Infectious mononucleosis, with the possible direct involvement of bone marrow and other blood-forming organs as causative factors, whooping cough, chickenpox, disseminated or miliary tuberculosis, and infectious lymphocytosis in children are all associated with lymphocytic leukemoid reactions. Rarely, one may see a monocytic leukemoid pattern associated with tuberculosis. Intoxications such as in severe burns, heavy-metal poisoning, and eclampsia are associated with the myelocytic or granulocytic leukemoid pattern, possibly caused by a toxic effect on marrow cells.

Tumors such as carcinoma or sarcoma especially, but not specifically with metastases or infiltration to the bone marrow, Hodgkin's disease, and multiple myeloma are observed with either myelocytic, granulocytic, or lymphocytic leukemoid patterns. Myeloproliferative disorders producing a leukemoid pattern and including such disorders as polycythemia vera, thrombocythemias, Di Guglielmo's syndrome, and myelosclerosis with myeloid metaplasia are associated with extramedullary hematopoiesis. Miscellaneous causes of leukemoid reactions are those associated with the stimulation of marrow such as occurs after severe hemorrhage, sudden hemolysis, thalassemia major, and, rarely, during the response to beginning therapy of megaloblastic anemias with vitamin B_{12} or folic acid. Also occasionally Sézary syndrome and questionably erythrodermic mycosis fungoides may be seen concomitantly with a leukemoid pattern.

Differential Diagnosis

If there is a transient peripheral blood leukemoid reaction, the clinical course may reveal whether or not the disorder is leukemia. However, differentiation may not be made even after necropsy study. If there is erythroid depression with hyperplasia and a shift of the myeloid elements to the left, the bone marrow pattern may resemble myelocytic leukemia. In these cases a heavily positive alkaline phosphatase stain of mature granulocytes in the peripheral blood will take place in the leukemoid reaction with a negative reaction in granulocytic leukemia. In addition, a positive PAS or periodic acid/salicyloyl hydrazide stain is diagnostic of acute leukemia.[26] A positive heterophil serologic test and an atypical lymphocytic pattern differentiate infectious mononucleosis from leukemia. Leukemic cell tissue infiltration does not occur in leukemoid reactions. At times one cannot be certain of the diagnosis and therefore occasionally one reads of so-called "cures" of leukemic-leukemoid patients.

DISEASES OF LEUKOPOIESIS

INFECTIOUS MONONUCLEOSIS

The symptom complex known as infectious mononucleosis usually has benign clinical findings and a good prognosis; it is supposedly of viral etiology. Prominent findings of this disease are irregular temperature elevation, lymphadenopathy, pharyngitis, splenomegaly, marked lymphocytosis (mature or atypical type), and marked elevation of heterophil antibodies against sheep erythrocytes. In 1889, this disease was described as "glandular fever" by Emil Pfeiffer in a description of a children's epidemic.[148] In 1909, a hematologic description of increased mononuclear leukocytes was made by Burns.[27] The present term was used in 1920 by Sprunt and Evans, who also described the blood pattern of atypical lymphocytes.[185] A more detailed description of this pattern was made in 1923 by Downey and McKinlay.[54] In 1932, there appeared the heterophil antibody test of Paul and Bunnel, describing the high concentration of sheep erythrocyte agglutinins in a patient's serum.[144]

Infectious mononucleosis is widely distributed geographically and has a greater preponderance in 15- to 30-year-old males. However, all ages and races may be involved, epidemics and sporadic forms being reported in young adults, especially from

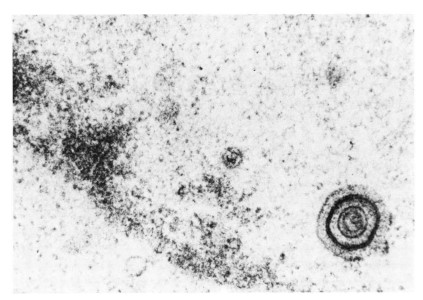

Fig. 13-12. Extracellular Epstein-Barr virus with intact envelope (× 150,000; Courtesy of P. Lai, M.D.)

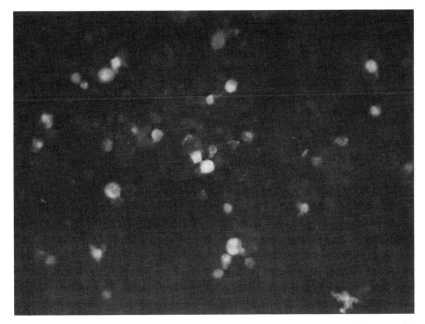

Fig. 13-13. Cells from laboratory maintained cell line are positive for Epstein-Barr viral capsid antigen in a case of infectious mononucleosis. The technique was indirect FITC immunofluorescence staining. (Courtesy of P. Lai, M.D.)

colleges and hospital personnel, with 10 to 15 per cent of the cases in 45- to 65-year age group. The Epstein-Barr (EB) herpes virus has now defintely been shown to be the etiologic agent, and the initial infection, often undiagnosed and mild, usually confers lasting immunity (Figs. 13-12; 13-13).[87, 88, 110] Drugs,[62] and protozoal, bacterial, and other agents have been implicated in some cases.

Pathology

Lymphoid hyperplasia of nasopharyngeal tissue and cervical node enlargement are frequently present grossly. Microscopically, the pattern runs the gamut from follicular hyperplasia to an effacement of lymphocytic and reticuloendothelial compartments in the corticomedullary areas occasionally resembling histologic changes of malignant lymphoma, but containing the atypical lymphocytic nuclear and cytoplasmic structures therein. Splenic changes are characterized by a soft pulpy structure with a thin, easily ruptured lymphocytic infiltrated capsule and trabeculae. The normal pattern is partially obscured and consists of normal and atypical lymphocytic infiltrates throughout with widely separated malpighian bodies. Perivascular abnormal and normal lymphocytes are seen in any and all tissue structures with associated periportal and subcapsular infiltrates associated with hepatomegaly and icterus. Skin rash and focal myocardial, pulmonary, renal, and central nervous system lesions are also seen. In the central nervous system lesions, meningoencephalitis occasionally develops, characterized by meningeal edema and congestion with mononuclear cells in the pia-arachnoid and perivascular spaces of intracerebral vessels. Guillain-Barré syndrome patients show swelling of the myelin sheath, and disruption and mononuclear cellular infiltration of the anterior nerve roots. Bone marrow fragments only occasionally show granulomatous lesions and lymphocytic infiltrates (possibly from sinusoidal dilution), but occasionally the cell pattern may be difficult to differentiate from leukemia.

Clinical Findings

Clinically, the disease is characterized by an incubation period varying from 2 to 3 days to 2 weeks, with early malaise, temperatures of 100 to 103° F, and sore throat and headache evident during the first 5 to 7 days. The pharyngitis may be delayed but finally observed with its associated injection, lymphoid hyperplasia, or membranous changes associated with petechiae in groups. Posterior and anterior cervical lymphadenopathy is prominent, with occasional other lymph nodes involved (axillary, inguinal, and mediastinal). Mesenteric lymphadenitis may simulate an acute condition within the abdomen. Firm, elastic, discrete nonsuppurating enlarged nodes may be associated with local heat and redness.

In half the cases, a splenomegaly of 2 to 3 cm. or more is found. Mild anicteric hepatitis associated with bilirubinemia frequently occurs, with or without hepatomegaly, between days 5 and 15 of the disease; rarely, acholic stools are seen. All types of exanthematous-like transient skin rashes may be seen, with a predominance of small pinkish to pinkish brown macular lesions involving the trunk and upper areas. Headache is common with rare cranial and peripheral nerve paralyses, nystagmus, toxic psychoses, ataxia, paresis of an extremity, papilledema, and skin hyperesthesias. Ascending paralysis with high cerebrospinal fluid protein may occur. Multiple peripheral nerve involvement and death are infrequently seen. Cardiac impairment and positive radiographic findings in the chest and associated bronchopulmonary symptoms are rare. Occasionally, red blood cells, albumin, and white blood cells are seen in the urine. Palpebral edema with narrowed visual fields may also occur. It is not uncommon for some degree of debility and lethargy to persist for two or three months after the acute symptoms have abated.

Hematologic Findings (Plates 47, 48)

The atypical lymphocytic pattern with associated small lymphocytes and monocytes appears by the fourth or fifth day and remains 2 to 10 weeks. In typical cases, the total leukocyte count may be normal or rise to 10,000 to 20,000 per cu.mm. with Downey cells seen in large numbers. Type I cells have oval, kidney-shaped or lobulated nuclei with vacuolated, foamy, and a granular cytoplasm; the nuclei of Type II cells have larger, less condensed nuclear chromatin and nonvacuolated more homogeneous cytoplasm; Type III nuclei contain one or two nucleoli and resemble lymphoblasts. Sixty to 90 per cent of mononuclear cells may be seen, although occasionally an excess of lymphocytes are seen in normal or leukopenic leukocyte counts.

Although the red blood cells and platelets are usually not involved, one may occasionally see acute hemolytic anemia[61, 192] with a positive or negative Coombs test as part of an autoimmune mechanism. Thrombocytopenia may possibly be similarly produced, and infectious mononucleosis may occur during remission of acute lymphocytic leukemia.[18] The bone marrow pattern shows a myeloid shift to the left with an increased number of myelocytes. Atypical lymphocytes are usually not present in the bone marrow; however, the myeloid hyperplasia may simulate the chronic myelocytic leukemic pattern at times.

Heterophil agglutinins (absorbed by beef erythrocyte antigen, but not completely by guinea pig antigen, which absorbs Forssman antibodies) appears from the first week. The highest titer usually occurs during the second to third week, and lasts up to 8 to 10 weeks. However, the initial appearance of the antibodies may be delayed beyond the first week, making repeated serologic testing important. The positive heterophil (Paul-Bunnell) test in typical clinical hematologic cases is diagnostic from 1:56 to 1:224 titer as minimum levels. Occasionally a nonspecific anamnestic elevation of heterophil antibodies occurs in unrelated illnesses. Another test approach reveals hemolysins against ox erythrocytes. Two recently described modifications of the Paul-Bunnel test are (1) a capillary 5-minute screening test for infectious mononucleosis[114] with a 98.7 per cent degree of sensitivity, and (2) a rapid 2-minute slide test for infectious mononucleosis[91] with a purported 99 per cent accuracy (Fig. 13-

14). Serologic false-positive tests for syphilis may occur in about 7 per cent of cases and may persist up to 2 to 3 months. The probability that these patients have a mixed infection (i.e., infectious mononucleosis together with syphilis) is about 33 per cent. In addition, a high proportion of infectious mononucleosis patients give a positive indirect Coomb's test, while anti-cold agglutinins (IgG and IgM) have been reported in 30 to 80 per cent. However, the direct Coomb's test is negative except when hemolytic anemia is present. In about 60 per cent of patients, rheumatoid factor (latex agglutination test) or antinuclear factors (immunofluorescence test) may be detected, while antiplatelet antibodies have also been reported in a small number (Fig. 13-15). Abnormal liver function tests (for example, the cephalin-cholesterol flocculation test, thymol turbidity test, the serum glutamic oxalic transaminase test, alkaline phosphatase, and the bromsulphalein excretion test) with associated hepatitis (with or without icterus) are fairly common, as are EKG changes with abnormal T-wave and prolonged P-R intervals. An elevated spinal fluid pressure with pleolymphocytosis may also be seen.

Differential Diagnosis

Because of its protean manifestations, infectious mononucleosis may be confused with febrile illnesses associated with typical and atypical lymphocytosis. The acute sore throat must be differentiated from streptococcal infection, aphthous stomatitis, diphtheria, and Vincent's angina. General infections with or without exanthemata may be confused with typhoid fever, brucellosis, influenza, measles, and others. Infectious hepatitis or homologous serum jaundice must also be differentiated. Neurologically, poliomyelitis, lymphocytic choriomeningitis, and encephalitis must be considered. Hematologically, leukemia or infectious lymphocytosis must be ruled out (the latter is not associated with lymphadenopathy, splenomegaly, atypical lymphocytes, or

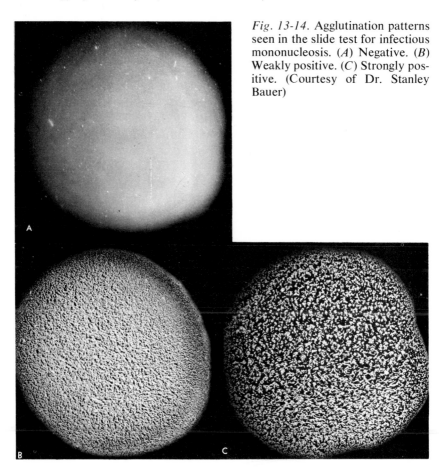

Fig. 13-14. Agglutination patterns seen in the slide test for infectious mononucleosis. (*A*) Negative. (*B*) Weakly positive. (*C*) Strongly positive. (Courtesy of Dr. Stanley Bauer)

positive serologic findings). Also, Epstein-Barr infections occasionally have hematologic patterns similar to those found in cytomegalovirus and adenovirus infections, measles, and toxoplasmosis. Since one-fourth of patients do not have Paul-Bunnell heterophil antibodies, serologic investigations are mandatory to rule out conditions that may simulate infectious mononucleosis. In addition, it is necessary to test for IgM antibody to EB virus or to assay for the increase or decrease in anti-EA (early antigen) titers in patients lacking Paul-Bunnel antibodies.

Treatment

The treatment of infectious mononucleosis is nonspecific. Secondary infections are treated with appropriate antimicrobial drugs; sore throat, with perborate mouth washes; analgesics and sedatives for fever and pain. Surgical intervention is indicated for abdominal pain and shock associated with splenic rupture. Steroids are given for tonsillar enlargement and glottic edema and rarely for the hemolytic and thrombocytopenic side reactions. Tracheotomy may be rarely indicated for tracheal occlusion. Liver complications are treated with diet and bed rest, and serial liver function tests are used to follow state of convalescence. Splenic rupture is to be avoided by careful splenic examination and enforced bed rest during the acute and convalescent periods. The prognosis is guarded when splenic rupture, neurologic sequelae, myocarditis, and glottic edema occur because they may be life-threatening. Infectious mononucleosis

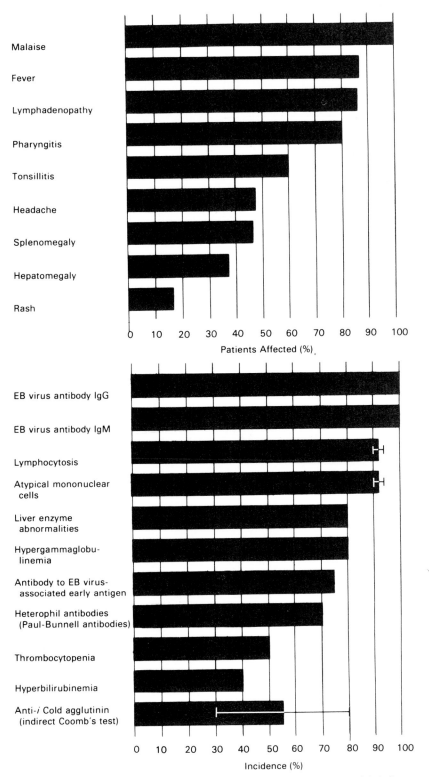

Fig. 13-15. (Top) Clinical features commonly found in patients with infectious mononucleosis are ranked in order of their frequency. Malaise is not only universally present but is likely to persist longest, after acute symptoms wane (usually within a month). (Bottom) Graph shows relative incidence of most common laboratory findings. (Courtesy of P. Lai, M.D.)

usually is characterized by a benign course, but fever lasts 1 to 3 weeks and may exacerbate with the usual postconvalescent asthenia, debility, and lethargy persisting for 2 to 3 months. Complete recovery usually occurs, and neurologic residuals are rare.

INFECTIOUS LYMPHOCYTOSIS

Infectious lymphocytosis is a benign, infectious, and contagious specific disease entity of unknown etiology occurring sporadically or in epidemic form. The incubation period is 12 to 21 days, and the disease is characterized by a hyperleukocytosis of small mature lymphocytes persisting for 2 to 7 weeks with mild or marked constitutional reaction without lymphadenopathy or splenomegaly.

Clinical Findings

The patients are usually 1 to 10 years of age, but infectious lymphocytosis may occur in young adults as multiple sporadic cases in families and in institutional epidemics with occasional associated upper respiratory and gastrointestinal distress (diarrhea). The leukocyte count ranges from 15,000 to 140,000 per cu.mm. with 63 to 97 per cent lymphocytes. Lymph nodes show a proliferation of lining reticuloendothelium with almost complete blockage of the sinuses by masses of these lymphocytic cells and degeneration of the lymph follicles. Occasionally fever, skin rashes and meningoencephalitic manifestations may be present. A deeply injected throat, upper respiratory tract infection, headache, irritability, and meningism may simulate polio, but it is differentiated by the high leukocyte count observed in infectious lymphocytosis. Clinically, infectious lymphocytosis must be differentiated from infectious mononucleosis (15 to 30 years of age, lymphadenopathy, splenomegaly, atypical lymph, and positive heterophil agglutination), acute lymphoblastic leukemia (10 to 20 years of age, fever, anemia, enlarged lymph nodes, splenomegaly, peripheral blood lymphoblasts, bone marrow lymphoblasts, and fatal outcome) and chronic lymphocytic leukemia (after 45 years of age, no fever, anemia, splenomegaly, lymphadenopathy, lymphocytes in bone marrow, and fatal outcome).

Hematologic Findings

The erythrocyte count, hemoglobin level, platelet count, and sedimentation rate are usually normal. The leukocyte count averages 40,000 to 50,000 per cu.mm. with 60 to 97 per cent mature lymphocytes whose nuclear chromatin is dark purple and of an overripe type. The duration of infectious lymphocytosis is 3 to 7 weeks, and the percentage of eosinophils is elevated usually at or following the peak of leukocytosis. The bone marrow shows normal myeloid and erythroid patterns with an increase in the total number of nucleated cells—that is, the percentage of small mature lymphocytes. The heterophil agglutination test is negative.

AGRANULOCYTOSIS (IMMUNE OR TOXIC NEUTROPENIA)

Agranulocytosis, an acute disease complex, is characterized by marked leukopenia and severe neutropenia with suddenly developing high temperature, chills, prostration, and oral, rectal and vaginal ulcerations. Septicemia is usually secondary to bacterial tissue infiltration. The disorder was first described by Werner Schultz[173] in 1922; then Kracke[107] in 1931 emphasized the relationship of the symptoms with the ingestion of drugs containing coal tar derivatives, especially in Germany and the United States. A hypersensitivity mechanism was later described by Madison and Squier,[121] Plum,[151] and others as the modus operandi of these drugs, especially amidopyrine. This was confirmed experimentally by Moeschlin.[132] Many other drugs have since been listed as suspected offenders in the production of agranulocytotic states.

Etiology

Sequentially, after the offending drugs and chemicals are ingested, 7 to 14 days, to weeks or months may pass by before sensitization and subsequent neutropenia develop to be followed by the appearance of infection. Amidopyrine-induced agranulocytosis occurs in a very small percentage of patients taking the drug (more common in females in a 2 to 3:1 ratio). However, in recovered patients, a single dose may produce an exacerbation. Moeschlin's experiments using amidopyrine revealed phenomena of immune agglutinative lysis, both in vitro and in vivo, of homologous and heterologous neutrophils, occurring perhaps largely in the lungs. Leukocyte agglutinins were also reported in conjunction with hemolytic anemia, with elevated cold agglutinin titers in virus pneumonia, in infectious mononucleosis, in Felty's syndrome, and other disorders. Although the amidopyrine agglutinins developed in the plasma of the sensitized patient, this plasma administered to the same patient or another patient, or tested in a test tube revealed clumping and subsequent lysis of the neutrophils soon thereafter.

No leukoagglutinins or leukolysins could be demonstrated in chlorpromazine neutropenia; only temporary aplasia occurs after ingestion of chlorpromazine. Peripheral granulocyte destruction and not marrow depression therefore must be a factor in the production of agranulocytosis. The marrow findings of maturation arrest, with a reduced percentage of myeloid elements (granulocytes) beyond the myelocyte stage, suggest exhaustion and depletion of the bone marrow in response to excessive peripheral leukocyte destruction and in response to damage of precursor granulocytic marrow elements by either the same or a different mechanism from that resulting in extramarrow leukocyte destruction. Drugs involved include amidopyrine, sulfa drugs, gold compounds, Tridione, phenylbutazone, thiouracil, propylthiouracil, dini-

trophenol, organic arsenicals, phenothiazine, chloramphenicol, chlorpromazine, pyribenzamine, quinine, acetanilid, barbiturates, Plasmochin, Apresoline, mercurial diuretics, procaine amide, and DDT. Although drugs and some infections produce most of the cases of agranulocytosis, there are some instances in which no recognizable agent can be etiologically related.

Pathology and Clinical Findings
(Plates 49, 50)

The pathologic findings include necrotic ulcerative dermal, oral, vaginal, and rectal lesions that are devoid of neutrophils, but full of bacteria. Abscesses form during hematologic remission. The bone marrow then shows a reduction in or absence of myelocytes and metamyelocytes with normal proportions of erythroid and megakaryocytic elements. Later, or in milder cases, there may be normal or hyperplastic granulopoiesis with a reduced number of polymorphonuclear cells, but excess quantities of myelocytes and metamyelocytes. Clinically, there is a sudden episode of chills, elevation of temperature and prostration, which is frequently associated with the developing neutropenia and therefore may be due to the agglutinogen-agglutinin reaction, followed by a period of rapid granulocytic destruction (a similar process may be seen after repeated transfusions due to agglutinins against homologous leukocytes in transfused blood). This process then recurs with associated headache, chills, fever, sepsis, and necrotic gray membrane ulcerations of mouth, vagina, and rectum. Finally, septicemia and bacteremia occur with a temperature of 104 to 105° F and associated mental confusion, stupor, and death from severe infection. Pyuria and bacilluria with abscess formation may occur if the polymorphonuclear cells return. Regional tender lymphadenopathy, splenomegaly, icterus, bone pain, pneumonitis, hypotension, and hyperventilation may supervene.

Hematologically, the leukocyte count ranges from 1000 to 4000 per cu.mm. with practically no neutrophils seen. The polymorphonuclear cells present show pyknotic nuclei, cytoplasmic vacuolization, and toxic granulation. The erythrocyte count and platelet count usually remain normal. Agranulocytosis persists for 5 to 10 days with the same marrow picture of maturation arrest described previously. The myelocytes and metamyelocytes return to the marrow before the polymorphonuclear cells appear in the peripheral blood and other tissues. Often the peripheral blood may show a few myelocytes (10–15%), and transient monocytosis may precede the return of normal white blood cells to be followed by leukocytosis.

Differential Diagnosis

One must consider aplastic anemia and aleukemic leukemia, both of which show peripheral blood anemia and thrombocytopenia plus a marrow pattern of leukemic cells in the latter and cytologic aplasia and hypoplasia in the former. Irradiation damage and toxic depression of the white blood cell series are associated with a history of exposure and the presence of multiple cytopenias. Infectious mononucleosis shows atypical lymphocytes, different bone marrow findings, and a positive heterophil agglutination test. Lymphoma, subacute bacterial endocarditis, and miliary tuberculosis have underlying disease findings. Drug or chemical history is often diagnostic.

Treatment

With early and proper antimicrobial therapy, and sometimes transfusions if anemia is present, most patients recover without residual hematopoietic damage. If no anemia is present, WBC mass (HLA-typed, preferably) transfusions may be used, provided no untoward reactions occur. Leukocyte counts below 1000 per cu.mm. in patients under 60 still indicate a grave condition. Associated with therapy is immediate withdrawal of the drug or chemical involved. Repeat cultures of ulcerated areas, blood, urine, and occasional cerebrospinal fluid determinations, with specific sensitivity testing, affords knowledge of the best antimicrobial agent to use. Usually the infected area is cultured first. Without waiting for results, 2,000,000 units of aqueous penicillin G, divided into four daily doses, and 0.5 g. of steptomycin are given every 12 hours intramuscularly. When bacterial sensitivities are known, the specific antibiotic agent is then used. Steroids may further depress resistance to infection, mask complications, and worsen the clinical condition. Dimercaprol may be used for neutropenia due to gold or arsenic, mouth washes are frequently used, constipation and anal abrasions are avoided and parenteral fluids are given if necessary.

LEUKEMIAS

Leukemias are general diseases of unknown etiology, usually characterized by qualitative and quantitative alterations in peripheral blood leukocytes and associated with a diffuse, abnormal, self-perpetuating growth of leukocyte precursors in the bone marrow and frequently in other hematopoietic tissues that eventually leads to anemia, thrombocytopenia, and death. It has not been definitely ascertained whether the lymphocytic leukemic processes originate from bone marrow lymphoid tissue or in extramedullary lymphoid tissues and secondarily infiltrate the bone marrow. This becomes apparent in comparison with the non-Hodgkin lymphoma group, which probably begins in lymph nodes and then subsequently may be associated with a blood pattern very similar to acute or chronic lymphocytic leukemia. Leukosarcoma or chronic lymphocytic lymphosarcoma is a term now used to name a known lymphomatous phase preceding blood invasion. The lymphoid group also includes hairy cell leukemia (leukemic reticuloendotheliosis), in which the monocytic-lymphocytic features are observed, and in

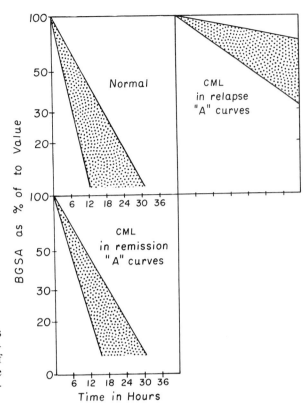

Fig. 13-16. Survival time of granulocytes in chronic myelocytic (granulocytic) leukemia. (Boggs, D. R., et al.: The effect of adrenal glucocorticosteroids upon the cellular composition of inflammatory exudates. Am. J. Pathol., *44:*763, 1964)

which there is some doubt as to the originating tissue. Also included in the leukemias are the red blood cell progenitor type (erythroleukemia) and the thrombocyte precursor variety (megakaryocytic leukemia). The proliferation rate (generation time) of single leukemic cells usually is slower than that for their normal counterparts; however, the massive total quantity of proliferating cells leads to an overall increase in WBC production. Some recent workers believe that a decreased rate of leukocytic cell removal or destruction may also be involved and possibly account for the increased leukocyte body mass (Fig. 13-16).

Classification

There are several ways of classifying the leukemias. They may be classified according to the *course* of the disease: (1) *Acute leukemia*, in which very primitive cell types predominate, and the life expectancy is usually 6 months or less. This type is frequently called stem-cell leukemia because blast forms may be too immature to allow any more specific label. (2) In *subacute leukemia*, a 6- to 12-month life duration may be expected, but there is a tendency for the disorder to be more acute than chronic in duration and also in cell maturity. (3) In *chronic leukemia*, the life expectancy is 12 months or more. Differentiation of acute from chronic leukemia is made preferably on the degree of predominant cell immaturity in the peripheral blood and bone marrow.

A second way in which the leukemias may be classified is according to *blood picture*, possibly related to cellular maturity, which often parallels the course and duration of the disease and correlated with the peripheral white blood cell count (e.g., *leukemic, subleukemic* and *aleukemic*). In the more common leukemic blood picture, the total white blood cell count is usually over 15,000 to 20,000 white blood cells per cu.mm. and there are immature lymphocytic and granulocytic cells in the peripheral blood. In the subleukemic pattern, the white blood cell may be normal or less than normal, but there are sufficient immature lymphocytes and granulocytes in the peripheral blood to suggest a diagnosis. In the aleukemic type, the peripheral leukocytic count is less than normal and there are no immature granulocytes or lymphocytes present.

Another way to classify leukemia is by *cell type* — that is, according to the identity and site of origin of the predominant cell type. Examples include: (1) *myelocytic leukemia* (myelogenous, myeloblastic, granulocytic); (2) *lymphocytic leukemia* (lymphogenous, lymphatic), which is normally found in nodes, but in the leukemia phase, the lymphatic cells are also seen in the marrow — in this group hairy cell leukemia (leukemia reticuloendotheliosis may be included with its doubtful origin and lymphocytic-monocytic features; (3) *monocytic leukemia,* of which there are two types. In the *Schilling type,* the monocyte develops from reticulum cells, histiocytic or clasmatocytic. In the *Naegeli type* (myelomonocytic), monocytes develop from myeloblasts. Some hematologists believe there is only one form of monocytic leukemia — that is, the abnormal proliferation involves monoblasts, and variations found in the clinical and hematologic patterns are part of the disease complex development variation; (4) *plasmacytic* (myeloma), *megakaryocytic,* and *erythroid leukemias.*

Theories of Etiology

The *infective* concept of etiology includes the oncogenic viruses, which may produce chromosomal abnormalities in laboratory animals — for example, fowl leukosis and mouse leukemia in certain strains.[129] Viruses may also evoke malignant transformations in tissue culture. In addition, cell-free extracts of brain tissue from human patients dying from leukemia, when injected into a spontaneously leukemic strain of mice, have been reported to hasten the development of leukemia. The electron microscopic study of blast cells in some patients with acute leukemia reveal virus-like particles. However, all laboratory evidence to date fails to reveal convincing evidence of a virus-like spread of leukemia in man. In fact, attempts to transmit human leukemia to other patients by cross-transfusion of bone marrow and other tissue injection have met with failure. However, it is still possible that an oncogenic virus may be present in a latent form in many persons, and that they become activated by irradiation, certain chemical cell poisons, and other unrecognized influences. Recent reports of familial transmission of acute leukemia[86] and myeloproliferative disease[160] help lend support to the concept of a viral etiology. In addition, the demonstration of reverse transcriptase in human leukemic cells seems to suggest the involvement of an "oncornavirus." WBCs (not normal) in human leukemic patients possess RNA nucleotide sequences like those observed in murine and simian oncornaviruses. Still, the etiology of human leukemia remains unknown.

Neoplastic and *irradiation* theories of leukemia development are based on current knowledge consistent with interpretation that the continuing reaction recognized as neoplasia or cancer involves some kind of damage to or interference with the basic stuff of life — namely, the nucleic acids, which program or implement the vital activities of all living cells. After sporadic case reports of leukemia in radiation workers and the experimental induction of the disease by exposing mice to radiographs, epidemiologic studies revealed that human leukemia can be radiation-induced. Most convincing in this regard have been the data from the survivors of the atomic bombing of Hiroshima and Nagasaki, among whom the leukemia rates were proportionate to the radiation dose received. Other studies indicate that sufficiently large partial-body exposures of radiation therapy are also leukemogenic. It is less certain that intrauterine exposures to diagnostic radiation can induce childhood leukemia. For the first time, a decline in leukemia mortality rates for the white population of the United States between the ages of 1 and 74 has been observed recently. Possible explanations include diminished exposure to medical radiographs following the release in the United States and Great Britain in 1956 of widely publicized reports on the biologic effects of ionizing radiation.[65]

Another development has been the addition of an *immunologic* concept in the proliferative etiology of leukemias.[168] Phytohemagglutinin (PHA), a substance derived from the jack bean, produces an effect on lymphocytes in vitro analogous to that produced by antigenic material in vivo. This serves to provide a model of normal lymphocytic response and also helps to elucidate the reaction of abnormal, particularly leukemic, lymphocytes. Because infectious mononucleosis (IM) and chronic lymphocytic leukemia (CLL) represent two types of proliferative disorders involving cells of the immunocyte complex, PHA was added, in vitro, to the peripheral lymphocytes isolated from patients with IM and CLL. Different growth patterns accompanied by specific alterations in nucleic acid metabolism were produced. Also, after exposure to PHA, normal mature lymphocytes are transformed through dedifferentiation into large, apparently immature blast cells, while no such transformation occurs in leukemic lymphocytes. These findings provide further proof that CLL is a disease of immunologically atypical and frequently incompetent lymphocytes and also helps to explain the accumulation of abnormal lymphocytes in large masses throughout the body.

Specific factors involved in the causes of leukemia include the extent to which *genetic* or *familial* (chromosomal) factors play a part in the etiology of human leukemia, factors which at present are uncertain. However, these prenatal influences are important in childhood leukemia. For example, the high degree of concurrence of mongolism and leukemia in the same child was recognized by epidemiologic studies before laboratory research revealed that in mongolism there is a visible chromosomal abnormality (trisomy-21) that may cause or predispose to leukemia. Common to mongolism, miscarriages, and childhood leukemia are (1) cytogenetic factors, (2) an increasing frequency as maternal age increases at childbirth, and (3) the tendency, small as far as mongolism and childhood leukemia are concerned, for multiple cases to occur in a sibship. One might also mention the detection of the Philadelphia (Ph') chromosome (Fig. 13-17) in certain patients with chronic myelogeneous leukemia.[137]

A recent study on marrow chromosomes of 23 preleukemic patients (13 with myeloproliferative syndrome and 10 with intractable anemia, leukopenia, or pancytopenia) revealed that five of 17 patients with a chromosome abnormality in the marrow died of leukemia in 3 months. Only two of 13 patients with marrow chromosome changes developed leukemia when followed up to 26 months. Therefore, a positive marrow chromosome study in an unirradiated preleukemic patient suggests that a leukemic phase is imminent. A negative study may indicate a protracted nonleukemic course.[135] However, bone marrow cytogenetic studies utilizing more advanced techniques are needed to establish whether specific chromosomal patterns that have unique prognostic significance exist, and whether they can be used to separate early leukemias from chronic myeloproliferative disorders such as agnogenic myeloid metaplasia, in which cytogenetic abnormalities may not carry the same ominous significance.[136]

Other laboratory techniques should also

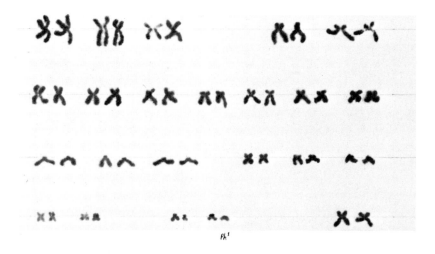

Fig. 13-17. Philadelphia chromosome (see Ph¹ in illustration). (Nowell, P. C., and Hungerford, D. A.: A minute chromosome in human granulocytic leukemia. Science, *132:*1497, 1960)

be considered in the recognition of the preleukemic state, colony-forming cell assays, cytochemistry, cell-enzyme studies, and electron microscopy. Finally, it is quite essential that one knows the natural history of the preleukemic state in order to determine whether the risks of therapy are warranted. The prospective study of suspected preleukemic patients suggests that this

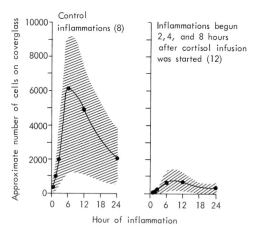

Fig. 13-18. Effects of steroids on granulocytes in inflammation. (Athens, J. W., et al.: Leukokinetic studies. X. Blood granulocyte kinetics in chronic myelocytic leukemia. J. Clin. Invest., *44:*765, 1965)

"preleukemic phase" of acute myelocytic leukemia is a serious situation and may lead to the patient's demise even in the absence of overt leukemic transition. Therefore, attempts to develop effective low-risk therapy protocols are indicated for patients with identified preleukemic disorders.

Various *chemical agents,* such as benzol, that damage bone marrow have also been etiologically associated with leukemia. Perhaps this damage is related to the aforementioned concept of abnormal chromosomal development, leading eventually to preleukemia and finally leukemia itself. *Hormonal* abnormalities or disordered metabolic functions have also been implicated in some experiments on leukemia production—that is, specific substances that produce myeloid and lymphoid maturation animals have been extracted from the urine of patients with leukemia.[126] Data have also been obtained supporting the concept that the failure of cell maturation in patients with leukemia is associated with a loss of factors that inhibit cell proliferation. Further evidence along the line of hormonal factors is work suggesting the isolation of a granulocytosis-promoting factor from CE 1460 tumors (possibly related to leukopoietin),

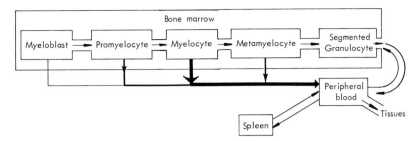

Fig. 13-19. Leukocyte kinetics concept in CML patients.

which is capable of inducing permeation of the spleen with large undifferentiated myeloid cells and the formation of multiple small foci of both immature and mature granulocytic forms in the liver.[46]

Recent leukokinetic studies reveal a marked delay in the generation time of myelocytes in acute myelocytic leukemia; the intermitotic interval in acute leukemia could be many times longer than that of normal precursors and still support a large number of potentially proliferative cells.[20] Athens and co-workers conclude that prolonged granulocyte survival in chronic leukemia and myelofibrosis is mainly attributable to the young age of the labeled cells.[9] These data, therefore, add support to the growing suspicion that the accumulation of long-lived, poorly-matured cells accounts for much of the deadly increase in leukocyte mass in leukemia (Fig. 13-18). A model (Fig. 13-19) for leukocyte kinetics in patients with chronic myelocytic leukemia (CML) reveals a newer concept.[147] In some acute leukemia patients, this prolonged cell survival, rather than an increased rate of proliferation, appears to be the principal mechanism.

PATHOLOGY OF LEUKEMIAS

In the United States, about 40 per cent of leukemias are acute. The acute lymphocytic type usually occurs during ages 1 to 20; from ages 20 to 45 chronic myelocytic leukemia is most common, and after 45 years of age chronic lymphocytic leukemia

predominates (approximately $2/3$–$3/4$ in males). The most common cell predominates in the peripheral blood and bone marrow, with associated marked replacement of normal bone marrow by the specific leukemic cell type. There is subsequent reduction in erythroid and megakaryocytic elements. The peripheral blood mirrors these changes by leukocytosis, the presence of a large number of mature or immature myeloid, monocytic, or lymphocytic cells, as a predominating type in most instances, with associated anemia and thrombocytopenia. Occasionally, there is an increase in the megakaryocytes early in chronic myelocytic leukemia.

The marrow pattern is altered and even reversed after spontaneous and therapeutic remission, the marrow itself showing an almost normal cytologic makeup. The lymph nodes and spleen show lymphocytic proliferation in the lymphocytic leukemias. In the other leukemias there is infiltration, and possibly de novo leukemic cellular changes in some cases. Other symptoms and signs in the leukemias result from infiltration, hemorrhage, or infection involving any portion of the body. The liver, spleen, and lymph nodes are most commonly involved by proliferation or infiltration with subsequent tumor production in these organs, resulting in associated pressure effects and the interference with function of these and adjacent organs. When osseous and surrounding structures are involved, the infiltrate may have a greenish color (chloroma).

The modified classification of leukemia,

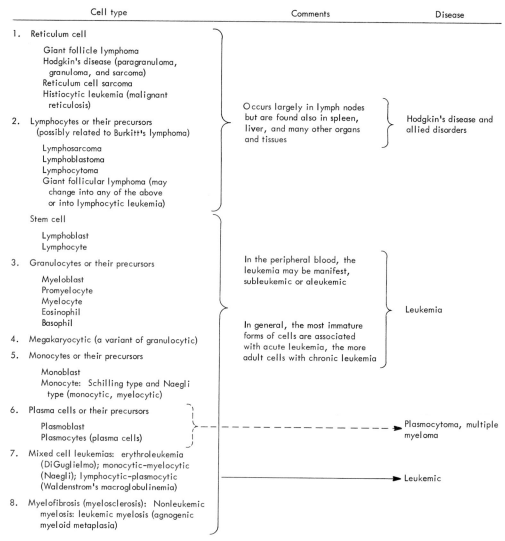

Fig. 13-20. Modified classification of leukemia, Hodgkin's disease, and allied disorders, using early nomenclature. (Page, L. B., and Culver, P. J.: Syllabus of Laboratory Examinations in Clinical Diagnosis. Cambridge, Harvard University Press, 1960)

Hodgkin's disease, and allied disorders shown in Figure 13-20 might be of some help in visualizing their close relationship.[142]

Strict criteria to define the subgroups of acute leukemia have recently been proposed. These are based on the premise that more direct and specific therapy would result in more accurate prognoses and longer remissions.[78] French, American, and British workers in one study state that the clinician and morphologist both assume that the morphologic differences on which classifications are based reflect basic biologic differences in the acute leukemias. By means of histochemical techniques and more specialized methods, such as electron microscopy, cytogenetics, and biochemical and immunologic markers, specific, significant, differentiating morphologic features have been sought and proposed. For example, the primary granules of the granulocytic series contain myeloproxidase and stain with Sudan Black B, factors that might be helpful in distinguishing undifferentiated leukemias. That is, in theory, uniform and constant assignment of positive cases to the myeloid category and of negative cases to the non-myeloid category should be possible. Ever since the classification was proposed, it has appeared increasingly probable that even in cells lacking lymphocyte markers, some still belong to a lymphoid-committed cell line, because they contain the enzyme terminal deoxynucleotidyl transferase. From these and other observations, it is obvious that morphology alone cannot provide evidence of the nature of undifferentiated blasts. Some types of what is currently called lymphoblastic leukemia may later prove to involve truly undifferentiated stem cells not yet committed to differentiation along either the lymphoid or myeloid pathway. The three categories of lymphoblastic leukemia are designated by the French, American, and British workers as L1 (exemplified by the common childhood type), L2 (the heterogeneous group, more common in adults), and L3 (the rare homogeneous group, with the cytomorphology of Burkett's lymphoma).

Blast-cell leukemias of myeloid origin, arising from a stem cell committed for differentiation along one or more of the granulocytic, monocytic, or erythrocytic pathways, have long been known to show marked morphologic variation. Some variants have distinctive hematologic features, and some have particular clinical manifestations (e.g. gum hypertrophy and skin infiltrates with monocytic and myelomonocytic leukemia, and the association of promyelocytic leukemia and intravascular coagulation). However, current chemotherapy schedules are not especially effective in most forms of acute myeloblastic leukemia. In an effort to be more specific in diagnosis and prognosis in this blast-leukemia group,

the French, American, and British group defined three variants of acute myeloid leukemia showing predominantly granulocytic differentiation: M1 as those with minimal evidence of differentiation, but no maturation along the granulocyte pathway; M2 as those showing clear evidence of maturation to the promyelocyte stages and beyond; M3 as those in which highly abnormal cells, packed with abnormal azurophilic granules or with numerous Auer rods, showing characteristic nuclear abnormalities (also called "hypergranular promyelocytic leukemia" and regularly associated with disseminated intravascular coagulation); M4 as the mixed and heterogeneous myelomonocytic leukemia or an associated form characterized by an essentially monocytic picture in the peripheral blood but a minimal monocytic component in the marrow; M5 as the "pure" monocytic leukemia which exists in two forms – in one, almost all the cells are blast, whereas in the other, a high proportion of the cells have matured beyond the promonocyte stage, at least in the peripheral blood; M6 as erythroleukemia and associated with a high proportion of bone marrow pronormoblasts, the severe dyserythropoiesis mirrored also by the appearance of many pronormoblasts in the peripheral blood. All of the above refer to blood and marrow samples from untreated patients and are not valid if they are applied to treated patients (Plate 51). An unequivocal diagnosis of acute leukemia may be made only when the lower limit of the combined percentage of blasts and promyelocytes is on the high side of 50 per cent. Acute leukemia usually occurs in dysmyelopoietic states (acquired idiopathic sideroblastic anemia, refractory anemia with excess of blasts, chronic myelomonocytic leukemia, aplastic anemia, paroxysmal nocturnal hemoglobinuria and bone marrow failure with cellular marrow) after a long static period; whereas the early stage of acute myeloid leukemia becomes apparent and clear after only a few weeks or months of observation.

Finally, many children and adults (approximately 75%) lack readily demonstrable B- or T-markers and are classified as having "null-acute lymphocytic leukemia." This is further differentiated into childhood (L1) and adult (L2) forms based on differences not only in the age of the patient, but also blast-cell morphology, reactivity with an antinull acute lymphocytic leukemia serum, clinical features, and response to treatment. This group and T-cell acute lymphocytic leukemia group are further characterized by the finding of high concentrations of terminal deoxynucleotidyl transferase; low levels of this enzyme are found in acute myeloid leukemia patients. The T-ALL (acute lymphocytic leukemia) group also is characterized by a positive acid-phosphatase stain, the presence of an anterior mediastinal mass, high leukocyte count, and high incidence in an older age group. The null-ALL group was also acid-phosphatase negative. In contrast to non-Hodgkin's lymphoma, B-cells are seldom seen in acute lymphocytic leukemia, and they probably represent the leukemic phase of poorly differentiated lymphomas. There are two morphologic types, the Burkitt type and the lymphosarcoma type. The former is more common in children and young adults and probably corresponds to the advanced stage of the so-called non-African sporadic or nonendemic Burkitt's lymphoma. In those patients, a leukemic evolution (bone marrow, blood, and central nervous system) is much more common than it is in African patients. Cells of the lymphosarcoma type, which are usually seen in patients older than 50 years of age, often are extremely undifferentiated by morphologic criteria.

The term "non-lymphocytic leukemia" includes all the French, American, and British group types M1 through M6. The confirming cytochemical stains show PAS positivity in circulating leukocytes; positive myeloperoxidase granulocytes and monocytes, but absent in lymphocytes (therefore in acute lymphocytic leukemia, the blast cells are peroxidase-negative, and when more than 3% of blast cells are positive, a patient is classified as having nonacute lymphocytic leukemia). Also, all patients with acute myeloid and acute myelomonocytic leukemia are peroxidase-positive, and 50 per cent of patients with acute monocytic leukemia are peroxidase-positive. With a nonspecific cytoplasmic esterase stain (naphthol-ASD acetate), acute monocytic leukemia cells invariably give an intense reaction that is strikingly reduced by sodium fluoride incubation (Plate 52).

It is difficult to determine whether a patient has a true acute myeloid leukemia or refractory anemia with excess of blasts. For practical purposes, continual and repeated examinations of blood and bone marrow are necessary. In patients with acute myeloid leukemia, myeloblastic proliferation becomes predominant after a relatively short time. In refractory anemia with excess of blasts, the hematologic condition remains relatively steady for many months or years without evidence of acute myeloid leukemia. There is now general agreement that all forms of leukemic chemotherapy must be avoided in this syndrome unless the patient has overt leukemia.[55]

ACUTE LEUKEMIAS

Clinical Findings

Clinical findings in acute leukemias are characterized by the usually abrupt onset in the younger age groups associated with fever, pallor, bone or joint pain, skin or mucous membrane bleeding, prostration, sudden lymphadenopathy, or oral cavity ulceration. In adults, one usually sees a more gradual development of symptoms, frequently preceded by a history of upper respiratory infection. This is followed by anorexia, pallor, progressive weakness, low-grade fever, prostration, and other symptoms—all within a 1- to 2-month period. Most of these findings are due to the proliferation and infiltration of leukemic cells in the peripheral blood and bone marrow with subsequent anemia, hemorrhage, and infection. The fever may be of any type and is frequently related to infection in the respiratory tract, kidneys, or blood stream, or to ulcerative processes. Pathogenic, nonpathogenic, and widespread mycotic infections occur – the latter two in patients with diminished host resistance and associated with therapy involving antimicrobial drugs, adrenal steroids, and antileukemic agents.

If the temperature elevation is not related to infection, it may be presumed to be due to the increased metabolic state of these patients, to excessive leukemic cell turnover, to normal cell necrosis, or to viral disease. Pallor or anemia may be attributed to one or more of the following: the failure of marrow red blood cell production to compensate for shortened erythrocyte survival,[22] a hemolytic component, an absolute reduction in erythrocytic production, and hemorrhage. The anemia, if severe, is accompanied by dyspnea, cardiac dilatation, and cardiac failure associated with high output. The manifestations of thrombocytopenia and bleeding usually are related (thrombocyte levels less than 25,000/cu.mm.). Occasionally the bleeding can be attributed to prolonged clotting time, a reduction in Factor V, active fibrinolysis, and, rarely, to a circulating anticoagulant.

Physical Findings

Among the physical findings is lymph node enlargement, commonly observed in the lymphocytic type, especially in about $1/3$ of patients, and also in the myelocytic type. The lymph nodes are discrete, soft or firm, tender, and approximately 2 to 4 cm. in size. This produces symptoms of pressure or abdominal pain in specific areas. The thymus, tonsils, or anterior mediastinal nodes may also enlarge and press on adjacent structures with or without hepatosplenomegaly of 2 to 3 cm. When the retroperitoneal space, facial bones, and ovaries are involved, Burkitt's lymphoma versus acute lymphocytic leukemia must be considered.[60]

Petechiae, purpura, and ecchymoses are frequently observed. In the monocytic and myelocytic forms, blisters, necrotic areas, or plaques with abscesses and associated regional lymphadenitis are seen. Nasal and oral bleeding and ulceration are also observed. The gums become swollen, spongy, and hyperplastic in the acute monocytic type. Retinal and conjunctival hemorrhages also occur in 75 to 90 per cent of cases. Subarachnoid and intracerebral hemorrhage may occur in thrombocytopenic patients with associated blastic crises and leukocytoses over 90,000 to 120,000 per cu.mm.

Leukemic infiltrations may consist of retrobulbar greenish (chloromatous) nodules, which occasionally lead to exophthalmos; pulmonary infiltrates with or without pleural effusion; gastrointestinal leukemic cell invasion, which leads to pain or ulceration; the formation of perirectal abscesses; genitourinary tract involvement with renomegaly and rarely priapism; and fetal death, if associated with pregnancy. Subperiosteal infiltration may occur producing bone and joint pain similar to that of arthritis, with subperiosteal or intramedullary nodules resulting in pathologic fractures. Sternal tenderness can be present. Meningeal (especially in males, usually with the lymphocytic type), cranial nerve, and spinal nerve root involvement may be associated with neurologic findings – for example, peripheral neuritis, ocular movement, and deafness. If the brainstem is involved, there may be an obstruction of cerebrospinal fluid flow with subsequent hydrocephalus and such associated signs and symptoms as pleocytosis and occasionally hypothalamic symptoms.

Hematologic Findings

The blood pattern in acute leukemia is that of a normochromic, normocytic anemia and thrombocytopenia; this varies in degree in each case. Leukocytosis occurs in 65 per cent, leukopenia in 20 per cent, and normal leukocyte counts in 15 per cent of cases. Eighty-five to ninety-five per cent of lymphocytic-like stem to blast cells are seen in the peripheral blood. Occasionally only a rare abnormal form is seen when the leukocyte count is normal. Sternal or iliac crest marrow aspirates show almost solid masses of young leukemic cell types with occasional normal nucleated red blood cells, megakaryocytes, or granulocytes, except during early acute myelocytic and monocytic leukemia, when normal erythropoiesis with megaloblastic-like cells are seen.

In this blood dyscrasia, the abnormality is present in the cell and not in the environment, a concept suggested by the findings in blood or marrow cultures in vitro. That is to say, when normal blood cells are cultured in semisolid media, colonies of 50 to 2000 neutrophils, eosinophils, or monocytes are produced within 10 days. Contrasted with those found when acute granulocytic patient blood cells are cultured, the cultures may reveal no growth, abnormally large numbers of clones or clusters (colonies of less than 50 cells), or occasionally large colonies of immature cells. The most logical theory explaining normal cell production failure is twofold; the clone of leukemic stem cells does not mature and the clone itself inhibits maturation and growth of residual normal stem cells. Therefore, studies of cytogenetic patterns in remission cases appear to demonstrate regrowth of normal cells rather than maturation of leukemic cells.

Acute Granulocytic Leukemia
(Plates 53, 54)

Acute granulocytic leukemia is specifically characterized by myeloblast nuclei that have fine vesicular reticulated noncondensed chromatin without nuclear membrane, but with one or more light grayish-blue nucleoli. There is a thin rim of homogeneous basophilic cytoplasm present without specific granules but with occasional azurophilic granules. Promyelocytes, myelocytes, and metamyelocytes are scarce,

producing a leukemic hiatus. If these cells are present with splenomegaly but without thrombocytopenia or purpura, then patients with symptoms of several months probably have an acute exacerbation of a chronic leukemia. The cell type (granulocytic, monocytic, or lymphocytic) is determined (from blood films using Wright's stain) by "the company (myelocyte, polymorphonuclear cell, monocyte or lymphocyte) the blast cells keep." Occasionally the presence of specific granules is determined in promyelocytes and myelocytes by the use of supravital or peroxidase stains. Auer bodies may help to identify the type of leukemia because they are found only in acute myelocytic or acute monocytic leukemia. These are reddish, peroxidase-positive, rodlike, homogeneous, crystalline cytoplasmic inclusions with blunt or pointed ends resembling acid-fast slivers. They are probably formed by granule coalescence and are found in the cytoplasm of myeloblasts and occasionally in myelocytes and monocytes. Bone marrow films show marrow and fat replacement with diffuse infiltration by undifferentiated blast cells. After therapy (remission), the marrow may appear normal. The morphologic variants of acute myeloid leukemia have mixed clinical differences, higher frequency of gum infiltration in the monocytic subgroups and the increased incidence of disseminated intravascular coagulation with the promyelocytic variant. Among the variegated morphologic subtypes, there is really no difference in prognosis or therapeutic response; infection is usually the cause of death with the chief clinical findings associated with a paucity of normal blood cells.

Acute Lymphocytic Leukemia
(Plates 55, 56)

In acute lymphocytic leukemia, the lymphoblast nuclei have condensed, thick nuclear membrane edges with coarser, granular, or stippled nuclear chromatin containing one to four indistinct nucleoli and frequent clear perinuclear zone with thin basophilic agranular homogeneous cytoplasm. Occasionally, the lymphoblasts show nuclear indentations, deep nuclear clefts or unusual lobulation. Nucleoli are usually present even in mature lymphocytes, but they are masked by the chromatin. This blood dyscrasia originates from the probable proliferation of a clone of cells derived from the thymus gland or, occasionally, from the more immunologically mature thymus-derived T-lymphocyte cells. T-cell membrane markers are observed on the lymphocytes of a few patients; most patients have "null" lymphocytes on which there is neither T- nor B-cell surface determinants.

Acute Monocytic Leukemia
(Plates 57, 58)

In acute monocytic leukemia, the monoblast nucleus has a very delicate, reticular, finely masked chromatin network that is frequently folded, indented, or coarsely and incompletely segmented. Nucleoli are less frequent and not prominent when they are present. The cytoplasm is relatively agranular and basophilic, with an irregular margin similar to a pseudopod. Occasionally, one sees a phagocytic type of pattern the cytoplasm of which contains red blood cells, pigment granules, or other cellular and nuclear particles. Monocytes in various stages of development are also seen; they have grayish blue, ground-glass cytoplasm containing innumerable purplish pink granules. Two forms are described: the Naegli type is derived from myeloblasts and contains many myeloblasts; it represents a monocytic form of myeloblastic leukemia, in which the percentages of monoblasts and monocytes vary daily, finally giving way to a preponderance of myeloblasts. The Schilling type or true monocytic or histiomonocytic leukemia is derived from the reticuloendothelial cell type (Plate 59).

Other laboratory test findings include elevated basal metabolic rate, and serum and urinary uric acid. The plasma α_2 globulin is also elevated, as are the serum vitamin

B_{12} level and the vitamin B_{12} binding capacity. Pleocytosis of the cerebrospinal fluid is also evident.

Differential Diagnosis

The differential diagnosis of acute leukemia is established in the following way: (1) When there is marked leukocytosis, the leukemoid pattern of various types must be considered, such as infectious mononucleosis, whooping cough, chickenpox, infectious lymphocytosis, or congenital syphilis. However, acute leukemia is associated with maximal peripheral blood and bone marrow cytologic immaturity. The leukemoid disease is of short duration with subsidence of lymphadenopathy and splenomegaly. The heterophil antibody test is positive in infectious mononucleosis. Metastatic adrenal or sympathetic neuroblastoma cells in the peripheral blood and bone marrow may resemble immature lymphocytic cells. (2) When the leukocyte count is normal or less than normal, few immature leukemic cells are seen in the peripheral blood, and marrow changes are typical. Anemia and thrombocytopenia occur early in these diseases, especially in hypoplastic anemia with a cellular marrow pattern. Some of these patients eventually develop acute myelocytic or monocytic leukemia. Also confusing are malignant lymphomas (including Burkitt's lymphoma), agranulocytosis (no anemia or thrombocytopenia), myelophthisic anemias, and multiple myeloma. Differentiation is made possible by lymph node or marrow study.

Treatment

Treatment is based on the principle of giving the patient as long and as normal a life as is possible under the circumstances.

The first drugs used in acute lymphocytic leukemia include Prednisone, 40 to 60 mg. per day in three or four spaced doses. Corticosteroids are lympholytic, interfere with mitosis, produce a sense of well-being, and temporarily enhance erythropoiesis and thrombopoiesis. This regimen was continued until fairly complete remission occurred in 6 to 8 weeks. The temperature returns to normal, anorexia disappears, a sense of well-being is established, hemorrhagic areas are reduced, the leukocyte count falls to 10,000 per cu.mm. or less within 1 to 2 weeks, the differential cell pattern returns to normal, the erythrocyte and platelet count come back to normal, and enlarged lymph nodes and spleen are reduced. Also used was 6-mercaptopurine; 2.5 mg. per kg. of body weight per day is given until the leukocyte count falls below 3000 per cu.mm. or the platelet level begins to decrease. The dose is then reduced by half until the effects of the bone marrow toxicity have subsided. If sign and symptoms of relapse appear, prednisone is then used. After a second course of prednisone, A-methopterin (1 to 5 mg./day) is substituted.

Selawry and associates believe that complete remission in childhood leukemia lasts five times longer in patients given methotrexate (30 mg./sq.M. twice a week intramuscularly) than in those receiving daily oral medication.[176] Moreover, intermittent methotrexate proved superior to any other single agent or combined simultaneous or sequential maintenance regimen studied previously, as measured by duration of remission and longevity of survival. However, it is difficult to tell from the data whether the superiority of the intermittent parenteral therapy is attributable to the intermittency, to the route of administration, or to the fact that larger doses were used parenterally (at least it eliminates dangerous gastrointestinal injury). If the leukocyte count is normal or reduced, one may occasionally use as guides the disappearance of blasts, the rise in erythrocyte and platelet levels, the clinical status of patient, and the cellular changes seen in the bone marrow.

Other more recent drugs and therapeutic concepts used in acute lymphocytic leukemia (all) therapy have produced major prognostic changes for most patients during the last 8 to 10 years. As is well known, most of these patients are less than 10 years old, and because of this they have a better therapeutic response and prognosis than do older patients. The objective of remission induction therapy is to restore the sick child to a state of well-being as quickly as possible using specific antileukemic and supportive therapy. This is much easier and safer to do than in acute myeloid leukemia since the three major drugs used to kill leukemic lymphoblasts usually do not injure normal myeloid tissue (e.g., vincristine, L-asparaginase, and adrenal glucocorticosteroids). Destruction of 99.9 per cent of the leukemia cell population will usually permit sufficient restoration of normal hematopoietic activity to result in a state of complete remission. That is, pancytopenia does not necessarily become more severe during induction treatment, and morbidity-mortality, from infection or hemorrhage or both, rarely occurs at this stage. The specific therapy of choice is a combination of prednisone and vincristine, which acts rapidly, has minimal toxicity, and permits restoration of normal hematopoiesis, inducing completely remission in 80 to 90 per cent of children with ALL. The addition of a third agent such as L-asparaginase or one of the anthracycline antibiotics, after 4 weeks of therapy, may not significantly increase the remission rate but may prolong the duration of remission or bring most of the initial failures into complete remission, perhaps as a result of the additional cytocidal effect provided.[82, 139, 182]

Supportive therapy with antibiotics, packed red cells, and, on occasion, preferably HL-A matched or sibling donated platelet transfusion, may be life-saving during the early weeks of treatment. Granulocyte transfusions are less often needed at this time in the treatment of children with ALL; care must be taken of all veins. The use of allopurinol, adequate hydration, and alkalinization of the urine to prevent uric acid nephropathy is frequently essential. Hygiene includes proper oral and anal care with early treatment of infection.

At the end of the above-described induction phase of therapy, with the absence of demonstrable leukemia activity and the restoration of normal hematopoietic function and well-being (i.e., a complete remission in which the temperature returns to normal, anorexia disappears, a sense of well-being is established, hemorrhagic areas are reduced, the leukocyte count falls to 10,000/ cu.mm., the differential cell pattern reveals a disappearance in blasts and a return to normal, the erythrocyte and platelet count come back to normal, and enlarged lymph nodes and spleen are reduced), there are usually still 10^9 leukemic cells remaining. This necessitates further intensive chemotherapy as well as treatment aimed at reaching leukemic cells situated in areas not readily reached by standard chemotherapy.

Specifically, in the majority of patients, some form of prophylactic therapy of the central nervous system is necessary to assure prolonged remission; the central nervous system leukemia will develop in the majority of patients during the first 2 years of bone marrow remission unless 2500 rads of radiographs are delivered to the craniospinal axis, or repeated intrathecal methotrexate is given with or without cranial irradiation.[10, 66, 92, 150]

Manipulation of the various aspects of induction and maintenance therapy is necessary for prolonged remission and has indeed led to a gradual and continuing increase in survival time. The basis of these continuing innovations is the utilization of 6-mercaptopurine 2.5 mg. per kg. of body weight per day administered until the leukocyte count falls below 3000 per cu.mm. or the platelet level begins to decrease. The dose is then reduced by half until the effects of the bone marrow toxicity have subsided. Intermittent methotrexate therapy is also used. "Consolidation" therapy is also, when indicated, added to maintenance regimens; an intensive short course of cytotoxic therapy is administered after the induction of a remission. "Reinduction"

therapy is also used; short courses of inducing agents are given periodically during remission. One of the most serious sequelae of most such regimens is immunosuppression with possible subsequent fatal opportunistic infections. Therapy is usually discontinued after $2\frac{1}{2}$ to 3 years of successful remission maintenance. With intensive therapy, 50 per cent of children can survive for at least 5 years from diagnosis; 25 per cent have prolonged survival without evidence of recurrence; occasional patients have relapsed after more than 10 years remission; and some children may have been cured.

Toxic side effects of drugs include: aplasia of marrow, produced by folic acid antagonists; Cushingoid facies and salt retention due to steroids; bile stasis with jaundice, caused by 6-mercaptopurine; painful stomatitis, gastrointestinal upset, and megaloblast marrow changes such as arrested mitoses, gigantism, nuclear fragmentation, and dissociation are all reversed by folinic acid;[109] that is, with the antileukemic effect gone, these effects are due to A-methopterin, vincristine, L-asparginase, prednisone, and so forth (Plate 81).

Drugs used in the treatment of acute myelocytic and monocytic leukemia include 6-mercaptopurine (or thioguanine) in 2.5 mg./kg. body weight dosage, cytosine arabinoside for 7 days, and daunomycin (or adriamycin) for 3 days. Prednisone (40–60 mg. daily), given in various combinations with two or all three of the above-mentioned drugs, is occasionally used; it must be borne in mind that occasionally some patients are made worse by steroids. When any of the above drugs are used as single medications, there is a poor remission rate; however, when two or all three are used in combination, there is frequently a remission rate exceeding 50 per cent. Usually better results are produced when daunomycin is included in the therapy. In order for treatment to be effective, it should be early and intensive from the start and the bone marrow must become hypoplastic and not contain obvious leukemic cells. When this stage is attained, normal cells usually (but not always) regenerate before leukemic cells. This occurs provided the patient survives—with such aid as various supportive medications—the severe pancytopenia which occurs 1 to 4 weeks later.

When remission occurs, an effective suitable regimen of maintenance chemotherapy must be given, or relapse will quickly recur. A fairly good program consists of periodic thrusts of cytosine arabinoside for 7 days or daunomycin for 3 days, often joined especially in chronic treatment, with 6-mercaptopurine. Radiation therapy is occasionally used for treatment of bone pain or leukemic meningitis (the latter sometimes treated prophylactically with intrathecal methotrexate). If so, oral therapy is withheld for 24 to 48 hours.

The response to the treatment outlined above in adults with AML is sufficient improvement so that remission can now be achieved regularly in at least half of all patients treated and in approximately $\frac{1}{3}$ of those over 60 years of age. The production of a complete hematologic and clinical remission is the major determinant of survival in this group of patients, but the median survival for all patients with AML is still less than 1 year.[37, 59]

The prognostic value of various pretreatment characteristics has been analyzed in many studies. In all analyses, the major elements of prognostic significance were the age of the patient, the pretreatment functional status, and the achievement of a remission. The WBC level, platelet count, and Hb concentration are of lesser importance, and the morphologic type of AML has also proved to be of little significance. The use of early intensive therapy rather than prolonged intermittent treatment or therapy with lower doses of effective chemotherapeutic agents leads to marrow aplasia for a shorter period of time (2–3 weeks), and it is during this time patients need adequate supportive treatment with platelets, granulocytes, and antibodies.[152, 194]

Transfusions are also used. Care must be taken of all veins, and subcutaneous and intramuscular injections should be avoided. Blood transfusions are given if chemotherapy does not work, and platelet transfusions are used to tide the patient over bleeding episodes, associated with the accompanying thrombocytopenic hemostatic defect observed when the platelet level reaches the serious level of 20,000 mm³. Platelet concentrates utilizing platelets obtained from one unit of blood suspended in 20 to 40 ml. of plasma are used. Although it is the practice to use randomly matched donors for acute bleeding episodes, it is probably wiser to select HLA-compatible donors. They prevent HLA immunization with the accompanying reduction in life span of the donor platelets; such typing of platelets need not be as selective as that required for tissue transplantation. The fresher the platelet suspension, the higher the circulating platelet yield and probably the more efficient the recipient's hemostatic function will be. Storage may be accomplished at 22° C (room temperature) for 1 to 2 days with satisfactory hemostasis in the platelet-poor recipient. Prophylactic use of platelets given three times per week is usually instituted when the thrombocyte count reaches levels of approximately 20,000 mm.³, especially in aplastic anemia and leukemia patients. Occasionally, frozen platelets utilizing dimethylsulfoxide, experimentally, as the cryopreservative, are used. Leukocyte transfusions (frequently from HLA-compatible donors) have been given to patients with acute leukemia resistant to chemotherapy or to patients who have been unable to take drugs because of severe neutropenia. Different types of temporary remissions occur in a third of the patients.[175]

The most recent therapeutic approach to the treatment of the acute leukemias has been the use of bone marrow transplantation. As is well known, it is possible successfully to transplant human bone marrow between genetically identical twins and also between non-twin siblings in whom the four major histocompatibility loci (HL-A loci) are identical.[40a] Although the identity of the HL-A loci is crucial to a successful marrow transplantation, it does not guarantee tissue compatibility since the latter is dependent on other loci as well. In the process, the acute leukemia patient (recipient) is given potentially lethal doses of whole-body irradiation or Cytoxan (Cyclophosphamide) prior to transplantation. This leads to immunosuppression and concomitantly diminishes the total leukemic cell mass.[189a] In the technique, normal marrow is aspirated in large volumes; then clumps are removed by filtration, and the resultant product is injected intravenously. Graft-versus-host disease may develop. If this occurs, steroid and methotrexate therapy are given; this may not help the patient, who may die following severe skin and liver damage (Plate 60).[182a] If the engraftment is successful, the patient usually develops marked pancytopenia for a period of time followed by growth of the new marrow to a functioning size. Complete remission may then occur; however, it is usually of short duration with quick recurrence of the leukemic process both within and without the engrafted marrow.[78a] Therefore, as a therapeutic process, bone marrow transplantation probably has a more successful potential in the treatment of bone marrow failure (aplastic anemia) patients and occasionally in immune deficiency patients (see pp. 214-216).

Hygiene includes proper oral and anal care with early treatment of infection; prophylactic antibiotic therapy should be avoided because of subsequent associated fungous infections. The median survival rate of most untreated acute leukemia patients is 3 to 6 months. Children with acute lymphocytic leukemia now survive for indefinite periods with some "cures" being reported, especially if the initial leukocyte count is less than 10,000 per cu. mm. The duration of the initial remission may determine the total increase in survival time. Death is usually due to infection and hemorrhage, usually in the central nervous system or gastrointestinal tract.

Acute promyelocytic leukemia was first described as a syndrome variant of acute leukemia associated with a tendency to severe bleeding, low fibrinogen levels, and a predominance of promyelocytes in the bone marrow and peripheral blood.[50, 72, 90, 143, 163a] It is characterized by a marrow pattern of myeloid hyperplasia with promyelocytes predominating, suggesting a type of maturation arrest. The course is rapid; death occurs in 3 to 12 months. The pathogenesis of fibrinogen deficiency is not clear; it is due either to accelerated fibrinogenolysis or increased intravascular coagulation. In support of increased intravascular coagulation were occasional observations that the blood clotted abnormally rapidly in vitro even in the presence of citrate, and also the apparent absence of increased fibrinogenolytic activity at all times[50, 72, 90, 143, 163a] (Plates 61, 62).

CHRONIC LEUKEMIAS

Chronic leukemias are clinically characterized by a gradual symptomless onset associated with the progressive loss of appetite, weakness and weight loss, with a subsequent variable severity of anemia, thrombocytopenia, and foci of leukemic proliferation and infiltration. A familial tendency is observed in chronic lymphocytic leukemia. Patients with trisomy-21 mongolism are 20 per cent more prone to develop leukemia. Chromosomal abnormality such as the Philadelphia (Ph') chromosome is seen in some cases (Figs. 13-21; 13-22). A relationship to radiation with possible chromosome damage is inferred.

Chronic Lymphocytic Leukemia and Chronic Granulocytic Leukemia

In Table 13-6, a brief comparison of chronic lymphocytic leukemia and chronic granulocytic leukemia is seen.

(Text continues on p. 470.)

Table 13-6. A Comparison of Characteristics of Chronic

	Chronic Lymphocytic Leukemia	Chronic Granulocytic Leukemia
Age peak	Majority of patients 45–75 years of age	30–39 years; more common in Jewish people
Fever	Fever a late manifestation because of reduced gamma globulin; patients are susceptible to infection; rarely cryoglobulinemia with Raynaud's disease and hypersensitivity to cold; smallpox vaccination contraindicated because of susceptibility to vaccinia gangrenosa	Late in disease
Lymphadenopathy	Commonly seen in most cases, marked early; firm, discrete, nontender, 2–5 cm.; mediastinal enlargement in 30% of cases with pressure; tonsillar hypertrophy; bilateral lachrymal and salivary glands (Mikulicz's syndrome)	Mild to moderate in only 20–30% of cases and late in disease
Splenomegaly	Slight to moderate	Marked, occurs in 90% of cases, producing heavy feeling in left upper abdomen with occasional pressure symptoms; occasionally shoulder pain is referred through diaphragmatic irritation; when infarction or perisplenitis occurs, there is friction rub with intense pain
Hepatomegaly	Slight to moderate	Moderate, firm, smooth, and nontender due to leukemic infiltration
Lungs	Occasional pulmonary infiltration or pleural effusion	Rarely affected
Gastrointestinal tract	Occasional flatulence, diarrhea, and hemorrhage with ileum and colon involvement	Occasional flatulence, diarrhea, hemorrhage, and abdominal pain (late) related to possible infarction or infiltration
Cardiovascular system	Symptoms rare; if present, secondary to anemia	Symptoms are secondary to anemia; also pericarditis with effusion and myocardial infiltration
Genitourinary	Occasional hematuria secondary to thrombocytopenia; occasional renal infiltration	Pain in lumbar region with associated renal infiltration; hematuria (15–20%); priapism
Gyn	Occasional abnormal menstrual bleeding or amenorrhea	More common
Bone	Occasional sternum-point tenderness	Common sternum-point tenderness; terminally, bone pain; gout is rare
Eyes, ears, nose, and throat	Occasional leukemic nodules in cornea and sclera Hemorrhagic infiltration along 8th cranial nerve may produce deafness, otitis media, or Meniere's syndrome	Same as under chronic lymphocytic leukemia plus rentinal hemorrhages with associated visual disturbances due to leukemia infiltration along optic nerve; bleeding from nose or bruises; may produce deafness, otitis media, or Meniere's syndrome
Central nervous system	Symptoms are the same as in myelogeneous leukemia but not as common or as marked	Infiltration with pressure from enlarged nodes or nodules with associated interference of vascular supply by thrombosis or hemorrhages (cranial nerve palsies, absent reflexes, and pyramidal tract signs)

Lymphocytic Leukemia and Chronic Granulocytic Leukemia*

	Chronic Lymphocytic Leukemia	Chronic Granulocytic Leukemia
Skin	Nonspecific leukemoid reactions or specific nodular infiltrations	Symptoms rare; when present, include sharply circumscribed cutaneous or subcutaneous brownish, slate gray, bluish plaques
Blood picture	Red blood cells and platelets remain normal for a time; anisocytosis and polychromatophilia	Same
Gross blood picture	In advanced cases, the blood moderately thickened and sticky, making it difficult to prepare smears; a thick layer of buffy coat seen in the hematocrit tube	The blood markedly thickened; in advanced cases, the buffy layer increased; the platelet layer broader especially early in the disease
Anemia	Uncommon until later stages when it is 100% normochromic, normocytic with associated decreased erythropoiesis; hemolytic component in 5–30% of cases with associated positive Coombs test (acquired hemolytic anemia); anemia persists or improves little with antileukemic treatment; however, anemia does respond to corticosteroid therapy if Coombs test positive, except terminally when there is no response	In early stages, moderate polycythemia seen just like the lymphocytic form; a variable combination of impaired erythropoiesis, accelerated erythrocyte destruction, and hemorrhage account for the anemia; anemia corrected when antileukemic treatment induces remission, except terminally when there is no response
Thrombocytopenia	Normal or reduced initially; decreased late; thrombocytopenia purpura responds to corticosteroid treatment early in disease and not to antileukemic treatment; thrombocytopenia unresponsive to treatment terminally	Thrombocytosis may occur early in chronic granulocytic leukemia with thrombocytopenia appearing later; thrombocytopenia responds to antileukemic treatment except in terminal cases
Leukocytes	Elevated generally between 20,000 and 200,000/cu. mm; small lymphocytes have very little cytoplasm, very few azurophilic granules, less dense nuclear chromatin; large lymphocytes occasionally show indentation; differential blood count reveals 75–90% small lymphocytes and reduction in gamma globulin late in disease; 30–60% of patients have acquired hypogammaglobulinemia; terminally, anemia, infection, and hemorrhage	Typically between 100,000 and 500,000/cu.mm; wide variety of granulocytes and precursors; 5–20% basophilic granulocytes; eosinophilia also common; nucleated red blood cells seen occasionally; terminally, resembles acute myelocytic leukemia clinically and hematologically
Bone marrow	Extensive predominance of small lymphocytes (frequently more than 90%); marrow may be so tightly packed that it aspirates with difficulty or a dry tap is obtained; may necessitate trephine biopsy or lymph node removal	Hyperplasia of granulocytic elements, high myeloid:erythroid ratio, some immaturity of myelocytes and increased percentage of eosinophilic and basophilic forms; sea-blue histiocytes occasionally found (i.e., an inert ceroid pigment staining bright blue); possibly due to an enzyme deficit that prevents normal lipid metabolism.[187]

* See Plates 63, 64, 65, 66.

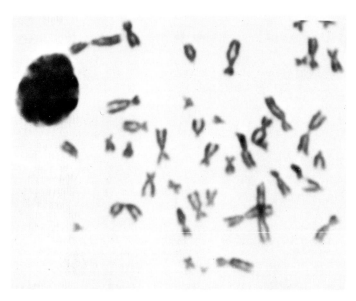

Fig. 13-21. Chromosomes in metaphase in chronic granulocytic leukemia before match pairing.

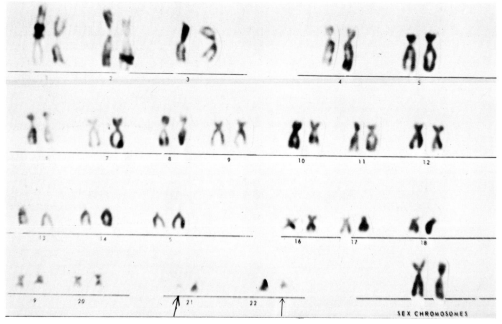

Fig. 13-22. Karyotype showing Philadelphia chromosome pattern in chronic granulocytic leukemia. Part of the long arm of chromosome 22 is missing, and chromosome 9 is missing chromatin.

The Use of Lymphocytic Markers in Chronic Lymphocytic Leukemia. Elsewhere in this text (p. 419), the immunopathology of the lymphocyte is dis-cussed in great detail. In this section are presented a brief recapitulation of the immunologic pattern of the lymphocyte in chronic lymphocytic leukemia, its differentiating features from other lymphocytosis moieties, and the correlation of morphologic criteria with clinical staging.[29]

As is now well known, peripheral blood mononuclear cells can be identified and distinguished by the presence of surface membrane markers.[3] B-cells are characterized by easily detectable surface immunoglobin (SIg), complement receptors (EAC), and Fc receptors of low affinity detected by binding of heat-aggregated IgG (Agg). T-cells are primarily identified by E rosette formation and by cytotoxicity with anti-T-cell antisera. Macrophages lack the ability to synthesize Ig but bind EAC and have high affinity Fc receptors that bind Agg and IgGEA. Cytochemical stains for acid phosphatase (AP), beta-glucoronidase (BG), and nonspecific esterase (EST) are also useful for identifying cell types.

CLL in 95 per cent of cases is a monoclonal proliferation of B-lymphocytes. The cells bear a single light chain type, usually IgM with or without IgD. The SIg is of low density and staining is typically very faint. Complement receptors are present but either qualitatively or quantitatively reduced; Agg receptors also are present. T-cells are reduced. In most cases the cells lack lysosomal enzymes (AP and BG). These features distinguish CLL from a variety of other processes presenting as lymphocytosis: (1) *Reactive lymphocytosis*. In most cases a reactive lymphocytosis will be composed predominantly of T-cells. The B-cells identified should be polyclonal, not of a single light chain type. (2) *T-cell CLL*. Approximately 2 per cent of cases of CLL are T-cell proliferations. The cells form E rosettes and react with anti-T-cell antisera, but respond poorly to mitogens. The cells have a high content of lysosomal enzymes (AP and BG). These cases have clinically distinctive features including massive splenomegaly, skin lesions, and neutropenia. (3) *Lymphosarcoma cell leukemia (LSCL)* or leukosarcoma. LSCL or peripheral blood involvement by a non-Hodgkin's lymphoma occurs with both nodular and diffuse, poorly differentiated lymphocytic lymphomas. These are usually monoclonal B-cell proliferations but the surface markers still differ from those of CLL (Plates 79, 80). The SIg is of high density with intense staining and frequent spontaneous capping. Complement receptors are present and binding of EAC is more avid than in CLL. (4) *Hairy cell leukemia (HCL)*. HCL does not often present with high peripheral counts. However, in such cases determination of surface markers would distinguish the proliferation from CLL. The cells may have abundant SIg, and IgG is more often identified than Igm. When the cells are freshly isolated, they frequently have a polyclonal distribution of SIg staining for both heavy and light chains. This feature is due to the high avidity Fc receptors present on these cells, which can also be detected by binding of IgGea. The cells also have a characteristic tartrate-resistant acid phosphatase. (5) *Sezary syndrome (SS)*. The characteristic erythroderma of the SS as well as the cerebriform nature of the cells should permit its recognition. However, the cells can also be distinguished from those of CLL by their T-cell characteristics and by their high content of AP and BG.

Within recent years attempts have been made to classify chronic lymphocytic leukemia (CLL) by morphologic features. Both prolymphocytic leukemia and leukemic reticuloendotheliosis (hairy cell leukemia) have been recognized as distinct clinical entities and have been separated from chronic lymphocytic leukemia. Chronic lymphosarcoma cell leukemia is another variant of CLL in which the cell nucleus is notched, and the cell is of a larger size than that of the more common form. This clinical subtype has also been excluded from the classic CLL entity. In general, however, morphologic features of CLL lymphocytes are not qualitatively distinguishable from the normal circulating small lymphocyte. In fact, patients with virtually identical morphologic lymphocyte characteristics may not have the same or even similar survival times. A number of techniques have been developed that have made possible the characterization of human lymphocytes as either (thymic-derived) T-cells or (bone marrow derived) B-cells. The major population of lymphocytes in CLL display B-cell surface markers with either IgM or IgG of monoclonal origin. Many patients, in addition, show the presence of IgD on these cells. In 5 to 10 per cent of patients with CLL, the majority of lymphocytes show T-cell surface characteristics. No simple correlation between cell surface marker and patient survival is generally accepted. Studies of other B-lymphocyte markers demonstrate that CLL lymphocytes show the presence of an Fc receptor as well as a complement receptor, but the number of these receptors in CLL lymphocytes is usually diminished when it is compared to normal lymphocytes. In addition, some reports have noted lymphocytes that form rosettes with sheep erythrocytes (S-RBC) and also demonstrate a receptor for complement and for a Fc fragment of IgG. These findings indicate the presence of a transitional type of lymphocyte as the predominant cell in some patients with CLL. Attempts have been made to correlate the clinical course of the disease with mean numbers of circulating T- and B-cells. Han and co-workers have reported that the total T-lymphocyte count correlated well with the duration of disease in CLL patients in remission and also correlated with the status of the delayed hypersensitivity response in these patients.[83] Silber has studied the plasma membrane enzyme 5' nucleotidase and has reported marked diminution of this enzyme in the lymphocytes of most patients with CLL.[181] Assessment of lysosomal enzymes has shown reduced total activity of acid phosphatase and beta glucuronidase in CLL lymphocytes. In addition, many investigators have found a diminished response to phytomitogen by CLL lymphocytes. Those

least responsive have been associated with more advanced disease.

At present it is generally agreed that CLL is a disease characterized by a progressively increasing accumulation of lymphocytes. It is not known, however, what proportion of the circulating T- and B-lymphocytes, if any, have normal function, and whether there is any progressive decrease in lymphocyte function with progression of this disease.

From a study of a large number of patients with CLL, it has been found that survival and presumably progression of disease may be correlated with a few simple clinical signs leading to the proposal of a clinical staging system for CLL (see below).[156]

Patients with only peripheral blood and bone marrow involvement (Stage O) had a median survival of 12 years compared to patients who were anemic or thrombocytopenic (Stages III and IV), whose median survival time was only 1.5 years.

There is question whether, in fact, such a clinical staging system represents differences in total body tumor load and whether progression in clinical staging parallels a progressive increasing accumulation of lymphocytes. In addition, it is won-

---

Clinical Staging of CLL*

Stage O: Absolute lymphocytosis of 15,000 lymphocytes $\times 10^6/1$ with bone marrow lymphocytosis

Stage I: Absolute lymphocytosis plus enlarged lymph nodes

Stage II: Absolute lymphocytosis plus enlarged liver or spleen†

Stage III: Absolute lymphocytosis plus anaemia (Hgb < 11 g./dl. in males; < 10 g./dl. in females)‡

Stage IV: Absolute lymphocytosis plus thrombocytopenia (platelet count $< 100,000 \times 10^6/L.$)‡

---

* Rai, K. R., et al.: Clinical staging of chronic lymphocytic leukemia. Blood, *46*:219, 1975. By permission of Grune and Stratton.
† Stage II patients may or may not have adenopathy.
‡ Stages III and IV patients may or may not have adenopathy or organomegaly.

dered whether the function of lymphocytes in the earlier stages of disease shows more normal portions of T- and B-cells (as measured by cell surface markers), whereas, with progressive accumulation of lymphocytes, more abnormal and decreased function of lymphocytes could be demonstrated.

Other studies have shown that patients with early clinical stages (O and I) of CLL showed minimal increased increments of total body potassium, whereas late-stage (III and IV) disease was characterized by a much higher total body potassium. Patients treated for CLL with subsequent clinical reduction in their leukemic mass also showed a decline in the total body potassium. In addition Stage O patients showed a predominance of B-cells of almost three times that found in the blood of normal patients with a mean T:B cell ratio of 15:75. On the other hand, Stage III and IV patients had fewer T-cells and more B-cells with a mean ratio of 10:85. Similarly, there was a progressive decrease in the serum immunoglobulin concentration in CLL patients with progression in clinical stage. There was little or no skin hypersensitivity reaction to the recall antigens by patients in clinical Stages III or IV.

In conclusion, it appears that although no morphologic or quantitative differences are apparent in the peripheral blood lymphocytes of patients with Stage O CLL when they are compared to those of patients with advanced disease, lymphocyte function is progressively impaired in later-stage disease. There is not enough data on hand to determine whether a significant reduction in body tumor load will result in return or improvement in lymphocyte function.

Chronic Monocytic Leukemia
(Plates 67, 68)

In chronic monocytic leukemia there are two forms not fundamentally related to one another. One rare variant, the Schilling or histiocytic type is characterized by primitive stemlike cells having the cytologic pattern of peripheral blood monocytes combined with the tissue form or histiocyte. The myelomonocytic or Naegeli type is considered to be related to myelocytic or granulocytic leukemia and makes up about 8 to 12 per cent of all leukemias. It usually presents as a preleukemic state with a refractory anemia, associated leukopenia, and a thrombocytopenia that may last up to 5 years. Hematologically, it is characterized by the presence of myelomonocytes of up to 30 per cent in the peripheral blood and 15 to 20 per cent in the bone marrow, with an increased number of myeloblasts. Clinically, chronic monocytic leukemia is associated with lymphadenopathy and splenomegaly. Microscopically, the myelomonocytes show the monocytic nuclear pattern and myeloid cytoplasmic features; there is a folded, delicate chromatin nuclear network with a minimal number of peroxidase-positive granules, even in the cytoplasm of the blast and problast forms. The myelomonocytes are devoid of pale myelocytic cytoplasmic zones; occasionally, Auer bodies are present.

Among other laboratory test findings in the chronic leukemias, the basal metabolic rate is elevated ($+20$–$+40$), as is the blood uric acid. The positive alkaline phosphatase-staining granulocytes are absent from the peripheral blood or nearly so. The serum vitamin B_{12} level is elevated (greater than 1000 μg./ml.). There is an increase in the urinary excretion of uric acid in myelocytic leukemia, but it is normal in lymphocytic leukemia.

Differential Diagnosis

Chronic lymphocytic leukemia should be differentiated from other malignant lymphomas such as lymphosarcoma. In chronic lymphocytic leukemia, the marrow is widely replaced or infiltrated by mature lymphocytes. However in subleukemic lymphocytic leukemia and hypoplastic anemia, 30 to 40 per cent of marrow cells may be lymphocytic. Lymph node biopsy

Table 13-7. Differential Diagnosis of the Common Forms of Leukemia*

Age in years	Acute Leukemia 1–20	Chronic Granulocytic Leukemia 20–40	Chronic Lymphocytic Leukemia 40–80
Splenomegaly	+	++++	++
Adenopathy	+	+	++++
Fever	++++	±	±
Bone pain	++++	±	±
WBC (10^3/mm.^{3})	1–200	100–800	30–400
Differential	Blasts	Myelocytes, metamyelocytes, PMN	Adult lymphocytes
Platelets anemia	++++ Markedly decreased	++ High early, decreased later	± Normal early, decreased late
Ph' (Philadelphia chromosome)	–	+	–
Histochemical stains	AGL – 1–3 + $\left(\begin{array}{c}\text{Sudan}\\\text{black}\end{array}\right)$ ALL – 0	1–3 + $\left(\begin{array}{c}\text{Peroxidase}\\\text{and Sudan black}\end{array}\right)$	0 $\left(\begin{array}{c}\text{Peroxidase}\\\text{and Sudan black}\end{array}\right)$

* Modified from Cartwright, G. E.: Diagnostic Laboratory Hematology, ed. 3. New York, Grune & Stratton, 1963.

should differentiate these two because in subleukemic lymphocytic leukemia there is effacement of the lymph follicle–germinal center pattern; in hypoplastic anemia the follicular pattern is distinctly maintained. Miliary tuberculosis may also produce a lymphocytic leukemoid pattern; however, isolation of the organism and the demonstration of *Mycobacterium tuberculosis* bacilli differentiates these two. Recent work on the morphological origination of the lymphocyte involved in chronic lymphocytic leukemia appears to suggest that it is due to the proliferation of an abnormal B-type lymphocyte clone, with subsequent loss of normal B-cell formation. As a result, the chief cause of the severe morbidity and mortality, bacterial, or fugal infection is the associated hypogammaglobulinemia and deficient humoral antibody production. The latter is directly related to subsequent development of the autoimmune hemolytic anemia or thrombocytopenia so frequently seen in this lymphoid blood dyscrasia.

Chronic granulocytic leukemia should be differentiated from myeloid metaplasia with associated myelofibrosis and late leukocy-totic, subnormal erythrocyte stages of polycythemia vera, which may in reality represent variants of chronic granulocytic leukemia. In most cases, marrow examination reveals tumor cells and fibrotic zones; the granulomatous pattern in various leukemoid states differentiates these entities. Furthermore, a greater alkaline phosphatase staining pattern of peripheral blood granulocytes and an elevation of serum vitamin B_{12} levels usually differentiate these nonleukemic syndromes from chronic granulocytic leukemia. Most difficult to differentiate is a hypoplastic or refractory anemia with a cellular bone marrow pattern from chronic granulocytic leukemia with a normal or subnormal leukocyte level. Further help in making a specific diagnosis is the presence of the Philadelphia chromosome (Ph'); this represents a translocation of a portion of the long arms of chromosome number 22 with the missing chromatin found on chromosome number 9. A poor prognosis and a poor response to therapy is found in those cases in which the Ph' chromosome is absent. A fibrous tissue increase in the bone marrow also implies a poor prognosis. A summary of the differential diagnosis of the common forms of leukemia is given in Table 13–7.

Treatment

Part of the treatment of chronic leukemias includes checking the blood counts every 1 or 2 months or oftener in order to determine the cellular levels and to note any evidence of marrow depression. In the case of chronic lymphocytic leukemia (CLL), one must remember that this dyscrasia may remain clinically quiescent for many weeks, months, or years and, therefore, require no special therapy. However, once symptoms begin, these are related to extensive lymphadenopathy and severe anemia with or without hemolysins (i.e. in 30% of cases, an autoimmune reaction develops associated with reticulocytosis, a positive Coombs test, and hypogammaglobulinemia). In these cases, prednisone (60–100 mg.) is given, in divided doses 1 day a week until erythrocyte values return to normal. This type of treatment also helps the thrombocytopenia until platelet resistance occurs; at that time either HL-A-matched platelet infusions or transfusions of fresh, viable platelet-rich blood occasionally may offer relief. If infection occurs, antibiotics and gamma globulin may be given; these should not be used prophylactically. Pregnancy and surgical conditions are treated accordingly. Specific therapy (e.g., alkylating agents such as chlorambucil or Cytoxan) is helpful. For example, chlorambucil may be given in an initial dose range of 0.1 to 0.2 mg. per kg. per day; 8 mg. is given as one dose 30 minutes before breakfast for 4 to 8 weeks; the dose is reduced when the leukocyte count falls below 15,000 per cu.mm. Fairly good partial remissions are observed in 55 to 75 per cent of patients with ionizing radiation inducing a marked resolution of lymphoid tumor masses. Combination chemotherapy with such drugs as vincristine, prednisone, and cyclophosphamide (Cytoxan) may indeed produce higher complete remission rates. However, these cases were not always documented by all the relevant criteria; evidence of lymphoid infiltration of any organs, complete normalization of the blood counts and blood and bone marrow differential counts, and increase in lymphoid nodules in sections of bone marrow fragments were lacking.[115] Recent chemotherapeutic trials, on Stages 2 to 4 CLL, consisted of a protocol called M-2 (vincristine, BCNU, cyclophosphamide, melphalan, and prednisone).[149] Preliminary observations suggest that, as in most neoplastic diseases, previously untreated patients respond best; 25 per cent have shown a complete response and 69 per cent have had either a complete or partial response. No patient with Stage 4 disease has yet had a complete response. It is still unclear how long treatment should be continued in those patients having complete remissions. The average survival time of chronic lymphocytic leukemia patients is approximately 5 years, with many patients surviving much longer. The exact role of antileukemic therapy or its relation to its influence on life span is not clear at this time. The atypical immune responses listed above are best treated as if they had occurred unrelated to the chronic lymphocytic leukemia. In fact, most hematologists probably do not offer therapy to the asymptomatic or mildly asymptomatic patient and only very conservative, cautious treatment to those who are more symptomatic. There is no therapeutic agent that will elicit a return to normal B-type lymphocyte function.

Therapy for chronic granulocytic leukemia includes the use of ^{32}P or busulfan in alternating fashion or until resistance occurs to one or the other. Because urinary excretion of uric acid increases, possibly causing ureteral obstruction by uric acid crystals, the urine should be made alkaline. ^{32}P in the form of oral sodium acid phosphate is administered in individual doses (in the fasting state) of 1 to 2.5 mc., depending on the leukocyte level. This is repeated 2 weeks later or before if the leukocyte count is above 100,000 per cu.mm. Busulfan, an alkylating agent that exerts its effect possibly by inactivating nuclear DNA, is usually given as a daily single dose of 4 to 6 mg. before breakfast until the leukocyte count falls to 10,000 per cu.mm. or less. When busulfan is given alone and in the usual dosage, it may be used during pregnancy without toxicity to the human fetus.[56] Some side effects occur with busulfan (see p. 477); subleukemic leukemias are also treated this way.

The question is often raised what role splenectomy has in chronic granulocytic leukemia (CGL). Except in rare instances of hypersplenism, splenectomy is discouraged because of the complications of the operation. In recent years, it has been reevaluated, especially in patients who sustain a prolonged pancytopenia following chemotherapy or in those whose disease proves difficult to control because of marked sensitivity of the platelet count to conventional doses of busulfan. The procedure has also been reconsidered because it has been shown that splenectomy can ameliorate some of the hematologic and clinical complications of CGL and can be performed with some benefit to the patient, even in the blastic phase of the disease. The possibility that the spleen may be a preferential site for the inception and acceleration of the blastic phase of the disease has generated some enthusiasm for the prophylactic removal of the spleen during the chronic phase of CGL. In addition, because of the risks of this operation late in the course of CGL, it may be desirable to perform a prophylactic splenectomy to avoid the pain and complications of massive splenomegaly after the inception of the blastic phase. In addition it may prove helpful in facilitating the transfusion of required blood products, such as RBCs and platelets, and thus improve the prospects of achieving some benefit from chemotherapy during this refractory phase of the disease. In conclusion, data to date suggest that splenectomy does not increase the response to the blastic

phase directed to chemotherapy, although there is a possibility that the quality of life may be improved.[28] Recent work has demonstrated that the blast cells of CGL may have some characteristics that suggest a "lymphoblastic" transformation of the disease. On the basis of number of nucleoli, nuclear: cytoplasmic ratio, lack of granularity, and PAS positivity, approximately $1/3$ of the patients are capable of responding to antilymphoblastic chemotherapy with vincristine and prednisone. The "lymphoblastic" conversion concept has been strengthened by the observation that an unusual DNA synthetic enzyme known as terminal deoxynucleotydl transferase (TdT) has been found in some patients in the blastic phase of CGL. TdT has been found in lymphoblastic cell lines, T lymphocytes, and in a high percentage of patients with ALL. Also, TdT positive blast cells react with rabbit antihuman ALL cell antiserum.[119]

In the 80 per cent of patients with terminal basic blastic phase, 6-mercaptopurine is used as described in the treatment of acute leukemia (pp. 463–467). An enzyme, terminal deoxynucleotide transferase, found in the thymus in normal patients and in very low bone marrow concentration, has been found in some of these terminal blastic phase patients. Its presence in these crises poses the question of lymphoblastic transformation, since the enzyme is usually found in most cases of acute lymphoblastic leukemia. Blood transfusions are rarely necessary until late in the course of the disease. Antibiotics are used as described above in the therapy of chronic lymphocytic leukemia. All patients to be placed on cytolytic drugs including irradiation should be prepared for such by ample hydration and urinary alkalinization. In patients who have hyperuricemia and uric acid nephropathy or in whom widespread cell destruction is anticipated, allopurinol (300–800 mg. daily) is recommended, beginning just prior to antineoplastic therapy.[108] Equivocal success has been attained when other types of chemotherapy (e.g., prednisone and vincristine) have been suggested singly and in combination with an attempt to improve survival (i.e., marrow hypoplasia is produced or splenectomy is performed).

Busulfan may manifest nonhematologic toxicity after prolonged treatment, for instance, amenorrhea in females, aspermia in males, and a dark pigmentation of the skin. The last resembles Addison's disease but is not accompanied by adrenal insufficiency. In addition, the so-called "bisulfan lung" occurs as a pulmonary fibrosing process and is only partially relieved by steroid therapy.

Remissions of chronic leukemias may last 1 to 2 years. The median survival time in chronic lymphocytic leukemia is 60 months, and in chronic granulocytic leukemia it is 54 months. Longer remissions are possible although therapeutic results in blast crises of chronic myeloid leukemia are even less satisfactory than for the acute disease. Because there is enormous variability in the clinical course of CLL with some patients dying within less than a year and others living 20 years or longer, it has been difficult to assess the effects of treatment or survival. The longer survival in some series has been attributed to inclusion of higher proportions of patients who have a more favorable prognosis. There is little solid evidence that single-agent chemotherapy has appreciably altered overall survival in CLL, although such treatment is widely recognized to be useful in controlling troublesome signs and symptoms. Immediate causes of death are usually hemorrhage, infection, visceral involvement, and congestive heart failure secondary to severe anemia.

ALEUKEMIC AND SUBLEUKEMIC LEUKEMIA

Symptoms and signs are the same as in other types of leukemia – that is, granulocytic if marrow depicts such and lymphocytic if such is demonstrated in the marrow.

Aleukemic leukemia is defined as a state in which the leukocyte count is less than normal and the peripheral blood supposedly contains no abnormal immature cells of the myeloid or lymphoid series. In subleukemic leukemia, on the other hand, the leukocyte count is less than normal, but there are enough immature atypical cells in the peripheral blood film to suggest a diagnosis of leukemia. In most cases, examination of a smear of the buffy coat of peripheral blood will reveal leukemic cells. Bone marrow examination will usually reveal the typical leukemic lymphocyte or immature granulocytic pattern and therefore establish the diagnosis (Plate 69).

Other Types of Leukemia or Leukemic-like Disorders – The Myeloproliferative Disorders

Because the classic leukemic pattern may be an end product of the various symptom complexes (myelofibrosis with myeloid metaplasia, polycythemia vera, essential thrombocythemia and the Di Guglielmo syndrome), Dameshek has placed these under one heading.[45] Thus, the cellular proliferative process in all the myeloproliferative disorders begins in the bone marrow or in extramedullary blood sites, and all are of unknown etiology. Most frequently one or more of the various marrow cell types – for example, fibroblastic-like cells derived from the reticulum, erythrocytic cells, myelocytic, and megakaryocytic cells – proliferate in and are observed in the spleen, liver, lymph nodes, and bone marrow.

Dameshek proposes that because megakaryocytic as well as granulocytic elements may be undergoing hyperplasia in polycythemia vera, myelocytic leukemia, and Di Guglielmo syndrome, because the bone marrow may also be hyperplastic early in myeloid metaplasia associated with myelofibrosis; and because myelofibrotic patterns may be seen in the late stages of polycythemia vera and granulocytic leukemia, enough overlapping or change occurs from case to case and in different stages of the same case to suggest that several or all of these symptom complexes may be varied manifestations of the same fundamental disturbance.[58]

Theories on the pathogenesis of myelofibrosis range from necrobiosis (due to the toxic action of benzene, radioactive phosphorus, radium, and other agents) and primary bone marrow failure (in which myeloid metaplasia is viewed as a compensatory process) to the current widely held theory that it is but one of a group of myeloproliferative disorders. Proponents of this last view believe that intramedullary and extramedullary changes stem from a common "myelostimulatory factor."

As just elicited, depending on the phase of the disease, or the form it takes in a particular patient, the myeloproliferative disorder might be manifested as polycythemia vera, myelogeneous leukemia, erythroleukemia of Di Guglielmo, myelofibrosis, or variants. Because most of the marrow patterns in this group are hypercellular but may be hypoplastic with many primitive forms; because the term "myelofibrosis" is restricted to one element, recent investigators prefer "panmyelosis" as more descriptive in most instances. Use of this word should emphasize that fibrosis is not the major finding in many instances and that distinction from leukemia is, many times, far from real. Nowell believes that a positive chromosome study in a patient with the myeloproliferative disorder who has not received therapeutic irradiation suggests that a frankly leukemic phase is imminent.[135]

Therefore, one must realize that patients develop transitions and variegated combinations of unorganized cell growth and that the hematologic entity includes a spectrum of proliferative abnormalities. Spontaneous remissions and interconversion from one entity to another does not occur; the same fundamental atypical blood pattern or combination of abnormal morphologic cells first observed in a patient usually continues and even becomes increasingly more severe

with acute exacerbations. Occasionally, one specific cell line in a myeloproliferative disorder may exacerbate acutely while another atypicality in another cell line may remain stationary or become chronic.

ERYTHREMIC MYELOSIS (ACUTE AND CHRONIC ERYTHROLEUKEMIA OR THE DI GUGLIELMO SYNDROME)
(Plates 71, 72)

Erythremic myelosis is the erythrocytic counterpart of acute leukemia characterized by a progressive and irreversible proliferation of neoplastic developing red cells.[161] The clinical manifestations of this rare disease are similar to those of the other acute leukemias but with more pronounced splenomegaly and hepatomegaly. Grossly, the erythrocytic leukemic infiltrates are a dark copper red with almost a metallic glint, unlike the lymphocytic or granulocytic forms. In patients past the first few days of life, the erythroblastosis (normoblastosis) exceeds that of the leukocytic components. Two other forms are both characterized by a failure of the intense normoblastosis to be manifested in the peripheral blood. In one group, peripheral blood shows a variable leukocyte count, persistent and unremitting anemia refractory to all therapy and marked by very low or even absent reticulocytosis, and by thrombocytopenia.

Examination of the marrow reveals an overgrowth of myeloblasts and developing normoblasts, to the exclusion of granulocytes and megakaryocytes. The normoblastic overgrowth permeates the connective tissue everywhere, but the normoblasts are obviously unproductive of adult red corpuscular products. In this first group, the myeloblasts are often also present with Auer bodies. In a second and most common variant, the peripheral blood presents a macrocytic picture sometimes marked by large, round macrocytes, but at times by large ovoid megalocytes and hypersegmented leukocytes, in which it is almost undistinguishable from the peripheral blood in pernicious anemia. However, the cell pattern does not respond to vitamin B_{12}, folic acid, or liver therapy.

Marrow aspiration reveals either a megaloblastic picture or a megaloblastoid overgrowth worsened by vitamin B_{12}—that is, either increased quantities or outright dedifferentiation of myeloblasts or blood-forming reticulum cells (primitive stem cells) occurs. One also sees hemoglobin-bearing tumor giant cells (monster cells) characterized by a size of 50 to 100 μ with multinucleation or hyperchromatic polymorphic giant nuclei and large cell bodies always showing evidence of the copper or pink color of hemoglobin. The spleen, lymph nodes, and liver are also enlarged and contain marked extramedullary infiltrations. Late in the disease, a stem cell leukemic picture may develop. Finkel has described immunologic abnormalities that include an overproduction of antibody protein (hypergammaglobulinemia) and an increased tendency to form rheumatoid factor, LE factor, positive serologic tests for syphilis, and erythrocytic autoantibodies and isoantibodies.[63]

Myelofibrosis with Myeloid Metaplasia (Agnogenic Myeloid Metaplasia)

Myelofibrosis with myeloid metaplasia affects the upper age groups as an atypical, bizarre, slowly evolving replacement of the bone marrow spaces by varying degrees of fibrosis or sclerosis with associated peripheral blood changes such as mature and immature leukocytosis, thrombocytosis (early), thrombocytopenia (late), and normoblastosis. Eventually splenic extramedullary hematopoiesis develops. The case of most cases is unknown although marrow intoxicants (radiation, phosphorus poisoning, and chronic benzene exposure), carcinomatosis of bone marrow, tuberculosis, and leukemoid reactions) as terminal part of polycythemia vera or myelocytic leukemia patterns) are involved.

Apparently the elevated plasma and urinary erythropoietin levels in this syndrome, and also in aplastic anemia, point toward a localized flat-bone marrow involvement. Thus, compensatory extramedullary hematopoiesis occurs in agnogenic myeloid metaplasia, and a generalized metabolic defect is observed in the bone marrow failure of aplastic anemia. Patchy, fatty, and hyperplastic marrow changes alternate with zones of osteosclerosis and fibrosis. Lymphadenopathy, marked hepatosplenomegaly, and associated hematopoiesis are noted in the sinusoids; occasionally splenic fibrosis and infarction are seen.

Clinical Findings

The enlarged splenic mass with its heavy dragging feeling, pallor, weakness, loss of weight, and increasing abdominal size due to the hepatosplenomegaly make up the main complaints of these patients. Symptoms of portal hypertension such as ascites, esophageal varices, and gastrointestinal hemorrhage, increased basal metabolic rate, severe anemia, thromboses (thrombocytosis), and petechiae (thrombocytopenia) also occur.

Hematologic Findings (Plates 73, 74, 75, 76)

Hematologically, the following are observed: moderate to severe normocytic anemia (polycythemia early or vice versa); anisocytosis and poikilocytosis (tear drop), and polychromasia; and normoblastosis with occasional reticulocytosis. The leukocyte count is elevated, usually with mature granulocytes, myelocytes, promyelocytes, and myeloblasts; the latter immature types increase late in the disease. Alkaline phosphatase stains are strongly positive in the neutrophilic leukocytes. Thrombocytosis occurs early with thrombocytopenia later. Morphologically, the platelets are very large with atypical shapes; occasionally one sees increased megakaryocytes and megakaryocytic fragments. Bone marrow aspirations are frequently characterized by dry taps. Trephine biopsy reveals fibrosis, sclerosis, carcinoma cells, or a granulomatous pattern, as in tuberculosis.

Other laboratory findings include extramedullary hematopoiesis observed in needle biopsy sections of liver or spleen and a high basal metabolic rate. Radiographs of bones show osteosclerosis in approximately half of patients. This disease complex must be differentiated from chronic granulocytic leukemia.

Treatment

Erythrocyte survival tests should be performed over the liver and spleen using ^{51}Cr to detect excess erythrocyte destruction, especially in the spleen. Splenectomy is a last resort for hemolysis and thrombocytopenia, especially if the patient is corticosteroid-resistant. However, anemia and platelet deficiency in myelofibrosis are better treated with 400 to 600 mg. a week of intramuscularly injected testosterone before resorting to splenic irradiation, busulfan, or splenectomy. Most patients live 3 to 5 years on the average, except a recently described case in an infant in which reversible myelofibrosis was asssociated with vitamin D deficiency rickets.[43]

POLYCYTHEMIA VERA (POLYCYTHEMIA RUBRA, ERYTHREMIA, OR PRIMARY POLYCYTHEMIA)

Polycythemia vera, chronic panmyelopathy[81] of unknown cause, is associated with bone marrow cellular hyperplasia involving all cytologic components, especially the nucleated erythrocytic elements. Polycythemia vera is characterized by peripheral blood findings of an abnormal increase in the erythrocyte mass, hemoglobin concentration, and frequently leukocytosis and thrombocytosis. Erythrocytosis is a term used to denote polycythemia, usually without excess granulocytes or platelets secondary to other pathologic phenomena (discussed later).

The etiology of polycythemia vera is unknown. It is not related to tissue anoxia, endocrine stimulus, or erythropoietin-like factors. It is found only occasionally in children and seldom in more than one member of a family. When it is familial, it has a benign course without elevated mature or immmature leukocyte and platelet levels. It is rare in Blacks, and its incidence is high in middle-aged Jewish males.

Pathologic Findings

The laboratory findings reveal that beta and gamma globulin levels are occasionally elevated. The blood histamine level is elevated probably owing to the increased number of basophils. Plasma vitamin B_{12} levels are elevated in some cases, just as in chronic granulocytic leukemia. Hyperuricemia is evident (5% of patients), leading to a secondary form of gout. This is caused by the increased formation and destruction of erythrocytes and leukocytes and to the increased metabolism of nucleic acids in the hematopoietic tissues with increased elaboration of intermediate products of purine metabolism.

Circulatory minute volume is reduced, but the circulation time may be prolonged with associated visceral stasis. The velocity of blood flow is greatly lowered. Arterial oxygen saturation of the blood is normal, but arterial oxygen tension is subnormal. There is also an increased basal metabolic rate and total blood volume. There is an increased blood viscosity, which is associated with an elevation of hematocrit above 60. Thrombocytosis occurs in this syndrome, and this together with increased blood viscosity leads to intravascular thromboses. There is a tendency to bleed from slight injuries, possibly owing to the increased blood volume and accompanying capillary and venous distention. Thromboplastin generation is abnormal, and platelet factor 3 levels are reduced in acute polycythemia vera.

Clinical Findings

Clinical findings reveal a reddish cyanotic plethoric hue to the skin and mucosa with concomitant frequent petechial hemorrhages. Hepatosplenomegaly is evident with left-sided abdominal heaviness. Hypertension is found with associated cephalalgia and fullness in the head. Visual disturbances occur with retinal and scleral venous distention, paresthesias, dyspnea, pruritus associated with hot baths, dizziness, weakness, and easy fatigability. Frequent complications are hepatic venous thrombosis and cirrhosis with esophageal, gastric, and rectal varices and bleeding therefrom. Duodenal ulceration is also common. Frequently polycythemia vera is characterized by a chronic course with termination in anemia, myelofibrosis, myeloid metaplasia, and a leukemoid to granulocytic or erythroleukemia pattern.[11]

Hematologic Findings (Plate 78)

Hematologically one observes an elevated red blood cell volume and mass (6,500,000–9,000,000/cu.mm.); the hematocrit is very high, frequently above 60. The MCV and MCH are low, and the total hemoglobin is elevated. The red blood cells appear normal and the reticulocyte percentage is normal, but the absolute number of reticulocytes is increased. The leukocyte count ranges from 12,000 to 55,000 per cu.mm. with an increased quantity of immature forms (metamyelocytes and occasionally myelocytes), slight basophilia, an elevated alkaline phosphatase of the granulocytes, and a thrombocytosis of 2,500,000 to 5,500,000 per cu.mm. with associated fibrinogenopenia and qualitative morphologic platelet irregularities. Disorganization of the platelet fibrin network has been observed in sections of platelet-plasma clots from polycythemia vera patients.[95] The possibility that red cells could easily slip through openings in the network was considered to be the cause of the erythrocyte dispersion out of clotted blood, long recognized as characteristic of the clot in polycythemia vera.[166]

A hemorrhagic tendency, paradoxically accompanied by a predisposition to thromboses when the platelet count is elevated, probably accounts for the increased risk of surgery in patients with uncontrolled polycythemia vera. The bone marrow pattern shows a megakaryocytosis with normoblastosis. The marrow is often devoid of fat and sometimes hard to tell from leukemic marrow.

Because of the frequent difficulties in the differential diagnosis of polycythemia vera, the following diagnostic protocol has been proposed:

Criteria A
1. Splenomegaly
2. Increased erythrocytic volume: $♀ = > 32$ ml./kg.; $♂ = > 36$ ml./kg.
3. Arterial oxygen saturation: $>92\%$

Criteria B
1. Elevated leukocyte alkaline phosphatase
2. Leukocytosis: $>12,000$ mm.[3]
3. Serum Vitamin $B_{12} > 900$ pg./ml.
4. Thrombocytosis $>400,000$/mm.[3]

If all of the findings under A are present, the diagnosis of polycythemia vera may be made. If an enlarged spleen is absent, the diagnosis may be made with A-2 and A-3 plus any two items from the B column. Increased usage of technetium nuclide scanning has permitted the diagnosis of an enlarged spleen more accurately and more frequently. Usually the hematocrit is greater than 52 per cent and, rarely, occult bleeding may confuse the diagnosis.

Opinion is divided on proper therapy: phlebotomy, alkylating agents (chlorambucil), and P[32]. A prospective, controlled therapy program utilizing these three modes reveals a treatment period with no obvious differences in survival rates. Termination in acute leukemia has occurred with each of the antimitotic agents; therefore all of the above methods are used since there is no defined optimal therapy and since there is no real evidence that the onset of leukemia is related to P[32] dosage. Decreased complications from hemorrhage and thromboembolism are associated with more prolonged periods of relatively normal blood values. Therefore, it is suggested that elective surgery not be performed until the blood values remain normal for weeks or months.

Differential Diagnosis

The differential diagnosis of primary polycythemia includes the elimination of relative polycythemia, secondary polycythemia, and myeloproliferative syndrome.

Relative polycythemia is due to plasma loss and hemoconcentration without associated loss of erythrocytes. It may be produced in several ways: a loss of fluid (water) and electrolytes due to diarrhea, excess sweating, vomiting, adrenal insufficiency, and hyposthenuria, excessive plasma loss seen in severe burns and traumatic shock, or reduced intake of fluid with subsequent reduced plasma volume. Relative polycythemia caused by reduced fluid intake is also seen in anxiety states; it is therefore called the stress type. Most of these patients are middle-aged, obese males with moderately elevated blood pressure, a hematocrit of 54 to 58 per cent, and increased CO Hb levels associated with smoking. Hematologically, there is a moderate leukocytosis, normal erythrocyte volume, and a hematocrit elevation of 10 to 25 per cent. Treatment of relative polycythemia with fluid and electrolytes restores the hematocrit and the leukocyte count to normal levels.

Familial polycythemia, a type of erythrocytosis, may suggest the presence of a mutant hemoglobin with increased oxygen affinity. As a group, unstable hemoglobins are frequently accompanied by amino acid substitutions that affect the "niche or pocket" where the heme portion is attached to the globin chains. They are characterized by precipitated denatured hemoglobin (forming Heinz bodies) and by abnormal breakdown of heme leading to urinary excretion of darkly pigmented dipyrroles. Therefore, abnormal hemoglobins may be associated with some cases of familial poly-

cythemia; other cases may be attributable to a familial increase in erythropoietin levels.

Secondary polycythemia is a symptom complex usually but not necessarily associated with tissue hypoxia. Thus there is increased oxygen-carrying power with an associated decrease in oxygen saturation. Hemoglobin is normal or slightly elevated; this is associated with the prolonged reduction of arterial oxygen tension. It is thought that this blood hypoxia is related to something in the plasma that acts on the kidneys and probably other organs, which in turn elaborate a humoral factor called erythropoietin. The juxtaglomerular apparatus of the kidney may be hyperplastic with many large, pale cells and a decrease in granularity.[131] Erythropoietin in turn stimulates the differentiation and maturation of normoblasts into mature red blood cells. In most patients, one can demonstrate increased erythropoietin levels, which appear to increase the rate and number of maturation of erythropoietin-responsive erythroid marrow cells. This specific erythroid marrow stimulation is usually seen without associated thrombocytosis or leukocytosis. The increased erythrocyte mass leads to increased blood viscosity and together with primary cardiac or pulmonary disease produces a decrease in oxygen delivery to tissues. Red cell mass measurements correlate better with arterial saturation. There may be increased oxygen unsaturation in the recumbent elderly patient, a position more suitable for collection of blood.

Conditions underlying secondary polycythemia are elevated altitudes, patent interventricular septum (right-to-left shunt), pulmonary arteriovenous fistula, and pulmonary hemangioma, cyanotic heart disease, lung disease with decreased alveolocapillary permeability (mitral stenosis), emphysema, silicosis, extreme obesity, metabolic abnormalities of red blood cells, large abdominal tumors with or without ascites leading to decreased pulmonary ventilation, methemoglobinemia, sulfhemoglobinemia, and carboxyhemaglobinemia. Cushing's syndrome, cerebellar cysts and hemangioma (Lindau-von Hippel disease), uterine fibroids, liver carcinoma,[25] and renal lesions (carcinoma, cystic kidney, hydronephrosis, hyperparathyroidism with nephrocalcinosis), cobalt ingestion, and adrenocorticosteroid treatment in large doses.

Clinically, at high altitudes, secondary polycythemia is characterized by dypsnea at rest, headache, anorexia, tinnitus, lethargy, and vomiting—all aggravated by exertion. If the disorder is of long standing, one sees an emphysematous chest, cyanosis, clubbing of terminal phalanges, and reduced pulmonary vital capacity. Hematologically, the blood volume is increased, with reticulocytosis, occasional bilirubinemia, and leukocytosis. When the patient returns to sea level, the erythrocyte count and hematocrit come back to normal. In pulmonary disease such as pulmonary arteriosclerosis, occasionally with emphysema, pulmonary fibrosis, and the eventual development of right-sided heart failure (Ayerza's disease), one also observes the symptoms just described. The hematocrit and hemoglobin levels are elevated, erythrocyte counts range from 7,500,000 to 9,000,000 per cu.mm. with slight reticulocytosis and hyperbilirubinemia. No leukocytosis occurs. Secondary polycythemia is diagnosed also by finding a lowered oxygen saturation of blood (less than 90%) without correlation of hematocrit and erythrocyte volume as occurs in true polycythemia vera. Oxygen administration in secondary polycythemia produces depression of the iron clearance rate, whereas it has no effect in polycythemia vera.

Bone marrow findings include occasional normoblastosis with a slight increase in myeloid forms. There is no increase in myeloblasts or promyelocytes; megakaryocyte and platelet levels are also satisfactory. Oxygen is given as part of therapy during periods of marked cyanosis. Any causative drugs are eliminated; cardiac and pulmonary diseases are treated. Phlebotomy is performed if the hematocrit rises above 65 to 75 per cent; this helps to lower the blood volume and viscosity.

Myeloproliferative Syndrome. The differential diagnosis also includes the myeloproliferative syndrome, especially chronic granulocytic leukemia. One sees reduced alkaline phosphatase staining of granulocytes and the presence of the Philadelphia chromosome in the marrow cells of some patients with chronic granulocytic leukemia, whereas this is not usually found in polycythemia vera. One also observes qualitative platelet deficiencies and fibrinogenemia usually not found in chronic granulocytic leukemia.

Treatment

The treatment of polycythemia vera is aimed at keeping the blood volume at normal levels (hematocrit below 50 to 55), decreasing blood viscosity, and reducing the platelet levels (see also p. 481). An increased plasma volume occurs as the erythrocyte mass decreases. This may persist for months even if the hematocrit is brought to normal. Therefore, it is necessary to continue phlebotomies for one to two more times than are necessary to bring the hematocrit to normal range. This frequently reduces headaches and other symptoms not otherwise relieved. If phlebotomies become more necessary and more frequent, the patient is given ^{32}P orally (4.5 to 6.5 mc.). No further treatment is necessary for 2 or 3 months, at which time 2.5 to 3 mc. of ^{32}P may be given orally again (in the interim the erythrocyte, leukocyte, and platelet levels are checked every week or so). No further treatment is necessary for 1 to 2 years. In this way, only an occasional phlebotomy may be necessary in the interim. This approach also reduces the possibility of the development of radiation-induced leukemia. According to Osgood, "most persons with polycythemia vera would rather run some risk of dying of leukemia at an advanced age than of dying younger without leukemia."[32] If the patient becomes refractory to ^{32}P therapy or develops severe leukocytosis or thrombocytosis, one may use nitrogen mustard, triethylene melamine, or busulfan with frequent checkups of the peripheral blood picture.[197] Splenic irradiation is performed only if the spleen produces abdominal pressure symptoms. When the polycythemia vera patient needs surgery, the platelet and hematocrit levels are reduced to low values, or ^{32}P is given and phlebotomy performed with concomitant rapid postoperative ambulation of the patient.

STEM CELL, HISTIOCYTIC, HAIRY CELL, PLASMACYTIC, AND MEGAKARYOCYTIC LEUKEMIAS

Stem cell leukemia is a hematologic process frequently found in children. It is characterized by a proliferation of a lymphocytic type of undifferentiated cell present both in the peripheral blood and bone marrow. Morphologically, the cells are of medium size and have ovoid nuclei, vesicular nuclear chromatin containing nucleoli, and a pale blue cytoplasm with frayed, taglike projections. Pallor, fever, normocytic anemia, leukocytosis or leukopenia, purpura with associated thrombocytopenia, bone pain, malaise, slight enlargement of the liver, spleen, and lymph nodes, and frequent central nervous system involvement are observed on varying occasions. Death usually occurs 2 to 8 weeks after diagnosis with but slight response to chemotherapeutic agents. Occasionally bone marrow aspiration results in a dry tap requiring surgical biopsy.

Histiocytic leukemia is characterized by a stellate cell type that in this disease process is the undifferentiated reticulum or mesenchymal cell. It has a round, slightly indented nucleus, fine nuclear chromatin, and a bluish agranular cytoplasm with filamentous fibrillar extensions. These cells are similar but not identical to those that have been labelled "hairy cells," and the symptom complex itself is rare and without any proven benefit from chemotherapy. Bone marrow aspiration is fraught with difficulties and biopsy may need be performed. Cytologically, the hematologic pattern is that of a leukemia closely related to Hodgkin's disease, reticulum cell sarcoma, nonlipid histiocytosis, and the Schilling variants of monocytic leukemia. Clinically, it acts chronically and insidiously in adults, but has a fulminating course in young adults with frequently associated normocytic anemia, purpuric thrombocytopenia, leukopenia, neutropenia, and splenomegaly. Therapy is the same as in monocytic leukemias, life expectancy is less than 12 months with an associated, accelerated rate of destruction of normal cells leading to pancytopenia; this complication is often reduced by splenectomy.

Hairy cell leukemia (*leukemic reticuloendotheliosis*) is a disease of middle-aged to elderly adults characterized by a proliferation of atypical mononuclear cells with fingerlike cytoplasmic processes ("hairy cells"). Although the cells are usually present in small numbers in the peripheral blood, they commonly infiltrate the bone marrow and the red pulp of the spleen. Patients frequently present themselves with fatigue, weakness, anemia, and splenomegaly associated with hypersplenism. Splenectomy may be of therapeutic value. It is a chronic indolent disease entity that must be distinguished from other leukemic forms since it does not require aggressive chemotherapy. The origin of the hairy cells are unclear; various studies have shown them to have features of both B-lymphocytes and monocytes (Plate 77).

Plasmacytic leukemia has a pattern practically identical with that of a leukemic variant of multiple (plasma cell) myeloma. The peripheral blood has plasmoblasts, proplasmacytes, and plasmacytes, the latter occasionally containing eosinophilic Russell bodies. The onset, course, and therapy are the same as in the myeloma variety (pp. 508–509).

Megakaryocytic leukemia (essential thrombocythemia) is a variant of chronic myelocytic leukemia and is characterized by hyperplasia of the marrow megakaryoblasts, promegakaryocytes, and megakaryocytes. When marrow fibrosis occurs, the disorder is considered to be a member of the myeloproliferative group (myelofibrosis). The peripheral blood contains fragments of megakaryocytes, and frequently an overwhelming thrombocytosis is observed with variation in platelet size and shape; rarely, only a few platelets are seen. Clinically, the course is that of other granulocytic leukemias with infiltration of liver, kidney, spleen, and lymph nodes by megakaryocytes and other myeloid cells.

Mast cell leukemia is a rare process associated with urticaria pigmentosa, hepatosplenomegaly, and a marked infiltration of mast cells in the bone marrow, spleen, peripheral blood, and other organs. This leukemic symptom complex is related to systemic mast cell disease[193] in the same manner that monocytic leukemia compares to reticulum cell sarcoma and leukosarcoma to lymphosarcoma. In the systemic process, one also observes a hematologic pattern of anemia, leukopenia, mastocytosis, thrombocytopenia, and occasional erythrophagocytosis. Widespread skeletal disease with bone marrow aspirations showing replacement of normal elements by mast cells with basophilic granules is also found. Very infrequently an abnormal proliferation of basophils may be observed that is consistent with a major manifestation of basophilic leukemia and therefore is unlike the basophilia observed in patients with chronic granulocytic leukemia (Plate 70).

LYMPHOMAS

The lymphoma is a progressively fatal neoplasm derived from one or more of the cellular elements of the lymphoreticular system and characterized by aggressive proliferation and eventual spread from the site of origin. All organs may eventually become involved. It is less common in non-Caucasians, males are affected twice as commonly as females. All ages are involved, with symptoms related to the areas at which lymph node enlargement and lymphoid tissue involvement is greatest and by the anatomic structures subjected to pressure, obstruction, and infiltration by the neoplastic tissue process. In the late stages, fever, anemia, hemorrhagic phenomena, cachexia, and susceptibility to infections frequently occur.

Rappaport states that "although many observations support the theory of the histogenetic unity of malignant lymphomas, the predominating cell type prevails throughout the course of the disease in the majority of the patients."[158] He also considers this sufficiently significant to justify retention of a cytologic classification that includes malignant lymphomas with follicular or nodular patterns. Although Rappaport's classification of systemic proliferative diseases and tumors of the hematopoietic tissues (Table 13–8) is based primarily on their cellular compositions, the systemic and the initially localized lesions are listed separately in order to emphasize that one or other of these listed clinical and gross morphologic patterns frequently prevails. This arrangement does not imply that sharp differentiation between the two forms of involvement can always be made.

PATHOLOGIC FINDINGS

Non-Hodgkin's Lymphoma (NHL)

Grossly, the lymph nodes involved in NHL are enlarged, grayish white, somewhat firm, and adhere to one another with thickening of the capsule. Microscopically, the individual follicles and their germinal centers lose their "starry-eyed" follicular pattern and appear as monotonous sheets of lymphoblasts, lymphocytes, or histiocytes (reticulum cells) with numerous mitoses. Occasionally, reticulum fibers are

Table 13-8. Classification of Systemic Proliferative Diseases and Tumors of the Hematopoietic Tissues*

Predominant Component Cell(s)	Systemic Proliferative Diseases (tumor formation may occur)	Initially Localized Tumors (systemic involvement occurs frequently)
Primitive reticular cell		Malignant lymphoma, undifferentiated†
Undifferentiated hematopoietic cell	Undifferentiated (stem cell) leukemia	
Monocyte	Monocytic leukemia, acute and chronic (also hairy cell leukemia)	
Histiocyte	Malignant histiocytosis	Malignant lymphoma, histiocytic (reticulum cell sarcoma)† Hodgkin's disease†
Histiocyte and lymphocyte		Malignant lymphoma, mixed cell (histiocytic-lymphocytic)†
Lymphocytic cells Lymphoblast	Acute lymphocytic leukemia	
Poorly differentiated lymphocyte		Malignant lymphoma, poorly differentiated lymphocytic†
Differentiated lymphocyte	Chronic lymphocytic leukemia Lymphoproliferative disease with dysproteinemia (including primary macroglobulinemia)	Malignant lymphoma, well differentiated lymphocytic† **Mycosis fungoide and Sézary syndrome**
Plasma cell	Myelomatosis (multiple myeloma)	Plasmacytoma
Tissue mast cell	Malignant tissue mast cell disease	Mastocytoma
Myelopoietic cells	Myeloproliferative diseases	
Granulocyte	Granulocytic leukemia, acute and chronic	Granulocytic sarcoma (chloroma)
Erythroblast	Erythremic myelosis	
Erythroblast and granulocyte	Erythroleukemia	
Megakaryocyte	Megakaryocytic myelosis Idiopathic thrombocythemia	
Erythroblast, granulocyte, and megakaryocyte	Polycythemia vera Myelosclerosis with myeloid metaplasia	

* Modified from Rappaport, H.: Tumors of the Hematopoietic System. Armed Forces Institute of Pathology, Fascicle 8, 1966.
† Malignant lymphomas that have follicular (nodular) patterns are designated by addition of "follicular" ("nodular") to the cytologically appropriate terms.

observed by silver staining, and invasion of the marginal and medullary sinuses is seen with eventual infiltration through the capsule of the lymph node to the surrounding tissues.

A more detailed and most commonly used microscopic Rappaport classification of NHL provides a unifying approach to the study of anatomic distribution, clinical course, and prognosis in the various histologic types. It is as follows:

Nodular and Diffuse
1. malignant lymphoma, undifferentiated type
2. malignant lymphoma, histiocytic type
3. malignant lymphoma, lymphocytic type, poorly differentiated
4. malignant lymphoma, lymphocytic type, well differentiated
5. malignant lymphoma, mixed (histiocytic-lymphocytic) type

Those with a nodular pattern are designated by the addition of the word "nodular"

Table 13-9. Histologic Classification of Malignant Lymphoma*

Predominating Cells	Rappaport Classification	Old Classification
Primitive reticulum cell	Malignant lymphoma, un-differentiated†	Large cell lymphosarcoma; reticulum cell sarcoma
Histiocyte	Malignant lymphoma, his-tiocytic†	
Histiocyte and lymphocyte	Malignant lymphoma, mixed-cell type†	Large cell lymphosarcoma; lymphoblastic lympho-sarcoma
Poorly differentiated lymphocyte	Malignant lymphoma, lym-phocytic type, poorly dif-ferentiated†	
Well-differentiated lymphocyte	Malignant lymphoma, lym-phocytic type, well dif-ferentiated†	Small-cell lymphosarcoma; lymphocytic lympho-sarcoma

* Ultmann, J. E., and Stein, R. S.: Non-Hodgkin's lymphoma—An approach to staging and therapy. CA—A Cancer Journal for Clinicians, 25:320, 1975.
† Both nodular and diffuse forms exist. Nodular lymphomas were previously termed (giant) follicular lymphomas.

Table 13-10. Relative Incidence of Histologic Types*

Histologic Type	Nodular	Diffuse
Well-differentiated lymphocytic lymphoma	Rare, usually chronic lymphocytic leukemia.	
Poorly differentiated lymphocytic lymphoma	30%	30%
Mixed-cell lymphoma	5%	5%
Histiocytic lymphoma	Rare	30%

* Ultmann, J. E., and Stein, R. S.: Non-Hodgkin's lymphoma—An approach to staging and therapy. CA—A Cancer Journal for Clinicians, 25:320, 1975.

preceding the cytologically appropriate terms and are probably the most important histologic criteria with respect to prognosis. Cell type and differentiation also have prognostic import. Tables 13–9 and 13–10 compare old and recent classification and relative incidence of histologic types.

Since the differences in nodularity, cell type, and cellular differentiation of the tissue are important in the ultimate response and prognosis of the patient, precise classification is mandatory. The interpretation of therapeutic responses must be made with particular care when there is evidence of disagreement over the underlying hematopathology.

With the advent of new immunologic, cytochemical, functional, and ultrastructural techniques, it has been possible to characterize the distribution of thymus-dependent (T) lymphocytes, bursa-equivalent (B) lymphocytes, and mononuclear-phagocytic cells of normal lymph nodes, and to some

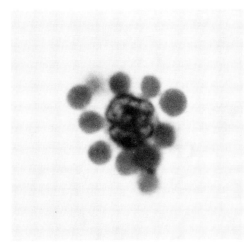

Fig. 13-23. Millipore-filter preparation of neoplastic lymphocytes forming IgMEAC (B-cell) rosettes shows prominent nuclear irregularities of neoplastic cell. (× 1000; Jaffe, E. S., Shevach, E. M., Frank, M. M., Berard, C. W., and Green, I.: Nodular lymphoma—Evidence for origin from follicular B lymphocytes. N. Engl. J. Med., 290:813, 1974, also from N.I.H.)

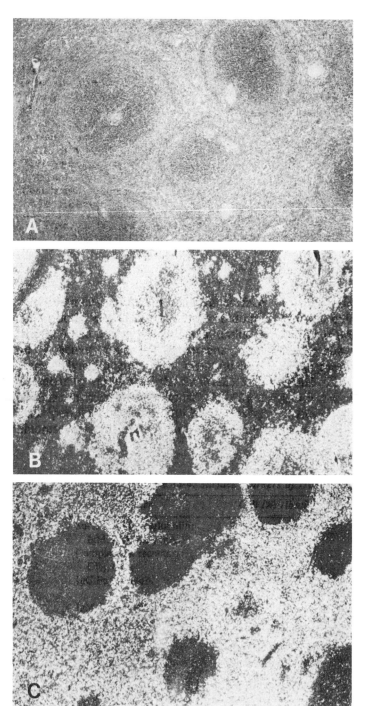

Fig. 13-24. (*A*) Spleen involved by nodular lymphoma —poorly differentiated lymphocytic type. White pulp regions are expanded and are replaced by neoplastic lymphocytes. (*B*) Frozen section of nodular lymphoma spleen treated with IgMEAC (dark field microscopy). Reagent RBCs adhere to neoplastic white pulp nodules as well as to small aggregates of neoplastic lymphocytes infiltrating the red pulp. (*C*) Frozen section of spleen of nodular lymphoma treated with IgGEA (dark field microscopy). Reagent RBCs adhere only to histiocytes in uninvolved red pulp. (*Continued on facing page*)

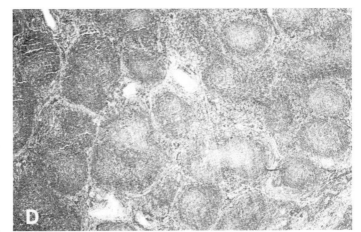

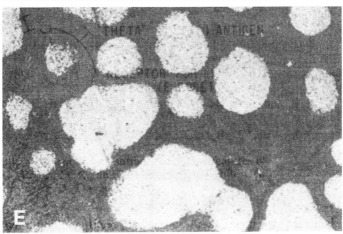

(*Continued*) (*D*) Lymph node — nodular lymphoma — mixed lymphocytic and histiocytic type. Neoplastic nodules composed of a mixture of small and large cells replace the lymph node. (*E*) Frozen section of 3D treated with IgMEAC (dark field microscopy). Reagent and RBCs bind diffusely to neoplastic nodules and spare normal appearing lymphocytes in compressed internodular cords. (× 25; Jaffe, E. S., Shevach, E. M., Frank, M. M., Berard, C. W., Green, I.: Nodular lymphoma — Evidence for origin from follicular B lymphocytes. N. Engl. J. Med., *290*:813, 1974. also from N.I.H.)

extent their pathologic counterparts.[23] From a study of B- and T-derived lymphocyte surface markers on these cells in tissue sections, (Figs. 13-23 and 13-24) 70 per cent of NHL involves malignant monoclonal tumors of the B-cells of the follicular center. It has been further found that small and large nondividing cleaved cells predominate in the nodular lymphoma, and noncleaved dividing cells predominate in the diffuse lymphoma. In the last-mentioned group, there is a greater range of cell size and a high proliferative rate. Morphologically, histiocytic lymphoma large cells look like transformed B-lymphocytes and only occasionally possess the biochemical characteristics of macrophages. True malignant disease of the mononuclear-phagocytic cell or malignant histiocytosis is rare; histiocytic medullary reticulosis is an example. T-cell markers are seen in the predominant diagnostic cell components of Sézary syndrome, mycosis fungoides, and a form of poorly differentiated "convoluted cell" lymphocytic non-Hodgkin's lymphoma of childhood. The last is more common in adolescence and frequently spreads to the marrow and leptomeninges. Further, all of the nodular lymphomas and many of the diffuse forms are composed of malignant lymphoid cells of "B" origin, mostly of follicular origin. In addition the vast majority of "histiocytic" and lymphocytic-histiocytic cell types lack monocytic-macrophage markers but bear surface immunoglobulins. As a result of these findings, new classifications are constantly being proposed.

Nodular Lymphoma Evidence for Origin from Follicular B-Lymphocytes

Nodular or follicular lymphomas make up a large percentage of malignant lymphomas with distinct clinical, therapeutic, prognostic, and pathologic features. Benign follicular hyperplasia has been described and differentiated from nodular lymphoma; however, the cytogenetic relation of the neoplastic nodules to normal or hyperplastic lymphoid follicles has remained nebulous. Immunologic techniques, newly developed, now permit elucidation of the morphogenesis of nodular lymphoas and may possibly allow classification of its cellular components as thymus-independent lymphocytes (B-cells), thymus-dependent lymphocytes (T-cells), or histiocytes. Most animals demonstrate B-cells, and, in addition to possessing easily demonstrable surface immunoglobulin and a receptor for the Fc portion of the immunoglobulin molecule, also have receptors for the third component of complement (C3). These are identified by their binding of RBCs coated with antibody and complement (EAC). Most monocytes, histiocytes, and macrophages also bear C3 receptors but also have additional receptors for cytophilic antibody and will bind RBCs coated with IgG (IgGEA). The Ig MEAC and IgGEA receptors can be identified on cells both in frozen tissue sections (Fig. 13-24B, C, E) and in suspensions. Human T-cells bear none of these receptors, but living cells in suspension may be identified by their ability to form nonimmune rosettes with sheep RBCs. Since recent work has indicated that all these receptors may also be identified on neoplastic lymphoreticular cells, Jaffe and co-workers believed that demonstration of their presence or absence might establish the origin of these neoplastic cells.[93a] They studied neoplastic cells from six patients with nodular lymphoma both in cell suspen-

sions and in frozen tissue sections for (1) the C3 receptor—RBCs coated with antibody and complement (IgMEAC)—of B-lymphocytes; (2) the receptor for cytophilic antibody—RBCs coated with IgG (IgGEA)—of histiocytes; and (3) spontaneous rosette formation with sheep RBCs characteristic of T-lymphocytes.[93a] A high proportion of the neoplastic lymphoma cells in suspension bound IgMEAC. They did not bind IgGEA and did not form sheep RBC rosettes. In tissue sections of nodular lymphomas the IgMEAC reagent bound to the neoplastic nodules (Fig. 13-24B, E). In control lymph nodes and spleens (Fig. 13-24C) these binding properties were demonstrated to be characteristic of the cells of the lymphoid follicle, thus suggesting a follicular B-cell origin for nodular lymphoma.

Cervical, axillary, or inguinal nodes are involved more commonly than tonsillar and nasopharyngeal tissue. Mediastinal and retroperitoneal nodes, spleen, liver, gastrointestinal tract, central nervous system, and bone may become involved with compression and involvement of adjacent nerves and other structures. Cytologic examination of pleural or ascitic fluid may show great numbers of lymphoblasts, lymphocytes, or histiocytes (reticulum cells). Lymphadenopathy and a symptom complex simulating those of malignant lymphoma can be produced by hydantoin (Dilantin) and hydantoin-like drugs.

In 1974, Frizzera and colleagues described a disease which they called "angioimmunoblastic lymphadenopathy" (AILD).[67] It usually began acutely in an elderly person with severe constitutional symptoms, generalized lymphadenopathy, hepatosplenomegaly, polyclonal hypergammaglobulinemia, and hemolytic anemia. Patients had a notable susceptibility to infections that may have been induced or aggravated by cytotoxic therapy[159] that seemed to respond to corticosteroid therapy that, if it was not rapidly fatal, permitted prolonged survival.

From the foregoing reports, as well as

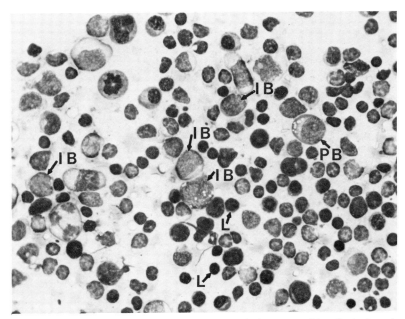

Fig. 13-25. Immunoblasts, lymphocytes, and plasmacytoid cells in lymph node imprint (× 635). IB = immunoblast; PB = plasmablast; L = Lymphocyte. (Courtesy of Adel A. Yunis, M.D.)

other writings on the subject, immunoblastic lymphadenopathy is probably a hyperimmune disorder of varying origin. It closely resembles the graft-versus-host reaction and may follow administration of drugs or vaccines or may accompany or follow other diseases.[53, 85, 171] Histologically, immunoblastic lymphadenopathy closely resembles a malignant lymphoma. Lymph nodes and other tissues display widespread disruption of lymphoid tissue by infiltration of immunoblasts and plasmacytes, capsular invasion, and vascular proliferation and deposits of amorphous eosinophilic material in lymph nodes (Figs. 13-25; 13-26; 13-27). The basic process appears to be a non-neoplastic hyperimmune proliferation of the B-cell system (involving an exaggeration of lymphocyte transformation to immunoblasts and plasma cells that may be triggered by a hypersensitivity reaction to therapeutic agents).

Many pathologists emphasize the tendency to misdiagnose the tissue findings as a malignant lymphoma (particularly Hodgkin's disease) and, therefore, stress the consequent importance of meticulous microscopical study and the potential misadventure when cytotoxic drugs are administered because of mistaken diagnosis. Some believe that the classification by Custer and Bernhard helps to clarify the interrelationships of lymphomas but is not therapy-oriented (Fig. 13-28).

Detailed clinical and surgical staging of lymphoma patients under the classification of Hodgkin's disease and non-Hodgkin's lymphoma (NHL) has allowed clear characterization of the differences in these two groups of patients. Patients with Hodgkin's disease are younger, have more frequent constitutional symptoms, less frequent involvement of Waldeyer's ring, the gastrointestinal tract, the bone marrow, the mesenteric nodes, and less advanced disease when they are first seen. They have more frequent involvement of mediastinal nodes than patients with non-Hodgkin's lym-

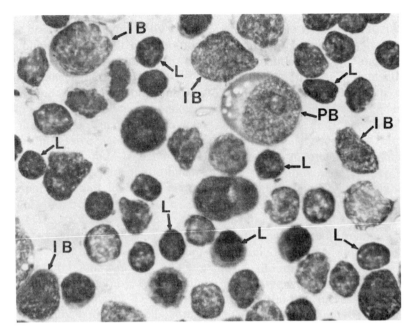

Fig. 13-26. Immunoblasts in lymph node imprint (× 1588). The immunoblast is a term commonly used for the large (15–25 μ) transformed lymphocyte (formerly called reticulum cells) of both the T-cell and the B-cell system in histologic sections with specific immunologic markers required to distinguish between the two. They have large, oval nuclei with finely dispersed pale, basophilic finely reticulated chromatin and one large or two to three smaller nucleoli, often situated on or near the nuclear membrane; there is a moderate amount of cytoplasm (IB = immunoblast; PB = plasmablast; L = lymphocyte; Courtesy of Adel A. Yunis, M.D.)

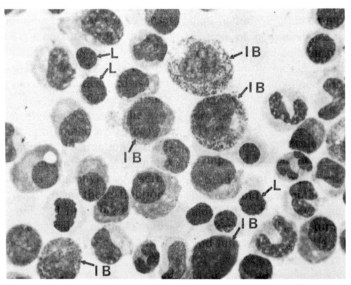

Fig. 13-27. Immunoblasts in bone marrow (× 1000). IB = immunoblast; L = lymphocyte. (Courtesy of Adel A. Yunis, M.D.)

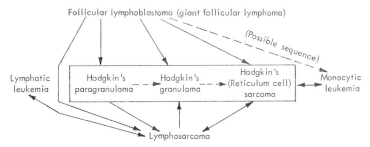

Fig. 13-28. The modified Custer and Bernhard classification of lymphomas. Dotted lines represent Parker's concept of Hodgkin's disease. (Custer, R. P., and Bernard, W. G.: The interrelationship of Hodgkin's disease and other lymphatic tumors. Am. J. Med. Sci., *216:*625, 1948)

phoma.[98] Table 13–11 compares the clinical features of these two diseases. Although they are similar in many respects, the non-Hodgkin's lymphoma that arises in extranodal sites (e.g., tonsil or bone) may be more curable than others in early stages but progresses rapidly if it is not controlled.

Mycosis Fungoides (MF) and Sézary Syndrome

Mycosis fungoides is a malignant lymphoma that primarily involves the skin in the early stages of disease. It is most common in adults over the age of 40 and affects males more often than females. Histologically, in the skin there is a bandlike dermal infiltrate of atypical, often cerebriform lymphocytes, admixed with histiocytes and other inflammatory cells. Collections of atypical cells in the epidermis (Pautrier's microabscesses) are commonly found. Peripheral lymph nodes draining the skin lesions may be enlarged and usually reveal dermatopathic lymphadenitis. For many

Table 13-11. Comparison of Selected Clinical Features in Previously Untreated Patients with Lymphoma*

Feature	Hodgkin's Disease %	Non-Hodgkin's Nodular %	Lymphoma Diffuse %
Systemic symptoms	40+	17	24
Involvement of:			
Waldeyer's ring	< 1	2	11
Mediastinal or hilar lymphadenopathy	40–60	18	24
Gastrointestinal tract	< 1	7	22
Bone marrow	5	24	14
Mediastinal skipping	9	40	20
Involvement at laparotomy of:			
Mesenteric nodes	1	34	14
Spleen	35	42	11
Liver	< 5	18	11
Localized extralymphatic involvement			
('E')	10	6	16
Contiguous spread (Stages II–III$_E$)	< 90	81	90
Localized (Stages I–II$_E$) †	50	6	30
Advanced (Stages III, III$_E$, IV) ‡	50	94	70

* Coltman, C. A., et al.: Lymphoma: Diagnosis and Management. Presented at the Education Program of the American Society of Hematology. San Diego, 1977.
  † Modified from Jones, S. E.: Clinics in Hematology, *3:*131, 1974.
  ‡ Modified from Chabner, B. A., et al.: Ann. Intern. Med., *85:*149, 1976.

years this disease may be limited to the skin. However, the prognosis is eventually poor, for visceral involvement of lymph nodes, liver, and other organs occur in 70 per cent of cases studied at autopsy.

A variant called the Sézary syndrome occurs, which is characterized by exfoliative dermatitis with mycosis fungoides-like skin lesions and a leukemic blood picture. The leukemic cells are cerebriform, have T-cell characteristics, and are similar to those seen in the mycosis fungoides skin lesions. Symptomatic relief is afforded by treatment, but it does not prolong the survival rate of less than 50 per cent at 5 years. Early skin lesions are controlled to some extent by topical steroids, topical nitrogen mustard, and electron beam therapy. Systemic chemotherapy is also used as in the therapy of lymphoid leukemia, but no large series have been reported as of this date.

Malignant Histiocytosis (Histiocytic Medullary Reticulosis)

Malignant histiocytosis is a rare, rapidly progressive and fatal disease that usually occurs in adults but may occur in children on occasion. Fever, lymphadenopathy, hepatosplenomegaly, anemia, and thrombocytopenia occur. Histologically, there is a neoplastic proliferation of true histiocytes primarily involving the sinuses of lymph nodes, the splenic red pulp, liver sinusoids, bone marrow, and skin. The histiocytes are atypical and usually show evidence of phagocytosis (frequently RBCs). Chemotherapy is the same as in monocytic and histiocytic leukemia, to which it may be very closely allied.

Hematologic Findings

Usually the bone marrow and peripheral blood are normal and thus merely serve to exclude leukemia in the differential diagnosis. In histiocytic lymphoma the bone marrow may contain histiocytic cells with occasional monocytic or reticulum-like cells in the peripheral blood. A normocytic, normochromic anemia occurs early in 5 to 10 per cent of cases and late in 90 to 100 per cent of cases. Platelets are normal or increased early and frequently decreased late in the disease. The leukocyte count is usually normal early, or a lymphocytic lymphosarcoma may be terminating in a pattern similar to that in acute lymphocytic leukemia, in which the bone marrow is replaced by lymphosarcoma cells, the white blood cells may rise to high levels, and most of the peripheral blood leukocytes are abnormal lymphocytes with associated severe anemia and thrombocytopenia. Occasionally the spleen is enlarged, and secondary hemolysins develop producing a hemolytic anemia and giving a positive Coombs test. Histiocytic lymphoma may occasionally terminate in acute leukemia[123] (Plates 79, 80).

Occasionally, lymphosarcoma and chronic granulocytic leukemia coexist.[202] A special type of poorly differentiated lymphosarcoma (Burkitt's tumor) with a high predilection for jaw, ovarian, and abdominal lymph nodes, and visceral involvement has been described mainly in children of central Africa with some cases described in the United States. Herpes-like viral particles and antibodies have been reported.[209] The blood uric acid and urea nitrogen levels become elevated, especially after treatment has been initiated. If bone is involved, alkaline phosphatase and serum calcium levels are elevated. The average survival time of the African patients is 2 to 2½ years from the time of onset of symptoms.

Prognosis and Treatment

Treatment options in non-Hodgkin's lymphoma (NHL) are multiple and undergoing constant revision. To a large extent, this is a direct consequence of the marked heterogeneity of the pathologic subtypes (e.g., bone lymphomas, gastrointestinal lymphomas, and skin lymphomas

Table 13-12. Relationship Between Histology and Stage of Disease at Presentation*†

Histology	Stage		
Non-Hodgkin's Lymphoma	Stages I and II (%)	Stage III (%)	Stage IV (%)
Poorly differentiated lymphocytic lymphoma—nodular	15	< 15	> 70
Poorly differentiated lymphocytic lymphoma—diffuse	15	< 15	> 70
Histiocytic lymphoma	< 50	> 50	

* Ultmann, J. E., and Stein, R. S.: Non-Hodgkin's lymphoma—an approach to staging and therapy. CA—A Cancer Journal for Clinicians, *25*:320, 1975.
† See Plate 82.

such as mycosis fungoides). These range from the lymphoblastic (convoluted or non-convoluted) lymphomas of children to the well-differentiated lymphocytic lymphomas of middle-aged adults. In addition, there is an apparent difference in survival among the histiocytic subtypes, including architectural pattern (nodular or diffuse) and cell type (lymphocytic or histiocytic). These prognostic features are of considerably more value in adults, where close to half of the lymphomas have a nodular pattern, than in children and adolescents, where virtually all of the lymphomas have a diffuse pattern. Certainly, current available data suggest that nodular lymphomas have, overall, a better prognosis and higher percent of survival than diffuse lymphomas.[172]

In the planning of therapy, staging is used (Table 13–12). Stage I represents the disease limited to a single lymph node group, and Stage II is limited to two or more lymph node groups either above or below the diaphragm. However, laparotomy and staging in NHL has not been widely used, since NHL tends to affect an older population with patients more likely to have advanced disease on initial presentation, and since NHL spreads in an unpredictable pattern and usually involves nodal sites (e.g., mesentery, etc.) outside the standard radiation fields. Therefore, in the staging procedures, bone marrow biopsy, lymphangiography, liver biopsy, laparoscopy, and laparotomy are utilized quite often, since at

least 80 per cent of patients have shown extranodal involvement with malignant classification in Stage III (disease above and below the diaphragm) and Stage IV (disseminated disease in lymphoid and nonlymphoid structures).[33] Thus, therapy for NHL, with rare exceptions, is designed for systemic rather than regional control and care. However, when patients present themselves with localized or regional nodal or extranodal disease (Stage I and II), local irradiation (3500 to 4500 rad) is generally indicated, although there is a high rate of relapse outside the treatment field with radiotherapy alone. The use of chemotherapy and local irradiation for Stages I and II disease is being studied. There is no evidence that extended-field irradiation or total nodal irradiation increases survival in localized disease.

In general, advanced systemic disease (Stages III and IV) should be treated with chemotherapy or by total-body irradiation. Certain histologic types of non-Hodgkin's lymphoma, such as diffuse lymphocytic, well differentiated, and nodular lymphocytic poorly differentiated, tend to grow slowly and may respond well to therapy with a single agent. These agents fall into several broad categories: alkylating drugs (cyclophosphamide, chlorambucil); vinca alkaloids (vincristine, vinblastine); antibiotics (bleomycin, adriamycin); nitrosureas (BCNU, CCNU); corticosteroids (prednisone) and miscellaneous agents (procarbazine, streptonigrin, hexamethylmelamine).[12]

The efficacy of cyclophosphamide (Cytoxan) was confirmed with a complete remission rate of 16 per cent in 1968; the unique advantage of vincristine over vinblastine derive from significantly less hematologic toxicity and the production of significant partial regression. There were no complete responses with prednisone.[13]

More aggressive disease, such as diffuse lymphocytic poorly differentiated or diffuse histiocytic non-Hodgkin's lymphoma, generally require combination chemotherapy. The effectiveness of cyclophosphamide (C), vincristine or Oncovin (V or O), and prednisone (P) has led to the use of the acronym COP or CVP in the medical literature. Complete remissions (CR) have been reported in the range of 35 to 57 per cent with median durations of 3 to greater than 18 months. Where the data are separated by histologic pattern, the CR percent is higher for nodular lymphomas than for diffuse lymphomas. It is important to separate relapse-free survival or the disease-free interval from survival. Although overall response rates for nodular and diffuse patterns are similar (60–80%), median survival is distinctly greater for nodular lymphomas, usually in excess of 6 years in contrast to under 2 years for diffuse lymphomas. In addition, treatment of nodular lymphomas with cytoxan or chlorambucil as compared with treatment utilizing CVP or CVP plus total nodal irradiation (150 rad in 5 weeks) produced complete remissions in 40 months (single agent) or 16 months (combined chemotherapy).

Diffuse histiocytic lymphomas are now being treated with either cyclophosphamide: prednisone (CP), CVP, or BCNU-CVP. Patients were treated for 9 cycles at 3-week intervals, and the median survival for the CVP group was 70.4 weeks; the largest survival of 143 weeks was in the mixed-cell type of diffuse lymphoma. Later on, regimens of cyclophosphamide, hydroxydaunomycin (Adriamycin), vincristine (Oncovin), and Prednisone (called CHOP) and bleomycin, Adriamycin, cyclophosphamide, Oncovin, and prednisone (called BACOP) both produced similar remission rates (5–30 months) and survival rates (approximately 2 years). The MOPP and C-MOPP (P = prednisone and procarbazine; M = nitrogen mustard) series therapeutic program produced a similar complete remission rate of 2 to 9 years after therapy with a median survival of more than 4 years. Total body irradiation studies reveal a 5-year survival figure for nodular lymphoma of 80 per cent and for diffuse lymphomas of 40 per cent, exclusive of histiocytic types. Relapse-free survivals were 25 per cent and 10 per cent respectively, indicating high relapse potential for both groups.

The use of immunotherapy in NHL is also under investigation in a number of centers. Preliminary data suggest that BCG may prolong the disease-free interval in patients achieving complete remission after induction chemotherapy.

Virtually no complete responses were observed when liver, bone marrow, or central nervous system involvement was present.

The pharmacologic concept behind the above-described chemotherapy (nitrogen mustard, triethylene melamine, chlorambucil, vincristine, or cytoxan) is related to their use when the systemic findings are severe with associated wide-spread disease, or when it is necessary to avoid edema due to radiotherapy, or when radiotherapy has lost its effectiveness. (2) Steroids (prednisone) are used to produce euphoria in a very sick patient, to increase his appetite, to reduce fever and lymph node size, and to decrease capillary bleeding and symptoms of atypical splenic activity. However, steroids may lead to the development of terminal tuberculosis and mycotic infection. (3) Transfusions are given for supportive therapy. (4) Surgery is used when lymph nodes are easily accessible; it is followed by radiotherapy.

Color Plates   75–92

Plate 75

MYELOFIBROSIS WITH MYELOID METAPLASIA
(Agnogenic Myeloid Metaplasia)
Bone Marrow, Lymph Node, and Spleen

Bizarre (biz), giant platelet (g Pl), juvenile (Juv), lymphocyte (L), megakaryocyte (Mgk), myeloblast (Myb), metamyelocyte (mMc), neutrophilic myelocyte (NMc), orthochromic normoblast (ONb), polychromatophilic normoblast (PcNb), polymorphonuclear neutrophil (PmN), prolymphocyte (prL), promonocyte (prM), promyelocyte (prMc), pronormoblast (prNb).

Diagnostic Features: Usually hypocellular, but occasionally normal or hypercellular; marrow fibrosis or excessive osseous tissue may be encountered with islands of hematopoiesis scattered throughout. It may be necessary to resort to marrow biopsy to demonstrate myelofibrosis or osteosclerosis. Fewer nucleated RBCs are seen than in the peripheral blood of the same patient. Large clumps and masses of platelets without a concomitant megakaryocytic increase in a hypocellular marrow is very suggestive of myelofibrosis. Splenic and lymph node imprints may demonstrate foci of hematopoiesis with immature myeloid and erythroid cells.

Fig. 1. Arrows show platelet clumps. Fig. 6. Lymph node imprint. Fig. 7. Spleen aspirate.

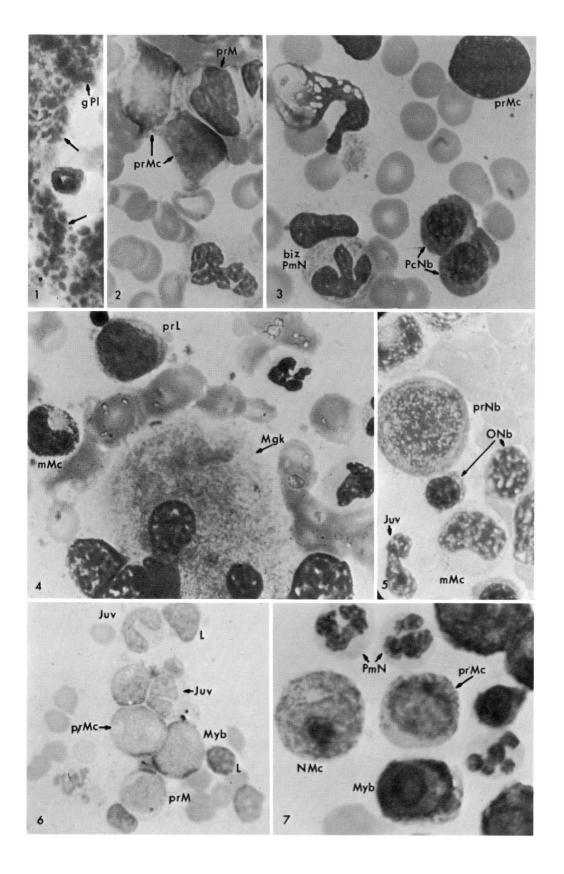

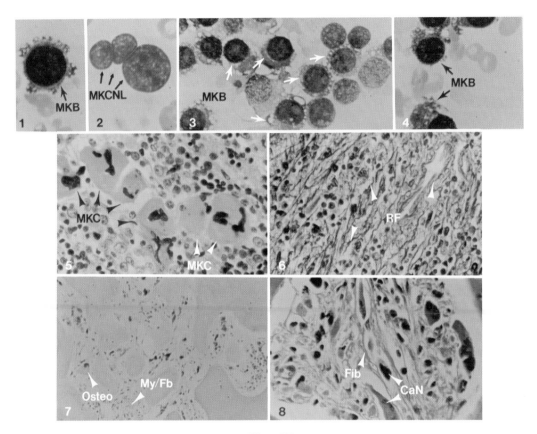

Plate 76

MYELOFIBROSIS WITH MYELOID METAPLASIA
(Agnogenic Myeloid Metaplasia, Acute Megakaryocytic Myelosis)
Bone Marrow

Varying patterns are observed ranging from hypocellular and fibrotic to hypercellular with islands of hematopoiesis and excess numbers of megakaryocytes. (MKB = megakaryoblast; MKCNL = megakaryocytic nuclear lobes; MKC = megakaryocyte; RF = reticulin fibers—reticulin stain; Osteo = osteosclerosis; My/Fb = myelofibrosis; CaN = cancer cell nucleus; Fib = fibrosis trichrome stain)

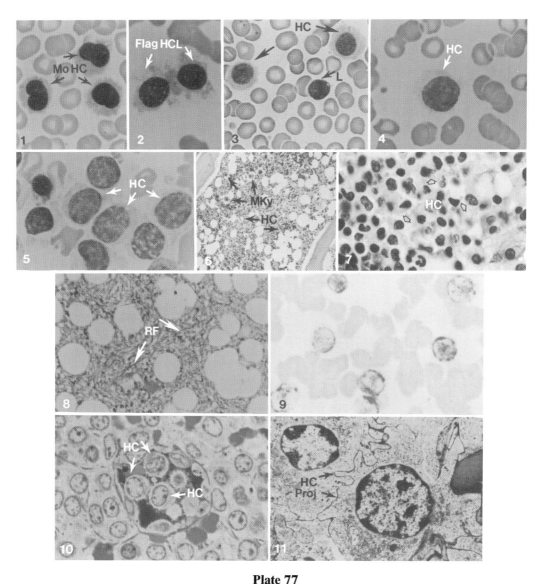

Plate 77

HAIRY CELL LEUKEMIA
(Leukemic Reticuloendotheliosis)

Diagnostic Features: Hairy cell leukemia is characterized by a variable WBC count, is often neutropenic, and is dependent upon the quantity of atypical mononuclear cells present (leukemic or aleukemic). The hematologic characteristic of "hairy" cells is owing to the irregular cytoplasmic villi that give the mononuclear cell a ciliated hairy appearance in electron microscopic or stained cellular patterns. It is approximately 15 to 30 μm. in diameter with a round or oval nucleus and has fairly abundant gray-blue cytoplasm. The nuclear chromatin is moderately clumped, and nucleoli are usually small or not visible. Histochemically, acid-phosphatase activity is prominent in these cells and is resistant to degradation by tartrate, characteristics common mostly to monocytoid cells. Hepato-splenomegaly, lymphadenopathy, and anemia occur, with marrow aspiration occasionaly associated with a "dry tap." Biopsy reveals a hypoplastic parenchyma with a moderate number of hairy cells. In tissues, the infiltration is differentiated from histiocytic lymphomatous infiltrates by being diffuse rather than nodular, and flagellated cells are seen in spleen and lymph nodes. Occasionally splenectomy may be helpful; other forms of therapy are usually not successful. Thick and thin electron microscopic patterns are also helpful. (MoHC = monocytoid hairy cell; FlagHCL = flagellated hairy cell lymphocytoid; L = lymphocyte; HC = hairy cell; MKy = megakaryocyte; HC foci = hairy cell foci; RF = reticulin fibers; HCPrj = hairy cell projections)

Plate 78

POLYCYTHEMIA VERA (POLYCYTHEMIA RUBRA, ERYTHREMIA OF PRIMARY POLYCYTHEMIA)
Peripheral Blood and Bone Marrow

Basophilic normoblast (Bnb), eosinophilic myelocyte (EMc), juvenile (Juv), lymphocyte (L), monocyte (M), megakaryocyte (Mgk), metamyelocyte (mMc), myeloblast (Myb), mitosis (mit), neutrophilic myelocyte (NMc), orthochromic normoblast (ONb), polychromatic normoblast (PcNb), polymorphonuclear eosinophil (PmE), promonocyte (prM), promyelocyte (prMc), platelets (Pl).

Diagnostic Features: Peripheral blood is dark red color with larger number of RBCs (hematocrit usually over 55). Frequently observe polychromatophilia and occasionally basophilic stippling and normoblasts. Occasionally see leukocytes with 1 to 2 per cent myelocytes and metamyelocytes; myeloid cells have positive alkaline phosphatase stain. Basophils and monocytes increased. Platelets are increased 5 to 10 times with frequent clumps of platelets. Bone marrow is dark red and hypercellular (all cells) with normal M:E ratio. Nucleated RBCs, myelocytes, myeloblasts and megakaryocytes are increased; frequently see increased number of eosinophilic and basophilic leukocytes. Fig. 1. Increased numbers of normoblasts. Fig. 4. (Inset) Polymorphonuclear neutrophil with alkaline phosphate stain. Fig. 5. Peripheral blood showing clumps of platelets and polychromatic RBCs (arrows).

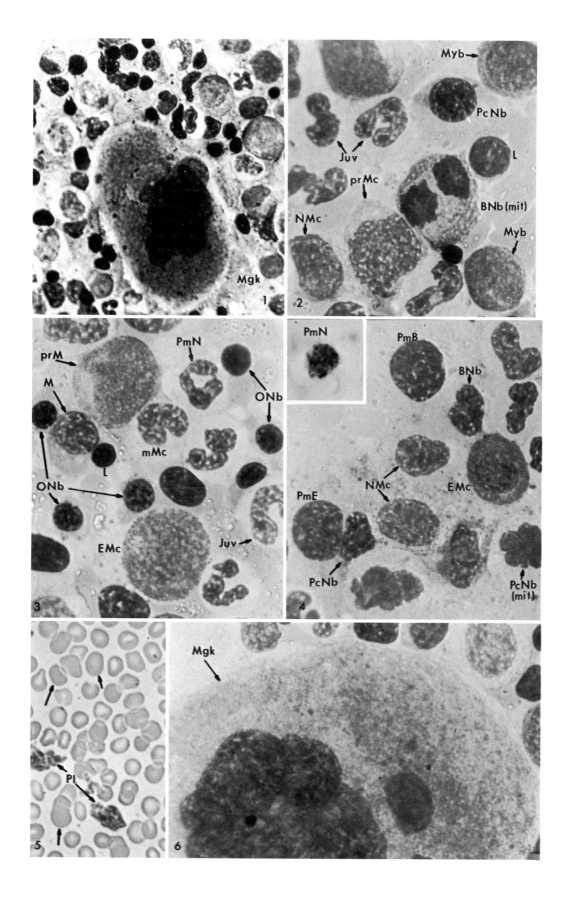

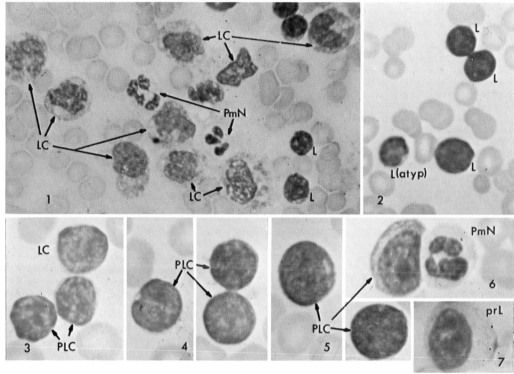

Plate 79

LEUKOSARCOMA
(Acute and Chronic Lymphosarcoma Cell Leukemia)
Peripheral Blood

Atypical (atyp), lymphocyte (L), leukosarcoma cell or atypical prolymphocyte (LC), polymorphonuclear neutrophil (PmN), primitive leukosarcoma cell (PLC), prolymphocyte (prL).

Diagnostic Features: This entity is frequently confused morphologically with acute monocytic leukemia and chronic lymphocytic leukemia. It differs from C.L.L. (chronic lymphocytic leukemia) in that C.L.C.L. (chronic lymphosarcoma cell leukemia) runs a rapid course in patients of a younger age group; the WBC count is lower than in C.L.L. (i.e., 20,000 to 80,000 per cu. mm.). The characteristic cell is an atypical prolymphocyte which is more mature than the primitive cell seen in the acute variety of lymphosarcoma cell leukemia and

resembles the monocyte and promonocyte. The lymphosarcoma cells (LC above) of the primitive type are usually large in size and possess oval, oblong, notched or round nuclei with spongy or reticular nuclear chromatin. There is usually a single prominent nucleolus eccentrically placed and obvious as a blue-colored area around which there is a dense rim of chromatin. The nuclear wall is distinct and there is sparse to abundant blue-grey, opaque cytoplasm occasionally containing a few nonspecific azurophilic granules. Therapeutically it responds like a lymphoma, with a short, rapidly downhill course unlike that of C.L.L. In more than half the cases the primary seat of the disease has been the anterior mediastinum.

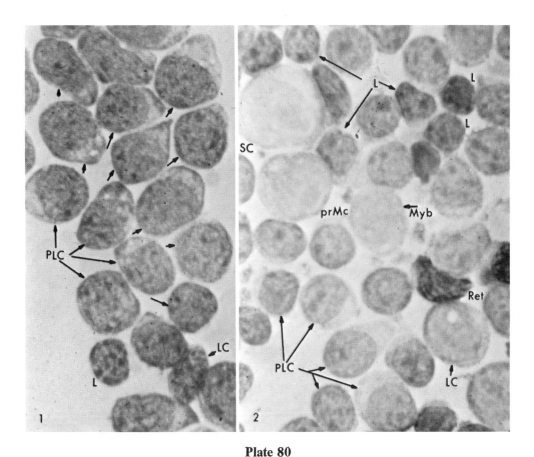

Plate 80

LEUKOSARCOMA
(Acute and Chronic Lymphosarcoma Cell Leukemia)
Bone Marrow

Lymphocyte (L), leukosarcoma cell (LC), myeloblast (Myb), primitive lymphosarcoma cell (PLC), promyelocyte (prMc), reticulum cell (ret), stem cell (SC).

Diagnostic Features: See peripheral blood description.

Plate 81

THE EFFECTS OF LEUKEMIA AND LYMPHOMA CHEMOTHERAPY
ON HEMATOPOIETIC CELLS
Bone Marrow Cytologic Changes

1. Cytoxan and Vinblastine. Orthochromic normoblast showing nuclear karyorrhexis with associated myelosuppression and thrombocytopenia (Nuc kar = nuclear karyorrhexis).

2. Methotrexate. Orthochromic (megaloblastoid type) normoblast with nuclear karyorrhexis and myeloid degeneration (Nuclear degeneration with associated vacuolation. Vac = vacuolation; Nuc degen = nuclear degeneration; Nuc. kar = nuclear karyorrhexis).

3, 4. Cytosine Arabinoside. Giant orthochromic megaloblastic normoblast with open nuclear chromatin pattern. Multilobulated giant megaloblastic orthochromic normoblast. Suppression of myelopoiesis and thrombopoiesis. (GON = giant orthochromic normoblast; Mult = multilobulated nuclei; OPEN = open nuclear chromatin pattern).

5–8. 6-Thioguanine and Cytosine Arabinoside. Binucleated polychromatophilic megaloblastic cells, vacuolated cytoplasm, and irregularities of chromatin clumping. Large neutrophil precursors show marked premature segmentation of nucleus. Giant metamyelocyte with monocytoid pattern with vacuolation of cytoplasm. Nuclear contortion of blast cells. Super-giant erythroid precursors. (BiN = binucleated; Vac = vacuoles; Monocyt = monocytoid; PerSeg = premature segmentation; Nuc cont = nuclear contortion; Sg Nuc Prec = super giant nuclear erythroid precursor; GC = giant metamyelocyte).

9. Vinblastine and Cytoxan. Multinucleated megaloblastoid orthochromic normoblasts with marked nuclear karyorrhexis and abnormal mitoses. Also leukopenia and thrombocytopenia. (Mult = multinucleated megaloblastoid normoblast; Nuc kar = nuclear karyorrhexis).

10. Hydroxyurea. Altered nuclei of myeloid cells and megaloblastoid nuclear changes. (Alt Nuc = altered metamyelocyte nuclei; GC = giant metamyelocyte).

11–13. Steroids and Vincristine and 6-Mercaptopurine. Lymphocytopenia (steroid effect); enlarged erythroid precursors with karyorrhexis of nuclear structures. Multinucleated giant normoblasts. (L Norm = large normoblast; Kar = karyorrhexis of nuclei; Mult GN = multinucleated giant normoblast).

14, 15. VAMP (vincristine, methotrexate, 6-mercaptopurine, and prednisone). Monocytoid nuclear pattern, vacuolated nuclei, and cytoplasm; atypical mitosis and large normoblast. (Mono = monocytoid nucleus; Vac = vacuoles; Atyp Mit = atypical mitosis; L Norm = large normoblast).

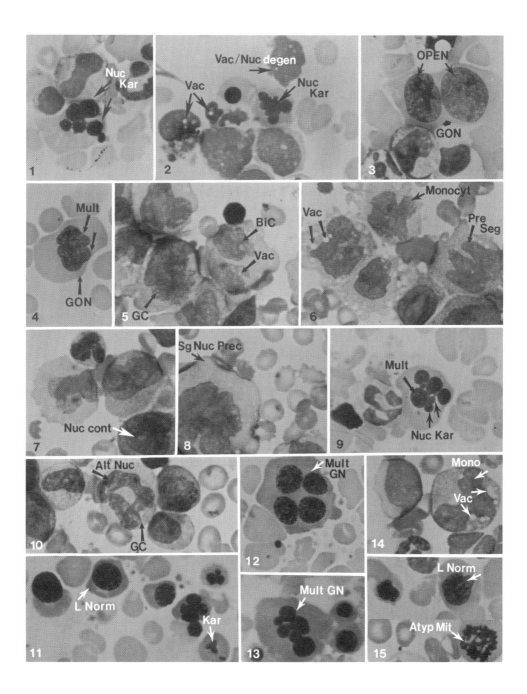

Plate 82

NON-HODGKIN'S LYMPHOMAS (NHL)
(Histopathologic Pattern in Lymph Nodes, Differentiated from Reactive Hyperplasia)
Lymph Node Pattern

1. Reactive Hyperplasia. Large paler-staining reaction (germinal) centers contain predominantly immature lymphocytes but are associated with plasma cells and varied numbers of histiocytes (GC(F) = germinal center; follicle; PF = parafollicular area; ×32).

2. This is a higher magnification of lymph node in Figure 1 (GC = germinal center; PF = parafollicular lymphocytes; ×470).

3. Nodular poorly differentiated lymphocytic type has ovoid nodular collections of lymphocytic-type cells with invasion of capsule (Nod = nodular; × 32).

4. This is a higher magnification of Fig. 3. The cellular proliferation is composed of small- to medium-size cells of variable size and configuration. The nucleus characteristically is irregular. There is typical loose nuclear chromatin; small nucleoli may be present. The quantity of cytoplasm in these cells is variable although never abundant, and the cells are often cohesive (Lymph PD = poorly-differentiated lymphocyte; ×470).

5. Nodular, (mixed) lymphohistiocytic-type (Rappaport) and mixed small and large lymphoid-type (Berard) are all follicular B-lymphocytes. There is compression of the intervening lymph node stromata in occasional areas (Nod = nodular; ×32).

6. This is a higher magnification of Figure 5. Small lymphocytes are cleaved, and irregular-looking; large lymphocytes may also be cleaved. The large lymphocytes are proliferating and the small ones nonproliferating. B-cell derivation is proven by ultrastructural, histochemical, and immuno-

logic studies (Large Lymph = large lymphocyte; Small Lymph = small lymphocyte; ×470).

7. Diffuse, well-differentiated histiocytic types have no differentiation of lymph node architecture into distinct follicles, with germinal centers and parafollicular lymphoid elements making up the cortex. In this photomicrograph, the normal lymph node pattern is effaced, and the nodular pattern is absent (Absence of Nod = absence of nodule formation; ×32).

8. This is a higher magnification of Figure 7. There is a diffuse proliferation of cells, paler and larger than lymphocytes, possessing fairly abundant granular cytoplasm, vesicular nuclei, and prominent nucleoli. Immunologically, it is a B-cell lymphocytic tumor (rare cases are composed of T-cells; Hist = histiocytic; ×100).

9. Diffuse, moderately well to poorly differentiated histiocytic type has an absence of follicular formation with no differentiation of lymph node architecture into cortex and medulla (Absence of Nod = absence of nodule; ×32).

10. This is a higher magnification of Figure 9. There is marked variation in morphologic appearance, even in a single lesion. The cells vary from poorly differentiated types with scanty cytoplasm to forms with large amounts of cytoplasm (histiocyte) or even pleomorphic forms (histiocyte). The nuclei are large and oval or pleomorphic and usually contain a prominent nucleolus. Phagocytized material may be present in the cytoplasm. On occasion, there is prominent reticulum fiber formation about individual cells (Hist = histiocyte; ×470).

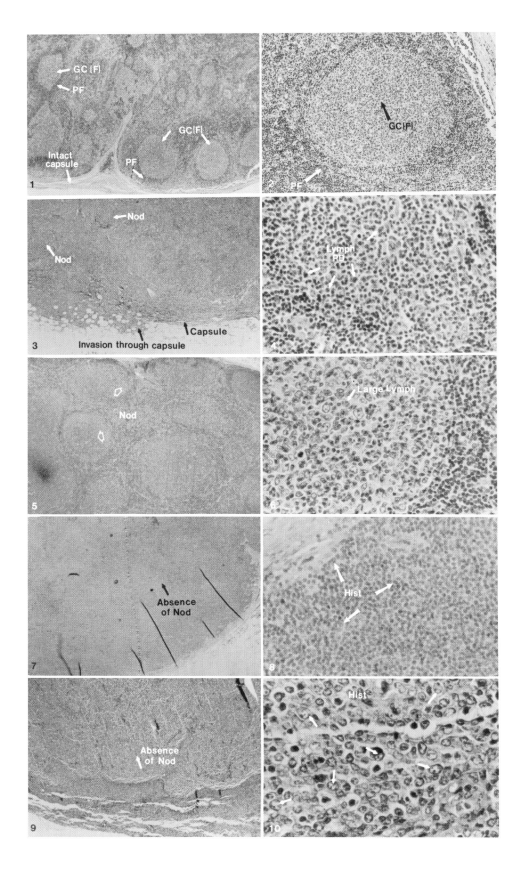

Plate 83

HODGKIN'S DISEASE
(Histopathologic Pattern in Lymph Nodes)

1. Lymphocyte predominance type. Cells are arranged in a diffuse, uniform fashion with lymphocyte proliferation. Numerous cytoplasmic histiocytes located within spaces are scattered throughout the predominantly lymphocyte background. Admixture of other cellular components or fibrosis is minimal, and necrosis is absent (CH = cytoplasmic histiocytes; Lymphs = lymphocytes; ×32).

2. This is a higher magnification of Figure 1. Polypoid cells without huge nucleoli are numerous; diagnostic Reed-Sternberg cells with prominent nucleoli are rare (RS = Reed-Sternberg cell; Ppd cell = polypoid cell; Lymph = lymphocytes; ×430).

3. Nodular Sclerosis Type. Collagen bands extend from the capsule into the node, circumscribing abnormal lymphoid tissue and forming a distinctive nodular pattern. The degree of collagen formation varies greatly from a single broad band to extensive degrees of sclerosis with a small amount of residual abnormal lymphoid tissue (CB = collagen band; ×32).

4. This is a higher magnification of Figure 3. It is characterized by the presence of a distinct variant of the Reed-Sternberg cell, the lacunar cell, with a sharply demarcated border, water-clear cytoplasm when it is fixed in formalin, and a variable number of nuclei. Occasional mixed cellularity (eosinophils, mononuclear and plasma cells) is also seen together with lymphocytes and degrees of sclerosis (LC = lacunar cell; ×430).

5. Mixed Cellularity Type. Lymph node pattern is partially or completely involved by cells of non-lymphocytic type in a diffuse pattern with reduction of lymphocytes (×32).

6. This is a higher magnification of Figure 5. Histiocytes, eosinophils, plasma cells, fibroblasts with numerous diagnostic Reed-Sternberg cells and diminished lymphocytes are seen (RS = Reed-Sternberg cell; Eos = eosinophil; H = histiocyte; Fib = fibroblast; ×430).

7. Lymphocyte Depletion Type. The lymph node is partially or entirely replaced by disorderly fibrillar connective tissue associated with a depletion of lymphocytes (Fib = fibrosis; ×32).

8. This is a higher magnification of Figure 7. It demonstrates an advanced degree of fibrosis with associated hypocellularity. Variable numbers of Reed-Sternberg cells are seen. Lymphocytes are markedly depleted (RS = Reed-Sternberg cell; Fib = fibroblast; Hist = histiocyte; Eos = eosinophil; ×430).

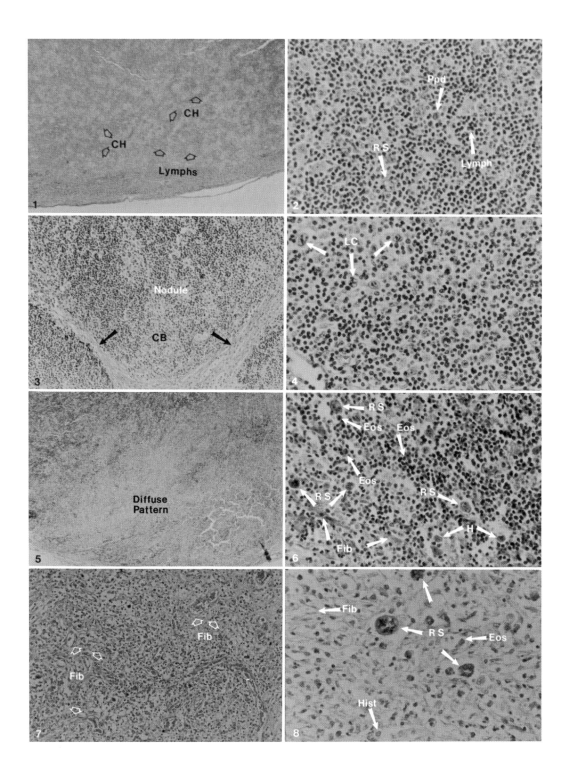

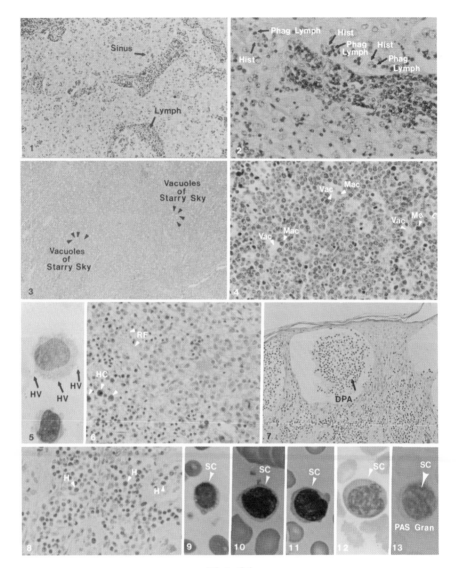

Plate 84

OTHER LYMPHOMATOUS AND NONLYMPHOMATOUS HISTOPATHOLOGIC PATTERNS
Lymph Node

1. Sinus Histiocytosis. Marked dilatation of lymphatic sinuses with almost complete architectural effacement (Sinus = dilated sinuses; Lymph = lymphocytes; ×32).

2. This is a higher magnification of Figure 1. Sinuses are filled with numerous histiocytes with large vesicular nuclei and a large amount of clear cytoplasm. The histiocytes often contain within their cytoplasm numerous phagocytosed lymphocytes, a feature of diagnostic significance. Most patients are African and West Indian Blacks (Hist = histiocyte; Phag Lymph = phagocytosed lymphocytes; × 430).

3. Burkitt's Lymphoma. The characteristic "starry-sky" appearance due to phagocytic histio-

cytes is demonstrated by punctate vacuolated areas diffusely present throughout a lymph node pattern devoid of well-delineated cortex, which shows no germinal centers (×32).

4. This is a higher magnification of Figure 3. There is marked uniformity of cells with a nuclear diameter similar to that of the macrophages in the "starry-sky" areas. Most of the cells are B-type cohesive primitive cells with round regular nuclei and small nucleoli. They are intensely pyrinophilic, and the vacuoles in the cytoplasm of Burkitt's cells are for the most part either neutral lipids or dilated mitochondria (Mac = macrophage; Vac = vacuole; ×430).

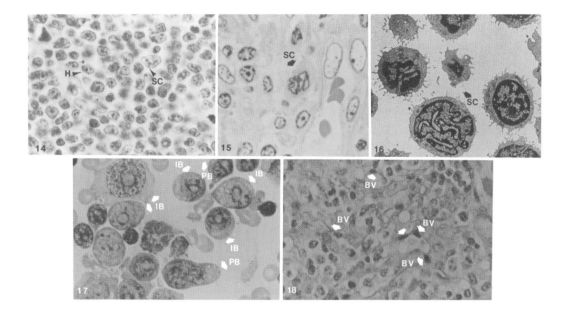

Peripheral Blood

5. Hairy or Ruffle Cells. Large (15–30 μm. in diameter) with round or oval nucleus and fairly abundant gray-blue cytoplasm. Nuclear chromatin is moderately clumped, and nucleoli are single and small. Irregular cytoplasmic filamentous-like villi project from the cell, and give it a flagellated appearance. These cells have characteristic monocytes under scanning electron microscopy ("ruffle" appearance) and can phagocytize. They have strong receptors for IgG and also have strong Fc receptors (HV = hairy villi; ×970).

Bone Marrow

6. Hairy or Ruffle Cell Leukemia (Leukemic Reticuloendotheliosis). Attempts to aspirate marrow frequently result in a dry tap. This is due to the tremendous amount of reticulin present. Biopsy usually reveals diffuse patches of uniform cells with scanty, pale, eccentrically located cytoplasm that exhibits no phagocytosis. The nuclei are open in appearance with a small single nucleolus (RF = reticulin fibers; HC = hairy cell).

Skin

7. Mycosis Fungoides shows acanthosis, parakeratosis, elongated rete pegs, spongiosis, and "Darier-Pautrier abscesses" which are intradermal clusters of histiocytes. Systemic lymphoma frequently develops in these patients (DPA = Darier-Pautrier abscess; ×100).

8. This is a higher magnification of Figure 7. Sézary cells are frequently seen in the peripheral blood of these patients (H = histiocytes; ×430).

Peripheral Blood

9. Sézary cell is characterized by a large convoluted nucleus with a condensed chromatin pattern and pale to dark blue cytoplasm, with occasional vacuoles distributed around the nucleus. These vacuoles (glycogen) are PAS-positive (SC = Sézary Cell; PAS Gran = PAS granule; ×970).

Bone Marrow and Lymph Node

14, 15. Sézary Cell (Epon-embedded thick section). This is a relatively small number of large (15–25 μmm. diameter) cells with irregular cytoplasmic borders and oval, round, or cleft containing, densely clumped nuclear chromatin, with a cerebriform nuclear pattern, on many occasions. Nucleoli usually are not apparent in Wright-stained smears (SC = Sézary cell; H = histiocyte; ×430).

16. Sézary Cell Electron Micrograph. Note convoluted gyriform, cerebriform nuclear configuration.

(Legend continues on overleaf)

Plate 84 *(Continued)*

OTHER LYMPHOMATOUS PATTERNS
Lymph Node

17. Immunoblastic Lymphadenopathy. The immunoblast is a term commonly used for the large (15–25 μ), transformed lymphocyte (formerly called reticulum cells) of both the T-cell and the B-cell system in histologic sections. Specific immunologic markers are required to distinguish between the two. They have large, oval nuclei with finely dispersed pale, basophilic, finely reticulated chromatin and one large or two to three smaller nucleoli; often situated on or near the nuclear membrane, there is a moderate amount of cytoplasm (IB = immunoblast; PB = plasmablast).

18. Immunoblastic Lymphadenopathy. The number and character of the typical proliferating vessels are dramatically demonstrated in PAS-stained sections. The vessels are typically small and arborizing, situated predominantly in the paracortical region and present in almost every field. The involved vessels are typically thickened by a deposit of amorphous PAS-positive material. Lymphocytes are occasionally arranged longitudinally within the vessel wall in the PAS-positive material. Endothelial cells are inconsistently hyperplastic. The outer margin of the vessels is frequently irregular and ill-defined (BV = blood vessel).

Immunolymphadenopathy is a hyperimmune entity resembling Hodgkin's disease, but it is a distinct disorder apparently of the B-cell system. It is characterized by a morphologic triad: (1) proliferation of arborizing small vessels; (2) prominent immunoblastic proliferations; and (3) amorphous acidophilic interstitial material. Clinically, it is manifested by fever, sweats, weight loss, occasionally a rash, generalized lymphadenopathy, and often hepatosplenomegaly. There is a consistent polyclonal hyperglobulinemia and often hemolytic anemia. The course of the disease is usually progressive, with a median survival of 15 months. The cellular proliferation appears benign morphologically in the pretherapy biopsies with occasional evolvement into a lymphoma of immunoblasts. The basic process appears to be a non-neoplastic hyperimmune proliferation of the B-cell system involving an exaggeration of lymphocyte transformation to immunoblasts and plasma cells that may be triggered by a hypersensitivity reaction to therapeutic agents. (From Lukes, R. J.. and Tindle, B. H.: Immunoblastic lymphadenopathy—A hyperimmune entity resembling Hodgkin's disease. N. Engl. J. Med., *292*:1, 1975)

Plate 85

LYMPHOMAS
(Hodgkin's Disease)
Bone Marrow

1. Reed-Sternberg Cell is a modified reticulum-like cell, large and multinucleated, bilobed or binucleated (mirror-image form) with huge inclusion-like nucleoli and abundant amphophilic cytoplasm. Bone marrow is often normal in Hodgkin's disease; Reed-Sternberg cells are observed in 5 per cent of cases. Occasionally, nonspecific granulomas may be found with or without fibrosis, eosinophilia, increased myeloid proliferation, and decreased erythroid production (RS = Reed-Sternberg cell).

2. Reed-Sternberg cell with acute granulocytic leukemia development is being reported more often in recent years; its relationship with Hodg-

kin's disease is uncertain (RS = Reed-Sternberg cell; PB = plasmablast).

3. Acute granulocytic leukemia pattern in Hodgkin's disease demonstrates myeloblastic proliferation in the bone marrow of a patient with proven Hodgkin's disease (MyB = myeloblast; Pr Mono = promonocyte; L = lymphocyte; Atyp Mit = atypical mitosis; Pro My = promyelocyte).

4. Reed-Sternberg cell with concomitant acute granulocytic leukemia is a huge Reed-Sternberg cell. Occasionally lacunar type of Reed-Sternberg cells are seen. It has very faint cytoplasmic staining and is separated from adjacent cells by an empty space or lacuna.

Burkitt's Lymphoma

5, 6. Peripheral blood. Burkitt cells (mostly B-type cohesive primitive lymphoid cells) with cytoplasmic and nuclear vacuoles. They are frequently described as medium-size primitive cells of remarkably uniform size and shape. The nucleus is round or oval with finely dispersed chromatin and contains a small indistinct nucleolus. There is a moderate amount of amphophilic cytoplasm (here basophilic) with cohesive borders (BC = Burkitt

cell).

7. Bone Marrow. B-type lymphoblastic Burkitt cells with vacuolated nuclei and cytoplasm (BC = Burkitt cell; L = lymphocyte).

8. Electron Micrograph shows clumped border nuclear chromatin with not many organelles in the cytoplasm of each cell and no cell contact specialization among cells (cc = clumped border chromatin).

Plate 85 *(Continued)*

LYMPHOMAS
Chronic Lymphosarcoma Cell Leukemia
Leukosarcoma or Well-Differentiated Lymphocytic Lymphosarcoma

9-11. Peripheral Blood. The cells of chronic lymphosarcoma are associated with a type of lymphocytic leukemia in which the leukemic stage is related to a lymphadenopathy possessing the histologic features of lymphosarcoma. The circulating lymphocytes are larger, reticulated, and unusually immature. The accompanying anemias may be the result of blood loss, hemolysis, or bone marrow infiltration. Monoclonal serum components are occasionally found (IgM) and may be associated with reduction in serum protein concentration (RIL = reticulated immature lymphocyte; CL = cleaved lymphocyte; SL = small lymphocyte).

12-14. Bone Marrow. These cells are, occasionally, morphologically indistinguishable from the lymphoblasts of acute lymphoblastic leukemia;

however, more commonly, the cells are larger with large nuclei possessing more cytoplasm than does nucleus of the typical lymphoblast. The nuclear chromatin is clumped and reticular with very large, often single, nucleoli present. These nuclei are round or oval, and may have deep clefts. The cytoplasm may stain lightly, deeply or gray-blue (CLSC = chronic lymphosarcoma cell; CC = cleaved or convoluted cell; CCC = cleaved and convoluted cell; H = histiocyte).

15. Lymph Node. This figure was made from the cut surface of fresh nodes to aid in the assessment of lymphocyte morphology, degree of immaturity, and accompanying cellular reaction (CC = cleaved or convoluted cell).

Histiocytic Lymphoma

16, 17. Peripheral Blood. Histiocytic lymphoma only occasionally is associated with a hematogenous presence of histiocytic cells. When they are present, the undifferentiated forms are relatively large (15–35 μm.), with varying amounts of cytoplasm that is frequently scanty and pale. A syncytial arrangement may be observed. The nucleus is vesicular and approximately 3 to 4 times as large as a lymphocyte. It is round, oval, or indented, and the chromatin appears delicate and is irregularly distributed. The nuclear membrane is thin and distinct, and there is usually a single, prominent, dark-staining nucleolus. The differentiated form is smaller (15–20 μm.), and the nucleus is often eccentric, oval, uniform, or horseshoe-shaped, and the cytoplasm has irregular borders suggesting ameboid properties (DHC =

differentiated histiocyte cell; ×970).

18–20. Pleural Fluid. These cells are desquamated in cases with mediastinal, pleural, or pulmonary involvement. The variation in cytoplasmic outline may be related to its desquamation into the pleural fluid and possibly accompanying ameboid and phagocytosing capabilities (AP = ameboid pseudopod; HC = histiocytic cell; Vac = vacuole; ×1000).

21, 22. Bone Marrow. Marrow involvement is found in approximately 10 per cent of cases. Lymphoblasts and reticulum-like "cells" are seen (HC = Histiocytic cell; L = lymphocyte; ON = orthochromic normoblast; ×970).

23. Spleen. Clumps of histiocytes are seen with typical vesicular nuclear chromatin pattern (×970).

Histiocytic Medullary Reticulosis (variant of Histiocytic Lymphoma, also called Histiocytic Leukemia and Aleukemic Reticuloendotheliosis)

24. Peripheral Blood. Histiocytic medullary reticulosis is a rare, fatal form of malignant lymphoma characterized by fever, lymphadenopathy, hepatosplenomegaly, purpura, anemia, and leukopenia. An unusual microscopic feature is the extensive histiocytic hyperplasia with associated erythrophagocytosis simulating a hemolytic pattern. The cell is typically large (10–50 μm.) and is related to the reticulum cell. Occasionally, they are cohesive and associated with fibrillar formation. The nucleus is irregular, distorted, oval, or oblong with a vesicular chromatin network and is occasionally convoluted and cleft with abundant cytoplasm with irregular borders (HC = histiocytic cell).

25–28. Bone Marrow. The bone marrow fre-

quently reveals syncytia with prominent eccentrically located vesicular chromatin in the nucleus and vacuolated abundant cytoplasm with or without erythrophagocytes. There is engulfing of granulocytes and platelets by abnormal histiocytes. Nuclei are occasionally folded (HC = histiocytic cell; LE = lymphocyte engulfed; Vac = vacuole; EP = erythrophagocytosis; ANAE gran = alpha naphthyl acetate esterase granules in histiocyte; PAS gran = PAS granules in histiocyte; PHAG = phagocytosis).

29. Electron Micrograph is characterized by large convoluted nucleus with typical lysosomal granule and occasionally Langerhan's structures (Conv. Nuc = convoluted nucleus; LG = lysosomal granules; LaS = Langerhan's structure).

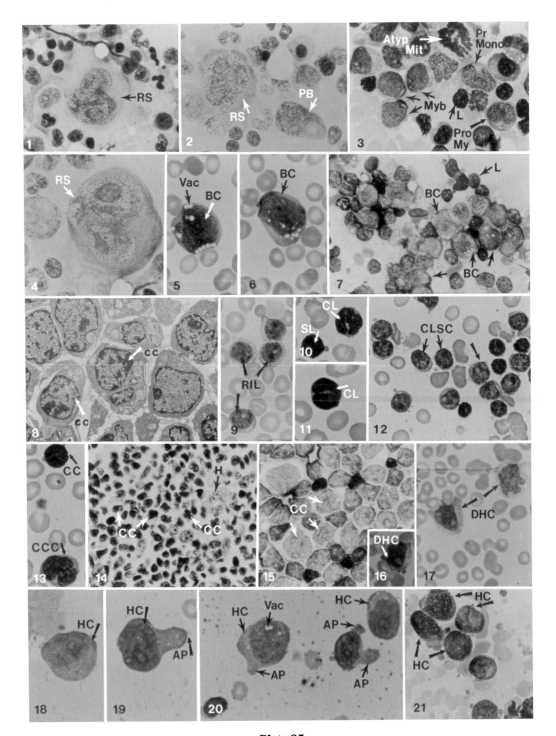

Plate 85

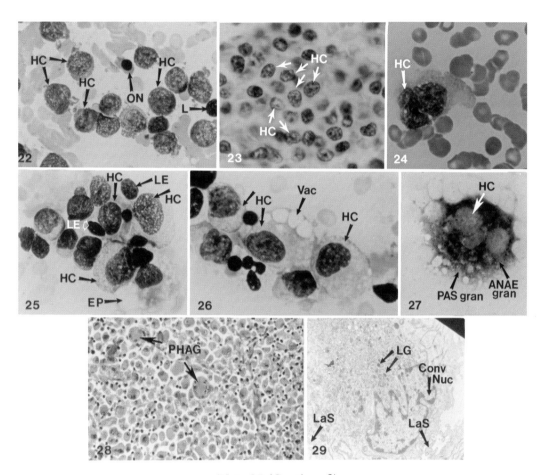

Plate 85 *(Continued)*

Plate 86

PLASMACYTIC MYELOMA
(Plasma Cell Myeloma, Multiple Myeloma)
Peripheral Blood

1. Rouleaux formation. 2. Plasma cell (PC), plasmablast (Plb). 3. Plasma cells (one binucleate). 4. Binucleate plasma cell. 5. Lymphocyte (L), atypical juvenile (Juv), proplasma cell (prPC), plasmablast (Plb).

Diagnostic Features: Normocytic, occasionally macrocytic anemia on a bluish-gray dysproteinemic background; rouleaux formation, increased polychromatophilia, slight reticulocytosis and occasional nucleated RBCs (especially in hemolysis). WBC pattern varies with a normal total count usually present (if WBC is above 50,000/cu.mm. with large numbers of myeloma-type plasma cells, it is consistent with plasma cell leukemia); a leukemoid pattern with myelocytes, lymphocytes, eosinophils, plasma cells and atypical mononuclear forms is also observed. Platelet count is usually normal; when reduced, it is indicative of marked marrow replacement of megakaryocytes. One may have difficulty in obtaining serum from myeloma patient's blood due to failure of clot retraction. Frequently there are abnormalities of the third stage of coagulation and increased blood viscosity with increased sedimentation rate. Petechiae are found when there is associated capillary damage. Electrophoretic pattern usually diagnostic in γ, β or "M" myeloma peaks (20% of patients have a normal pattern); ultracentrifugation reveals S value of 7 or less.

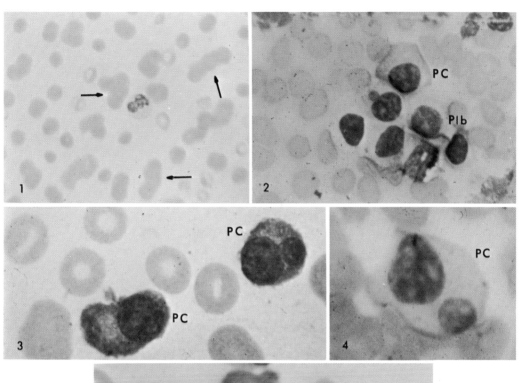

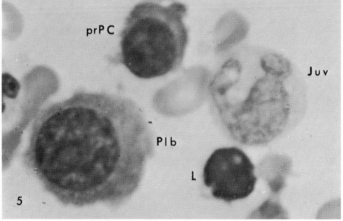

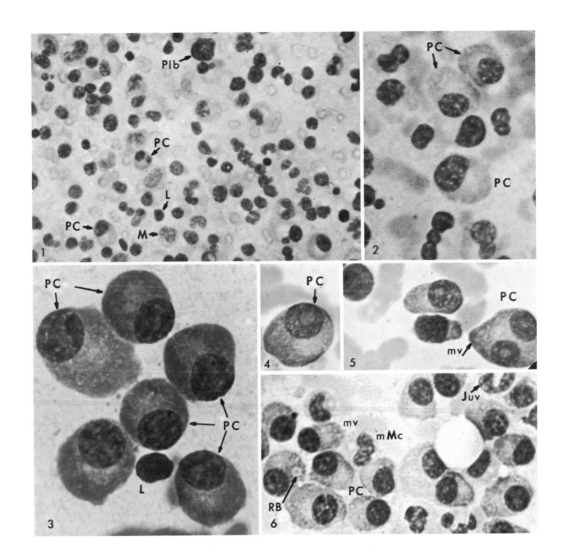

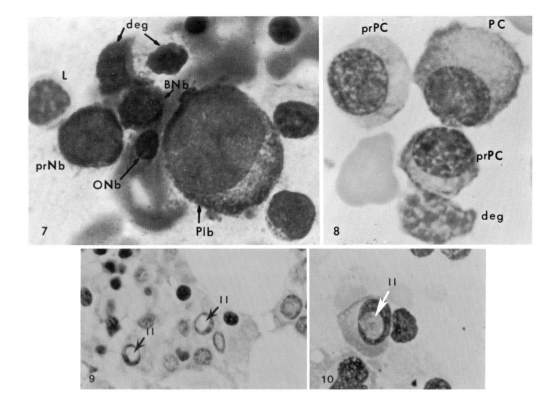

Plate 87

PLASMACYTIC MYELOMA
(Plasma Cell Myeloma, Multiple Myeloma)
Bone Marrow

Basophilic normoblast (BNb), degenerating cells (deg), juvenile (Juv), lymphocyte (L), metamyelocyte (mMc), monocyte (M), Mott vacuoles (mv), orthochromic normoblasts (ONb), plasmablast (Plb), plasma cells (PC), pronormoblast (prNb), proplasma cells (prPC), Russell body (RB), intranuclear inclusion (II).

Diagnostic Features: Characterized by atypical immature plasma cells, i.e., a 15 to 30 μ cell with round or ovoid nuclei measuring 5 to 7 μ; the latter are eccentrically placed and may have 1 to 2 nucleoli located in the nuclear chromatin, especially in the plasmoblast type. The nuclear chromatin is not as fine as in the myeloblast nor as coarse as in the normal plasma cell. The nuclei do *not* have the wheel-spoke chromatin arrangement observed in normal or tissue plasma cells. Cytoplasm of the myeloma plasma cell is basophilic and frequently bright blue and may contain few azure granules, acidophilic inclusions (Russell bodies) or clear globules or vacuoles (Mott bodies). Myeloma elements are located focally and therefore repeat marrow punctures may be necessary on many occasions.

9. PAS positive intranuclear inclusion IgA type immunoglobulin.

10. Intranuclear inclusion resembling large nucleolus.

Plate 88

PRIMARY MACROGLOBULINEMIA (Waldenstrom's Syndrome)

Lymphocyte (L), monocyte (M), orthochromic normoblast (oNb), atypical plasmacytoid lymphocyte (aty PIL), polymorphonuclear basophil (PmB), spherocytes (Sph), plasmacytoid lymphocyte (PlL), promyelocyte (PrMy), PAS positive intranuclear inclusion (PAS II).

Diagnostic Features: Neurologic findings are observed; also associated retinal hemorrhages and exudates, skin petechiae and purpura most frequently in 50- to 70-year-old males. There is a moderate to severe normocytic normochromic anemia present with associated hemolytic phenomena. The latter consists of polychromasia, reticulocytosis, spherocytosis, nucleated RBCs in the peripheral blood with or without a positive direct Coombs test. The WBC and platelet counts vary; there is neutropenia, with relative or slight absolute lymphocytosis frequently present, which progresses to pancytopenia in some cases; occasionally one sees thrombocytopenia with massive bleeding. Rouleaux formation is striking when it occurs. The Sia test is usually positive.

To perform the Sia test, add one drop of plasma to 10 ml. of distilled water, A positive test is present when there is a moderate to heavy precipitate forming within 10 seconds. The photograph shows No. 1, a positive control, No. 2, a positive test using patient's plasma and No. 3, a negative control with normal plasma. Protein electrophoresis resembles the myeloma type; there is increased serum viscosity present with ultra-centrifugation revealing S values of 15 or higher. The bone marrow contains up to 30 per cent lymphoid type cells or "plasmacytoid" type lymphocytes with very little basophilic cytoplasm—they may resemble small lymphocytes or atypical plasma cells. Naked nuclei are present, with cytoplasmic shedding frequently seen; mast cells may also be seen, also basophils and/or eosinophils. Normal myelocytes, etc., are decreased.

5. Bone Marrow. Numerous plasmycytoid lymphocytes and immature myeloid cells.

6. Bone Marrow. Intranuclear inclusions stain orange red with PAS and are associated with IgM immunoglobulin.

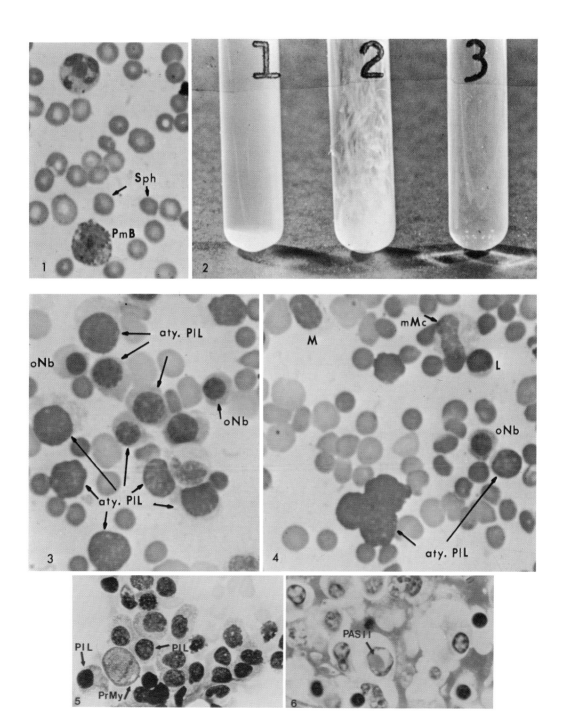

Plate 89

PATHOLOGIC CYTO-PROTEIN MOIETIES

Basophilic normoblast (bNb), lymphocyte (L), neutrophilic myelocyte (NMc), plasma cells (PC), polymorphonuclear neutrophil (PmN).

Diagnostic Features: Cyto-protein abnormalities are frequently associated with disorders of hepatic metabolism (cirrhosis), hypergammaglobulinemia, plasma cell proliferations and lymphocytic proliferations (e.g., acute lymphocytic leukemia is frequently associated with alpha globulin increase and decreased albumin levels; chronic lymphocytic leukemia is associated in 35% of the cases with hypogammaglobulinemia and 20% of the cases have hypergammaglobulinemia; lymphomas may be associated with decreased albumin, increased globulin or rarely hypogammaglobulinemia). Granulocytic-monocytic proliferative diseases (granulocytic and myelomonocytic leukemias) may be associated with increased gamma globulins. Plasma cells and lymphocytoid cells in plasmacytic myeloma and primary macroglobulinemia respectively are usually associated with specific hyperglobulinemias ("M," beta, and gamma type in plasma cell myeloma and 15S and 20S type in Waldenstrom's macroglobulinemia). Collagen diseases (especially systemic lupus erythematosus) are associated with hypergammaglobulinemia. Boeck's sarcoid is also associated with hyperglobulinemia. Hypogammaglobulinemic diseases may be leukemias, lymphomas, thymic diseases, and congenital lymphocytic-plasmacytic deficiencies. Immuno-electrophoresis detects specific immunoglobulins (IgA, IgC, and IgM types).

1. Plasma cells with eccentric nuclei making up the bone marrow picture of part of a nonspecific hypergammaglobulinemia.

2. A bone marrow with reactive plasmacytosis making up a portion of the cytologic picture of cirrhosis of the liver.

3. A Prussian blue stained bone marrow smear of a patient with hemochromatosis, associated cirrhosis of the liver and hypergammaglobulinemia. Iron retention is seen in the mononuclear cells of bone marrow, liver and spleen and shows as the bluish particulate deposits (arrows) in these marrow mononuclear cells.

4. A typical L. E. cell in which the polymorphonuclear structure surrounds the basophilic homogeneous nucleoprotein material.

5. The bone marrow of a case of hypogammaglobulinemia in which no plasma cells are seen. The rest of the bone marrow is active with orderly maturation of the myeloid and erythroid series.

6. The L. E. cells as seen in 4; also the L. E. phenomenon in which there is a rosette of the nucleoprotein surrounded by the nuclear material of the poly and mononuclear cell.

7a. A normal pattern of protein immunoelectrophoresis. In this the gamma globulin fraction is situated in the left-hand side of the figure as a semicircular curve.

7b. An immunoelectrophoretic pattern with the gamma globulin fraction missing, indicative of hypogammaglobulinemia.

7c. A similar process depicted in a serum protein electrophoretic pattern in which the gamma globulin is missing indicative of hypogammaglobulinemia.

7d. A normal protein electrophoretic pattern in which one sees the gamma globulin fraction to be present in the left-hand side of the figure.

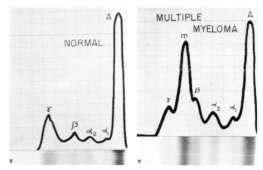

8. Normal protein electrophoretic pattern, depicted graphically and with paper electrophoretic mobility pattern stained with blue dye.

9. Protein electrophoretic pattern of multiple myeloma.

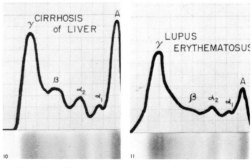

10 & 11. These protein electrophoretic patterns show one of cirrhosis of the liver with an enlarged gamma globulin fraction depicted graphically as well as on the paper electrophoretic mobility pattern stained with the blue dye. The lupus erythematosus fraction also shows an elevated gamma globulin and a flattened beta globulin fraction. The alpha fraction is reduced correspondingly; the blue dye mobility pattern is shown at the bottom of the L. E. graph.

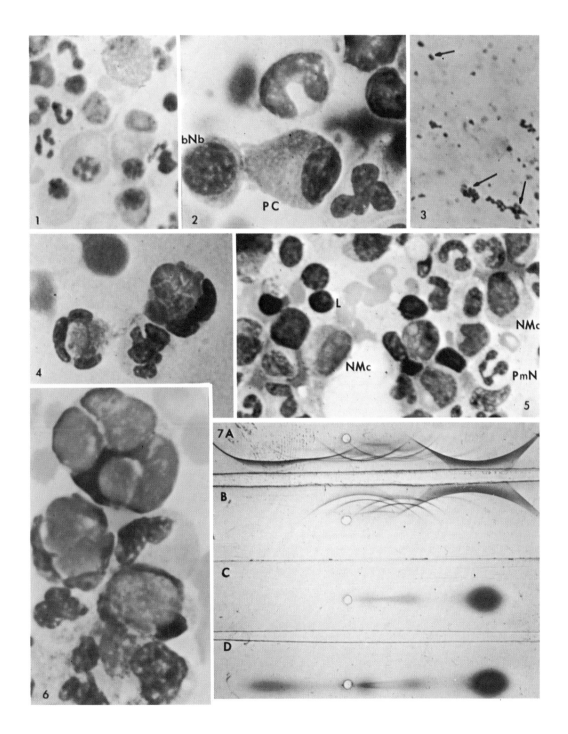

Plate 90

SYSTEMIC LUPUS ERYTHEMATOSUS (S.L.E.)
Fluorescent Antibody Stains

1. Homogeneous Pattern. Total nuclear fluorescence is observed and is due to an antibody directed against the nucleoprotein. This is most common in S.L.E.

2. Peripheral (Rim and Fibrillar) Pattern. There is fluorescence about the edges of the nucleus with a fibrillar or shaggy appearance. Anti-DNA antibodies produce this pattern; this tends to vary considerably with the different sources of nuclei. It is common in S.L.E.

3. Speckled Pattern. This results from an antibody directed against different nuclear antigens. The antibody is directed against soluble material (S_m antigen), a nonchromatin antigen extracted from nuclei with dilute phosphate buffer. It is found in some S.L.E. patients. Patients with Raynaud's phenomenon and progressive systemic sclerosis may give this pattern with antibody directed against nuclear material other than S_m antigen.

4. Nucleolar Pattern. This is thought to result from an antibody directed against a specific RNA configuration of the nucleolus or is antibody-specific for proteins necessary for maturation of nucleolar RNA. It is usually seen in patients with progressive systemic sclerosis (isothiocyanate fluorescein stain).

The major sequela of the L.E. cell configuration in systemic lupus erythematosis (S.L.E.) has been the demonstration that these antinuclear antibodies are the factors that lead to the production of the L.E. cell and the indirect immunofluorescent methodology. Whole nuclei of human origin (WBC smears or tumor imprints) or cryostat sections of animal liver, kidney, thyroid, or thymus are used as antigen. One may purchase tissue culture cells growing in monolayers. In the technique, the tissue or whole cells are fixed to the slide and then overlaid with appropriate dilutions of the patient's serum. Following incubation and washing of the slide, a solution of fluorescein-labeled antihuman immunoglobulin antiserum (reactive against all three of the main immunoglobulin classes) is laid over the cells and incubated. Finally, the preparation is examined under the ultraviolet microscope for nuclear fluorescence.

Four main patterns of fluorescence within the nuclei are identified, which correspond to the localization of specific antigenic components. By using individual nuclear constituents as antigens, these comparisons and correlations can be defined by other serologic methods (e.g., complement fixation, immunodiffusion, passive agglutination, etc.). The patient's disease process may be roughly correlated with the pattern, although combined or mixed fluorescent patterns occurring in some sera make this difficult. To obviate this, one may serially dilute the serum, and one pattern may disappear before the other at high dilutions. It is thought that the sera contain distinct antibody sets, each with separate antigen specificity.

Antinuclear antibody patterns and titers may show variation, possibly owing to differences in antigen or technique used. This has been corrected by the use of horseradish-peroxidase conjugated antihuman immunoglobulin serum to label the antinuclear antibodies on cell nuclei. When the slides are finally treated with diaminobenzidine and hydrogen peroxide, the conjugate takes on a brown color that is easily visible with the light microscope, and the patterns described above are identified with fluorescence antibody techniques.

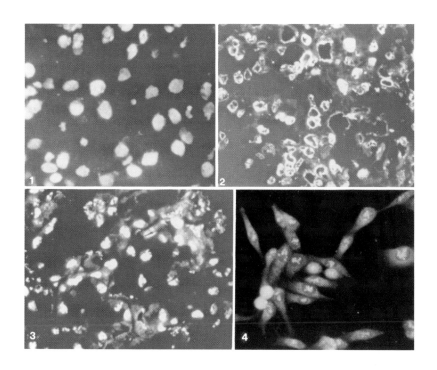

Plate 91

DIFFERENTIAL CYTOLOGIC PATTERNS IN MARROW SECTIONS

Diagnostic Features:

1. Normal marrow with section of blood vessel ($\times$430). Note variation in quantitation of myeloid and erythroid elements (4:1).

2. Moderate marrow hyperplasia ($\times$430). Note the increase in the total number and variety of cells with no special preponderance or predominance of any one cell type.

3. Hypoplasia of bone marrow. Note the reduction in the total number of cells with the widening of the marrow fat spaces.

4. Lymphosarcoma marrow (focal). Observe the marked increase in the total number of marrow cells, especially the lymphocytic type with reduction in marrow fat spaces.

5. Multiple myeloma marrow. Observe the increase in the number of plasma cells arranged in clumps or clones throughout the marrow proper.

6. Granulomatous lesion in the bone marrow (? Boeck's sarcoid). Observe concentric semiovoid focal collection of giant cells, epitheliod cells, histiocytes, and lymphocytes but without the presence of caseation necrosis.

7. Pernicious anemia marrow section. Note the large cells with large nuclei involving both myeloid and erythroid series of cells.

8. Chronic granulocytic leukemia marrow section. Observe the monotonous preponderance of large myeloid type cells.

9. Chronic monocytic leukemia. Note the monotonous preponderance of large monocytic type cells with irregular nuclear and cystoplasmic borders.

10. Myelofibrosis marrow section. Observe replacement of marrow elements by giant cells and fibroblastic tissue.

11. Hemosiderosis in marrow section (H & E stain). Note the deposition of brownish hemosiderin granules both intracellularly and extracellularly.

12. Hemosiderosis marrow section (Prussian blue stain). Observe the selective affinity of the Prussian blue stain for iron in the hemosiderin granules observed in the mononuclear cells or phagocytes (dark, chunky, blue-staining granules).

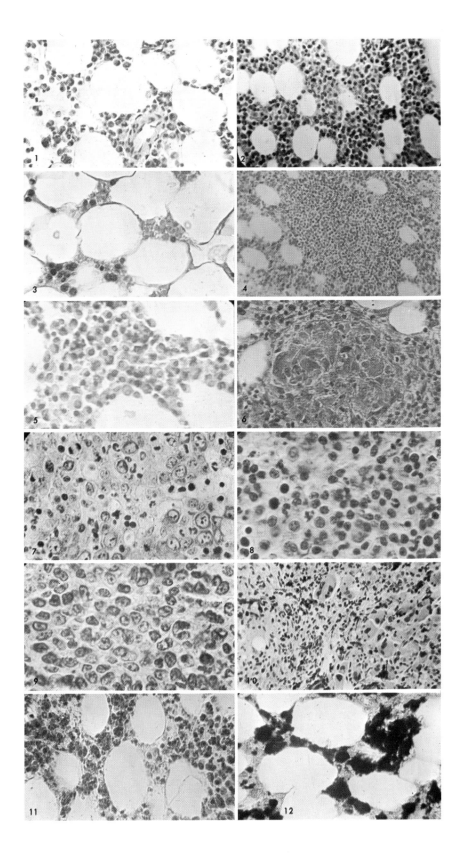

Plate 92

SPECIAL STAINS

1. *Peroxidase stain* (Diaminobenzidine). *Peripheral Blood.* Auer bodies, 1° granules. Acute granulocytic leukemia (AB = Auer body; Per G = peroxidase granules).

2. *Peroxidase stain* (Kaplow). *Peripheral Blood.* Auer bodies, 1° granules. Acute granulocytic leukemia (Ab = Auer body; Per G = peroxidase granule).

3. *PAS stain. Bone Marrow.* Positive acute lymphoblastic leukemia cells (PAS + = PAS granules in cytoplasm of lymphoblast).

4. *Nonspecific esterase stain. Peripheral Blood.* Positive pinkish-orange granules in acute monocytic leukemia cell (NSpE = nonspecific esterase granules).

5. *Alpha Naphthyl Propionate Esterase stain. Peripheral Blood.* Positive blackish granules in acute monocytic leukemia cell (ANPE = alpha naphthyl propionate esterase granules in monoblastic cytoplasm).

6. *Sudan Black B stain. Peripheral Blood.* Auer bodies and granules in acute granulocytic leukemia (Ab = Auer body; SBb = Sudan Black B granules).

7. *Acid-phosphatase stain. Peripheral Blood.* Chronic lymphocytic leukemia with Auer-like bodies (Alb = Auer-like body; AP = Acid phosphatase granule in cytoplasm of lymphoblast or immature lymphocyte).

8. *Leukocytic Alkaline Phosphatase stain* (LAP). Reddish granules in neutrophil cytoplasm, markedly increased in polycythemia vera (LAP = leukocytic alkaline phosphatase granules in cytoplasm of polys).

9. *Leukocytic Alkaline Phosphatase stain* (LAP). Light-staining granules in cytoplasm of monocytes in case of acute granulocytic leukemia (LAP = leukocytic alkaline phosphatase granules in cytoplasm of polys).

10. *Reticulin stain.* Increased bluish-black reticulin fibers throughout bone marrow in agnogenic myeloid metaplasia (RF = reticulin fibers separating cells of bone marrow).

11. *Trichrome stain. Bone Marrow.* Reddish-orange protein crystals in case of multiple myeloma with normal serum protein.

12. *Prussian Blue stain. Bone Marrow.* Increased stainable iron (blue) smear of patient with chronic illness (Fe = iron granules).

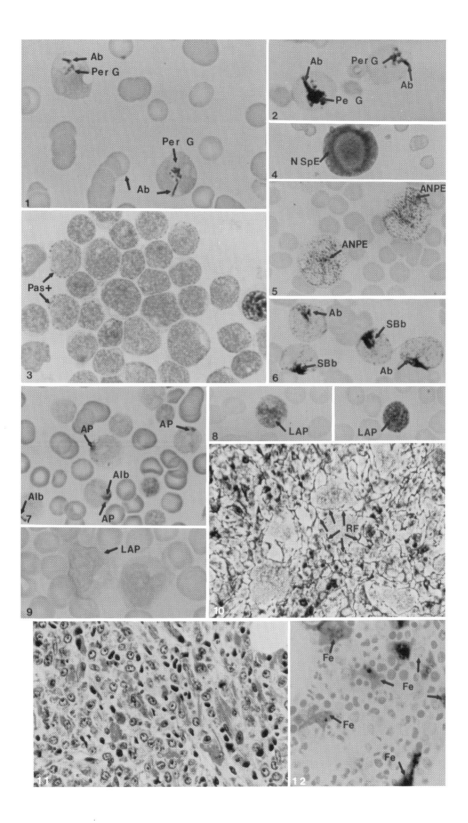

Table 13-13. Histopathologic Classification of Hodgkin's Disease*†

Type	Features	Relative Prognosis
Lymphocyte predominance (LP)	Abundant lymphocytic stromata sparse Reed-Sternberg (R-S) cells**	Most favorable
Nodular sclerosis (NS)	Nodules of lymphoid tissue of varying size, separated by bands of collagen and containing "lacunar" cell-variants of R-S cells	Favorable
Mixed cellularity (MC)	More numerous R-S cells in pleomorphic stromata rich in eosinophils, plasma cells, fibroblasts, and lymphocytes	Guarded
Lymphocyte depletion (LD)	Paucity of lymphocytes; diffuse, irregular fibrosis in some instances; bizarre, anaplastic R-S cells usually numerous	Least favorable

* Kaplan, H. S., and Rosenberg, S. A.: Hodgkin's disease: Current recommendations for management. CA—A Journal for Clinicians, *25*:307, 1975.

† See Plate 83.

** R-S cells are essential for diagnosis of Hodgkin's disease, but are not pathognomonic; they may be seen in infectious mononucleosis, metastatic breast cancer, and other conditions. It is therefore important to observe them in appropriate stromata.

HODGKIN'S DISEASE

The definition and etiology of Hodgkin's disease are similar to those of lymphocytic lymphosarcoma and histiocytic lymphoma with the histiocytic cells more specifically involved than are the lymphocytes. The disease is characterized by fever, pruritus, and the histologic landmark of Sternberg-Reed cells occurring more commonly than in other lymphomas. There is a greater incidence in young male adults, 35 to 55 years of age, with a definite older age shift toward the female population. An association between infectious agents such as spirochetes, protozoa, bacteria, avian tubercle bacilli, cryptococci, and viruses has been proposed by many because of the known alteration in immunity that exists in the disorder. Many investigators have demonstrated a cutaneous anergy,[89] which extends to many allergens and is mediated by the delayed or cellular type of hypersensitivity mechanism.[169]

Pathologic Findings

Pathologic findings include firm, discrete to matted lymph nodes, which on cut-section have a suet-like gross appearance (especially in the spleen), which develop multicentrically, and which extend to surrounding structures. Early in the disease, there is usually a destroyed normal pattern with cellular pleomorphism consisting of polymorphonuclear cells, eosinophils, plasma cells, reticulum cells, lymphocytes, and Sternberg-Reed cells. Sternberg-Reed cells must be present for specific diagnosis. These cells are 15 to 45 μ in size with folded or multilobulated unistructured or multistructured nuclei, coarse chromatin, prominent nucleoli, and abundant eosinophilic or basophilic cytoplasm. Necrosis and fibrosis also occur in the larger lymph nodes, spleen, and occasionally in the liver.

Nearly 12 years of field testing have provided convincing evidence that the Rye histopathologic classification does indeed correlate well with prognosis.[117] Although most cases can be readily classified among the four categories in Table 13–13, approximately 15 per cent of patients present with features that make classification difficult; when therapeutic management depends on the outcome, consultation, preferably with hematopathologists, should be sought.

Clinical Findings

Clinical findings consist of pruritus and fever, frequently of irregular Pel-Ebstein type, with symptoms related to anemia, weakness, and lassitude. Organ involvement occurs with or without pressure by enlarged lymph nodes. There is frequent secondary infection (for example, tuberculosis) related to the leukopenia and associated antibody impairment. Also there is pain, which is apparently alcohol-induced. Diagnosis is made by lymphangiography and the biopsy of involved large, deep lymph nodes.[174]

Although it is usually both feasible and desirable to complete the diagnostic workup before undertaking treatment, not infrequently a modified approach is indicated.[99] For example, the patient with massive mediastinal or hilar lymphadenopathy is not a good candidate for either lymphangiography or staging laparotomy until the thoracic lymph node masses have been appreciably reduced in size. A diagnostic workup* follows:

A. Careful history, with special attention to unexplained fever, night sweats, weight loss of more than 10 per cent in prior 6 months
B. Physical examination, emphasizing peripheral lymph node chains, liver, spleen, and bony tenderness
C. Chest radiograph; whole-lung tomography if mediastinal/hilar adenopathy present
D. Bilateral lower extremity lymphangiography; identification of suspicious nodes
E. Laboratory tests, especially CBC and platelet count, serum alkaline phosphatase, ESR, and serum Cu^{++}
F. Staging laparotomy (except when Stage IV disease is apparent); splenectomy and biopsy of suspicious paraaortic, celiac, porta hepatis, splenic hilar or iliac nodes, liver, and iliac crest bone marrow
G. Radioisotopic scans (optional): ^{67}Ga, $^{99m}TcEHDP$, $^{111}In\ Cl_3$
H. Delayed hypersensitivity skin tests (optional): natural intradermal antigens, DNCB

* Kaplan, H. S., and Rosenberg, S. A.: Hodgkin's disease: current recommendations for management. CA — A Journal for Clinicians, *25*:308, 1975.

Hematologic Findings

Hematologic manifestations are not specific. The peripheral blood is characterized by moderate leukocytosis, an increase in granulocytes and monocytes, and occasionally by eosinophilia and lymphopenia. Anemia, occurring more commonly late in the disease, is normocytic, normochromic with associated anisocytosis and poikilocytosis. The anemic pattern is throught to be caused both by depressed erythropoiesis and accelerated erythrocyte destruction. Thrombocytopenia and hemolytic changes are associated with dyssplenism. Bone marrow occasionally shows Sternberg-Reed cells with the concomitant appearance of myelocytes and normoblasts in the peripheral blood. The sedimentation rate is usually rapid; hyperglobulinemia is occasionally observed; elevated serum alkaline phosphatase occurs when bones are osteoblastically involved; and the basal metabolic rate is increased. Occasionally, chronic lymphocytic leukemia and Hodgkin's disease coexist.[138]

Prognosis and Treatment

Prognostic information involving this symptom complex was markedly affected by the 1966, Rye, New York, histopathologic classification. In general, lymphocyte predominance and nodular sclerosis have longer survival rates than histologies with mixed cellularity and lymphocytic depletion. Nodular sclerosis behaves somewhat differently from the other histologic types for it tends to affect females, has a predilection for the mediastinum, tends to spread by contiguity, and is unlikely to transform into a different histologic type. Although the nature and origin of the Reed-Sternberg cells in this disease are not clear, it has been suggested that the degree of lymphocyte predominance is a reflection of host reaction to a malignant cell population.

Hodgkin's Disease: Ann Arbor Modfication of Rye Staging System (1971)*†

Stage I   Involvement of a single lymph node region (I) or of a single extralymphatic organ or site (I_E)

Stage II   Involvement of two or more lymph node regions on the same side of the diaphragm (II) or localized involvement of an extralymphatic organ or site and of one or more lymph node regions on the same side of the diaphragm (II_E)

Stage III   Involvement of lymph node regions on both sides of the diaphragm (III), which may also be accompanied by localized involvement of an extralymphatic organ or site (III_E) or by involvement of the spleen (III_S) or both (III_{SE})

Stage IV   Diffuse or disseminated involvement of one or more extralymphatic organs or tissues with or without associated lymph node enlargement; reasons for classifying the patient as Stage IV should be identified

---

* Ultmann, J. E., and Stein, R. S.: Non-Hodgkin's lymphoma—an approach to staging and therapy. CA A Cancer Journal for Clinicians, 25:321, 1975.

† In Hodgkin's disease, all patients are subclassified A or B to indicate the absence or presence, respectively, of (1) unexplained weight loss of more than 10 per cent body weight; (2) unexplained fever with temperatures above 38° C; (3) night sweats. Biopsy-documented involvement of Stage IV sites is also denoted by letter suffixes: marrow = M+; lung = L+; liver = H+; pleura = P+; bone = O+; skin and subcutaneous tissue = D+; E = localized nodal lesions.

Staging laparotomy is a useful means of planning logical therapy and as a valuable adjunct to the evaluation of patients or situations where the presence of abdominal disease would influence treatment decisions. In addition to splenectomy and liver biopsy, this procedure includes careful search for nodes beyond the midline chain (mesenteric, peripancreatic, porta hepatic) that would fall outside the usual treatment fields for radiotherapy. Laparoscopy is now advocated instead of laparotomy, and bone marrow biopsies (large ones) appear to yield increasing evidence of H.D. in initial staging procedures, depending on the number of sites sampled.

Treatment and more prolonged survival are related directly to an increasingly aggressive approach.

Stages I and II. Radiotherapy (4000 to 4500 rads) is given to involved and extended fields. For disease above the diaphragm, extended fields usually include an upper mantle and a para-aortic portal down to the level of aortic bifurcation. Some oncologists favor total nodal irradiation for symptomatic (B) disease. Patients with Stage I and II below the diaphragm have, in general, been treated with inverted Y (para-aortic and pelvic) portals or with total nodal irradiation. The addition of combination chemotherapy to radiotherapy in the treatment of Stage I and II disease has resulted in significantly fewer recurrences; however, thus far, there has not been improvement in survival. A current cooperative study suggests that survival is the same for involved-field and extended-field irradiation, although the relapse rate is higher with involved-field treatment.

Stage III. There is controversy regarding the optimal management of Stage III A and III B disease; no definite results have been reported on random trials comparing radiotherapy alone, chemotherapy alone, and a combination of both modes of therapy in Stage III disease.

Stage IV. The management of this stage of Hodgkin's disease is principally that of high-dose intermittent combination chemotherapy. Since the classic basic studies of DeVita and associates with MOPP chemotherapy[47] a number of other combinations have been tested, (1) MOPP plus bleomycin; (2) CVPP (cyclophosphamide, vinblastine, procarbazine, and prednisone); and (3) ABVD (adriamycin, bleomycin, vincristine and imidazole carboxamide). They have been reported to be as good or better than MOPP alone for remission induction of Hodgkin's disease. No combinations, however, have been clearly proven to be better than MOPP in head-to-head comparison. Some of these combinations are said to produce fewer side effects than MOPP.[19] The optimal duration of therapy is yet to be defined. It would seem that somewhere between 6 and 12 months of intermittent therapy, with complete response documented by systematic restaging, should approach the optimal degree of treatment in patients with disseminated Hodgkin's disease. The NCI data[208] as well as the most recent follow-up of the Southwest Oncology Group experience[40] fail to show an advantage for maintenance therapy for those in documented complete remission. The use of radiotherapy in Stage IV disease has been limited to kidney disease and, in some cases, to have involved the liver.

Use of careful staging has resulted in 5-year survivals for Stages I, II, III, and IV of 86, 94, 81 and 39 per cent, respectively. It has been claimed, but with some disagreement, that extranodal disease, which represents an extension of nodal disease (E disease), does not confer a less favorable prognosis, provided the extranodal disease is included in the field of treatment. Several groups have reported (with ominous confirmation) a greater than twenty-fold increased risk of second tumors arising in patients who have received both radiotherapy and combination chemotherapy (i.e., out of 18 second malignancies, 11 were found to be acute myeloid leukemia with correlation directly related to intensity of treatment).[6, 190]

Since cell surface markers appear to be of some significance in differentiating the various lymphoreticular malignancies, the following summary may be helpful in categorizing immunologic patterns and origins.*

---

1. Well-differentiated lymphocytic malignancies, B-lymphocytic (chronic lymphocytic leukemia, well-differentiated lymphocytic lymphoma, Waldenström's macroglobulinemia)

---

* Modified from Mann, R. B.: Diseases of Hematopoietic and Lymphoid Tissue. Pathology Lecture. Baltimore, Johns Hopkins University School of Medicine, Nov. 21 and 22, 1977.

2. Nodular lymphoma, B-lymphocytic
3. Burkett's lymphoma, B-lymphocytic
4. Mycosis fungoides and Sézary syndrome, T-lymphocytic
5. Lymphocytic lymphoma, T-lymphocytic (Acute lymphocytic leukemia; 25%)
6. Hodgkin's disease, T-lymphocytic†
7. Histiocytic lymphoma, Variable
8. Malignant histiocytosis, Histiocytic
9. Hairy cell leukemia, B-lymphocytic – monocytic

---

† The bulk of clinical immunologic data suggests a T-lymphocyte abnormality. Recent evidence indicates that Reed-Sternberg cells are derived from lymphocytes rather than reticulum cells or histiocytes.

THE EFFECTS OF LEUKEMIA AND LYMPHOMA CHEMOTHERAPY ON HEMATOPOIETIC CELLS

Drugs used in the treatment of the leukemias and lymphomas may produce striking morphologic alterations in hematopoietic cells (Plate 81). There is a close relationship between the effects on normal hematopoiesis and the action of these drugs on malignant cells. Those actions, although different for the various groups of drugs, depend on the fact that malignant cells have a high rate of proliferation and consequently are susceptible to agents that interfere with cell replication and maturation. The normal tissues in the body that resemble malignant cells by having a high proliferative capacity (i.e., the bone marrow, gastrointestinal epithelium, and hair follicles) are susceptible to the same effects of antineoplastic agents as malignant cells and bear the brunt of the toxicity of these drugs. Because of the deleterious effects of anticancer drugs on these normal tissues, the limitations on the use of these agents are, in good part, determined by the extent of acceptable damage to the susceptible normal tissue, particularly the bone marrow. Table 13-14 summarizes the effects of chemotherapeutic drugs on hematopoietic cells.

Table 13-14. Summary of the Effects of Chemotherapeutic Drugs on Hematopoietic Cells*

Drug	Effects on Hematopoietic Tissue
Alkylating agents Mechlorethamine (Mustargen)	Rapid onset of cell destruction, chromosomal fragmentation, clumping, and bridging occur; lymphocytopenia begins in 24 hours; nadir occurs in 6–8 days; granulocytopenia begins in 2–3 days; nadir occurs in 10–21 days; platelet and red cell decrease occurs in 2nd and 3rd weeks.
Cyclophosphamide (Cytoxan)	Myelosuppressive, but thrombocytopenia is not as striking as with other alkylating agents
Chlorambucil	Moderate degree of myelosuppression
Melphalan	Moderate degree of myelosuppression
Busulfan (Myleran)	Selective depression of granulocytopoiesis at low dosage; platelets affected by relatively small doses; erythroid elements affected as dosage increased; continued therapy will result in pancytopenia
Antimetabolites Folic acid analogs Methotrexate	Rapid degeneration of myeloid tissue; megaloblastic alterations occur in erythroid cells in 24 hours; marrow becomes hypoplastic in 48–96 hours
Pyrimidine analogs 5-Fluorouracil	Early evidence of megaloblastosis followed by granulocytopenia and thrombocytopenia
Cytosine Arabinoside	Striking megaloblastic changes at 48 hours; suppression of leukopoiesis; thrombopoiesis may appear within 14 days
Purine analogs 6-Mercaptopurine	Megaloblastic changes occur early; marrow injury develops gradually; pancytopenia may be delayed for several weeks
6-Thioguanine Natural products Vinca alkaloids Vinblastine (Velban)	Leukopenia, low point at 4–10 days; at high doses reticulocytopenia and thrombocytopenia occur; at 24 hours 10–50% of erythroid precursor cells exhibit mitotic arrest; multinucleated erythroid cells and erythroid cells with nuclear fragments are found 15–28 hours after the drug is given
Vincristine	Leukopenia; relatively little effect on erythroid cells and platelets; marrow changes similar to vinblastine; maturation should be essentially normoblastic; few megaloblastic changes may be present; by 72–96 hours after drug administered, number of mitotic figures should be normal
Antibiotics Daunomycin	Potent marrow suppressant; affects all myeloid elements; development of marrow hypoplasia and pancytopenia may begin at 24–48 hours and may persist for several days; low point on days 9–11; by day 14 some evidence of recovery usually present
Enzymes L-asparaginase	Anemia and leukopenia reported in some experimental animals
Miscellaneous agents Hydroxyurea (Hydrea)	Megaloblastic changes develop in 24–48 hours; leukopenia and thrombocytopenia occur
Procarbazine	Leukopenia and thrombocytopenia occur; suppression of mitoses in interphase; Heinz body hemolytic anemia may develop
Steroids	No depressant effect on myeloid elements other than eosinophils; neutrophilia may occur; lymphocytopenia develops rapidly

* Brunning, R. D.: The effects of leukemic and lymphoma hemotherapy on hematopoietic cells. Am. J. Med. Tech., *39*:165–174, 1973.

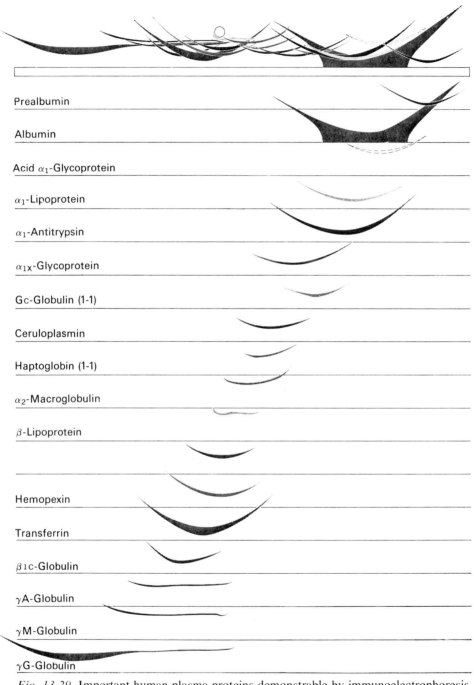

Prealbumin

Albumin

Acid α_1-Glycoprotein

α_1-Lipoprotein

α_1-Antitrypsin

α_{1x}-Glycoprotein

Gc-Globulin (1-1)

Ceruloplasmin

Haptoglobin (1-1)

α_2-Macroglobulin

β-Lipoprotein

Hemopexin

Transferrin

β_{1c}-Globulin

γA-Globulin

γM-Globulin

γG-Globulin

Fig. 13-29. Important human plasma proteins demonstrable by immunoelectrophoresis. (Courtesy of Hoechst Pharmaceuticals, Inc.)

Table 13-15. Abnormal Globulins*

Physicochemical Characteristics	Gamma-2 (7S)	Macro (19S)	Gamma-1A ($\beta_2 A$)
Sedimentation coefficient	7	19	7
Molecular weight (ultra-centrifugation)	160,000	1,000,000	160,000
Electrophoretic mobility	Gamma globulin	Fast gamma globulin	β globulin
Carbohydrate content (glycoprotein)	2.5%	10–12%	8.5%
Diseases associated with paraprotein	Myeloma, cryoglobulinemia, and some lymphomas.	Macroglobulinemia & some lymphomas	Myeloma
Antibodies associated therewith	Antibacterial and antiviral.	Isohemagglutinins, Rh antibodies, cold agglutinins, Rheumatoid factor	Diphtheria & tetanus toxin antibodies, typhoid O agglutinins, paratyphoid B antibodies

* From Gellhorn, A.: Abnormal globulins: paraproteinemias. In Beeson, P. B., and McDermott, W. (eds.): Cecil-Loeb Textbook of Medicine. Philadelphia, W. B. Saunders, 1963.

PARAPROTEINEMIAS—PLASMACYTIC MYELOMA (MULTIPLE MYELOMA) AND MACROGLOBULINEMIA (WALDENSTRÖM'S)

Monoclonal gammopathies constitute a variety of clinical disorders associated with increased production of a homogeneous globulin recognized as a "peak" on serum or urine electrophoresis. In about 5 per cent of patients with multiple myeloma and about 50 per cent of patients with localized plasmacytoma, an abnormal peak cannot be demonstrated.

Classification

Monoclonal gammopathies may be classified in the following manner (p. 504):

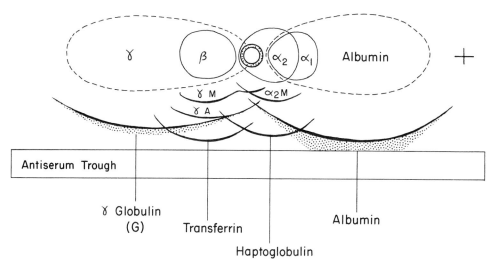

Fig. 13-30. Schematic representation of major serum components that can be separated by microimmunoelectrophoresis.

Monoclonal Gammopathies	Approximate frequency (% of "peaks")
1. Plasma cell myeloma	
a. Multiple myeloma— symptomatic	55
b. Multiple myeloma— asymptomatic and indolent	5
c. Localized plasmacytoma (1–2 lesions)	5
2. Macroglobulinemia of Waldenström	10
3. Heavy chain disease	1
4. Primary amyloidosis (without myeloma)	1
5. Idiopathic monoclonal peak	25

Plasmacytic Myeloma

Plasmacytic myeloma may be defined as a malignant progressive proliferation of abnormal plasma cells (10% immature) originating in the bone marrow from stem cells[74] or immature lymphoid-type cells and seen most frequently in the 55- to 70-year age group. Principal consequences of this myelomatosis are (1) the development of progressive destructive lesions of the skeleton resulting in pain, pathologic fractures, and orthopedic deformities; (2) progressive replacement of the bone marrow resulting in varying degrees of hemopoietic insufficiency; and (3) longstanding proteinuria, hypercalcemia, and hypercalciuria with resulting renal damage. In addition, the myeloma cells produce one or more distinctive paraproteins. These form a major constituent of the so-called immunoglobulins, which are separable by microimmunoelectrophoresis and other related techniques into the major serum components[71] shown in Table 13–15 (Figs. 13-29 and 13-30).

Anderson and Vye speculate that their case of coexistent myeloma-like dysproteinemia and thymoma may both be expressions of a single immunologic disturbance—that is, the face that the thymus plays a major role in establishing the immunologic response of the organism together with the belief that myasthenia gravis, erythroid aplasia, and acquired hypogammaglobulinemia may represent autoimmune disorders.[5] Furthermore, Miller states that the thymus is necessary to create an adequate population of immunologically competent lymphoid cells.[128] He believes that once these cells are formed, their behavior in response to antigen is normal whether the thymus is present or not.

The pathogenesis of plasmacytic (multiple) myeloma includes the consideration that the myeloma cell probably is derived from the reticulum stem cell or immature lymphoid-type cell and varies morphologically from a small cell with scant, lightly basophilic cytoplasm and an eccentrically placed nucleus closely resembling a normal plasma cell to the large cell type with abundant vacuolated lightly basophilic cytoplasm and an eccentric nucleus with one or more nucleoli (Fig. 13-31). Diagnosis is made by a film study of bone marrow aspirate in which the marrow puncture is frequently characterized by a sudden give during the puncture (Plates 86, 87).

Clinical and Pathologic Findings. Early Stages of Myeloma. A small fraction of patients present with unequivocal multiple myeloma that is asymptomatic with the diagnosis established following a series of screening studies (most frequently by an electrophoresis of serum with a high total protein on a SMA scan). A few of these patients may remain in stable health for months or years before increasing myeloma proteins or symptoms indicate the need for chemotherapy.

Patients with a localized plasmacytoma are being recognized more frequently. No more than two bone lesions, absence of bone marrow plasmacytosis in other areas, low level or absent myeloma peaks, and normal levels for nonmyeloma immunoglobulins are usually present. Treatment with radiotherapy alone will control the disorder in most patients, who frequently remain stable for many years. Some patients may be incorrectly staged as

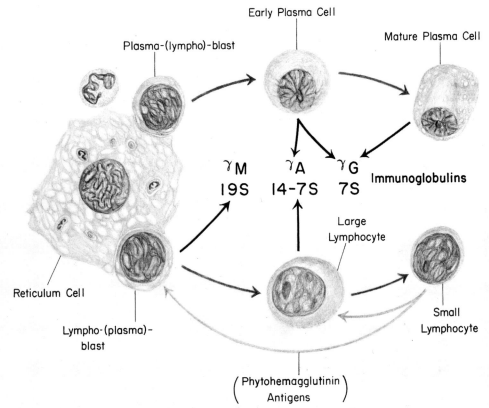

Early Plasma Cell

Plasma-(lympho)-blast

Mature Plasma Cell

γM 19S γA 14-7S γG 7S Immunoglobulins

Large Lymphocyte

Reticulum Cell

Lympho-(plasma)-blast

Small Lymphocyte

(Phytohemagglutinin)
Antigens

Fig. 13-31. Cellular origin of immunoglobulins.

"localized" when their diagnosis is made during an early proliferative phrase of overt multiple myeloma.

Idiopathic monoclonal peaks occur in about 0.5 per cent of normal patients older than 30. These patients have no symptoms attributable to myeloma, a serum peak less than 4.0 g. per cent, no lytic bone lesions, no Bence Jones protein, and normal levels of nonmyeloma immunoglobulins. No treatment is justified. Less than 2 per cent of these patients will ever develop myeloma.

A serum peak higher than 4.0 g. per cent is almost always due to multiple myeloma, macroglobulinemia, or heavy chain disease; the presence of Bence Jones protein by unequivocal studies usually signifies myeloma (localized or multiple), macroglobulinemia or primary amyloidosis.

Skeletal changes in plasmacytic myeloma consist of demineralization of bones including general bone pain, pathologic fractures, and back pain; multiple osteolytic lesions of cancellous bone of the pelvis, spine, sternum, ribs, and skull; erosion of local myeloma tumor nodules through the cortex of bone into surrounding soft tissues; and occasionally spinal cord compression by extradural pressure. A combination of immobilization and active bone destruction leads to hypercalcinuria and hypercalcemia, the latter causing muscle weakness, decreased glomerular filtration rate, and azotemia. The high concentration of calcium in the nephron also causes impairment of water reabsorption owing to a direct effect on the tubular cells.

A study of the hematopoietic system reveals severe anemia due to marrow re-

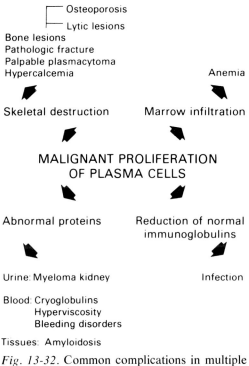

Osteoporosis
Lytic lesions
Bone lesions
Pathologic fracture
Palpable plasmacytoma
Hypercalcemia   Anemia

Skeletal destruction   Marrow infiltration

MALIGNANT PROLIFERATION
OF PLASMA CELLS

Abnormal proteins   Reduction of normal
                           immunoglobulins

Urine: Myeloma kidney   Infection

Blood: Cryoglobulins
       Hyperviscosity
       Bleeding disorders

Tissues: Amyloidosis

Fig. 13-32. Common complications in multiple myeloma. (Redrawn and modified from Alexanian, R.: Plasma cell neoplasms. Ca—A Cancer Journal for Clinicians, *26*:38, 1976)

placement by excess abnormal plasma cell proliferation and occasionally by increased hemolysis; leukopenia, the presence of immature granulocytes, normoblasts, and plasma cells in the circulating blood, rapid sedimentation rate, autoagglutination and rouleaux formation, and thrombocytopenia are also present.

Metabolic changes in plasmacytic myeloma consist of the following (Fig. 13-32):

1. *Diffuse Renal Disease.* Uremia follows precipitation of Bence Jones protein within the nephron; this occurs in 55 per cent of cases. Bence Jones protein is precipitated when the acidified urine is heated to 44° to 50° C, and the precipitate dissolves as the temperature is raised to 95° C; Bence Jones protein is also detected by electrophoresis of urine. This protein precipitates in the tubules producing hyaline casts that are surrounded by foreign body giant cells, the tubular epithelium becomes vacuolated and

may disappear. Similar changes may be seen in the endothelial cells of the glomerular capillaries.

A protein-paper-extraction test differentiates Bence Jones protein from uroglobulins.[133] The following technique is used. Five milliliters of clear urine (with 1+ or more protein reaction or 10 ml. with greater than 1+ reaction) is precipiated with 0.5 or 1.0 ml., respectively, of 50 per cent weight-to-volume trichloracetic acid, and centrifuged at 2500 r.p.m. for 10 minutes. The supernatant is discarded. The precipitate is stirred with 1 to 3 drops of 27 per cent ammonium hydroxide, and the suspension is absorbed on a one-eighth sector of a 9 cm. filter paper circle. The filter paper is dried in air, rolled into a tight cylindrical wad, and dropped into 1.5 ml. of hot sodium chloride-acetate buffer.* After 10 minutes in a boiling water bath, the tube is cooled by immersion in cold water, the paper is removed, and 3 drops of sulfosalicylic acid (20% w/v) is added. A cloudy buffer filtrate indicates the presence of Bence Jones protein. Clear fluids indicate the absence of Bence Jones protein regardless of any nonextractable uroglobulins. The limit of sensitivity for this test is approximately 27 mg. per 100 ml. compared with 45 mg. per 100 ml. for the heat filtration test and about 75 mg. per ml. for the sulfosalicylic acid heat test.[133]

2. *Para-amyloidosis* is the accumulation of glycoprotein deposits that do not stain well with metachromatic stains, but which possess variable affinity for Congo red. In a patient with this proteinaceous material, the amyloid fibrillar protein is thought to consist of homogenous immunoglobulin light chain (either intact or the variable portion) and has been demonstrated to possess an amino acid sequence identical to the

---

* Prepared by mixing 100 ml. of 10 per cent sodium chloride, 14 ml. of 2 M sodium acetate (272.1 g. of the trihydrated salt-liter of distilled water), 36 ml. of 2 M acetic acid (114.6 ml. of glacial acetic acid/liter of distilled water), adding water to 1000 ml. and adjusting *p*H to 4.3.

Bence Jones protein. However, the relationship between myeloma and amyloidosis is still unclear. Signs and symptoms are related to the sites of deposition (myocardium with cardiac decompensation, gastrointestinal tract with malabsorption, peripheral neuropathy, and joint capsule involvement).

3. *Immunologic Abnormality.* The serum protein concentration is variable; abnormal globulins are diagnostic, especially the M type, and occasionally gamma, beta and alpha globulins and cryoglobulins are observed. The cryoglobulins are associated with IgM–IgG complexes.[145] Normal gamma globulin production is depressed leading to a deficiency of circulating antibodies and therefore poor immunologic response with recurrent attacks of pyogenic infections and bacterial pneumonias.

It is important to differentiate this entity from benign monoclonal gammopathy, since the latter usually remains stable and rarely evolves into a malignant pattern. Benign monoclonal gammopathy presents itself in 3 per cent of patients over 70 years of age and is most frequently associated with low levels of circulating monoclonal protein ($<$1.0 g./dl.), normal concentrations of polyclonal immunoglobulins, small numbers of mature-appearing bone marrow plasma cells, and usually without lytic bone lesions.

4. *Abnormal bleeding* is associated with thrombocytopenia and occurs secondary to bone marrow replacement with abnormal plasma cells. Interference with blood coagulation is due to the low concentration of prothrombin and accelerator globulins plus interference with the conversion of fibrinogen to fibrin. Some patients develop a cryoglobulinemia that leads to peripheral capillary thromboses. Hemorrhage is due to endothelial membrane damage.

5. *Hyperuricemia* is due to an increased rate of purine metabolism secondary to the formation and degradation of plasma cell nucleic acids with uric acid being the final step in purine catabolism, occasionally leading to secondary gout and the obstructive deposition of urate crystals in kidneys.

The differential diagnosis of plasmacytic myeloma includes consideration of skeletal metastases from carcinoma, postmenopausal and senile osteoporosis, hyperparathyroidism (elevated alkaline phosphatase), lymphosarcoma, and primary amyloidosis.

Staging of Myeloma. The "average" patient with multiple myeloma has about 10^{12} cells/M^2, a level probably reached within 4 years, during which there is a progressive slowing of the growth rate with increasing tumor mass. The extent of disease in patients may be assessed from a combination of routine laboratory tests. The following represents a simple staging system now used in myeloma patients treated in the Southwest Oncology Group (SWOG):

High tumor mass ($> 1.2 \times 10^{12}$ plasma cells/M^2) is confirmed when any of the following is present:
1. Hemoglobin $<$ 8.5 g. %
2. Corrected calcium $>$ 11.5 mg. %*
3. Serum IgG peak $>$ 7 g. % or
   Serum IgA peak $>$ 5 g. %

Low tumor mass ($<0.6 \times 10^{12}$ plasma cells/M^2) is confirmed when all of the following are present:
1. Hemoglobin $>$ 10.5 g. %
2. Corrected calcium $<$ 11.5 mg. %*
3. Serum IgG peak $<$ 5 g. % or
   Serum IgA peak $<$ 3 g. %
4. None or few lytic bone lesions

Intermediate tumor mass ($0.6 - 1.2 \times 10^{12}$ plasma cells/M^2)
All other patients

The following represents correlations of tumor mass grade with prognosis in 635 SWOG patients:

	High	Intermediate	Low
Frequency (%)	44	31	23
Response rate (% evaluable)	50	55	54
Survival (median months)	17	27	42

* Corrected calcium (mg./100 ml.) = serum calcium (mg./100 ml.) − serum albumin (g./100 ml.) + 4.0.

Thus, the response rate was not affected by the tumor mass grade, but increasing tumor mass was associated with a shorter life span. In most patients responding to melphalan-prednisone chemotherapy, a one-log reduction in cell number was associated with a short plateau phase before eventual relapse of a resistant cell population.

Treatment. Supportive and Ancillary Therapy. Increased physical activity should be expedited with the rational use of analgesics, corsets, and walkers. Back braces are often not well tolerated. Radiation therapy is useful for disabling osteolytic bone pain from pathologic fractures, and for prevention of these fractures and is recommended for severe pain persisting after the first course of chemotherapy. Internal surgical fixation of long bone fractures and artificial hip prostheses may assist in reducing pain and allowing ambulation. Adequate hydration is essential in myeloma patients who may have high serum osmolalities, viscosities, and calcium levels. Dehydration must be avoided in preparing patients for radiologic procedures. After tumor masses are identified by prompt myelography, immediate radiotherapy to areas of cord compression may prevent the need for decompressive laminectomy. Corticosteroids may prevent edema when the spinal cord is receiving emergency radiation therapy. Hypercalcemia must be managed vigorously and is usually controlled by a high fluid intake, diuretics, and corticosteroids. However, in previously untreated patients, alkylator-prednisone therapy should not be delayed since hypercalcemia is almost always reversed by such treatment. Control of hypercalcemia is unlikely in disabled patients with drug-resistant myeloma, but mithramycin may provide brief control. Short-term hemodialysis may be useful for severe renal failure due either to "myeloma kidney" or amyloidosis; provided a remission has been achieved, long-term hemodialysis has been continued in some patients symptomatic only from chronic uremia. Androgens may be useful in selected patients with chronic anemia. Prophylactic gamma globulin has no value in the prevention of infection. Sodium fluoride 50 mg. ½ hour before meals and calcium lactate 0.9 to 1.8 g. 2 hours after meals continue under study for their utility in increasing bone calcification and reducing bone pain. Of greatest importance is the recognition that supportive and ancillary therapy is of little value unless the myeloma itself is adequately treated and controlled.

Chemotherapy. For symptomatic patients with plasmacytic myeloma or in asymptomatic patients with rising myeloma proteins, chemotherapy is required. Serial evaluations of myeloma protein levels are essential in the evaluation of tumor mass change. Response to chemotherapy is confirmed when there has been a 75 per cent or greater reduction in serum myeloma protein production and disappearance of Bence Jones proteins. Combination chemotherapy with vincristine, melphalan, cyclophosphamide, prednisone, and BCNU produced a 55 per cent response rate and a median survival time of about 40 months. More recently, patients treated at 3-week intervals with a VMCP combination of vincristine (1 mg. IV on day 1), melphalan (5 mg./M²/day × 4 days), cyclophosphamide (100 mg./M²/day × 4 days), prednisone (60 mg./M²/day × 4), or a vincristine-cyclophosphamide-adriamycin (25 mg./M² IV on day 1)-prednisone combination (VCAP) had response rates of about 60 per cent with a median survival of about 35 months. Another cooperative group concluded that combinations of different alkylating agents without vincristine were no more effective than treatment with melphalan-prednisone. In the above group of chemotherapeutic agents, prednisone given in the initial phase of therapy decreases the rate of hemolysis and promotes a sense of well-being, and melphalan (L-phenylalanine mustard) is a bone marrow depressant and, therefore, necessitates careful attention to the peripheral blood pattern. It is toxic in the presence of uremia, and therefore it must be withheld until renal failure is corrected as well as possible. Melphalan should also be withheld during radiotherapy and during persistent neutropenia and thrombocytopenia.

After one year of treatment for responding patients, one study indicated no apparent value from indefinite alkylator-prednisone therapy; patients must be followed closely because reinstitution of melphalan-prednisone therapy produced second remissions in about 80 per cent of relapsing patients. In view of the 6 per cent incidence of acute leukemia in responding patients living longer than 2 years, unmaintained remissions appear indicated for selected myeloma patients likely to experience long remissions, such as those with a low tumor mass or with disappearance of their myeloma protein. Long-term maintenance therapy with intermittent courses of MCBP (melphalan - cyclophosphamide - BCNU - prednisone) or of azathioprine-prednisone with periodic MCBP reinforcement did not prolong survival time in comparison with patients having no therapy. With only a 20 per cent death rate for registered patients, preliminary analyses have not yet indicated any significant benefit from a 1-year chemoimmunotherapy program using alternating courses of intermittent Pasteur-strain BCG and an alkylator-prednisone combination. During remission, certain drugs such as cytosine arabinoside, methotrexate, azathioprine, and actinomycin have been ineffective in producing further reductions in tumor mass. In some patients relapsing after melphalan-prednisone, an adriamycin-prednisone combination or a vincristine-BCNU-adriamycin-prednisone combination (VBAP) has produced second remissions in about 25 per cent of patients, but neither cyclophosphamide or BCNU alone was active. Although occasional remissions have been observed, the role of cis-platinum remains to be defined.[4, 14]

Because these patients also have de-pressed gamma globulin levels and associated poor immunologic response, plasma itself might be indicated as part of the therapy. Plasma is advocated instead of commercial gamma globulin because it contains all three immune globulins, provides greater quantities of gamma (G) globulin than can be given by intramuscular injections, and is more acceptable to the patient. Because of the risk of serum hepatitis, this mode of therapy in the routine management of hypogammaglobulinemia and agammaglobulinemia is endorsed only if special precautions are taken.[188] The survival of patients with this condition is adversely affected by the severity of the anemia, the amount of renal impairment, and the extent of the hypoalbuminemia. Hyperviscosity occurs usually if the paraprotein concentrations are above 5 g. per dl. The average survival for myeloma patients is 2 to 4 years, and many patients on previous prolonged melphalan therapy appear to also develop acute myelogenous leukemia.

Macroglobulinemia (Plate 88)

Macroglobulinemia (Waldenström's) may be defined as a chronic progressive, idiopathic, neoplastic disturbance of the reticuloendothelial system characterized by the proliferation of an abnormal cell generally described as a "lymphocytoid" plasma cell, which is probably responsible for the production of serum macroglobulins—high molecular weight globulins that are quite homogeneous on electrophoresis.

The clinical diagnosis of Waldenström's macroglobulinemia includes ophthalmologic findings of decreased visual acuity with increased retinal vein distention and tortuosity; multiple retinal hemorrhages; neurologic findings of myelitis, radiculitis, and increased spinal fluid protein; lymphadenopathy; and hepatosplenomegaly. Hematologically, this symptom complex is characterized by an increased number of atypical blast forms (lymphocytoid and plasmacytoid) in the peripheral blood and bone marrow. The sedimentation rate is elevated and the serum viscosity is increased with an associated hyperglobulinemia. Weakness and the tendency to bleed are also noted. Atypical lymphocytic infiltration is also seen in the portal triad area of the liver. Suggestive diagnostic laboratory tests include the Sia water dilution test and electrophoresis, which gives a characteristic pattern. Specific diagnostic tests include ultracentrifugation and immunoelectrophoresis with the demonstration of sharp-peak macroglobulins having a molecular weight of 400,000 to 1,000,000 in a 5 per cent or greater concentration.

The pathogenesis of this abnormal protein moiety involves macroglobulins derived from small lymphocyte-type cells. These are probably in turn derived from reticulum cells. Conjugation of the patient's serum proteins and macroglobulins prevents the normal coagulation of blood. Shortened erythrocyte life and increased sedimentation rate are related to the coating of the erythrocyte with this protein combination. Vascular thromboses result from the increased serum viscosity and sedimentation rate.

The differential diagnosis of Waldenström's macroglobulinemia includes consideration of multiple myeloma (no macroglobulins), purpura hyperglobulinemia (broad-hump macroglobulins), malignant lymphoma, and lymphatic leukemia (rarely associated macroglobulins).

Treatment. Treatment consists of penicillamine, which depolymerizes macroglobulins into smaller protein moieties that in themselves do not produce serum alterations and pathologic changes. Plasmapheresis over a period of 2 to 3 weeks removes plasma macroglobulins, and steroids improve the secondary hemolytic anemias. Continuous 1-phenylalanine mustard[154] and cyclophosphamide[21] have produced excellent remissions. Occasionally malignant transformation to reticulum cell sarcoma occurs.[196]

Heavy chain disease is a malignant proliferative disorder of the reticuloendothelial system in which the asynchronous production of an excess of heavy (H) chains of a myeloma-type protein or macroglobulin occurs. The other chains, that is, light (L) chains may also be produced. If this type of production exceeds H chain formation, the thermal and solubility properties of Bence Jones protein appear in the urine. Clinically, most patients have been male, 43 to 71 years of age, and they have exhibited lymphadenopathy, splenomegaly, fever, and anemia. Occasionally, hepatomegaly, leukopenia, and thrombocytopenia occur with associated poor resistance to infection due to decreased normal immunoglobulins, unusual erythema, and edema of the palate. Laboratory study shows the presence of predominantly atypical immature plasma cells admixed with atypical lymphocytes, plasma cells, reticulum cells, and eosinophils in bone marrow aspirate and lymph node sections. Urine examination reveals negative Bence Jones protein and electrophoretic abnormal homogeneous protein with fast gamma or slow beta mobility. Normal gamma globulin is decreased. The abnormal serum and urine proteins have a molecular weight of approximately 53,000 and are related immunologically to 75 γ G globulins—not similar antigenically to 7S γ A, or Bence Jones protein. Treatment is by external irradiation with short-term improvement by nitrogen mustard, cyclophosphamide, and steroids.[64, 141]

REFERENCES

1. Abernathy, M. R.: Döhle bodies associated with uncomplicated pregnancy. Blood, *27:*380, 1966.
2. Aisenberg, A. C., and Bloch, K. J.: Immunoglobulins on the surface of neoplastic lymphocytes. N. Engl. J. Med., *287:*272, 1972.
3. Aiuti, F., et al.: Identification, enumeration, and isolation of B and T lymphocytes from human peripheral blood. Special technical report. Scandinavian Journal of Immunology, *3:*521, 1974.
4. Alexanian, R., Salmon, S., Bonnet, J., Gehan, E., Haut, A., and Weick, J.: Combination therapy for multiple myeloma. Cancer, *40:*2765, 1977.
5. Anderson, E. T., and Vye, M. V.: Dysproteinemia of the myeloma type associated with a thymoma. Ann. Intern. Med., *66:*141, 1967.

6. Arseneu, J. C., et al.: Non-lymphomatous malignant tumors complicating Hodgkin's disease, possible association with favorable histologies. N. Engl. J. Med., *287:*1119, 1976.

7. Athens, J. W.: Hematology — sustained explosion of knowledge. J.A.M.A., *198:*38, 1966.

8. Athens, J. W.: Leukocyte physiology. J.A.M.A., *198:*38, 1966.

9. Athens, J. W., Raab, S. O., Haab, O. P., Boggs, D. R., Ashenbrucker, H., Cartwright, G. E., and Wintrobe, M. M.: Leukokinetic studies. X. Blood granulocyte kinetics in chronic myelocytic leukemia. J. Clin. Invest., *44:*765, 1965.

10. Aur, R. J. A., et al.: A comparative study of central nervous system irradiation and intensive chemotherapy early in remission of childhood acute lymphocytic leukemia. Cancer, *29:*381, 1972.

11. Bank, A., Larsen, P. R., and Anderson, H. M.: DiGuglielmo's syndrome after polycythemia. New Engl. J. Med., *275:*489, 1966.

12. Bennett, J., et al.: The Chemotherapy of Non-Hodgkin's Lymphoma: The Eastern Cooperative Oncology Group Experience. Cancer Treatment Reports, *61:*1079, 1977.

13. Bennett, J. M.: The Chemotherapy of non-Hodgkin's Lymphoma — Cancer Chemotherapy — Hahnemann Symposium, Phila. — April 19, 1977 — p. 3 brochure.

14. Bergsagel, D., et al.: Treatment of plasma cell myeloma with prednisone and sequential alternating or concurrent schedules of melphalan, cyclophosphamide and carmustine. Proceedings of the 13th Annual Meeting ASCO, Denver, Colorado, May, 1977.

15. Bergsma, D. (ed.): Immunodeficiency in Man and Animals. National Foundation, March of Dimes, XI. Sunderland, Massachusetts, Sinauer Associates, 1975.

16. Beutler, E.: Drug-induced "aplastic anemia." J.A.M.A., *198:*38, 1966.

17. Block, M., Jacobson, L. O., and Bethard, W. F.: Preleukemic acute human leukemia. J.A.M.A., *152:*1018, 1953.

18. Blom, J.: Infectious mononucleosis in acute lymphocytic leukemia. J.A.M.A., *194:*139, 1965.

19. Bloomfield, D. C., et al.: Combined chemotherapy with cyclophosphamide, vinblastine, procarbazone, and prednisone (CVPP) for patients with advanced Hodgkin's disease. An alternative program to MOPP. Cancer, *38:*42, 1976.

20. Boll, I., and Kühn, A.: Granulocytopoiesis in human bone marrow cultures studies by means of kinematography. Blood, *26:*449, 1965.

21. Bouroncle, B. A., Datta, P., and Frajola, W. J.: Waldenström's macroglobulinemia: report of three patients treated with cyclophosphamide. J.A.M.A., *189:*729, 1964.

22. Bowie, E. J. W., Tauxe, W. N., Kiely, J. M., and Stickney, J. M.: Erythrokinetic studies in acute leukemia before and after remission: report of case. Mayo Clin. Proc., *39:*245, 1964.

23. Braylan, R. C., Jaffee, E. S., and Berard, C. W.: Malignant lymphomas: current classification and new observations. Pathol. Annu., *10:*213, 1975.

24. Brouet, J. K., Toben, H. R., Chevalier, A., and Seligmann, M.: T and B membrane markers on blast cells in 69 patients with acute lymphoblastic leukemia. Ann. Inst. Pasteur (Paris), *125c:*691, 1974.

25. Brownstein, M. H., and Ballard, H. S.: Hepatoma associated with erythrocytosis: report of 11 cases. Am. J. Med., *40:*204, 1966.

26. Burns, J., and Neame, P. B.: Staining of blood cells with periodic acid/salicyloyl hydrazide (PA-SH): a fluorescent method for demonstrating glycogen. Blood, *28:*674, 1966.

27. Burns, J. E.: Glandular fever: report of an epidemic in the children's ward of the Union Protestant Infirmary. Arch. Intern. Med., *4:*118, 1909.

28. Canellos, G. P., DeVita, V. T., Whang-Peng, J., Chabner, P., Schein, P., and Young, R. C.: Chemotherapy of the blastic phase of chronic granulocytic leukemia: hypodiploidy and response to therapy. Blood, *47:*1003, 1976.

29. Canellos, G. P., Jaffe, E., Sawitsky, A., and Clarkson, B.: Chronic Lymphocytic Leukemia. Presented at the Education Program of the American Society of Hematology. San Diego, 1977.

30. Carpentieri, U., Thorpe, L., and Sordahl, L. A.: An improved method for purification of lymphocytes. Am. J. Clin. Pathol., *68:*763, 1977.

31. Cartwright, G. E.: Diagnostic Laboratory Hematology. ed. 3, p. 124. New York, Grune & Stratton, 1963.

32. Castle, W. B.: Polycythemias: Yearbook of Medicine. Chicago, Yearbook Publishers, 1966–67.

33. Chabner, B. A., et al.: Sequential non-surgical and surgical staging of non-Hodgkin's lymphoma. Ann. Intern. Med., *85:*149, 1976.

34. Chase, M. W.: Cellular transfer of cutaneous hypersensitivity to tuberculosis. Proc. Soc. Exp. Biol. Med., *59:*134, 1965.

35. Chin, A. H., Saiki, J. H., Trujillo, J. M., and Williams, R. C., Jr.: Peripheral blood T and B lymphocytes in patients with lymphoma and acute leukemia. Clinical Immunology and Immunopathol., *1:*499, 1973.

36. Choi, Y. S., Biggar, W. D., and Good, R. A.: Biosynthesis and secretion of immunoglobulins by peripheral blood lymphocytes in severe hypogammaglobulinema. Lancet, *1:*1149, 1972.

37. Clarkson, B. D., Dowling, M. D., Gee, T. S., Cunningham, I. B., and Burchenal, J. A.: Treatment of acute leukemia in adults. Cancer, *36:*775, 1975.

38. Cohen, P.: Fluoride and calcium therapy for myeloma bone lesions. J.A.M.A., *198:*583, 1966.

39. Coltman, C. A., et al.: Lymphoma: Diagnosis and Management. Presented at the Education Program of the American Society of Hematology. San Diego, 1977.

40. Coltman, C. A., Jr., Frei, E., III, and Moon, T. E.: MOPP maintenance vs. unmaintained remission for MOPP induced complete remission of advanced Hodgkin's disease. Proc. American Society of Clinical Oncology, *17:*289, 1976.

40a. Congdon, C. C.: Bone marrow transplantation. Science, *171:*1116, 1971.

41. Coons, A. H., Leduc, K. H., and Connolly, J. M.: Studies on antibody production I.A. Method for the histochemical demonstration of specific antibody and its application to a study of the hyperimmune rabbit. J. Exp. Med., *102:*49, 1955.

42. Cooper, M. D., Peterson, R. D. A., Soyth, M. A., and Good, R. A.: The functions of the thymus system and the bursa system in the chicken. J. Exp. Med., *123:*75, 1966.

43. Cooperberg, A. A., and Singer, O. P.: Reversible myelofibrosis due to vitamin D deficiency rickets. Can. Med. Assoc. J., *94:*392, 1966.

44. Cronkite, E. P., and Fliedner, T. M.: Granulocytopoiesis. New Engl. J. Med., *270:*1347, 1964.

45. Dameshek, W.: Some speculations on the myeloproliferative syndrome. Blood, *6:*372, 1951.

46. Delmonte, L., and Liebelt, R. A.: Granulocytosis—promoting extracts of mouse tumor tissue, partial purification. Science, *148:*521, 1965.

47. DeVita, V. T., Jr., Serpick, A., and Carbone, P. O.: Combination chemotherapy in the treatment of advanced Hodgkin's disease. Ann. Intern. Med., *73:*881, 1970.

48. Dickler, H. B., Adkinson, N. F., and Terry, W. D.: Evidence for individual human peripheral blood lymphocytes bearing both B and T cell markers. Nature, *247:*213, 1974.

49. Dickler, H. B., and Kunkel, H. G.: Interaction of aggregated-globulin with B lymphocytes. J. Exp. Med., *136:*191, 1972.

50. Didisheem, P., Trumbold, J. S., Vandervoort, R. L. E., and Meboshan, R. S.: Acute promyelocytic leukemia with fibrinogen and Factor V deficiencies. Blood, *23:*717, 1964.

51. Dimitrov, N., and Stjernholm, R. L.: Metabolic deviations in lymphoproliferative disorders. Presented at the American Society of Hematology, 9th annual meeting, 1966.

52. Dorfman, R. F.: Childhood lymphosarcoma in St. Louis, Missouri, clinically and histologically resembling Burkitt's tumor. Cancer, *18:*418, 1965.

53. Dorfman, R. F., and Warnke, R.: Lymphadenopathy simulating the malignant lymphomas. Hum. Pathol., *5:*519, 1974.

54. Downey, H., and McKinlay, C. A.: Acute lymphadenosis compared with acute lymphatic leukemia. Arch. Intern. Med., *32:*82, 1923.

55. Dreyfus, B.: Preleukemic states. I Definition and Classification. II Refractory anemia with excess of myeloblasts in the bone marrow (smoldering acute leukemia). Nouv. Rev. Fr. Hematol., Blood Cells, *17*(1–2):33, 1976.

56. Dugdale, M., and Fort, A. T.: Busulfan treatment of leukemia during pregnancy. J.A.M.A., *199:*131, 1967.

57. Ebbe, S. N.: The megakaryocyte: Maturation and self-renewal. Pathologic physiology and anatomy of the platelet. Presented at the Int'l. Academy of Pathologists. San Francisco, 1969.

58. Editorial: Myelofibrosis (panmyelosis) in Hiroshima. J.A.M.A., *189:*165, 1964.

59. Ellison, R. R.: Management of acute leukemia in adults. Medical and Pediatric Oncology, *1:*149, 1975.

60. Epstein, M. A., Henle, G., Achong, B. G., and Barr, Y. M.: Morphological and biological studies on a virus in cultured lymphoblasts from Burkitt's lymphoma. J. Exp. Med., *121:*761, 1965.

61. Fekete, A. M., and Kerpelman, E. J.: Acute hemolytic anemia complicating infectious mononucleosis. J.A.M.A., *194:*158, 1965.

62. Fieve, R. R., Blumenthal, B., and Little, B.: The relationship of atypical lymphocytes, phenothiazines, and schizophrenia. Arch. Gen. Psychiatry, *15:*529, 1966.

63. Finkel, H. E., Brauer, M. J., Taub, R. N., and Dameshek, W.: Immunologic aberrations in the DiGuglielmo syndrome. Blood, *28:*634, 1966.

64. Franklin, E. C., Lowenstein, J., Bigelow, B., and Meltzer, M.: Heavy chain disease. A new disease of serum γ globulins. Am. J. Med., *37:*332, 1964.

65. Fraumeni, J. F., Jr., and Miller, R. W.: Leukemia mortality: downturn rates in the United States. Science, *155:*1126, 1967.

66. Freeman, A. I., et al.: High dose MTX (HDM) in acute lymphocytic leukemia (ALL). Proceedings American Society of Clinical Oncology, *16:*232, 1975.

67. Frizzera, G., Moren, E. M., and Rappaport, H.: Angio-immunoblastic lymphadenopathy with dysproteinemia. Lancet, *1:*1070, 1974.

68. Gajl-Peczalski, K. J., Bloomfield, C. D., Coccia, P. F., Sosin, H., Brunning, R. D., and Kersey, J. H.: B and T cell lymphomas: analysis of blood and lymph nodes in 87 patients. Am. J. Med., *59:*674, 1975.

69. Gajl-Peczalska, K. J., Biggar, W. D., Park, B. D., and Good, R. A.: B Lymphocytes in DiGeorge syndrome. Lancet, *1:*1344, 1972.

70. Gajl-Peczalska, K. J., Hansen, J. A., Bloomfield, C. D., and Good, R. A.: B lymphocytes in untreated patients with malignant lymphoma and Hodgkin's disease. J. Clin. Invest., *52:*3064, 1973.

71. Gellhorn, A.: Abnormal globulins: paraproteinemias. *In* Beeson, P. B., and McDermott, W. (eds.): Cecil-Loeb Textbook of Medicine. Philadelphia, Saunders, 1963.

72. Ghitis, J.: Acute promyelocytic leukemia. Blood, *21:*237, 1963.

72a. Giordino, G. F., and Lichtman, M. A.: Marrow cell egress: central interaction of barrier pore size and cell maturation. J. Clin. Invest., *52:*1154, 1973.

73. Glick, B., Chang, T. S., and Jaap, R. G.: The bursa of Fabricus and antibody production. Poult. Sci., *35:*224, 1956.

74. Goldberg, G. M.: Plasma cell "myeloma," a lymphoproliferative disease. Bulletin of Pathology, *7:*108, 1966.

75. Good, R. A., Dalmosio, A. P., Martinez, C., Archer, O. K., Pierce, J. C., and Papermaster, B. W.: The role of the thymus in development of immunologic capacity in rabbits and mice. J. Exp. Med., *116:*773, 1962.

76. Gowans, J. L.: Immunobiology of the small lymphocyte. Hospital Practice, *3*:34, 1968.

77. Gowans, J. L., McGregor, D. D., and Cohen, D. M.: The role of small lymphocytes in the rejection of monografts of skin. *In* Wolstenholme, G. E. W., and Knight, J. (eds.): Ciba Foundation Study Group on the Immunologically Competent Cells. pp. 20-29. London, Little, Brown & Co., 1963.

78. Gralnick, H. R., Galton, D. A. G., Catovsky, D., Fulton, C., and Bennett, J. M.: Classification of acute leukemia. Ann. Intern. Med., *87*:740, 1977.

78a. Graw, R. G., et al.: Bone marrow transplantation from HL- A matched donors to patients with acute leukemia. Toxicity and antileukemic effect. Transplantation, *14*:79, 1972.

79. Greaves, M. F., Owen, J. J. T., and Raff, M. C.: T and B Lymphocytes: Origins, Properties, and Roles in Human Responses. New York, American Elsevier Publishing Co., 1974.

80. Guerry, D., IV, Dale, D. C., Omene, M., Perry, S., and Wolff, S. M.: Periodic hemopoiesis in human cyclic neutropenia. J. Clin. Invest., *52*:3220, 1973.

81. Gurney, C. W.: Polycythemia vera and some possible pathogenetic mechanisms. Annu. Rev. Med., *16*:169, 1965.

82. Hagbin, M., et al.: Intensive chemotherapy in children with acute lymphoblastic leukemia (L-2 protocol). Cancer, *33*:1491, 1974.

83. Han, T., Moyeri, H., and Minowada, J.: T-N-B lymphocytes in chronic lymphocytic leukemia correlation with clinical and immunologic status of the disease. J. Natl. Cancer Inst., *57*:497, 1976.

84. Haron-Ghera, N., and Peled, A.: Thymus and bone marrow derived lymphatic leukemia in mice. Nature, *241*:396, 1973.

85. Hartsock, R. J.: Postvaccinial lymphadenitis. Hyperplasia of lymphoid tissue that simulates malignant lymphomas. Cancer, *21*:632, 1968.

86. Heath, C. W., Jr., and Moloney, W. C.: Familial leukemia: five cases of acute leukemia in three generations. New Engl. J. Med., *272*:882, 1965.

87. Henle, W., and Henle, G.: Epstein-Barr virus: The cause of infectious mononucleosis. Oncogenesis and Herpes viruses. *In* Biggs, P. M., de-The, G., and Payne, L. N. (eds.): IARC Publication No. 2. p. 269. Lyon, France, 1972.

88. Henle, W., Henle, G., and Diehl, V.: Relationship between infectious mononucleosis and a herpes-type virus. Medical Tribune, *1*:1, 1968.

89. Hersh, E. M., and Oppenheim, J. J.: Impaired in vitro lymphocyte transformation in Hodgkin's disease. New Engl. J. Med., *273*:1006, 1965.

90. Hillestad, L. K.: Acute promyelocytic leukemia. Acta Med. Scand., *159*:189, 1957.

91. Hoff, G., and Bauer, S.: A new rapid slide test for infectious mononucleosis. J.A.M.A., *194*:351, 1965.

92. Hustu, H. D., et al.: Prevention of central nervous system leukemia by irradiation. Cancer, *32*:585, 1973.

93. Hoover, R., and Fraumeni, J. F., Jr.: Risk of cancer in renal-transplant recipients. Lancet, *2*:55, 1973.

93a. Jaffe, E. S., Sherach, E. M., Frank, M. M., Berard, C. W., and Green, I.: Nodular lymphoma—Evidence for origin from follicular B lymphocytes. N. Engl. J. Med., *290*:813, 1974.

94. James, K. K.: Lymphocytes: a new dimension. Laboratory Medicine, *7*:37, 1976.

95. James, T. N., Johnson, S. A., and Monto, R. W.: Physiology and morphology of blood coagulation in polycythemia vera. J. Appl. Physiol., *15*:1049, 1960.

96. Jankovic, B. O., and Isvaneski, M.: Experimental allergic encephalomyelitis in thymectomized, bursectomized, and normal chickens. Int. Arch. Allergy Appl. Immunol., *2*:188, 1963.

97. Jondal, M., Holm, G., and Wigzell, H.: Surface markers on human T and B Lymphocytes. A large population of lymphocytes forming nonimmune rosettes with sheep red blood cells. J. Exp. Med., *136*:207, 1972.

98. Jones, S. E., et al.: Clinical features and course of the non-Hodgkin's lymphomas. Clinics in Hematology, *3*:131, 1974.

98a. Kaplan, H. S.: On the natural history of the murine leukemias. Cancer Res., *27*:1325, 1967.

99. Kaplan, H. S., Dorfman, R. F., Nelson, T. S., and Rosenberg, S. A.: Staging laparatomy and splenectomy in Hodgkin's disease: analysis of indications and patterns of involvement in 285 consecutive, unselected patients. Natl. Cancer Inst. Monogr., *36*:291, 1973.

100. Kaplan, J., Mastrangelo, R., and Peterson, W. D., Jr.: Childhood lymphoblastic lymphoma, a cancer of thymus-derived lymphocytes. Cancer Res., *34*:521, 1974.

101. Kerbel, R. S., and Davies, A. J. S.: The possible biological significance of Fc receptors on mammals in lymphocytes and tumor cells. Cell, *3*:105, 1974.

102. Kersey, J. H., and Gajl-Peczalska, K. J.: T and B lymphocytes in humans. Am. J. Pathol., *81*:446, 1975.

103. Kersey, J. H., Nesbit, M. E., Hallgren, H., Yunis, E. J., and Gajl-Peczalski, K. J.: Evidence for origin of certain childhood acute leukemias and lymphomas in thymus-derived lymphocytes. Cancer, *36*:1348, 1975.

104. Kersey, J. H., Sabad, A., Gajl-Peczalska, K., Hallgren, H. M., Yunis, E. J., and Nesbit, M. E.: Acute lymphoblastic leukemic cells with T (Thymus-derived) lymphocyte markers. Science, *182*:1355, 1973.

105. Kersey, J. H., Spector, B. D., and Good, R. A.: Primary immunodeficiency diseases and cancer: the immunodeficiency-cancer registry. Int. J. Cancer, *12*:333, 1973.

106. Kersey, J., Spector, B., and Good, R. A.: Immunodeficiency and Cancer, Advances in Cancer Research. New York, Academic Press, 1973.

107. Kracke, R. R.: Recurrent agranulocytosis: report of an unusual case. Am. J. Clin. Pathol., *1*:385, 1931.

108. Krakoff, I. H., and Meyer, R. L.: Prevention of hyperuricemia in leukemia and lymphoma: use of

allopurinol, a xanthine oxidase inhibitor. J.A.M.A., *193:*1, 1965.

109. Kündel, D. W., and Nies, B. A.: Morphologic abnormalities of bone marrow cells induced by chemotherapeutic agents during treatment of leukemia. Am. J. Clin. Pathol., *44:*146, 1965.

110. Lai, P.: Infectious mononucleosis: recognition and management. Hospital Practice, *12:*47, 1977.

111. Lajtha, L. G., Oliver, R., and Gurney, C. W.: Kinetic model of bone marrow stem-cell population. Br. J. Haematol., *8:*443, 1962.

112. Lau, P., Brody, J. I., and Beizer, L. H.: Developmental potential of bone marrows from patients with neutropenia. American Society of Hematology, 9th annual meeting, 1966.

113. Lay, W. H., and Nussenzweig, V.: Receptors for complement on leukocytes. J. Exp. Med., *128:*991, 1968.

114. Lee, C. L., Davidsohn, I., and Mih, N. L.: A capillary screening test for infectious mononucleosis. Am. J. Clin. Pathol., *44:*162, 1965.

115. Liepman, M., and Votaw, M. L.: Chronic lymphocytic leukemia treated with COP. Proceedings American Society of Clinical Oncology, *18:*281, 1977.

116. Lohmann, H. J.: Prognostic significance of histopathology in Hodgkin's granuloma. Acta Pathol. Microbiol. Scand., *64:*16, 1965.

117. Lukes, R. J., Craver, L. F., Hall, T. C., Rappaport, H., and Rubin, P.: Report of the nomenclature committee. Cancer Res., *26:*1311, 1966.

118. McArthur, W. P., Chapman, J., and Thorbecke, G. J.: Immunocompetent cells of the chicken. I. Specific surface antigenic markers on bursa and thymus cells. J. Exp. Med. *134:*1036, 1971.

119. McCaffrey, R., et al.: Biochemical and immunological evidence and lymphoblastic conversion in chronic myelogenous leukemia. Blood, *46:*1043, 1976.

120. McFarland, W., and Heilman, D. H.: Lymphocyte foot appendage: its role in lymphocyte function and in immunologic reactions. Nature, *205:*887, 1965.

121. Madison, F. W., and Squier, T. L.: The etiology of primary granulocytopenia (agranulocytic angina). J.A.M.A., *102:*755, 1934.

122. Maldonado, J. E., and Hanlon, D. G.: Monocytosis: a current appraisal. Mayo Clin. Proc., *40:*248, 1965.

123. Marin-Padilla, M., Fabimi, H. D., and Moloney, W. C.: Leukemic reticulum-cell sarcoma (reticulum-cell sarcoma terminating in acute leukemia). Am. J. Clin. Pathol., *41:*402, 1964.

124. Martinez, C., Kersey, J., Papermaster, B. W., and Good, R. A.: Skin homograft survival in thymectomized mice. Proc. Soc. Exp. Biol. Med., *109:*193, 1962.

125. Metcalf, D., and Moore, M. A. S.: Hematopoietic Cells: Their Origin, Migration and Differentation. Amsterdam, North Holland Publishing Co., 1971.

126. Miller, F. R., and Turner, D. L.: The action of specific stimulators on the hematopoietic system. Am. J. Med. Sci., *206:*146, 1943.

127. Miller, J. F. A. P.: Immunologic function of the thymus. Lancet, *2:*748, 1961.

128. Miller, J. F. A. P.: Response to antigens by cells independent of thymus hormone. Med. Trib., *8:*1, 1967.

129. Miller, R. W.: Radiation, chromosomes and viruses in the etiology of leukemia. N. Engl. J. Med., *271:*30, 1964.

130. Minnich, V.: Identification and differentiation of blood and bone marrow cells stained with Wright's stain. Washington University School of Medicine, Hematology Notes, 1965.

131. Mitus, W. J., Gollerheri, M., and Gailbraith, P. R.: Experimental production of erythrocytosis in rabbits. Tufts N. Engl. Med. Cent. Sci. News, *1:*2, 1964.

132. Moeschlin, S., Meyer, H., Israels, L. G., and Tarr-Gloor, E.: Experimental agranulocytosis: its production through leukocytic agglutination by antileukocytic serum. Acta Haematol., *11:*73, 1954.

133. Naumann, H. N.: Differentiation of Bence-Jones protein from uroglobulins. Am. J. Clin. Pathol., *44:*413, 1965.

134. Norman, A., Sasaki, M. S., Ottoman, R. E., and Fingerhut, E. G.: Lymphocyte lifetime in women. Science, *147:*745, 1965.

135. Nowell, P. C.: Prognostic value of marrow chromsome studies in human "preleukemia" Arch. Pathol., *80:*205, 1965.

136. Nowell, P. C., Gardner, F., Murphy, S., Chaganti, R. S., and German, J.: Chromosome studies in "preleukemia." III. Myelofibrosis. Cancer, *38:*1873, 1976.

137. Nowell, P. C., and Hungerford, D. A.: A minute chromosome in human granulocytic leukemia. Science, *132:*1497, 1960.

138. Oberfield, R. A.: Coexistence of chronic lymphocytic leukemia and Hodgkin's disease. J.A.M.A., *195:*865, 1966.

139. Ortega, J., et al.: L-asparaginase, vincristine and prednisone for induction of first remission in acute lymphocytic leukemia (ALL). Proc. Am. Assoc. Cancer Res., *16:*140, 1975.

140. Osserman, E. F., and Lawlor, D. P.: Abnormal serum and urine proteins in thirty-five cases of multiple myeloma, as studied by filter paper electrophoresis. Am. J. Med., *18:*462, 1955.

141. Osserman, E. F., and Takatsuki, K.: Clinical and immunochemical studies of four cases of heavy (Hγ^2) chain disease. Am. J. Med., *37:*351, 1964.

142. Page, L. B., and Culver, P. J.: Syllabus of Laboratory Examinations in Clinical Diagnosis. p. 171. Cambridge, Harvard University Press, 1960.

143. Parker, M. G., and Lowney, J. F.: Acute promyelocytic leukemia. Mo. Med., *62:*374, 1965.

144. Paul, J. R., and Bunnell, W. W.: The presence of heterophile antibodies in infectious mononucleosis. Am. J. Med. Sci., *183:*90, 1932.

145. Peetoom, F., and Van Loghem-Langereis, E.: I$_G$M-I$_G$G (β_2-M-7Sγ) cryoglobulinemia: Autoimmune phenomenon. Vox Sang., *10:*281, 1965.

146. Pernis, B., Ferarini, M., Forni, L., and Amante, L.: Immunoglobulins on lymphocyte mem-

branes. *In* Amos, B. (ed.): Progress in Immunology. pp. 95-106. New York, Academic Press, 1971.

147. Perry, S., Godwin, H. A., and Zimmerman, T. S.: Physiology of the Granulocyte, Part 2. J.A.M.A., *203:*1025, 1968.

148. Pfeiffer, E.: Drusenfieber. Jahrb. F. Konderh., *29:*257, 1889.

149. Phillips, E. A., Kempin, S., Passe, S., Milhe, V., and Clarkson, B.: Prognostic factors in chronic lymphocytic leukemia and their implications for therapy. Clinics in Hematology, *6:*203, 1977.

150. Pinkel, D., et al.: Drug dosage and remission duration in childhood lymphocytic leukemia. Cancer *27:*247, 1971.

151. Plum, P.: Agranulocytosis due to amidopyrine. An experimental and clinical study of seven new cases. Lancet, *1:*14, 1935.

152. Powles, R. L.: Immunotherapy in the management of acute leukemia. Br. J. Hematol., *32:*145, 1976.

153. Preud'homme, J. L., and Flandrin, G. J.: Identification by peroxidase staining of monocytes in surface immunofluorescence tests. J. Immunol., *113:*1650, 1974.

154. Raab, S., and Dahlke, M.: The treatment of multiple myeloma and macroglobulinemia of Waldenström with the continuous administration of L-phenylalanine mustard. Scientific program. p. 5. American College of Physicians, October, 1965.

155. Rabellino, E., and Grey, H. M.: Immunoglobulins at the surface of lymphocytes. J. Immunol. *106:*1418, 1971.

156. Rai, K. R., et al.: Clinical staging of chronic lymphocytic leukemia. Blood, *46:*219, 1975.

157. Rall, D. P.: Research findings of potential value to the practitioner – New prednisone regimen in myasthenia gravis. MAMA, *237:*635, 1977.

158. Rappaport, H.: Tumors of the Hematopoietic System. Section III. fascicle 8. pp. F8–98, 12, 13, 161. Armed Forces Institute of Pathology, Washington, D.C., 1966.

159. Rappaport, H., and Moran, E. M.: Angio-immunoblastic (immunoblastic) lymphadenopathy. N. Engl. J. Med., *292:*42, 1975.

160. Randall, D. L., Reiquam, C. W., Githens, J. H., and Robinson, A.: Familial myeloproliferative disease: new syndrome closely simulating myelogenous leukemia in childhood. Am. J. Dis. Child., *110:*479, 1965.

161. Rebuck, J. W.: Hematology check sample No. H-21 (C.C.E. – A.S.C.P.). October, 1964.

162. Robbins, J. H.: Tissue culture studies of the human lymphocyte. Science, *146:*1648, 1654, 1964.

163. Rosenacen W., and Tsoukas, C. D.: Lymphotoxin, a review and analysis. Am. J. Pathol., *84:*580, 1976.

164. Ross, G. D., Polley, M. J., Rabellino, E. M., and Grey, H. M.: Two different complement receptors on human lymphocytes. One specific for C3$_b$ and one specific for C3$_b$ inactivator-cleaved C3$_b$. J. Exp. Med., *138:*798, 1973.

165. Ross, G. D., Rabellino, E. M., Polley, M. J., and Grey, H. M.: Combined studies of complement receptor and surface immunoglobulin-bearing cells and sheep erythrocyte rosette-forming cells in normal and leukemic human lymphocytes. J. Clin. Invest., *52:*377, 1973.

166. Rosenthal, R. L.: Blood coagulation in leukemia and polycythemia: value of heparin clotting time and clot retraction rate. J. Lab. Clin. Med., *34:*1321, 1949.

167. Rosenthal, R. L.: Acute promyelocytic leukemia associated with hypofibrinogenemia. Blood, *21:*495, 1963.

168. Rubin, A. D., Havemann, K., Kochwa, S., and Dameshek, W.: Differences in nucleic acid metabolism of PHA-stimulated lymphocytes from patients with infectious mononucleosis and chornic lymphocytic leukemia (abstract). Presented at the 9th annual meeting of the American Society of Hematology, 1966.

169. Rubin, P.: Hodgkin's disease. J.A.M.A., *190:*910, 1964.

170. Saarni, M. I., and Linman, J. W.: Preleukemia: Hematologic syndrome preceding acute leukemia. Am. J. Med., *55:*38, 1973.

171. Saltzstein, S. L., and Ackerman, L. V.: Lymphadenopathy induced by anticoagulant drugs and mimicking clinically and pathologically malignant lymphomas. Cancer, *12:*164, 1959.

172. Schein, P. S., et al.: Potential for prolonged disease-free survival following combination chemotherapy of non-Hodgkin's lymphomas. Blood, *43:*181, 1974.

173. Schultz, W.: Über eigenartige Halserkrankungen (a) monozytenangina (b) gangrinezierende Prozesse und Defekt des Granulozytensystems. Dtsch. Med. Wochenschr., *48:*1495, 1922.

174. Schwarz, G.: The role of lymphangiography (in Hodgkin's disease). J.A.M.A., *190:*912, 1964.

175. Schwarzenberg, L., et al.: Attempted adoptive immunotherapy of acute leukemia by leucocyte transfusions. Lancet, *2:*365, 1966.

176. Selawry, O. S., et al.: New treatment schedule with improved survival in childhood leukemia: intermittent parenteral vs. daily oral administration of methotrexate for maintenance of induced remission. J.A.M.A., *194:*75, 1965.

177. Seligmann, M., Preud'Homme, J. L., and Brouet, J. C.: B and T cell markers in human proliferative blood diseases and primary immunodeficiencies with special reference to membrane bound immunoglobulins. Transplant Rev., *16:*85, 1973.

178. Sen, L., and Borelli, L.: Clinical importance of lymphoblasts with T markers in childhood acute leukemia. N. Engl. J. Med., *292:*828, 1975.

179. Shelley, W. B., and Parnes, H. M.: The absolute basophil count. J.A.M.A., *192:*108, 1965.

180. Shevoch, E. M., Jaffe, E. S., and Green, I.: Receptors for complement and immunoglobulin on human and animal lymphoid cells. Transplant Rev., *16:*3, 1973.

181. Silber, R., Comklyn, M., Grusky, G., and Zucker, F. D.: Human lymphocytes: 5' nucleotidase positive and negative subpopulations. J. Clin. Invest., *56:*1324, 1975.

181a. Silverstein, M. N. et al.: The syndrome of the sea-blue histiocyte. N. Engl. J. Med., *282*:1, 1970.

182. Simone, J.: Factors that influence haematological remission duration in acute lymphocytic leukemia. Br. J. Haematol., *32*:465, 1976.

182a. Slavin, R. E., and Santos, G. W.: The graft versus host reaction in man after bone marrow transplantation: pathology, pathogenesis, clinical features and implications. Clinical Immunology and Immunopathol., *1*:472, 1973.

183. Smith, R. W., Terry, W. D., Buell, D. N., and Sell, K. W.: An antigenic marker for human thymic lymphocytes. J. Immunol., *110*:884, 1973.

184. Speed, D. E., Galton, D. A. G., and Swan, A.: Melphalan in treatment of myelomatosis. Br. Med. J., *1*:1664, 1964.

185. Sprunt, T. P., and Evans, F. A.: Mononuclear leukocytosis in reaction to acute infections (infectious mononucleosis). Bull. Johns Hopkins Hosp., *31*:410, 1920.

186. Stein, H., Lennert, K., and Parwaresch, M. R.: Malignant lymphomas of B-cell type. Lancet, *2*:855, 1972.

187. Steinberg, M. H., and Dreiling, B. J.: Chronic granulocytic leukemia: Prolonged survival, muscle infiltration and sea blue histiocytes. Am. J. Med., *55*:93, 1973.

188. Stiehm, E. R., Vaerman, J. P., and Fudenberg, H. H.: Plasma infusions in immunologic deficiency states: metabolic and therapeutic studies. Blood, *28*:918, 1966.

189. Strober, S.: T and B-cells in immunologic diseases. Am. J. Clin. Pathol., *68*:671, 1977.

189a. Thomas, E. D., and Rainer, S.: Technique for human marrow grafting. Blood, *37*:507, 1970.

190. Toland, D. M., and Coltman, C. A., Jr.: Second malignancy complicating Hodgkin's disease. The Southwest Group experience. Proc. ASCO, *18*:351, 1977.

191. Trentin, J. J.: Relationships between lymphocytes and other hemic cells. The stem cell concept. Symposium: The Lymphocyte in Health and Disease, American Assoc. of Pathologists and Bacteriologists. San Francisco, Calif., March 11, 1969.

192. Troxel, D. B., Innella, F., and Cohen, R. J.: Infectious mononucleosis complicated by hemolytic anemia due to anti-i. Am. J. Clin. Pathol., *46*:625, 1966.

193. Ultmann, J. E., Mutter, R. D., Tannenbaum, M., and Warner, R. R. P.: Clinical cytologic and biochemical studies in systemic mast cell disease. Ann. Intern. Med., *61*:326, 1964.

194. Volger, W. R., and Chan, Y. K.: Prolonging remission in myeloblastic leukemia by Tice-strain bacillus Calmette-Guerin. Lancet, *2*:128, 1974.

195. Waldmann, T. A., et al.: Role of suppressor T cells in pathogenesis of common variable hypogammaglobulinemia. Lancet, *2*:609, 1974.

196. Wanebo, H. J., and Clarkson, B. D.: Essential macroglobulinemia: report of a case including immunofluorescent and electron microscopic studies. Ann. Intern. Med., *62*:1025, 1965.

197. Ward, H. N., Konikov, N., and Reinhard, E. H.: Cytologic dysplasia occurring after Myeleran therapy. Ann. Intern. Med., *63*:654, 1965.

198. Warner, N. L.: Membrane immunoglobulins and antigen receptors on B and T lymphocytes. Adv. Immunol., *19*:67, 1974.

199. Warner, N. L., Szenberg, A., and Burnet, F. M.: The immunological role of different lymphoid organs in the chicken. I. Dissociation of immunological responsiveness. Aust. J. Exp. Biol. Med. Sci., *40*:373, 1962.

200. WHO/IARG Sponsored Workshop on Human B and T cells: Identification, enumeration and isolation of B and T lymphocytes from human peripheral blood. Scand. J. Immunol., *3*:521, 1974.

201. Williams, R. C., DeBoard, J. R., Mellbye, O. J., Messner, R. P., and Lindstrom, F. K.: Studies of T and B lymphocytes in patients with connective tissue diseases. J. Clin. Invest., *52*:283, 1973.

202. Wilson, D., and Van Slyck, E. J.: Coexistent lymphosarcoma and chronic granulocytic leukemia. Scientific program. American College of Physicians, October 7, 1965.

203. Wilson, J. D., and Nossal, G. J. V.: Identification of human T and B lymphocytes in normal peripheral blood and in chronic lymphocytic leukemia. Lancet, *2*:788, 1971.

204. Wu, L. Y. F., Lawton, A. R., and Cooper, M. D.: Differentation capacity of cultured B lymphocytes from immunodeficient patients. J. Clin. Invest., *52*:3180, 1973.

205. Wybran, J., Carr, M. C., and Fudenberg, H. H.: The human rosette-forming cell as a marker of a population of thymus-derived cells. J. Clin. Invest., *51*:2537, 1972.

206. Wybran, J., and Fudenberg, H. H.: Thymus-derived rosette-forming cells in various human disease states: Cancer, lymphoma, bacterial and viral infections and other diseases. J. Clin. Invest., *52*:1026, 1973.

207. Yoffey, J. M.: The lymphocyte. Annu. Rev. Med., *15*:125, 1964.

208. Young, R. C., et al.: Maintenance chemotherapy for advanced Hodgkin's disease in remission. Lancet, *1*:1139, 1973.

209. Ziegler, J. L., and Carbone, P. P.: Burkitt tumor in the United States: diagnosis, treatment and prognosis (abstract). Presented at the 9th annual meeting of the American Society of Hematology, 1966.

AUDIOVISUAL AIDS*

Acute Leukemia. Set N2. [35 mm. transparencies, audiotape, manual]. A.S.H. National Slide Bank, HSLRC T-252 (SB-56), University of Washington, Seattle, Washington 98195.

Acute Leukemia. Part III. CDC-77-12. Marguerite Candler Ballard, M.D. [36 (35 mm.) transparencies plus handout, 12 pp., and standard audiocassette, $65.10.]. Communications in Learning, Inc., 2929 Main Street, Buffalo, New York 14214.

---

* Films unless otherwise stated.

Acute Leukemias, Megaloblastic Anemias. Tape 47. Southern Audio-Visual Exhibition Service, 550 Meridian Ave., Miami Beach, Florida 33139.

Agar-gel and Immunoelectrophoresis. ASCP Seminar 212-3. [35 mm. transparencies, audio-tape]. ASMT Education and Research Fund, Inc. 5555 West Loop South, Bellaire, Texas 77401.

B&T Cell Interaction in the Immune Response. 247401. [14 (35 mm.) transparencies and standard audiocassette, $23.10.]. Richard H. Zeschke, Ph.D., Communications in Learning, Inc., 2929 Main Street, Buffalo, New York 14214.

Chronic Leukemias. [Self-Teaching Slide Review 20], University of Miami School of Medicine, Department of Internal Medicine (Hematology), Miami, Florida 33136.

Chronic Leukemias, Lymphoma. Tape 48. Southern Audio-Visual Exhibition Service, 550 Meridian Ave., Miami Beach, Florida 33139.

Clinical Management of Acute Leukemia. (1958). Schering Corporation, Audio-Visual Department, 1011 Morris Avenue, Union, New Jersey 07083.

The Differential Diagnosis of Leukocyte Abnormalities by Morphologic Examination of the Peripheral Blood. The Myeloproliferative Syndrome, T-2612; *The Lymphoproliferative Syndrome and Other Lymphocytic Disorders,* T-2613; *Congenital Anomalies of Leukocytes and Unusual Acquired Conditions,* T-2614; *The Acute Leukemias,* T-2615; National Medical Audiovisual Center (Annex), Station K, Atlanta, Georgia 30324. (1972)

Histocompatibility Testing. 247502. Elias Cohen, Ph.D., Joseph Gerbasi, M.D., and Shirley Gregory, M.A. [13 (35 mm.) transparencies and standard audiocassette, $29.35]. Communications in Learning, Inc., 2929 Main Street, Buffalo, New York 14214.

Hodgkin's Disease: Differential Diagnosis and Staging. (1978). [videocassette program]. American Society of Clinical Pathologists, P.O. Box 12073, Chicago, Illinois 50512.

Infectious Mononucleosis. [Self-Teaching Slide Review 22]. University of Miami School of Medicine, Department of Internal Medicine (Hematology), Miami, Florida 33136.

Immunoglobulin Structure and Function, Monoclonal Gammopathies, Infectious Mononucleosis, Hemorrhagic Diseases. Tape 50. Southern Audio-Visual Exhibition Service, 550 Meridian Ave., Miami Beach, Florida 33139.

Laboratory Diagnosis of Immunoglobulin Disorders. Set M1. [35 mm. slides, transparencies, audiotape, manual]. A.S.H. National Slide Bank, HSLRC T-252 (SB-56) University of Washington, Seattle, Washington 98195.

The Leukemias. 27. James W. Linman, M.D. [100 color transparencies (35 mm.) plus descriptive booklet, $65.00]. MedCom, Inc., 2 Hammerskjold Plaza, New York, New York 10017.

Malignant Lymphomas. Self-Teaching Slide Review 19. University of Miami School of Medicine, Department of Internal Medicine (Hematology), Miami, Florida 33136.

Myeloproliferative Diseases, Myeloid Metaplasia, Polycythemia, Thrombocytothemia, RBC Production Defects, Granulocyte Production Defects. Self-Teaching Slide Review 23. University of Miami School of Medicine, Department of Internal Medicine (Hematology), Miami, Florida 33136.

Non-Hodgkin's Lymphomas. [videocassette program]. American Society of Clinical Pathologists, P.O. Box 12073, Chicago, Illinois 60612.

Normal and Leukemic White Cells of Human Blood. International Society for Hematology, James L. Tullis, M.D., 110 Francis Street, Boston, Massachusetts 02215.

Polycythemia and Myeloid Metaplasia, RBC Production Defects, WBC (Granulocytic) Production Defects, Essential Thrombocythemia. Tape 44. Southern Audio-Visual Exhibition Service, 550 Meridian Ave., Miami Beach, Florida 33139.

Proliferative Disorders of Plasma Cells and Lymphocytes (Myeloma and Lymphoma). [TV and audiotape]. University of Miami School of Medicine, Department of Internal Medicine (Hematology), Miami, Florida 33136.

T & B Lymphocytes: Their Identification in Peripheral Blood and Solid Tissue. (1978). [videocassette program]. American Society of Clinical Pathologists, P.O. Box 12073, Chicago, Illinois 60612.

14 *Special Stains in Hematology*

There are special stains that can be used with great success in the various hematologic laboratory procedures. Some of these have been reproduced on color plates 52, 89, 91, and 92.

PEROXIDASE STAIN

Principle of Stain

One may differentiate the various immature myeloid cells from the younger lymphoid forms by demonstrating an oxidizing enzyme in the cytoplasm of the myeloid cells and, to a lesser extent, in monocytic cells. The oxidizing enzyme in the myeloid cells brings about the oxidation of benzidine by hydrogen peroxide; this oxidized benzidine compound is then deposited in the cell cytoplasm. Because the source of oxygen is hydrogen peroxide, the term "peroxidase staining" is used. Peroxidase-positive granules are found in neutrophils, eosinophils, monocytes, and myelocytes. Lymphocytes, plasma cells, and all forms of blast cells are peroxidase-negative. Histiocytes are also peroxidase-negative, but they may contain phagocytosed material that is peroxidase-positive.

Review of Methods and Interpretation

Fresh blood films are used because the enzyme fades with age.

Sato-Schiya Copper Peroxidase Method. A fresh air-dried smear is flooded with 0.5 per cent copper sulfate solution for 1 minute; the solution is poured off without washing. The smear is then flooded with a saturated solution of benzidine for 2 minutes (0.2 g. of benzidine and 200 ml. of distilled water; filter and add 4 drops of 3% H_2O_2 and store in dark. The solution is tested by mixing 1 ml. of 0.5% $CuSO_4$ and 1 ml. of the benzidine solution; a blue color should develop. If no blue color occurs, its absence is usually due to an incompletely saturated benzidine solution). The smear is washed well with distilled water, then dried and counterstained for 2 minutes with 1 per cent safranin; then it is washed and dried. Peroxidase-positive granules stain bluish green; eosinophil and basophil granules take a deeper blue as contrasted with the light blue staining small granules in monocytes. Lymphocytes take up reddish counterstain color. Red blood cells do not appear distinctly.

Goodpasture Method. A fresh air-dried smear is flooded with one part of the nitroprusside benzidine basic fuchsin solution for 1 minute (0.05 g. of sodium nitroprusside in 2 ml. of distilled water plus 100 ml. of absolute ethyl alcohol. Add 0.05 g. of basic fuchsin and 0.05 g. of benzidine). One part of H_2O_2 (1:200 HO_2 in distilled water) solution is added and allowed to stand for 4 minutes. The smear is then washed well and dried. Peroxidase-positive granules are deep blue; eosinophilic granules are darker blue; basophilic granules do not stain. The nuclei of cells are red, cytoplasm is pink, and red blood cells have a buff color.

Washburn Method Modified by Osgood and Ashworth. A fresh air-dried smear is flooded with 10 drops of benzidine. Sodium nitroprusside solution (0.3 benzidine base dissolved in 99 ml. of absolute ethyl alcohol plus 1 ml. of saturated aqueous solution of sodium nitroprusside) is added and allowed to stand for 1 to 1½ minutes. Five drops of diluted H_2O_2 solution is added and allowed to stand for 3 to 4 minutes (make fresh each time by adding 0.3 ml. of fresh 3% H_2O_2 to 25 ml. of distilled water). The smear is washed thoroughly in tap water for 3 to 4 minutes and is then counterstained with Wright's stain. Neutrophilic granules are plentiful, large and bluish black; myelocytic granules are reduced in number, small and bluish green; monocytic granules are even less in number and bluish green; eosinophils have large bronze granules; basophilic granules appear partially "empty."

Jacoby Method. A fresh air-dried smear is flooded with a mixture of 1 part of 40 per cent formaldehyde and 9 parts of absolute ethyl alcohol for 3 minutes. The smear is washed in tap water, and then 4 drops of H_2O_2 solution (4 volumes) is added to 5 ml. of aqueous 0.05 per cent 2,6 dichlorophenol-indophenol solution (keep in refrigerator). This is put on the smear and allowed to stand for 5 minutes. The smear is washed thoroughly in tap water for 3 minutes and counterstained with a 0.5 per cent neutral red solution. Peroxidase-positive granules of myeloid cells stain deep purple-violet, especially in eosinophils; monocytes contain a moderate number of fine, small lilac granules.

Simplified Myeloperoxidase Stain That Uses Benzidine Dihydrochloride.[5] *Technique.* (1) Use fresh smears of blood or bone marrow or organ imprints. Activity may be preserved for as long as 3 weeks if the preparations are stored in the dark. Venous or peripheral blood is equally acceptable. Heparin, oxalate, and EDTA are not inhib-

itory. (2) Fix slides in a 10 per cent formalin-ethanol mixture for 60 seconds. (3) Wash in running tap water for 15 to 30 seconds. Shake off excess water, but do not dry. (Reaction will not take place if slides are dry.) Wash in distilled water. (4) Incubate mixture at room temperature for 30 to 45 seconds. (5) Wash in running tap water for 5 to 10 seconds and distilled water (2 changes). (6) Stain in neutral red for 1 minute. (For greater nuclear detail, counterstain in 1% crystal violet for 1 min. or freshly prepared Giemsa for 10 min.) (7) Distilled water (2 changes). (8) Blot and air dry. (9) Mount with permount.

Solutions. 10 per cent formalin-ethanol mixture is 40 per cent formalin, 10 ml., and 100 per cent ethyl alcohol, 90 ml.

The incubation mixture is 30 per cent ethyl alcohol, 200 ml.; benzidine dihydrochloride, 0.6 g.; 0.132 M (3.8% W/V) $ZnSO_4$. ($7H_2O$), 2.0 ml.; sodium acetate, 2.0 g.; 3% H_2O_2, 1.4 ml.; 1.0 N NaOH, 3.0 ml.; and safranin O, 0.4 g.

The reagents should be added in the order listed, mixing well with each addition. The benzidine salt may contain a small amount of inert residue that will not go into solution. A precipitate forms upon the addition of the remaining reagents. The final pH is 6.00 ± .05, on a pH meter. The solution should be filtered and stored in a capped Coplin jar at room temperature. (The same solution can be used over and over again for as long as 6 months.)

The buffered 1 per cent neutral red solution is Neutral Red 1 g. and 1N acetate buffer pH 5.0 100 ml. Mix well. Filter and store at room temperature. (The 1N acetate buffer pH 5.0 is sodium acetate, 4.797 g.; 1N acetic acid, 14.75 ml.; and distilled water q.s., 1,000 ml. Adjust pH to 5.0; 1N acetic acid is glacial acetic acid, 6 ml. and distilled water, 994 ml.) Always use a control slide, which may be any fresh normal blood smear.

Results. Peroxidase azure granules (lysosomes) of neutrophils and monocytes become *bluish*-black. These granules may be scattered and are said to be positive in granulocytic leukemia.

Federal regulations now prohibit the use of benzidine and its derivatives in concentrations above 0.1 per cent, unless rigorously defined safety precautions are taken.[2] This is because benzidine is supposed to be carcinogenic for rats. The safety rules include the washing of hands frequently in the laboratory, the prohibition of eating in the laboratory, and so on. These and other requirements are too complex and demanding for many clinical laboratories and manufacturing laboratories may also find compliance very difficult. Thus, it is probable that benzidine and its derivatives will shortly become unavailable, and their use in detecting occult blood and in staining leukocytes for myeloperoxidase activity will soon cease.

Among alternative methods, one technique modified from the work of two groups has yielded consistent and satisfactory results.[3, 11] The method is as follows: Fix thin blood smears in buffered formalin acetone for 15 seconds at room temperature. Wash gently and incubate slides for 2½ minutes at room temperature in a filtered mixture containing: 3-amino-9-ethylcarbazole,* 10 mg.; dimethylsulfoxide, 6 ml.; .02 M acetate buffer, (pH 5.0-5.2), 50 ml.; and 0.3 per cent hydrogen peroxide, 0.4 ml. The final pH is 5.5.

Wash gently in running tap water and counterstain with Mayer's hematoxylin for 8 minutes. Wash, dry, mount in glycerol-gelatin, and examine. Peroxidase activity is represented by red-brown granular deposits. The distribution of dye is identical to that seen with benzidine stains.

Nonspecific Esterase Stain (alpha naphthyl butyrate).[12] (1) Fix smears in cold formalin acetone at pH 6.6 for 10 to 15 minutes. (2) Air dry. (3) Mix alpha naphthyl substrate solution (keep refrigerated): (A) 0.125 ml. pararosanalin; (B) 0.125 ml. 4% $NaNO_2$;

Mix well. Wait 1 to 2 minutes. Develops light straw color. (C) To this add 47.5 ml. of M/15 phosphate buffer pH 6.3. (D) Weigh out 50.0 mg. of alpha naphthyl butyrate and place in 100 ml. beaker. (Store alpha NB in freezer.) (E) To this, add 2.5 ml. of ethylene glycol. (4) Add solution I to solution II (cloudy). Mix well, and filter with No. 40 Whatman. (5) Incubate for 45 minutes at room temperature. (6) Rinse in water. (7) Counterstain 20 minutes in Mayer's Hematoxylin. (8) Wash well for 30 minutes in water. (9) Dry, dip in xylol, and mount with permount.

Always use a control slide. Counterstaining is very difficult and sometimes impossible. Enzyme activity is seen as red-brown granules in the cytoplasm of monocytes, histiocytes, megakaryocytes, platelets, and stain also differentiates monocytes from lymphocytes. The stain granule can be erased with fluoride; however, histiocyte granules are not erased, and, therefore, it is a good differential stain for this.

Solutions. For pararosanalin, dissolve 1.0 g. pararosanalin in 20 ml. water and 5 ml. concentration HCl with gentle warming. Filter. Store at room temperature.

For M/15 Buffer pH 6.3, dissolve 2.366 g. Na_2HPO_4 and 6.798 g. KH_2PO_4 in distilled water q.s. 1000 ml. Adjust pH to 6.3, with 1N HCl or 1N NaOH.

Sudan Black B Stain for Smears.[114] *Technique.* (1) Fix air dried smears in formalin vapor for 10 minutes. (2) Air dry for 10 minutes. (3) Sudan Black B (working solution) for 30 minutes. (4) 100 per cent ethyl alcohol, two changes for 2 minutes each. (5) Distilled water two changes. (6) Giemsa (working solution) for 5 minutes. (7) Distilled water for 10 to 15 minutes. (8) Blot dry and air dry. (9) Mount in permount.

Solutions. For Sudan Black B stock solution, add 0.3 g. of Sudan Black B to 100 ml. of 100 per cent ethyl alcohol. Shake vigorously and frequently for 1 or 2 days or until the dye is dissolved, filter.

For buffer, mix 16 g. pure phenol crystals in 30 ml. of 100 per cent ethyl alcohol with

---

* Aldrich Chemical Co., Inc., Milwaukee, Wisconsin 53233.

a solution of 0.119 g. Na_2HPO_4 in 100 ml. of water.

For Sudan Black B working solution, mix 30 ml. of Sudan Black B stock solution with 20 ml. of buffer. Filter under suction on double No. 1 filter paper. Mixture should be neutral or slightly alkaline. Do not keep for use for more than 3 weeks.

For working Giemsa, 1 ml. of stock Giemsa plus 49 ml. distilled water.

For fixative, drop 10 or more drops of full strength 37 to 40 per cent formalin on a piece of gauze placed at the bottom of a Coplin jar. Smears are then placed in the jar and covered. Care must be taken not to wet the slides with fixative.

Results. Phospholipids on particular granules of the granulocytic series stain black. This stain is as specific as the peroxidase stain; in fact it stains intensely bluish black with less background material than the peroxidase stain.

Acid Phosphatase and Tartrate-Resistant Acid Phosphatase for Smears.[4, 6, 7, 9, 13, 14]

Procedure. For smears and imprints, fix in cold buffered methanol-acetone solution for 30 seconds, wash in distilled water 3 changes and air dry. (1) Incubate in freshly mixed substrate solution at 37° C for 90 minutes. (Use control slide of normal prostate). Substrate solution is 0.1M Acetate buffer *p*H 5.0, 38.0 ml.; freshly hexazotized New Fuchsin (HPR), 0.2 ml.; naphthol AS-BI phosphoric acid sol., 2.0 ml. For the tartrate solution, add 300 mg of L(+) tartaric acid to the equivalent of the above substrate solution and adjust the *p*H to 5.0. (2) Distilled water for 2 to 3 changes. (3) Counterstain with Mayer's hematoxylin for 4 to 5 mintues. (4) Running tap water for 20 minutes. (5) Air dry. Dip in xylene and mount in Permount or glycerin jelly.

Reagents. The fixative for smears is 10 per cent methanol in 60 per cent acetone, buffered with 0.03M citrate at *p*H 5.4. (Solution is composed of methanol, 10 ml.; 60 per cent acetone in 0.03M citrate buffer, 90 ml.; adjust *p*H to 5.4 with 1N NaOH or 1N HCl. This is stable for one month).

Table14-1. Cytochemical Profile (Leukemia)*

Stains	AGL	AMML	ALL	CGL	CLL
Peroxidase	1–3+	1–3+	0	3+	0
P.A.S.	0	1–2+	0–3+		2+
Naphthol AS-D-chloroacetate esterase	1–2+	1–2+	0	1–3+	0
Alpha naphthyl butyrate esterase	0	1–3+	1+	0	0–1+
Sudan black	1–3+	1–3+	0	1–3+	0

Key: AGL = acute granulocytic leukemia; AMML = acute myelomonocytic leukemia; CGL = chronic granulocytic leukemia; CLL = chronic lymphocytic leukemia; Scale: 0–3+.
* The peroxidase stain is a short stain and easy to do. The PAS stain is best in cases of acute erythroleukemia. The naphthol AS-D-chloroacetate esterase stain is helpful in differentiating acute granulocytic leukemia from lymphomas and is similar to the peroxidase stain.

For fresh 4 per cent sodium nitrite solution, dissolve 1 g. $NaNO_2$ in 25 ml. distilled water.

For New Fuchsin solution, dissolve 1 g. New Fuchsin in 25 ml. of hot, not boiling, 2 N HCl. Filter when cool.

For freshly hexazotized New Fuchsin use equal amounts, Sodium Nitrite, 0.15 ml.; New Fuchsin solution, 0.15 ml.

For naphthol AS-BI phosphoric acid solution, dissolve 40 mg. of Naphthol AS-BI phosphoric acid into 2 ml. of N,N-dimethyl formamide. Store tightly stoppered in freezer until used.

For 0.1M acetate buffer *p*H5.0, dissolve 4.797 g. of sodium acetate $CH_3COONa \cdot 3H_2O$ in 14.75 Ml of 1N acetic acid (6 ml. glacial acetic acid in 994 cc distilled water). Add distilled water to make a final volume of 1,000 ml.

Results. Enzyme activity is seen as bright red granules in the cytoplasm of the blood cells. The presence of tartrate in the incubating medium almost completely inhibits enzyme activity in all types of blood cells. The neoplastic "reticulum cells" (hairy cells) of leukemic reticuloendotheliosis and a rare histiocyte from spleen and lymph node imprints from patients with other diseases have tartrate-resistant acid phosphatase activity. That is, reddish-orange granules are observed at the edge of the hairy cells, which appear to be a cross between a lymphocyte and monocyte. Under the scanning electron microscope, these cells have cornflake-like ruffles on their surface.

The reaction product is very chromagenic and insoluble in organic solvents. It forms no crystals, even in specimens with very strong activity. It is most useful in marrow and imprint materials. The method is not very sensitive, and smears older than 3 days will show appreciable decrease in activity.

Supplies. New Fuchsin (C.I. 42520) is available from Allied Chemical Co., Inc., P.O. Box 431, Morristown, New Jersey 07960.

Naphthol AS-BI phosphoric acid is available from Sigma Chemical Co., 3500 DeKalb Street, St. Louis, Missouri 63118.

N,N-Dimethyl formamide is available from Fisher Scientific Co., Fairlawn, New Jersey 07410.

FEULGEN REACTION

Principle, Results of Stain, and Clinical Application

Two main types of nucleic acid are found in blood cells, and they are differentiated by the type of sugar linked to the acid radical. One type of sugar is ribose, which when linked to nucleic acid forms ribonucleic acid (RNA). The other type of sugar is deoxyribose, which when linked to nucleic acid forms deoxyribonucleic acid (DNA). RNA and DNA have a strong affinity for basic dyes (Schiff's reagent), which are retained when they are linked with proteins. The Feulgen reaction is specific for DNA —that is, acid hydrolysis frees the aldehyde groups of the deoxyribose (sugar) component of DNA. The aldehyde groups then react with the leukobasic fuchsin in Schiff's

reagent to produce a pink-purple color where DNA is present. The Feulgen nuclear reaction therefore stains white blood cells and normoblasts according to the concentration of DNA in the nucleus. It is of special use in distinguishing between mature and immature cells—for example, lymphocytes versus micromyeloblasts.

Nucleoli contain RNA and appear distinctly as Feulgen-negative spaces in the nucleus surrounded by bands of deeply-stained nuclear chromatin material, and the nucleoli therefore can be counted. Lymphoblasts contain one to two nucleoli and myeloblasts frequently contain two to four nucleoli. Megaloblasts are usually Feulgen-negative, but all cells of the normoblastic series are Feulgen-positive. The cell is said to be Feulgen-negative when the nucleus stains a diffuse pale pink and the nucleoli appear as cellular spaces surrounded by bands of deeply-stained (purplish) material. The nuclei of Feulgen-positive cells stain deep pinkish-purple, arranged in clumps and thick strands. When light green is used as a counterstain, the red blood cells and the cytoplasm of all cells appear light green.

Technique

A fresh air-dried blood film is fixed for 10 minutes in fixative (absolute methyl alcohol, 15 parts; 5% acetic acid, 5 parts; 40% formalin, 1 part; and 5 parts of distilled water). The film is washed with tap water for 20 minutes and then in distilled water for 2 minutes. It is then dipped in N/1 HCl at 60° C for 10 minutes. The film is then rinsed in distilled water; it is stained with Schiff's reagent and allowed to stand for 20 minutes (Schiff's reagent is made as follows: dissolve, with shaking, 1 g. of basic fuchsin in 200 ml. of boiling distilled water; cool to about 50° C, add 2 g. of sodium bisulfate and 1 ml. of concentrated HCl and allow to stand in a glass-stoppered bottle for 24 hrs., at which time it should be pale yellow; add 0.5 g. of charcoal; shake and allow to stand for a few minutes and then filter. The filtrate should be colorless. Store in a refrigerator). The film is then dipped in two or three changes of sulfurous acid solution (5 ml. of 10% HCl and 100 ml. of 0.5% potassium metabisulfite). The film is washed in tap water and counterstained with 0.5 per cent aqueous light green solution; it is then dehydrated in 40 per cent, 80 per cent, and absolute alcohol for 5 minutes each. The film is then cleared with xylol and mounted with Permount.

To summarize, Feulgen-positive cells include metamyelocytes, granulocytes, lymphocytes, normoblasts, and LE cells; Feulgen-negative cells include myeloblasts, lymphoblasts, myelocytes, monocytes, megaloblasts, and promegakaryocytes.

HISTOCHEMICAL TECHNIQUE FOR LEUKOCYTIC ALKALINE PHOSPHATASE

The histochemical technique for leukocyte alkaline phosphatase, a hematologic, semiquantitative measurement of enzymatic concentration in leukocytes, is of differential diagnostic significance. Two methods popularly used are the Gomori method and the Kaplow technique.

Gomori Method

In the modified Gomori method, alkaline phosphatase demonstration depends on the formation of a colored precipitate at the site of hydrolysis of the substrate. This modified Gomori method depends on incubating smears with glycerophosphate at pH 9 in the presence of magnesium and calcium ions. Calcium phosphate is precipitated and formed at the site of reaction, visualization occurring after conversion to black cobalt sulfide. Some feel that this method is inferior to the Kaplow technique.

The method as it is used at the University of Rochester Medical Center is as follows: (1) Concentrated leukocyte push smears are made by mixing 5 cc. of venous blood with a very small amount of powdered dipotassium EDTA. As soon as possible, the blood is placed into two Wintrobe

hematocrit tubes and spun in a centrifuge at 1800 r.p.m. for 6 minutes. The supernatant plasma is decanted, and the buffy layer and an equal amount of plasma are taken off. They are mixed on a paraffin-coated watchglass. A drop of the mixture is placed on each of several slides, and push smears are made. One smear is stained with Wright's stain to use as a standard to estimate the approximate number of neutrophilic cells per oil immersion field, because on low alkaline phosphatase smears it may be impossible to be certain of the cell type.

(2) For best results, the dried concentrated smears are allowed to stand for at least 24 hours. They may then be fixed in 0.25 per cent celloidin solution (0.25 g. of celloidin mixed with 50 cc. of absolute alcohol; then add 50 cc. of ether. Shake until dissolved) for 5 seconds. This step can be successfully ignored if the smears are allowed to stand for 2 days or more before staining. (3) The smears are dipped into 95 per cent ethyl alcohol for 5 seconds (in and out about five times). The smears are tapped on a dry sponge to remove the excess alcohol. (4) The smears are dipped in and out of distilled water 10 to 20 times, until alcohol traces are removed. (5) The smears are transferred to solution X, which is made by using 10 cc. of 3.2 per cent sodium glycerophosphate·$5H_2O$; 10 cc. of 10 per cent sodium barbital; 10 cc. of N/10 magnesium sulfate (24.7 g. of $MgSO_4$·$7H_2O$ dissolved in 12.0 ml. distilled water); 15 cc. of 2 per cent $Ca(NO_3)_2$ (28.8 g. of $Ca(NO_3)_2$/L. of distilled water); and 55 cc. of distilled water. The smears are incubated in this solution at 37° C for 15 hours.

(6) The slides are washed in a Coplin jar of distilled water containing 5 cc. of $Ca(NO_3)_2$ solution by dipping the slides in and out five to ten times. (7) The slides are tapped on dry gauze and transferred to 2.5 per cent cobalt nitrate solution for 5 minutes (32 g. of $Co(NO_3)_2$ dissolved in 1000 cc. of distilled water). (8) The slides are

washed thoroughly in running tap water by filling an empty Coplin jar 5 times. (9) The slides are put into a Coplin jar that is filled with a solution of tap water plus 3 drops of $(NH_4)_2S$ for 30 seconds. All windows should be opened and all fans turned on before this step. (10) Repeat Step 8.

(11) The slides are air dried, mounted with immersion oil, and examined under the oil immersion field. (12) The slides are then read. First the Wright's stained slide is examined, the number of neutrophilic cells (metamyelocytes and polymorphonuclear neutrophils) are estimated per oil immersion field. It is then determined if the alkaline phosphatase smear appears to have the same number. The cells are classified with respect to their content of alkaline phosphatase; this is done on 100 cells — for example, 0 = no stain, 1+ = whitish gray, 2+ = gray, 3+ = grayish black, and 4+ = black. Many laboratories stain two smears from each sample of blood and count 200 cells on each smear; the results are then averaged. (13) The number of cells in each group is multiplied by the number of positives (+'s) then totaled to obtain the final index. For example:

Classification	(Number of cells of that classification in the total of 100 cells)	
0	×	13 = 0
1+	×	9 = 9
2+	×	13 = 26
3+	×	14 = 42
4+	×	51 = 204

281 = alkaline phosphatase index

The normal range = 80 – 185 (mean is 140). Very low results are observed in chronic myeloid leukemia. Very high results are seen in agnogenic myeloid metaplasia, leukemoid reaction, or polycythemia vera.

Kaplow Alkaline Phosphatase Technique

This method uses fixation in a solution of 10 per cent formalin in absolute methyl alcohol at 0° C, sodium alpha naphthyl phosphate is the substrate, and fast blue

RR as the diazonium salt. The results are thought to be clearer than Gomori method and more reproducible. The procedure is as follows: (1) Dry, unstained blood smears are prepared as in Steps 1 and 2 in the Gomori method. (2) The slides are dipped in the fixative solution (10 ml. of 39% formalin and 90 ml. of absolute methyl alcohol; mix and refrigerate) for 30 seconds at 0 to 4° C. (3) The slides are washed in running tap water for 10 seconds. (4) They are then incubated in substrate mixture (prepare immediately before use) for 10 minutes at room temperature. The substrate mixture has a pH of 9.6. It contains the following ingredients:

A. Sodium acid naphthyl phosphate, 35 mg.

B. Fast blue RR, 35 mg.

C. Propanediol, buffer solution (0.05 M), 35 ml.

1. Propanediol stock solution (0.2 M), 25 ml.:

2 amino 2 methyl 1, 3 propanediol, 10.5 g.

Distilled water, 500 ml.

(Mix and store in refrigerator)

2. 0.1N HCl, 5 ml.

3. Distilled water is added to make a volume of 100 ml. (Store in refrigerator)

D. Filter and use at once.

(5) The smears are washed in running water for 10 seconds. (6) They are then counterstained with Mayer's hematoxylin for 3 to 4 minutes. This solution consists of two parts. Solution A is made from 1.0 g. of hematin and 50 ml. of 90 per cent ethyl alcohol; it is incubated 24 hours at 37° C. Solution B is made from 50 g. of potassium alum sulfate and enough distilled water to make 1 liter. Solutions A and B are mixed and placed in sunlight for 3 to 4 weeks. (7) The smears are washed in running water for 10 seconds and air dried. (8) They are mounted in immersion oil and examined under microscope. (9) The slides are read in the following manner: The metamyelocytes and the polymorphonuclear forms are the only cells that become pale brown to deep

black. They are graded on intensity and the appearance of the precipitated dye in the cytoplasmic granules: 0 = no stain; 1+ = diffuse, pale brown cytoplasm with no granules; 2+ = brown cytoplasm with or without occasional clumps of brownish black precipitate; 3+ = brownish black, unevenly distributed granular precipitate; 4+ = uniform deep black granular precipitate. The scoring is done as in the Gomori method (p. 524). The leukocyte alkaline phosphatase (LAP) score increases as the total leukocyte count increases in nonleukemic patients (infections, polycythemia vera, and myelofibrosis). In normal adults and children, approximately 75 per cent of all neutrophils and metamyelocytes remain unstained, and the remaining 25 per cent show mild activity. In leukocytosis due to infection, more than 50 per cent of neutrophils and metamyelocytes show marked phosphatase activity.

Clinical Applications

Abnormally low alkaline phosphatase indices are found in chronic granulocytic leukemia, cirrhosis of the liver, congestive heart failure with passive congestion of the liver, diabetes mellitus, and gout. Because the biochemical abnormality shared by these diseases is a high serum level of vitamin B_{12}, there is the possibility that there might be a connection between blood levels of vitamin B_{12} and leukocyte alkaline phosphatase activity.[8] Another possibility is that the leukocyte alkaline phosphatase index is controlled by a gene in chromosome 21, for leukocyte alkaline phosphatase activity is abnormally high in children with mongolism and abnormally low in patients with chronic myelogeneous leukemia, both diseases characterized by an aberration of chromosome 22 (Philadelphia chromosome).[10] Also leukocyte alkaline phosphatase levels often are elevated later in chronic granulocytic leukemia, particularly in connection with infection, remissions due to treatment, or changes in the nature of leukemia. Abnormally high leukocyte

alkaline phosphatase values are seen in leukemoid reactions, polycythemia rubra vera (normal in other types of polycythemia), infections, and other leukemias.

PERIODIC ACID/SALICYLOYL HYDRAZIDE (PA–SH) STAIN

The periodic acid-Schiff stain is generally accepted as the fluorescent method of choice for demonstrating glycogen in blood cells. Because glycogen is a common constituent of certain normal and abnormal blood cells, and because its presence in some primitive cells has been used as a diagnostic aid in the differentiation of leukemias, the periodic acid/salicyloyl hydrazide staining method was tried to see if it could be used for demonstrating glycogen in peripheral blood and bone marrow cells. After much testing, it was found that the PA–SH stain could be used to replace existing Schiff fluorescent methods and would probably prove to be a useful technique in the diagnosis of blood conditions such as acute leukemia in which PAS positivity occurs.

MISCELLANEOUS STAINS USED IN HEMATOLOGY

Periodic Acid-Schiff Reaction for Carbohydrates (PAS)

0.5 Per Cent Periodic Acid and Schiff's Leuco-Fuchsin. Basic Fuchsin, 1 g., should be dissolved by boiling in 200 cc. of distilled water. Cool to 50° C. Filter. Add 1 Normal HCl (20 cc.; HCl concentration: Sp. Gr.− 1.19, 83.5 cc.; distilled water, 916.5 cc.). Cool. Add anhydrous sodium bisulfite, 1.0 g. Store in dark 24 to 48 hrs. (straw-colored). Add activated charcoal, approximately 0.3 g. Shake for 1 minute.

Filter (discard first drops). Reagent should be colorless. When pink tint appears, discard. Store in refrigerator.

For Celestine blue (Celestine Blue B or R) Stain use Celestine blue, 1 g.; concentrated sulphuric acid, 0.5 ml.; 2.5 per cent fresh aqueous alum, containing 14 ml. of glycerol, 100 ml.

The solution is prepared by titrating 1 g. celestine blue with 0.5 ml. concentrated sulphuric acid until effervescence ceases, then adding, with constant stirring, 100 ml. of 2.5 per cent fresh aqueous ferric alum, containing 14 ml. of glycerol at 50° C. The resulting dye dispersal is cooled to room temperature and filtered. The staining time will have to be tested with each batch. It may vary from 2 to 15 minutes. If a background color is noticed, differentiation in 1 per cent acid-alcohol will be necessary. If there is no background staining, a 1 to 3 minutes wash in tap water will be necessary. This stain is stable and will last 4 to 6 weeks with use.

Mayer's Hematoxylin. In 500 ml. distilled water, dissolve with heating (do not boil) aluminum ammonium sulfate, 50.0 g. In 500 ml. distilled water, dissolve chloral hydrate, 50.0 g.; citric acid, 1.0 g.; sodium iodate, 0.2 g. In 10 ml absolute alcohol, dissolve 1.0 g. of hematoxylin.

Mix the above three solutions. Ripening is not necessary. It will last 2 to 3 months.

PAS Stain

(1) Fix in 10 per cent formal-methanol for 10 to 15 minutes; (2) Running tap water for 15 minutes; (3) 1 per cent periodic acid (or 0.5% periodic acid) for 20 minutes; (4) Distilled water 3 to 4 times; (5) Schiff's reagent for 20 minutes; (6) Running tap water for 15 minutes; (7) Counterstain in Mayer's hematoxylin for 10 to 15 minutes or Celestine Blue* 3 minutes; (8) Rinse in very dilute NH_4OH (3-5 drops NH_4OH in 50 ml. H_2O); (9) Tap water for 20 minutes;

(10) Air dry or dehydrate, and mount in permount.

Results. Material containing carbohydrates stains red. That is, glycogen is a common constituent of certain normal and abnormal blood cells, and because its presence in some primitive cells has been used as a diagnostic aid in the differentiation of leukemias, the PAS stain is used to demonstrate glycogen in peripheral blood and bone marrow cells. In the stain technique, one may reincubate the PAS stained smear with 0.5 per cent diastase for 20 to 30 minutes in a 37° incubator. Rinse in running tap water for 10 minutes and rinse with distilled water. Proceed with Step 3 and restain. If the previously stained red material (glycogen) is now negative, this is corroborative proof of the presence of glycogen. Acetate may also be used instead of diastase. In acute lymphoblastic leukemia with a clear background (polys have a hazy background), the cytochemistry must be interpreted in the light of all information available. In erythroleukemia (DiGuglielmo's syndrome), PAS stains pronormoblasts with vacuoles in the cytoplasm, staining as chunky red lakes and granules with clear background; normoblasts are granular and with a hazy background. In Waldenstrom's macroglobulinemia, in which IgM is secreted, one observes intranuclear (pale pink) and occasionally intracytoplasmic granules; therefore, with the PAS stain (hexose) red granules are observed in the plasmacytoid lymphocytes. In Alpha chain disease (heavy chain of IgA dark red material), one sees plasma-like cells stuffed with brilliant red material (e.g., lymphoma of small intestines).

Naphthol AS-D Chloroacetate Esterase Stain for Granulocytes and Mast Cells (N.C.A.)[12]

Technique. For smears and imprints, fix in cold buffered formalin—acetone solution for 30 seconds, wash in distilled water and air dry. (1) Incubate smears in freshly mixed substrate solution at room tempera-

---

* Step 8 may be omitted when Celestine Blue is used, or the following abbreviated stain procedure may be used, (1) periodic acid for 5 minutes; (2) Distilled water (drain off excess, wipe back of slide dry); (3) Schiff's stain for 15 minutes; (4) running tap water for 10 minutes; (5) Celestine Blue for 3 minutes; (6) Tap water for 5 minutes; (7) Dehydrate, clear, and mount.

ture for 10 to 30 minutes, until pink or rose color is obtained. (Use control slide to monitor staining.) The substrate solution consists of Phosphate buffer, M/15, *p*H 7.4, 38 ml; Freshly hexazotized new fuchsin, 0.2 ml.; Naphthol AS-D chloroacetate solution, 2.0 ml. (2) Wash with distilled water 2 to 3 times. (3) Counterstain with Mayer's hematoxylin 4 to 5 minutes. (4) 'Blue' in running tap water for 20 minutes. (5) Air dry, dip in xylene, and mount in permount.

Reagents. For buffered formalin-acetone fixative, dissolve 20 mg. Na$_2$HPO$_4$ and 100 mg. KH$_2$ PO$_4$ in 45 ml. acetone and 30 ml. water and 25 ml. of 40 per cent formalin. Mix well and store in refrigerator. The final *p*H is about 6.6.

For fresh 4 per cent sodium nitrite solution, dissolve 1 g. NaNO$_2$ in 25 ml. distilled water.

For new fuchsin solution, dissolve 1 g. new fuchsin in 25 ml. of hot (not boiling) 2 N HCl. Filter when cool. Hexazotize with an equal amount of 4 per cent sodium nitrite solution just before use.

For naphthol AS-D chloroacetate solution, dissolve 10 mg. of naphthol AS-D chloroacetate in 5 ml. of N,N-dimethyl formamide. Store tightly stoppered in freezer until used.

For M/15 phosphate buffer *p*H 7.4, dissolve 7.572 g. Na$_2$HPO$_4$ and 1.814 g. KH$_2$ PO$_4$ in 1000 ml. distilled water. Adjust to *p*H 7.4 with either 1N HCl or 1N NaOH.

Results. Enzyme activity is seen as bright red granules in the cytoplasm of mast cells, neutrophilic granulocytes, including promyelocytes and many myeloblasts. Chloroacetate esterase is inhibited by many chemicals. Poor or false-negative results may occur if slides are overheated while drying. All solutions are stable in the refrigerator for 1 month, except the sodium nitrite, which is stable for 1 week at 4° C.

Supplies. New Fuchsin (C.I. 42520) is available from Allied Chemical Co., Inc., P.O. Box 431, Morristown, New Jersey 07960. Naphthol AS-D chloroacetate is available from Sigma Chemical Co., 3500 DeKalb Street, St. Louis, Missouri 63118. N,N-Dimethyl Formamide is available from Fisher Scientific Co., Fairlawn, New Jersey 07410.

Methyl Green-Pyronin Stain for RNA and Plasma Cells

Solutions. Methyl Green-Pyronin Reagent (MGP) is Pyronine Y, 0.25 g.; Methyl green, 0.75 g.; and Phosphate buffer, *p*H 5.3, 100.0 cc.

To this add 0.5 per cent phenol soln, 0.5 cc. and 1.0 per cent resorcinol (fresh) 2.5 cc.

MGP reagent is relatively stable. It requires 2 to 3 days to ripen, and will last 3 to 6 months at room temperatures. It can be reused if it is kept refrigerated when not in use.

Phosphate Buffer Mixture is M/5 disodium phosphate (Na$_2$HPO$_4$), 52.5 cc. and M/10 citric acid, 47.5 cc. (Both the above made up in 25% methyl alcohol to prevent mold growth.) If these proportions do not produce a *p*H of 5.3, it must be adjusted to *p*H 5.3.

Use control slide.

Technique. (1) Fix in 10 per cent formalin methanol for 10 minutes. (2) Wash in distilled water twice. (3) Air dry 10 to 15 minutes. (4) MGP for 5 minutes. (5) Wash in distilled water twice. (6) Wash in Acetone 2 times. (7) Dip in 50/50 acetone/xylene. (8) Dip in Xylene. (9) Mount in permount.

Results. For cytoplasmic and nucleolar RNA, red plasma cell cytoplasm will stain red, which is especially striking in cases of multiple myeloma. In this stain, methyl green stains the DNA in the nucleus while pyronin stains the RNA of the cytoplasm and nucleolus a red color; the cytoplasm is involved in protein synthesis and production of antibodies. In lymph node sections and imprints, the MGP may be used to differentiate reactive processes from Hodgkin's disease, which possesses large eosinophilic, usually bilobed, nucleoli. The immunoblasts of infectious mononucleosis also possess similar reddish nucleoli-like granules. However, mononuclear Reed-Sternberg cells of Hodgkin's disease are only weakly positive with the MGP stain, whereas the immunoblast of infectious mononucleosis is strongly positive. This stain may also be used routinely and is an excellent contrast for Gram's stain (i.e., intracellular bacteria are red and the nuclei of cells are blue to reddish-purple). It also is used to demonstrate red Döhle inclusion bodies in the blood. Because it colors lymphocyte cytoplasm and basophilic granules bright red, it may be used as a differential stain for these cells. It is also satisfactory for the study of red blood cells, especially in polychromatophilia.

Giemsa Stain

Giemsa stain is prepared in the following manner:

a. Azure I plus methylene blue makes Azure II, 0.8 g.; Azure II plus equal parts of eosin makes Azure II-eosin, 3 g. Or, use Giemsa powder, 3.8 g.

b. Glycerine, 200 ml.

c. Methyl alcohol (absolute), 300 ml.

Dissolve Azure II-eosin mixture (3.8 g.) or Giemsa powder (3.8 g.) in glycerine (200 ml.) by holding at 55° C to 60° C for 1½ to 2 hours. Then add the absolute methyl alcohol (300 ml.). This makes the stock staining solution. Before using, dilute 1 ml. of stock staining solution with 10 ml. of distilled water.

Technique. Thin blood smears are made, air dried, and fixed in methyl alcohol for 3 minutes. To this is added 1:10 diluted Giemsa stain; it is allowed to stand for 15 to 30 minutes (20 min. average). The slide is kept on its edge to prevent the precipitate from settling on the slide. The slide is washed off with distilled water, dried, and examined.

Giemsa stain is good for staining large numbers of slides simultaneously. Also it is valuable in hot climates because evaporation is retarded by the glycerin. It is useful in laking and the staining of thick films and in the diagnosis of parasitic diseases (malaria). Giemsa stain is not as good as Wright's stain for routine blood smears because the staining time is longer, preliminary fixation is required, and neutrophilic granular detail is not as good. The combination of the Wright and May-Grünwald stains is useful in bringing out nuclear and cytoplasmic detail and for permanent stained smears.

Pappenheim Methyl Green Pyronine Stain

Pappenheim methyl green stain is made from 1 g. of methyl green (50% dye concentration), 0.25 g. of pyronine, 5 ml. of ethyl alcohol (95%), 20 ml. of glycerine, and 100 ml. of phenol (2% aqueous). This stain is good for routine use; is an excellent contrast for Gram's stain (intracellular bacteria are red and the nuclei of cells are blue to reddish purple. It is also used to demonstrate red Döhle inclusion bodies in the blood. Because it colors lymphocyte cytoplasm and basophilic granules bright red, it is used as a differential stain for these cells. It is also satisfactory for the study of red blood cells, especially in polychromatophilia.

Thin blood smears are made, air dried, or heat fixed, and cold stain is allowed to stand on the smears for ½ to 5 minutes.

Jenner Stain

This stain is also called May-Grünwald or Pappenheim panoptic stain. It is made by dissolving 0.5 g. of eosinate of methylene blue (in tablet or powder) in 100 ml. of acetone-free, neutral absolute methyl alcohol. It also may be purchased in solution form. The unfixed blood film is covered with the staining solution; after 3 to 5 minutes, the film is rinsed with water, dried in air, and mounted. This stain is good for differential counting; however, it stains nuclei poorly and is not as good as the Wright or Giemsa stain in the detection of malarial parasites because it does not produce Romanowsky staining.

Prussian Blue Reaction

In this method, which is especially useful in detecting siderocytes, a thin blood film is prepared and air dried. It is fixed for 5 to 10 minutes in absolute methyl alcohol, dried, and immersed for 10 minutes in a fresh mixture of equal parts of 2 per cent aqueous KCN solution and N/5 HCl (1.7 ml. of concentrated HCl with enough distilled water to make 100 ml.). The blood film is rinsed in distilled water and then counterstained 1 to 2 minutes with a 0.1 per cent aqueous eosin or safranin solution. The film is then rinsed and dried.

Iron-containing granules (small and blue) are seen in red blood cells (called siderocytes) in certain refractory, postsplenectomy, and other unusual anemias. A minimal quantity of siderotic granules are normally present in bone marrow normoblasts, possibly representing iron not immediately bound into heme. These granules are not found in the normoblasts of iron deficiency anemia patients. This is of major interest in the differential diagnosis of hematologic disorders. Prussian blue may be used as a counterstain with Wright's stain to detect stainable iron in the erythroid cell series in marrow material. Another technique involves aspirating 3 ml. of an EDTA solution (1 mg./ml.) into a 20 cc. Tomac plastic syringe together with 3 ml. of mixed blood and marrow; the entire mixture is placed on a large watchglass. Particles of marrow are identified, teased out, and smeared on coverglasses. Unstained, the hemosiderin appears as minute golden-yellow refractile granules. The smear is fixed in methyl alcohol, stained with concentrated Prussian blue solution (4 g. of potassium ferrocyanide in 20 ml. of iron-free distilled water. Concentrated HCl is added until a white precipitate forms. The solution is filtered, and the filtrate is used) for 30 minutes and counterstained 1 to 2 minutes with a 0.1 per cent aqueous eosin or safranin solution.

Iron granules appear blue; the protein granules of hemosiderin, containing absorbed bilirubin but not iron, stain pale yellow. Normal marrow usually has a few small bluish granules diffusely dispersed throughout the smear, and a reduced number of bluish granules is seen in iron deficiency (reduced iron storage). An increased number of bluish granules is seen in the marrow films of patients with large amounts of iron storage — for example, in infection, cirrhosis, hemochromatosis (Plates 89, 91), pernicious anemia, malignant neoplasia, uremia, hemolytic anemia, and refractory sideroblastic anemia.

REFERENCES

1. Burns, J., and Neame, P. B.: Staining of blood cells with periodic acid/salicyloyl hydrazide (PA–SH). A fluorescent method for demonstrating glycogen. Blood, *28*:674, 1966.
2. Federal Register 39, No. 20. pp. 3756–3797. Jan. 29, 1974.
3. Graham, R. C., Jr., Lundholm, U., and Karnovsky, M. J.: Cytochemical demonstration of peroxidase activity with 3-amino-9-ethylcarbazole. J. Histochem. Cytochem., *13*:150, 1965.
4. Hayhoe, F. G. J., and Cawley, J. C.: Acute leukemia: cellular morphology, cytochemistry and fine structure. Clin. Hematol., *1*:49, 1972.
5. Kaplow, L.: Simplified myeloperioxidase stain using benzidine dihydrochloride. Blood, *26*:215, 1965.
6. Katayama, I., Li, C. Y., and Yam, L. T.: Histochemical study of acid phosphatase isoenzyme in leukemic reticuloendotheliosis. Cancer, *29*:157, 1972.
7. Li, C. Y., et al.: Acid phosphatase isozyme in human leukocytes in normal and pathologic conditions. J. Histochem. Cytochem., *18*:473, 1970.
8. Martinez-Maldonado, M., Menendez-Corrada, R., and DeSala, A. -R.: Diagnostic value of alkaline phosphatase in leukocytes. Am. J. Med. Sci., *248*:175, 1964.
9. Mover, S., Li, C. Y., and Yam, L. T.: Semiquantitative evaluation of tartrate resistant acid phosphatase activity in human blood cells. J. Lab. Clin. Med., *80*:711, 1972.
10. Robinson, J. C., Pierce, J. C., and Goldstein, D. P.: Leukocyte alkaline phosphatase electrophoretic variants associated with chronic myelogenous leukemia. Science, *150*:58, 1965.
11. Schaefer, H. E., and Fischer, R.: Peroxidase detection in smear preparations and tissue sections after decalcification and paraffin embedding. Klin. Wochenschr., *46*:1228, 1968.

11A. Sheehan, H. J.: An improved method of staining leucocyte granules with Sudan Black B. J. Pathol., *59:*336, 1947.

12. Yam, L. T., Li, C. Y., and Crosby, W. H.: Cytochemical identification of monocytes and granulocytes. Am. J. Clin. Pathol., *55:*283, 1971.

13. Yam, L. T., Li, C. Y., and Lam, K. W.: Acid phosphatase isoenzyme in human leukocytes in normal and pathologic conditions. J. Histochem. Cytochem., *13:*473, 1970.

14. ———: Tartrate-resistant acid phosphatase isoenzyme in the reticulum cells of leukemic reticuloendotheliosis. N. Engl. J. Med., *284:*357, 1971.

15 L.E. Phenomenon, Continuation of Bone Marrow Study, and Electrophoresis

L.E. PHENOMENON

L.E. cell is a mature neutrophilic or eosinophilic leukocyte that has phagocytosed or surrounded a large purplish hyaline, homogeneous mass. The nucleus of the neutrophil is tightly adjacent to the peripheral portion of the inclusion body. The inclusion body varies from 7 μ to 21 to 28 μ and is round or oval, granular, smoky or pale lavender, homogeneous in appearance, and without a visible chromatin network. The L.E. structures take a purplish to reddish brown stain and are not as prominent as the host nucleus. Also found in the positive smear is the L.E. phenomenon, which includes the formation of clumps or rosettes — central homogeneous masses surrounded by neutrophilic leukocytes and easily seen under low power (Plates 42, 89).

It is believed that the production of L.E. cells and phenomenon depends on an immunocellular reaction occurring in the lupus erythematosus disease complex, which requires that at least three factors be brought together in vitro and that adequate time elapse for the reaction. The three factors are: (1) the nucleolytic agent, or L.E. factor(s) that dwells antigenically distinct in the serum gamma globulin fraction, (2) a source of nuclear protein to react with the lytic factor (that is, cell nuclei, usually from neutrophils or lymphocytes, with which the L.E. factor reacts), and (3) viable phagocytic neutrophilic leukocytes, which engulf the lysed nuclear material.

Rotation of the slightly heparinized (too much will inhibit the test) blood in glass beads, or maceration of the blood clot through a fine sieve, produces the trauma necessary to obtain nuclear protein (extruded nuclei). The material is then incubated to permit phagocytosis of any lysed nuclear protein; the serum L.E. factor then attaches itself to extruded nuclei and causes lysis of the nuclear chromatin with subsequent phagocytosis of the nuclear chromatin by viable neutrophils.

The tart cell represents phagocytosis of unlysed or partially lysed nuclear protein. Nucleophagocytosis is seen frequently and can be differentiated from the L.E. phenomenon; the tart cell has a phagocytosed, frequently eosinophilic nucleus with an almost intact nuclear pattern, is frequently vacuolated, and has conspicuous, condensed chromatin, especially around its circumference.

There are four common techniques for making L.E. preparations. In order of decreasing sensitivity, they are: rotating glass beads (most sensitive), wire trauma of microhematocrit, the collection in heparinized vacutainer, and the mashed clot technique. The mashed clot method destroys cellular morphology. The heparinized Vacutainer tube contains too much heparin, which inhibits the formation of L.E. cells. The Davidsohn microhematocrit method is satisfactory, but it is not as sensitive or reproducible as the rotating glass bead method. The glass bead system, with controlled amounts of heparin, gives a superior smear requiring only a few minutes of scanning to give a positive or negative answer.[6-8]

Rotary Method Technique

(1) Add 10 glass beads (2–3 mm.) and 5 drops of ammonium heparinate; a No. 25 needle is held horizontally to a 10 ml. test tube fitted with a tight clear stopper (1% ammonium heparinate*). (2) Add 10 ml. of freshly drawn blood to the tube and mix. A disposable syringe is used to draw the blood. (3) Incubate at room temperature for 30 minutes. (4) Rotate for 30 minutes in a rotator with tubes in vertical position. (5) Incubate at room temperature for 30 minutes. (6) Centrifuge for 5 minutes in a clinical centrifuge. (7) Remove the plasma. (8) Transfer the buffy layer (with a few RBCS) to a Wintrobe hematocrit tube and centrifuge in a clinical centrifuge for 5 minutes. (9) Remove the buffy layer and prepare smears. (10) Stain with Wright's stain. (11) Screen two slides under the high dry objective.

Many physicians are in the habit of ordering three times the amount of L.E. preparations they need, and these are usually done three times in a row, a habit developed when methods with poor sensitivity were widely used. This is probably a waste of time because if a sufficiently sensitive L.E. method is used, daily repeats are not indicated. It is far wiser to repeat every month or every few months if there is continued clinical suspicion of lupus erythematosus. With the rotating glass bead method, positive L.E. preparations are usually loaded with L.E. cells, and many free nuclear bodies are seen.

Interpretations and Limitations of Positive L.E. Tests

A positive report should not be made when only one L.E. cell is seen; one must observe several absolutely typical L.E. cells because in positive smears many L.E.

cells and rosettes are usually observed. When there is severe leukopenia, the test may be falsely negative owing to an absence or decrease in phagocytic cells in the presence of the plasma factor. In these cases it is suggested that 5 ml. of patient's serum be incubated with 5 ml. of washed cells obtained from a normal subject.

A positive test is usually diagnostic of disseminated lupus erythematosus; however, one may occasionally observe L.E. cells or phenomenon in patients with periarteritis nodosa, dermatomyositis, scleroderma, drug hypersensitivity, rheumatoid arthritis, hepatitis, and the hydralazine syndrome. In the hydralazine syndrome, no Blacks were involved in a recent report of 14 of 32 patients on hydralazine therapy. In addition, there was no significant difference in the total dose of hydralazine or in the duration of exposure for the groups with and without antinuclear antibodies as demonstrated by immunofluorescence.[5] A negative L.E. test does not rule out disseminated lupus erythematosus because the blood from some patients with obviously active lupus erythematosus does not show L.E. cells. Also approximately 50 per cent of lupus erythematosus patients with positive L.E. cell tests show negative L.E. test results 2 or more months after adrenocorticosteroid treatment.

BONE MARROW EXAMINATION

For a review of bone marrow techniques of aspiration, the medical technologist's role in assisting the pathologist, and bone marrow differential with general considerations for good films and staining, see the description in Chapter 1, including the discussion of the Jamshidi technique of aspiration and biopsy, which provides improved specimens from the iliac crest (pp. 11–16).

Tabulating the Bone Marrow Differentials

First, the marrow film is examined under low power. In this way the cellularity of the

---

* Produced by Scientific Products Co., No. B2950.

specimen is noted, the number of mega-karyocytes is estimated and the qualitative presence of neoplastic cells, lipid histiocytic cells, and atypical megakaryocytes may be picked out because they may be few and located only in focal areas — for example, in the thick part and edge of marrow film. Further study under oil immersion may follow. For quantitative differential estimation, an area should be picked out in which the cells almost touch one another, an area that is not too thick or too thin. The erythrocyte precursors, including the number and maturity, are surveyed, and megaloblastic or normoblastic erythropoiesis is noted. The myeloid series is then reviewed as to total number and increase in myeloblasts, promyelocytes, macropolycytes, and giant metamyelocytes. The number and maturity of megakaryocytes and the qualitative evidence of platelet function are noted. Reticulum cells, histiocytes, plasma cells, and other cells are studied for number and immaturity, and also for cytoplasmic inclusions. An estimate is also made of the number of lymphocytes. The presence of any tumor cells or abnormal, unidentifiable cells is also noted. A total number of 200 to 400 cells is counted, and the results for each cell type are counted as a percentage of total cells counted. Although a normal bone marrow differential is tabulated in Chapter 1, the simpler norm shown in Table 15-1 is quite satisfactory and practical.

The myeloid-erythroid (M:E) ratio is obtained by dividing the number of myeloid cells (myeloblasts, promyelocytes, myelocytes, metamyelocytes, and polymorphonuclear neutrophils) recorded by the total number of erythroid cells (pronormoblasts and normoblasts) recorded. If only myeloid-erythroid ratio results are wanted, one may group all myeloid cells into one group and the erythroid cells into another. The non-myeloid cells and the specific stage of erythroid and myeloid maturation of cells may be ignored. Normal values observed in bone marrow films are given in Table 15-1.

Table 15-1. Myelogram*

	Patient in	
Cell Type	Mean Percentage	Range Percentage
Myeloblasts	2.0	0.3– 5.0
Promyelocytes	5.0	1.0– 8.0
Myelocytes		
Neutrophilic	12.0	5.0–19.0
Eosinophilic	1.5	0.5– 3.0
Basophilic	0.3	0.0– 0.5
Metamyelocytes	22.0	13.0–32.0
Polymorphonuclears		
Neutrophilic	20.0	7.0–30.0
Eosinophilic	2.0	0.5– 4.0
Basophilic	0.2	0.0– 0.7
Lymphocytes	10.0	3.0–17.0
Plasma cells	0.4	0.0– 2.0
Monocytes	2.0	0.5– 5.0
Reticulum cells	0.2	0.1– 2.0
Mitotic cells	0.0	0.0– 2.0
Megakaryocytes	0.4	0.0– 3.0
Pronormoblasts	4.0	1.0– 8.0
Normoblasts	18.0	7.0–32.0
Megaloblasts	0.0	0.0– 0.0
Myeloid: Erythroid ratio (WBC: Nucleated RBC ratio)	3:1	2:1–5:1

* Cartwright, G. E.: Diagnostic Hematology, ed. 3. New York, Grune & Stratton, 1963; and Burtner, O. W.: Bone marrow examination in clinical medicine: a study of 500 cases. J. Florida M.A., *41*:726, 1955.

Other Uses of Bone Marrow Study

Maturation Curves. Occasionally, one may plot a maturation curve for the myeloid or erythroid series of cells by adding up the total number of cells counted in the series and calculating the percentage of each cell type within the series. The percentages are then plotted.

Volumetric Data. Place 1 cc. of the bone marrow sample into a paraffin-lined vial containing a small amount of heparin or sodium EDTA. Mix gently but well. Make marrow films (pp. 17–18). Then pipette 1 cc. of the anticoagulated marrow sample into a Wintrobe hematocrit tube, and centrifuge for 8 minutes at 2500 r.p.m. Note the percentage of the various layers (reading down): fat layer, mixed layer, plasma layer, M:E layer, and mature erythrocyte layer. Normally the fat layer is 1 to 3 per cent of the total volume and the M:E layer is 5 to 8 per cent. Plasma and erythrocyte volumes vary because in this technique and in instances of less centrifugation, the erythrocyte volume is usually more than the hematocrit. Furthermore, because of the frequent admixture of sinusoidal blood and bone marrow, the proportions of the different fractions may be markedly altered. Because of this, these volumetric marrow determinations may not correlate with the morphologic appearance of fixed bone marrow sections, and, therefore, in individual cases the variation in the number of nucleated cells is too great to serve as a reliable diagnostic aid.

Megakaryocyte Counts. Because of the tendency for megakaryocytes to accumulate in the thick end or edge of the smear, one should survey these areas under low magnification. At best, quantitative estimation of the exact number of megakaryocytes is not accurate; one can only say that they are apparently increased, normal, or apparently decreased. After study of 25 to 50 megakaryocytes, one can assess qualitative variations—evidence of immaturity, cytoplasmic granulation, vacuolization or hyalinazation of cytoplasm, and the absence of peripheral fragmentation or platelet production.

Histologic Structures. One may section the aspirated particles, the M:E layer of the centrifuged specimen, or the fragments obtained by surgical biopsy.[11] Although this method is not as good as the smear method for study of cytologic details, it does give a much better picture of the overall marrow pattern. Conditions in which a marrow biopsy is nearly mandatory for a histologic diagnosis include aplastic anemia, granulomatous disease of the marrow (including sarcoidosis, miliary tuberculosis, and fungal diseases), myelophthisic anemias (whether due to myelofibrosis or to primary or metastatic malignant disease), malignant lymphoma (including Hodgkin's disease), and thrombotic thrombocytopenic purpura. Biopsies may also be of value in diseases with increased marrow cellularity, a condition often difficult to assess on aspirated smears. The biopsy technique also offers a way to follow the effect of chemotherapeutic agents on the bone marrow, both in clinical and research areas (Plates 89, 91).[2]

Fat: Cell Ratios. Low fat values and high M:E values without peripheral leukocytosis suggest marrow hyperplasia; high fat values and low M:E values suggest marrow hypoplasia. If the M:E layer is less than 2 per cent and fat is absent, the marrow material is probably mainly sinusoidal blood.

Comparative Study of Combined Bone Marrow Films and Sections.[1] A routine aspiration, using an 18-gauge (University of Illinois) bone marrow needle or the Powsner type,[15] is performed at the site the operator prefers—the sternum, iliac crest, or the vertebral bodies proper. The Powsner B-D needle consists of a 13-gauge stock trocar and stylet, modified as in Figure 15-1. The needle can be drilled into the ilium with only moderate hand pressure; penetration of dense bone is best accomplished with clockwise rotation. The laterally directed holes seldom become plugged with bone. The tip of the needle must be properly sharpened at all times (Fig. 15-2). Because normal bone marrow is an admixture of loosely fixed cells and free cells, within as well as outside of vascular channels, sampling by aspiration of 0.5 to 1.0 ml. of marrow involves tearing the fixed marrow tissue loose from its moorings. Once this separation has been effected, large vascular channels are opened, and the material becomes increasingly diluted with blood as more marrow material is removed. Therefore, as soon as 0.5 ml. of marrow material is obtained, the syringe is removed from the aspirating needle, which is temporarily left in place, and the syringe contents are quickly expelled onto a clean glass slide. From this pool of liquid material, successive spreads

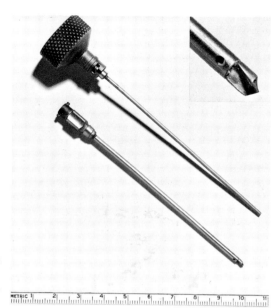

Fig. 15-1. Powsner's trocar-type B.M. needle with laterally directed holes. (Powsner, E. R.: Letter to Editor. Am. J. Clin. Pathol., *43*:85, 1964)

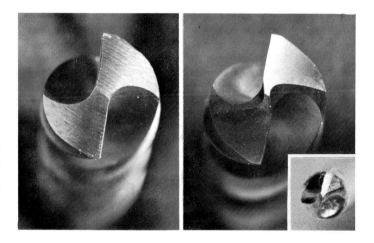

Fig. 15-2. Tips of Powsner's B.M. needles with clockwise rotary effect. Drilling accomplished with only moderate hand pressure. (Powsner, E. R.: Letter to Editor. Am. J. Clin. Pathol., *43*:85, 1964)

are prepared by touching clean edges of slides or coverslips to the marrow specimens and transferring the material to another clean slide or coverslip. Spreading is then carried out in the same way it is done in preparing slide or coverslip films of peripheral blood.

This preparation of 8 to 12 slides and coverslips is done rapidly before the marrow pool has had time to clot. The films are Wright-stained. The pool of bone marrow material is then allowed to clot. The stylus of the aspirating needle is stirred in the clot, and the clot particles are brought together. As a result of this maneuver, the clot contains practically all the marrow units, leaving behind a pool of blood that is almost devoid of marrow units, that is, a concentration technique. The clot is then transferred to 10 per cent formalin or Zenker-acetic acid fixative solution. From here on, the specimen is treated in a manner similar to that used routinely for surgical biopsy tissues.[1]

IMMUNOELECTROPHORETIC TECHNIQUE AND USE IN HEMATOLOGIC DIAGNOSES

In order to make a more accurate and rapid diagnosis of blood dyscrasias associated with protein disorders—for example, multiple myeloma, Waldenström's macroglobulinemia, hypergammaglobulinemia, hypogammaglobulinemia, and agammaglobulinemia—new techniques facilitating the separation of serum proteins have been developed. The techniques have rapidly improved, starting with moving-boundary electrophoresis, paper electrophoresis, ultracentrifugation, and more recently, immunoelectrophoresis (Plate 89).

In the technique, electrophoretic separation of serum fractions is first performed. Subsequently, antiserum—for example, antihuman serum antiserum—is applied parallel to the separated serum fractions. Both the serum fractions and the antiserum diffuse toward each other, and at the point of contact an antigen-antibody reaction takes place with the formation of visible, individual precipitin lines. In the original technique of Graber and Williams, an agar-covered large glass plate was used for electrophoresis, thus enabling the antigens (serum proteins) to separate out according to their different electrophoretic mobility.[9]

Basically, the electrophoretic pattern of serum proteins on agar gel is similar to that obtained by paper electrophoresis. After the completion of the process, the antigen (the individual separated serum protein fractions) then diffuse radially outward. A trough parallel to the separated protein fractions is cut and an antibody solution (antiserum containing antibodies against the separated individual serum proteins) is applied. This is allowed to diffuse laterally and inward toward the antigens. After several hours to several days, each antigen can be identified by its reaction with the specific antibody resulting in the formation of specific curved precipitin lines (Figs. 13-11, 13-12; Plate 89). A new modified micro-

method of immunoelectrophoresis has been devised utilizing ordinary microscope slides.[10]

REFERENCES

1. Agress, H.: Comparative study of spreads and sections of bone marrow. Am. J. Clin. Pathol., *27*:282, 1957.
2. Burney, S. W.: Bone marrow examination. J.A.M.A., *195*:859, 1966.
3. Burtner, O. W.: Bone marrow examination in clinical medicine: a study of 500 cases. J. Florida M.A., *41*:726, 1955.
4. Cartwright, G. E.: Diagnostic Hematology. ed 3. p. 237. New York, Grune & Stratton, 1963.
5. Condemi, J. J., Moore-Jones, D., Vaughan, J. H., and Perry, H. M.: Antinuclear antibodies following hydralazine toxicity. N. Engl. J. Med., *276*:486, 1967.
6. Dubois, E. L., Drexler, E., and Arterberry, J. D.: A latex nucleoprotein test for the diagnosis of systemic lupus erythematosus. J.A.M.A., *177*:141, 1961.
7. Dubois, E. L., and Freeman, V.: A comparative evaluation of the sensitivity of the L. E. cell test performed simultaneously by different methods. Blood, *12*:657, 1957.
8. Gambino, S. R.: L.E. cell tests. Summary report. Council on Clinical Chemistry (A.S.C.P.). III (No. 18, issue 42). pp. 1, 2. Jan., 1966.
9. Graber, P., and Williams, C. A., Jr.: Méthode permettant l'étude conjugée des propriétés electrophoretiques et immunochimiques d'un mélange de proteines. Application au sérum sanguin. Biochim. Biophys. Acta, *10*:193, 1953.
10. Lawrence, M.: The techniques of immunoelectrophoresis. Am. J. Med. Techn., *30*:209, 1964.
11. Martin, R. S.: An aid to bone marrow biopsy. N. Engl. J. Med., *272*:1172, 1965.
12. Powsner, E. R.: Letter to the editor (an improved needle for aspiration of marrow from dense bone). Am. J. Clin. Pathol., *36*:598, 1966; Am. J. Clin. Pathol., *43*:85, 1964.

AUDIOVISUAL AIDS*

Bone Marrow Interpretation in the Leukemias. [videocassette program]. American Society of Clinical Pathologists, P.O. Box 12073, Chicago, Illinois 12073.

Bone Marrow Interpretation in Selected Anemias. [videocassette program]. American Society of Clinical Pathologists, P.O. Box 12073, Chicago, Illinois 12073.

Immunodiagnostic Tests for Autoimmune Diseases. CDC-76-01. Joseph Cavallero, Ph.D. [14 (35 mm.) transparencies plus handout, 20 pp., and standard

---

* Films unless otherwise stated.

audiocassette, $34.80]. Communications in Learning, Inc., 2929 Main Street, Buffalo, New York 14214.

Introduction to Bone Marrow Morphology. Set B5. HSLRC T252 (SB-56). [35 mm. transparencies, manual, audiotape] A.S.H. National Slide Bank, University of Washington, Seattle, Washington 98195.

L.E. Formation. (1962). FACSEA, 927 Fifth Avenue, New York, New York 10021.

Method for Rapid Electrophoresis. M-1015. (1966). National Medical Audiovisual Center (Annex), Station K, Atlanta, Georgia 30324.

Normal and Abnormal Marrow Elements. Set B2. HSLRC T252 (SB-56). [35 mm. transparencies, manual] A.S.H. National Slide Bank, University of Washington, Seattle, Washington 98195.

Systemic Lupus Erythematosus. Geigy Pharmaceuticals, Division of Geigy Chemical Corporation, Ardsley, New York 10502.

16

Electron Microscopy of Blood Cells and Chromosome Abnormalities in Hematologic Disorders

ELECTRON MICROSCOPY OF BLOOD CELLS

Because detailed study of diseases of the hematopoietic and reticuloendothelial systems must include an analysis of the fine normal structure of cells and tissues, electron microscopy, producing magnifications up to 100,000, has been used to demonstrate new details of the internal structure and molecular arrangement of erythrocytic, leukocytic, and thrombocytic cells. Reconstruction of the hematopoietic cell components, or organelles, is fraught with many technical obstacles because of the normal thickness of blood cells; objects cannot be examined under the electron microscope if they are thicker than about 0.2 μ. Thus, in electron microscopy, resolution is best extended to about 80.2 angstroms.

Another difficulty in electron microscopy is that the techniques used in cytologic examination require special fixation and preparation of the cell for ultimate study under an elevated vacuum. Therefore, interpretation of the final hematopoietic image is somewhat difficult. However, when the final preparation shows good resolution, the structure of nucleoproteins and large molecules can be perceived. Furthermore, electron microscopy and allied techniques have enabled visualization of numerous cellular components whose existence was not even suspected when cellular structure was studied by the light microscope with its limita-

tions (Figs. 16-1 and 16-2). A current list of cellular organelles and structures, which have now been described in great detail, would include the following: plasma membrane and its modifications, such as cilia, microvilli, and desmosomes; pinocytic vesicles; endoplasmic reticulum and ergastoplasm; glycogen; microtubules; lipids; myelin figures; pigments; inclusions such as ferritin; fibrils (extracellular, contractile, and others); and nuclei.[19]

Braunsteiner and Pakesch,[10] closely followed by Low and Freeman,[33] were among the first to describe the inner details of the hematopoietic tissues by the electron microscopic technique. Many other investigators have since described the individual blood constitutents and have clarified their respective organelle systems, functions, and in some cases, alterations in fine structure associated with specific diseases.[6, 19, 21] They have demonstrated that hematopoietic cells—erythrocytes, leukocytes, platelets, and most of their precursors—possess organelles also observed in other body cells, such as mitochondria, lysosomes, endoplasmic reticulum, and the Golgi apparatus. However, there is still a void in descriptive specific identification for the multipotential stem cells of bone marrow.

Various electron micrographs with photomicrographic inserts are provided herein for comparative microscopic detail and study (Figs. 16-3 to 16-16). Although no

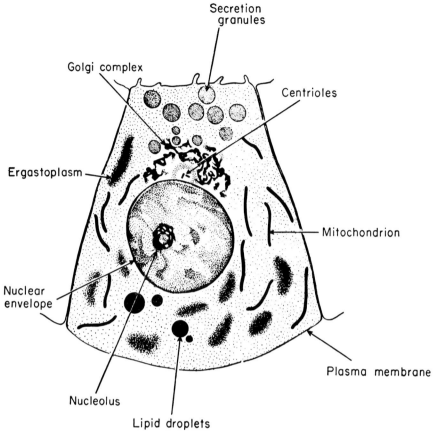

Secretion granules

Golgi complex

Centrioles

Ergastoplasm

Mitochondrion

Nuclear envelope

Nucleolus

Lipid droplets

Plasma membrane

Fig. 16-1. The cell: old version. Components of the cell, in light microscope view, are few and relatively simple. (Medical World News, Feb. 2, 1962)

detailed examples of erythrocytic ultramicroscopic structures appear in this series of electron microscopic patterns, much information is available concerning the normal erythrocyte surface, the erythrocyte ghosts and their stromater, and the erythrocytic surface changes associated with agglutination. In erythrocytes, ribosomes, without associated unit membranes, synthesize hemoglobin for use within the cell. In diseases characterized by defective hemoglobin synthesis, such as thalassemia, iron may accumulate in mitochondria of pronormoblasts.[20] The Golgi complex is entirely lacking in mature erythrocytes. Crater-like pits are observed on the erythrocyte surface when the imprint

method is used. These pits vary in size and quantity in different erythrocytes, and they possibly represent immune specific group loci, where antigen-antibody reactions occur. During hemolysis, there is an increase in the quantity of these surface craters (Fig. 8-8).[50] In addition, traumatized erythrocytes occasionally possess filamented processes called "myelin forms," which are seen under the electron microscope as prominent threadlike connections between agglutinated erythrocytes.

On the other hand, leukopoietic cells have some of the following characteristics:[6] (1) *Neutrophils* show a scalloped cell surface, and a three- to four-lobed nucleus, having many cytoplasmic granules, rodlike

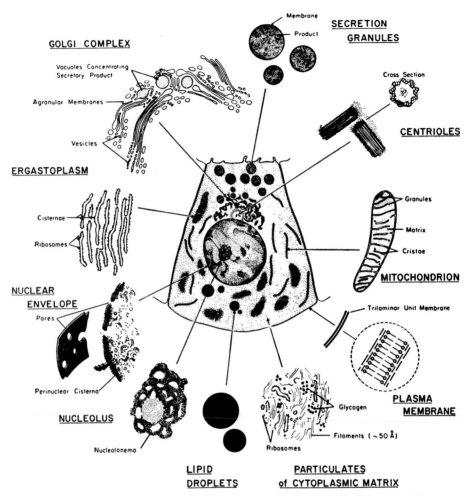

Fig. 16-2. The cell: new perspective. The complex structure of its living, working parts is revealed by the electron microscope. (Medical World News, Feb. 2, 1962)

mitochondria with cristae, endoplasmic reticulum represented as light granules with a denser periphery, vesicular larger pale areas, and a matrix of finely granular cytoplasmic protein with other small granules of varying density and strands connecting lobes of the double-walled nuclear membrane. The endoplasmic reticulum also synthesizes hydrolytic enzymes (lysosomes), which remain in the cell as membrane-bound granules. (2) *Eosinophils* contain a nucleus and many cytoplasmic granules with dense multiple inclusions of varying form. The mitochondria and other structures resemble those seen in the neutrophil.

(3) *Lymphocytes* possess a large nucleus with few large prominent mitochondria containing distinct cristae. The Golgi complex is small or poorly developed. The cytoplasm is frequently reduced in amount and usually has very few granules other than the mitochondria. The nuclear wall is a double membrane as in the neutrophils. (4) *Monocytes* have a nucleus-cytoplasm ratio lower than that in lymphocytes, and a distinct Golgi apparatus may be observed in the hof of the double-membraned nucleus. The size of the Golgi apparatus diminishes with decreasing functional capacity.

(*Text continues on p. 545.*)

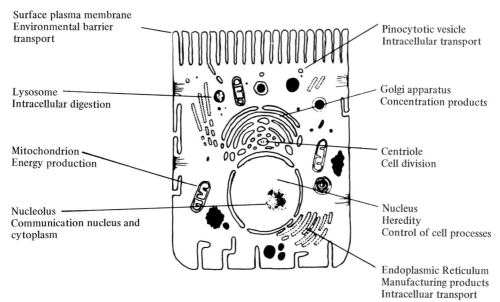

Surface plasma membrane
Environmental barrier
transport

Pinocytotic vesicle
Intracellular transport

Lysosome
Intracellular digestion

Golgi apparatus
Concentration products

Mitochondrion
Energy production

Centriole
Cell division

Nucleolus
Communication nucleus and
cytoplasm

Nucleus
Heredity
Control of cell processes

Endoplasmic Reticulum
Manufacturing products
Intracelluar transport

Fig. 16-3. Modern concept of epithelial cell pattern relating morphologic structure and function.

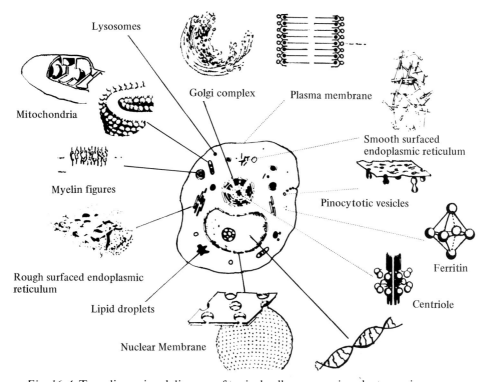

Lysosomes

Golgi complex

Plasma membrane

Mitochondria

Smooth surfaced
endoplasmic reticulum

Myelin figures

Pinocytotic vesicles

Ferritin

Rough surfaced endoplasmic
reticulum

Centriole

Lipid droplets

Nuclear Membrane

Fig. 16-4. Two-dimensional diagram of typical cell as seen using electron microscopy.

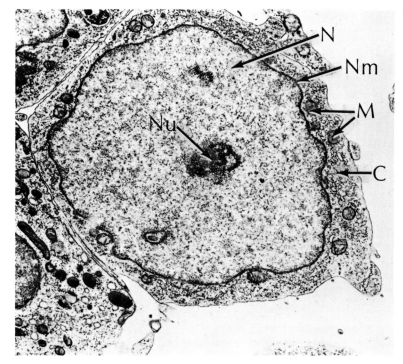

Fig. 16-5. Blast cell. Nu = nucleolus; M = mitochondria; N = nucleus; Nm = nuclear membrane; C = cytoplasm.

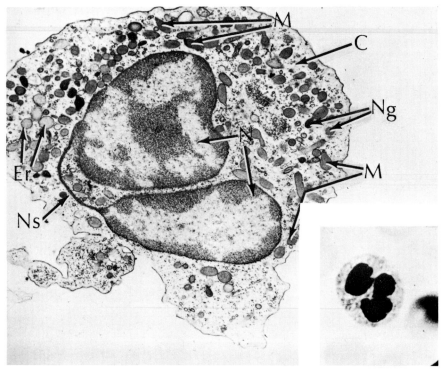

Fig. 16-6. Neutrophil (inset shows light-microscopy outline of neutrophil). N = nucleus; Ns = nuclear strand; Ng = nuclear granules; Er = endoplasmic reticulum; M = mitochondria; C = cytoplasm.

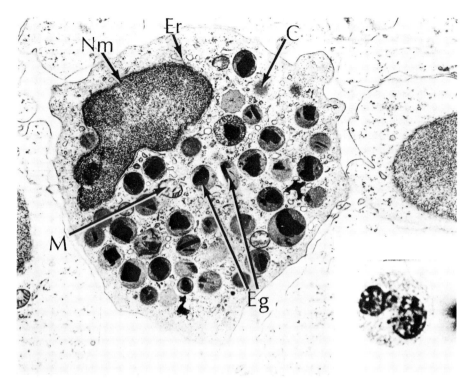

Fig. 16-7. Eosinophil (inset shows light-microscopy outline of eosinophil), Eg = eosinophilic granules; Er = endoplasmic reticulum; M = mitochondria; C = cytoplasm; Nm = nuclear membrane.

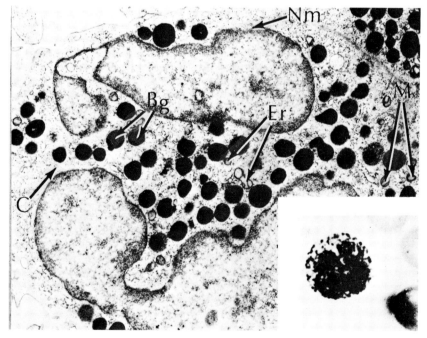

Fig. 16-8. Basophil (inset shows light-microscopy outline of basophil). Bg = basophilic granules; Er = endoplasmic reticulum; M = mitochondria; Nm = nuclear membrane; C = cytoplasm.

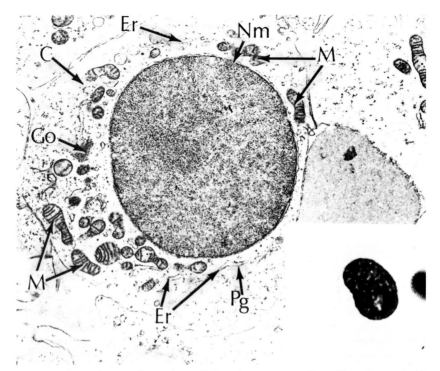

Fig. 16-9. Lymphocyte (inset shows light-microscopy outline of lymphocyte). M = mitochondria; Er = endoplasmic reticulum; C = cytoplasm; Nm = nuclear membrane; Go = Golgi zone; Pg = Palade granules.

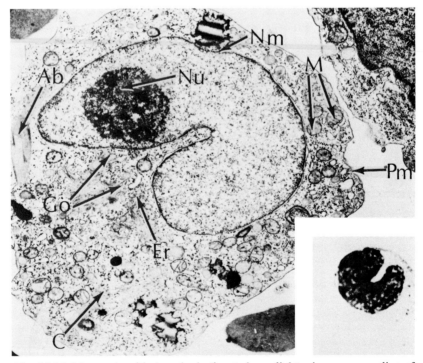

Fig. 16-10. Monocyte with Auer body (inset shows light-microscopy outline of monocyte with Auer body). Nu = nucleolus; M = mitochondria; Er = endoplasmic reticulum; Go = Golgi zone (indistinct); C = cytoplasm; Nm = nuclear membrane; Pm = plasma membrane; Ab = Auer body.

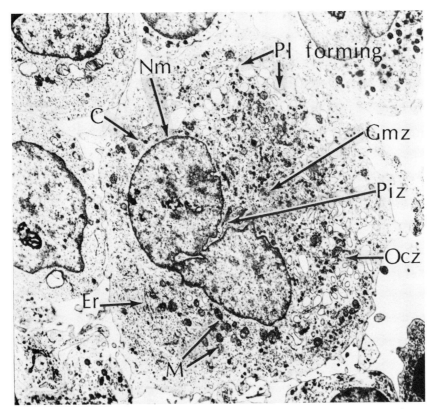

Fig. 16-11. Megakaryocyte. C = cytoplasm; Nm = nuclear membrane; Piz = perinuclear inner zone; Gmz = granular middle zone; Ocz = outer cytoplasmic zone; Er = endoplasmic reticulum; M = mitochondria; Pl = platelet forming from coalescence, demarcation and dislodging of cytoplasm.

(5) *Platelets* frequently occur in groups and show fairly uniform dense granules. A few vesicles and spicules are also present. Electron microscopy of thrombocytes is excellent and reproducible because they tend spontaneously to flatten out on foreign surfaces. Normally (without contact and in the circulation) the platelet is round or oval without processes, with an inner granulomere, and with a clear outer hyalomere. As soon as contact is made with a foreign surface, numerous pseudopods form, and the granulomere condenses into a central nucleus-like structure. During early blood coagulation, the hyalomere begins to disintegrate; later during blood coagulation, the granulomere forms a retraction point in the fibrin network. During blood clotting, beginning with platelet exposure to thrombin, the following changes take place: the platelet changes from a round circulating form to a spread-out form with pseudopods, disintegration begins at the periphery, fibrillary processes form, the hyalomere disappears eventually leaving an amorphous mass representing the original granulomere. With the release of the granulomere components (platelet factors), thrombus formation occurs. (6) *Megakaryocytes* contain a large lobulated nucleus surrounded by cytoplasm divided into three distinct zones: a perinuclear inner zone, a middle zone consisting of numerous granules and a well developed membranous system, and a thin outer cy-

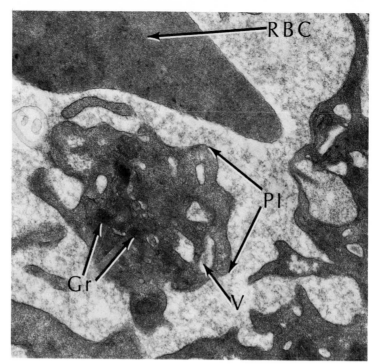

Fig. 16-12. Platelets and portion of normal erythrocyte (upper left). RBC = erythrocyte with uniform texture and little evidence of cell membrane; Pl = platelet; V = vesicle; Gr = granules.

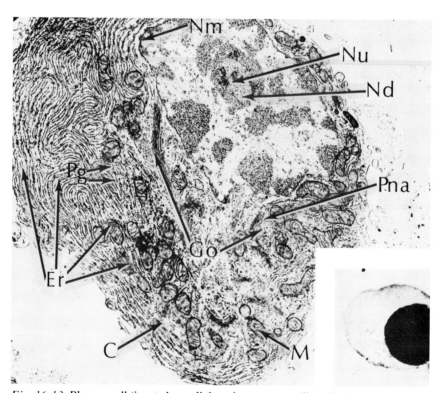

Fig. 16-13. Plasma cell (inset shows light-microscopy outline of plasma cell). Er = endoplasmic reticulum; Pg = Palade granules; M = mitochondria; Pna = paranuclear area (part of Go); Go = Golgi zone; C = cytoplasm; Nd = nucleoplasm; Nm = nuclear membrane; Nu = nucleolus.

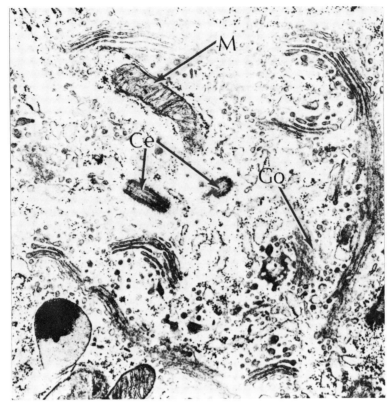

Fig. 16-14. Golgi apparatus and centrioles of plasma cell (prominent in plasma cells). M = mitochondrion; Ce = centriole; Go = Golgi zone.

toplasmic zone. Platelets normally are formed in the bone marrow by the partitioning of the membranous portion – that is, vesicles of smooth endoplasmic reticulum coalesce to demarcate and dislodge portions of cytoplasm to form platelets.[14]

Clinically, there are certain ultrastructural abnormalities noted in the various hematopoietic disorders. For example in sideroblastic anemia, ferritin accumulation is marked, both as an exaggeration of the normal cytoplasmic granules[5] and within mitochondria.[56] This morphologic collection is also present in thalassemia.[26] Heinz body anemia is an acquired hemolytic anemia characterized by large accumulations of altered hemoglobin within the erythrocytes,[56] the end result of interference with the protective mechanisms

that normally restrict irreversible hemoglobin oxidation. Deficiencies of vitamin B_{12}, folic acid, and pyridoxine are megaloblastic states characterized by asynchrony of maturation and nuclear pleomorphism visible in electron micrographs.[26]

In idiopathic thrombocytopenic purpura and thrombasthenia, qualitative changes in the platelet granulomere are frequently observed. Platelets in these disorders are less "sticky" than normal, remain round, unaltered, and insensitive to contact with a foreign surface. Also, normal platelets suspended in serum in thrombocytopenic purpura often do not spread out and disintegrate. However, currently, none of the alterations in the fine structure of platelets can be specifically considered pathognomonic of any disease.[38] The leukemias are

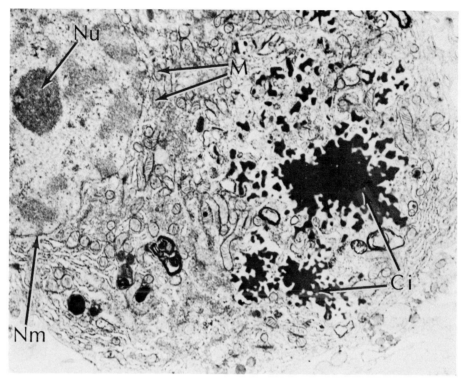

Fig. 16-15. Plasma cell in dysglobulinemia (cytoplasmic inclusions not seen in all dysglobulinemias). Nm = nuclear membrane; Nu = nucleolus; M = mitochondria; Ci = cytoplasm inclusions in cisternae.

not characterized by any specific electron microscopic morphologic differences; normal granulocytes and lymphocytes do not seem to differ from similar cells observed in chronic granulocytic and lymphocytic leukemias. The Philadelphia chromosome therefore is the only morphologic change unique to chronic granulocytic leukemia.[43] However, other chromosomal alterations are also found (pp. 567–569). Electron microscopic patterns, like those of the light microscopic type of acute leukemias, reveal nuclear pleomorphism (often atypical), nuclear and nucleolar hypertrophy, abnormal mitoses, and asynchrony of nuclear and cytoplasmic maturation.[6, 33] The lymphomas contain only one bizarre structure visualized by electron microscopy—the diagnostic Sternberg-Reed cell of Hodgkin's disease, with its bilobate nucleus and prominent multiple nucleoli.[4]

Burkitt's lymphoma reveals herpes-like virus particles in some of the suspension-cultured cells. These are visualized by electron microscopy, but no virus particles have ever been isolated.[44] The tumor cells are characterized by a prominent nucleolus, a ribosome-rich cytoplasm, and a scanty elongated endoplasmic reticulum with narrow cisternae. The herpes-like virus particles are intranuclear, have a single outer membrane, and measure about 90 $\mu\mu$. The cytoplasmic particle has a double membrane and measures $150 \times 32,500$ mμ.

In multiple myeloma, electron microscopy reveals many disturbances in organelle morphology—profile changes in the rough endoplasmic reticulum.[57] An addi-

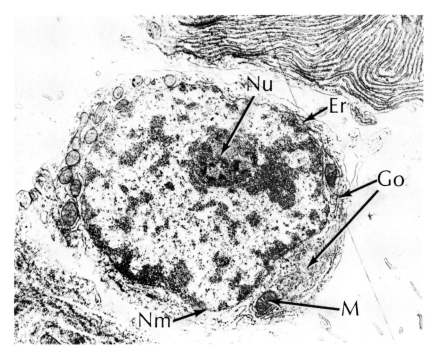

Fig. 16-16. Plasmablast (myeloma). Nm = nuclear membrane; M = mitochondrion; Nu = nucleolus; Er = endoplasmic reticulum; Go = Golgi zone.

tional finding is the accumulation of proteinaceous material within cisternae, as a single large cytoplasmic inclusion, or within the nucleus. Current investigators believe there may be some correlation between these protein accumulations and the dysproteinemias — as precursors of the myeloma globulin.[37] The lipoidoses, especially Niemann-Pick disease, are characterized by distinctive electron microscopic patterns of the metabolically-disturbed bone marrow lipid reticuloendothelial cell. A typical cell shows vacuoles filled with tubular, lamellar, or crystalline structures, microvilli present at the cell surface, and a fanlike structure of the lipid in the granules.[58]

(7) *Leukemic reticuloendotheliosis cell (LRE; hairy cell)* demonstrates numerous long microvilli and pseudopods, whereas the immediately fixed lymphocytes and monocytes in the same patient demonstrate fewer, shorter microvilli and no pseudopods. Nuclear pockets are rare in hairy cells but frequent in lymphocytes, and the inclusions of ribosome-lamella complexes are more prevalent in LRE cells. This differential is mentioned since it is less well appreciated that lymphocytes change their surface topology in vitro with the production of pseudopods and microvilli, and this may simulate LRE cells closely (Fig. 16-17).[25]

(8) *Sezary cell* is associated with a disease having features clinically and histologically quite similar to mycosis fungoides. It is characterized by typical serpentine and lobulated nuclear changes. Dense heterochromatin is irregularly distributed along the nuclear membrane and is clumped throughout the nucleus. The cytoplasm appears normal. In other views, the nucleus is cerebriform and composed of highly convoluted folds (Fig. 16-18).[34]

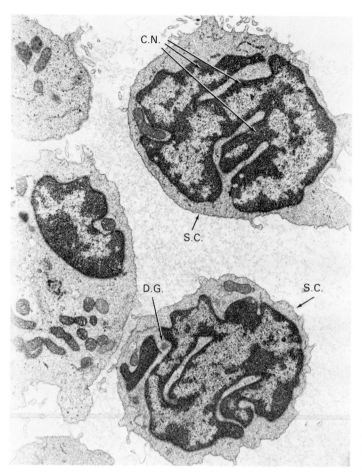

Fig. 16-17. Leukemic reticuloendotheliosis cell (hairy cell) from peripheral blood. S.C. = Sézary cell; D.G. = dense granules; C.N. = convoluted or cerebriform nucleus. (15 K ×) (Katayama, I., and Schneider, G.B.: Further ultrastructural characterization of hairy cells of leukemic reticuloendotheliosis. Am. J. Pathol., *86:*163, 1977)

SCANNING ELECTRON MICROSCOPY (SURFACE MORPHOLOGY) OF WHITE BLOOD CELLS IN NORMAL AND PATHOLOGIC STATES

Study of the structure of the leukocyte surface has just begun in recent years. It utilizes the scanning electron microscope (SEM). This instrument has a great depth of focus, provides a 3-dimensional view of cell surface topography, and permits examination of a large number of cells, which provides an overall view of the surface features of a population of cells. At the same time, it shows details of each individual cell surface at a good resolution of 200 Å. Surface morphology is well preserved when cells are prepared for SEM by the freeze-drying or critical-point drying techniques.[9, 46]

The critical-point drying technique allows cells to dry without the distorting effect of surface tension; it is superior to air drying, which produces distortion of the surface architecture and loss of microvilli. Variation in techniques of collection, concentration, fixation, and air-drying probably accounts for the loss of a certain number of microvilli, which at best are transient labile structures. Also, different modes of harvesting cells including differences in types of substrate used, varying intervals prior to fixation, plus different techniques in separation of cells, may explain the variable degrees of adhesions to the different substrates used. These lead to selective loss of

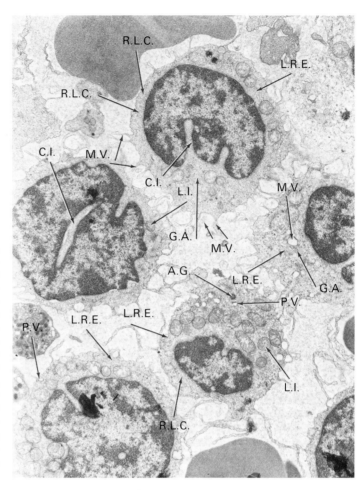

Fig. 16-18. Sézary cell. L.R.E. = leukemic reticuloendotheliosis cell or hairy cell; R.L.C. = ribosome-lamella complexes; L.I. = lysosomal inclusions; G.A. = golgi apparatus; P.V. = pinocytic vesicles; C.I. = cytoplasmic inclusions; A.G. = Azurophil granules; M.V. = microvilli. (10 K ×; Lutzner, M. A., Hobbs, J. W., and Horvath, P.: Ultrastructure of abnormal cells in Sézary syndrome, mycosis fungoides, and parapsoriasis en plaque. Arch. Dermatol., *103:*375, 1971)

cells. Finally, cell cycle, temperature changes, cell contact and interaction in vitro are thought to influence the morphology of the surface of the cell. The method of critical-point drying, described by Pollack and associates, harvests cells onto a silver membrane and is applicable to the study of blood samples and cell suspensions.[46] Furthermore, cells, particularly monocytes and granulocytes, collected onto this type of substrate rather than another, are more likely to retain their natural contours as a result of the spreading attachment to a glass surface.

Morphologic Surface Features of Normal Leukocytes

Granulocytes. The WBCs of the granulocyte series do not possess surface characteristics that would allow their differentiation into neutrophils, eosinophils, or basophils. However, the granular white cells as a group can be identified. They average 10 μ in diameter and possess a very irregular contour, which in many cases is elongated into definite cell protuberances and processes. In addition, the surface appearance is very finely irregular, small ridges separating adjacent troughs on the cells' surface membrane (i.e., convoluted surface structures with thickened ridge-like profiles and ruffled membranes, which sometimes attach to the filter substrate). The pattern of the nucleus is difficult to outline through the cell surface membrane (Fig. 16-19).

Granulocyte precursors can be distinguished from mature granulocytes, but the

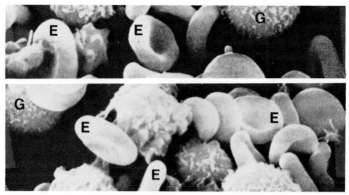

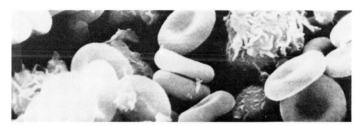

Fig. 16-19. Granulocyte (G) and erythrocyte (E). (Courtesy of Aaron Polliack, M.D., Associate Professor of Medicine, Department of Hematology, Hadassah University Hospital and Hebrew University Medical School, Jerusalem, Israel)

Fig. 16-20. Myelocyte in upper right-hand corner with nuclear bulge, indicating cell division, in cell beneath it. (Clarke, J. A., Salsbury, A. J., and Rowland, G. F.: Surface ultrastructure of human leukocytes. Br. J. Haematol., *14:*533, 1968)

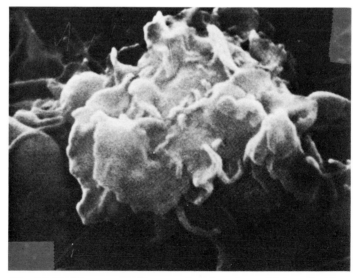

Fig. 16-21. Monocyte with convoluted surface, thickened ridge-like profile and ruffled membrane. Some are attached to the substrate. (Polliack, A., Lampen, N., Clarkson, B., and DeHarven, E.: Scanning electron microscopy of human leukocytes — A comparison of air-dried and critical point dried cells. Isr. J. Med. Sci., *10:*1075, 1974)

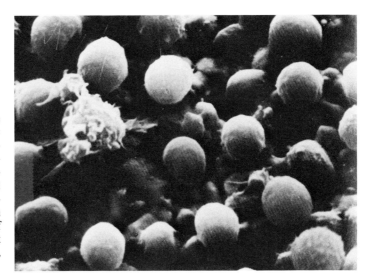

Fig. 16-22. Lymphocytes are spherical cells with relatively smooth contours, slight surface irregularity, and few microvilli. (Polliack, A., Lampen, N., Clarkson, B., and DeHarven, E.: Scanning electron microscopy of human leukocytes— A comparison of air-dried and critical point dried cells. Isr. J. Med., Sci., *10:*1075, 1974)

distinction between such cells as promyelocytes and myelocytes cannot be ascertained. Several characteristic features can be observed, however; for example, in contrast to mature granulocytes, the outline of the nucleus inside the cell is visible on many occasions. Also, the margin of the cell displays numerous small processes of varying length, and there appears to be a transition of surface membrane characteristics that range from a surface that is relatively "smooth," and featureless to one on which there are numerous irregularities similar to the surface characteristics of peripheral granular WBCs. The cells are larger (15–20μ) than the mature granulocyte. No difference between granulocyte precursors in normal marrow and in marrow from cases of chronic myelogenous leukemia can be observed (Fig. 16-20).

Monocytes. The outline of the monocyte is very irregular; it appears more flattened and in close proximity to RBCs or other WBCs. It seems to be engulfing these cells since definite cytoplasmic processes from the monocytes can be observed partly encircling them. The surface is convoluted with thickened ridge-like profiles and ruffled membranes, some of which are attached to the substrate (Fig. 16-21).

Lymphocytes. Most circulating lymphocytes are spherical (4.0–5.0 μm. in diameter) and have a relatively smooth contour with slight surface irregularity and few microvilli. About 20 per cent of normal lymphocytes are generally larger (5.1–6.4 μ in diameter) and have a more complex villous pattern with much of the exposed surface covered by microvilli of varying lengths (Fig. 16-22).

Lymphocytes from a few patients with chronic lymphocytic leukemia are spherical in shape. Many of these cells have moderate to markedly villous surfaces, and most of them, previously identified as B-cells by immunologic methods, have a surface architecture similar to that of normal circulating B-lymphocytes (Fig. 16-23).

Lin, Cooper, and Wortis examined thymus-derived (T) cells and thymus-independent (B) cells by virtue of the ability of T-cells to form rosettes with sheep red cells and for some B-cells to form rosettes with complement-coated human RBCs.[32] The rosettes were glutaraldehyde-fixed and subsequently examined by scanning electron microscopy. Lymphocytes, both rosetting and nonrosetting, had multiple, surface microvilli compared to rosetting B-cells; rosetting T-cells were generally smaller and smoother with fewer, shorter microvilli. Microvilli appeared to be the sole cell-cell contact point between T-cells and sheep RBCs; B-cells made contact through both

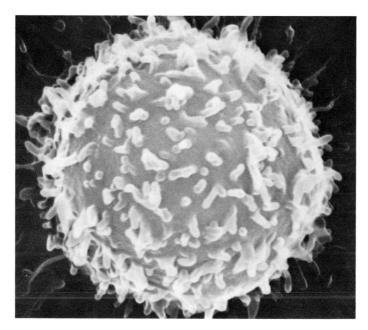

Fig. 16-23. Chronic lymphocytic leukemia patient has B-lymphocyte with marked villous surface. (Polliack, A., Lampen, N., Clarkson, B., and DeHarven, E.: Scanning electron microscopy of human leukocytes—A comparison of air-dried and critical point dried cells. Isr. J. Med. Sci., *10:*1075, 1974)

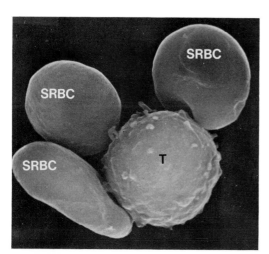

Fig. 16-24. Sheep red blood cell (SRBC) rosetting lymphocyte (T-cell) with smooth surface and a few stud-like microvilli that make contact with the edges of the SRBC. (× 8000; Lin, P. S., Cooper, A. G., and Wortes, H. H.: Scanning electron microscopy of human T-cell and B-cell rosettes. N. Engl. J. Med., *289:*548, 1973)

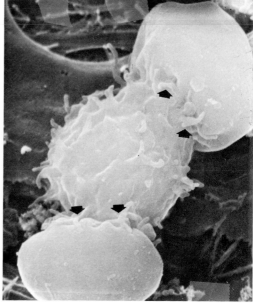

Fig. 16-25. B-cell with surface undulations. The microvilli appear mainly at the areas of contact with the C3 HRBC. The microvilli appear to be deeply invaginating the red-cell surface. (× 10,000; Lin, P. S., Cooper, A. G., and Wortes, H. H.: Scanning electron microscopy of human T-cell and B-cell rosettes. N. Engl. J. Med., *289:*548, 1973)

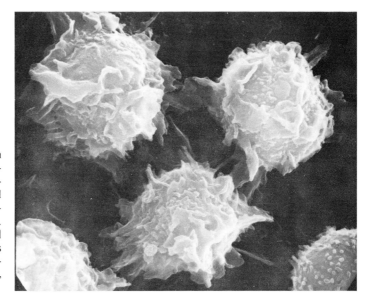

Fig. 16-26. Hairy cell with numerous cytoplasmic projections, short stubble-like microvilli, long microvilli, and ruffled membranes. (Katayama, I., and Schneider, G. B.: Further ultrastructural characterization of hairy cells of leukemic reticuloendotheliosis. Am. J. Pathol., *86:*163, 1977)

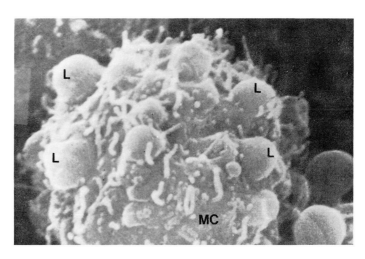

Fig. 16-27. Myeloma cell (MC) and lymphocyte (L). (Polliack, A., Lampen, N., Clarkson, B., and DeHarven, E.: Scanning electron microscopy of human leukocytes—A comparison of air-dried and critical point dried cells. Isr. J. Med. Sci., *10:*1075, 1974)

villous and nonvillous areas (Figs. 16-24; 16-25).

Hairy cells or leukemic reticuloendotheliosis cells measure 5 to 8 μm. in diameter with a range of 5.0 to 6.8 μ. They demonstrate numerous cytoplasmic projections: short, stubble-like microvilli, long microvilli; and ruffled membranes. The stublike microvilli are similar in size and shape to those seen in normal and chronic lymphocytic leukemic lymphocytes. The long microvilli measure 1.0 to 1.8 μ in length, and the ruffled membranes 1.5 to 3.5 μ at their base and 1.0 to 2.5 μ in length (Fig. 16-26).[25]

Myeloma cells characteristically display multiple surface blebs. These blebs do not appear to be a function of the cell. Similar surface features are also encountered on malignant plasma cells obtained from patients with plasma cell leukemia (Fig. 16-27).

CHROMOSOME ABNORMALITIES IN HEMATOLOGIC DISORDERS

The use of antibiotics and tissue culture techniques has made it possible to investigate intrinsic cell structure. Every cell has chromosomes and genes at some point during its development, but the chromosomes

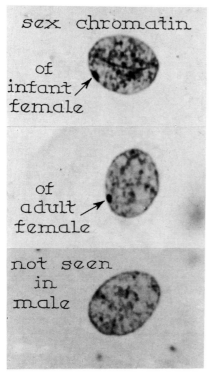

sex chromatin

of
infant
female

of
adult
female

not seen
in
male

Fig. 16-28. Photomicrographs of epithelial cells from the oral mucosa stained with cresyl-echt violet (× 2,000). The upper two nuclei have Barr bodies, which are indicated by arrows. (Moore, K. L., and Barr, M. L.: Lancet, 2:57, 1955)

are distinguishable only during cell division. An exception to this rule may be the Barr sex chromatin body (Fig. 16-28),[2] which is thought to represent part of one of the X chromosomes.[35, 53] Chromosomes are defined as the microscopic structures that organize from the nucleus of a cell when the cell is dividing. A chromosome is made up of a tightly coiled molecule of deoxyribonucleic acid (DNA). DNA is composed of a phosphate-sugar backbone bridged together by four base pairs (two purines and two pyrimidines). The purine guanine is always linked to the pyrimidine cytosine, and the purine adenine is always linked to the pyrimidine thymine.

The arrangement of molecules making DNA, by their very physicochemical nature, forms a double helix much like a tightly coiled spring (Fig. 16-29). A gene is

thought to be a region of this coil containing many thousands of these base pairs arranged in specific sequence for the different genes. Millions of such areas, and therefore millions of genes, are the mechanisms responsible for the supply of information needed to produce the ultimate growth and characteristic development of an individual in a species. The sequence of base pairs that help to make up the DNA molecule is known as the genetic code. When the genetic code is quantitatively or qualitatively violated, an abnormality develops, and a hereditary genetic defect results. Many defects are caused by DNA changes that cannot be satisfactorily demonstrated. Some defects, however, produce microscopically observable changes in the chromosomes.

The visual microscopic study of chromosomes has been carried on in plants and animals for years. It was first determined that different species have different num-

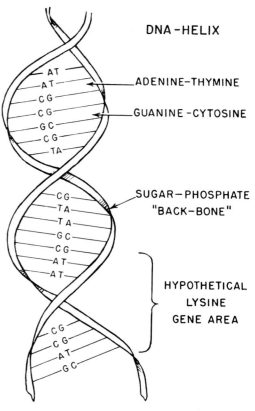

DNA-HELIX

ADENINE–THYMINE

GUANINE–CYTOSINE

SUGAR–PHOSPHATE "BACK-BONE"

HYPOTHETICAL LYSINE GENE AREA

Fig. 16-29. Deoxyribonucleic acid helix.

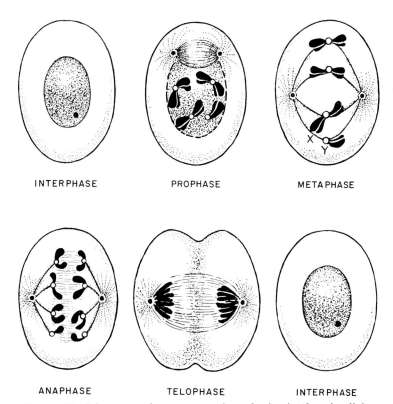

INTERPHASE   PROPHASE   METAPHASE

ANAPHASE   TELOPHASE   INTERPHASE

Fig. 16-30. Diagrammatic representation of mitosis (for simplicity, four chromosomes are used here). During interphase the major metabolic functions of the cell take place, and the nuclear chromatin is diffuse. In prophase the chromatin begins to condense and form chromosomes, and the centriole divides to form the spindle fibers and poles. By metaphase, the nuclear membrane has disappeared, and the chromosomes are lined up singly on the equatorial plate. During anaphase the chromosomes split and half migrate to each pole. The cell wall begins to divide during telophase. Two daughter cells are formed (only one is illustrated), and each begins interphase. (Adapted from Hampton, C. L.: Understanding chromosome analysis. Am. J. Med. Technol., *30:*321, 1964).

bers of chromosomes and that this number is species-specific. In 1956, Tijo devised a practical and relatively simple method that allowed a detailed visual study of the number and morphologic appearance of human chromosomes.[62] Until this method was developed, the human chromosome number was thought to be 48. Tijo's technique and its revision by other workers confirmed the presence of 46 chromosomes in the cells of normal humans.[12, 18] At that time, most workers believed that abnormalities that were obvious enough to be evident in chromosomes would be lethal. Lejeune and co-

workers however, demonstrated the non-lethal chromosomal abnormality present in mongolism.[30] Eggen in a lucid summary subsequently reviewed and discussed other chromosomal aberrations.[16]

Chromosomal demonstration and observation depend on the process of cell division. It is only during the metaphase stage of cell division that chromosomes can be seen as bodies distinct enough to be analyzed. Study of the diagrammatic representation of mitosis helps one understand chromosomal analysis (Fig. 16-30). Actively dividing cells are not seen frequently enough in most normal body tissues; therefore tissue culture techniques are utilized to furnish metaphase stages in sufficient numbers to be valuable for study. Leukocytes from peripheral blood, bone marrow, and skin may be readily grown in tissue culture. Usually, peripheral blood is drawn into heparin and the leukocyte-rich plasma is incubated in tissue culture media for 3 days and allowed to grow. When the cells reach an actively dividing phase, colchicine or a related drug is added to the culture and incubated 6 more hours. These drugs stop the formation of spindle fibers or, expressed differently, arrest cell division in the metaphase stage. The cells are washed and then placed in hypotonic saline solution, which causes them to swell and allows the chromosomes to spread. The cells are then fixed in an alcohol mixture, smeared on slides, and stained. These metaphase slides or plates are then ready for study.

Culture of Leukocytes

1. Draw 10 to 15 ml. of blood in a sterile syringe, and add it to a sterile, screw-cap, 15 ml. centrifuge tube containing 1.0 ml. of heparin (Liquaemin, 1000 units/ml.). Do not use heparin with phenol. Invert the tube several times to mix the blood with the heparin. Allow the blood to settle (30–60 min.).

2. Using a sterile pipette, transfer the plasma supernate to the sterile tube. Perform a standard leukocyte count on an aliquot of this supernate.

3. Prepare the culture bottles. In some laboratories, the small, flat-sided bottles that can be incubated in a horizontal position are used. The total culture volume should be 10 ml. The desired cell concentration is 2,000,000 per ml. (20,000,000/bottle). This cell concentration can usually be obtained in a volume of 1 to 3 ml. of plasma. Because a serum protein concentration of 15 to 30 per cent (20% optimal) is preferred in some laboratories, calf serum is added to maintain this range if the cell count is very high. For example, if the cell count is 20,000, 1 ml. of plasma, 8 ml. of medium, and 1 ml. of calf serum would be used to total 10 ml.

For a medium, mixture 199* in 400 ml. bottles may be used with sodium bicarbonate. To each fresh bottle of medium add 180,000 units of penicillin G (45,000 units/100 ml.) and 0.2 g. of streptomycin (0.05 g./ml.).

4. As a final step in the preparation of the culture bottles, add 0.3 ml. of Phytohemagglutinin P stock working solution, cap the bottles, and incubate at 37° C for 68 to 72 hours. Phytohemagglutinin P and its buffer powder may be ordered.† The buffer powder can be dissolved in 1 liter of sterile distilled water and stored at 4° C indefinitely. To one bottle of phytohemagglutinin P add 5 ml. of phytohemagglutinin buffer. This concentrated solution should be stored frozen. To make stock working solution, add 1 ml. of the concentrate to 9 ml. of phytohemagglutinin buffer. This stock solution may be stored at 4° C for up to 2 weeks.

Neoplastic cells (e.g., leukemic leukocytes) grow in vitro without stimulation and divide earlier. The peak of cell division occurs at 24 to 48 hours of cell culture. This point is important in the study of patients with hematologic disorders. For example, if a 72-hour phytohemagglutinin- (PHA) stimulated culture of peripheral blood is requested from a patient with chronic granulocytic leukemia, it is apt to be negative for the Philadelphia chromosome since the cells examined are normal lymphocytes that do not contain the abnormality. If an unstimulated culture is harvested at 24 or 48 hours, cells with the Philadelphia chromosome will be obtained. Likewise, in studying lymph node material in patients with malignant lymphoma, PHA-stimulated cultures are apt to be normal, while unstimulated short-term or direct preparations may show distinctive abnormalities.

---

* Sold by Microbiological Associates, Bethesda, Maryland.
† From Difco Laboratories.

5. At the end of the incubation period, add Colcemide* to each culture bottle. The stock solution of this contains 2 mg. per 100 ml. of solution. This may be stored indefinitely at 4° C. Use 0.10 ml. (2.0 μg.) of Colcemide solution for each 10 ml. in the culture bottle (0.5 micromolar). The culture with the Colcemide should be incubated at 37° C for 3 to 4 hours.

A disadvantage of the culture method is that the conditions in vitro may selectively favor growth of one cell line and lead to an erroneous impression of the prevalence of certain cell types. In addition, cell culture may induce chromosome abnormalities under some conditions.

Harvest of Leukocytes

In all of the subsequent steps, sterile technique is not required.

6. After incubating the Colcemide and culture bottle, remove the bottles from the incubator, and transfer the contents to screw-cap centrifuge tubes. Use a disposable capillary pipette with gentle agitation to assist in removing all the culture material from the glass. Centrifuge for 10 minutes at 900 r.p.m.

7. Remove the supernate by aspiration. To each tube add 10 ml. of warm Hank's solution. Resuspend the cells, and then centrifuge for 10 minutes at 900 r.p.m.

8. Remove the supernate by aspiration. To each tube add 10 ml. of warm (37° C) sodium citrate solution (1.1%). Immediately resuspend the cells and incubate in a 37° C water bath for 13 minutes, followed by 7 minutes of centrifuging at 900 r.p.m. so that the total cell exposure to citrate solution does not exceed 20 minutes.

9. Pour the supernate off carefully; the cell pellet is very soft at this point. Invert the tubes carefully, and drain off the excess moisture. Wipe out the tube with a small roll of paper to remove as much moisture as possible without disturbing the cells.

10. To each tube add 10 ml. of ice-cold fixative. Without resuspending the cells in

the pellet, cap the tubes and refrigerate for 30 minutes. The fixative is made from 3 parts of absolute ethanol to 1 part of glacial acetic acid. This should be made fresh for each harvest and kept in the refrigerator.

11. After fixation, resuspend the cells in the pellet, and centrifuge at 900 r.p.m. for 10 minutes.

12. Pour off the supernate, and resuspend the cells in 5 to 10 ml. of ice-cold fixative. Centrifuge at 900 r.p.m. for 10 minutes.

13. Repeat Step 12 two or three times. Finally, pour off the supernate, and resuspend the cells in the pellet in 0.5 ml. of fixative.

14. Make slides by adding a small drop of cell suspension to the slide surface; spread with gentle blowing and tipping of the slide. Air dry. The slides are ready to stain when they are dry, but they may be stored unstained until later. They should be kept free of dust. Photomicrographs are made under oil immersion, and karyograms are prepared.

15. Giemsa stain is used for 10 to 15 minutes. The slides are rinsed in acetone, 7 to 10 dips until no further blue color runs off the slide. Then a rinse made from 1 part of acetone and 1 part of xylene is used for 5 minutes. Next the slides are rinsed in xylene for five to eight dips, and then the slides are left in xylene rinse for five minutes. The slides are then mounted with coverslips and allowed to dry. The Giemsa stain used here is made from 27 ml. of Giemsa stain liquid concentrate plus 373 ml. of phosphate buffer (*p*H 7.4). The phosphate buffer is made from 80.3 ml. of M/15 Na_2HPO_4 plus 19.7 ml. of M/15 $NaH_2PO_4 \cdot H_2O$ plus 900 ml. of distilled water. The buffer may be stored at room temperature.

Bone Marrow Preparation

1. Aspirate 0.5 to 1.5 ml. of marrow in a separate syringe. Immediately transfer the sample to 20 ml. of Colcemid solution in a 40 ml. centrifuge tube.

---

* Produced by CIBA.

2. Incubate the tube in slanted position under a 60-watt incandescent bulb 45 to 60 minutes.

3. Centrifuge at 500 r.p.m. for 10 minutes; then aspirate supernate, which may be turbid.

4. Add 10 ml. of a 0.77 per cent sodium citrate solution, previously warmed to 37° C to the cell button. Disperse the cell button gently with a Pasteur pipette. Incubate under an incandescent bulb as in Step 2 for 20 minutes.

5. Centrifuge at 500 r.p.m. for 10 minutes; then aspirate supernate.

6. Carefully add 10 ml. of freshly prepared Carnoy's fixative,* layering it into the tube without disturbing the cell button.

7. After the cell button turns brown, but not longer than 5 minutes, disperse the button gently with a Pasteur pipette.

8. Centrifuge at 500 r.p.m. for 10 minutes; then aspirate the supernate.

9. Add 10 ml. of Carnoy's fixative and disperse the button with a Pasteur pipette. Allow the dispersion to stand 5 minutes.

10. Centrifuge at 500 r.p.m. for 10 minutes; then aspirate the supernate.

11. Repeat Steps 9 and 10 until the supernate is colorless. Usually no more than four times is needed.

12. After the last centrifugation and aspiration, there should be a cell button in the tube that is clear to white. There may also be larger brown particles that are waste, at the very tip of the tube.

13. Add enough Carnoy's fixative to make a turbid solution, approximately 0.5 to 1.5 ml.

14. Use clean slides stored in cold 20 per cent ethanol. Place 2 drops of turbid solution on each cold, alcohol-wet slide, and forcefully blow the solution along the long axis of the slide.

15. Quickly heat the slide moderately over a bunsen burner until the alcohol solu-

tion beads. Do not boil the solution. Shake off the excess alcohol, and the slide should dry rapidly. Make 10 to 20 slides.

16. Place the dry slides in Giemsa stain for 15 minutes.

17. Dip the slides seven times in fresh acetone.

18. Place the slides in fresh acetone and xylene for 5 minutes.

19. Dip the slides seven times in xylene.

20. Place the slides in xylene for 5 minutes.

21. Cover the xylene-wet slides with coverslips using Permount. Photomicrographs are made under oil immersion, and karyograms are prepared.

Since 1972, a variety of special staining techniques have been perfected that take advantage of the fact that various regions of the chromosome stain according to their heterochromatin content. This gives the chromosomes a banded appearance. The numbers and appearances of the bands are specific for each of the human chromosomes. Special stains have therefore made it possible to categorize specifically each of the human chromosomes and to recognize small, previously indistinguishable abnormalities of the individual chromosome. Examples of the special staining techniques include quinicrine, fluorescent staining (Q banding), Giemsa banding (G banding), reverse staining (R banding), and centromeric staining (C banding).[17, 64]

Findings

The chromosome number is determined by counting the chromosomes in at least ten but preferably 50 to 100 metaphase plates. Because chromosomes are so small, even under oil immersion, their morphologic aspects are studied from enlarged photomicrographs made of selected metaphase plates. The chromosomes are cut from a photomicrograph, and these are arranged in an orderly fashion called a karyotype. Each body cell contains 46 chromosomes, and these are paired. Twenty-two pairs are autosomes, and one pair, the sex chromo-

---

* Carnoy's fixative is made from 3 parts of absolute ethanol and 1 part of glacial acetic acid. Approximately 80 ml. is enough for marrow preparation.

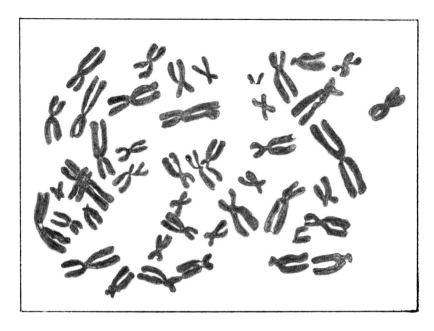

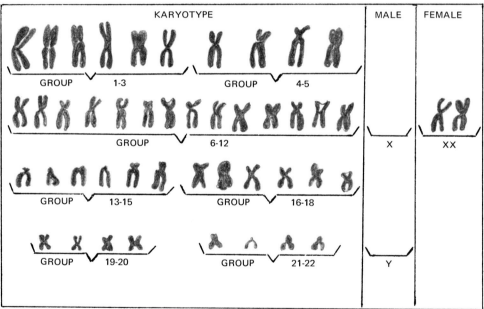

Fig. 16-31. (Top), Metaphase plate (normal female). *(Bottom)*, Female karyotype made from metaphase plate. The chromosome preparations were Giemsa-stained (approximately 2500 ×; Adapted from Hampton, C. L.: Understanding chromosome analysis. Am. J. Med. Technol., *30:*321, 1964)

somes. A human female has XX as her sex chromosome complement and 22 pairs of autosomes (Fig. 16-31). The male has XY as his sex chromosome complement and of course also the 22 pairs of autosomes (Fig. 16-32). In the process of karyotyping, the chromosomes are paired according to decreasing size and the position of their cen-

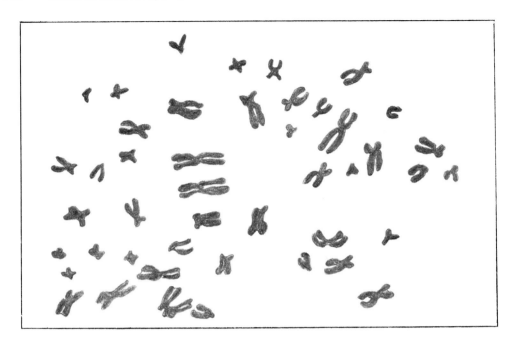

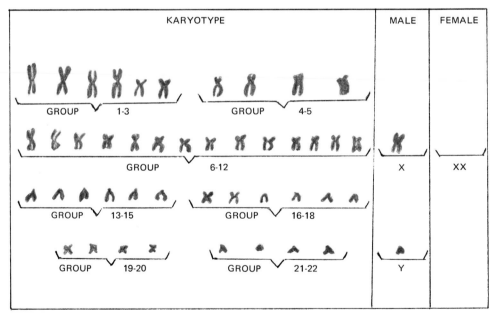

Fig. 16-32. (Top), Metaphase plate (normal male). *(Bottom),* Male karyotype made from metaphase plate, Giemsa stain was used (approximately 2500 ×; Adapted from Hampton, C. L.: Understanding chromosome analysis. Am. J. Med. Technol., *30:*321, 1964)

tromeres. The centromere is the constricted area on the chromosome. Most have median or submedian centromeres, but a few have terminal centromeres (acro-centrics). These acrocentric chromosomes are associated with the nucleolus and are subject to considerable mechanical stress. The autosomes are assigned numbers from

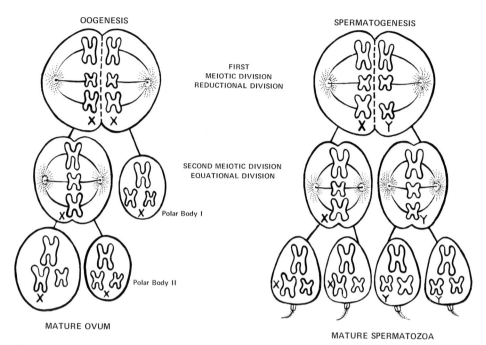

OOGENESIS

SPERMATOGENESIS

FIRST
MEIOTIC DIVISION
REDUCTIONAL DIVISION

SECOND MEIOTIC DIVISION
EQUATIONAL DIVISION

Polar Body I

Polar Body II

MATURE OVUM

MATURE SPERMATOZOA

Fig. 16-33. Meiosis, the maturation of ova and spermatozoa. Meiosis is somewhat different from mitosis; the process is pictured with the cell starting to divide at the metaphase stage. Note that chromosomes line up in pairs in the first division, resulting in half the normal chromosome number. The spermatozoa are the determiners of the sex of the offspring. Half the spermatozoa carry the X, and half carry the Y. Ova carry only X. (Adapted from Hampton, C. L.: Understanding chromosome analysis. Am. J. Med. Technol., *30:*321, 1964)

1 to 22 (Denver system). Most workers do not attempt to give absolute identity to any one chromosome or pair of chromosomes. For this reason they are grouped and labeled Group 1-3, Group 6-12, and so on.

Chromosomal abnormalities are of two kinds, of *number* or of *morphology,* or occasionally of both. To understand the mechanism of the abnormalities, one must be familiar with the production of ova and spermatozoa by meiosis (Fig. 16-33). In meiosis the chromosome number is reduced by half—the haploid number. Figure 16-34 shows that by fertilization a new individual starts life by receiving half the chromosome complement from each parent—that is, 22 autosomes, one member from each pair, and one sex chromosome from each parent join to form a cell capable of growing into an individual.

Chromosomal abnormalities occurring in the parent cell will persist in the body cells of the offspring, owing to the ability of the chromosomes to produce exact replicas of themselves during cell division. Sometimes an error occurs in meiosis and a chromosome fails to disjoin in the first meiotic division. In this instance the ovum or spermatozoon, as the case may be, carries an extra chromosome. This is called *nondisjunction* (Fig. 16-35). Union of such an abnormal cell with a normal sex cell produces an abnormal chromosome constituent and hence an abnormal person. Specific abnormalities occur when chromosomes are deficient, deformed, or present in excess. Some of the more common chromosomal abnormalities involve numbers—that is, 47 instead of 46, as occurs in mongolism. The extra chromosome is called a trisomy;

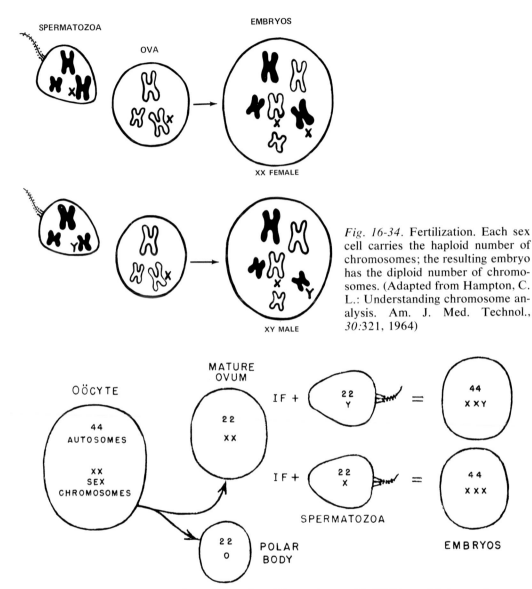

Fig. 16-34. Fertilization. Each sex cell carries the haploid number of chromosomes; the resulting embryo has the diploid number of chromosomes. (Adapted from Hampton, C. L.: Understanding chromosome analysis. Am. J. Med. Technol., *30:*321, 1964)

Fig. 16-35. Mechanism of nondisjunction. The embryo with XXY would demonstrate Klinefelter's syndrome. The embryo with XXX would demonstrate the triple X syndrome. (Adapted from Hampton, C. L.: Understanding chromosome analysis. Am. J. Med. Technol., *30:*321, 1964)

hence, mongolism is sometimes called trisomy-21 (Fig. 16-36). It seems to be the rule that the human body can tolerate an extra autosome, a trisomy, but that the loss of an autosome is incompatible with life. The body, on the other hand, seems to be able to tolerate the loss of a sex chromo-some and also the presence of supernumerary sex chromsomes.

Errors in chromosome morphology also occur. These are rarer than errors in number, possibly because of our technical limitations. The morphologic errors usually involve a translocation consisting of a

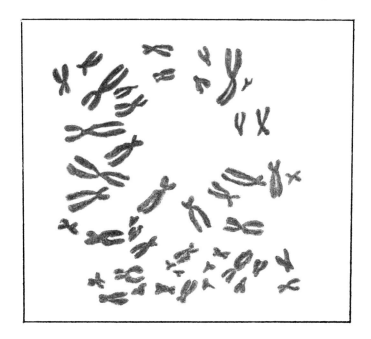

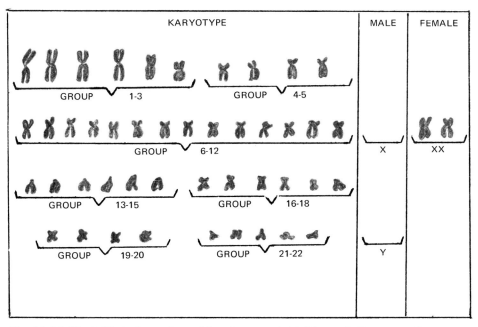

Fig. 16-36. (Top), Metaphase plate of female mongoloid. (*Bottom*), Karyotype from metaphase plate. Note the extra chromosome in group 21-22. (Adapted from Hampton, C. L.: Understanding chromosome analysis. Am. J. Med. Technol., *30:*321, 1964)

chromosome or part of a chromosome attached to another chromosome (Fig. 16-37). Errors of this type are transmitted from generation to generation.

Among the better known erythrocytohematologic chromosomal deviations are hereditary spherocytosis (an example of an autosomal dominant disorder), and four X-

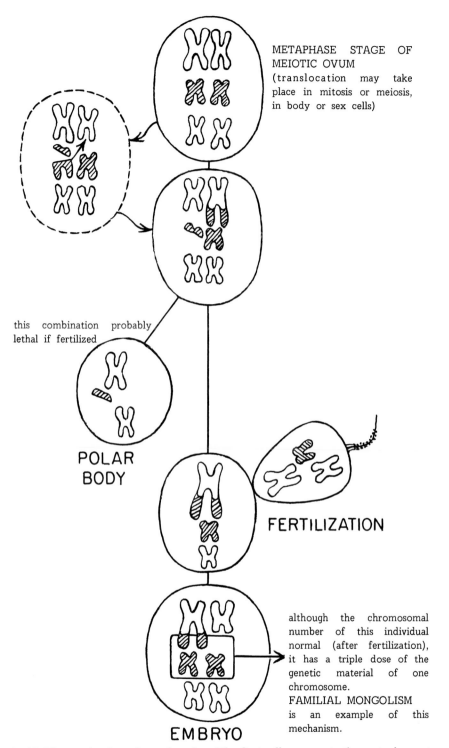

METAPHASE STAGE OF MEIOTIC OVUM (translocation may take place in mitosis or meiosis, in body or sex cells)

this combination probably lethal if fertilized

POLAR BODY

FERTILIZATION

although the chromosomal number of this individual normal (after fertilization), it has a triple dose of the genetic material of one chromosome. FAMILIAL MONGOLISM is an example of this mechanism.

EMBRYO

Fig. 16-37. The mechanism of translocation. The first cell represents the metaphase stage of a meiotic ovum (the second meiotic stage is not shown). The ovum fertilized by a normal spermatozoon results in an embryo possessing the normal chromosome number but a morphologically abnormal chromosome and triple the amount of genetic material of one chromosome (pictured as cross-hatched). Familial mongolism is an example of this mechanism. (Adapted from Hampton, C. L.: Understanding chromosome analysis. Am. J. Med. Technol., *30:*321, 1964)

Fig. 16-38. Karyotype of a metaphase plate from peripheral blood in congenital erythroid hypoplasia — the Blackfan-Diamond syndrome. The arrow indicates achromatic areas on the chromatid of a member of chromosome pair 1. (Tartaglia, A. P., et al.: Chromosome abnormality and hypocalcemia in congenital erythroid hypoplasia — Blackfan-Diamond syndrome. Am. J. Med., *41:*990, 1966)

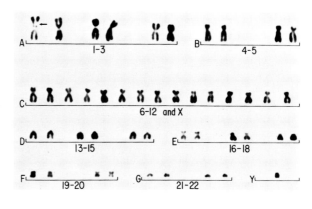

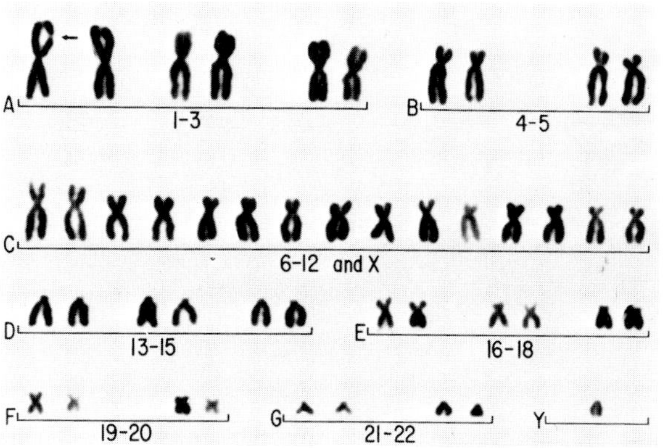

Fig. 16-39. Karyotype of a metaphase plate from peripheral blood taken 4 months later than in Figure 16-38 from patient with congenital erythroid hypoplasia. Note achromatic area on chromosome pair 1. (Tartaglia, A. P., et al.: Chromosome abnormality and hypocalcemia in congenital erythroid hypoplasia — Blackfan-Diamond syndrome. Am. J. Med., *41:*990, 1966)

linked (sex-linked) disorders — hemophilia A (Classic hemophilia), hemophilia B (Christmas disease), agammaglobulinemia (Bruton type), and certain enzyme deficiencies, the best known of which is glucose-6-phosphate dehydrogenase (G-6-PD) deficiency (favism, sensitivity to primaquine and other drugs). Tartaglia and colleagues reported a patient with chronic erythroid hypoplasia (Blackfan-Diamond syndrome) characterized by a marked decrease in bone marrow erythropoiesis, hypocalcemia, and a persistent chromosome abnormality consisting of an achromatic area always in the distal portion of one specific chromatid (Figs. 16-38 and 16-39).[59]

The best known and most thoroughly documented hematologic chromosomal deviation is that found in chronic granulocytic leukemia — the Philadelphia chromosome (Ph'). This was thought to represent a partial deletion of the long arm of one of the members of the twenty-first pair of autosomes. However, recent work reveals it to be a translocation of the long arm of the number 22 chromosome to chromosome number 9. It has also been described by other researchers in other locations.[51] On occasion, if bone marrow is not available, a direct preparation done on the buffy coat of the peripheral blood may be successful in demonstrating the Philadelphia chromosome. That is, since in chronic granulocytic leukemia there are many mitotable myeloid cells circulating, it is also possible to do short-term unstimulated cultures of the peripheral blood and obtain Philadelphia chromosome-positive cells. This technique may also be used to advantage where samples must be mailed to a reference laboratory. It is possible to obtain Philadelphia chromosome-positive cells from peripheral blood samples that are several days old. The diagnostic importance of the Philadelphia chromosome is so significant that its absence raises a question as to whether the

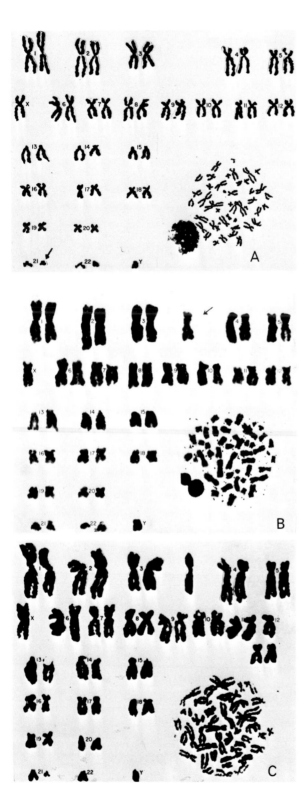

Fig. 16-40. (*A*) Karyotype of cell showing Ph′ chromosome as its only gross abnormality. (*B*) Arrow indicates karyotype of cell without Ph′ chromosome but with abnormal metacentric extra chromosome. (*C*) Karyotype showing abnormal submetacentric chromosome, a Ph[1] chromosome, an extra number 12 chromosome, and a missing group C chromosome. (Ritzmann, S. E., et al.: Coexistent chronic myelocytic leukemia, monoclonal gammopathy and multiple chromosomal abnormalities. Am. J. Med., *41*:981, 1966)

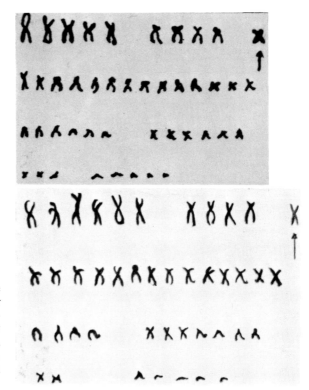

Fig. 16-41. Two karyotypes from a case of multiple myeloma, with modal number of 44 chromosomes. Morphologic abnormalities are seen throughout, especially medium-sized metacentric chromosome, which the arrow indicates. (Castoldi, G. L., et al.: Chromosomal imbalance in plasmacytoma. Lancet, *1*:829, 1963)

hematopoietic disorder is really chronic granulocytic leukemia[60] (Fig. 16-40). Also important is the fact that the Philadelphia chromosome is found in almost all dividing cells (myeloid, erythroid, and megakaryocytic) of the marrow in chronic granulocytic leukemia.[63, 66] This may mean that a single stem or precursor cell is the source for the granulocyte, erythrocyte, and megakaryocyte series. A less likely alternative is that simultaneous cytogenetic events have taken place in each of the three purportedly separate systems in chronic granulocytic leukemia.

The Ph' study is also useful in the diagnosis of patients with early chronic granulocytic leukemia (CGL) and in distinguishing typical from atypical CGL. These cytogenetic studies may also be used in the demonstration or prediction of the blast transformation of CGL, since clonal evolution, with the appearance of additional cytogenetic abnormalities, frequently occurs prior to the onset of the blast crisis.[29]

The fact that leukocyte alkaline phosphatase (LAP) is decreased in chronic granulocytic leukemia and increased in mongolism, in which triplication of chromosome 22 is found, has given rise to the suggestion that the structural gene for this enzyme (LAP) may be on chromosome 22.[1] Strong evidence against this concept lies in the fact that subsequently normal[7] or even elevated[61] LAP levels can be found in the presence of the Ph' chromosome. Furthermore, it has been shown that other enzymes, even G-6-PD, which is X-linked, are increased in mongolism.[39] This Ph' chromosome abnormality, in conclusion, is unique for chronic granulocytic leukemia, and it has not been observed in any other myeloproliferative disorder. In fact, it is limited to the myeloid, erythroid, and megakaryocytic cells in mitosis of this disease and has not been found in other cells including lymphocytes.[13]

Ritzmann and co-workers described a case of coexistent chronic myelocytic leukemia, monoclonal gammopathy, and mul-

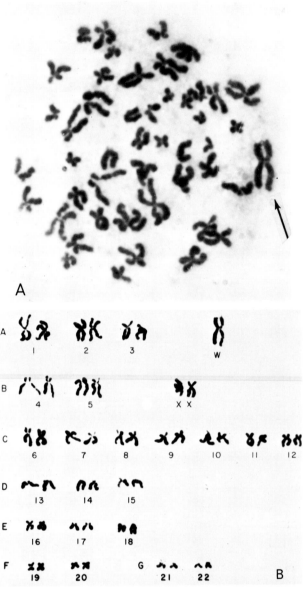

Fig. 16-42. (*A*) Metaphase plate taken from blood culture in Waldenström's macroglobulinemia. Arrow indicates excessively long chromosome. (*B*) Karyotype from blood culture in Waldenström's macroglobulinemia. Note *w*, excessively long chromosome. *(Figure continues on facing page.)*

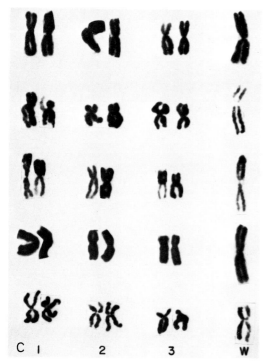

Fig. 16-42 Continued. (C) Waldenström's macroglobulinemia, showing group A chromosomes of five karyotypes with (w) excessively long chromosome. The centromere is more central. (Benirschke, K., Brownhill, E., and Ebaugh, F. G.: Chromosomal abnormalities in Waldenström's macroglobulinemia. Lancet, *1:*594, 1962)

tiple chromosomal abnormalities.[48] The chromosomal abnormalities consisted of Ph' anomalies, the presence of large extra chromosomes, and pair 12 abnormalities indistinguishable from those frequently associated with primary macroglobulinemia (Waldenström's)[3] and myeloma[31] (Fig. 16-41). In macroglobulinemia, all spreads with 47 chromosomes contained one excessively large chromosome, which stained less darkly and appeared less contracted. The Group A chromosomes of five such karyotypes have an additional marker chromosome (w; Fig. 16-42). This abnormal chromosome is excessively long and its centromere is much more centrally located. It is thought that such abnormal cells produce the abnormal globulins, implying that cells cultured from the peripheral blood (lymphocytes and monocytes perhaps) are capable of protein synthesis.

Castoldi described a clear modal number of 44 in his chromosomal report on myeloma.[11] He also described in all cells an abnormal karyotype characterized by an aberrant medium-sized metacentric chromosome (Fig. 16-41). Lewis and colleagues described chromosomal abnormalities in two cases of multiple myeloma but not in the third case.[31] After communication with two other investigators, who also had negative chromosomal findings, he concludes that the positive chromosomal abnormalities noted in his first two cases are derived from malignant cells and finding them in significant numbers may conceivably give an indication of the degree of malignancy.

Bottura believes that chromosome abnormalities in multiple myeloma have been inconstant and that no two published examples have been the same (Fig. 16-43). Therefore, with a relatively constant pattern in the related Waldenström's macroglobulinemia, there appears to be a clear distinction, chromosomally, between macroglobulinemia and myeloma. However, in a study of 24 patients with monoclonal gammopathies (γM-MG, γA-MG, and γG-MG), evidence was obtained suggesting that certain chromosomal abnormalities are common to all three types of monoclonal gammopathies (Fig. 16-44).[24] All this may be interpreted alternatively as a reflection of a primary disturbance of immunocompetent cells, which may permit the emergence of a myeloproliferative syndrome, or as a perversion of immunocompetent cells resulting from the occurrence of a myeloproliferative disorder. Although these studies have demonstrated marker chromosomes (M chromosomes) in a relatively high proportion of patients with myeloma or macroglobulinemia, there has been little application of chromosome banding

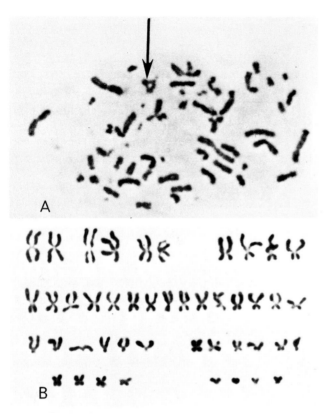

Fig. 16-43. (A) Metaphase plate of bone marrow in multiple myeloma, showing at least 51 chromosomes and four or five fragments. A complex chromosome aberration is indicated by the arrow. (B) Karyotype of a metaphase cell in multiple myeloma, showing 45 chromosomes. One small acrocentric autosome is missing. (Bottura, C.: Chromosomal abnormalities in multiple myeloma. Acta Haematol., *30:*274, 1963)

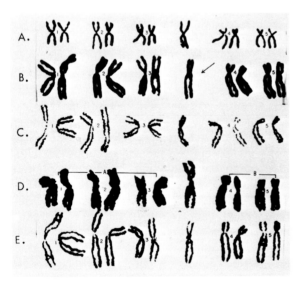

Fig. 16-44. Composite of group A and group B chromosomes showing MG chromosomes. (A) MG chromosome from the marrow in γM monoclonal gammopathy. (B) MG chromosome from the blood of the same patient as in A. (C) MG chromosome from the blood in γG monoclonal gammopathy. (D) MG chromosome from the blood in γG monoclonal gammopathy and chronic myelocytic leukemia. (E) MG chromosome from the blood in γA monoclonal gammopathy. (Houston, E. W., Ritzmann, S. E., and Levin, W. C.: Chromosomal aberrations common to three types of monoclonal gammopathies. Blood, *29:*214, 1967)

studies to myeloma. Cytogenetic studies have potential value in the evaluation of patients with suspected myeloma, since the demonstration of a clonal chromosomal abnormality would exclude the diagnosis of a reactive plasma-cell disorder.

Chromosomal analysis of both peripheral blood and bone marrow in acute granulocytic leukemia has failed to reveal any characteristic abnormality, except that leukemia occurs 30 to 50 times as often in children with mongolism. The most common change is hyperdiploid aneuploidy, an alteration in the number of chromosomes—that is, a mode of 92 or more. It has been noted, however, that the aneuploid cells may also be replaced by normal diploid cells in association with hematologic remissions. Therapy that induces remission in acute leukemias results in the disappearance of the abnormal karyotypes, which reappear before imminent relapse of the disease. Also, although as a group the acute leukemias do not show any consistent karyotypic abnormality (however, group C-9 more commonly has an extra autosome), individual patients frequently show the same cytogenetic abnormalities during each relapse —that is, many patients with acute leukemia exhibit abnormalities of chromosome number or morphology in the affected (leukemic) cells, which may be constant in any one patient but may vary considerably from one patient to another.

Sandberg and associates found that the chromosome group most frequently involved in the aneuploidy of acute leukemia is Group C (Fig. 16-45).[55] Trisomies of Group C have also been observed in several other cases of acute granulocytic leukemia (Fig. 16-46) and other myeloproliferative conditions[67]. If standard Giemsa stains are used, approximately 50 per cent of patients will show abnormalities. If more refined techniques, such as banding studies, are utilized, approximately 60 per cent of patients will show abnormalities. To date, it has not been possible to utilize cytogenetic

studies in the classification of acute leukemias, although, in general, acute lymphoblastic leukemias show a hyperdiploid pattern, whereas the acute nonlymphocytic leukemias may show hypodiploid, hyperdiploidy, or pseudodiploidy patterns. A wide variety of chromosomal abnormalities have been described in patients with acute leukemia, and there are several specific chromosomal patterns in acute leukemia that have been described, such as the 8-21 translocation with associated sex chromosome loss described by Rowley.[51a] The presence or absence of cytogenetic abnormalities does correlate with prognosis for survival and response to therapy. Winkelstein and co-workers have described a patient with an atypical myeloproliferative syndrome. characterized by leukocytosis with myeloid immaturity, ineffective extramedullary hematopoiesis, overt hemolysis, low leukocyte alkaline phosphatase activity, and a trisomy in Group C bone marrow metaphase chromosomes (Fig. 16-47).[67] They cite two additional cases—one of a patient with myeloid metaplasia and possible leukemia who showed a C-9 trisomy[54] and another of a patient with myeloid metaplasia and subacute leukemia who was shown to have a group C trisomy and an absence of one Group F chromosome resulting in a pseudodiploid state.[42]

Because there is an overlapping of chromosomal patterns in certain of these cases and those described by others (Fig. 16-48)[28] —such as myelofibrosis with myeloid metaplasia and atypical panmyelosis, together with the uncertainty of making a definite clinical diagnosis in some of them—the concept of myeloproliferative syndrome as an interrelated disorder may be fortified. Although it is presumed that these chromosome abnormalities are related to the neoplastic behavior of leukemic cells,[47] the precise role of such changes in the evolution of leukemia remains to be determined. Direct evidence bearing on this issue would

(*Text continues on p. 576.*)

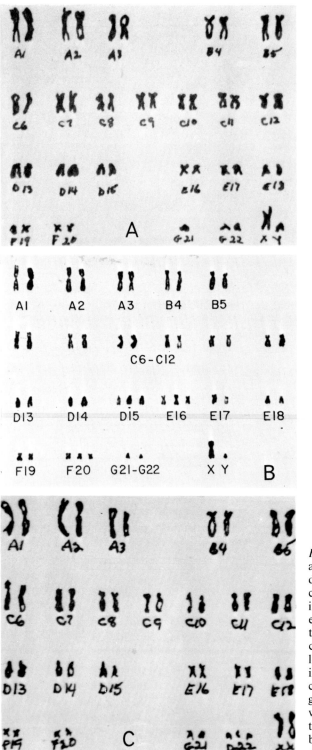

Fig. 16-45. Chromosomal alterations in acute leukemia. (*A*) Karyotype of pseudodiploid character. The number of chromosomes is 46 because of a missing autosome in group G and the presence of the M chromosome. (*B*) Karyotype of hypodiploid modal cells with 45 chromosomes in acute myeloblastic leukemia. Two chromosomes are missing from groups C and G; one extra chromosome is present in each of groups D, E, and F. (*C*) Karyotype with 47 chromosomes from an untreated patient. The extra chromosome belongs to group G. *(Figure continues on facing page.)*

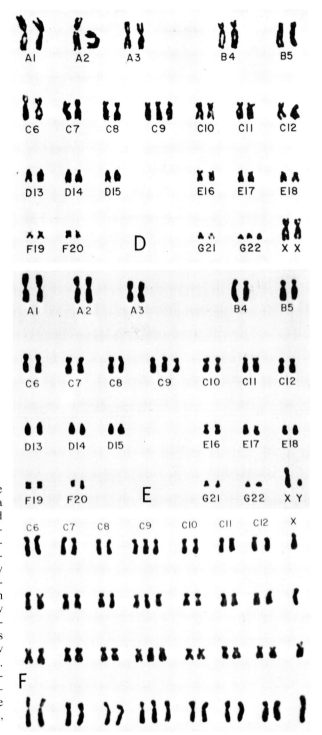

Fig. 16-45 Continued. (*D*) Karyotype with 48 chromosomes. The two extra chromosomes belong to groups C and G. (*E*) Abnormal hyperdiploid karyotype of modal cell with 47 chromosomes from bone marrow in acute myeloblastic leukemia. The hyperdiploidy is due to an extra autosome in group C-9. (*F*) Four rows of chromosomes in group C from four different marrow cells with 47 chromosomes, demonstrating the trisomy of group C-9. This finding is very common in the marrow cells of patients with acute leukemia. (Sandberg, A. A., Ishihara, T., Kihuchi, Y., and Crosswhite, L. H.: Chromosome differences among the acute leukemias. Ann. N.Y. Acad. Sci., *113*:663, 1964)

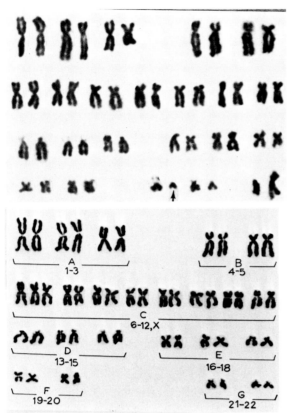

Fig. 16-46. Karyotype of bone marrow in chronic granulocytic leukemia. Arrow indicates the Philadelphia chromosome, a loss of part of the long arm of one member of the twenty-second chromosome pair. (Courtesy of Dr. Raymond L. Teplitz)

Fig. 16-47. Trisomy of group C in a myeloproliferative disorder as shown in a karyotype of a 47 chromosome metaphase plate. The extra chromosome is arbitrarily included with the first pair of the group C chromosomes. (Winkelstein, A., Sparkes, R. S., and Craddock, C. G.: Trisomy of group C in a myeloproliferative disorder. Blood, *27:*722, 1966)

accrue from systematic analyses of chromosome constitution, beginning with the presumably normal subject, progressing through the preleukemic phase, and culminating in the overtly leukemic stage of affected patients. However, such evidence is difficult to come by, especially when one realizes that acute leukemia is not recognized before the full-blown diagnostic stage. The closest one can come to this situation is that described by Rowley and colleagues—who investigated 15 potentially leukemic patients manifesting obscure anemia, leukopenia, thrombocytopenia, or thrombocytosis.[52] They found that three of these patients had abnormal chromosome members, and none had yet developed leukemia. The abnormality was confined to Group C chromosomes with a different alteration in each

instance of aplastic anemia, idiopathic sideroachrestic anemia and idiopathic thrombocythemia (Fig. 16-49, pp. 576–578).

In summary, one may postulate that cytogenetic studies may be of value in the diagnosis of suspected preleukemic patients. If the term "preleukemia" is restricted to patients with hematologic abnormalities secondary to the presence of a leukemic stem cell line in their bone marrow (i.e., an early or preclinical phase of acute leukemia), then cytogenetic study may demonstrate abnormalities in approximately 50 per cent of these patients. The presence of cytogenetic abnormalities in a patient with suspected preleukemia confers a greater risk for the evolution of acute leukemia than in a patient without it, and gives a poorer prognosis for survival. The

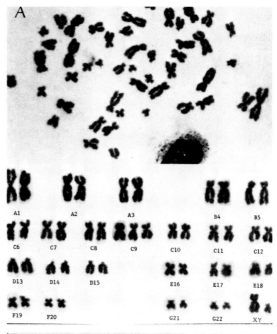

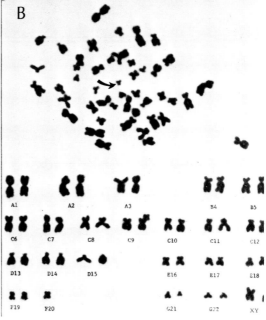

Fig. 16-48. (A) Myelofibrosis with myeloid metaplasia. The metaphase plate shows 47 chromosomes. The karyotype shows an extra chromosome in group C, the C trisomy. (B) Atypical myeloproliferative disorder. The metaphase plate contains 46 chromosomes. The Ph' chromosome (*arrow*) is shown in the karyotype. (C) Atypical myeloproliferative disorder. The metaphase plate shows 47 chromosomes. The karyotype shows an extra chromosome in group C (C trisomy; Kiossoglou, K. A., Mitus, W. J., and Dameshek, W.: Cytogenic studies in the chronic myeloproliferative syndrome. Blood, 28:241, 1966)

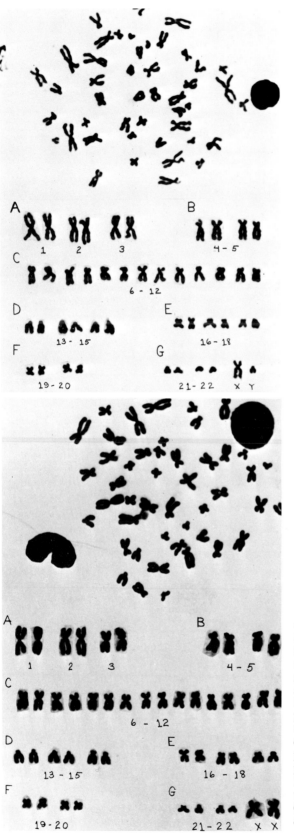

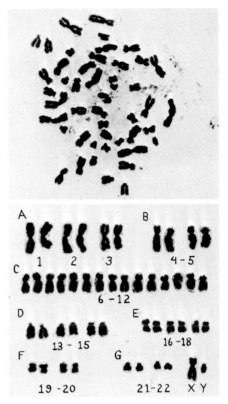

Fig. 16-49. (*Upper Left*) Aplastic anemia. (*Top*) Metaphase plate from bone marrow, using phase contrast. (*Bottom*) Karyotype containing 45 chromosomes with one group C chromosome missing. (*Upper Right*) Sideroachrestic anemia. (*Top*) Metaphase plate from bone marrow, using phase contrast. (*Bottom*) Karyotype showing 47 chromosomes. There is one extra group C chromosome. (*Left*) Idiopathic thrombocythemia. (*Top*) Metaphase plate from bone marrow. (*Bottom*) Karyotype containing 48 chromosomes with two extra C group chromosomes. (Courtesy of Dr. Janet D. Rowley; *figure continued on facing page.*)

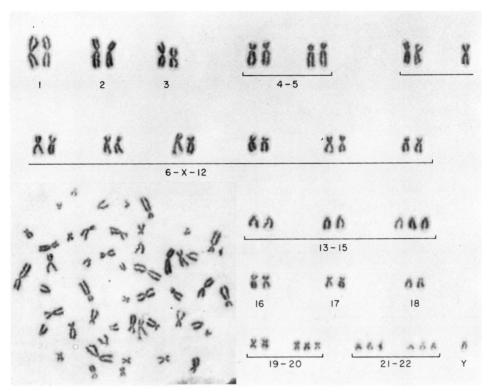

(Fig. 16-49) Continued. Dividing cell from bone marrow of patient with Down's syndrome (mongolism), showing trisomy in group 21-22, an extra chromosome in group 13-15, an extra chromosome in group 19-21, and an extra chromosome in group 21-22. The blood pattern of leukemia appeared several weeks after this marrow sample was obtained. (DeMayo, A. P., et al.: A marrow chromosomal abnormality preceding clinical leukemia in Down's syndrome. Blood, *29*:233, 1967)

cytogenetic abnormalities observed in patients with preleukemia are similar to those observed in the overt stage, since one is merely looking at the early stage of the disease.[45]

Another example is described by DeMayo and associates, who discovered a minor line of cells with a complement of 50 chromosomes during a routine diagnostic cytogenetic study of the marrow and peripheral blood of a child with Down's syndrome (mongolism).[15] The predominant cell in marrow and blood had 47 chromosomes with the standard trisomy in Group 21-22 (Fig. 16-49, p. 579). Leukemia appeared several weeks later. Because these conditions tend to terminate in leukemia, the ob-

servation of these chromosome abnormalities is important in any hypothesis relating aneuploidy and leukemia. Rowley and coworkers postulate that a stable aneuploid stem line does not of itself produce neoplasia but rather that this alteration of the genome may provide a more favorable milieu for the action of some transforming agent.[52] Because of the frequent occurrence of Group C abnormalities in these cases of marrow disorders, Winkelstein and associates further postulate that genes on one or more C chromosomes might be responsible for the homeostatic control of hemopoiesis, and that a change in genetic balance involving a Group C chromosome(s) coupled with a transforming agent might result in leuke-

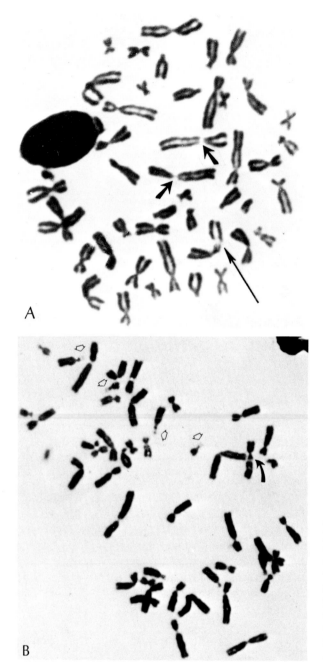

Fig. 16-50. Marrow cells in vitamin B_{12} and folate deficiency. (*A*) Metaphase plate showing a prominent secondary constriction in a group A chromosome (*long arrow*) and prominent centromeric constrictions, shown by short arrows. (*B*) Metaphase plate showing prominent satellites on group D and G chromosomes (*light arrows*) and a secondary constriction in a group C chromosome, shown by solid arrows. *(Figure continues on facing page.)*

mia in a greater proportion of patients than aneuploidy of some other chromosomal group.

Little information has, until recently, been available on the functional derangement accompanying the structural abnormalities in erythrocyte or leukocyte precursors in vitamin B_{12} and folic acid deficiency or in the way in which such malfunction leads to the underproduction of erythrocytes, leukocytes and platelets. Menzies and associates have attempted to clarify the functional defect in these deficiencies by means of chromosome studies, au-

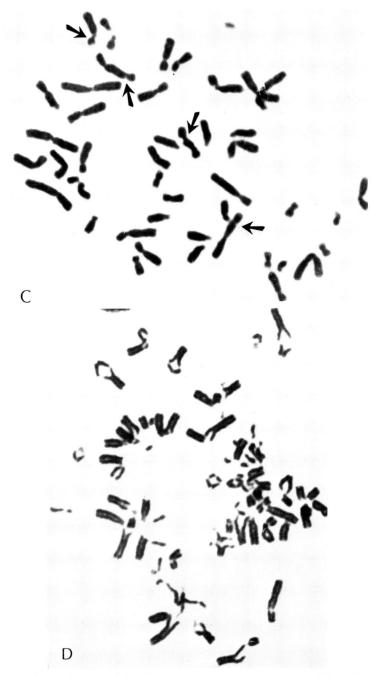

C

D

Fig. 16-50 Continued. (*C*) Metaphase plate showing chromatid breaks, with arrows. (*D*) Metaphase plate showing multiple breaking of chromosomes, especially near the centromeres, and the separation of the chromatids, (Menzies, R. C., et al.: Cytogenetic and cytochemical studies on marrow cells in B$_{12}$ and folate deficiency. Blood, *28*:581, 1966)

toradiography, and DNA measurements in individual cells.[40] They found that there were no numerical changes in mitoses in pernicious anemia, but there were numerous morphologic abnormalities of the chromosomes. These abnormalities included: (1) The centromeric constrictions were of exaggerated size. (2) Chromatid breakage was very common. (3) A number of cells showed thin, elongated chromosomes, possibly resulting from either reduced contraction or despiralization. (4) Some metaphases had abnormally small and poorly defined chromosomes whose chromatids had separated; others showed more pronounced degeneration of the chromosomes. (5) There were sizable numbers of mitoses in prophase, up to 50 per cent compared to 15 per cent in a normoblastic marrow (Fig. 16-50).

Kiossoglou and co-workers demonstrated numerical and morphologic chromosomal aberrations in nine cases of pernicious anemia (six cases of which were reported later) in relapse.[27] The morphologic abnormalities, including chromatid breaks, gaps, and giant chromosomes, were reduced in remission following vitamin B_{12} therapy (Fig. 16-51). The numerical changes consisted of aneuploidy (45 and 44 chromosomes) with the most common finding encountered (6 to 100 per cent of the cells) being monosomy involving the G-21 chromosome. This chromosome was present, not only in the marrow cells, but also in other tissues—for example, in peripheral blood and possibly in skin fibroblasts, thus suggesting a more general disorder. The numerical anomalies persisted in remission. The authors postulated that the structural anomalies—namely, chromatid breaks, gaps, acentric fragments, and giant chromosomes—are related to vitamin B_{12} deficiency and are correctable.

The cause of the aneuploidy, because it was not correctable by treatment, is not clear. Because the patients were not studied before the disease had begun, a congenital or acquired predisposition to megalo-blastosis on the basis of G-21 monosomy cannot be excluded. The origin and significance of the extra chromatin material translocated onto the short arms of G-21 chromosomes cannot be explained. Because these chromosome changes were closely similar to those produced by known inhibitors of DNA synthesis, this appears to be strong evidence that they themselves were expressions of deficient DNA synthesis. Also, the appearance of significant number of prophases and metaphases indicates that mitosis was not only disordered but also prolonged or at times abortive. These same changes were also reported by others,[27] as were frequent aneuploidies not observed by Menzies and co-workers.[40]

There is increasing interest in the use of cytogenetics in the classification and clinical management of patients with malignant lymphoma. Since non-Hodgkin's malignant lymphomas have a very high incidence of cytogenetic abnormalities, cytogenetic studies are potentially useful in the diagnosis of malignant lymphoma where the histologic diagnosis is questionable. The demonstration of a clonal cytogenetic abnormality in lymph nodes or splenic tissue almost certainly establishes a diagnosis of neoplasm, whereas the lack of cytogenic abnormalities does not exclude the possibility of malignancy.

A second area of interest in application of cytogenetics to lymphoma is in staging. Cases have been reported in which histologic staging was negative, but cytogenetic study of the apparently uninvolved nodes revealed abnormalities consistent with malignant lymphoma.

One type of malignant lymphoma, the Burkitt lymphoma, has a characteristic cytogenetic abnormality involving a translocation from the number 8 chromosome to the number 14 chromosome.[69] The application of chromosome banding techniques to the study of malignant lymphomas may eventually establish specific chromosomal abnormality patterns in the malignant lymphomas. Careful prospective studies will be

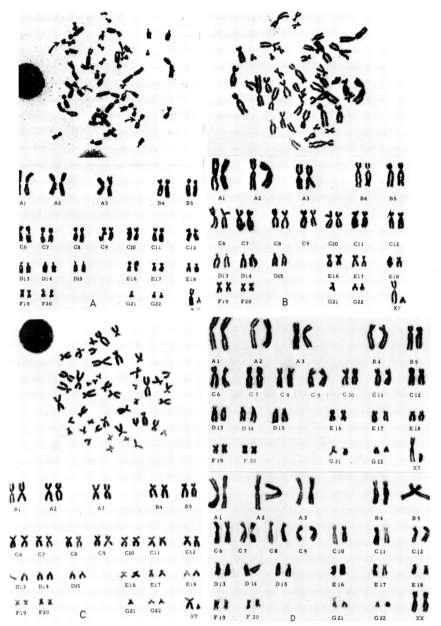

Fig. 16-51. Chromosomal aberrations in pernicious anemia. (*A*) In relapse, the metaphase bone marrow plate and karyotype show 45 chromosomes with G-21 monosomy. Extra chromatin material is translocated onto the short arms of the twenty-first chromosome. Arrows point to chromatid breaks, and chromatid and isochromatid gaps. (*B*) In relapse, the metaphase bone marrow plate and karyotype show the same characteristics as *A* plus "giant" chromosomes with imperfect coiling. (*C*) In remission, the metaphase bone marrow plate and karyotype show the same characteristics as *A* and *B* except that the breaks, gaps, and "giant" chromosomes seen in relapse are no longer present. (*D*) In remission, the karyotypes are of two diploid cells from a peripheral blood leukocyte culture. One of the G-21 chromosomes in each of the cells is abnormally large. (Kiossoglou, K. A., Mitus, W. J., and Dameshek, W.: Chromosomal aberrations in pernicious anemia. Blood, *25*:662, 1965)

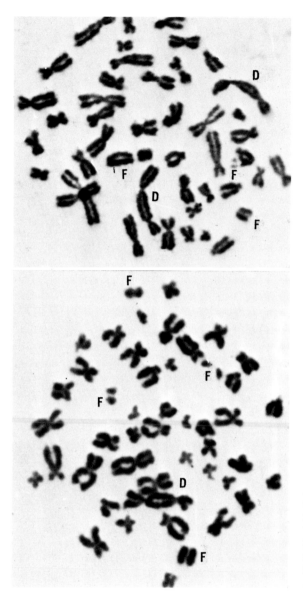

Fig. 16-52. Metaphase plate demonstrating fragments (*F*) and dicentric chromosomes. (*D*) from blood culture of patient after radiographic therapy. (Warren, S., and Meisner, L.: Chromosomal changes in leukocytes of patients receiving irradiation therapy. J.A.M.A., *193:*352, 1965)

required to determine whether the presence or absence of cytogenetic abnormalities or specific abnormalities correlate with survival, classification of lymphoma, or response to therapy.

Therapeutic irradiation used in the treatment of both hematologic and nonhematologic malignant disorders produces a chromosomal aberration that can be assessed by analysis of lymphoid cells from peripheral blood culture. Initially there is a marked in-crease in the frequency of cells with chromosome numbers deviating from the normal complement of 46. After conclusion of radiographic therapy, the incidence of aneuploidy tends to return to normal levels in about 1 year. Structural chromosome aberrations increase with the dose throughout the course of radiographic therapy. At lower doses, these changes consist of fragments and dicentric chromosomes; at higher doses, atypical and ring chromo-

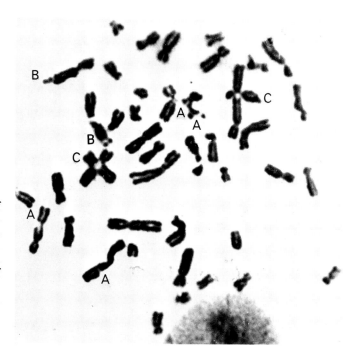

Fig. 16-53. Metaphase plate of patient with nonleukemic internal disease. Illustration shows chromatid (*A*) and isochromatid (*B*) breaks, and two interchanges in chromosomes (*C*) after use of Thio-Tepa, a cytostatic agent. (Hampel, K. E., et al.: The action of cytostatic agents on the chromosomes of human leukocytes in vitro. Blood, *27:*816, 1966)

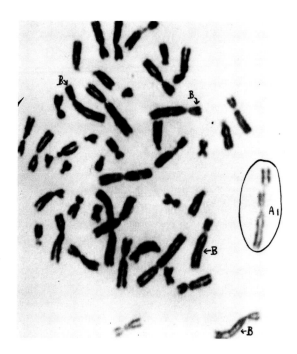

Fig. 16-54. Metaphase plate of patient with polycythemia after therapy with ^{32}P, showing chromatid break in the encircled chromosome A, and chromosome B (dicentric; MacDiarmid, W. D.: Chromosomal changes following treatment of polycythemia with radioactive phosphorus. Q. J. Med., *34:*133, 1965)

somes are observed (Fig. 16-52). Aberrations persisting longest after the end of radiographic therapy are those involving the larger chromosomes, particularly aberrations of chromosomes 1 or 2.[65]

Because various cytostatic agents are also used in the treatment of malignant nonhematopoietic and hematopoietic disorders, a quantitative analysis of the chromosomal injuries following in vitro addition of

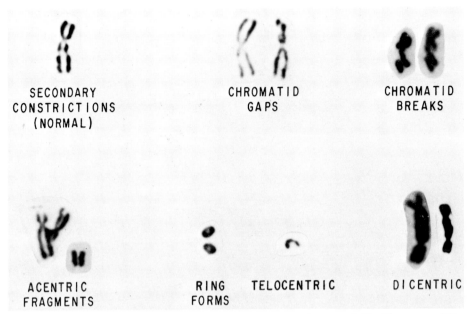

SECONDARY
CONSTRICTIONS
(NORMAL)

CHROMATID
GAPS

CHROMATID
BREAKS

ACENTRIC
FRAGMENTS

RING
FORMS

TELOCENTRIC

DICENTRIC

Fig. 16-55. Some abnormal chromosomes resulting from the use of ³²P. (Courtesy of Dr. W. D. MacDiarmid)

these chemotherapeutic drugs to short-term leukocyte cultures was used to reveal a cytogenetic pattern similar to the action of these drugs when administered therapeutically to man. TEM, thio-TEPA, cyclophosphamide, A2ASTA, Amethopterin, and FUDR were used to produce chromatid and isochromatid breaks and interchanges in human chromosomes (Fig. 16-53). In addition, damage to chromosomes has been shown to occur after treatment with ³²P in patients with polycythemia vera, whose chromosomes are like those of normal subjects before treatment.[36] Such effects may indicate some enhancement by ³²P of the risk of leukemia in these patients. There seems to be a tendency for the higher initial levels of damage to become less after a time, probably owing to the death of damaged cells. The incorporation of ³²P into DNA as a strategically situated link in the molecular chain may explain the marked effect of a rather low dose of irradiation (Figs. 16-54; 16-55). On the other hand, recent work has clearly demonstrated clonal cytogenetic abnormalities in patients with polycythemia vera and agnogenic myeloid metaplasia.[68]

REFERENCES

1. Alter, A. A., Lee, S. L., Pourfar, M., and Dobkin, G.: Leukocyte alkaline phosphatase in mongolism; a possible chromosome marker (Abstract). J. Clin. Invest., *41*:1341, 1962.
2. Barr, M. L., and Bertramy, E. G.: A morphologic distinction between the neurones of the male and female, and the behaviour of the nucleolar satellite during accelerated nucleoprotein synthesis. Nature, *163*:676, 1949.
3. Benirschke, K., Brownhill, L., and Ebaugh, F. G.: Chromosomal abnormalities in Waldenström's macroglobulinemia. Lancet, *1*:594, 1962.
4. Bernhard, W.: Some problems of fine structure in tumor cells. Prog. Exp. Tumor Res., *3*:1, 1963.
5. Bessis, M. C., and Breton-Gorius, J.: Iron metabolism in the bone marrow as seen by electron microscopy: a critical review. Blood, *19*:635, 1962.
6. Bessis, M., and Thiery, J. P.: Electron microscopy of human white blood cells and their stem cells. Int. Rev. Cytol., *12*:199, 1961.
7. Block, J. B., Carbone, P. P., Opphein, J. J., and Frei, E., III: The effect of treatment in patients with chronic myelogenous leukemia. Biochemical studies. Ann. Intern. Med., *59*:629, 1963.
8. Bottura, C.: Chromosomal abnormalities in multiple myeloma. Acta Haematol., *30*:274, 1963.

9. Boyde, A., Weiss, R. A., and Vesely, P.: Scanning electron microscopy of cells in culture. Exp. Cell. Res., *71:*313, 1972.

10. Braunsteiner, H., and Pakesch, F.: Electron microscopy and the functional significance of a new cellular structure in plasmocytes: a review. Blood, *10:*650, 1955.

11. Castoldi, G. L., Ricci, N., Punturieri, E., and Bosi, L.: Chromosomal imbalance in plasmacytoma. Lancet, *1:*829, 1963.

12. Chu, E. H. Y., and Giles, N. H.: Human chromosome complements in normal somatic cells in culture. Am. J. Hum. Genet., *11:*63, 1959.

13. Court-Brown, W. M., and Tough, I. M.: Cytogenetic studies in chronic myeloid leukemia. *In* Advances in Cancer Research. Haddow, A., and Weinhouse, S., (eds).: vol. VII. New York, Academic Press, 1963.

14. David-Ferreira, J. F.: The blood platelet: electron microscopic studies. Int. Rev. Cytol., *17:*99, 1964.

15. DeMayo, A. P., Kiossoglou, K. A., Erlandson, M. E., Notterman, R. F., and German, J.: A marrow chromosomal abnormality preceding clinical leukemia in Down's syndrome. Blood, *29:*233, 1967.

16. Eggen, R. R.: Cytogenetics. Am. J. Clin. Pathol., *39:*3, 1963.

17. Finaz, C., and De Grouchy, J.: Identification of individual chromosomes in the human karyotype by their banding pattern after proteolytic digestion. Humangenetik, *15:*249, 1972.

18. Ford, C. E., and Hamerton, J. L.: The chromosomes of man. Nature, *178:*1020, 1956.

19. Freeman, J. A.: Cellular fine structure. Bull. Pathol., *6:*194, 1965.

20. ————: Cellular fine structure (mitochondria). Bull Path., *7:*148,, 1966.

21. Goodman, J. R., Reilly, E. B., and Moore, R. E.: Electron microscopy of formed elements of human blood. Blood, *12:*428, 1957.

22. Hampel, K. E., Kober, B., Rösch, D., Gerhartz, H., and Meinig, K. H.: The action of cytostatic agents on the chromosomes of human leukocytes in vitro (preliminary communication). Blood, *27:*816, 1966.

23. Hampton, C. L.: Understanding chromosome analysis. Am. J. Med. Technol., *30:*321, 1964.

24. Houston, E. W., Ritzmann, S. E., and Levin, W. C.: Chromosomal aberrations common to three types of monoclonal gammopathies. Blood, *29:*214, 1967.

25. Katayama, I., and Schneider, G. B.: Further ultrastructural characterization of hairy cells of leukemic reticuloendotheliosis. Am. J. Pathol., *86:*163, 1977.

26. King, D. W.: Ultrastructural Aspects of Disease. p. 213. New York, Hoeber Medical Division (Harper & Row), 1966.

27. Kissoglou, K. A., Mitus, W. J., and Dameshek, W.: Chromosomal aberrations in pernicious anemia. Study of 3 cases before and after therapy. Blood, *25:*662, 1965.

28. ————: Cytogenetic studies in the chronic myeloproliferative syndrome. Blood, *28:*241, 1966.

29. Krompotic, E., Lewis, J. P., and Donnelly, W. J.: Chromosome aberrations in two patients with chronic granulocytic leukemia undergoing acute transformation. Am. J. Clin. Pathol., *49:*161, 1968.

30. Lejune, J., Turpin, R., and Gantier, M.: Le mongolisme premier example d'aberration autosomique humaine. Ann. Genet., *1:*41, 1949.

31. Lewis, F. J., Crow, R. S., MacTaggart, M., and Willis, M. R.: Chromosomal abnormalities in multiple myeloma. Lancet, *1:*1183, 1963.

32. Lin, P. S., Cooper, A. G., and Wortes, H. H.: Scanning electron microscopy of human T-cell and B-cell rosettes. N. Engl. J. Med., *289:*548, 1973.

33. Low, F. N., and Freeman, J. A.: Electron Microscopic Atlas of Normal and Leukemic Human Blood. New York, McGraw-Hill, 1958.

34. Lutzner, M. A., Hobbs, J. W., and Horvath, P.: Ultrastructure of abnormal cells in Sezary syndrome, Mycosis fungoides and Parapsoriasis en Plaque. Arch. Dermatol., *103:*375, 1971.

35. Lyon, M. F.: Gene action in the X-chromosome of the mouse (mus. musculus L.). Nature, *190:*372, 1961.

36. MacDiarmid, W. D.: Chromosomal changes following treatment of polycythemia with radioactive phosphorus. Q. J. Med., *34:*133, 1965.

37. Maldonado, J. E., Bayrd, E. D., and Brown, A. L., Jr.: The flaming cell in multiple myeloma. Am. J. Clin. Path., *44:*605, 1965.

38. Marcus, A. J., and Zucker-Franklin, D.: Studies on subcellular platelet particles. Blood, *23:*389, 1964.

39. Mellman, W., Oski, F., Tedesco, T., Mauera-Coelko, A., and Harris, H.: Leucocyte enzymes in Down's syndrome. Lancet, *2:*674, 1964.

40. Menzies, R. C., Crossen, P. E., Fitzgerald, P. H., and Gunz, F. W.: Cytogenetic and cytochemical studies on marrow cells in B$_{12}$ and folate deficiency. Blood, *28:*581, 1966.

41. Nowell, P. C., and Hungerford, D. A.: Chromosome studies in human leukemia. II. Chronic granulocytic leukemia. J. Nat. Cancer Inst., *27:*1013, 1961.

42. ————: Chromosome studies in human leukemia. IV. Myeloproliferative syndrome and other atypical myeloid disorders. J. Nat. Cancer Inst., *29:*911, 1962.

43. ————: Chromosome changes in human leukemia and a tentative assessment of their significance. Ann. N. Y. Acad. Sci., *113:*654, 1964.

44. O'Conor, G. T., and Rabson, A. S.: Herpes-like particles in an American lymphoma: preliminary note. J. Nat. Cancer Inst., *35:*899, 1965.

45. Pierre, R. V.: In American Society of Hematology Education Program, San Diego, 1977, p. 62.

46. Polliack, A., Lampen, N., Clarkson, B., and De Harven, E.: Scanning electron microscopy of human leukocytes — A comparison of Air Dried and Critical Point Dried Cells. Israel J. Med. Sci., *10:*1075, 1974.

47. Reisman, L. E., Zuelzer, W. W., and Thompson, R. I.: Further observation on the role of aneuploidy in acute leukemia. Cancer Res., *24:*1448, 1964.

48. Ritzmann, S. E., Stoufflet, E. J., Houston, E. W., and Levin, W. C.: Coexistent chronic myelocytic leukemia, monoclonar gammopathy and multiple chromosomal abnormalities. Am. J. Med., *41:*981, 1966.

49. Rodman, N. F., Jr., Mason, R. G., McDevitt, N. B., and Brinkhous, K. M.: Morphologic alterations of human blood platelets during early phases of clotting: electron microscopic observations of thin sections. Am. J. Path., *40:*271, 1962.

50. Roose, W. F., Dourmashkin, R., and Humphrey, J. H.: Immune lysis of normal human and paroxysmal nocturnal hemoglobinuria (PNH) red blood cells. III. The membrane defects caused by complement lysis. J. Exp. Med., *123:*969, 1966.

51. Rowley, J. D.: Population Cytogenetics of Leukemia *In:* Porter, I. H., Hook, E. B. ,eds..: Population Cytogenetics. New York, Academic Press, 1976.

51a. Rowley, J. D., and Potter, D.: Chromosomal banding patterns in acute nonlymphocytic leukemia. Blood, *47:*705, 1976.

52. Rowley, J. D., Blaisdell, R. K., and Jacobson, L. O.: Chromosome studies in preleukemia. Blood, *27:*782, 1966.

53. Russell, L. B.: Mammalian X-chromosome action. Science, *140:*976, 1963.

54. Sandberg, A. A., Ishihara, T., and Crosswhite, L. H.: Group C-trisomy myeloid metaplasia with possible leukemia. Blood, *24:*716, 1964.

55. Sandberg, A. A., Ishihara, T., Kihuchi, Y., and Crosswhite, L. H.: Chromosome differenences among the acute leukemias. Ann. N. Y. Acad. Sci., *113:*663, 1964.

56. Sorenson, G. D.: Electron microscopic observations of bone marrow from patients with sideroblastic anemia. Am. J. Path., *40:*297, 1962.

57. ———: Electron microscopic observations of bone marrow from patients with multiple myeloma. Lab. Invest., *13:*196, 1964.

58. Tanaka, Y., Brecher, G., and Frederickson, D. S.: Cellules de la maladie de Niemann-Pick et de quelques autres lipoidoses. Nouv. Rev. Franc. Hemat., *3:*5, 1963.

59. Tartaglia, A. P., Propp, S., Amarose, A. P., Propp, R. P., and Hall, C. A.: Chromosome abnormality and hypocalcemia in congenital erythroid hypoplasia (Blackfan-Diamond syndrome). Am. J. Med., *41:*990, 1966.

60. Teplitz, R. L., and Beutler, E.: Mosaicism, chimerism and sex-chromosome inactivation. Blood, *27:*258, 1966.

61. Teplitz, R. A., Rosen, R. B., and Teplitz, M. R.: Granulocytic leukemia, Philadelphia chromosome and leukocyte alkaline phosphatase. Lancet, *2:*418, 1965.

62. Tjio, J. H., and Levan, A.: The chromosome number of man. Hereditas, *42:*1, 1956.

63. Trujillo, J., and Ohno, S.: Chromosomal alteration of erythropoietic cells in chronic myeloid leukemia. Proc. 9th Int. Cong. Hematol., Mexico City, 1962, Acta Haemat., *29:*311, 1963.

64. Wang, H. C., and Federoff, S.: Banding in human chromosomes treated with trypsin. Nature New Biol., *235:*52, 1972.

65. Warren, S., and Meisner, L.: Chromosomal changes in leukocytes of patients receiving irradiation therapy. J.A.M.A., *193:*352, 1965.

66. Whang, J., Frei, E., Tjio, J. H., and Carboni, P. P.: Distribution of the Philadelphia (Ph¹) chromosome in patients with chronic myelogeneous leukemia. Clin. Res., *11:*35, 1963.

67. Winkelstein, A., Sparkes, R. S., and Craddock, C. G.: Trisomy of group C in a myeloproliferative disorder. Report of a case. Blood, *27:*722, 1966.

68. Wurster-Hill, D. et al.: Cytogenetic studies in polycythemia vera. Seminars in Hematology, *13:*13, 1976.

69. Zeck, L., Haglund, V., Nilsson, K., and Klein, G.: Characteristic chromosomal abnormalities in biopsies and lymphoid-cell lines from patients with Burkitt and non-Burkitt lymphomas. International J. Cancer, *17:*47, 1976.

AUDIOVISUAL AIDS*

Biochemical Genetics and Genetics in Cancer. [Self-Teaching Slide Review No. 25]. University of Miami School of Medicine, Department of Internal Medicine (Hematology), Miami, Florida 33136.

Electron Microscopy of normal and Leukemic Leukocytes. International Society for hematology, James L. Tullis, M.D., 110 Francis St., Boston, Massachusetts 02215.

Human Chromosomes and How they are Studied. T-2025. (1970). National Medical Audiovisual Center (Annex) Station K, Atlanta, Georgia 30324.

Medical Genetics. Association Films, 600 Grand Avenue, Ridgefield, New Jersey 07657.

Monoclonal Gammopathies. [Self-Teaching Slide Review No. 21]. University of Miami School of Medicine, Department of Internal Medicine (Hematology), Miami, Florida 33136.

Normal and Pathological Erythrocytes of Human Blood. I; *Normal and Leukemic White Cells of Human Blood.* II; *Cytological Aspects of Immunohematology.* III. International Society for Hematology, James L. Tullis, M.D., 110 Francis St., Boston, Massachusetts 02215.

Numerical Abnormalities of Human Chromosomes. T-2031. (1969). National Medical Audiovisual Center (Annex), Station K, Atlanta, Georgia 30324.

Structural Abnormalities of Human Autosomes. T-2033. (1970). National Medical Audiovisual Center (Annex), Station K, Atlanta, Georgia 30324.

_____

* Films unless otherwise stated.

17 Diagnostic Hematologic-Clinical Pathology Summaries

Normal Blood and Bone Marrow

Normal blood and bone marrow are characterized by normal hematocrit, hemoglobin, and erythrocyte, leukocyte, and platelet counts with normal blood indices; normal distribution of granulocytes, lymphocytes, and monocytes. The qualitative appearance of erythrocytes, leukocytes, and platelets are within the limits of normal variability. Bone marrow pattern shows a normal distribution of cell types for the age of patient. For example, the M:E ratio is 1.8:1 at birth with low lymphocyte percentage; 2 weeks later it may be as high as 9 to 11:1 with 30 to 40 per cent lymphocytes; during first year it gradually decreases to 3:1 with gradual reduction in lymphocytic percentage to adult level during and after the second year of life. The normal M:E ratio for adults varies from 2.5 to 5:1.

Infections (Acute and Chronic)

Infections are hematologically characterized by normal hematocrit, a slightly reduced hemoglobin, a normal erythrocyte count, a leukocyte count increased to 14,000 to 20,000 per cu. mm. with a shift to left and frequent increase in stab forms. Occasionally, there are moderate to severe vacuolization and toxic granules in polymorphonuclear neutrophils. Serum iron and iron-binding capacity are lowered. In chronic infections, hemoglobin, hematocrit, and red blood cells may be moderately re-

duced with shortened erythrocyte life span, as determined by the ^{51}Cr procedure. The bone marrow pattern shows an increased M:E ratio; there is a neutrophilic increased associated with a slight shift to right of the maturation curve. In severe infections, especially in miliary tuberculosis, the bone marrow differential shows an increase in band forms to marked proliferation of metamyelocytes and myelocytes. The severe infection produces a leukemoid pattern, occasionally both in peripheral blood and bone marrow. In chronic infection, there is also normoblastic hyperplasia and increased iron depots in the bone marrow (Prussian blue stain is used to determine the latter).

Hemorrhage (Acute and Chronic)

In acute hemorrhage the clinical pattern depends on the volume of blood lost and the duration of time in which the loss occurs. The peripheral blood shows a leukocytosis of 10,000 to 20,000 per cu.mm. with a shift to the left revealing metamyelocytes, myelocytes, and even an occasional myeloblast. The platelets increase to levels of approximately 1,000,000 per cu.mm. The erythrocyte pattern is that of a normocytic anemia that in 24 to 48 hours is associated with a 5 to 15 per cent reticulocytosis, normoblasts, polychromatophilia, and eventually macrocytosis; if hypochromia is evident, it probably indicates previous hemorrhage. The bone marrow reveals a normal active pattern with fatty and gelatinous areas adjacent thereto.

Microscopically, one sees a minimal to moderate increase in polychromatophilic normoblasts and myelocytes with a reduced M:E ratio. The degree of M:E ratio reduction depends on the degree of blood loss, the rate of blood loss, and the interval of time between the blood loss and the marrow examination. In 3 to 4 days, leukocyte levels are normal; in 2 weeks the peripheral blood and marrow erythroid patterns are also normal. If bleeding into an open cavity occurs, the leukocytosis is more marked and of longer duration. Serum iron in acute hemorrhage is within normal levels and is occasionally reduced; iron-binding capacity is increased.

Chronic blood loss is associated with continuous, prolonged bleeding, leading to a continued high level of reticulocytosis, with associated hypochromia and microcytosis, and subsequently a serum iron deficiency. The iron content of the marrow and other depots is also reduced. The marrow pattern is one of normoblastic hyperplasia, representing an attempt to compensate for the hemoglobin mass deficiency. There is usually no peripheral blood leukocytosis or thrombocytosis.

Hypochromic Microcytic Anemia

Hypochromic microcytic anemia is associated with premature infants, pregnancy, hookworm, chlorosis, malnutrition, and chronic blood loss. There is a hemoglobin reduction that is out of proportion to the lowering of the erythrocyte count and hematocrit level. The peripheral blood shows erythrocytes with exaggerated central pallor, microcytes, poikilocytes of elongated elliptical form, occasional polychromatophilic macrocytes; a reduction in reticulocytes, and occasionally normoblasts. White blood cells are normal or slightly reduced in number with few multisegmented neutrophils found. A slight absolute granulocytopenia and a relative lymphocytosis are observed in longstanding cases. Eosino-

philia is found in hookworm patients. Platelets are normal in number, but small. The bone marrow is hyperplastic with a relative as well as absolute increase in normoblasts. The increase in normoblasts is roughly proportional to the degree of anemia. Polychromatophilic normoblasts predominate with a tendency for the maturation curve to be shifted slightly to the right. Serum iron is low and iron-binding capacity is increased. Bone marrow hemosiderin and siderocytes are usually absent. The polychromatophilic normoblasts increase after iron therapy.

Normocytic to Microcytic Anemia of Infection and Chronic Systemic Disease

The peripheral blood may show normocytic or microcytic red blood cells and occasionally hypochromic ones that are indicative of hemoglobin deficiency. The number of red blood cells and hematocrit are usually reduced. The serum iron and iron-binding capacity are frequently diminished. There is also moderate anisocytosis with slight poikilocytosis, and occasionally polychromatophilia, especially in severe chronic renal disease. The leukocytic picture depends on the nature of the causative disorder. For example, polymorphonuclear cells increase with frequent toxic granules in acute coccal and bacterial infections; lymphocytosis with occasional vacuoles and monocytosis are found in typhoid and viral infections; monocytosis is seen in tuberculosis and brucellosis; and eosinophilia is seen in parasitic infestations, allergic disorders, scarlet fever, polyarteritis nodosa, and occasionally in other collagen disorders. The marrow pattern varies somewhat; in chronic infections, there is hyperplasia of the leukocytic elements with a qualitative shift to younger normoblasts. The marrow pattern, however, frequently shows a predominance of neutrophils and a slight shift of the maturation curve to the right, if at all. The M:E ratio in infection is usually greatly increased. In renal insufficiency, there is a decrease in the ratio of nucleated erythrocytes to leukocytes, owing to leukocytic and megakaryocytic hyperplasia rather than to the reduction of normoblasts with a shift to the left of myeloid series (myelocytes, histiocytes, plasma cells, phagocytic cells, and eosinophils with karyorrhexis of normoblastic nuclei). The staining of the bone marrow with Prussian blue for iron is frequently increased.

Anemia of Chronic Liver Disease

The peripheral blood pattern in anemia related to chronic liver disease usually shows a normocytic, normochromic, and frequently macrocytic anemia with or without hemolytic aspects. Frequently, a slight reticulocytosis and decreased erythrocyte survival time (^{51}Cr) are seen. Anemia may occur secondary to hypervolemia, acute or chronic blood loss (eosophageal or rectal varices), folic acid deficiency, or impaired hepatic function, in which there are elevated values in tests for serum bilirubin, bromsulphalein retention, SGPT (Serum glutamic pyruvic transaminase), and alkaline phosphatase. The bone marrow patterns depend on associated sequelae. If the total erythrocyte mass is normal, peripheral blood and marrow are normal. If there is associated acute or chronic blood loss, the pattern is the same as in acute posthemorrhagic anemia or iron deficiency anemia. If there is an associated folic acid deficiency, one sees megaloblasts in marrow. If liver disease is uncomplicated by any of the disorders just mentioned, one sees normoblastic marrow hyperplasia with a predominance of large polychromatophilic normoblasts. One also frequently observes 5 to 20 per cent plasma cell increase in the marrow, which correlates with the peripheral blood hyperglobulinemia. The number of iron granules in the bone marrow frequently is increased. If liver disease is secondary to alcoholism, vacuoles are seen in myeloid nuclei and cytoplasm.

Nonspecific Hemolytic Anemias

Included in nonspecific hemolytic anemias are those due to infections and burns, acquired hemolytic anemias, and autohemolysis and paroxysmal types. The peripheral blood pattern may be normocytic or macrocytic, the blood morphology being dependent on the severity of the process. If the hemolytic process is due to autoantibody formation, agglutination or clumping of red blood cells can be observed. Anisocytosis is usually marked with Heinz-Ehrlich bodies frequently seen in the red blood cells. Very little poikilocytosis is seen except spherocytosis and schistocytosis in this nonspecific group. A reticulocytosis of 10 to 25 per cent or higher is seen in acute cases, less in cases associated with chronic liver disease. Polychromatophilia is common. Normoblasts of all types are observed; all are macrocytic, as are the red blood cells. Erythrophagocytosis by monocytes occurs with associated leukocytosis and a shift to left—that is, metamyelocytes, myelocytes, and occasionally myeloblasts are found. Platelets are numerous, large, and bizarre.

Laboratory tests useful in the diagnosis of nonspecific hemolytic anemias are: the autohemolysis test[4]; morphologic studies, especially of elliptocytosis, leptocytosis, and basophilic stippling; hemoglobin electrophoresis, also for nonsickle cell patterns; and staining to detect parasites and inclusion bodies. The Donath-Landsteiner test used in paroxysmal hemoglobinuria, the detection of hemosiderin and hemoglobin in urine, the detection of heme pigments in serum, Ham's acid serum test, and the thrombin test are all of use in paroxysmal nocturnal hemoglobinuria. Spot[2] and screening tests[3, *] are used in the diagnosis of glucose-6-phosphate dehydrogenase deficiency and pyruvate kinase deficiency.[1] The tests for decreased erythrocyte survival time (^{51}Cr and the Ashby technique), the tests for antibodies (indirect an-

---

* Fairbanks, V. F.: A tetrazolium stain for quantitative estimation of G6PD in individual erythrocytes and for the identification of weakly expressed heterozygotes for G6PD deficiency (personal communication).

tiglobulin test, tests for warm and cold autoantibodies and isoantibodies) and tests for fecal and urine urobilinogen are all increased in the hemolytic anemias. Iron-binding capacity is also decreased.

Bone marrow films usually show a high degree of hyperplasia; approximately 25 to 60 per cent of the cells are normoblastic with the increase roughly proportional to the severity of the hemolytic process. Thus, instead of the normal 20 per cent, the M:E ratio shifts from 4 or 5:1 to 1:1 or less. Polychromatophilic normoblasts are preponderant. In excessive hemolysis and when the regenerative index is rapid, basophilic normoblasts make up the major portion. These nucleated red blood cells do not have the nuclear chromatin scrollwork pattern seen in pernicious anemia and related macrocytic anemias. Numerous mitoses are seen. The white blood cells are normal myelocytes and metamyelocytes with a slight shift to myelocytic type (shift to left). No bizarre leukocyte forms are seen (as in pernicious anemia). Bone marrow hemosiderin granules, visualized by the use of Prussian blue stain, are increased.

Specific Hemolytic Anemias

Hereditary Spherocytosis. The laboratory test of most significance is the saline osmotic fragility test when it is associated with a positive hereditary background and microspherocytosis. Normally, red blood cells show no hemolysis until the salt concentration is reduced to approximately 0.45 per cent with hemolysis complete at approximately 0.3 per cent of NaCl. In congenital hemolytic icterus, red blood cells begin to hemolyze at 0.75 per cent; the process is complete at 0.4 per cent of saline concentration. Peripheral blood and bone marrow are the same as in other hemolytic anemias. In the chronic stage, there is an increase in lymphocytes, monocytes, plasma cells, and basophils.

Sickle Cell Disease. Peripheral blood findings are the same as in other hemolytic anemias except for hereditary background and

its frequency in Blacks. The anemia is marked to severe. If the blood is taken in an acute crisis and stained immediately, one observes round or oval erythrocytes, tiny microcytes, and occasional macrocytes. There are also elongated and narrow erythrocytes with rounded or pointed ends, occasional target cells, one to ten normoblasts per 100 white blood cells, polychromatophilia, basophilic stippling, Howel-Jolly bodies, and occasionally sickled normoblasts and reticulocytosis. Only a few sickle cells are seen immediately after preparation of the coverslip film. However, within 2 to 6 hours, using one of the partial anoxia techniques (petrolatum rim, bisulfite technique, *Bacillus subtilis* technique, and others) a maximal sickle effect is seen including bizarre shapes with elongated and pointed filaments. Severe leukocytosis is seen, especially in crisis, with a shift to the left revealing myelocytes. Also seen are eosinophilia, monocytosis with erythrophagocytosis. Platelets are increased with bizarre forms. Laboratory tests reveal S-S hemoglobin (homozygous) in the classic disease. Hemoglobin combinations may occur. For example, sickle cell trait (Hb A and Hb S), sickle-cell thalassemia (Hb S and Hb A plus Hb F), sickle cell hemoglobin C disease (Hb S plus Hb C plus Hb F), and sickle-cell D, E, J, and N diseases (Hb S plus D, E, J, or N) hemoglobins are all found. Other laboratory tests for hemolytic anemias may also be used (for example, shortened erythrocyte life span, and others).

In the bone marrow pattern, orthochromic normoblasts are preponderant (50–70% of all nucleated red blood cells in marrow) with some polychromatophilic and basophilic normoblasts. There is a moderate myeloid shift to the left with numerous eosinophils. Megakaryocytes are increased; monocytosis with erythrophagocytosis is evident. Nuclear fragments and pigment granules are seen, and occasionally there are sickle normoblasts and long, filamentous erythrocyte cytoplasmm In sickle cell trait, it may take 24 hours for bizarre red blood cells to appear under the coverslip with reduced oxygen tension. Clinically, in the trait pattern one sees no hemolytic anemia and no signs of active erythrocyte regeneration; iron deficiency with occasional elliptical or spherocytic cells is observed. With the aid of electrophoresis, hemoglobin AS is observed.

Thallassemia Major (Cooley's Anemia). Peripheral blood of patients with thalassemia major shows hypochromic, microcytic red blood cells with occasional macrocytes. All erythrocytes show a thin colorless peripheral membrane. Target cells are common with occasional thin bridges of hemoglobin joining the periphery and the target areas. Occasionally, red blood cells are ridged; edges are occasionally folded over. Many normoblasts and microblasts (15 μ) are present with deep blue cytoplasm and granular nuclear chromatin. Also many polychromatophilic and stippled red blood cells may be seen with occasional Howell-Jolly bodies. Reticulocytosis is evident. The leukocyte pattern shows marked leukocytosis and marked myeloid stimulation, including myelocytes and myeloblasts. Monocytosis with lymphocytosis is found in infants. Platelets are normal.

Laboratory tests show the following: In homozygous disease, the patient's red blood cells contain 40 to 100 per cent of Hb F with up to 40 per cent of Hb F in heterozygous patients. The alkali denaturation test is the simplest test for Hb F. Hemoglobin A_2 also is found in most cases of thalassemia (Hb A plus Hb F plus Hb A_2). The Hb A_2 levels are increased in thalassemia minor (Hb A plus Hb F plus increased Hb A_2). Thus, electrophoretically there are really two common types of thalassemia—those with increased Hb A_2 and little Hb F, and those with a normal level of Hb A_2 and a high level of Hb F. Occasionally, one sees combinations with the sickle cell fraction (Hb S) or with hemoglobins C, D, or E. Falciparum malaria rarely occurs in patients having Hb F and Hb S. Also, excess urobilinogen is seen in the urine and feces. Excess deposits of iron are also observed in the skin and other organs of the body.

Bone marrow examination reveals a hyperplastic marrow with many parent stem cells, numerous normoblasts, myelocytes, megakaryocytes, phagocytosis with hemosiderin (a Prussian blue stain of 6+ intensity), foam cells in small islands, and a PAS-positive substance found in the marrow normoblasts.

Thalassemia Minor (and Minima). In the peripheral blood, hemoglobin values are usually normal and AA_2, with slight increase in HBg F in beta type, or there is evidence of a moderate hypochromic microcytic anemia with a MCV of less than 75 cu. μ. There are a slight reticulocytosis, and marked anisocytosis and poikilocytosis. Hypochromia is variable; target erythrocytes and numerous stippled erythrocytes are found. There are no nucleated erythrocytes in the peripheral blood. Schistocytes are occasionally seen, and a relative polycythemia may be seen with associated increased ^{51}Cr RBC survival. In fact, morphologic changes of the red blood cells are out of proportion to the degree of anemia found. Bone marrow examination shows marked normoblastosis of the marrow foci, but there usually are no hemosiderin-laden phagocytes in the marrow. The electrophoresis pattern is as above.

Hemolytic Disease of Newborn (HDN), or Erythroblastosis Fetalis. Hemolytic disease of newborn is the term preferred because hydrops and normoblastosis ("erythroblast" is not used in our nomenclature of erythrocyte development) do not always occur in every case. Large nucleated erythrocytes are observed in every stage of maturation with associated marked polychromatophilia. Also seen are red blood cells with nuclear fragments, large numbers of reticulocytes, and macrocytic erythrocytes. There is little to no spherocytosis if HDN is due to Rh antigens, and there is no increase in osmotic fragility. Moderate to marked sperocytosis is seen if the HDN is due to ABO antigens, and there is a marked increase in osmotic fragility of the red blood cells. Leukocytosis is observed with an increase in the number of immature granulocytes and lymphocytes. Platelets are normal to reduced.

Laboratory findings show that 95 per cent of the cases are associated with anti-Rh$_0$ antibody formation and severe normoblastosis. The rest of the cases are caused by sensitization to other antigens and their antibodies—for example, anti-rh', anti-rh'', anti-hr', anti-B, anti-A, anti-S, and anti-Kell with mild or absent normoblastosis. The serum bilirubin is usually above 3 mg. per 100 ml.; an exchange transfusion is usually not indicated until the serum bilirubin is 20 mg. per 100 ml. or above. Normoblastosis is not diagnostic because it is also associated with septicemia (including cytomegalic virus inclusion disease), congenital syphilis, heart disease, and with the icterus-kernicterus complex of prematurity.

Serologic studies are absolutely necessary for determining the etiology—for example, blood groups and genotypes of the mother, fetus, and father, especially if antibodies are found, and immune antibodies are detected by direct and indirect antiglobulin tests. The direct antiglobulin (Coombs') test on cord blood is usually positive except in ABO sensitization, in which it is almost always negative. A positive indirect antiglobulin (Coombs') test on cord blood demonstrates the presence of free immune antibodies; the use of an erythrocyte panel specifically identifies the antibody involved. If HDN is due to ABO incompatibility, the presence and titer of immune anti-A and anti-B antibodies in the mother must be determined. If the mother is not sensitized, she will have neither anti-A nor anti-B; if she is sensitized, the group O mother usually forms immune anti-A (A$_1$) antibodies and rarely anti-B. The presence of immune antibodies does not prove that HDN is present, only that sensitization has occurred.

Bone marrow findings indicate marked hyperplasia of all elements, especially normoblasts of all types. The pattern is like that observed in severe acute hemolytic anemia.

Megaloblastic Macrocytic Anemias

The most important member of the group of megaloblastic macrocytic anemias is pernicious anemia, with achlorhydria and possible neurologic changes necessary in order to differentiate it from other members of this group. Also included in this group are anemias associated with sprue, idiopathic steatorrhea, celiac disease, intestinal abnormalities, nutritional macrocytic anemia, *Diphyllobothrium latum* infestation, megaloblastic anemia of infancy or pregnancy, the administration of antimetabolites, and the administration of anticonvulsants.

Pernicious Anemia (P.A.). The peripheral blood in cases of pernicious anemia usually shows macrocytosis, anisocytosis, poikilocytosis, diffuse or punctate basophilia, Howell-Jolly bodies, Cabot rings, polychromasia, macropolycytosis of polymorphonuclear neutrophil nuclei, occasionally giant metamyelocytes, and myelocytes that are poorly granulated. Occasionally eosinophilia is found, and leukopenia is fairly common, as is thrombocytopenia with bizarre giant platelets.

Laboratory findings. The MCV is usually above 100 cu.μ; the MCH is usually above 31 $\mu\mu$g.; the MCHC is never above 36 per cent. The reticulocyte percentage is less than 2 per cent; gastric analysis shows a reduced volume of gastric juice, free HCl is absent after histamine stimulation. Stools are soft and mucoid, and urobilinogen is increased in the feces and urine. The serum iron is high, and the iron-binding capacity is normal or slightly decreased. The serum bilirubin is slightly elevated (slightly above 4 mg./100 ml.), especially the indirect type. Serum cholesterol is slightly reduced. The erythrocyte survival rate (^{51}Cr method) is decreased. The Schilling test, or urinary excretion of ^{60}Co vitamin B$_{12}$, reveals less than 5 per cent is excreted (when intrinsic factor is added, 8% or more of ^{60}Co vitamin B_{12} dose given is excreted).

Bone marrow studies reveal 30 to 50 per cent of nucleated cells in the erythrocyte series are present, especially megaloblasts, which are larger than normoblasts and show early hemoglobinization. The scroll chromatin network in nuclei and the deeply basophilic cytoplasm are also evident. Promegaloblasts are noted. Polychromatophilic and acidophilic megaloblasts are seen in groups of three to six with many mitoses and reticulocytes. The presence of megaloblasts is of itself not diagnostic of pernicious anemia; their presence confirms the diagnosis of P.A. when supported by clinical and other laboratory evidence. Giant bizarre metamyelocytes are observed, having doughnut nuclei with vacuoles and poor staining; the cytoplasm is light blue to basophilic and relatively agranular. Reticulum or Ferrata cells and lymphocytes are seen. The megakaryocytes are reduced or possibly abnormal. A deficiency of hemopoietic factor is also seen in the morphologic abnormalities of leukocytes and megakaryocytes just described; therefore, involvement of all marrow elements suggests a complete defect in hematopoiesis, producing a pattern in the peripheral blood of anemia, leukopenia, and thrombocytopenia. After 6 to 24 to 48 hours of treatment with vitamin B_{12}, one observes reticulocytosis in the peripheral blood, and a reduction in total number of nucleated cells in the bone marrow witht he disappearance of megaloblasts and the appearance of basophilic, polychromatophilic, and orthochromic normoblasts.

Sprue. Patients with sprue are usually from a subtropical country, and the disorder is usually associated with polychromasia and anisocytosis in cells of the peripheral blood. The MCH and MCV are elevated; the MCHC is normal or a little reduced. Characteristically, this syndrome is representative of a macrocytic anemia that is occasionally hypochromic and microcytic. Other cellular elements display a pattern of leukopenia with macropolycytosis and giant metamyelocytes containing broad, tortuous, vacuolated nuclei. Also relative lymphocytosis and thrombocytopenia are observed. Free acid is present in the gastric juice, and neurologic abnormalities are absent. In idiopathic steatorrhea, one sees achlorhydria in a small percentage of cases (acid returns after treatment). In celiac disease, one observes a hypochromic microcytic pattern. Both show an increase in normoblasts. In mixed types, the hypochromic microcytic pattern changes to a macrocytic pattern. The serum iron is normal or high. The iron-binding capacity is depressed, and bone marrow hemosiderin is greatly increased. After treatment with folic acid, the macrocytic picture becomes microcytic with associated marked reticulocytosis.

The bone marrow pattern is usually hyperplastic and megaloblastic, similar to that described in pernicious anemia, especially if macrocytic anemia is evident in the peripheral blood. If the peripheral blood is hypochromic and microcytic, there is a normoblastic marrow pattern. However, when the MCV is normal, the marrow pattern is mixed.

Macrocytic Anemias of Infancy and Pregnancy. The description of the peripheral blood and bone marrow is the same as in sprue (just described).

Cirrhosis of Liver. The peripheral blood is usually thin with macrocytic or normocytic erythrocytes. The blood is not hypochromic unless gastric hemorrhage is present. In 60 to 90 per cent of cases, the anemia present is due to acute or chronic blood loss, hypervolemia, impaired liver function, or folic acid deficiency. Depending on the etiology of the anemia, one may therefore see, respectively, a peripheral blood or marrow pattern the same as that in either acute posthemorrhagic anemia or iron deficiency, a megaloblastic marrow picture, or a macrocytic picture with slight reticulocytosis and apredominance of large polychromatophilic normoblasts (macronormoblasts) in the marrow. Vacuolated cytoplasm and nuclei are observed in marrow myeloid cells when cirrhosis of the liver is associated with alcoholism. The lymphocytes and platelets are reduced in number. The plasma cells are increased in number, varying directly with the globulin elevation in the peripheral blood. Other findings are increased fibrinolytic activity and hypoprothrombinemia. Bone marrow and liver biopsies may show an increased amount of stainable iron if there is an associated hemochromatosis. Erythrocyte life-span, determined by use of ^{51}Cr, is shortened.

Polycythemia Vera

The peripheral blood pattern of polycythemia vera shows a marked increase in all cellular components. Polycythemia vera should be suspected in a plethoric patient who also has splenomegaly, hypertension, and an absence of cardiopulmonary disease. The hematocrit is elevated to 55 to 65 per cent or higher. The blood is dark red and frequently viscous. The hemoglobin and erythrocyte values are also elevated. The MCHC is 30 to 35 per cent; the MCV is 60 to 80 cu.μ (the higher the count, the smaller the red blood cells). The total blood volume is two to three times normal. The red blood cells show marked polychromatophilia; there is occasional basophilic stippling, and normoblasts are present. Leukocytosis is seen with an increase in myelocytes of 1 to 2 per cent; metamyelocytes, basophils, and monocytes are also increased. Because the syndrome may terminate as a chronic myelogenous leukemia, the leukocyte alkaline phosphatase stain may be used to differentiate the two (elevated in polycythemia vera and decreased in chronic myelogenous leukemia). The platelets may be increased five to ten times the normal levels. The serum uric acid is frequently elevated; this helps to differentiate polycythemia vera from secondary polycythemia.

The bone marrow is dark red and cellular; in fact, there is hyperplasia of all cells, but with a normal M:E ratio. Nucleated cells of the erythrocyte series may be moderately elevated (orthochromic or polychromatophilic types), and usually there is a shift to the left in the myeloid series with increased quantities of myelocytes and myeloblasts. Also there is an increase in eosinophilic and basophilic leukocytes. Megakaryocytes are numerous and are frequently found in clumps. This syndrome is considered to be related to the myeloproliferative disorders.

Bone Marrow Failure

Included in bone marrow failure are the idiopathic type (those of unknown etiology) and the secondary type, which is etiologically related to bone marrow poisons. These disorders are also called refractory, hypoplastic, aplastic, and aregenerative anemias.

Peripheral blood studies show a total erythrocyte count of less than 2,000,000 and usually less than 500,000 per cu.mm. The erythrocytes are usually normocytic, but they occasionally are macrocytic with minimal anisocytosis and poikilocytosis. The MCV is often elevated; the MCHC is normal or slightly lowered. Leukopenia is usually noted with a reduction in polymorphonuclear neutrophils to 20 per cent level or less. Lymphocytosis occurs with lymphopenia late in the disease. Thrombocytopenia is frequently observed with a prolonged bleeding time and poor clot retraction. If normoblasts are seen in the peripheral blood, one may also observe immature myeloid cells. In familial cases, a reticulocytosis of 6 to 10 per cent may be seen. If the aplasia is of the pure erythrocytic type, there is usually no leukopenia or thrombocytopenia. The serum iron is elevated in early cases and is of diagnostic significance.

The bone marrow in the aplastic type is grossly yellowish white and fatty. Fat, fibrous tissue, reticulum cells, red blood cells, and lymphocytes are visible microscopically, especially in bone marrow sections. The marrow may also be normal or hyperplastic, with occasional sporadic "nests" of marrow cells aspirated. Characteristically, although there is a relative increase in lymphocytes, monocytes, and plasma cells and the megakaryocytes are decreased, the marrow differential may not be very abnormal; thus, the M:E ratio may still be normal. In the pseudoaplastic type, the normoblastic cytoplasm is usually poorly formed, with an excess of large siderotic granules or megaloblastic-like cells having bizarre chromatin in the normoblasts (see refractory sideroblastic anemia described on Plate 26). Occasionally, hyperplasia of mast cells is seen. In the hyperplastic cases (secondary to irradiation, drugs such as chloramphenicol, amimopyrine, sulfa drugs, and benzol), one may not see the excess of lymphoblasts or myeloblasts seen in leukemic states.

Variants of Refractory Anemias. *Congenital Hypoplastic Anemia (Fanconi's Syndrome).* This is a hereditary, closely-linked, autosomal, recessive, genetic disorder characterized by one or more congenital defects, such as small stature, skeletal abnormalities, and renal defects. Hematologically, a peripheral blood pancytopenia and marrow hypoplasia are seen. Bone marrow failure occurs at 2 to 6 years with a progressive downhill course. Death results from bleeding, infection, or transfusion hemosiderosis.

Congenital Erythrocytic Hypoplasia (Blackfan-Diamond Syndrome). This disorder is usually evident at 3 to 5 months of age, suggestive of a congenital origin; there is a possible associated defect in tryptophan metabolism. Hematologically, there is a normocytic, normochromic anemia and reticulocytopenia without other abnormalities. The bone marrow shows a marked reduction in normoblasts with a normal myeloid percentage; 30 per cent of patients have spontaneous remissions. Transfusion hemosiderosis may occur.

Refractory Sideroblastic Anemia. The exact classification of this syndrome is dubious. Some classify this disease as an idiopathic hypochromic anemia. The secondary type is related to infection, lead poisoning, thalassemia, or pyridoxine deficiency. The essential type contains a hereditary hypochromic sideroachrestic or hereditary iron-loading anemia that is frequently sex-linked and most common in boys. The acquired type is commonly called refractory sideroblastic anemia.

The peripheral blood reveals a double population of erythroid cells—that is, hypochromia of a portion of the normoblasts and mature red blood cells. Anisocytosis and poikilocytosis are also evident. The leukocyte count varies with associated monocytosis and hyposegmented polymorphonuclear leukocytes, which have a poor supply of granules and occasional Döhle inclusion bodies. The serum iron is high, and the iron-binding capacity is largely saturated.

The bone marrow shows a minimal increase in myeloblasts with a nucleus-cytoplasm asynchrony suggestive of early myelocytic leukemia; thus, there is a persistence of nucleoli as in later granulocytic forms. There is also a hypochromic normoblastic hyperplasia with a partial maturation arrest (megaloblastoid). The bone marrow shows an increase in sideroblasts (perinuclear) with no cytoplasmic hemoglobin and occasional cytoplasmic vacuoles in these normoblasts.

Myeloproliferative Disorders

Myelofibrosis (Myelosclerosis, Agnogenic Myeloid Metaplasia). Peripheral blood studies show the variable anemia to be frequently normocytic, normochromic with macrocytosis and spherocytosis, especially when hemolytic phenomena are present. There is a variable polycythemia in the early stages of some cases. Poikilocytosis with tear-drop, comma, and tailed forms are seen, as are polychromasia, anisocytosis, and nucleated erythrocytes. The leukocyte count is frequently moderately increased, with an excess of myeloid elements (especially neutrophils). Occasionally, myelocytes, promyelocytes, and myeloblasts are seen. Lymphocytosis is not present, whereas it is in hypoplastic and aplastic anemias. The leukocytic alkaline phosphatase is usually normal, but it may be increased in patients with a polycythemic pattern. Platelets are usually increased, although normal or moderately reduced levels are also observed. Large platelets with pale-staining chromomeres and hyalomeres are seen. These bizarre giant platelets may also be accompanied by megakaryocytic fragments and even by peripheral blood megakaryoblasts.

The bone marrow is frequently gritty when the needle is introduced into the sternum or iliac creast; very little actual marrow material may be obtained. Because of the hypocellularity, one sees fewer nucleated erythrocytes than in the peripheral blood. Normal, aplastic, and occasional hyperplastic foci are seen, but if hyperplastic foci are present, they usually are not of the florid leukemic variety. It may be necessary to make multiple marrow aspirations from different loci to finally obtain representative marrow patterns. Marrow biopsies of the iliac crest frequently reveal fibroblastic proliferation (fibrosis) or sclerosis with an increase in the number of bony trabeculae and replacement of marrow spaces with a loose fairly cellular connective tissue containing a few islands of hematopoietic tissue (especially large clumps of thrombocytes without an increase in megakaryocytes). One may also see necrosis of partly matured erythroid and myeloid marrow with reactive overgrowth of immature cells and reticulum, leading eventually to ossification. If the peripheral blood shows a myeloid reaction, the M:E ratio may be increased. The M:E ratio is decreased if a hemolytic process is present.

Splenic aspiration (when the syndrome is suspected) will reveal normally developing marrow components but with lymphocytes making up to 20 to 50 per cent of all nucleated cells. Roentgenography may demonstrate increased bone density. The serum uric acid is elevated. The ^{51}Cr test shows decreased erythrocyte survival time. Coomb's test is negative (even with hemolysis), and serum acid phosphatase is elevated in patients with elevated platelet levels.

Myelophthisic Anemia. In this type of anemia, also called leukoerythroblastic anemia, blood production is impaired, usually secondary to space-occupying lesions of the marrow. The peripheral blood pattern is similar to that of myelofibrosis. This anemia is most commonly associated with the finding of tumor cells from primary carcinoma of the prostate, lung, breast, kidney, adrenal gland (neuroblastoma), and thyroid; it occasionally is secondary to myeloma or lymphoma of the marrow. However, although the marrow cells may be crowded out with subsequent anemia, leukopenia, and thrombocytopenia, the peripheral blood picture may be normal to hypercellular, owing to irritative phenomena. Thus, the anemia is probably due to the same cause as the anemia seen in malignant tumors that do not involve the marrow. The differential blood films show an increase in macrocytic red blood cells and nucleated red blood cells out of proportion to the anemia per se. Reticulocytosis, polychromatophilia, and stippling also occur. A normal or reduced leukocyte count and an occasional leukemoid pattern are seen, associated with the presence of immature myelocytes and a decrease in the number of lymphocytes. Platelets are normal to reduced with the same bizarre platelets seen in myelofibrosis.

The bone marrow pattern usually reveals metastatic carcinoma cells, which frequently are larger than the largest myeloid cells. They have a tendency to occur in sheets (examine first under low power magnification). Under oil immersion, the nuclei appear to occupy most of the cell with one or two unusually large blue nucleoli. The cytoplasm is frequently vacuolated, disrupted, and degenerating. One may see carcinoma cells surrounded by areas of active blood formation—that is, normoblasts, megakaryocytes, and a few leukocytes. One may also observe cells of primary xanthomatoses—the large foam cells containing lipid, as in Hand-Schüller-Christian disease and in Gaucher's disease. These cells are 20 to 80 μ in diameter with abundant very pale and poorly visualized cytoplasm. In fact,the nuclei may appear to be devoid of cytoplasm and appear to rest in an open space set apart from other cells. Fibrillae are present in the cytoplasm, and one or many nuclei are found with a fine, reticulum, cell-like chromatin pattern and usually without nucleoli. In Niemann-Pick disease, cells are 40 μ in diameter with many small, cytoplasmic, hyaline droplets that are stained by Sudan IV. These cells have a honeycomb or foamy appearance; one or two nuclei are present, rarely more. Occasionally, the myelophthisic marrow-peripheral blood pattern is the result of granulomatous lesions, as in tuberculosis and histoplasmosis.

Thrombocytopenic Purpura (Idiopathic)

The peripheral blood in the thrombocytopenic purpura syndrome most characteristically reveals a marked reduction in the number of giant or very small, deeply stained platelets. Characteristic are a prolonged bleeding time, impaired clot retraction, and a positive capillary fragility test. Occasionally, portions of megakaryocytes are seen. The erythrocytic and leukocytic pattern depends on the acuteness and severity of the blood loss. Thus, it is usually normocytic, but if blood loss is of long duration, severe, or continuous, a hypochromic, microcytic anemia is seen. If the blood loss is recent, severe, or acute, a macrocytic anemia with reticulocytosis and nucleated red blood cells is observed. Similarly, the leukocyte count is usually normal,

but if hemorrhage is severe, a leukocytosis with a shift to the left may be seen. If bleeding is long standing, there is a lymphocytosis and slight leukopenia with some atypical lymphocytes, as in infectious mononucleosis, but without splenomegaly or lymphadenopathy.

Eosinophilia is occasionally observed and may or may not be attributable to intracutaneous hemorrhage. When neutropenia with or without anemia occurs, an immune phenomenon is thought to exist, possibly with hypersplenism. Results of laboratory procedures on peripheral blood include a shortened serum prothrombin time, a normal coagulation time and one-stage prothrombin time, and an elevated serum acid phosphatase (the latter probably because of the large amount of acid phosphatase that is liberated on the destruction of platelets). Platelet agglutinins are found in chronic idiopathic thrombocytopenic purpura (not acute).

The bone marrow pattern reveals no changes in the myeloid or erythroid pattern unless there is a severe recent hemorrhage, in which normoblastic hyperplasia is evident. In hypersplenic states, one may see hyperplasia of the myeloid elements with an occasional maturation arrest at the myelocytic-metamyelocytic stage. Occasionally marrow eosinophilia with peripheral eosinophilia is seen. The number of megakaryocytes is usually increased, particularly in the immature forms. These forms show degenerative changes in the nuclear chromatin and cytoplasm; they are rounded with sharply demarcated borders, single nuclei, relatively little or only moderately abundant cytoplasm, and little or no evidence of granulation (platelet formation or budding). Normally, platelets form from the cytoplasm of at least 50 per cent of the megakaryocytes; in ITP, platelets form from less than 20 per cent of the megakaryocytes. Occasionally, small megakaryocytes or very large megakaryocytes with nonlobulated nuclei, many vacuoles and only a few granules in the cytoplasm are seen.

None of these changes distinguish secondary thrombocytopenic purpura (acute leukemia and aplastic anemia) from the ITP form except that most frequently one sees morphologically normal megakaryocytes in the secondary type; however, they are reduced in number. One should not suggest splenectomy if marrow shows few or no megakaryocytes; however, before this conclusion is reached, one must be sure that the amegakaryocytosis is not due to a sampling error.

Primary thrombocythemia usually occurs during the 50- to 60-year-age period and is frequently associated with hematuria and gastrointestinal bleeding. There is a thrombocytosis of over 1 million, with an accompanying leukocytosis and increasing hemorrhagic complications as the platelet count rises. Because of the loss of blood, patients frequently develop an anemia that does not respond to iron therapy. If the iron therapy produces an increased red cell mass and elevated hematocrit, the diagnosis of polycythemia vera should be considered. There is an accompanying qualitative platelet dysfunction, with associated atypical bleeding time and incomplete platelet aggregation, indicated by ADP and epinephrine testing in vitro. Because of the unreliability and lack of reproducibility of this procedure, only abnormal results can confirm the diagnosis of primary thrombocythemia.

Disseminated intravascular coagulation (DIC) is a hemorrhagic diathesis accompanied by hypofibrinogenemia and thrombocytopenia and associated with variable deficiencies of other coagulation factors (e.g., Factors V and VIII). It is also characterized by erythrocyte fragmentation and schistocytic RBCs plus other peripheral blood film findings that are probably due to intravascular deposition of fibrin strands and subsequent mechanical trauma to the red cells.

In this symptom complex, there is intravascular activation of prothrombin to thrombin, with possible involvement by other enzymes. Platelet and fibrinogen consumption, with destruction of the labile coagulation Factors V and VIII, is easily explained if thrombin is the predisposing agent. At the same time as the intravascular coagulation develops, activation of the fibrinolytic process occurs, possibly as a defense mechanism. The hemostatic defect is exacerbated by fibrinogen (lysis of fibrin), which releases degradation products that inhibit coagulation of blood and interfere with thrombocyte functions. The thrombin time is elevated, which is important in detecting the circulating fibrin degradation products that prolong it. These products can also be measured directly using immunologic techniques. Clinically, disseminated intravascular coagulation may be characterized by extensive bleeding from multiple sources (e.g., venipuncture sites, etc.). Purpura fulminans with associated thrombosis may occur; or hematologic abnormalities associated with coagulation may occur without any significant clinical findings.

Hemophilia

Hemophilia is associated with a bleeding defect inherited as a sex-linked recessive trait. Affected males usually show active bleeding phenomena, and females are usually carriers, but rarely do females show active bleeding. The anemia is of the acute or chronic hemorrhage type with their leukocyte pattern. The platelet count is usually normal, except that a slight increase is observed when tissue damage and hemorrhage occurs. The bone marrow findings are the same as those found in acute and chronic hemorrhage. The laboratory findings include prolonged coagulation time, abnormal prothrombin consumption time, and an abnormal thromboplastin generation test. Fibrinogen concentration is normal, and the level of AHF factor (VIII) is decreased. Family history and capillary weakness are important cofactors in the specific diagnosis. Christmas disease should be considered in the differential diagnosis.

Von Willebrand's Disease

Von Willebrand's disease is a hemorrhagic diathesis inherited as an autosomal dominant trait and characterized by an abnormal platelet retention (adhesiveness) on glass beads, a prolonged bleeding time, and a diminution of plasma Factor VIII activity. Unlike hemophilia A, there is simultaneous reduction in Factor VIII_{VWF} and Factor VIII_{AGN}, as well as Factor VIII_{AHF}. This bleeding disorder is probably observed with greater frequency than classical hemophilia A.

Agranulocytosis

Agranulocytosis is caused by a neutropenia secondary to an idiopathic etiology, drug hypersensitivity, or an autoimmune response with associated variable marrow pattern. The peripheral blood picture depends on the etiologic factor involved. If hypersplenic or drug-induced neutropenia is present, the platelet and erythrocyte values are normal. However, if the disorder is secondary to an associated lymphomatous process, there may be an accompanying anemia. The leukocyte count is usually reduced to values less than 2000 per cu.mm. with associated relative and absolute neutropenia, relative lymphocytosis, and an occasional monocytic cell increase. The granulocytes frequently have pyknotic nuclei and vacuolated cytoplasm with poorly stained granules. Myelocytes are occasionally seen in the peripheral blood when recovery begins. Occasionally, Türk irritation leukocytes are seen. Leukocyte agglutinins may be demonstrated, especially if the patient has received multiple transfusions.

The bone marrow pattern is slightly variable. If the disorder is etiologically related to hypersplenism, one sees normal or increased numbers of granulocytic precursors. In marrow changes due to drug-induced hypersensitivity, one usually observes normal erythroid and megakaryocytic cells, but hypoplasia of the myeloid elements, resulting in impaired production with so-called maturation arrest at the promyelocyte and myeloblastic stages. The pattern reveals diminished numbers of polymorphonuclear forms, metamyelocytes, and myelocytes in this sequence. Plasma cells, lymphocytes, and reticulum cells are increased in the marrow. Quantitatively, the M:E ratio is reduced; the type of myeloid cell predominating depends on the duration of action and potency of the offending agent.

Infectious Mononucleosis

The peripheral blood pattern in infectious mononucleosis rarely involves the erythroid or platelet series of cells. The leukocyte count is usually leukopenic in the beginning and slowly increases during the second to fifth day — 4000 to 15,000 leukocytes per cu.mm. in 80 per cent of cases. In 75 to 95 per cent of cases, more than 50 per cent of the peripheral blood leukocytes are atypical lymphocytes reaching a maximum percentage from the sixth to eleventh day and persisting for 16 to 22 days. These large atypical (mononuclear) lymphocytes have an oval or kidney-shaped nucleus, sometimes slightly lobulated. Occasionally, mitosis is seen. The cytoplasm is nongranular, vacuolated, or foamy. The nuclear chromatin forms a coarse network of strands and masses and cannot be differentiated from the parachromatin. The three types most commonly described are Type I just described; Type II, which is larger than Type I, and in which the nuclear chromatin is not as condensed, has homogeneous cytoplasm, and is nonvacuolated; and Type III, which looks like lymphoblasts with sieve-like chromatin, one or two nucleoli, is vacuolated, and has basophilic cytoplasm. A slight increase in metamyelocyte and stab forms is occasionally seen, and a 3 to 7 per cent eosinophilia may occur in convalescence.

The bone marrow pattern may only be necessary in unusual cases to rule out the possibility of leukemia, especially if a lymph node has been previously examined histologically. There is a moderate left shift of myelocytes and the presence of an occasional to moderate number of the aforementioned atypical lymphocytes. Also observed occasionally are eosinophils and leukocytoid lymphocytes, and rarely granulomata with associated epithelial cells.

Serologically, heterophil antibodies are found in titers over 1:56 in 92 per cent of patients on the eighth to twenty-second day of illness; these remain elevated 3 to 7 weeks. Diagnostically, they are not absorbed by guinea-pig kidney antigen, but are absorbed by beef erythrocytes. A small percentage of patients with this disease also manifest a false-positive serologic test for syphilis. One also sees an abnormal bromsulphalein excretion, and elevated serum glutamic oxaloacetic transaminase (SGOT), alkaline phosphatase, and serum lactic dehydrogenase values.

The diagnosis of infectious mononucleosis is based on (1) the clinical pattern (splenomegaly, lymphadenopathy, and oral lesions), (2) a rising serologic reaction, and (3) the cytologic study of the blood. An occasional diagnosis is made if the clinical pattern and cytologic study are definite with an associated negative serologic finding. An essential condition is always the finding of the aforementioned atypical lymphocytes. The differential diagnosis must rule out acute lymphocytic leukemia, viral disorders, lymphomata, acute infectious lymphocytosis, infectious hepatitis, chronic lymphatic leukemia with leukocytoid lymphocytes, the "post-pump" syndrome occurring 3 weeks after open-heart surgery or similar procedures, macroglobulinemia, and heavy chain disease.

Leukemoid Reaction

Leukemoid reaction includes any alteration in the total leukocyte count—that is, leukocytosis (50,000/cu.mm. and above) or leukopenia with an increase in young myeloid or lymphocytic forms in the peripheral

blood and bone marrow. The most common associated diseases are pertussis, infections of any type, intoxications (severe burns, eclampsia, malignant neoplasia with bone metastases), severe hemorrhage with sudden hemolysis, acute infectious lymphocytosis, infectious mononucleosis, and miliary tuberculosis involving marrow with associated monocytosis resembling acute monocytic leukemia and in which Auer bodies may be seen. Most commonly, there is a shift to immature neutrophilic granulocytes (myelocytes, metamyelocytes, and occasionally promyelocytes and myeloblasts). In infants, one may occasionally observe normoblasts. The leukocytic alkaline phosphatase deposition is high in the polymorphonuclear forms of leukemoid reaction, whereas it is practically absent in leukemic states. Leukocytic alkaline phosphatase granulation is reduced in polymorphonuclear forms found in infectious mononucleosis, collagen diseases, pernicious anemia, and refractory or aplastic anemias.

Bone marrow and splenic aspirates do not show the maturation abnormalities diagnostic of leukemic states; there is no hiatus leukaemicus in leukemoid states; in fact, one sees all transition forms of immature cells from promyelocytes, myelocytes, and metamyelocytes to polymorphonuclear forms, especially the last without the monotonous pattern of predominant myeloblasts, myelocytes, or lymphoblasts. In newborn infants it is impossible to differentiate between congenital leukemia with sepsis and leukemoid patterns without tissue infiltration studies. Tissue infiltration is associated with leukemia but is not observed in leukemoid reaction.

Acute Leukemia

Most commonly lymphocytic cases of acute leukemia occur in children under 6 years of age, and the rest occur in adults. The peripheral blood findings reveal at first a slight normocytic normochromic anemia, which becomes increasingly severe as the disease progresses. Occasionally, one sees a moderate to marked anisocytosis, poikilocytosis, and shortened erythrocyte lifespan (^{51}Cr test) especially in the Naegeli type. Depending on the degree of involvement of marrow erythroid tissue, one may find a varying percentage of normoblasts in the peripheral blood. Approximately 20 to 40 per cent of patients have leukocyte counts from 8000 to 3000 per cu.mm. The rest have a leukocytosis varying between 12,000 and 100,000 per cu.mm. The percentage of lymphoblasts, myeloblasts, monoblasts, stem cells, and leukosarcoma cells varies in each diagnostic entity. Rodlike pink cytoplasmic Auer bodies are occasionally seen in myeloblasts and monoblasts. Occasionally, a leukemic hiatus revealing absence or marked reduction of myelocytes and metamyelocytes is seen.

In leukosarcoma and lymphoblastic leukemia, one sees a reduced percentage of mature polymorphonuclear leukocytes. In the Naegeli type myeloblastic and monoblastic processes, no reduction in peripheral blood lymphocytes is seen. The leukocytic alkaline phosphatase content of polymorphonuclear leukocytes is reduced markedly in acute myeloblastic leukemia. Thrombocytopenia with prolonged bleeding times and clot retraction, and a positive Rumpel-Leede test are seen. Occasionally, bizarre large platelets are observed. Fibrinogen deficiency has been described in acute promyelocytic leukemia. Hemorrhage, infection (frequently the nonresponsive type of the upper respiratory tract), and variable degrees of lymphadenopathy or hepatosplenomegaly are seen, depending on the cell type involved. Gingival hypertrophy, other organomegalies, and bizarre manifestations also occur variably.

The bone marrow pattern is usually characterized by a monotonous blastform pattern (50% or more in most cases), with a shift of the maturation curve far to the left and a markedly elevated M:E ratio. Labeling of the blast cell type will be most frequently made by the "company" kept (e.g., lymphoblasts and lymphocytes; myeloblasts and myelocytes-polys; monoblasts and monocytes).

Cytologically, lymphoblasts are usually 10 to 18 μ but are frequently smaller, and have an even smooth border. The nuclei are usually oval with a wider area of cytoplasm on one side of the cell. The nuclear membrane is coarse, and the nuclear chromatin is moderately coarse with some aggregation and condensation of the strands, particularly near the inner surface of the membrane. Only one or two inconspicuous nucleoli are seen, or are entirely absent. The cytoplasm is basophilic and without granules. Most of the cells other than the lymphoblasts are lymphocytes. Occasionally, azurophilic granules are present, but they do not give a peroxidase stain, and no Auer bodies are seen.

Myeloblasts are usually 10 to 18 μ in diameter; occasionally a micromyeloblastic variant is seen that is difficult to distinguish from lymphocytes. The presence of other immature myeloid cells helps to classify them as myeloblasts. The myeloblasts have a smooth, even border, and the nucleus is usually oval with a wider area of cytoplasm on one side of cell. The nuclear membrane is smooth, fine, and even; the nuclear chromatin is even, diffuse, delicate, and shows little condensation. The two to five nucleoli are prominent. The cytoplasm is basophilic and without granules. Few promyelocytes and more mature myeloid forms are seen. The peroxidase stain gives positive results for the granules of promyelocytes and myelocytes. Auer bodies are occasionally seen in the cytoplasm.

Monoblasts are usually 12 to 20 μ in diameter, and the outline of the cells is frequently irregular or serrated, with or without pseudopodia. The nucleus is centrally placed and is frequently indented, kidney-shaped, folded over, or even lobular. The nuclear chromatin is fine, reticular, and lacy with a smooth, even, fine nuclear membrane. Two to five nucleoli may be indistinct. The cytoplasm is grayish blue with many very fine and larger dustlike reddish pink granules. Many monocytes may be present, and they occasionally give positive results with peroxidase stains. Auer bodies are only occasionally present in the cytoplasm.

Occasionally seen is a mixed type of myeloid and monocytoid elements (Naegeli type). Erythroid and megakarycytoid proliferation is decreased in acute myelocytic and monocytic leukemias. There is a variation of Naegeli monocytic leukemia in which atypical erythroid and megakaryocytic multinuclear, lobular, reticular cells may be seen. Other laboratory findings include increased serum and urine uric acid levels and variable serum protein levles. The basal metabolic rate may be increased. Radiographs of long bones frequently reveal marrow horizontal lines of reduced density proximal to the metaphyses. Osteoporosis and osteolytic lesions are occasionally seen. If meningeal symptoms are present, one may find leukemic cells in the spinal fluid. Blood glucose levels are occasionally reduced.

Chronic Leukemias

Chronic Myelocytic or Granulocytic Leukemia. This type of leukemia is most common between 25 and 55 years of age, and it is characterized by weakness, pallor, easy fatigue, heat intolerance, hepatosplenomegaly, and, rarely, lymphadenopathy. Peripheral blood findings usually are characterized by progressively normocytic normocrhomic anemia with slight polychromasia. Occasionally normoblasts are seen with a 2 to 5 per cent reticulocytosis. The leukocyte count averages 80,000 to 250,000 per cu.mm., frequently with an increase in polymorphonuclear cells and an associated eosinophilia or basophilia. Promyelocytes and myeloblasts increase as the disease terminates; the alkaline phosphatase concentration of the polymorphonuclear cells is subnormal. Platelet levels are increased early and decreased terminally. Fragments of megakaryocytes and

atypical platelet forms are occasionally seen.

Bone marrow patterns are cellular with a slight to moderate left shift and an increase M:E ratio. Myelocytes and metamyelocytes predominate with a variable increase in basophilic and eosinophilic myelocytic forms. Later on, blast and promyelocyte forms predominate. Megakaryocytes are increased at first and reduced later. The erythroid pattern is depressed. The Philadelphia (Ph') chromosome frequently is seen in the marrow cells of many patients. The basal metabolic rate, serum uric acid level, vitamin B_{12} level, and B_{12} binding capacity are elevated.

Chronic Lymphocytic Leukemia. This type of leukemia is most common between 55 and 70 years of age. It is twice as common in males as females. Lymphadenopathy, minimal to moderate hepatosplenomegaly, weakness, fatigue, weight loss, and skin lesions, especially herpes zoster, are increased. Heat intolerance is found, and occasionally (10% of cases) hemolytic phenomena are present early with associated polychromasia, increased numbers of normoblasts, and reticulocytes, spherocytosis, and atypical erythrocyte osmotic fragility.

Peripheral blood reveals normocytic normochromic anemia early, becoming severe as the disease progresses. The leukocyte count varies between 25,000 to 250,000 per cu.mm. with 55 to 95 per cent of lymphocytes characterized by larger, denser, clumps of nuclear chromatin and accentuated parachromatin. Occasionally, immature granulocytes are found. Later in the disease, platelet deficiency occurs with petechial and other hemorrhagic findings.

Most of the leukemic cells have been shown by immunofluorescence to be B-type lymphocytes. There is decreased production of humoral antibodies associated with and related to reduced levels of immunoglobulins. In addition, there are frequent defects of response to certain immunologic stimuli, with a particular susceptibility to encapsulated coccal organisms that leads to recurrent pneumococcal pneumonia and septicemia. Significantly, there is an increased incidence of autoimmune disorders, related to the ability of these leukemic B lymphocytes to elaborate humoral antibodies that react with antigens of the patient's own cells (e.g., neutropenia, hemolytic anemia, and thrombocytopenia described above).

The bone marrow shows 50 per cent or more lymphocytes with an increasing reduction in the other marrow elements as the disease progresses. Occasionally, a combination of lymphocytes and normoblastic hyperplasia is seen. Among other laboratory findings is the fact that 20 per cent of cases show increased serum gamma globulin levels. Thirty-five per cent of advanced disease cases have reduced gamma globulin levels. The BMR is often increased. Radiographs reveal osteolytic and osteoporotic changes. Patients with a secondary hemolytic process frequently have a positive indirect Coombs test; occasionally, leukocyte and platelet antibodies are seen. The serum bilirubin is elevated with an increase in the excretion of urine and fecal urobilinogen.

Chronic Monocytic Leukemia. This leukemia is usually of the Nageli type; it is unusual to find the pure monocytic type. Also uncommon is the chronic form of monocytic leukemxia; usually the acute type is seen. Remission may be induced by a natural attack of infectious mononucleosis. Oropharyngeal and gastrointestinal ulceration is frequently described with acute exacerbation associated with gingival hypertrophy. Normochromic or hypochromic, normocytic or macrocytic anemia frequently is present with reduced hemoglobin and hematocrit. The initial leukocyte counts are generally lower than in other leukemias (15,000–45,000/cu.mm.); aleukemic variants occur.

The peripheral blood shows a 50 to 90 per cent monocytosis early; later on, the disorder becomes histiocytic in pattern as acute exacerbation occurs. Cells in aleuke-

mic phase frequently contain fine azure granules with vacuoles in cytoplasm or nuclei. Erythrophagocytosis is frequently seen. The bone marrow pattern is frequently mixed; the preleukemic phase occurs in half the cases, which may last for months to years. Occasionally an "aplastic anemia" pattern is seen with hypercellular marrow having a megaloblastoid type of erythropoiesis and giant platelets. Also, the pattern may vary from monocytic to monolastic or myeloblastic to the reticulum or stem cell type. The erythroid cell series and mature granulocytic forms are depressed terminally, and an acute monocytic pattern is seen. Other laboratory findings include hypergammaglobulinemia with an occasionally normal concentration of heterophil antibodies.

Leukosarcoma. In this leukemia-like syndrome, the duration of the disease and the therapy response are varied, justifying its differentiation from chronic lymphocytic leukemia—for example, the younger the age, the shorter the duration. The leukocyte count is lower (15,000–85,000/cu.mm.). The cell type is an atypical prolymphocyte with large, round, oval, or notched nuclei having a distinct nuclear wall. The nuclear chromatin is reticulated or spongy, and there is a single large prominent nucleolus surrounded by clumpy chromatin. The cytoplasm contains variable amounts of blue-gray, opaque cytoplasm with occasional azurophilic granules.

These patients do not respond as well as patients having chronic lymphocytic leukemia, and the course of the disease is shorter than in chronic lymphocytic leukemia. Hodgkin's disease occasionally shows Sternberg-Reed cells in the bone marrow Lymphosarcoma shows an occasio ripheral lymphocytosis an phocytosis, but they ar chronic lymphocy gans may also be i

Erythroleukemia (L This disorder is se males (2:1), with symp lar to those in chronic granulocytic leukemia. There is a severe to moderate normochromic and normocytic or slightly macrocytic pattern. Leukopenia and a normal leukocyte count are not uncommon. The platelet count is normal or reduced. Reticulocytes are commonly 2 to 4 per cent, normoblasts and myeloblasts are usually seen. The red blood cells may show anisocytosis and poikilocytosis. The bone marrow pattern reveals a marked hyperplasia of the erythroid precursors; large basophilic multinucleated immature pronormoblasts or stem cells, and some typical and atypical megaloblasts are seen. Occasionally, Auer bodies are seen in the myelocytes. Terminally, myeloblasts predominate in the peripheral blood and bone marrow. Other laboratory findings reveal an elevated serum vitamin B_{12} level with normal vitamin B_{12} absorption. The fecal urobilinogen is increased, and erythrocyte survival (^{51}Cr) is decreased. Plasma clearance of ^{59}Fe is increased, and the utilization or incorporation of radioactive iron into circulating erythrocytes is decreased.

Plasmacytic (Multiple or Plasma Cell) Myeloma

Plasmacytic myeloma, a dyscrasia, is most freqeuntly seen in males (2:1) between 40 and 70 years of age. It is characterized by bone pain (focal and diffuse) and is fairly commonly associated with osteolysis and pathologic fractures. Weakness, weight loss, fever, paraplegia, peripheral neuropathy, episodes of abnormal bleeding, uremia, hypercalcemia, and para-amyloidosis with possible cardiac and nephrotic patterns are also seen. Occasionally, cryoglobulinemia and extramedullary tumors are present.

Hematologically, this disorder is characterized by slight to moderate normochromic, normocytic anemia becoming progressively more severe when there is an associated uremic or hemolytic pattern; the anemia may be due to hemolysis associated cold or warm antibodies or to blood loss or chronic renal disease with a decrease in erythropoietin activity. Red blood cells show moderate polychromasia, rouleau formation, and a slight reticulocytosis with occasional normoblasts, especially with varying degrees of hemolysis. Blood films take a grayish blue underlying color, presumably because of an associated dysproteinemia. The sedimentation rate is increased. The leukocyte count varies from slightly decreased to slightly increased levels, occasionally with myelocytes, metamyelocytes, and eosinophilia, and foci of plasma cells seen in the peripheral blood in many cases. If the formation of foci of plasma cells is excessive, with leukocyte counts of over 60,000 per cu.mm., some consider the possibility of plasmacytic leukemia. Thrombocyte levels are usually within normal range unless myelophthisic changes are seen secondary to an excess of myeloma cells in the marrow; then thrombocytopenia may be observed. Purpura may also be the result of amaloidosis in the blood vessels or an increase in blood viscosity leading to capillary damage. Atypical coagulation defects with circulating anticoagulants also may be seen.

Bone marrow is characterized by the presence of the myeloma cell, which in different cases varies from very immature, anaplastic forms to very mature plasma cells that cannot be differentiated from the adult plasma cells seen in normal bone marrow. An average of 20 per cent (5–100% range) of these type cells are seen usually focally (clumps, syncyntia, or large sheets) distributed at the lesser percentage levels. The immature myeloma cells average 15 to 30 μ, are round or ovoid, and possess a round, eccentrically placed nucleus approximately 5 to 7 μ in diameter with one or more prominent deep blue nucleoli. The nuclear chromatin is delicate and reticular; the cytoplasm is pale blue without granules except occasionally for sliver-shaped azurophilic inclusion bodies. These larger immature cells may be confused with osteoblasts (Plate 70). However, the immature myeloma cells, although relatively large, have nuclei with one or two nucleoli, and a reticular chromatin network showing a sharp contrast between the basichromatin and parachromatin. The cytoplasm is basophilic and abundant, and frequently contains a rounded pale area distinct from the perinuclear clear zone. These cells are found normally in the bone marrow of infants and children. In adults, these cells are frequently associated with bone disorders —for example, metastatic malignant neoplasia.

The more mature myeloma cell is approximately 7 to 12 μ in diameter, is usually ovoid, and is more pointed on one end than the other. The nucleus is also eccentrically placed, with coarse, dense, cartwheel-type chromatin. Some think the absence of the cartwheel arrangement is more typical. No nucleoli are seen. The cytoplasm is deep blue varying in intensity in different cells and different parts of the same cell, especially the perinuclear clear zone on one side of nucleus. No granules are seen, but small cytoplasmic vacuoles (Russell protein globule bodies) are frequently observed.

Laboratory findings include hyperglobulinemia in 50 to 70 per cent of cases with a reversal of the A:G ratio. Abnormal serum electrophoretic and immunoelectrophoretic patterns are seen in 80 per cent of cases as a sharp slim homogeneous spike migrating as gamma globulin in 55 per cent of cases, and beta globulin in 20 per cent of cases. The M pattern (between gamma and beta) is seen in 10 per cent of cases, and 5 per cent of cases show paraproteins migrating as alpha globulins (some with two peaks) and 20 per cent with normal patterns, usually cases with one or few bony foci or extramedullary areas. Bence Jones proteinuria is observed in 50 per cent of cases; negative Bence Jones proteinuria is associated with hyperglobulinemia and vice versa. Seventy per cent of urines have an abnormal protein with globulin mobility between the gamma and alpha regions.

Serum cryoglobulins precipitate on refrigeration and dissolve on warming. Also found in these patients are hypercalcemia of 18 to 20 mg. per 100 ml. in 25 per cent of cases. The serum uric acid is elevated. If renal insufficiency is present, the BUN and serum phosphorus levels are elevated. The alkaline phosphatase is normal unless fracture and callus formation occurs. In 90 per cent of cases, focal and diffused punched-out lytic areas are seen without osteoblastic changes.

The malignant clone of plasma cells synthesizes varying quantities of light and heavy chains; that is, a monoclonal protein reveals itself as a complete immunoglobulin, a free light chain, or both. Therefore, three specific abnormalities are observed, (1) equal portions of one type of heavy chain and one type of light chain, which is found as a single homogeneous immunoglobulin in the peripheral blood and as a monoclonal spike on serum electrophoresis (urine is negative for free light chains); (2) an excessive production of light chains and a variable lesser amount of heavy chains (monoclonal serum spike). The light chains are found in the urine and demonstrated as a monoclonal spike on urine electrophoresis. (3) A homogeneous light chain is found only in both serum and urine. The manufacture of reduced normal immunoglobulins results in an increased susceptibility to infections.

Waldenström's (Primary) Macroglobulinemia

Waldenström's macroglobulinemia, which is rare, usually occurs in 50- to 70-year-old males, running an indolent course with associated mild degrees of lymphadenopathy and hepatosplenomegaly, visual disturbances (retinal hemorrhages), weakness, skin ulcerations and petechiae, recurrent bacterial infection due to a decrease in the production of normal immunoglobulins, and cold sensitivity (Raynaud's phenomenon). Secondary macroglobulinemia, 5 to 15 per cent macroglobulins or less in total

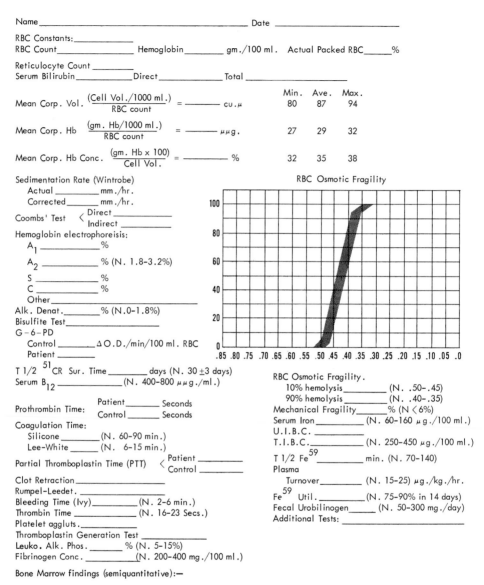

Name_____ Date _____

RBC Constants:_____
RBC Count_____ Hemoglobin_____ gm./100 ml.   Actual Packed RBC_____%

Reticulocyte Count _____
Serum Bilirubin_____Direct_____ Total _____

		Min.	Ave.	Max.
Mean Corp. Vol. $\frac{\text{(Cell Vol./1000 ml.)}}{\text{RBC count}}$ = _____ cu.μ		80	87	94
Mean Corp. Hb $\frac{\text{(gm. Hb/1000 ml.)}}{\text{RBC count}}$ = _____ μμg.		27	29	32
Mean Corp. Hb Conc. $\frac{\text{(gm. Hb x 100)}}{\text{Cell Vol.}}$ = _____ %		32	35	38

Sedimentation Rate (Wintrobe)
   Actual _____ mm./hr.
   Corrected_____ mm./hr.
Coombs' Test ⟨ Direct _____
              Indirect _____
Hemoglobin electrophoreisis:
  A_1 _____%
  A_2 _____ % (N. 1.8-3.2%)
  S _____ %
  C _____ %
  Other_____
Alk. Denat._____% (N.0-1.8%)
Bisulfite Test_____
G – 6 – PD
  Control _____ΔO.D./min/100 ml. RBC
  Patient _____
T 1/2 ^{51}CR Sur. Time_____ days (N. 30 ±3 days)
Serum B_{12} _____(N. 400-800 μμg./ml.)

Prothrombin Time: Patient_____ Seconds
             Control _____ Seconds
Coagulation Time:
  Silicone_____(N. 60-90 min.)
  Lee-White_____(N. 6-15 min.)
Partial Thromboplastin Time (PTT) ⟨ Patient _____
                            Control _____
Clot Retraction_____
Rumpel-Leedet. _____
Bleeding Time (Ivy)_____(N. 2-6 min.)
Thrombin Time _____(N. 16-23 Secs.)
Platelet aggluts._____
Thromboplastin Generation Test _____
Leuko. Alk. Phos. _____ % (N. 5-15%)
Fibrinogen Conc. _____(N. 200-400 mg./100 ml.)

Bone Marrow findings (semiquantitative):—

RBC Osmotic Fragility

RBC Osmotic Fragility.
  10% hemolysis_____ (N. .50-.45)
  90% hemolysis_____ (N. .40-.35)
Mechanical Fragility_____% (N <6%)
Serum Iron_____(N. 60-160 μg./100 ml.)
U.I.B.C. _____
T.I.B.C._____ (N. 250-450 μg./100 ml.)
T 1/2 Fe^{59}_____ min. (N. 70-140)
Plasma
  Turnover_____ (N. 15-25) μg./kg./hr.
Fe^{59} Util. _____(N. 75-90% in 14 days)
Fecal Urobilinogen_____ (N. 50-300 mg./day)
Additional Tests: _____

Fig. 17-1. Hematology consultation sheet. (Modified from Hematology Department, Washington University School of Medicine, St. Louis, Missouri)

serum proteins, may occur in association with lymphomas, chronic lymphocytic leukemia, plasmacytic myeloma, other malignant neoplasias, chronic infections, collagen disease, cirrhosis, and the nephrotic syndrome.

Hematologically, a moderate to severe normocytic normochromic anemia, associated with decreased erythropoiesis and hemolysins is seen. When hemolysins are present, erythrocytic polychromasia, reticulocytosis, and normoblasts are observed in the peripheral blood. An increased sedimentation rate with associated rouleau formation also is found. The leukocyte and thrombocyte levels are normal to decreased with progression to pancytopenia in some cases. A relative or moderate absolute lymphocytosis commonly occurs. Bone marrow aspirates reveal infiltration by 40 per cent or more of lymphocyte type cells with a lymphoplasmacytic pattern — that is, the cytoplasm is like that of a plasma cell and nucleus like that of a lymphocyte. These morphologic patterns are related to the transformation of normal B-type lymphocytes into plasma cells (i.e., appearing like transitional cells containing features of both cell lines). Naked nuclei are plentiful and cytoplasmic shedding may also be seen. Mast cells are also often increased. The percentage of normal myeloid elements is decreased.

Laboratory tests reveal an increase in the total protein level, especially the macroglobulin fraction (15 per cent or higher). A rather sharp peak, on serum paper electrophoresis, is seen in the beta or gamma region, making this disorder indistinguishable electrophoretically from plasmacytic myeloma. A specific diagnosis is usually made either by ultracentrifugal analysis, which reveals one or more protein constituents with sedimentation constants of 5 per cent or more of the 15S or 20S variety. The diagnosis can also be made by the use of serum protein immunoelectrophoresis on agar gel, which reveals a dense gamma M band (I_GM). Macroglobulins can also be identified in starch gel to which 2-mercaptoethanol has been added; this depolymerizes them to the lower weight 7S globulins, therefore enabling them to be seen as sharp peaks similar to those of the myeloma globulins.

Cryoglobulinemia and Bence Jones proteinuria are present in approximately 10 per cent of cases. The Sia water test (for any type of hyperglobulinemia) is usually positive (Plate 88); a moderate to heavy precipitate forms within 10 seconds after a drop of plasma is added to 10 ml. of distilled water. Radiographs of skeletal areas may show a general demineralization (diffuse osteoporosis), but focal punched-out lytic lesions and bone pain are usually not observed. The serum uric acid is elevated, and flocculation tests may be abnormal.

Heavy Chain Disease

Heavy chain disease, an unusual monoclonal protein complex, is formed from a single type of heavy chain without associated light chains; the coupling area in the heavy chain is deleted. The proteinaceous material is found in both urine and serum, leading to the development of H-chain or γ-chain disease (a lymphoma-like moiety with urinary free γ-chains), alpha-chain disease characterized by severe malabsorption, and an abdominal lymphoma and μ-chain disease somewhat similar to chronic lymphocytic leukemia.

As an aid in hematologic diagnosis, a completed consultation sheet (Fig. 17-1), together with a good clinical history, physical examination, peripheral blood and bone marrow study, is very important in helping one arrive at an accurate hematologic diagnosis.

REFERENCES

1. Beutler, E.: A series of new screening procedures for pyruvate kinase deficiency, glucose-6-phosphate dehydrogenase deficiency and glutathione reductase deficiency. Blood, *28:*553, 1966.
2. Fairbanks, V. F., and Beutler, E.: A simple method for detection of erythrocyte glucose-6-phosphate dehydrogenase deficiency (G-6-PD spot test). Blood *20:*591, 1962.
3. Jacob, H. S., and Jandl, J. H.: A simple visual screening test for glucose-6-phosphate dehydrogenase deficiency employing ascorbate and cyanide. N. Engl. J. Med., *274:*1162, 1966.
4. Young, L. E., Izzo, M. J., Altman, K. I., and Swisher, S. N.: Studies on spontaneous in vitro autohemolysis in hemolytic disorders. Blood, *11:*977, 1956.

AUDIOVISUAL AIDS*

Atlas of Abnormal Hematology. L. W. Diggs, M.D., and Ann Bell. [140 or more 2 × 2 Kodachrome transparencies]. American Society of Clinical Pathologists, P.O. Box 12073, Chicago, Illinois 60612.

---

* Films unless otherwise stated.

Basic Hematology. 24. Edward L. Amorosi, M.D. [100 color (35 mm.) transparencies plus description booklet, $65.00]. MedCom, Inc., 2 Hammerskjold Plaza, New York, New York 10017.

Color Atlas and Textbook of Hematology. A Slide Presentation. William R. Platt, M.D. [170 color transparencies (35 mm.) plus descriptive booklet, $170.00.]. J. B. Lippincott, East Washington Square, Philadelphia, Pennsylvania 19105.

Correspondence Course in Hematology. Sloan J. Wilson, M.D., and Thomas R. Walters, M.D. [Basic, Advanced, and Pediatric]. Department of Postgraduate Medical Education, University of Kansas School of Medicine, Kansas City, Kansas.

Hematology. (ASCP, 1950). M 1350. [24 stained blood film slides]. Director, AFIP, Scientific Direc-

tor, American Registry of Pathology, Washington, D.C. 20305.

Hematology. [Kodachrome 2 × 2 transparencies]. Harwyn Medical Photographers, 4814 Larchwood Avenue, Philadelphia, Pennsylvania 19143.

MR Hematology. [130 Kodachrome 2 × 2 transparencies]. Clay-Adams Corporation, 141 E. 25th St., New York, New York 10010.

New Developments in Hematology. [audiocassettes]. The Institute of Continuing Education, Sawyer, Michigan 49125.

Pediatric Hematology. 25. Sergio Piomelli, M.D., and Lawrence M. Corash, M.D. [100 color (35 mm.) transparencies plus descriptive booklet, $65.00]. MedCom, Inc., 2 Hammerskjold Plaza, New York, New York 10017.

Index

Numerals in *italics* indicate a figure; *t* following a page number indicates a table.